DIAGNOSTIC ULTRASOUND

FOURTH EDITION

Carol M. Rumack, MD, FACR
Professor of Radiology and Pediatrics
University of Colorado Denver School of Medicine
Denver, Colorado

Stephanie R. Wilson, MD, FRCPC
Clinical Professor of Radiology
University of Calgary
Staff Radiologist
Foothills Medical Centre
Calgary, Alberta, Canada

J. William Charboneau, MD, FACR
Professor of Radiology
Mayo Clinic College of Medicine
Consultant in Radiology
Mayo Clinic
Rochester, Minnesota

Deborah Levine, MD, FACR
Professor of Radiology
Harvard Medical School
Associate Radiologist-in-Chief of Academic Affairs
Director of Ob/Gyn Ultrasound
Beth Israel Deaconess Medical Center
Boston, Massachusetts

ELSEVIER
MOSBY

ELSEVIER
MOSBY

1600 John F. Kennedy Blvd.
Ste 1800
Philadelphia, PA 19103-2899

DIAGNOSTIC ULTRASOUND, FOURTH EDITION   ISBN: 978-0-323-05397-6
Copyright © 2011 by Mosby, Inc., an affiliate of Elsevier Inc.

Notices

Previous editions copyrighted 2005, 1998, 1993 by Mosby, Inc.

Library of Congress Cataloging in Publication Data
Diagnostic ultrasound / [edited by] Carol M. Rumack ... [et al.].—4th ed.
      p. ; cm
   Includes bibliographical references and index.
   ISBN 978-0-323-05397-6 (hardcover : alk. paper)   1. Diagnostic ultrasonic imaging.   I. Rumack, Carol M.
[DNLM: 1. Ultrasonography. WN 208]
RC78.7.U4D514 2011
616.07'543—dc22   2010034851

Acquisitions Editor: *Rebecca Gaertner*
Developmental Editor: *Lisa Barnes*
Publishing Services Manager: *Patricia Tannian*
Team Manager: *Radhika Pallamparthy*
Senior Project Manager: *John Casey*
Project Manager: *Anitha Sivaraj*
Designer: *Steven Stave*

Printed in United States of America

Last digit is the print number: 9 8 7 6 5 4 3 2 1

About the Editors

Carol M. Rumack, MD, is Professor of Radiology and Pediatrics at the University of Colorado Denver School of Medicine in Denver, Colorado. Her clinical practice is based at the University of Colorado Hospital. Her primary research has been in neonatal sonography of high-risk infants, particularly 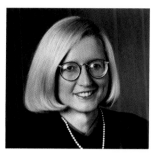 the brain. Dr. Rumack has published widely in this field and lectured frequently on pediatric ultrasound. She is a fellow and past president of the American College of Radiology, a fellow of both the American Institute of Ultrasound in Medicine and the Society of Radiologists in Ultrasound. She and her husband, Barry, have two children, Becky and Marc.

Stephanie R. Wilson, MD, is Clinical Professor of Radiology at the University of Calgary where she heads a specialty ultrasound clinic at the Foothills Medical Centre devoted primarily to the imaging of diseases of the gastrointestinal tract and gynecologic organs. With support from the 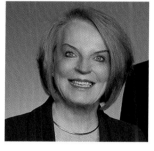 Canadian Institute of Health Research (CIHR), Dr. Wilson worked with Dr. Peter Burns in Toronto on the characterization and detection of focal liver masses with contrast-enhanced ultrasound (CEUS) and is an established authority in this field. A recognized expert on ultrasound of the gastrointestinal tract and abdominal and pelvic viscera, she is the recipient of many university teaching awards and is a frequent international speaker and author. Dr. Wilson was the first woman president of the Canadian Association of Radiologists (CAR) and is the current president-elect of the International Contrast Ultrasound Society (ICUS). She has received the gold medal from CAR in recognition of her contribution to radiology. A golf enthusiast, she and her husband Ken, have two children, Jessica and Jordan.

J. William Charboneau, MD, is Professor of Radiology at the Mayo Clinic in Rochester, Minnesota. His current research interests include image-guided tumor biopsy and ablation, as well as sonography of the liver and small parts. He is coauthor of over 200 publications, assistant editor of the 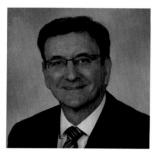 Mayo Clinic Family Health Book, and an active lecturer nationally and internationally. He is a fellow in the American College of Radiology and the Society of Radiologists in Ultrasound. He and his wife, Cathy, have three children, Nick, Ben, and Laurie.

Deborah Levine, MD, is Professor of Radiology at Beth Israel Deaconess Medical Center, Boston, and Harvard Medical School. At Beth Israel Deaconess Medical Center she is Associate Radiologist-in-Chief of Academic Affairs, Co-Chief of Ultrasound, and Director of Ob/Gyn Ultrasound. Her 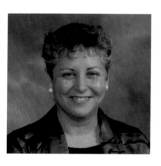 main areas of clinical interest are obstetric and gynecologic ultrasound. Her research has focused on fetal magnetic resonance imaging as an aid to improving ultrasound diagnosis. Dr. Levine is an American College of Radiology Chancellor, Chair of the American College of Radiology Commission on Ultrasound, a fellow of the American Institute of Ultrasound in Medicine and Society of Radiologists in Ultrasound. She and her husband, Alex, have two children, Becky and Julie.

Contributors

Jodi F. Abbott, MD
Associate Professor
Boston University School of Medicine
Director of Antenatal Testing
Boston Medical Center
Boston, Massachusetts

Jacques S. Abramowicz, MD, FACOG
Frances T. & Lester B. Knight Professor
Rush University
Director, Ob/Gyn Ultrasound
Rush University Medical Center
Co-Director, Rush Fetal and Neonatal Medicine Program
Rush University
Chicago, Illinois

Ronald S. Adler, PhD, MD
Professor of Radiology
Weill Medical College of Cornell University
Chief, Division of Ultrasound and Biology Imaging
Department of Radiology and Imaging
Hospital for Special Surgery
Attending Radiologist
Department of Radiology
New York Presbyterian Hospital
New York City, New York

Amit R. Ahuja, MD
Diagnostic Imaging Resident
Foothills Medical Centre
Calgary, Alberta, Canada

Jean M. Alessi-Chinetti, BS, RDMS, RVT
Technical Director
Vascular Laboratory
Tufts Medical Center
Boston, Massachusetts

Thomas Atwell, MD
Assistant Professor of Radiology
Mayo Clinic College of Medicine
Consultant in Radiology
Mayo Clinic
Rochester, Minnesota

Diane S. Babcock, MD
Professor of Radiology and Pediatrics
University of Cincinnati College of Medicine
Professor of Radiology and Pediatrics
Cincinnati Children's Hospital Medical Center
Cincinnati, Ohio

Carol E. Barnewolt, MD
Assistant Professor of Radiology
Harvard Medical School
Director, Division of Ultrasound
Children's Hospital Boston
Boston, Massachusetts

Daryl J. Barth, RVT, RDMS
Ultrasound Assistant
Department of Sonography
OSI St. Francis Medical Center
Ultrasound Assistant
Central Illinois Radiological AssociatesPeoria, Illinois

Beryl Benacerraf, MD
Clinical Professor of Obstetrics and Gynecology and
 Radiology
Brigham and Women's Hospital
Massachusetts General Hospital
Harvard Medical School
Boston, Massachusetts

Carol B. Benson, MD
Professor of Radiology
Harvard Medical School
Director of Ultrasound and Co-Director of High Risk
 Obstetrical Ultrasound
Brigham and Women's Hospital
Boston, Massachusetts

Raymond E. Bertino, MD, FACR, FSRU
Medical Director of Vascular and General Ultrasound
OSF Saint Francis Medical Center
Clinical Professor of Radiology and Surgery
University of Illinois College of Medicine
Peoria, Illinois

Edward I. Bluth, MD, FACR
Clinical Professor
Tulane University School of Medicine
Chairman Emeritus Radiology
Ochsner Health System
New Orleans, Louisiana

J. Antonio Bouffard, MD
Senior Staff Radiologist
Henry Ford Hospital
Detroit, Michigan
Consultant Radiologist
James Andrews Orthopedics and Sports Medicine Center
Pensacola, Florida

Bryann Bromley, MD
Clinical Associate Professor of Obstetrics and Gynecology
Massachusetts General Hospital
Clinical Associate Professor of Obstetrics and Gynecology
 and Radiology
Brigham and Women's Hospital
Boston, Massachusetts

Dorothy I. Bulas, MD
Professor of Radiology and Pediatrics
George Washington University Medical Center
Pediatric Radiologist
Children's National Medical Center
Washington, District of Columbia

Peter N. Burns, PhD
Professor and Chairman
Department of Medical Biophysics
University of Toronto
Senior Scientist
Department of Imaging Research
Sunnybrook Health Sciences Centre
Toronto, Ontario, Canada

Barbara A. Carroll, MD
Professor Emeritus of Radiology
Department of Radiology
Duke University Medical Center
Durham, North Carolina

J. William Charboneau, MD, FACR
Professor of Radiology
Mayo Clinic College of Medicine
Consultant in Radiology
Mayo Clinic
Rochester, Minnesota

Humaira Chaudhry, MD
Fellow in Abdominal Imaging
Duke University Medical Center
Durham, North Carolina

Tanya P. Chawla, MD, FRCPC
Assistant Professor
University of Toronto
Toronto, Ontario, Canada

David Chitayat, MD, FABMG, FACMG, FCCMG, FRCPC
Professor
University of Toronto
Prenatal Diagnosis and Medical Genetics Program
Department of Obstetrics and Gynecology
Mount Sinai Hospital
Toronto, Ontario, Canada

Peter L. Cooperberg, MD
Chief of Radiology
St. Paul's Hospital
Chief of Radiology
University of British Columbia
Vancouver, British Columbia, Canada

Peter M. Doubilet, MD, PhD
Professor of Radiology
Harvard Medical School
Senior Vice Chair
Department of Radiology
Brigham and Women's Hospital
Boston, Massachusetts

Julia A. Drose, BA, RDMS, RDCS, RVT
Associate Professor of Radiology
University of Colorado at Denver Health Sciences Center
Chief Sonographer
Divisions of Ultrasound and Prenatal Diagnosis & Genetics
University of Colorado Hospital
Aurora, Colorado

Beth S. Edeiken-Monroe, MD
Professor of Radiology
Department of Diagnostic Radiology
The University of Texas Houston Medical School
MD Anderson Cancer Center
Houston, Texas

Judy Estroff, MD
Associate Professor of Radiology
Harvard Medical School
Division Chief, Fetal Neonatal Radiology
Children's Hospital Boston
Radiologist
Department of Radiology
Beth Israel Deaconess Medical Center
Radiologist
Department of Radiology
Brigham and Women's Hospital
Boston, Massachusetts

Amy Symons Ettore, MD
Consultant
Department of Radiology
Mayo Clinic College of Medicine
Rochester, Minnesota

Katherine W. Fong, MBBS, FRCPC
Associate Professor of Medical Imaging and Obstetrics and Gynecology
University of Toronto Faculty of Medicine
Co-director, Centre of Excellence in Obstetric Ultrasound
Mount Sinai Hospital
Toronto, Ontario; Canada

Bruno D. Fornage, MD
Professor of Radiology and Surgical Oncology
M. D. Anderson Cancer Center
Houston, Texas

J. Brian Fowlkes, PhD
Associate Professor
University of Michigan
Department of Radiology
Ann Arbor, Michigan

Phyllis Glanc, MDCM
Assistant Professor
Department of Medical Imaging
University of Toronto
Assistant Professor
Department of Obstetrics & Gynecology
University of Toronto
Site Director
Body Imaging
Women's College Hospital
Toronto, Ontario, Canada

Brian Gorman, MB, BCh, FRCR, MBA
Assistant Professor of Radiology
Mayo Clinic College of Medicine
Consultant in Radiology
Mayo Clinic
Rochester, Minnesota

S. Bruce Greenberg, MD
Professor
University of Arkansas for Medical Sciences
Professor
Arkansas Children's Hospital
Little Rock, Arkansas

Leslie E. Grissom, MD
Clinical Professor of Radiology and Pediatrics
Department of Radiology
Thomas Jefferson Medical College
Thomas Jefferson University Hospital
Philadelphia, Pennsylvania;
Chair, Medical Imaging Department
Medical Imaging Department—Radiology
Alfred I. DuPont Hospital for Children
Wilmington, Delaware;
Pediatric Radiologist
Medical Imaging Department—Radiology
Christiana Care Health System
Newark, Delaware

Benjamin Hamar, MD
Instructor of Obstetrics, Gynecology, and Reproductive
    Biology
Beth Israel–Deaconess Medical Center
Boston, Massachusetts

Anthony E. Hanbidge, MB, BCh, FRCPC
Associate Professor
University of Toronto
Head, Division of Abdominal Imaging
University Health Network
Mount Sinai Hospital and Women's College Hospital
Toronto, Ontario, Canada

H. Theodore Harcke, MD, FACR, FAIUM
Professor of Radiology and Pediatrics
Jefferson Medical College
Philadelphia, Pennsylvania
Chief of Imaging Research
Department of Medical Imaging
Alfred I. DuPont Hospital for Children
Wilmington, Delaware

Ian D. Hay, MD
Professor of Medicine
Dr. R. F. Emslander Professor in Endocrinology Research
Division of Endocrinology and Internal Medicine
Mayo Clinic
Consultant in Endocrinology and Internal Medicine
Department of Medicine
Mayo ClinicRochester, Minnesota

Christy K. Holland, PhD
Professor
Departments of Biomedical Engineering and Radiology
University of Cincinnati
Cincinnati, Ohio

Caroline Hollingsworth, MD
Assistant Professor of Radiology
Duke University Medical Center
Durham, North Carolina

Bonnie J. Huppert, MD
Assistant Professor of Radiology
Mayo Clinic College of Medicine
Consultant in Radiology
Mayo Clinic
Rochester, Minnesota

E. Meridith James, MD, FACR
Professor of Radiology
Mayo Clinic College of Medicine
Consultant in Radiology
Mayo Clinic
Rochester, Minnesota

Susan D. John, MD
Professor of Radiology and Pediatrics
Chair, Department of Diagnostic and Interventional
    Imaging
University of Texas Medical School at Houston
Houston, Texas

Neil D. Johnson, MBBS, MMed, FRANZCR
Professor, Radiology and Pediatrics
Cincinnati Children's Hospital Medical Center
Cincinnati, Ohio

Korosh Khalili, MD, FRCPC
Assistant Professor
University of Toronto
Staff Radiologist
University Health Network
Toronto, Ontario, Canada

Beth M. Kline-Fath, MD
Assistant Professor of Radiology
Cincinnati Children's Hospital Medical Center
Cincinnati, Ohio

Clifford S. Levi, MD, FRCPC
Section Head
Health Sciences Centre
Professor
University of Manitoba
Winnipeg, Manitoba, Canada

Deborah Levine, MD, FACR
Professor of Radiology
Harvard Medical School
Associate Radiologist-in-Chief of Academic Affairs
Director of Ob/Gyn Ultrasound
Beth Israel Deaconess Medical Center
Boston, Massachusetts

Bradley D. Lewis, MD
Associate Professor of Radiology
Mayo Clinic College of Medicine
Consultant in Radiology
Mayo Clinic
Rochester, Minnesota

Ana Lourenco, MD
Assistant Professor of Diagnostic Imaging
Alpert Medical School of Brown University
Providence, Rhode Island

Edward A. Lyons, OC, FRCPC, FACR
Professor of Radiology
Obstetrics & Gynecology and Anatomy
University of Manitoba
Radiologist
Health Sciences Center
Winnipeg, Manitoba, Canada

Giancarlo Mari, MD
Professor and Vice-Chair, Department of Obstetrics and
    Gynecology
Director, Division of Maternal-Fetal Medicine
University of Tennessee Health Science Center
Memphis, Tennessee

John R. Mathieson, MD, FRCPC
Medical Director and Chief Radiologist
Vancouver Island Health Authority
Royal Jubilee Hospital
Victoria, British Columbia, Canada

Cynthia V. Maxwell, MD, FRCSC, RDMS, DABOG
Assistant Professor
Obstetrics and Gynecology
University of Toronto
Staff Perinatologist
Obstetrics and Gynecology
Division of Maternal Fetal Medicine
Toronto, Ontario, Canada

John McGahan, MD
Professor and Vice Chair of Radiology
University of California Davis Medical Center
Sacramento, California

Tejas S. Mehta, MD, MPH
Assistant Professor of Radiology
Beth Israel Deaconess Medical Center
Boston, Massachusetts

Christopher R. B. Merritt, BS, MS, MD
Professor
Thomas Jefferson University
Philadelphia, Pennsylvania

Norman L. Meyer, MD, PhD
Associate Professor, Division of Maternal-Fetal Medicine
Vice Chair, Department of OBGYN
University of Tennessee Health Science Center
Memphis, Tennessee

Derek Muradali, MD, FRCPC
Head, Division of Ultrasound
St. Michael's Hospital
Associate Professor
University of Toronto
Toronto, Ontario Canada

Sara M. O'Hara, MD, FAAP
Associate Professor of Radiology and Pediatrics
University of Cincinnati
Director, Ultrasound Division
Cincinnati Children's Hospital Medical Center
Cincinnati, Ohio

†Heidi B. Patriquin, MD
Department of Medical Imaging,
Sainte-Justine Hospital
Quebec, Canada

Joseph F. Polak, MD, MPH
Professor of Radiology
Tufts University School of Medicine
Chief of Radiology
Tufts Medical Center
Research Affiliation
Director, Ultrasound Reading Center
Tufts University School of Medicine
Boston, Massachusetts

Philip Ralls, MD
Radiology Professor
University of Southern California
Keck School of Medicine
Los Angeles, California

Cynthia T. Rapp, BS, RDMS, FAIUM, FSDMS
VP of Clinical Product Development
Medipattern
Toronto, Ontario, Canada

Carl C. Reading, MD, FACR
Professor of Radiology
Mayo Clinic College of Medicine
Consultant in Radiology
Mayo Clinic
Rochester, Minnesota

Maryam Rivaz, MD
Post Doctoral Fellow
Department of Obstetrics and Gynecology
University of Tennessee Health Science Center
Memphis, Tennessee

Julie E. Robertson, MD, FRCSC
Fellow
Division of Maternal Fetal Medicine
Obstetrics and Gynecology
University of Toronto
Toronto, Ontario, Canada

Henrietta Kotlus Rosenberg, MD, FACR, FAAP
Professor of Radiology and Pediatrics
The Mount Sinai School of Medicine
Director of Pediatric Radiology
The Mount Sinai Medical Center
New York, New York

Carol M. Rumack, MD, FACR
Professor of Radiology and Pediatrics
University of Colorado Denver School of Medicine
Denver, Colorado

---

†Deceased.

Shia Salem, MD, FRCPC
Associate Professor
University of Toronto
Radiologist
Mount Sinai Hospital
University Health Network
Women's College Hospital
Department of Medical Imaging
Mount Sinai Hospital
Toronto, Ontario, Canada

Nathan A. Saucier, MD
R4 Resident
Diagnostic Radiology
University of Illinois College of Medicine at Peoria
Peoria, Illinois

Eric E. Sauerbrei, BSc, MSc, MD, FRCPC
Professor of Radiology, Adjunct Professor of Obstetrics
    and Gynecology
Queen's University
Director of Ultrasound
Kingston General Hospital and Hotel Dieu Hospital
Director of Residents Research
Queen's University
Kingston, Ontario, Canada

Joanna J. Seibert, MD
Professor of Radiology and Pediatrics
Arkansas Children's Hospital
University of Arkansas for Medical Sciences
Little Rock, Arkansas

Chetan Chandulal Shah, MBBS, DMRD, MBA
Assistant Professor
Arkansas Children's Hospital
University of Arkansas for Medical Sciences
Little Rock, Arkansas

Rola Shaheen, MB, BS, MD
Radiology Instructor
Harvard Medical School
Chief of Radiology and
Director of Women's Imaging
Harrington Memorial Hospital
Boston, Massachusetts

William E. Shiels II, DO
Chairman, Department of Radiology
Nationwide Children's Hospital
Clinical Professor of Radiology, Pediatrics, and
    Biomedical Engineering
The Ohio State University College of Medicine
Columbus, Ohio;
Adjunct Professor of Radiology
The University of Toledo Medical Center
Toledo, Ohio

Thomas D. Shipp, MD
Associate Professor of Obstetrics, Gynecology, and
    Reproductive Biology
Harvard Medical School
Boston, Massachusetts
Associate Obstetrician and Gynecologist
Brigham & Women's Hospital
Boston, Massachusetts

Luigi Solbiati, MD
Director, Department of Diagnostic Imaging
General Hospital of Busto Arsizio
Busto Arsizio, (VA) Italy

Elizabeth R. Stamm, MD
Associate Professor of Radiology
University of Colorado at Denver Health Sciences Center
Aurora, Colorado

A. Thomas Stavros, MD, FACR
Medical Director, Ultrasound Invision
Sally Jobe Breast Center
Englewood, Colorado

George A. Taylor, MD
John A. Kirkpatrick Professor of Radiology (Pediatrics)
Harvard Medical School
Radiologist-in-Chief
Children's Hospital Boston
Boston, Massachusetts

Wendy Thurston, MD
Assistant Professor
Department of Medical Imaging
University of Toronto
Chief, Diagnostic Imaging
Department of Diagnostic Imaging
St. Joseph's Health Centre
Courtesy Staff
Department of Medical Imaging
University Health Network
Toronto, Ontario, Canada

Ants Toi, MD, FRCPC
Associate Professor of Radiology and Obstetrics and
    Gynecology
University of Toronto
Staff Radiologist
University Health Network and Mt. Sinai Hospital
Toronto, Ontario, Canada

Didier H. Touche, MD
Chief Radiologist
Centre Sein Godinot
Godinot Breast Cancer Center
Reims, France

Mitchell Tublin, MD
Professor of Radiology
Chief, Abdominal Imaging Section
Department of Radiology
University of Pittsburgh School of Medicine
Pittsburgh, Pennsylvania

Rebecca A. Uhlmann, MS
Program Administrator
Obstetrics and Gynecology
University of Tennessee Health Science Center
Memphis, Tennessee

Sheila Unger, MD
Clinical Geneticist
Institute of Human Genetics
University of Freiburg
Freiburg, Germany

Marnix T. van Holsbeeck, MD
Professor of Radiology
Wayne State University School of Medicine
Detroit, Michigan
Division Head, Musculoskeletal Radiology
Henry Ford Hospital
Detroit, Michigan

Patrick M. Vos, MD
Clinical Assistant Professor
University of British Columbia
Vancouver, British Columbia, Canada

Dzung Vu, MD, MBBS, Dip Anat
Senior Lecturer
University of New South Wales
Sydney, New South Wales, Australia

Wendy L. Whittle, MD
Maternal Fetal Medicine Specialist
Department of Obstetrics and Gynecology
Mount Sinai Hospital
University of Toronto
Toronto, Ontario, Canada

Stephanie R. Wilson, MD, FRCPC
Clinical Professor of Radiology
University of Calgary
Staff Radiologist
Foothills Medical Centre
Calgary, Alberta, Canada

Rory Windrim, MD, MSc, FRCSC
Professor
Department of Obstetrics & Gynecology
University of Toronto
Staff Perinatologist
Mount Sinai Hospital
Toronto, Ontario, Canada

Cynthia E. Withers
Staff Radiologist
Department of Radiology
Santa Barbara Cottage Hospital
Santa Barbara, California

*In memory of **my parents, Drs. Ruth and Raymond Masters,** who encouraged me to enjoy the intellectual challenge of medicine and the love of making a difference in patients' lives.*

CMR

*To a lifetime of **clinical colleagues, residents, and fellows** who have provided me with a wealth of professional joy. And **to my wonderful family,** for your love and never-ending support.*

SRW

*To **Cathy, Nicholas, Ben, and Laurie,** for all the love and joy you bring to my life. You are all I could ever hope for.*

JWC

*To **Alex, Becky, and Julie**—your love and support made this work possible.*

DL

Preface

The fourth edition of *Diagnostic Ultrasound* is a major revision. Previous editions have been very well accepted as a reference textbook and have been the most commonly used reference in ultrasound education and practices worldwide. We are pleased to provide a new update of images and text with new areas of strength. For the first time we are including video clips in the majority of chapters. The display of real-time ultrasound has helped to capture those abnormalities that require a sweep through the pathology to truly appreciate the lesion. It is similar to scrolling through images on a PACS and has added great value to clinical imaging. Daily we find that cine or video clips show important areas between still images that help to make certain a diagnosis or relationships between lesions. Now we rarely need to go back to reevaluate a lesion with another scan, making patient imaging more efficient.

We are pleased to announce that a new editor, Deborah Levine, has joined us, providing expertise in fetal imaging, in both obstetrical sonography and fetal MRI. Prenatal diagnosis is one of the frontiers of medicine that continues to grow as a field and has pushed our understanding of what happens to the fetus before we see a lesion at birth. These antecedents of disease in children and adults help us to arrange care for patients long before the mother goes into labor.

Approximately 90 outstanding new and continuing authors have contributed to this edition, and all are recognized experts in the field of ultrasound. We have replaced at least 50% of the images without increasing the size of the two volumes, so new value has been added to all of the chapters, particularly for obstetrics and gynecology. The fourth edition now includes over 5000 images, many in full color. The layout has been exhaustively revamped, and there are highly valuable multipart figures or key figure collages. These images all reflect the spectrum of sonographic changes that may occur in a given disease instead of the most common manifestation only.

The book's format has been redesigned to facilitate reading and review. There are again color-enhanced boxes to highlight the important or critical features of sonographic diagnoses. Key terms and concepts are emphasized in boldface type. To direct the readers to other research and literature of interest, comprehensive reference lists are organized by topic.

Diagnostic Ultrasound is again divided into two volumes. Volume I consists of Parts I to III. Part I contains chapters on physics and biologic effects of ultrasound, as well as more of the latest developments in ultrasound contrast agents. Part II covers abdominal, pelvic, and thoracic sonography, including interventional procedures and organ transplantation. Part III presents small parts imaging including thyroid, breast, scrotum, carotid, peripheral vessels, and particularly MSK imaging. Newly added is a chapter on musculoskeletal intervention.

Volume II begins with Part IV, where the greatest expansion of text and images has been on obstetric and fetal sonography, including video clips for the first time. Part V comprehensively covers pediatric sonography.

Diagnostic Ultrasound is for practicing physicians, residents, medical students, sonographers, and others interested in understanding the vast applications of diagnostic sonography in patient care. Our goal is for *Diagnostic Ultrasound* to continue to be the most comprehensive reference book available in the sonographic literature with a highly readable style and superb images.

Carol M. Rumack
Stephanie R. Wilson
J. William Charboneau
Deborah Levine

Acknowledgments

Our deepest appreciation and sincerest gratitude:

To all of our outstanding authors who have contributed extensive, newly updated, and authoritative text and images. We cannot thank them enough for their efforts on this project.

To Sharon Emmerling in Denver, Colorado, whose outstanding secretarial and communication skills with authors and editors have facilitated the review and final revision of the entire manuscript. Her enthusiastic attention to detail and accuracy has made this our best edition ever.

To Gordana Popovich and Dr. Hojun Yu for their artwork and schematics in Chapter 8, The Gastrointestinal Tract.

To Dr. Hojun Yu for his schematics on liver anatomy in Chapter 4, The Liver.

To Lisa Barnes, developmental editor at Elsevier, who has worked closely with us on this project from the very beginning of the fourth edition. We also thank the enthusiastic participation of many other Elsevier experts including **Rebecca Gaertner**, Elsevier's guiding hand overseeing the project. She has patiently worked with us through all the final stages of development and production. It has been an intense year for everyone, and we are very proud of this superb edition of *Diagnostic Ultrasound.*

Contents

Online Video Contents

Part IV

Obstetric Sonography

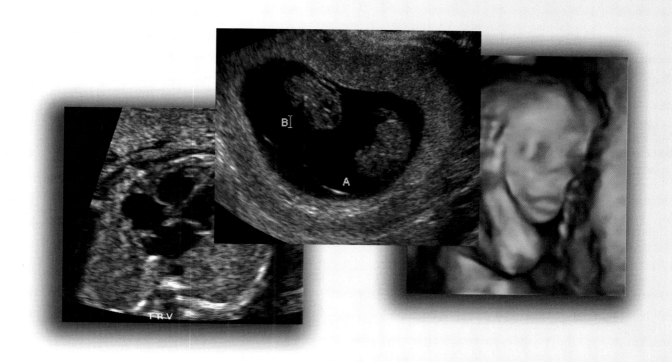

CHAPTER 28

Overview of Obstetric Imaging

Deborah Levine

Chapter Outline

There were more than 4.2 million live births in the United States in 2008.[1] It is estimated that obstetric ultrasound was used in 68% of pregnancies in 2002, up from 48% in 1989.[2] Given the upward trend in ultrasound use, it is likely that an even higher percentage of pregnant women undergo ultrasound evaluation currently in the United States. Ultrasound use is even higher in countries where it is considered a part of routine obstetric care, as opposed to the United States, where this is still a contentious issue.

Indications for ultrasound during the **first trimester** include pregnancy dating, assessment of women with bleeding or pain, and assessment of nuchal translucency in screening for aneuploidy. In the **second trimester**, ultrasound is used for pregnancy dating, assessment of interval growth, assessment of patients with abnormal pain or bleeding, assessment of size-to-dates discrepancy, routine survey of fetal anatomy, and assessment of maternal indications related to age, drug use, or history of prior abnormalities.

In cases of multiple gestations, ultrasound is used to assess growth and complications of twinning. In women with history of cervical incompetence, ultrasound is used to screen for cervical changes that put a patient at risk for preterm delivery. In the **third trimester**, ultrasound is predominantly used to assess fetal growth and well-being. Ultrasound is increasingly used for fetal procedures such as testing for aneuploidy, fetal drainage, and guidance for fetal surgery. Ultrasound is well recognized as the screening modality of choice, but additional information may be needed beyond that available with ultrasound. In many of these cases, especially those with fetal central nervous system abnormalities, fetal magnetic resonance imaging (MRI) can help clarify the diagnosis.

Part IV of this textbook focuses on obstetric ultrasound and reviews specific fetal organ system anatomy and pathology, with chapters also on safety of ultrasound in pregnancy, assessment of twins, and growth. Fetal MR and three-dimensional ultrasound images are added throughout to illustrate the benefit of these techniques in select cases.

TRAINING, PERSONNEL, AND EQUIPMENT

Obstetric ultrasound diagnosis is critically dependent on examiner training and experience.[3,4] Physicians and sonographers performing obstetric ultrasound examinations should have completed appropriate training and should be appropriately credentialed and boarded. Accreditation of ultrasound laboratories improves compliance with published minimum standards and guidelines.[5] Ultrasound practitioners should be knowledgeable regarding the basic physical principles of ultrasound, equipment, record-keeping requirements, indications, and safety of using ultrasound in pregnancy. Studies should be conducted with real-time scanners using a transabdominal and/or transvaginal approach, depending on the gestational age and the region of interest. The choice of transducer frequency is a trade-off between beam penetration and resolution. In general, a 3 to 5–MHz transducer frequency provides sufficient resolution with adequate depth penetration in all but the

INDICATIONS FOR FIRST-TRIMESTER ULTRASOUND

To confirm the presence of an intrauterine pregnancy.
To evaluate a suspected ectopic pregnancy.
To define the cause of vaginal bleeding.
To evaluate pelvic pain.
To estimate gestational (menstrual) age.
To diagnose or evaluate multiple gestations.
To confirm cardiac activity.
As an adjunct to chorionic villus sampling, embryo transfer, and localization, and removal of an intrauterine device.
To assess for certain fetal anomalies, such as anencephaly, in high-risk patients.
To evaluate maternal pelvic masses and/or uterine abnormalities.
To measure nuchal translucency when part of a screening program for fetal aneuploidy.
To evaluate a suspected hydatidiform mole.

From American College of Radiology. ACR practice guideline for the performance of antepartum obstetrical ultrasound. In *ACR practice guidelines and technical standards.* Philadelphia, 2007, ACR, pp 1025-1033.

INDICATIONS FOR SECOND- AND THIRD-TRIMESTER ULTRASOUND

Estimation of gestational (menstrual) age
Evaluation of fetal growth
Vaginal bleeding
Abdominal or pelvic pain
Cervical insufficiency
Determination of fetal presentation
Suspected multiple gestation
Adjunct to amniocentesis or other procedure
Significant discrepancy between uterine size and clinical dates
Pelvic mass
Suspected hydatidiform mole
Adjunct to cervical cerclage placement
Suspected ectopic pregnancy
Suspected fetal death
Suspected uterine abnormality
Evaluation of fetal well-being
Suspected amniotic fluid abnormalities
Suspected placental abruption
Adjunct to external cephalic version
Premature rupture of membranes and/or premature labor
Abnormal biochemical markers
Follow-up evaluation of a fetal anomaly
Follow-up evaluation of placental location for suspected placenta previa
History of previous congenital anomaly
Evaluation of fetal condition in late registrants for prenatal care
To assess for findings that may increase the risk for aneuploidy
Screening for fetal anomalies

From American College of Radiology. ACR practice guideline for the performance of antepartum obstetrical ultrasound. In *ACR practice guidelines and technical standards.* Philadelphia, 2007, ACR, pp 1025-1033.

extremely obese patient. During early pregnancy, a 4 to 7–MHz abdominal transducer or a 5 to 10–MHz vaginal transducer may provide superior resolution while still allowing adequate penetration. Higher-frequency transducers are most useful in achieving high-resolution scans, and lower-frequency transducers are useful when increased penetration of the sound beam is necessary. Use of Doppler ultrasound and three-dimensional (3-D) and four-dimensional (4-D) imaging depends on the specific indication. As in all imaging studies, complete documentation of the images and a formal written interpretation are essential for quality assurance, accreditation, and medicolegal issues.

ULTRASOUND GUIDELINES

First Trimester

The current guidelines of the American College of Radiology (ACR) and American Institute of Ultrasound in Medicine (AIUM) for the performance of first-trimester obstetric ultrasound examination include documentation of the location of the pregnancy (intrauterine vs. extrauterine), documentation of the appearance of the maternal uterus and ovaries (Fig. 28-1), and assessment of **gestational age,** either by measurement of mean sac diameter (before visualization of embryonic pole; Fig. 28-2) or by embryonic/fetal pole crown-rump length (Fig. 28-3).[6] Another important structure to assess is the **yolk sac.** An image of the heart rate is taken using M-mode ultrasound. It is important to use M-mode

GENERAL SURVEY GUIDELINES FOR FIRST-TRIMESTER ULTRASOUND

Gestational sac
    Location of pregnancy: intrauterine vs. extrauterine
Gestational age (as appropriate)
    Mean sac diameter
    Embryonic pole length
    Crown-rump length
Yolk sac or embryo/fetus
Cardiac activity on M-mode ultrasound
Fetal number (amnionicity/chorionicity)
Maternal anatomy: uterus and adnexa

Modified from American College of Radiology. ACR practice guideline for the performance of antepartum obstetrical ultrasound. In *ACR practice guidelines and technical standards.* Philadelphia, 2007, ACR, pp 1025-1033.

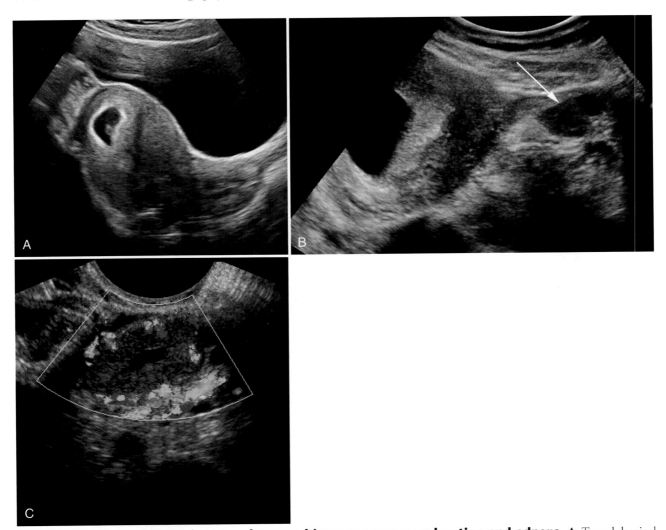

FIGURE 28-1. Normal first-trimester ultrasound images: pregnancy location and adnexa. A, Transabdominal sagittal sonogram shows an intrauterine gestational sac. **B,** Transverse image to the left of uterus shows normal appearance for the ovary *(arrow).* **C,** Transvaginal color Doppler image shows normal hypervascular rim around corpus luteum.

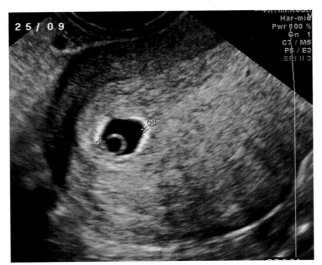

FIGURE 28-2. Normal first-trimester ultrasound images: mean sac diameter. Transvaginal sagittal image shows sagittal measurement of sac diameter *(calipers)*. Measurements in three orthogonal planes are averaged to calculate the mean sac diameter. Note yolk sac within the gestational sac.

rather than spectral Doppler ultrasound on the embryo to limit power deposition. Late in the first trimester, dating can be performed with measurement of the biparietal diameter and head circumference, rather than crown-rump length. Chapters 30 and 42 discuss the first-trimester examination and gestational dating in pregnancy, respectively.

In cases of multiple gestation, first-trimester scans should document the fetal number as well as the amnionicity and chorionicity (Fig. 28-4). Chapter 32 discusses the assessment of multifetal pregnancies.

It is increasingly common to assess for risk of **aneuploidy** (e.g., trisomy 21, 18, or 13) by measuring **nuchal translucency** between 11 and 14 weeks of gestation (see Fig 28-3, *I*). This measurement, in conjunction with maternal age and serology, can be used to determine an individualized risk of fetal aneuploidy (see Chapter 31). Increased use of first- and second-trimester ultrasound has reduced the number of interventional procedures to

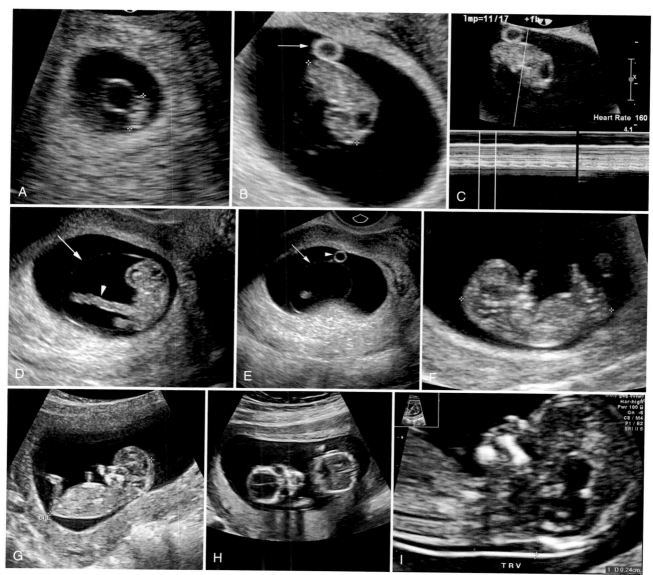

FIGURE 28-3. First-trimester ultrasound images: embryo and fetus. A, Normal embryo at 6.5 weeks' gestation. Note embryonic pole *(calipers)* adjacent to yolk sac. **B,** Normal embryo at 8 weeks' gestation. Note embryo *(calipers)* and adjacent yolk sac *(arrow).* **C,** M-mode ultrasound from same embryo as in **B.** Note normal heart rate of 160 beats/min. **D,** Normal embryo at 9 weeks' gestational age. Note embryo within amnion *(arrow)* and umbilical cord *(arrowhead).* **E,** Just lateral to image in **D,** note yolk sac *(arrowhead)* is located outside the amnion *(arrow).* **F,** Sagittal ultrasound at 10.5 weeks' gestation. **G,** Sagittal ultrasound at 11.5 weeks' gestation. **H,** Coronal view of face at 13 weeks' gestation. **I,** Sagittal ultrasound of nuchal translucency *(calipers)* at 13 weeks' gestation.

detect aneuploidy while increasing the prenatal diagnosis of aneuploidy.[7] Given the increased scanning late in the first trimester, it is also increasingly common for a limited anatomic survey to be conducted in the late first trimester. Anomalies that should be detected this early include **anencephaly** (Fig. 28-5) and **omphalocele** (Fig. 28-6). Although substantial information can be obtained at this time, first-trimester anatomic survey is unlikely to replace the second-trimester anatomic survey, since many structures are difficult to visualize completely early in the second trimester, particularly the heart, cardiac outflow tracts, posterior fossa, and distal spine.

Second and Third Trimesters

The current ACR/AIUM guidelines for the performance of the second- and third-trimester obstetric ultrasound examinations describe the **standard** sonographic examination.[6] It is important to understand that the guidelines were written to maximize detection of many fetal abnormalities, but are not expected to allow for detection of all structural abnormalities.[6]

The terminology **level I** and **level II** examinations refer to "standard" or "routine" (level I) and "high risk," "specialized," or "detailed" (level II) obstetric ultrasound. The concept of these two levels of scanning is that the

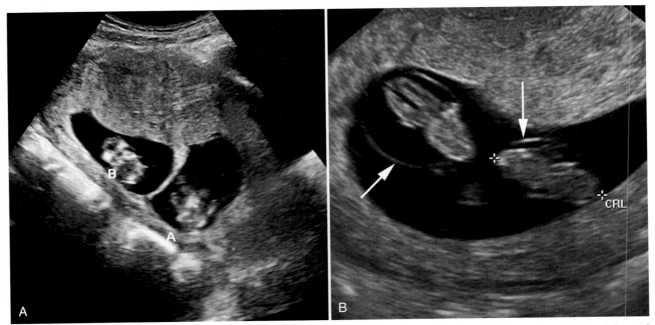

FIGURE 28-4. Multiple gestations. Be sure to examine the entire gestational sac to identify multiple gestations. **A,** Transabdominal image of **diamniotic dichorionic twins.** Note the thick, dividing membrane. **B,** Transvaginal image of **diamniotic monochorionic twins** at 8 weeks' gestational age (*calipers* denote crown rump length) with two thin membranes (*arrows, amnion*) still close to embryonic poles.

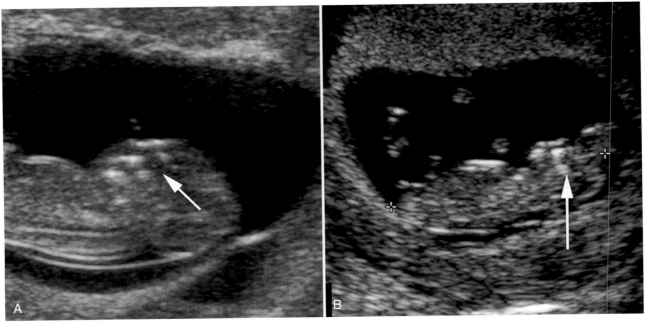

FIGURE 28-5. Anencephaly. A, Sagittal ultrasound at 10 weeks' gestation. **B,** Sagittal ultrasound in a different fetus at 12 weeks' gestation. Note the orbits *(arrow)* with absent ossified cranium above this level with angiomatous stroma.

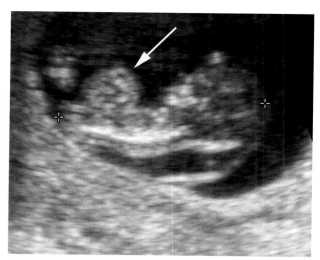

FIGURE 28-6. Omphalocele at 11 weeks' gestational age. Sagittal view of fetus *(calipers)* shows a large, abdominal wall defect *(arrow).*

standard, basic, routine, or level I examination is performed routinely on pregnant patients (Figs. 28-7 to 28-16). The methods to obtain all the required images are described in detail in subsequent chapters. This chapter provides a collage of figures as a guide for the anatomic survey and common additional views obtained during a fetal survey.

In general, the "standard fetal anatomic survey" refers to the **second-trimester scan,** typically performed between 16 and 22 weeks of gestation. When anatomic surveys are performed at 20 to 22 weeks' gestational age, there is less need for repeat scans to document normal anatomy compared to studies performed earlier in pregnancy.[8] However, there are practical considerations when determining the optimal timing of studies. In well-dated pregnancies in women who are unlikely to want amniocentesis, a survey at 20 to 22 weeks' gestation is optimal. However, if a pregnancy is not well dated, an earlier scan may be needed both to establish accurate dates for the pregnancy and to assess the anatomy. Some centers offer the scan at 16 weeks' gestation to coincide with performance of genetic amniocentesis and/or midtrimester quadruple serum screening.

 The level I examination consists of investigation of the maternal uterus and ovaries, the cervix, and placenta (Fig. 28-7; **Video 28-1**), as well as a systematic review of fetal anatomy. **Adnexal cysts** are common in pregnant women. In early pregnancy a cyst is most likely the corpus luteum. If a cyst appears atypical or enlarges beyond the middle second trimester, it should be further assessed. Leiomyoma position and size should be documented. If the myometrium appears thin in the lower uterine segment (e.g., <3 mm in woman with prior cesarean section), the myometrium should be measured because this puts the woman at risk for **uterine dehis-**

SURVEY GUIDELINES FOR SECOND- AND THIRD-TRIMESTER ULTRASOUND

GENERAL SURVEY
Cardiac activity: document with M-mode
Presentation: cephalic, breech, transverse, variable
Fetal number: for multiples, amnionicity/chorionicity, concordance with size, amniotic fluid
Maternal anatomy: uterus, adnexa, and cervix
Gestational age and fetal weight assessment
    Biparietal diameter
    Head circumference
    Abdominal circumference
    Femur length
Amniotic fluid
    Estimate as normal
    If abnormal, qualify if high or low
Placenta: position

FETAL ANATOMIC SURVEY
Head, Face, and Neck
Cerebellum
Choroid plexus
Cisterna magna
Lateral cerebral ventricles
Midline falx
Cavum septi pellucidi
Upper lip

Chest
Four-chamber view
Outflow tracts "if technically feasible"

Abdomen
Stomach (presence, size, and situs)
Kidneys, bladder
Umbilical cord insertion site into fetal abdomen
Umbilical cord vessel number

Spine
Cervical, thoracic, lumbar, and sacral

Extremities
Legs and arms: presence or absence

Gender (Sex)
Medically indicated in low-risk pregnancies only for evaluation of multiple gestations

Modified from American College of Radiology. ACR practice guideline for the performance of antepartum obstetrical ultrasound. In *ACR practice guidelines and technical standards.* Philadelphia, 2007, ACR, pp 1025-1033.

cence or **rupture**. It is helpful to begin the examination with a sagittal midline view to assess the cervix. If the cervix appears abnormally short or if placenta previa is suspected, a vaginal scan can then be performed.

Transverse and longitudinal scans of the entire uterine cavity are then performed for assessment of **fetal cardiac**

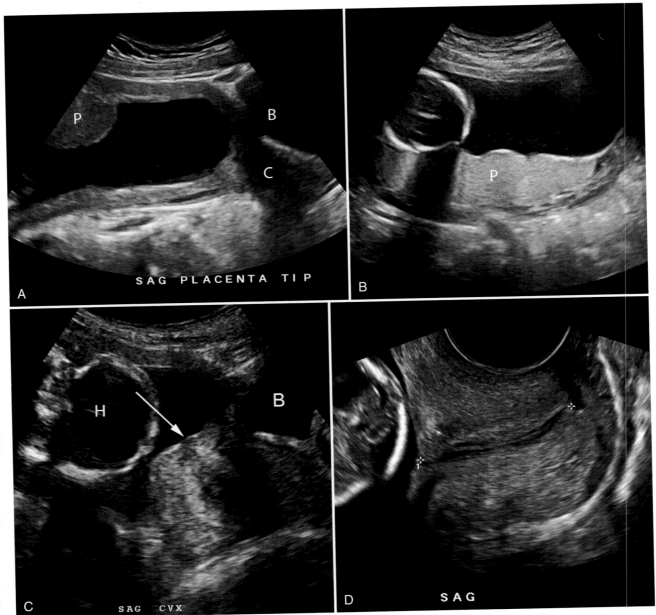

FIGURE 28-7. Overview of uterus, cervix, and fetal position. A, Sagittal sonogram of uterus shows a normal-appearing cervix *(C)* and an anterior placenta *(P),* with the placental tip far away from the internal cervical os; *B,* bladder. **B,** Transverse sonogram of posterior placenta *(P).* **C,** Transabdominal image of normal-appearing cervix *(arrow* on internal os). Note bladder *(B)* and fetal head *(H).* With the head as the presenting part, the fetus is in cephalic position. **D,** Transvaginal sonogram of normal-appearing cervix *(calipers).*

activity, amniotic fluid volume, localization of the placenta, and determination of **fetal presentation** and **situs** (Fig. 28-8). Knowledge of the plane of section across the maternal abdomen, combined with the position of the fetal spine and right-sided and left-sided structures within the fetal body, allows accurate determination of fetal position and identification of normal and pathologic anatomy. Some congenital anomalies, such as dextrocardia, will be recognized only if a structure is identified as "abnormal" by virtue of its atypical position related to the lie and presentation of the fetus.

Biometry is performed, both to estimate gestational age and to estimate fetal weight (Fig. 28-9).

The high-risk, targeted, detailed, or level II scan should have a specific indication that requires a detailed fetal sonogram, performed by a clinician with expertise in obstetric imaging.[9] This high-risk scan is performed when an anomaly is suspected because of maternal medical or family history, or if abnormal results are suspected on a routine scan. Additional views in routine obstetric sonography include the head (Fig. 28-10; **Video 28-2**), face (Fig. 28-11), heart

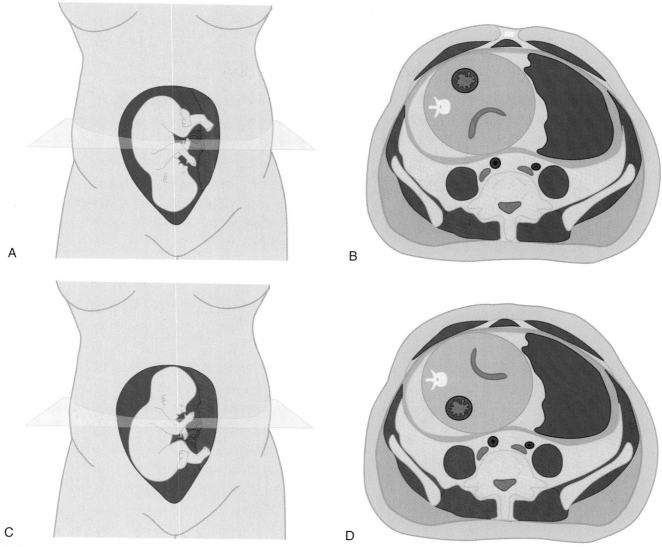

FIGURE 28-8. Determination of situs. A, Scan plane, and **B,** transverse scan diagram. With fetus in cephalic position and spine on the maternal right side, the left-sided stomach is "up" on the side closest to the transducer. **C,** Scan plane, and **D,** with the fetus in breech position and spine on the maternal right side, the left-sided stomach is "down" on the side farthest away from the transducer.

ADDITIONAL VIEWS FOR TARGETED FETAL SONOGRAMS*

Corpus callosum
Cerebellar vermis
Outflow tracts
Orbits
Extremities, including hands and feet
Profile/chin
Nuchal fold (at appropriate gestational age)
Individual long-bone measurements
Hands and feet

*These are not established imaging guidelines but rather the author's suggestions regarding views that are helpful in most targeted scans. Additional views may be needed depending on the indications for the obstetric/fetal examination.

(Fig. 28-12; **Video 28-3**), abdomen and pelvis (Fig. 28-13; **Videos 28-4** and **28-5**), spine (Fig. 28-14), extremities (Fig. 28-15), and umbilical cord (Fig. 28-16). Other specialized sonographic examinations include fetal Doppler sonography, biophysical profile, fetal echocardiography, and additional biometric measurements.

ROUTINE ULTRASOUND SCREENING

Estimation of Gestational Age

Determination of the **expected date of delivery** (EDD) is especially important in obstetric practice because it is

Text continued on p. 1055.

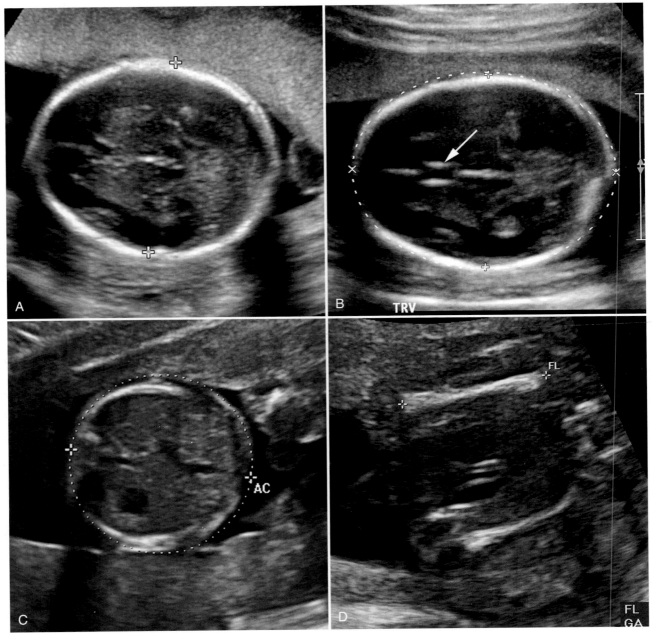

FIGURE 28-9. Second-trimester biometry. A, Biparietal diameter. Note the level of this ultrasound image at the thalamus and third ventricle. The calipers are placed from the outer skull in the near field to the inner skull in the far field. **B, Head circumference.** Note how circumference is measured around the outside of the skull. Arrow depicts cavum of the septum pellucidum. **C, Abdominal circumference.** Note the curve of the portal vein and stomach on this transverse image, with circumference drawn around the outside of the skin. **D, Femur length.** Note that the "upside" femur should be measured, with the shaft of the bone as near to perpendicular to the scan plane as possible, excluding the distal femoral epiphysis.

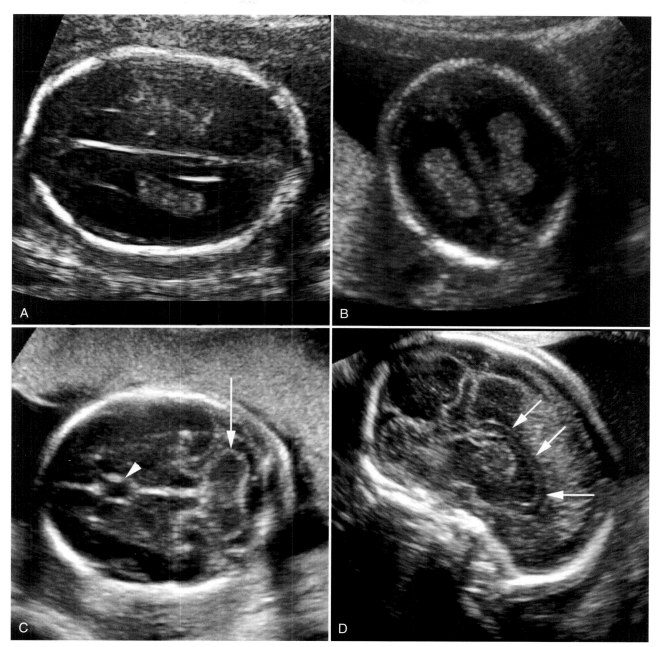

FIGURE 28-10. Routine sonographic views of fetal head. In addition to the biparietal diameter and head circumference, required views of the head include images of the **cerebral ventricles, cerebellum, cavum of the septum pellucidum,** and **midline falx.** Additional views that can be obtained are angled views to demonstrate both sides of the choroid plexus, and views through the anterior fontanelle or midline sutures to demonstrate the corpus callosum. **A,** Axial image shows cerebral ventricles filled with **choroid plexus. B,** Angled axial view shows both ventricles with choroid plexus. **C,** Axial image shows cerebellum *(arrow)* and cavum of the septum pellucidum *(arrowhead)*. **D,** Transvaginal sagittal view of the corpus callosum *(arrows)*.

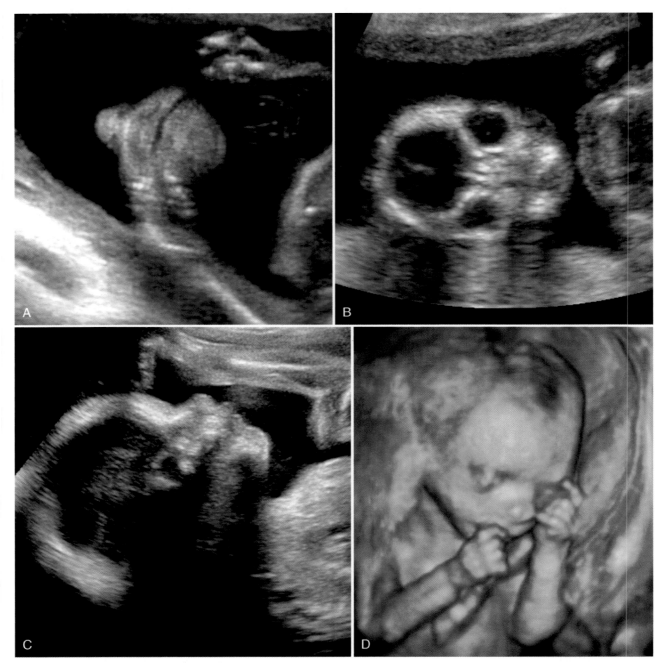

FIGURE 28-11. Views of fetal face. Required view of the face is of the nose and lips. Additional views include orbits and profile. **A,** Coronal view of nose and lips. **B,** Coronal view of orbits. **C,** Sagittal view of facial profile. **D,** 3-D image of fetal face.

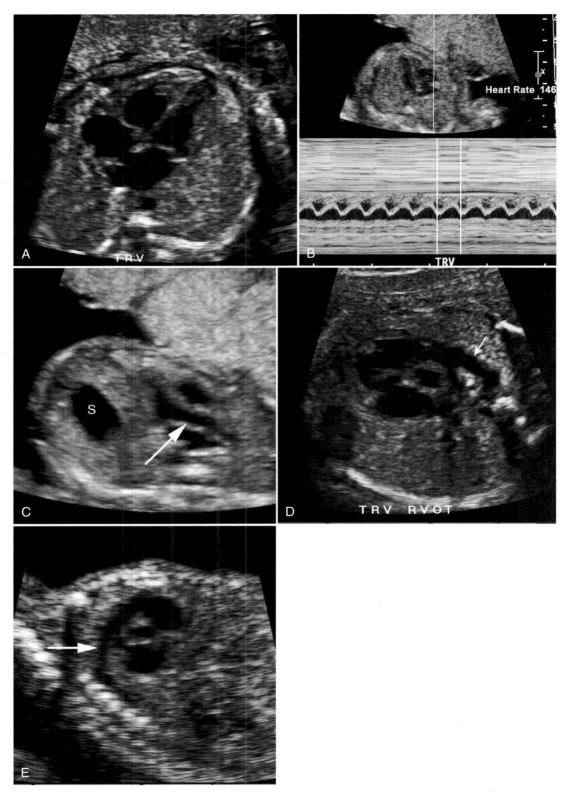

FIGURE 28-12. Views of fetal heart and outflow tracts. Required views include demonstration of normal situs, with heart and stomach on left side, four-chamber view of the heart, documentation of normal heart rate, and outflow tracts "if possible". **A,** Axial image shows normal four-chamber view of fetal heart. Note the normal axis of the heart, at about 60 degrees from midline. **B,** M-mode ultrasound. Note normal heart rate (146 beats/min). **C,** Angled view shows left ventricular outflow tract *(arrow)* with heart and stomach(s) on the same side of the fetus. **D** and **E,** Right ventricular outflow tract in oblique axial **(D)** and oblique sagittal **(E)** views with ductus arteriosus *(arrow)* extending posteriorly to aorta.

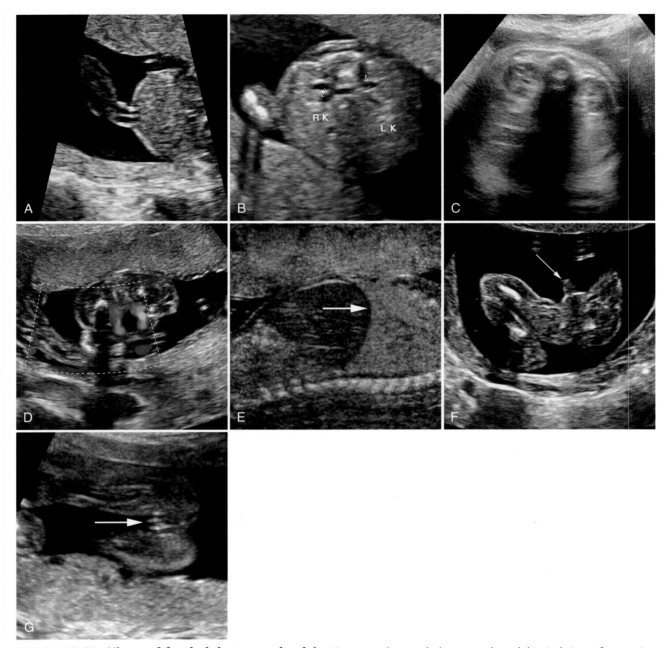

FIGURE 28-13. Views of fetal abdomen and pelvis. Note normal stomach documented on abdominal circumference view (Fig. 28-9, *C*). Other required views are cord insertion, kidneys, and bladder. Additional views document the diaphragm and fetal gender. **A,** Cord insertion site in the anterior abdominal wall. **B** and **C,** Transverse views of **kidneys** at 18 and 28 weeks' gestation. A small amount of central renal pelvic dilation (2 mm in this fetus) is a normal finding. **D,** Transverse image of **bladder.** Note umbilical arteries on either side of bladder. **E,** Sagittal view shows liver, diaphragm *(arrow)*, and lungs. Note how the liver is of lower echogenicity than the lungs. **F,** Male genitalia. **G,** Female genitalia.

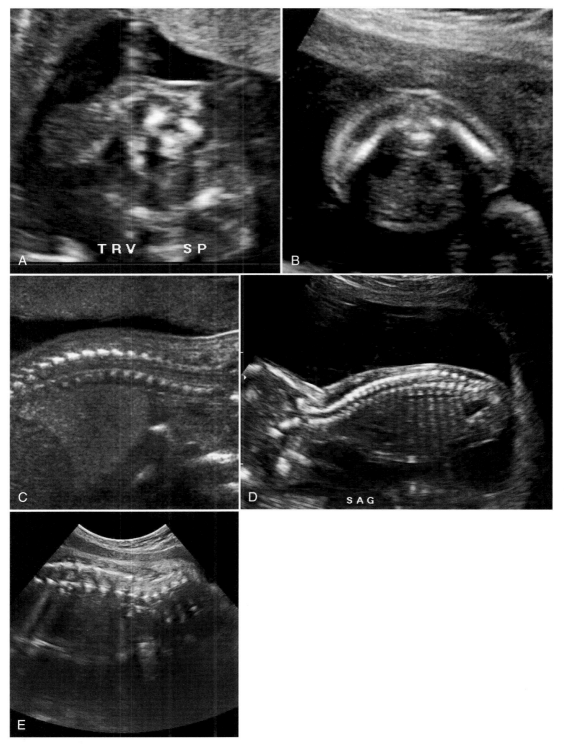

FIGURE 28-14. Views of fetal spine. Note transverse image of thoracic spine on four-chamber view (Fig. 28-12, *A*) and transverse image of lumbar spine between the kidneys (Fig. 28-13, *B* and *C*) and umbilical cord insertion site (Fig. 28-13, *A*). **A,** Transverse image of cervical spine. **B,** Transverse view of lumbosacral spine. Note how the posterior elements point towards each other and the skin covers the distal spine. **C,** Oblique sagittal image of cervical and thoracic spine. **D,** Oblique sagittal view of entire spine. **E,** Sagittal view focused on the distal spine. Note how the spinal canal narrows and has a gentle upturn distally. (See also Video 28-4.)

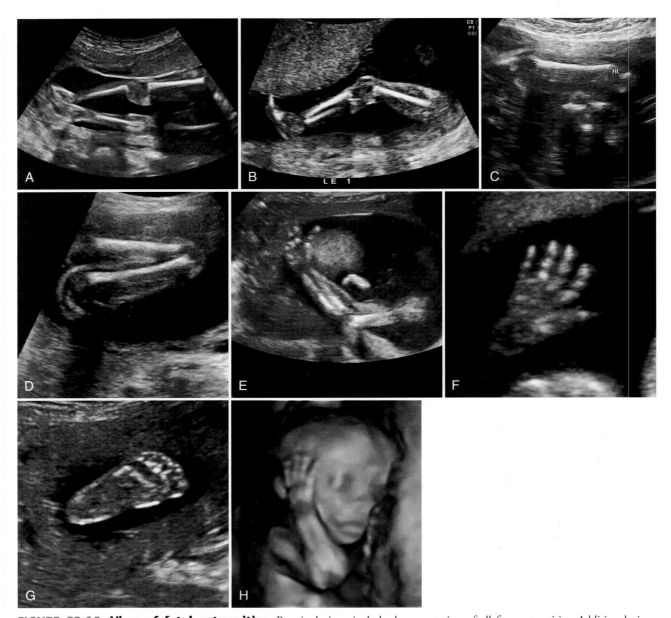

FIGURE 28-15. View of fetal extremities. Required views include documentation of all four extremities. Additional views include measurements of all the long bones and demonstration of the fingers and toes. **A** and **B,** Lower extremities. **C, D,** and **E,** Upper extremities. **F,** Hand. Note four fingers with thumb partially out of the field of view. **G,** Foot. **H,** 3-D view of upper extremity. (See also Fig. 28-11, *D,* for 3-D view of hands.)

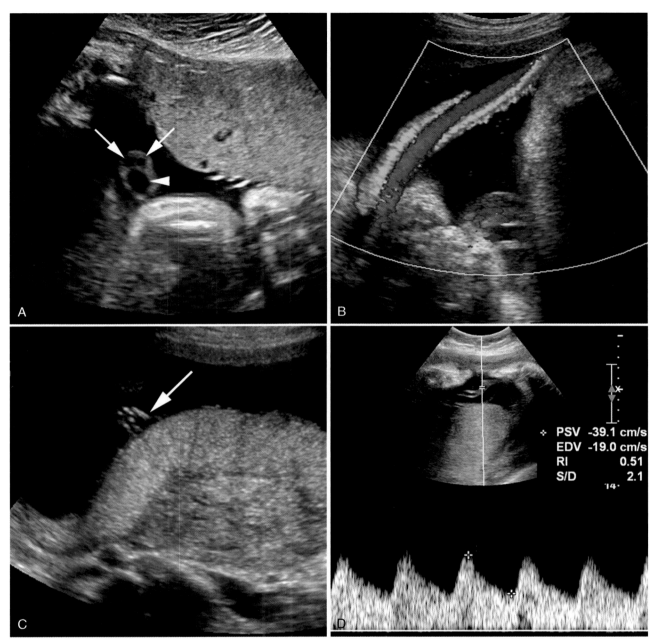

FIGURE 28-16. Views of umbilical cord. Required views include cord insertion site into the anterior abdominal wall (see Fig. 28-13, *A*) and documentation of number of vessels in the umbilical cord. Additional views include cord insertion site into the placenta and Doppler examination of the cord. **A,** Transverse image of **three-vessel umbilical cord.** Note two arteries *(arrows)* that are smaller than the single vein *(arrowhead).* (See also Video 28-5 and Fig. 28-13, *D.*) **B,** Color Doppler longitudinal image of three-vessel cord. **C,** **Cord insertion *site* (*arrow*)** into the placenta. **D,** Spectral Doppler image documents normal umbilical arterial systolic/diastolic ratio in third-trimester fetus.

used to intervene in pregnancies considered to be "growth restricted" and in postterm pregnancies. Multiple studies have demonstrated that routine use of ultrasound results in more accurate assessment of the EDD than last menstrual period (LMP) dating or physical examination, even in women with regular and certain menstrual dates.[10-13] **Pregnancy dating** is most accurately performed in the first half of pregnancy. **Fetal growth** should be assessed by comparison to earlier scans in

pregnancy. In a Cochrane review of nine trials of routine ultrasound in early pregnancy, routine use of early ultrasound and the subsequent adjustment of the EDD led to a significant reduction of postterm pregnancy.[14]

A rule of thumb is that in the first trimester, LMP dating should be maintained unless ultrasound yields an EDD more than 7 days off; in the second trimester, ultrasound should be used to change EDD if it is off by more than 2 weeks (and follow-up is then needed to ensure appropriate interval growth); and in the third trimester, a 3-week discrepancy between LMP and ultrasound dating is allowed, but needs to be taken into the clinical context, with assessment for growth restriction or macrosomia, if appropiate. It is important to recognize that if a pregnancy is redated after the first trimester, follow-up is needed to assess for appropriate interval growth (see Chapter 42).

Identification of Twin/Multiple Pregnancies

A major benefit of routine ultrasound screening is early identification of multiple gestations.[4,11,15-17] Randomized clinical trials comparing routine second-trimester ultrasound examination with sonography performed for clinical indications have shown that a substantial number of twin pregnancies are not recognized until the third trimester or delivery in women who do not undergo routine ultrasound. The improved diagnosis of twins leads to improved perinatal outcome because of a reduced incidence of low birth weight, smallness for gestational age, prematurity, depressed Apgar scores, and stillbirths.[15]

Screening and Perinatal Outcomes

The value of a routine second-trimester scan in apparently normal pregnancies to identify those at high risk for unsuspected problems is controversial. Many countries perform one, two, or even three sonograms as part of routine obstetric care.[16,18,19]

BENEFITS OF ROUTINE SECOND-TRIMESTER ULTRASOUND SCREENING

- More accurate gestational age
- Detection of major malformations before birth
- Earlier detection of multiple pregnancy
- Fewer low-birth-weight singleton births
- Lower incidence of induction for postterm pregnancy
- Early detection of placenta previa
- Reassurance of a normal pregnancy

It can be difficult to interpret the results of studies designed to assess the impact of routine screening.[4,11,16] Not only do anomalies need to be detected by ultrasound, but to show the benefit of ultrasound, there must be a documented difference in outcome, either in termination of pregnancies, potentially leading to decreased perinatal mortality from loss of anomalous fetuses, or improved perinatal care. Because these studies do not necessarily control for these outcomes, the benefit of screening, in particular the importance of parental under-

standing of fetal anomalies when pregnancies with fetal anomalies are continued, are difficult to demonstrate.

The Helsinki trial reported a significant decrease in perinatal mortality among the ultrasound-screened group, from 9 to 4.6 per 1000.[16] This was attributed to the relatively high rate of detection of fetal anomalies in that study (58% of major malformations were detected before 24 weeks) with subsequent termination of fetuses with anomalies.

In the Routine Antenatal Diagnostic Imaging with Ultrasound (RADIUS) trial, the investigators did not find a significant difference in "adverse perinatal outcome," defined as fetal death, neonatal death, or neonatal morbidity, in the screened versus control groups. The explanation for the lack of improved outcome was the limited sensitivity of routine sonography in the detection of congenital abnormalities (16.6% before 24 weeks and 34.8% before 40 weeks) coupled with a low rate of pregnancy termination once the diagnosis had been made.[4] A subsequent meta-analysis based on four randomized clinical trials with data on 15,935 women (7992 were allocated to routine sonography vs. 7943 to selective scanning) found the perinatal mortality rate was significantly lower in patients allocated to routine scanning, again because of the early detection of fetal abnormalities that led to induced abortions.[20] The authors concluded that routine ultrasound scanning is effective and useful as a screening test for malformations.

Fetal Malformations: Diagnostic Accuracy

The incidence of major congenital abnormalities at birth in the general population is 2% to 3%, yet these abnormalities are responsible for 20% to 25% of perinatal deaths and an even higher percentage of perinatal morbidity. Prenatal detection of an anomaly increases the options for pregnancy management, and in select cases the disorder may be amenable to intrauterine treatment. For these reasons, offering routine ultrasound as a screening test for congenital abnormalities is an attractive concept. However, the performance of screening ultrasound in detecting abnormalities in the low-risk population is variable, with sensitivity and specificity ranging from 14% to 85% and 93% to over 99%, respectively.[4,19,21-27] The wide range in sensitivity can be partially explained by what authors used as the definition of an "anomaly" and the experience of the individuals performing and interpreting the studies.[19,26] Another factor is the type of anomaly. In the Eurofetus study,[28] the best detected abnormalities were of the urinary system (88.5%) and central nervous system (88.3%). Cardiac abnormalities were not well detected, whether major (38.8%) or minor (20.8%), and the lowest rates of detection were for minor abnormalities of the musculoskeletal system (18% vs. 73.6% for major defects) and cleft lip and palate (18%).[28] Another important issue is the gestational age at which the study is performed. In the Eurofetus Study, for example, 38.5% of the anomalies were diagnosed after 29 weeks' gestation. Other factors influencing sensitivity of prenatal sonography include the quality of equipment, prevalence of a particular defect, maternal body habitus, and examination protocol.[19,28,29]

Many of the benefits of ultrasound are nonquantifiable. Having time to adjust prenatally to information about an anomaly can improve both the clinician's and the parents' approach to the pregnancy and birth, as well as their abilities to make decisions about prenatal and postnatal treatment.[30] It is important for patients and their physicians to understand the limitations of ultrasound. Not all abnormalities can be detected. The accuracy of prenatal ultrasound is variable and often depends on where and by whom it is being performed.

Three- and Four-Dimensional Ultrasound

In addition to two-dimensional (2-D) images, 3-D and 4-D imaging allow for reconstructed images in planes that were not previously available. This allows for improved visualization of facial anomalies[31] and anomalies of the hands, feet, and spine.[32] In addition, 3-D images may be more comprehensible to the patient, allowing for better understanding of the abnormality.[31,32] Cervical assessment is also thought to be more complete with volume imaging.[33] **Volume imaging** can be used to assess the lungs,[34,35] which is used in fetuses with suspected pulmonary hypoplasia. Reconstructed images can be helpful to image portions of the brain.[36] Subsequent chapters integrate 3-D and 4-D images as appropriate.

Prudent Use of Ultrasound

The AIUM, ACR, and American College of Gynecologists (ACOG) collaborative guidelines state that "Fetal ultrasound should be performed only when there is a valid medical reason, and the lowest possible ultrasonic exposure settings should be used to gain the necessary diagnostic information."[6] Although there is no reliable evidence of physical harm to human fetuses from diagnostic ultrasound imaging using current technology, public health experts, clinicians, and industry representatives agree that casual use of sonography, especially during pregnancy, should be avoided. The U.S. Food and Drug Administration (FDA) views the promotion, sale, or lease of ultrasound equipment for making "keepsake" fetal videos as an unapproved use of a medical device.[37] Medically indicated obstetric imaging can easily integrate making copies of key images for parents who want an early view of their baby.

MAGNETIC RESONANCE IMAGING

Ultrasound is the screening modality of choice for fetal imaging. However, when additional information regarding fetal anatomy or pathology is needed, fast MR imaging is increasingly being used as a correlative imaging modality in select cases (Fig. 28-17). MRI is useful in these cases because it has no ionizing radiation, provides excellent soft tissue contrast, has multiple planes for reconstruction, and has a large field of view, allowing for improved depiction of many complex fetal abnormalities.

It is important to tailor the examination to answer specific questions raised either by patient history or by prior sonographic examination. In the past decade, software and hardware have allowed for fetal MR images to be obtained in about 400 milliseconds. This allows for fetal imaging to be performed without maternal or fetal sedation. The ease of performing these examinations and the superb contrast resolution afforded by T2-weighted MRI have popularized the use of this imaging tool to improve prenatal diagnosis.

There are no known biologic risks from MRI. The MR procedure is not believed to be hazardous to the fetus.[38-50] No delayed sequelae from MR examination have been encountered, and it is expected that the potential risk for any delayed sequelae is extremely small or nonexistent.

Gadolinium is the contrast typically used for MR studies, but it is not recommended for fetal examination. Gadolinium crosses the placenta and appears within the fetal bladder soon after intravenous administration. The contrast is excreted from the fetal bladder into the amniotic fluid, where it is then swallowed and potentially reabsorbed from the gastrointestinal tract. Because of this reabsorption, the half-life of gadolinium in the fetal circulation is not known.[51] This drug has been shown to have adverse effects on the fetus in animal models. **Gadopentetate dimeglumine** has been shown to impair development slightly in rats (at 2.5 times the human dose, 0.1 mmol/kg), and in rabbits (at 7.5 times the human dose).[52,53] It is considered a **pregnancy category C** drug, meaning that it should be given only if potential benefit outweighs the risk; animal studies have revealed adverse effects, but no controlled studies have been performed in humans.[52] Therefore, we do not use contrast for fetal examinations at our institution.

CONCLUSION

Ultrasound is a readily available, noninvasive, and safe means of evaluating fetal health, determining gestational age, and assessing the intrauterine environment. It is an indispensable tool for the practice of obstetrics.

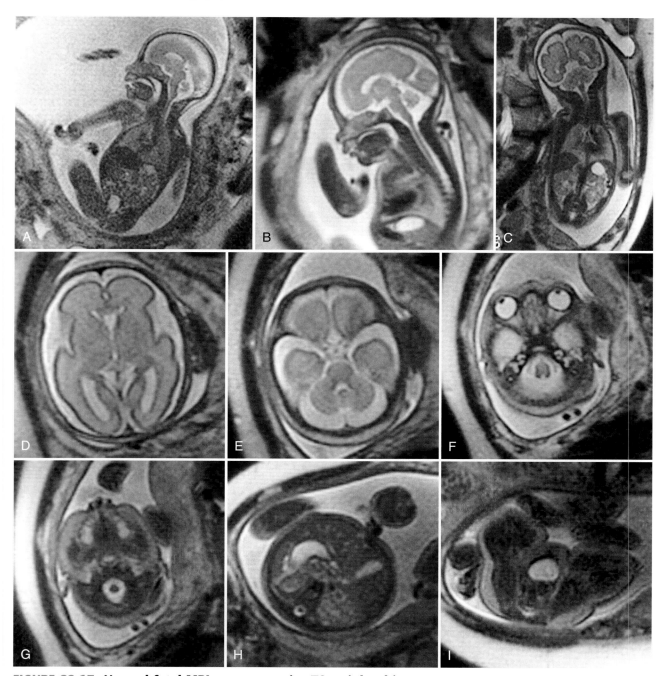

FIGURE 28-17. Normal fetal MRI: representative T2-weighted images. A, Sagittal view of fetal head with fetal body in coronal plane. **B,** Sagittal view of fetal head. Note normal appearance of corpus callosum and soft palate, with fluid outlining the soft palate above the tongue. **C,** Coronal view of the brain, chest, and abdomen. Note normal appearance to the lungs, diaphragm, stomach, and kidneys. **D,** Axial view of brain with normal-appearing lateral ventricles. **E,** Oblique axial view of brain shows normal cerebellar hemispheres and vermis. **F,** Axial view at level of globes. Note the dark lens in each globe. **G,** Axial view at level of palate. Note that majority of the alveolar tooth-bearing ridge is well depicted. **H,** Axial view at level of stomach and gallbladder. Note spinal cord outlined by fluid in thecal sac. **I,** Axial view at level of bladder.

Ultrasound is also a screening test, yielding results that must be interpreted and integrated in a knowledgeable way. As with physical examination, the ultrasound study is most helpful when performed in a consistent and reproducible fashion, carefully documenting positive and negative findings important in clinical decision making. The information gained from routine obstetric ultrasound may provide reassurance, guide therapy, or identify a pathologic condition that merits further investigation.

References

1. Centers for Disease Control and Prevention. National Vital Statistics Report: births, marriages, divorces, and deaths: provisional data for August 2008. Atlanta: CDC; 2009. p. 57.
2. Martin JA, Hamilton BE, Sutton PD, et al. Births: final data for 2002. Natl Vital Stat Rep 2003;52:1-113.

Training, Personnel, and Equipment

3. Levi S. Ultrasound in prenatal diagnosis: polemics around routine ultrasound screening for second trimester fetal malformations. Prenat Diagn 2002;22:285-295.
4. Ewigman BG, Crane JP, Frigoletto FD, et al. Effect of prenatal ultrasound screening on perinatal outcome. RADIUS Study Group. N Engl J Med 1993;329:821-827.
5. Abuhamad AZ, Benacerraf BR, Woletz P, Burke BL. The accreditation of ultrasound practices: impact on compliance with minimum performance guidelines. J Ultrasound Med 2004;23:1023-1029.

Ultrasound Guidelines

6. American College of Radiology. ACR practice guideline for the performance of antepartum obstetrical ultrasound. In: ACR practice guidelines and technical standards. Philadelphia, 2007, ACR, p. 1025-1033.
7. Benn PA, Egan JF, Fang M, Smith-Bindman R. Changes in the utilization of prenatal diagnosis. Obstet Gynecol 2004;103:1255-1260.
8. Schwarzler P, Senat MV, Holden D, et al. Feasibility of the second-trimester fetal ultrasound examination in an unselected population at 18, 20 or 22 weeks of pregnancy: a randomized trial. Ultrasound Obstet Gynecol 1999;14:92-97.
9. Filly RA. Level 1, level 2, level 3 obstetric sonography: I'll see your level and raise you one. Radiology 1989;172:312.

Routine Ultrasound Screening

10. Mongelli M, Wilcox M, Gardosi J. Estimating the date of confinement: ultrasonographic biometry versus certain menstrual dates. Am J Obstet Gynecol 1996;174:278-281.
11. Eik-Nes SH, Salvesen KA, Okland O, Vatten LJ. Routine ultrasound fetal examination in pregnancy: the "Alesund" randomized controlled trial. Ultrasound Obstet Gynecol 2000;15:473-478.
12. Bennett MJ, Little G, Dewhurst J, Chamberlain G. Predictive value of ultrasound measurement in early pregnancy: a randomized controlled trial. Br J Obstet Gynaecol 1982;89:338-341.
13. Waldenstrom U, Axelsson O, Nilsson S, et al. Effects of routine one-stage ultrasound screening in pregnancy: a randomised controlled trial. Lancet 1988;2:585-588.
14. Neilson JP. Ultrasound for fetal assessment in early pregnancy. Cochrane Database Syst Rev 1998:CD000182.
15. Hughey MJ, Olive DL. Routine ultrasound scanning for the detection and management of twin pregnancies. J Reprod Med 1985;30:427-430.
16. Saari-Kemppainen A, Karjalainen O, Ylostalo P, Heinonen OP. Ultrasound screening and perinatal mortality: controlled trial of systematic one-stage screening in pregnancy. The Helsinki Ultrasound Trial. Lancet 1990;336:387-391.
17. Bakketeig LS, Eik-Nes SH, Jacobsen G, et al. Randomised controlled trial of ultrasonographic screening in pregnancy. Lancet 1984;2:207-211.
18. Blondel B, Ringa V, Breart G. The use of ultrasound examinations, intrapartum fetal heart rate monitoring and beta-mimetic drugs in France. Br J Obstet Gynaecol 1989;96:44-51.
19. Levi S, Hyjazi Y, Schaapst JP, et al. Sensitivity and specificity of routine antenatal screening for congenital anomalies by ultrasound: the Belgian Multicentric Study. Ultrasound Obstet Gynecol 1991;1:102-110.
20. Bucher HC, Schmidt JG. Does routine ultrasound scanning improve outcome in pregnancy? Meta-analysis of various outcome measures. BMJ 1993;307:13-17.
21. Lys F, De Wals P, Borlee-Grimee I, et al. Evaluation of routine ultrasound examination for the prenatal diagnosis of malformation. Eur J Obstet Gynecol Reprod Biol 1989;30:101-109.
22. Rosendahl H, Kivenen S. Antenatal detection of congenital malformations by routine ultrasonography. Obstet Gynecol 1989;73:947-951.

23. Shirley IM, Bottomley F, Robinson VP. Routine radiographer screening for fetal abnormalities by ultrasound in an unselected low-risk population. Br J Radiol 1992;65:564-569.
24. Luck CA. Value of routine ultrasound scanning at 19 weeks: a four-year study of 8849 deliveries. BMJ 1992;304:1474-1478.
25. Chitty LS, Hunt GH, Moore J, Lobb MO. Effectiveness of routine ultrasonography in detecting fetal structural abnormalities in a low-risk population. BMJ 1991;303:1165-1169.
26. Levi S, Montenegro NA. Eurofetus: an evaluation of routine ultrasound screening for the detection of fetal defects—aims and method. Ann NY Acad Sci 1998;847:103-117.
27. Fadda GM, Capobianco G, Balata A, et al. Routine second trimester ultrasound screening for prenatal detection of fetal malformations in Sassari University Hospital, Italy: 23 years of experience in 42,256 pregnancies. Eur J Obstet Gynecol Reprod Biol 2009;144:110-114.
28. Grandjean H, Larroque D, Levi S. The performance of routine ultrasonographic screening of pregnancies in the Eurofetus Study. Am J Obstet Gynecol 1999;181:446-454.
29. Crane JP, LeFevre ML, Winborn RC, et al. A randomized trial of prenatal ultrasonographic screening: impact on the detection, management, and outcome of anomalous fetuses. The RADIUS Study Group. Am J Obstet Gynecol 1994;171:392-399.
30. Berwick DM, Weinstein MC. What do patients value? Willingness to pay for ultrasound in normal pregnancy. Med Care 1985;23:881-893.
31. Johnson DD, Pretorius DH, Budorick NE, et al. Fetal lip and primary palate: three-dimensional versus two-dimensional ultrasound. Radiology 2000;217:236-239.
32. Dyson RL, Pretorius DH, Budorick NE, et al. Three-dimensional ultrasound in the evaluation of fetal anomalies. Ultrasound Obstet Gynecol 2000;16:321-328.
33. Bega G, Lev-Toaff A, Kuhlman K, et al. Three-dimensional multiplanar transvaginal ultrasound of the cervix in pregnancy. Ultrasound Obstet Gynecol 2000;16:351-358.
34. Gerards FA, Engels MA, Twisk JW, van Vugt JM. Normal fetal lung volume measured with three-dimensional ultrasound. Ultrasound Obstet Gynecol 2006;27:134-144.
35. Jani J, Cannie M, Sonigo P, et al. Value of prenatal magnetic resonance imaging in the prediction of postnatal outcome in fetuses with diaphragmatic hernia. Ultrasound Obstet Gynecol 2008;32:793-799.
36. Zalel Y, Yagel S, Achiron R, et al. Three-dimensional ultrasonography of the fetal vermis at 18 to 26 weeks' gestation: time of appearance of the primary fissure. J Ultrasound Med 2009;28:1-8.
37. US Food and Drug Administration. Fetal keepsake videos. Washington, DC, 2005, FDA.

Magnetic Resonance Imaging

38. Wolff S, Crooks LE, Brown P, et al. Tests for DNA and chromosomal damage induced by nuclear magnetic resonance imaging. Radiology 1980;136:707-710.
39. Kanal E, Gillen J, Evans JA, et al. Survey of reproductive health among female MR workers. Radiology 1993;187:395-399.
40. Baker PN, Johnson IR, Harvey PR, et al. A three-year follow-up of children imaged in utero with echo-planar magnetic resonance. Am J Obstet Gynecol 1994;170:32-33.
41. Chew S, Ahmadi A, Goh PS, Foong LC. The effects of 1.5T magnetic resonance imaging on early murine in-vitro embryo development. J Magn Reson Imaging 2001;13:417-420.
42. Clements H, Duncan KR, Fielding K, et al. Infants exposed to MRI in utero have a normal paediatric assessment at 9 months of age. Br J Radiol 2000;73:190-194.
43. Glover P, Hykin J, Gowland P, et al. An assessment of the intrauterine sound intensity level during obstetric echo-planar magnetic resonance imaging. Br J Radiol 1995;68:1090-1094.
44. Kok RD, de Vries MM, Heerschap A, van den Berg PP. Absence of harmful effects of magnetic resonance exposure at 1.5 T in utero during the third trimester of pregnancy: a follow-up study. Magn Reson Imaging 2004;22:851-854.
45. Levine D, Zuo C, Faro CB, Chen Q. Potential heating effect in the gravid uterus during MR HASTE imaging. J Magn Reson Imaging 2001;13:856-861.
46. Merkle EM, Dale BM, Paulson EK. Abdominal MR imaging at 3T. Magn Reson Imaging Clin N Am 2006;14:17-26.

47. Myers C, Duncan KR, Gowland PA, et al. Failure to detect intrauterine growth restriction following in utero exposure to MRI. Br J Radiol 1998;71:549-551.

48. Schwartz JL, Crooks LE. NMR imaging produces no observable mutations or cytotoxicity in mammalian cells. AJR Am J Roentgenol 1982;139:583-585.

49. Shellock FG, Crues JV. MR procedures: biologic effects, safety, and patient care. Radiology 2004;232:635-652.

50. US Food and Drug Administration. Guidance for content and review of a magnetic resonance diagnostic device 510 (k) application. Washington, DC: FDA; 1988.

51. Shellock FG, Kanal E. Bioeffects and safety of MR procedures. In: Edelman RR, Hesselink JR, Zlatkin MB, editors. Clinical magnetic resonance imaging. 2nd ed. Philadelphia: Saunders; 1996. p. 429.

52. Magnevist product information. Wayne, NJ: Berlex Laboratories; 1994.

53. Runge VM. Safety of approved MR contrast media for intravenous injection. J Magn Reson Imaging 2000;12:205-213.

CHAPTER 29

Bioeffects and Safety of Ultrasound in Obstetrics

Jacques S. Abramowicz

Chapter Outline

*H*alf a century of extensive use in clinical obstetric and radiologic practice has shown that ultrasound does not cause major abnormalities in the fetus. Ultrasound is a form of energy, however, and one must consider whether subtle effects are possible when such energy penetrates living tissues. Although some effects have been described in animals, no immediate human correlation can be made. Conversely, "no effects detected so far" does not necessarily means "no effect." Only large, epidemiologic studies can solve this problem. In the United States, most women who receive prenatal care are referred for at least one ultrasound scan; in many other countries, almost 100% of these women are exposed to ultrasound. Multiple examinations are often performed, with or without clear indication. Because of this near-universal exposure of pregnant women and their unborn child to ultrasound, the issues of possible effects and safety need to be addressed.[1]

Whether short-term or long-term adverse bioeffects to the fetus may result from exposure to ultrasound is a major issue. It is well established that under certain conditions, ultrasound can have undesirable side effects.[2-25] Two conflicting points need clarification: (1) to date, no evidence has been found of harmful effects of ultrasound in humans at clinical exposure levels, but (2) all available published epidemiologic data are from before 1992. Since then, acoustic output of diagnostic systems for fetal use was increased by a factor of almost 8, from 94 mW/cm^2 to 720 mW/cm^2, and, in reality, a factor of 16 (from 46 mW/cm^2) based on earlier regulations.[26] Additional concerns follow:

- An increasing number of fetuses in the first trimester, a time of maximal susceptibility to external insults, are exposed to ultrasound, particularly spectral Doppler.[27]
- "Entertainment" ultrasound, scanning to obtain pictures or videos of the fetus (fetal "keepsake" video) without a medical indication has burgeoned[28] despite calls for avoidance of unnecessary exposure.[29-31]
- Clinical users of obstetric ultrasound appear to have limited knowledge and awareness of bioeffects and safety.[32]

Thus the main goals of this chapter are as follows:
1. Summarize the literature on bioeffects in experimental settings as well as the available knowledge on bioeffects in the human fetus.
2. Analyze changes that occurred over time in energy levels of ultrasound machines and the regulations involved.
3. Describe how manipulation of many instrument controls alters acoustic energy and thus exposure.
4. Educate sonographers and physicians on how best to minimize fetal exposure without sacrificing diagnostic quality.

INSTRUMENT OUTPUTS

Over the years, output of ultrasound instruments has increased.[33] Furthermore, many machine controls can alter the output. For example, keeping in mind that the degree of temperature elevation is proportional to the product of the amplitude of the sound wave times the pulse length and the pulse repetition frequency, it

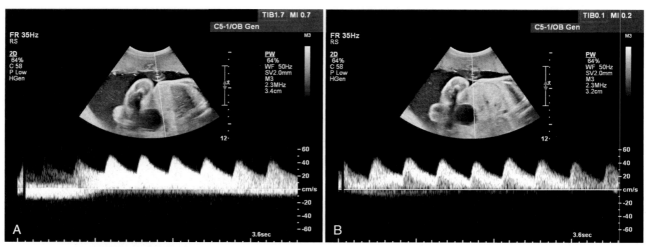

FIGURE 29-1. Effect of changing power setting on thermal index of bone (TIB) during spectral Doppler velocity measurements of umbilical artery. A, The output power is high, and the thermal index (TI) is 1.7 (see highlighted gray box, upper right). **B,** The power has been lowered; the TI is now 0.1, and the tracing is still diagnostic.

becomes immediately evident why any change (augmentation) in these characteristics can add to the risk of elevating the temperature, a potential mechanism for bioeffects. Three important parameters under end-user control are the (1) scanning/operating mode (including transducer choice), (2) system setup and output control, and (3) dwell time.

Scanning Mode

When comparing modes, the spatial peak, temporal average intensity (I_{SPTA}) increases from B-mode (34 mW/cm^2, average) to M-mode to color Doppler to spectral Doppler (1180 mW/cm^2, average).[34] Average I_{SPTA} values are 1 W/cm^2 in Doppler mode but can reach 10 W/cm^2. Caution is therefore recommended when applying this mode. Color Doppler has higher intensities than B-mode but is still much lower than spectral Doppler, mainly because of the mode of operation: sequences of pulses, scanned through the area of interest ("box"). High pulse repetition frequencies (PRFs) are used in pulsed Doppler techniques, generating greater temporal average intensities and power than B-mode or M-mode and thus greater heating potential. Also, because the beam needs to be held in relatively constant position over the vessel of interest in spectral Doppler ultrasound, temporal average intensity may further increase. This is particularly concerning in first-trimester applications. In addition, **transducer choice** is important because it will determine: frequency, penetration, resolution, and field of view.

System Setup

Starting or **default output power** is another important ultrasound parameter. Some manufacturers "boot" their

machines with high power, which supposedly produces a better image, and the sonographer must act to decrease that power. Other systems boot up with low power and, only if judged necessary, the sonographer will increase that power. In Figure 29-1, for example, the Doppler signal in *A* was obtained with a high power, whereas in *B* the power was greatly reduced, and the image is still diagnostic. Also, the examiner fine-tunes to optimize the image, influencing output but with no visible effect, except to change **thermal index** (TI) and **mechanical index** (MI), as discussed in Chapter 2.

Controls that regulate output include **focal depth**, usually with greatest power at deeper focus but occasionally with highest power in the near field; **increasing frame rate;** and **limiting the field of view,** as by high-resolution magnification or certain zooms. In Doppler mode, changing **sample volume** and **velocity range** (to optimize received signals) will change output. In Figure 29-2, only the size of the color box is smaller, which caused increased TI on the output. It should be remembered that **receiver gain** often has similar effects as these controls on the recorded image, but no effect on the output of the outgoing beam, and therefore it is completely safe to manipulate.

Dwell Time

Dwell time is the **actual scanning time** and thus directly under control of the examiner. Dwell time is not taken into account in the calculation of the safety indices and generally is not reported in clinical or experimental studies. However, it takes only one pulse to induce cavitation, and about a minute to raise temperature to its peak. Directly correlated with dwell time is **examiner experience:** knowledge of anatomy, bioeffects, instrument controls, and scanning techniques.

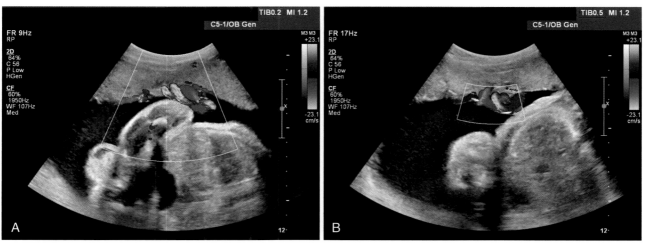

FIGURE 29-2. Effect of changing size of color box on thermal index of bone (TIB) during color Doppler examination of umbilical cord. Changing the size of the box from large (**A**) small (**B**) changes the TI *(red squared number at top right)* from 0.2 to 0.5.

THERMAL EFFECTS

Thermal changes induced by ultrasound have been demonstrated in various animals, with hyperthermia clearly shown to be teratologic to many species.[35-44] Elevated maternal temperature, whether from illness or exposure to heat, can produce teratogenic effects.[17,38,40-43,45-58] A rise less than 2° C is thought to be safe,[59] although any temperature increase for any amount of time may have some effect,[48,60] and a rise of 2.5° C may be considered significant.[61] A major question is whether diagnostic ultrasound can induce a rise in temperature in the fetus that could reach dangerous levels.[19,59,62] Temperature elevation in the human fetus cannot be exactly measured but can be estimated fairly accurately.[63,64] For prolonged ultrasound exposures, temperature elevations of up to 5° C have been obtained.[59] Thus, *any* temperature increment for *any* period of time has *some* effect; the higher the temperature differential or the longer the temperature increment, the greater is the likelihood of producing an effect. Although these assumptions cannot be demonstrated in diagnostic ultrasound and no human data exist, clinicians should keep these facts in mind when performing obstetric ultrasound. This also forms part of the argument against nonmedical or nonindicated ultrasound examinations.

As with any external influence on the pregnancy, **gestational age** is a vital factor. **Milder** (in time or intensity) exposures during the preimplantation period (very early gestational age) could have similar or worse consequences than **more severe** exposures during embryonic and fetal development and could result in fetal demise and abortion or structural and functional defects. Such a dose analysis is not available. As for many other **terato-gens**, the central nervous system (CNS) is most at risk because of a lack of compensatory growth by undamaged neuroblasts. In experimental animals the most common defects associated with temperature increase are of the neural tube (**anencephaly, microencephaly**) and the eyes (**microphthalmia, cataract**). Associated with CNS defects are functional and behavioral problems.[46] Other organ defects secondary to hyperthermia include defects of craniofacial development(e.g., clefts[65]) and anomalies of the axial and appendicular skeleton,[66] the body wall, teeth, and heart.[67]

Gestational age is critical when considering heat dispersion. In midterm, there was no significant difference when guinea pig fetal brains were exposed, alive (perfused) or postmortem (non-perfused), in the focal region of the ultrasound beam. However, a significant cooling effect of vascular perfusion was observed when the fetuses reached the stage of late gestation near term, when the cerebral vessels were well developed.[68] In early human pregnancy, less than 6 weeks, the minimal fetal perfusion may reduce heat dispersion.[69] The increased sensitivity of Doppler devices suggests evidence of blood flow within embryonic vesicles after heart formation, with the simultaneous development of a uterine circulatory pathway in the developing placenta. The flow is often termed "nonpulsatile" or "percolating"[70,71] with near-minimal Doppler-measured velocities, as opposed to later in pregnancy. At about week 12 of gestation, the plugs of the spiral arteries are "loosened" and allow for freer blood circulation.[72,73]

Thus, perfusion status is far from approaching that for normal tissue levels (as assumed in the TI algorithm) for much of the first trimester. Only later, when "free circulation" is established (about week 11-12 of gestation), does the tissue become normally perfused, when the embryonic circulation actually links up with the maternal circulation.[73] This absence of perfusion may result in underestimation of the actual ultrasound-induced temperature in early gestation. This warrants extreme caution in first-trimester scanning, particularly with the recent increase in utilization of Doppler in the first trimester.[74-77]

Also, the issue of **transducer heating** may be particularly relevant in the first trimester, if performing endovaginal scanning.[76,78] A mitigating factor is motion (even very small) of the examiner's hand, as well as the patient's breathing and body movements (in obstetric ultrasound, both mother and fetus), which tend to spread the region being heated. However, for spectral (pulsed) Doppler studies, it is necessary to have the transducer as steady as possible. Because the intensity and acoustic power associated with Doppler ultrasound are the highest of all the general-use categories, time spent scanning with Doppler ultrasound mode is crucial. Ziskin[79] reported that average duration of 15,973 Doppler ultrasound examinations was 27 minutes (longest, 4 hours!). It is clear that temperature increases of 1° C are easily reached in routine scanning.[80] Elevation of up to 1.5° C were obtained in the first trimester and up to 4° C in the second and third trimesters, particularly with the use of pulsed Doppler.[81] In many clinical machines, TI values of 5 or 6 can be obtained in Doppler mode.

MECHANICAL EFFECTS

Although effects have been described in neonates or adult animals, because gas bubbles are not present in fetal lung or bowel, it is assumed that the risk from mechanical effect secondary to cavitation is minimal.[10] Several other mechanical effects do not appear to involve cavitation, such as **tactile sensation** of the ultrasound wave, **auditory response, cell aggregation,** and **cell membrane alteration. Hemolysis** has also been reported,[82] although some cavitation nuclei must be present for hemolysis to occur. Such microbubbles would be provided by the introduction of ultrasound **contrast agents** to the area under ultrasound examination. However, there is currently no clear clinical indication for the use of these agents in fetal ultrasound.[83,84] In addition, fetal stimulation caused by pulsed ultrasound insonation has been described, with no apparent relation to cavitation.[85] This effect may be secondary to radiation forces associated with ultrasound exposures. No harmful effects of diagnostic ultrasound secondary to nonthermal mechanisms have been reported in human fetuses. However, because of these known mechanical effects of ultrasound in living tissues, and because pressures in Doppler propagation are much higher than in B-mode, further caution is recommended in the use of ultrasound, particularly in the first trimester.[86]

BIOEFFECTS OF ULTRASOUND

Animal Research

Multiple studies have shown effects of ultrasound in a wide variety of species.[87-90] Studies of gross effects on the brain and liver of cats showed well-defined lesions and demyelination in the brain[91] and tissue damage in the liver[92] resulting from ultrasound exposure of a few seconds at 1 and 3 MHz, respectively. Other observed effects include limb paralysis, as a result of spinal cord injury in the rat,[93,94] as well as lesions in the liver, kidney, and testes of rabbits.[95] Changes in fertility were demonstrated in male mice after in utero ultrasound exposure of the testes.[96] Although some effects are likely caused by mechanical processes, very high temperature elevations (much higher than with diagnostic ultrasound) may be more directly involved with the tissue damage. It took acoustic pressures generated by lithotripsy to obtain effects in muscles,[97] as well as hemorrhage in bowel[98] and lungs.[99] These intensities are much higher than in diagnostic ultrasound but are helpful in understanding the mechanisms involved with possible bioeffects of ultrasound.

Several major clinical end points for bioeffects in animals that could have direct relevance to human studies include fetal growth and birth weight, effects on brain and CNS function, and change in hematologic function. High-level exposures were associated with decreased body weight at birth in exposed monkeys compared with controls, but all showed catch-up growth when examined at 3 months of age.[100] Decreased birth weight after prenatal exposure to ultrasound has also been reported in mice,[101,102] but not convincingly in rats.[103] Clear species differences therefore seem to exist,[104] making it difficult to extrapolate to the human. In a report of 30 pregnancies in monkeys, half were exposed to ultrasound.[100] The scanned fetuses had lower birth weights and were shorter than the control group. No significant differences were noted in rate of abortions, major malformations, or stillbirths. Moreover, all showed catch-up growth when examined at 3 months of age. In-situ intensities were higher than routinely used in clinical obstetric imaging in the human. Studies in mice have shown increased mortality, and decreased body weight after in utero exposure to diagnostic ultrasound.[105,106] Gross lesions have been described in the central nervous system[107] and the spine[94] in mammals.

Neurologic or behavioral findings may be sensitive markers of teratogenic effect.[87,108] Pregnant Swiss albino mice were exposed to diagnostic ultrasound for 10, 20, or 30 minutes on day 14.5 (fetal period) of gestation and compared with sham-exposed controls.[109] Significant behavioral alterations in the exposed groups included decreased locomotor and exploratory activity and more trials needed for learning. No changes were observed in physiologic reflexes or postnatal survival. The authors concluded that ultrasound exposure during the early fetal period can impair brain function in the adult mouse.[109] In another study, the same authors found increased anxiolytic activity and learning latency in ultrasound-treated animals.[110] Pregnant Swiss albino mice were exposed to similar diagnostic levels of ultrasound for 10 minutes on days 11.5 or 14.5. Behavioral tests at 3 and 6 months postpartum showed more pronounced effects in the 14.5-day than in the 11.5-day group. The authors concluded that exposure to diagnostic ultrasound during the late organogenesis period or early fetal period in mice may cause changes in postnatal behavior.[110]

A very intriguing paper was published on memory changes in chicks after being insonated in ovo with various levels of Doppler ultrasound.[111] Exposure was to 5 or 10 minutes of B-mode, or to 1, 2, 3, 4, or 5 minutes of pulsed Doppler ultrasound. Two hours after hatching, chicks were trained to recognize certain colors in relation to some feeding procedures. B-mode exposure on day 19 (of a 21-day gestation) did not affect memory. However, significant memory impairment occurred after 4 and 5 minutes of pulsed Doppler exposure, as expressed by the inability to discern the colors. Short-, intermediate- and long-term memory was equally impaired, suggesting an inability to learn. The chicks were still unable to learn with a second training session. While there are major differences in terms of length of gestation, amount of "energy received," and other technical issues when compared with human fetal exposure, these findings raise important questions on the potential effect of pulsed Doppler ultrasound in utero exposure on cognitive function.

As mentioned previously, ultrasound induces thermal changes in various animals, and hyperthermia clearly is teratogenic to many species.[35-44,68] In guinea pigs, mean temperature increases of 4.9° C close to parietal bone and 1.2° C in the midbrain were recorded after 2-minute ultrasound exposures, although at exposure conditions higher than usually employed in clinical examinations.[68] After only 2 minutes of insonation with an ISPTA of 2.9 W/cm^2 (about four times higher than the current FDA allowance for diagnostic use), mean maximum temperature increases varied from 1.2° C at 30 days to 5.2° C at 60 days. Importantly, 80% of the mean maximum temperature increase occurred within 40 seconds. This rapid rate of heating is relevant to the safety of clinical examinations in which the dwell time may be an important factor. Because maximal ultrasound-induced temperature increase occurs in the fetal brain near bone, worst-case heating will occur later in pregnancy, when the ultrasound beam impinges on bone, and less will occur earlier in pregnancy, when bone is less mineralized. This is one of the justifications to utilize **thermal index for bone** (TIB) late in pregnancy and **thermal index for soft tissue** (TIS) earlier.

In 2006, Ang et al.[112] evaluated the effect of ultrasound insonation in pregnant mice on neuronal position within the embryonic cerebral cortex of the fetuses. Neurons generated at embryonic day 16 that normally migrate to the superficial cortical layers were chemically labeled. A small but statistically significant number of neurons remained scattered within inappropriate cortical layers and in the subjacent white matter, failing to acquire their proper position when exposed to ultrasound for a total of 30 minutes or longer during their migration. However, several major differences exist between this experimental setup and clinical ultrasound in humans,[113] most notably the length of exposure (up to 7 hours). No real mechanistic explanation was given for the findings, there was no real dose-response effect, and scans were performed over a short period of several days. The experimental setup was such that embryos received whole-brain exposure to the beam, which is rare in humans (although possible very early in pregnancy), and the small brains of mice develop over days. Thus, although the study merits repeating, the applicability to human embryology is questionable.[113]

These animal studies suggest precaution with obstetric ultrasound. However, the animal studies to date do not implicate ultrasound used at daily clinical exposure levels with major adverse fetal effects.

Human Studies

Several epidemiologic studies on obstetric ultrasound exposure have been published,[21,51,114-117] although some have serious limitations, such as lack of a testable hypothesis for causation of the studied effect, small samples, poorly matched controls, and most often, lack of information on acoustic output and exact quantification of exposure (number of episodes, duration of exposure, and inability to calculate "dose"). These limitations are a major problem when analyzing published data,[118] particularly with new imaging modalities that have potentially high energy levels and new applications of existing modalities. Typical examples are spectral Doppler ultrasound analysis of the tricuspid artery at 11 to 14 weeks' gestation in screening for Down syndrome[27] and studies of the fetal heart anatomy and function during the first trimester.[75,119-122] There is no epidemiologic or other information on levels of exposure or possible effects at these early, particularly susceptible gestational ages. Several "epidemiologic" reports are actually case-control studies and require caution in interpretation. The effects being studied (e.g., low estimated fetal weight) may be the same as the clinical indication for performing the ultrasound examination ("suspected intrauterine growth delay"). Thus an association may exist between the ultrasound and the growth delay, but not a causal relationship.

A further crucial confounding factor is that major congenital anomalies occur in 3% to 5% of the general human population. An increment of 1% to 2% over this "background" incidence would be a major clinical effect but might go undetected as an individual finding in routine clinical practice, and would be detectable only after prolonged observation in large populations. Also, some underreporting occurs; for example, a certain number of birth defects is expected in any ultrasound study in relatively large (>1000) populations. Often, however, these studies describe no anomalies in the study group or in the control population; in a survey of more than 121,000 patients among 68 examiners, combining 292 institute-years of experience, 3000 to 5000 anomalies would be expected as background rate, but none were reported.[123]

In fact, rigorous epidemiologic studies of the adverse bioeffects of ultrasound are scarce. Several biologic end points have been analyzed in the human fetus or neonate to determine whether prenatal exposure to diagnostic ultrasound had observable effects: intrauterine growth restriction (IUGR) and low birth weight,[124] delayed speech,[125] vision and hearing,[126] dyslexia,[127] neurologic and mental development or behavioral issues,[128,129] malignancies,[130] and non-right-handedness.[131,132] Most findings have never been duplicated, and the majority of studies have been negative for any association, with the possible exception of low birth weight.

There are no epidemiologic studies related to the output display standard (thermal and mechanical indices) and clinical outcomes. Only a few clinical studies describe routine scan,[133] first-trimester scan,[134] particularly, **nuchal translucency** screening,[135] as well as Doppler[136] and 3-D/4-D ultrasound.[137] Furthermore, although some studies address the issue of repeat scans,[138,139] it was not as an analysis of potential cumulative effects for which no information is available.

Birth Weight

In one often-quoted study in of more than 2000 infants, a small (116 grams at term) but statistically significant lower mean birth weight was found in the half exposed to ultrasound compared with the nonexposed group.[140] However, information was collected several years after exposure, with no indications known and no exposure information available. Moreover, in a later study, the authors concluded that the relationship of ultrasound exposure to reduced birth weight may be caused by **shared common risk factors,** which lead to both exposure and a reduction in birth weight,[141] an association but not a causal relationship.

A twice-greater risk of low birth weight was reported in another retrospective study after four or more exposures to diagnostic ultrasound.[21] These results were not reproduced in another retrospective study with a large population, originally of 10,000 pregnancies exposed to ultrasound matched with 500 controls and with 6-year follow-up.[142] No increased congenital malformations, chromosomal abnormalities, infant neoplasms, speech or hearing impairment, or developmental problems were observed in this latter study.

In a randomized controlled trial of more than 2800 pregnant women, about half received five ultrasound imaging and Doppler flow studies at 18, 24, 28, 34, and 38 weeks of gestation, and half received a single ultrasound imaging at 18 weeks.[143] An increased risk of IUGR was detected in those exposed to frequent Doppler ultrasound examinations, possibly through effects on bone growth. However, when children were examined at 1 year of age, there were no differences between the study and control groups. In addition, after examining their original subjects after 8 years, the investigators found no evidence of adverse neurologic outcome.[139] Similarly, other randomized studies found no harmful effect of one or two prenatal scans on growth.[144,145] Curiously, in some studies, birth weight was slightly higher in the scanned group, but not significantly, except in one group of newborns exposed to ultrasound in utero who weighed on average 42 g (75 g in reported smokers) more than the control group.[145]

Although extensively analyzed, ultrasound exposure in utero does not appear to be associated with reduced birth weight, although Doppler ultrasound exposure may have some risks.[116]

Delayed Speech

To determine if an association exists between prenatal ultrasound exposure and delayed speech in children, Campbell et al.[125] studied 72 children with delayed speech and found a higher rate of ultrasound exposure in utero than the 144 control subjects. However, this retrospective study used records more than 5 years old, with neither a dose-response effect nor any relationship to time of exposure. A much larger study of more than 1100 children exposed in utero and 1000 controls found no significant differences in delayed speech, limited vocabulary, or stuttering.[146]

Dyslexia

Dyslexia has been extensively studied. Stark et al.[127] compared more than 4000 children (ages 7-12 years) exposed to ultrasound in utero to matched controls, analyzing outcome measures **at birth** (Apgar scores, gestational age, head circumference, birth weight, length, congenital abnormalities, neonatal/congenital infection) or **in early infancy** (hearing, visual acuity/color vision, cognitive function, behavior). No significant differences were found, except for a significantly greater proportion of dyslexia in children exposed to ultrasound. Given the design of the study and the presence of several possible confounding factors, the authors indicated that dyslexia could be incidental.

Subsequently, long-term follow-up studies of more than 600 children with various tests for dyslexia (e.g., spelling, reading) were performed.[147-151] End points included evaluation for dyslexia along with examination of non-right-handedness, said to be associated with dyslexia. No statistically significant differences were found between ultrasound-exposed children and controls for reading, spelling, arithmetic, or overall performance, as reported by teachers. Specific dyslexia tests showed similar incidence rates among scanned children and controls in reading, spelling, and intelligence scores and no discrepancy between intelligence and reading or spelling. Therefore the original finding of dyslexia was not confirmed in subsequent randomized controlled trials.

It is considered unlikely that routine ultrasound screening can cause dyslexia.

Non-Right-Handedness

A possible link between prenatal exposure to ultrasound and subsequent non-right-handedness at age 8 to 9 years in children exposed to ultrasound in utero was first reported in 1993 from Norway.[150] According to the authors, however, the difference was "only barely significant at the 5% level" and was restricted to boys.[152] A second group of researchers (including Salvesen, main author of the first study), studying a new population of over 3000 children from Sweden, reported similar findings of a statistically significant association between ultrasound exposure in utero and non-right-handedness in males.[131] Evidence is insufficient to infer a direct effect on brain structure or function, or even that non-right-handedness is an adverse effect.

Neurologic Development and Behavioral Issues

Neurons of the cerebral neocortex in mammals, including humans, are generated during fetal life in the brain proliferative zones and then migrate to their final destination by following an inside-to-outside sequence. This neuronal migration occurs in the human fetal brain mainly from 6 to 11 weeks of gestation,[153] but continue until 32 weeks. It has long been thought that external factors such as ultrasound may theoretically affect this process.[154] In another study, only two of 123 variables were found to be disturbed at birth, but not at 1 year of age, in children exposed in utero: **grasp reflex** and **tonic neck reflex.**[155] The significance was not elaborated, and some doubts exist regarding statistical validity. In a paper previously mentioned,[127] vision and intelligence scores were identical among 425 exposed infants and 381 controls. A large report found no association between routine exposure to prenatal ultrasound and school performance (deficits in attention, motor control, perception, vision, and hearing).[156] In more than 4900 children age 15 to 16 years, no differences were found in school performance between exposed and nonexposed children, except for a lower score for exposed boys in physical education.[157]

Behavioral changes may be a more sensitive marker of subtle brain damage than obvious structural alterations.[158] Such changes have been described in animals,[87,108] although often transient.[100] No changes have been reported in humans. In particular, schizophrenia and other psychoses have not been found to be associated with prenatal ultrasound exposure.[159]

Congenital Malformations

In humans, prenatal ultrasound has not been shown to result in an increased incidence of congenital anomalies, as found in animals.

Childhood Malignancies

No association has been found between ultrasound exposure in utero and the later development of leukemia[160,161] or solid tumors in children.[130,162-166]

Again, although some of these studies were published in 2007 or 2008, the populations studied were exposed to ultrasound in utero 20 to 30 years ago, that is, with instruments generating lower outputs and with minimal or no information available on exposure conditions.

SAFETY GUIDELINES

It is difficult to issue precise safety recommendations because of the multitude of ultrasound instruments, each with a selection of transducers and used in a variety of applications. Patient characteristics further complicate the task.[167] An easy way to reduce exposure is to reduce the thermal and mechanical indices (TI, MI), using the appropriate controls, and/or reduce the dwell time. The 1999 statement of the British Medical Ultrasound Society (BMUS), reconfirmed in 2009, declares[168]:

> For equipment for which the safety indices are displayed over their full range of values, the TI should always be less than 0.5 and the MI should always be less than 0.3. When the safety indices are not displayed, T_{max} should be less than 1° C and MI_{max} should be less than 0.3. Frequent exposure of the same subject is to be avoided.

The BMUS has strict recommendations for maximum allowed exposure time (T_{max}), depending on the TI (Table 29-1). Interested readers are strongly encouraged to go to the BMUS website for more detailed recommendations in obstetric and other ultrasound.[169] Miller and Ziskin[59] demonstrated a logarithmic relationship between exposure duration and temperature elevation in producing harmful bioeffects in animal fetuses. For temperatures below 43° C, the exposure time necessary for every 1° C increase in temperature was decreased by a factor of 4. Using a maximum "safe" exposure time of 4 minutes for a temperature elevation of 4° C, based on these calculations, the following maximal exposure times are allowable with no obvious risks: 4 minutes at 4° C, 16 at 3° C, 64 at 2° C and 128 at 1° C. General recommendations from major organizations follow:

1. A diagnostic ultrasound exposure that produces a maximum in situ temperature rise of no more than 1.5° C above normal physiologic levels (37° C) may be used clinically without reservation on thermal grounds.[170]

2. A diagnostic ultrasound exposure that elevates embryonic and fetal in situ temperature above

TABLE 29-1. DURATION OF OBSTETRIC ULTRASOUND AS A FUNCTION OF THERMAL INDEX

THERMAL INDEX (TI)	RECOMMENDED UPPER LIMIT
0.7	60 minutes
1	30 minutes
1.5	15 minutes
2	4 minutes
2.5	1 minute

Modified from British Medical Ultrasound Society. Guidelines for the safe use of diagnostic ultrasound equipment. 2000, reconfirmed 2009. http://www.bmus.org/ultras-safety/us-safety04.asp.

41° C (4° C above normal temperature) for 5 minutes or more should be considered potentially hazardous.[170,171] In this regard, maternal temperature elevation (e.g., from viral disease) should be considered because body temperature of the fetus will also be increased above normal.[50]

3. The risk of adverse effects is increased with the duration of exposure (dwell time).[172]
4. Based on available information, there is no reason to withhold scanning in B-mode for medical indications. The risk of thermal damage secondary to heating appears to be negligible.[170]
5. M-mode ultrasound appears to be safe and not to cause thermal damage.[50]
6. Spectral Doppler ultrasound may produce high intensities, and routine Doppler examination during the embryonic period is rarely indicated.[173]
7. Education of ultrasound operators is crucial; the responsibility for the safe use of ultrasound devices is shared between the users and the manufacturers, who should ensure the accuracy of the output display.[173]
8. The American Institute of Ultrasound in Medicine (AIUM) advocates the responsible use of diagnostic ultrasound and strongly discourages the nonmedical use of ultrasound for "entertainment" purposes. The use of ultrasound without a medical indication to view the fetus, obtain a picture of the fetus, or determine the fetal gender is inappropriate and contrary to responsible medical practice. Ultrasound should be used by qualified health professionals to provide medical benefit to the patient.[29]
9. Examinations should be kept as short as possible and with as low MI and TI outputs as possible, but without sacrificing diagnostic accuracy. Follow the **as low as reasonably achievable** (ALARA) principle.[174]

CONCLUSION

Diagnostic ultrasound has been used in medicine in general and obstetrics and gynecology in particular for more than half a century. No confirmed biological effects have been described in patients as a result of exposure to diagnostic ultrasound. However, such effects have been described in animals, often at exposure levels higher than, but also occasionally equivalent to, those used in clinical practice. Epidemiologic information available is from studies performed on instruments with acoustic output much lower than current machines. Often, exposure data are insufficient and number of subjects too small. Furthermore, "no reported effects" does not mean "no effects," and such biologic effects may be identified in the future. Prudent use of ultrasound in fetal scanning, following the ALARA principle, is therefore recommended. Based on known mechanisms, there is no contraindication to the use of B-mode, M-mode, 3-D/4-D, and color Doppler ultrasound, when clinically indicated. However, special precaution is necessary when applying pulsed Doppler ultrasound, particularly in the first trimester.

References

1. Donald I. The safety of using sonar. Dev Med Child Neurol 1974;16:90-92.
2. Hellman LM, Duffus GM, Donald I, Sunden B. Safety of diagnostic ultrasound in obstetrics. Lancet 1970;1:1133-1134.
3. Dewhurst CJ. The safety of ultrasound. Proc R Soc Med 1971; 64:996-997.
4. Nyborg WL. Safety of ultrasound diagnosis. Science 1974;186: 1074.
5. Lele PP. Safety and potential hazards in the current applications of ultrasound in obstetrics and gynecology. Ultrasound Med Biol 1979;5:307-320.
6. Meyer RA. Diagnostic ultrasound: hazardous or safe? Appl Radiol 1982;11:71-74.
7. Stratmeyer ME, Christman CL. Biological effects of ultrasound. Women Health 1982;7:65-81.
8. Kremkau FW. Biological effects and possible hazards. Clin Obstet Gynaecol 1983;10:395-405.
9. Brown BS. How safe is diagnostic ultrasonography? CMAJ 1984;131:307-311.
10. Carstensen EL, Gates AH. The effects of pulsed ultrasound on the fetus. J Ultrasound Med 1984;3:145-147.
11. Muggah HF. The safety of diagnostic ultrasonography. CMAJ 1984;131:280, 282.
12. Andrews M, Webster M, Fleming JE, McNay MB. Ultrasound exposure time in routine obstetric scanning. Br J Obstet Gynaecol 1987;94:843-846.
13. Wells PN. The prudent use of diagnostic ultrasound. Ultrasound Med Biol 1987;13:391-400.
14. Desai BB, Sosolik RC, Ciaravino V, Teale JM. Effect of fetal exposure to ultrasound on B cell development in BALB/c mice. Ultrasound Med Biol 1989;15:567-573.
15. Reece EA, Assimakopoulos E, Zheng XZ, et al. The safety of obstetric ultrasonography: concern for the fetus. Obstet Gynecol 1990; 76:139-146.
16. Salvesen KA, Eik-Nes SH. Is ultrasound unsound? A review of epidemiological studies of human exposure to ultrasound. Ultrasound Obstet Gynecol 1995;6:293-298.
17. Barnett SB, Rott HD, ter Haar GR, et al. The sensitivity of biological tissue to ultrasound. Ultrasound Med Biol 1997;23:805-812.
18. Miller MW, Brayman AA. Biological effects of ultrasound: the perceived safety of diagnostic ultrasound within the context of ultrasound biophysics—a personal perspective. Echocardiography 1997;14:615-628.
19. Abramowicz JS. Ultrasound in obstetrics and gynecology: is this hot technology too hot? J Ultrasound Med 2002;21:1327-1333.
20. Kieler H, Cnattingius S, Haglund B, et al. Ultrasound and adverse effects. Ultrasound Obstet Gynecol 2002;20:102-103.

21. Marinac-Dabic D, Krulewitch CJ, Moore Jr RM. The safety of prenatal ultrasound exposure in human studies. Epidemiology 2002;13:S19-S22.

22. Bly S, van den Hof MC. Obstetric ultrasound biological effects and safety. J Obstet Gynaecol Can 2005;27:572-580.

23. Church CC, Miller MW. Quantification of risk from fetal exposure to diagnostic ultrasound. Prog Biophysics Mol Biol 2007;93:331-353.

24. Duck FA. Hazards, risks and safety of diagnostic ultrasound. Med Eng Physics 2008;30:1338-1348.

25. Safety issues in fetal ultrasound. 2007. http://fetalultrasoundsafety.net/. Accessed August 2008.

26. Miller MW, Brayman AA, Abramowicz JS. Obstetric ultrasonography: a biophysical consideration of patient safety—the "rules" have changed. Am J Obstetr Gynecol 1998;179:241-254.

27. Ndumbe FM, Navti O, Chilaka VN, Konje JC. Prenatal diagnosis in the first trimester of pregnancy. Obstet Gynecol Surv 2008;63:317-328.

28. Simonsen SE, Branch DW, Rose NC. The complexity of fetal imaging: reconciling clinical care with patient entertainment. Obstet Gynecol 2008;112:1351-1354.

29. American Institute of Ultrasound in Medicine. AIUM official statement: prudent use in obstetrics. 2007. http://www.aium.org/publications/statements. Accessed September 2008.

30. Wells PN. The prudent use of diagnostic ultrasound. British Institute of Radiology 1986 Presidential Address. Br J Radiol 1986;59:1143-1151.

31. Ziskin MC. The prudent use of diagnostic ultrasound. J Ultrasound Med 1987;6:415-416.

32. Sheiner E, Abramowicz JS. Clinical end users worldwide show poor knowledge regarding safety issues of ultrasound during pregnancy. J Ultrasound Med 2008;27:499-501.

Instrument Outputs

33. Duck FA, Martin K. Trends in diagnostic ultrasound exposure. Phys Med Biol 1991;36:1423-1432.

34. Duck FA, Henderson J. Acoustic output of modern instruments: is it increasing? In: Barnett SB, Kossoff G, editors. Safety of diagnostic ultrasound. New York: Parthenon; 1998. p. 147.

Thermal and Other Effects

35. Chance PF, Smith DW. Hyperthermia and meningomyelocele and anencephaly. Lancet 1978;1:769-770.

36. Edwards MJ. Congenital defects in guinea pigs: following induced hyperthermia during gestation. Arch Pathol 1967;84:42-48.

37. Graham Jr JM, Edwards MJ, Edwards MJ. Teratogen update: gestational effects of maternal hyperthermia due to febrile illnesses and resultant patterns of defects in humans. Teratology 1998;58:209-221.

38. Halperin LR, Wilroy Jr RS. Maternal hyperthermia and neural-tube defects. Lancet 1978;2:212-213.

39. Li Z, Ren A, Liu J, et al. Maternal flu or fever, medication use, and neural tube defects: a population-based case-control study in Northern China. Birth Defects Res 2007;79:295-300.

40. Lipson AH, Edwards MJ. Maternal sauna and hyperthermia during pregnancy and cardiovascular and other malformations in offspring. Eur J Epidemiol 1993;9:676-678.

41. Little BB, Ghali FE, Snell LM, et al. Is hyperthermia teratogenic in the human? Am J Perinatol 1991;8:185-189.

42. Milunsky A, Ulcickas M, Rothman KJ, et al. Maternal heat exposure and neural tube defects. JAMA 1992;268:882-885.

43. Shaw GM, Todoroff K, Velie EM, Lammer EJ. Maternal illness, including fever and medication use as risk factors for neural tube defects. Teratology 1998;57:1-7.

44. Shiota K. Induction of neural tube defects and skeletal malformations in mice following brief hyperthermia in utero. Biol Neonate 1988;53:86-97.

45. Dombrowski SC, Martin RP, Huttunen MO. Association between maternal fever and psychological/behavior outcomes: a hypothesis. Birth Defects Res 2003;67:905-910.

46. Edwards MJ, Saunders RD, Shiota K. Effects of heat on embryos and foetuses. Int J Hyperthermia 2003;19:295-324.

47. Layde PM, Edmonds LD, Erickson JD. Maternal fever and neural tube defects. Teratology 1980;21:105-108.

48. Miller MW, Nyborg WL, Dewey WC, et al. Hyperthermic teratogenicity, thermal dose and diagnostic ultrasound during pregnancy: implications of new standards on tissue heating. Int J Hyperthermia 2002;18:361-384.

49. Moretti ME, Bar-Oz B, Fried S, Koren G. Maternal hyperthermia and the risk for neural tube defects in offspring: systematic review and meta-analysis. Epidemiology 2005;16:216-219.

50. European Committee for Medical Ultrasound Safety (ECMUS). Thermal teratology. Eur J Ultrasound 1999;9:281-283.

51. National Council on Radiation Protection and Measurements. Exposure criteria for medical diagnostic ultrasound. II. Criteria based on all known mechanisms. Report No 140. Bethesda, Md: NCRP; 2002.

52. Acs N, Banhidy F, Puho E, Czeizel AE. Maternal influenza during pregnancy and risk of congenital abnormalities in offspring. Birth Defects Res 2005;73:989-996.

53. Cleves MA, Malik S, Yang S, et al. Maternal urinary tract infections and selected cardiovascular malformations. Birth Defects Res 2008;82:464-473.

54. Kleinebrecht J, Michaelis H, Michaelis J, Koller S. Fever in pregnancy and congenital anomalies. Lancet 1979;1:1403.

55. Miller MW, Church CC, Miller RK, Edwards MJ. Fetal thermal dose considerations during the obstetrician's watch: implications for the pediatrician's observations. Birth Defects Res C Embryo Today 2007;81:135-143.

56. Peterka M, Tvrdek M, Likovsky Z, et al. Maternal hyperthermia and infection as one of possible causes of orofacial clefts. Acta Chir Plast 1994;36:114-118.

57. Smith DW, Clarren SK, Harvey MA. Hyperthermia as a possible teratogenic agent. J Pediatr 1978;92:878-883.

58. Superneau DW, Wertelecki W. Similarity of effects: experimental hyperthermia as a teratogen and maternal febrile illness associated with oromandibular and limb defects. Am J Med Genet 1985;21:575-580.

59. Miller MW, Ziskin MC. Biological consequences of hyperthermia. Ultrasound Med Biol 1989;15:707-722.

60. Miller MW, Miller HE, Church CC. A new perspective on hyperthermia-induced birth defects: The role of activation energy and its relation to obstetric ultrasound. J Therm Biol 2005;30:400-409.

61. Brent RL. Is hyperthermia a direct or indirect teratogen? Teratology 1986;33:373-374.

62. Barnett SB. Can diagnostic ultrasound heat tissue and cause biological effects? In: Barnett SB, Kossoff G, editors. Safety of diagnostic ultrasound. New York: Parthenon; 1998. p. 30.

63. Nyborg WL, Steele RB. Temperature elevation in a beam of ultrasound. Ultrasound Med Biol 1983;9:611-620.

64. Nyborg WL, O'Brien WD. An alternative simple formula for temperature estimate. J Ultrasound Med 1989;8:653-654.

65. Toneto AD, Lopes RA, Oliveira PT, et al. Effect of hyperthermia on rat fetus palate epithelium. Braz Dent J 1994;5:99-103.

66. Martinez-Frias ML, Garcia Mazario MJ, Caldas CF, et al. High maternal fever during gestation and severe congenital limb disruptions. Am J Med Genet 2001;98:201-203.

67. Tikkanen J, Heinonen OP. Maternal hyperthermia during pregnancy and cardiovascular malformations in the offspring. Eur J Epidemiol 1991;7:628-635.

68. Horder MM, Barnett SB, Vella GJ, et al. Ultrasound-induced temperature increase in guinea-pig fetal brain in utero: third-trimester gestation. Ultrasound Med Biol 1998;24:1501-1510.

69. Jauniaux E, Gulbis B, Burton GJ. The human first trimester gestational sac limits rather than facilitates oxygen transfer to the foetus: a review. Placenta 2003;24(Suppl A):86-93.

70. Carbillon L, Perrot N, Uzan M, Uzan S. Doppler ultrasonography and implantation: a critical review. Fetal Diagn Ther 2001;16:327-332.

71. Kurjak A, Kupesic S. Doppler proof of the presence of intervillous circulation. Ultrasound Obstet Gynecol 1996;7:463-464.

72. Jauniaux E. Intervillous circulation in the first trimester: the phantom of the color Doppler obstetric opera. Ultrasound Obstet Gynecol 1996;8:73-76.

73. Makikallio K, Tekay A, Jouppila P. Uteroplacental hemodynamics during early human pregnancy: a longitudinal study. Gynecol Obstet Invest 2004;58:49-54.

74. Wloch A, Rozmus-Warcholinska W, Czuba B, et al. Doppler study of the embryonic heart in normal pregnant women. J Matern Fetal Neonatal Med 2007;20:533-539.

75. Russell NE, McAuliffe FM. First-trimester fetal cardiac function. J Ultrasound Med 2008;27:379-383.

76. Duck FA. Is it safe to use diagnostic ultrasound during the first trimester? Ultrasound Obstet Gynecol 1999;13:385-388.

77. Smythe GE, MacRae DJ. Doppler ultrasound and fetal hazard (letter). Lancet 1975;2:134.

78. Calvert J, Duck F, Clift S, Azaime H. Surface heating by transvaginal transducers. Ultrasound Obstet Gynecol 2007;29:427-432.

79. Ziskin MC. Intrauterine effects of ultrasound: human epidemiology. Teratology 1999;59:252-260.

80. O'Brien WD, Siddiqi TA. Obstetric sonography: the output display standard and ultrasound bioeffects. In: Fleischer AC, Manning FA, Jeanty P, Romero R, editors. Sonography in obstetrics and gynecology: principles and practice. 6th ed. New York: McGraw-Hill; 2001. p. 29-48.

81. Bly SH, Vlahovich S, Mabee PR, Hussey RG. Computed estimates of maximum temperature elevations in fetal tissues during transabdominal pulsed Doppler examinations. Ultrasound Med Biol 1992;18:389-397.

Mechanical Effects

82. Dalecki D, Raeman CH, Child SZ, et al. Hemolysis in vivo from exposure to pulsed ultrasound. Ultrasound Med Biol 1997;23:307-313.

83. Abramowicz JS. Ultrasonographic contrast media: has the time come in obstetrics and gynecology? J Ultrasound Med 2005;24:517-531.

84. Miller MW, Brayman AA, Sherman TA, et al. Comparative sensitivity of human fetal and adult erythrocytes to hemolysis by pulsed 1 MHz ultrasound. Ultrasound Med Biol 2001;27:419-425.

85. Fatemi M, Ogburn Jr PL, Greenleaf JF. Fetal stimulation by pulsed diagnostic ultrasound. J Ultrasound Med 2001;20:883-889.

86. Duck FA. Acoustic streaming and radiation pressure in diagnostic applications: what are the implications? In: Barnett SB, Kossoff G, editors. Safety of diagnostic ultrasound. New York: Parthenon; 1998. p. 87-98.

Bioeffects of Ultrasound

87. Jensh RP, Brent RL. Intrauterine effects of ultrasound: animal studies. Teratology 1999;59:240-251.

88. Harvey EN, Loomis AL. High-frequency sound waves of small intensity and their biological effects. Nature 1928;121:622-624.

89. Sikov MR. Effect of ultrasound on development. Part 1. Introduction and studies in inframammalian species. Report of the Bioeffects Committee of the American Institute of Ultrasound in Medicine. J Ultrasound Med 1986;5:577-583.

90. Sikov MR. Effect of ultrasound on development. Part 2. Studies in mammalian species and overview. J Ultrasound Med 1986;5:651-661.

91. Fry FJ, Kossoff G, Eggleton RC, Dunn F. Threshold ultrasonic dosages for structural changes in the mammalian brain. J Acoust Soc Am 1970;48(Suppl 2):1413.

92. Frizzell LA, Carstensen EL, Davis JD. Ultrasonic absorption in liver tissue. J Acoust Soc Am 1979;65:1309-1312.

93. Frizzell LA, Lee CS, Aschenbach PD, et al. Involvement of ultrasonically induced cavitation in the production of hind limb paralysis of the mouse neonate. J Acoust Soc Am 1983;74:1062-1065.

94. Borrelli MJ, Frizzell LA, Dunn F. Ultrasonically induced morphological changes in the mammalian neonatal spinal cord. Ultrasound Med Biol 1986;12:285-295.

95. Frizzell LA, Linke CA, Carstensen EL, Fridd CW. Thresholds for focal ultrasonic lesions in rabbit kidney, liver, and testicle. IEEE Trans Biomed Eng 1977;24:393-396.

96. Carnes KI, Hess RA, Dunn F. The effect of ultrasound exposure in utero on the development of the fetal mouse testis: adult consequences. Ultrasound Med Biol 1995;21:1247-1257.

97. Hynynen K. The threshold for thermally significant cavitation in dog's thigh muscle in vivo. Ultrasound Med Biol 1991;17:157-169.

98. Dalecki D, Raeman CH, Child SZ, Carstensen EL. Intestinal hemorrhage from exposure to pulsed ultrasound. Ultrasound Med Biol 1995;21:1067-1072.

99. Dalecki D, Child SZ, Raeman CH, et al. Ultrasonically induced lung hemorrhage in young swine. Ultrasound Med Biol 1997;23:777-781.

100. Tarantal AF, Hendrickx AG. Evaluation of the bioeffects of prenatal ultrasound exposure in the cynomolgus macaque (Macaca fascicularis): II. Growth and behavior during the first year. Teratology 1989;39:149-162.

101. Hande MP, Devi PU. Effect of in utero exposure to diagnostic ultrasound on the postnatal survival and growth of mouse. Teratology 1993;48:405-411.

102. O'Brien WD. Dose-dependent effects of ultrasound on fetal weight in mice. J Ultrasound Med 1983;2:1-8.

103. Vorhees CV, Acuff-Smith KD, Schilling MA, et al. Behavioral teratologic effects of prenatal exposure to continuous-wave ultrasound in unanesthetized rats. Teratology 1994;50:238-249.

104. O'Brien Jr WD, Januzik SJ, Dunn F. Ultrasound biologic effects: a suggestion of strain specificity. J Ultrasound Med 1982;1:367-370.

105. Hande MP, Devi PU. Effect of prenatal exposure to diagnostic ultrasound on the development of mice. Radiat Res 1992;130:125-128.

106. Rao S, Ovchinnikov N, McRae A. Gestational stage sensitivity to ultrasound effect on postnatal growth and development of mice. Birth Defects Res 2006;76:602-608.

107. Borrelli MJ, Bailey KI, Dunn F. Early ultrasonic effects upon mammalian CNS structures (chemical synapses). J Acoust Soc Am 1981;69:1514-1516.

108. Norton S, Kimler BF, Cytacki EP, Rosenthal SJ. Prenatal and postnatal consequences in the brain and behavior of rats exposed to ultrasound in utero. J Ultrasound Med 1991;10:69-75.

109. Devi PU, Suresh R, Hande MP. Effect of fetal exposure to ultrasound on the behavior of the adult mouse. Radiat Res 1995;141:314-317.

110. Hande MP, Devi PU, Karanth KS. Effect of prenatal ultrasound exposure on adult behavior in mice. Neurotoxicol Teratol 1993;15:433-438.

111. Schneider-Kolsky ME, Ayobi Z, Lombardo P, et al. Ultrasound exposure of the foetal chick brain: effects on learning and memory. Int J Dev Neurosci 2009;27(7):677-683.

112. Ang ESBC, Gluncic V, Duque A, et al. Prenatal exposure to ultrasound waves impacts neuronal migration in mice. Proc NY Acad Sci 2006;103:12903-12910.

113. Abramowicz JS. Prenatal exposure to ultrasound waves: is there a risk? Ultrasound Obstet Gynecol 2007;29:363-367.

114. Kieler H. Epidemiological studies on adverse effects of prenatal ultrasound: which are the challenges? Prog Biophysics Mol Biol 2007;93:301-308.

115. Newman PG. Studies of ultrasound safety in humans: clinical benefit vs. risk. In: Barnett SB, Kossoff G, editors. Safety of diagnostic ultrasound. New York: Parthenon; 1998.

116. Salvesen KA. Epidemiological prenatal ultrasound studies. Prog Biophys Mol Biol 2007;93:295-300.

117. Ziskin MC, Petitti DB. Epidemiology of human exposure to ultrasound: a critical review. Ultrasound Med Biol 1988;14:91-96.

118. Edmonds PD, Abramowicz JS, Carson PL, et al. Guidelines for Journal of Ultrasound in Medicine authors and reviewers on measurement and reporting of acoustic output and exposure. J Ultrasound Med 2005;24:1171-1179.

119. Carvalho JS. Fetal heart scanning in the first trimester. Prenat Diagn 2004;24:1060-1067.

120. Makikallio K, Jouppila P, Rasanen J. Human fetal cardiac function during the first trimester of pregnancy. Heart (Br Cardiac Soc) 2005;91:334-338.

121. Becker R, Wegner RD. Detailed screening for fetal anomalies and cardiac defects at the 11-13-week scan. Ultrasound Obstet Gynecol 2006;27:613-618.

122. Vinals F, Ascenzo R, Naveas R, et al. Fetal echocardiography at 11 + 0 to 13 + 6 weeks using four-dimensional spatiotemporal image correlation telemedicine via an Internet link: a pilot study. Ultrasound Obstet Gynecol 2008;31:633-638.

123. Ziskin MC. Survey of patients exposed to diagnostic ultrasound. In: Reid JM, Sikov MR, editors. Interactions of ultrasound and biological tissues. Proceedings of a workshop, Battelle Seattle Research Center, Seattle, 1971. Rockville, Md: Bureau of Radiological Health, US Department of Health, Education and Welfare; 1973. p. 203-206.

124. Newnham JP, Evans SF, Michael CA, et al. Effects of frequent ultrasound during pregnancy: a randomised controlled trial. Lancet 1993;342:887-891.

125. Campbell JD, Elford RW, Brant RF. Case-control study of prenatal ultrasonography exposure in children with delayed speech. CMAJ 1993;149:1435-1440.

126. Kieler H, Haglund B, Waldenstrom U, Axelsson O. Routine ultrasound screening in pregnancy and the children's subsequent growth, vision and hearing. Br J Obstet Gynaecol 1997;104:1267-1272.

127. Stark CR, Orleans M, Haverkamp AD, Murphy J. Short- and long-term risks after exposure to diagnostic ultrasound in utero. Obstet Gynecol 1984;63:194-200.

128. Bricker L, Neilson JP, Dowswell T. Routine ultrasound in late pregnancy (after 24 weeks' gestation). Cochrane Database Syst Rev (Online) 2008:CD001451.

129. Kieler H, Haglund B, Cnattingius S, et al. Does prenatal sonography affect intellectual performance? Epidemiology 2005;16:304-310.

130. Cartwright RA, McKinney PA, Hopton PA, et al. Ultrasound examinations in pregnancy and childhood cancer. Lancet 1984;2: 999-1000.

131. Kieler H, Axelsson O, Haglund B, et al. Routine ultrasound screening in pregnancy and the children's subsequent handedness. Early Hum Dev 1998;50:233-245.

132. Salvesen KA. Ultrasound and left-handedness: a sinister association? Ultrasound Obstet Gynecol 2002;19:217-221.

133. Sheiner E, Freeman J, Abramowicz JS. Acoustic output as measured by mechanical and thermal indices during routine obstetric ultrasound examinations. J Ultrasound Med 2005;24:1665-1670.

134. Sheiner E, Shoham-Vardi I, Hussey MJ, et al. First-trimester sonography: is the fetus exposed to high levels of acoustic energy? J Clin Ultrasound 2007;35:245-249.

135. Sheiner E, Abramowicz JS. Acoustic output as measured by thermal and mechanical indices during fetal nuchal translucency ultrasound examinations. Fetal Diagn Ther 2008;25:8-10.

136. Sheiner E, Shoham-Vardi I, Pombar X, et al. An increased thermal index can be achieved when performing Doppler studies in obstetric sonography. J Ultrasound Med 2007;26:71-76.

137. Sheiner E, Hackmon R, Shoham-Vardi I, et al. A comparison between acoustic output indices in 2D and 3D/4D ultrasound in obstetrics. Ultrasound Obstet Gynecol 2007;29:326-328.

138. Bellieni CV, Buonocore G, Bagnoli F, et al. Is an excessive number of prenatal echographies a risk for fetal growth? Early Hum Dev 2005;81:689-693.

139. Newnham JP, Doherty DA, Kendall GE, et al. Effects of repeated prenatal ultrasound examinations on childhood outcome up to 8 years of age: follow-up of a randomised controlled trial. Lancet 2004;364:2038-2044.

140. Moore Jr RM, Barrick MK, Hamilton TM. Effect of sonic radiation on growth and development. Am J Epidemiol 1982;116:571.

141. Moore Jr RM, Diamond EL, Cavalieri RL. The relationship of birth weight and intrauterine diagnostic ultrasound exposure. Obstet Gynecol 1988;71:513-517.

142. Lyons EA, Dyke C, Toms M, Cheang M. In utero exposure to diagnostic ultrasound: a 6-year follow-up. Radiology 1988;166: 687-690.

143. Newnham JP, Evans SF, Michael CA, et al. Effects of frequent ultrasound during pregnancy: a randomized controlled trial. Lancet 1993;342:887-891.

144. Saari-Kemppainen A, Karjalainen O, Ylostalo P, Heinonen OP. Ultrasound screening and perinatal mortality: controlled trial of systematic one-stage screening in pregnancy. The Helsinki Ultrasound Trial. Lancet 1990;336:387-391.

145. Waldenstrom U, Axelsson O, Nilsson S, et al. Effects of routine one-stage ultrasound screening in pregnancy: a randomised controlled trial. Lancet 1988;2:585-588.

146. Salvesen KA, Vatten LJ, Bakketeig LS, Eik-Nes SH. Routine ultrasonography in utero and speech development. Ultrasound Obstet Gynecol 1994;4:101-103.

147. Bakketeig LS, Eik-Nes SH, Jacobsen G, et al. Randomised controlled trial of ultrasonographic screening in pregnancy. Lancet 1984;2:207-211.

148. Eik-Nes SH, Okland O, Aure JC, Ulstein M. Ultrasound screening in pregnancy: a randomised controlled trial. Lancet 1984;1:1347.

149. Salvesen KA, Bakketeig LS, Eik-nes SH, et al. Routine ultrasonography in utero and school performance at age 8-9 years. Lancet 1992;339:85-89.

150. Salvesen KA, Vatten LJ, Eik-Nes SH, et al. Routine ultrasonography in utero and subsequent handedness and neurological development. BMJ Clin Res 1993;307:159-164.

151. Salvesen KA, Vatten LJ, Jacobsen G, et al. Routine ultrasonography in utero and subsequent vision and hearing at primary school age. Ultrasound Obstet Gynecol 1992;2:243-247.

152. Salvesen KA, Eik-Ness SH, Vatten LJ, et al. Routine ultrasound scanning in pregnancy [authors'reply]. BMJ 1993;307:1562.

153. Sidman RL, Rakic P. Neuronal migration, with special reference to developing human brain: a review. Brain Res 1973;62:1-35.

154. Mole R. Possible hazards of imaging and Doppler ultrasound in obstetrics. Birth 1986;13(Suppl):23-33.

155. Scheidt PC, Stanley F, Bryla DA. One-year follow-up of infants exposed to ultrasound in utero. Am J Obstet Gynecol 1978;131: 743-748.

156. Salvesen K. Routine ultrasonography in utero and development in childhood. In: Tejani N, editor. Obstetrical events and developmental sequelae. 2nd ed. Boca Raton, Fla: CRC Press; 1994.

157. Stalberg K. Prenatal ultrasound and x-ray-potentially adverse effects on the CNS. Upsalla, Sweden: Upsalla Universitet; 2008.

158. Coyle I, Wayner MJ, Singer G. Behavioral teratogenesis: a critical evaluation. Pharmacol Biochem Behav 1976;4:191-200.

159. Stalberg K, Haglund B, Axelsson O, et al. Prenatal ultrasound scanning and the risk of schizophrenia and other psychoses. Epidemiology 2007;18:577-582.

160. Shu XO, Potter JD, Linet MS, et al. Diagnostic x-rays and ultrasound exposure and risk of childhood acute lymphoblastic leukemia by immunophenotype. Cancer Epidemiol Biomarkers Prev 2002;11: 177-185.

161. Naumburg E, Bellocco R, Cnattingius S, et al. Prenatal ultrasound examinations and risk of childhood leukaemia: case-control study. BMJ Clin Res 2000;320:282-283.

162. Kinnier Wilson LM, Waterhouse JA. Obstetric ultrasound and childhood malignancies. Lancet 1984;2:997-999.

163. Bunin GR, Buckley JD, Boesel CP, et al. Risk factors for astrocytic glioma and primitive neuroectodermal tumor of the brain in young children: a report from the Children's Cancer Group. Cancer Epidemiol Biomarkers Prev 1994;3:197-204.

164. Sorahan T, Lancashire R, Stewart A, Peck I. Pregnancy ultrasound and childhood cancer: a second report from the Oxford Survey of Childhood Cancers. Br J Obstet Gynaecol 1995;102:831-832.

165. Salvesen KA, Eik-Nes SH. Ultrasound during pregnancy and birthweight, childhood malignancies and neurological development. Ultrasound Med Biol 1999;25:1025-1031.

166. Stalberg K, Haglund B, Axelsson O, et al. Prenatal ultrasound and the risk of childhood brain tumour and its subtypes. Br J Cancer 2008;98:1285-1287.

Safety Guidelines

167. Kossoff G, Griffiths KA, Garrett WJ, et al. Thickness of tissues intervening between the transducer and fetus and models for fetal exposure calculations in transvaginal sonography. Ultrasound Med Biol 1993;19:59-65.

168. British Medical Ultrasound Society. Guidelines for the safe use of diagnostic ultrasound equipment. 2000, reconfirmed 2009. http://www.bmus.org/ultras-safety/us-safety03.asp. Accessed January 2010.

169. British Medical Ultrasound Society (BMUS): Guidelines for the safe use of diagnostic ultrasound equipment. Prepared by the Safety Group of BMUS. Ultrasound 2010;18:52-59.

170. World Federation for Ultrasound in Medicine and Biology (WFUMB) Symposium on Safety and Standardization in Medical Ultrasound. Issues and recommendations regarding thermal mechanisms for biological effects of ultrasound. Ultrasound Med Biol 1992;18:748.

171. Barnett SB. WFUMB Symposium on Safety of Ultrasound in Medicine. Conclusions and recommendations on thermal and non-thermal mechanisms for biological effects of ultrasound. Ultrasound Med Biol 1998;24.

172. Canada Minister of Public Works and Government Services. Guidelines for the safe use of diagnostic ultrasound. 2001. http://www.hc-sc.gc.ca/ewh-semt/pubs/radiation/01hecs-secs255/index-eng.php. Accessed December 2008.

173. Abramowicz JS, Kossoff G, Marsal K, Ter Haar G. Safety statement, 2000 (reconfirmed 2003). International Society of Ultrasound in Obstetrics and Gynecology (ISUOG). Ultrasound Obstet Gynecol 2003;21:100.

174. Barnett SB, Ter Haar GR, Ziskin MC, et al. International recommendations and guidelines for the safe use of diagnostic ultrasound in medicine. Ultrasound Med Biol 2000;26:355-366.

CHAPTER 30

The First Trimester

Clifford S. Levi and Edward A. Lyons

Chapter Outline

*T*he first trimester of pregnancy is a period of rapid change that spans fertilization, formation of the blastocyst, implantation, gastrulation, neurulation, the embryonic period (weeks 6-10), and early fetal life.[1] First-trimester sonographic diagnosis traditionally focused on evaluation of growth by serial examination to differentiate normal from abnormal gestations. This has changed radically since the advent of transvaginal sonography (TVS), which affords enhanced resolution over transabdominal sonography (TAS), with earlier visualization of the gestational sac and its contents,[2] earlier identification of embryonic cardiac activity,[3] and improved visualization of embryonic and fetal structures. As investigators have gained experience with high-resolution TAS and TVS, reliable indicators of early pregnancy failure have been identified, making serial examination necessary in only a minority of patients, resulting in decreased morbidity and patient anxiety.

Despite these technologic improvements, it is important to set clinically relevant and realistic goals for first-trimester sonographic diagnosis. Most examinations are requested because the patient has presented with vaginal bleeding or pain, or a palpable mass has been identified on physical examination. The referring physician usually requests the ultrasound examination to exclude a nonviable pregnancy or an ectopic pregnancy.

The goals of first-trimester sonography include (1) visualization and localization of the gestational sac (intrauterine or ectopic pregnancy) and (2) early identification of embryonic demise and other forms of nonviable gestation. It also seeks to identify those embryos that are still alive but at increased risk for embryonic or fetal demise. In multifetal pregnancies, first-trimester ultrasound determines the number of embryos and the chorionicity-amnionicity, estimates the duration or menstrual/gestational age of the pregnancy, and assists in early diagnosis of fetal abnormalities, including identification of embryos more likely to be abnormal, based on secondary criteria (e.g., abnormal yolk sac).

Current trends in ultrasound late in the first trimester focus on **nuchal translucency** screening combined with maternal age and maternal serum screening to determine the risk of chromosomal abnormalities and structural anomalies. Associated with the increased emphasis on late-first-trimester ultrasound and first-trimester screening, there is an opportunity to visualize fetal anomalies earlier than at the time of the standard 18 to 20–week scan. First-trimester diagnosis of specific anomalies is discussed in the chapters covering those organ systems. This chapter discusses basic principles in the diagnosis of anomalies in the first trimester.

As experience with early first-trimester ultrasound evolves, there is controversy over the use of ultrasound parameters to diagnose early pregnancy failure or embryonic demise on a single examination.[4] Current practice is based on the use of reliable sonographic indicators of ectopic pregnancy and embryonic demise. The accuracy of some sonographic signs used as indicators of the presence of a live embryo or of embryonic demise depends on the use of modern, high-resolution ultrasound equipment and the operator's expertise. Published values in the literature based on data using high-frequency transducers cannot be applied to lower-resolution 5.0-MHz transducers.[5,6] The transvaginal signs listed in this chapter assume the use of modern equipment with a transducer frequency of at least 7 to 8 MHz, with meticulous scanning technique. Furthermore, published values cannot be used as "absolute" values, and allowing at least a few millimeters leeway is critical when using these numbers. Nyberg and Filly[4] emphasize that experienced physicians who interpret ultrasound rarely rely on a single parameter and simultaneously consider multiple variables to create a diagnostic impression.

Transvaginal color flow Doppler sonography became available in the early 1990s. Some authors have suggested that color Doppler TVS provides improved diagnostic accuracy over gray-scale TVS in the identification of early intrauterine and ectopic pregnancies and may allow more definitive diagnoses at the initial examination.[7] However this exposes the early **intrauterine pregnancy** (IUP) to the increased power deposition of Doppler scanning (see Chapter 29).

MATERNAL PHYSIOLOGY AND EMBRYOLOGY

All dates presented in this chapter are in **menstrual age** or **gestational age,** in keeping with the radiologic and obstetric literature, rather than in embryologic age, as used by embryologists. This can be counted as follows:

Gestational age = Conceptual age + 2 weeks

Early in the menstrual cycle, the pituitary secretes rising levels of follicle-stimulating hormone (FSH) and luteinizing hormone (LH), which cause the growth of 4 to 12 primordial follicles into **primary ovarian follicles**[1] (Fig. 30-1). When a fluid-filled cavity or antrum forms in the follicle, it is referred to as a **secondary follicle.** The primary oocyte is off to one side of the follicle and surrounded by follicular cells or the **cumulus oophorus.** One follicle becomes dominant, bulges on the surface of the ovary and becomes a "mature follicle" or **graafian**

follicle. It continues to enlarge until ovulation, with the remainder of the follicles becoming atretic. The developing follicles produce estrogen. The estrogen level remains relatively low until 4 days before ovulation, when the dominant or active follicle produces an estrogen surge, after which an LH and prostaglandin surge results in ovulation. Ovulation follows the LH peak within 12 to 24 hours. Actual expulsion of the oocyte from the mature follicle is aided by several factors, including the intrafollicular pressure, possibly contraction of the smooth muscle in the **theca externa** stimulated by prostaglandins, and enzymatic digestion of the follicular wall.[8]

Ovulation occurs on approximately day 14 of the menstrual cycle with expulsion of the secondary oocyte from the surface of the ovary. In women with a menstrual cycle longer than 28 days, this ovulation occurs later, so that the secretory phase of the menstrual cycle remains at about 14 days. After ovulation, the follicle collapses to form the **corpus luteum,** which secretes progesterone and, to a lesser degree, estrogen. If a pregnancy does not occur, the corpus luteum involutes. In pregnancy, involution of the corpus luteum is prevented by **human chorionic gonadotropin** (hCG), which is produced by the outer layer of cells of the gestational or chorionic sac (syncytiotrophoblast).

Before ovulation, **endometrial proliferation** occurs in response to estrogen secretion (Fig. 30-1). After ovulation, the endometrium becomes thickened, soft, and edematous under the influence of progesterone.[9] The glandular epithelium secretes a glycogen-rich fluid. If pregnancy occurs, continued production of progesterone results in more marked hypertrophic changes in the endometrial cells and glands to provide nourishment to the blastocyst. These hypertrophic changes are referred to as the **decidual reaction** and occur as a hormonal response regardless of the site of implantation, intrauterine or ectopic.

Oocyte transport into the fimbriated end of the fallopian tube occurs at ovulation as the secondary oocyte is expelled with the follicular fluid and is "picked up" by the fimbria. The sweeping movement of the fimbria, the currents produced by the action of the cilia of the mucosal cells, and the gentle peristaltic waves from contractions of the fallopian musculature all draw the oocyte into the tube.[10]

The mechanism of **sperm transport** is not completely understood. From 200 to 600 million sperm and the ejaculate fluid are deposited in the vaginal fornix during intercourse. Sperm must move through the cervical canal and its mucous plug, up the endometrial cavity, and down the fallopian tube to meet the awaiting oocyte within the distal third or ampullary portion of the fallopian tube. Sperm were thought to move primarily using their tails, although they travel at 2 to 3 mm per minute, which would take about 50 minutes to travel the 20 cm to their destination. Settlage et al.[10] found motile sperm within the ampulla between 5 and 10

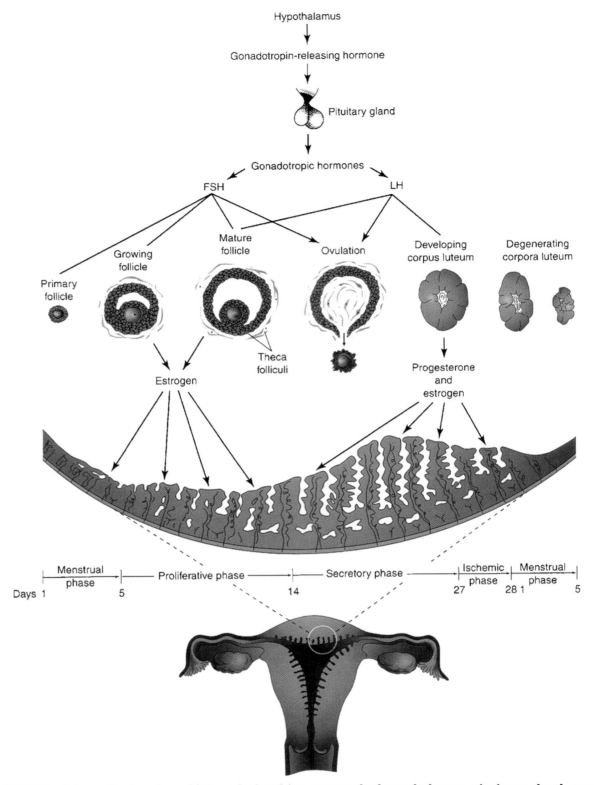

FIGURE 30-1. Schematic drawing of interrelationships among the hypothalamus, pituitary gland, ovaries, and endometrial lining. *FSH,* Follicle-stimulating hormone; *LH,* luteinizing hormone. *(From Moore KL, Persaud TVN, editors. The developing human: clinically oriented embryology. 6th ed. Philadelphia, 1998, Saunders.)*

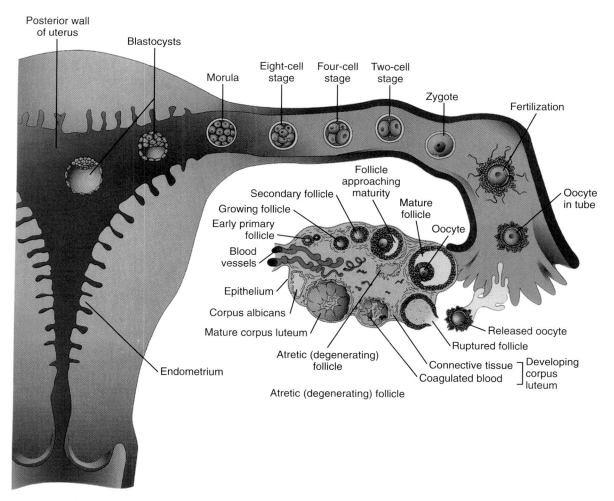

FIGURE 30-2. Diagram of ovarian cycle, fertilization, and human development to the blastocyst stage.
(From Moore KL, Persaud TVN, editors. The developing human: clinically oriented embryology. *6th ed. Philadelphia, 1998, Saunders.)*

minutes after deposition near the external cervical os. If inert particles such as radioactive macroaggregates or carbon particles are placed near the external os, they too will be picked up and transported up the uterus and down the tubes. Contractions of the inner layer of myometrium probably create a negative pressure strong enough to suck up particles and move them up the endometrial canal. We have demonstrated these contractions in nonpregnant women and shown that they increase in strength and frequency to peak at 3.5 contractions per minute at ovulation.[11]

Fertilization occurs on or about day 14 as the mature ovum and sperm unite to form the **zygote** in the outer third of the fallopian tube (Fig. 30-2). Cellular division of the zygote occurs during transit through the fallopian tube. By the time the conceptus enters the uterus, about day 17, it is at the 12- to 15-cell stage **(morula).** By day 20, the conceptus has matured to the **blastocyst stage.** The blastocyst is a fluid-filled cyst lined with trophoblastic cells that contain a cluster of cells at one side called the **inner cell mass.** On day 20, the blastocyst at the site of the inner cell mass burrows through the endometrial

membrane into the hyperplastic endometrium, and implantation begins[12] (Fig. 30-3, *A*).

Implantation is completed by day 23 as the endometrial membrane re-forms over the blastocyst (Fig. 30-3, *B*). During implantation, the **amniotic cavity** forms in the inner cell mass. A bilaminar embryonic disk separates the amniotic cavity from the exocoelomic cavity. The **primary (primitive) yolk sac** forms at about 23 days of gestational age as the blastocyst cavity becomes lined by the exocoelomic membrane and hypoblast (Fig. 30-4). As the extraembryonic coelom forms (Fig. 30-4, *A*), the primary yolk sac is pinched off and extruded, resulting in the formation of the **secondary yolk sac** (Fig. 30-4, *B* and *C*). Standard embryology texts indicate that the secondary yolk sac actually forms at approximately 27 to 28 days of menstrual age (MA), when the mean diameter of the gestational sac is approximately 3 mm. It is the secondary yolk sac, rather than the primary yolk sac, that is visible with ultrasound. For the remainder of this chapter, the term **yolk sac** is used to refer to the *secondary* yolk sac. The extraembryonic coelom becomes the **chorionic cavity.**

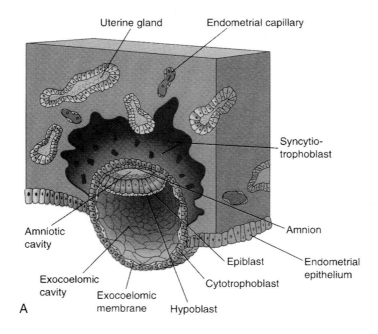

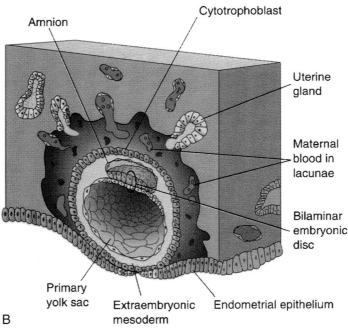

FIGURE 30-3. Implantation of the blastocyst into endometrium. Entire conceptus is approximately 0.1 mm at this stage. **A,** Partially implanted blastocyst at approximately 22 days. **B,** Almost completely implanted blastocyst at about 23 days. *(From Moore KL, Persaud TVN, editors.* The developing human: clinically oriented embryology. *6th ed. Philadelphia, 1998, Saunders.)*

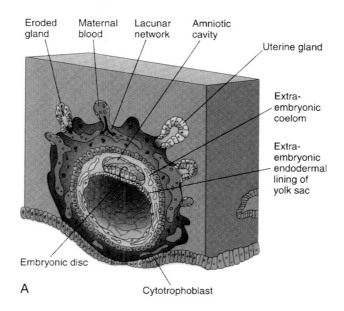

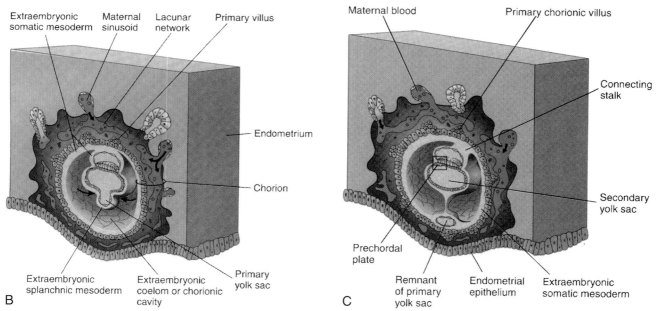

FIGURE 30-4. Formation of secondary yolk sac. A, Approximately 26 days: formation of cavities within extraembryonic mesoderm. These cavities will enlarge to form extraembryonic coelom. **B,** About 27 days, and **C,** 28 days: formation of secondary yolk sac with extrusion of primary yolk sac. Extraembryonic coelom will become chorionic cavity. *(From Moore KL, Persaud TVN, editors.* The developing human: clinically oriented embryology. *6th ed. Philadelphia, 1998, Saunders.)*

Later, because of differential growth, the yolk sac comes to lie between the amnion and chorion. During week 4, there is rapid proliferation and differentiation of the **syncytiotrophoblast,** forming primary **chorionic villi.** Traditional thinking that the syncytiotrophoblastic cells invade the maternal endometrial vessels, leaving maternal blood to bathe the trophoblastic ring, has been challenged. Hustin[12] compared transvaginal imaging to hysteroscopy of the placenta, chorionic villous sampling tissue, and hysterectomy specimens with an early pregnancy in situ. Before 12 weeks, the intervillous space contains no blood, only clear fluid, and on histologic examination, the villous tissue is separated from the maternal circulation by a continuous layer of trophoblastic cells. Only after the third month does the trophoblastic shell become broken and the maternal circulation become continuous with the intervillous space. Further, at weeks 8 and 9 of gestation, the trophoblastic shell forms plugs within the spiral arteries, allowing only filtered plasma to permeate the placenta.[13] In two thirds of abnormal pregnancies, the trophoblastic shell is thinner and fragmented, and the trophoblastic invasion of the spiral arteries is reduced or absent.[14]

Vascularization of the placenta occurs at the beginning of the fifth week. Oh et al.[15] showed significant increases in sac size from 5 weeks onward in normal pregnancies versus pregnancy failures. The rationale for placental vascularization was based on early work by Folkman,[16] who showed that tumors can grow to a size of 3 mm being nourished only by diffusion. To exceed this size, cells must recruit host blood vessels, or the cells at the center will receive inadequate nutrition. Similarly, the rapidly growing embryonic implantation must be vascularized by the 3-mm stage that occurs at 5 weeks' gestation.

During the fifth week, the embryo is converted by the process of **gastrulation** from a bilaminar disk to a trilaminar disk with the three primary germ cell layers: ectoderm, mesoderm, and endoderm. During gastrulation, the primitive streak and notochord form. The primitive streak gives rise to the **mesenchyme,** which forms the connective tissue of the embryo and stromal components of all glands.

The formation of the neural plate and its closure to form the neural tube is referred to as **neurulation.** This process begins in the fifth week in the thoracic region and extends caudally and cranially, resulting in complete closure by the end of the sixth week (day 42). Failure of closure of the neural tube results in neural tube defects.

During the fifth week, two cardiac tubes (the primitive heart) develop from splanchnic mesodermal cells. By the end of the fifth week, these tubes begin to pump into a primitive paired vascular system. By the end of the fifth week, a vascular network develops in the chorionic villi that connect through the umbilical arteries and vein to the primitive embryonic vascular network.

Essentially all internal and external structures present in the adult form during the **embryonic period,** which ends at 10 menstrual weeks. By the end of the sixth week, blood flow is unidirectional, and by the end of the eighth week, the heart attains its definitive form. The peripheral vascular system develops slightly later and is completed by the end of the tenth week. The primitive gut forms during week 6. The midgut herniates into the umbilical cord from week 8 through the end of week 12. The rectum separates from the urogenital sinus by the end of week 8, and the anal membrane perforates by the end of week 10. The **metanephros,** or primitive kidneys, ascend from the pelvis, starting at approximately week 8, but do not reach their adult position until week 11. Limbs are formed with separate fingers and toes. Almost all congenital malformations except abnormalities of the genitalia originate before or during the embryonic period. External genitalia are still in a sexless state at the end of week 10 and do not reach mature fetal form until the end of week 14.

Early in the **fetal period,** body growth is rapid and head growth relatively slower, with the crown-rump length doubling between weeks 11 and 14.

SONOGRAPHIC APPEARANCE OF NORMAL INTRAUTERINE PREGNANCY

Gestational Sac

Implantation usually occurs in the fundal region of the uterus between day 20 and day 23.[17] In a study of early implantation sites in 21 patients it was found that implantation occurs most frequently on the uterine wall ipsilateral to the ovulating ovary and least often on the contralateral wall.[17] In addition, in a study of predominant sleeping positions in the peri-implantation period, Magann et al.[18] found that the 33% of women who slept prone were most likely to have a high or fundal implantation than those who slept on their back or side. The latter groups predominantly had implantations corresponding to their resting posture.

At 23 days, the entire conceptus measures approximately 0.1 mm in diameter and cannot be imaged by TAS or TVS techniques. The earliest sonographic sign of an IUP was described by Yeh et al.,[19] who identified a focal echogenic zone of decidual thickening at the site of implantation at about 3½ to 4 weeks of gestational age. This sign is nonspecific and of limited diagnostic value.

The first reliable gray-scale evidence of an IUP is visualization of the gestational sac within the thickened decidua. Yeh et al.[19] originally identified this sign, referred to as the **intradecidual sign** (Fig. 30-5). An intradecidual gestational sac should be eccentrically

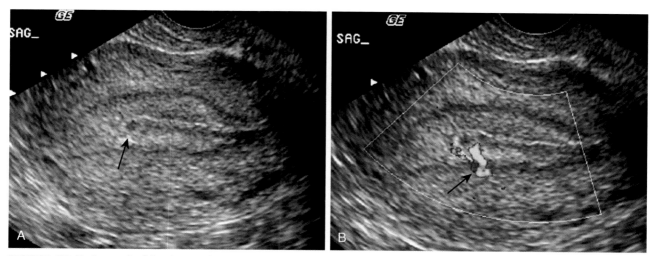

FIGURE 30-5. Intradecidual sac sign. A, Sagittal scan at 4 weeks, 4 days shows implantation site as a 2-mm focal thickening of posterior endometrium *(arrow)*. The chorionic fluid in the sac is just barely visible. The mass slightly displaces the endometrial stripe and has a slightly echogenic rim. **B,** Color Doppler image shows prominent terminal portion of a spiral artery *(arrow)* extending up to the sac.

located within the endometrium and should abut the endometrial canal. It is important to ensure that the sac abuts the endometrial canal to distinguish an intrauterine gestational sac from a decidual cyst.[19]

As a general rule, it is possible to demonstrate an early IUP as a small intradecidual sac between $4\frac{1}{2}$ and 5 weeks' gestational age using TVS (Fig. 30-6). Oh et al.[15] used a high-frequency (7.5-10 MHz) transvaginal transducer and were able to identify a gestational sac in all 67 patients scanned between 28 and 42 days' gestational age; mean sac diameter between 28 and 35 days was 2.6 mm.

In a literature review, Nyberg and Filly[4] noted the importance of the appropriate use of a threshold level and a discriminatory level for the appearance of a gestational sac. The **threshold level** identifies the earliest one can expect to see a sac (4 weeks, 3 days), and the **discriminatory level** identifies when one should always see the sac (5 weeks, 2 days). Although the menstrual history provides useful information early in a woman's obstetric care, because of the variability in the timing of ovulation and the unreliability of menstrual history, discriminatory levels based on history are of limited clinical use. Discriminatory levels using the serum beta subunit of human chorionic gonadotropin (β-hCG) provide a more reproducible value that can help guide management in clinical practice.

The serum β-hCG level becomes positive shortly after implantation, long before the gestational sac is visualized sonographically. A disproportionately low β-hCG is an indicator of a poor prognosis.[20] Although many earlier studies (from the 1970s) use the Second International Standard (IS) for serum β-hCG, the World Health Organization (WHO) First International

Reference Preparation (IRP) has been developed more recently and is in common usage. The IRP/IS preparations differ by a factor of approximately 2:1, although this ratio varies among laboratories. To convert from the Second IS to the First IRP, the following formula can be used:

$$\beta\text{-hCG (IRP)} \div \beta\text{-hCG (2nd IS)} = 2$$

A gestational sac can often be visualized sonographically at low serum β-hCG levels. Extensive effort has been made to identify a discriminatory level for the serum β-hCG above which it is abnormal not to be able to identify a gestational sac with ultrasound. Using TAS, Nyberg et al.[21] demonstrated gestational sacs in 36/36 patients with normal IUP in whom serum β-hCG was greater than 1800 mIU/mL (Second IS).

In a subsequent article by Nyberg et al.,[22] TVS correctly identified intrauterine gestational sacs in 20% of patients with β-hCG levels below 500 mIU/mL (Second IS), four of five patients with β-hCG levels of 500 to 1000 mIU/mL, and all 17 with β-hCG levels greater than 1000 mIU/mL. Bree et al.[23] identified a discriminatory level of 1000 mIU/mL (IRP) for TVS.

In a series of 60 patients whose ovulation was timed by ultrasonic follicle monitoring, Sengoku et al.[24] assessed sac appearance, size, and levels of β-hCG. Only 10 sacs were seen with a β-hCG of less than 1000 mIU/mL (IRP), five of six sacs with levels of 1000 to 2000 mIU/mL, and all sacs with levels above 2000 mIU/mL.

Keith et al.[25] found that the β-hCG level above which a singleton sac was always seen with TVS was 1161 mIU/mL (Third International Standard). This

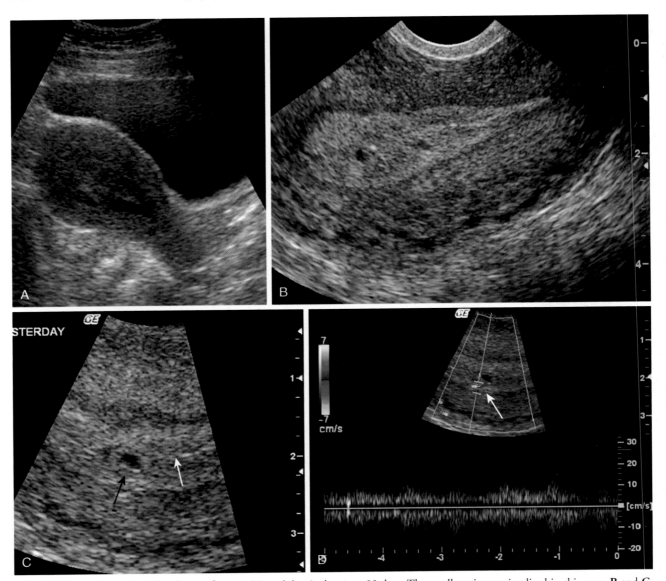

FIGURE 30-6. Intradecidual sac sign. A, Transabdominal scan at 32 days. The small sac is not visualized in this scan. **B** and **C,** Transvaginal scans the same day showing the echogenic ring of the sac *(black arrow)* implanted just below the endometrial interface *(white arrow).* **D,** Color Doppler flow of a feeding spiral artery adjacent to the sac with low-velocity flow of 10 cm/sec.

increased to 1556 mIU/mL in twins and 3372 mIU/mL in triplets. When applying discriminatory levels in clinical practice, it is important to remember that the actual discriminatory level depends of the (1) resolution of the ultrasound scanner, (2) patient's body habitus, (3) position of the uterus, and (4) type of hormonal assay. Keith's data emphasize that the use of discriminatory levels in isolation to effect clinical decision making ignores multifetal gestation. Discriminatory levels can be used to guide management but cannot be used as absolute indicators that the absence of a sonographically demonstrable gestation sac is abnormal. In a study of pregnancies achieved by assisted reproductive techniques, Pellicer et al.[26] found that an embryonic sac could be visualized at 37 to 38 menstrual days.

The **double-decidual sign** was previously described by Nyberg et al.[27] as a method of differentiation between an early IUP and the pseudosac of an ectopic pregnancy. The endometrium in the pregnant state is actually called the decidua capsularis, decidua vera, and decidua basalis (Figs. 30-7, 30-8, and 30-9). The double-decidual sign is based on visualization of the gestational sac as an echogenic ring formed by the decidua capsularis and chorion laeve eccentrically located within the decidua vera (Fig. 30-7), forming two echogenic rings. The outer ring is formed by the echogenic endometrium of the lining of the uterus. The decidua basalis–chorion frondosum (future placenta) may also be visualized as an area of eccentric echogenic thickening. The double-decidual sign can usually be identified by about 5.5 to 6 weeks'

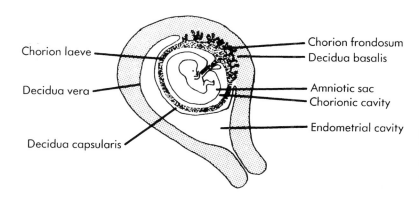

Chorion laeve

Decidua vera

Decidua capsularis

Chorion frondosum
Decidua basalis

Amniotic sac
Chorionic cavity

Endometrial cavity

FIGURE 30-7 Double-decidual sign. Diagram of anatomic basis showing three layers of decidua and endometrial cavity. *(From Lyons EA, Levi CS. The first trimester.* Radiol Clin North Am *1982; 20:259.)*

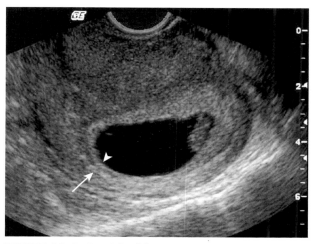

FIGURE 30-8. Decidual layers. Sagittal transvaginal sonogram at 7 weeks shows the gestational sac *(arrowhead)* and the maternal decidua *(arrow)* as separate echogenic bands.

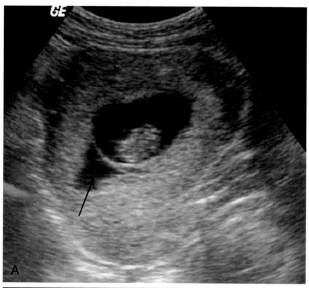

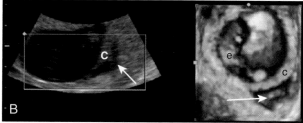

FIGURE 30-9. Subchorionic hemorrhage. A, Transabdominal scan at 10 weeks. The sac and embryo are seen as well as a fluid collection *(arrow)* behind the chorion, a subchorionic hemorrhage. *(arrow)* **B,** Transvaginal sagittal and 3-D scans show the fluid collections *(arrows); e,* embryo; *c,* chorion.

gestational age, at approximately the same time that the yolk sac becomes visible with TVS. A well-defined double-decidual sign is an accurate predictor of the presence of an intrauterine gestational sac. A vague or absent double-decidual sign may be seen in some patients with a fluid-filled pseudosac associated with an ectopic pregnancy and should be considered nondiagnostic.

The double-decidual sign was originally described as specific for an early IUP. Yeh et al.[19] clearly saw the double-decidual sign in 30.6%, vaguely in 33.3%, and not at all in 36.1% of IUPs at 3½ to 7 weeks' gestational age. They identified a double-decidual sign in two of five ectopic pregnancies, casting doubt on the usefulness of this sign. In our experience, a clear double-decidual sign is useful in predicting the presence of an IUP. A vague or absent double-decidual sign is considered nondiagnostic. Parvey et al.[28] found a double-decidual sac in only 53% of early pregnancies with no yolk sac or embryo present. They also assessed visualization of the echogenic chorionic rim alone as a sign of IUP and found its presence in 64% of cases. It was more clearly defined in later pregnancies with a higher β-hCG level (mean,

16,082 mIU/mL) and thin, less clearly defined or even absent in the earliest pregnancies. The pseudo–gestational sac may occasionally appear as a double-decidual sac or chorionic rim sign, but further scanning should differentiate the two.

Using a higher-frequency 10-MHz transvaginal transducer in scanning patients who had a positive pregnancy test and only a small (<1 cm) intrauterine "fluid collection" seen with a 6- to 7-MHz transducer, Benacerraf et al.[29] were able to improve their diagnostic confidence in all eight patients with an IUP. This demonstrates the need to scan transvaginally with a high-frequency transducer when an early pregnancy is in question.

The **normal gestational sac** is round in the very early stages and implants immediately beneath the thin, echogenic endometrial stripe (see Fig. 30-6, *C*). As it enlarges, the sac often has a somewhat oval shape because of the pressure exerted by the muscular uterine walls. It can be distorted during the transvaginal examination by compressing the uterus with the vaginal probe. The gestational (or chorionic) sac is filled with extracoelomic or **chorionic sac fluid** that is normally weakly reflective and more echogenic than the amniotic fluid. This difference is best appreciated if the system gain is increased. The low-level echoes within the chorionic fluid are accentuated, and yet the amniotic fluid remains echo free[30] (Fig. 30-10). The low-level echoes are likely caused by the relatively thick proteinaceous material in chorionic fluid.[31]

Transvaginal color flow Doppler sonography may be helpful in identifying the presence of an early intrauterine gestational sac (see Figs. 30-5, *B,* and 30-6, *D*). It has also proved helpful in distinguishing a normal from a failed intrauterine gestation and in the detection of an ectopic pregnancy through the exclusion of an IUP.[32] Emerson et al.[32] found that the detection of peritrophoblastic flow of high velocity and low impedance increased the sensitivity of detection of IUP from 90% to 99%. Even before a sac is seen, flows of 8 to 30 cm/sec were found in the endometrium at the implantation site. Parvey et al.[28] found that 15% of IUPs without the presence of a sac had high-velocity, low-impedance, intradecidual arterial-type flow. A specificity and positive predictive value of 95% could be achieved in diagnosing an intrauterine gestation by using a peak systolic intradecidual flow velocity of 15 cm/sec or more and a resistive index (RI) of 0.55 or less. As mentioned previously, however, use of Doppler ultrasound on the early gestational sac increases the amount of power deposition compared to gray-scale imaging and therefore is infrequently used.

Yolk Sac

The yolk sac is the first structure to be seen normally within the gestational sac. Using TAS, it is often seen when the **mean gestational sac diameter** (MSD) is 10 to 15 mm and should always be visualized by an MSD of 20 mm.[33] Transvaginal techniques allow earlier and more detailed visualization of the yolk sac (Fig. 30-11), which should always be visualized by an MSD of 8 mm.[34]

The demonstration of a yolk sac may be critical in differentiating an early intrauterine gestational sac from a pseudosac.[34] Although the double-decidual sign is not 100% specific for presence of an IUP, the identification of a yolk sac within the early gestational sac is diagnostic of IUP (Fig. 30-12). The yolk sac plays an important role in human embryonic development.[1] While the placental circulation is developing, the yolk sac has a role in **transfer of nutrients** to the developing embryo in the third and fourth weeks. **Angiogenesis** (blood vessel formation) occurs in the wall of the yolk sac in the fifth week. The mesenchymal cells or angioblasts aggregate to form "blood islands"; a cavity forms within these islands, which fuse with others to form networks of endothelial channels. Vessels extend into adjacent areas by endothelial budding and fusion with other vessels. This vascular network in the wall of the yolk sac eventually joins the fetal circulation via the paired vitelline arteries and veins through a stalk called the **vitelline duct. Hematopoiesis** (blood cell formation) occurs first in the well-vascularized extraembryonic mesoderm covering the yolk sac wall in the fifth week, in the liver in the eighth week, and later in the spleen, bone marrow, and lymph nodes. The dorsal part of the yolk sac is incorporated into the embryo as **primitive gut** (foregut, midgut, and hindgut) in the sixth week. The yolk sac remains connected to the midgut by the vitelline duct. In some cases the vitelline duct can be demonstrated sonographically (Figs. 30-13 and 30-14).

Lindsay et al.[35] reported that the yolk sac grows at a rate of 0.1 mm per millimeter of MSD growth when the MSD is less than 15 mm, then slows to 0.03 mm. The upper limit of normal for yolk sac diameter between 5 and 10 weeks of gestational age is 5.6 mm.

The number of yolk sacs present can be helpful in determining **amnionicity** of a multifetal pregnancy (Fig. 30-15). In general, if the embryos are alive, the number

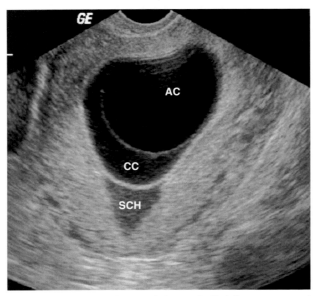

FIGURE 30-10. Echogenicity of fluids. Transvaginal sonogram of a 12-week sac with the echo-free amniotic fluid *(AC),* mildly echogenic chorionic fluid *(CC),* and more echogenic blood in the subchorionic space *(SCH).*

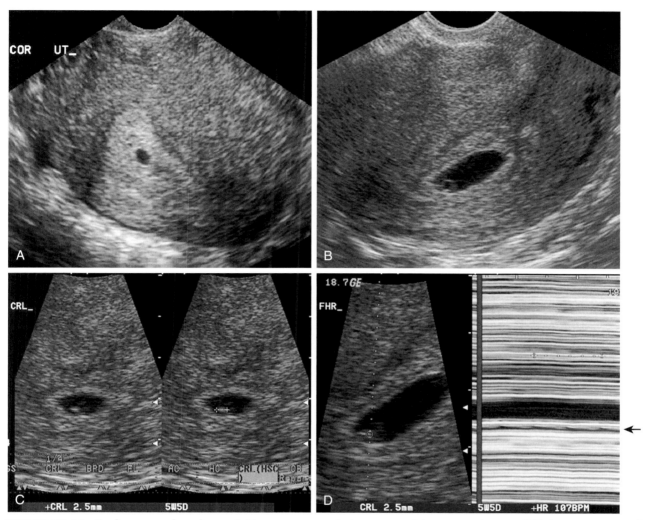

FIGURE 30-11. Early sac and embryo. A, Transverse transvaginal sonogram of the anteverted uterus *(UT)* demonstrates a small gestational sac at 4 weeks, 3 days. **B,** Sonogram at 5 weeks, 6 days shows an enlarging gestational sac with the appearance of a 2-mm yolk sac *(arrow)*. **C,** Magnified view of the sac reveals a 2.5-mm embryo *(calipers); CRL,* crown-rump length. **D,** M-mode ultrasound shows cardiac motion at a fetal heart rate *(FHR)* of 107 beats/min *(arrow)*.

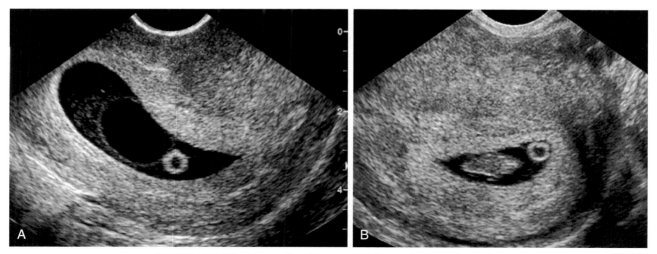

FIGURE 30-12. Normal yolk sac. A, Nine weeks. **B,** Eight weeks.

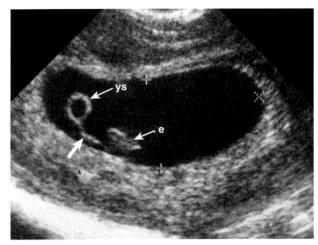

FIGURE 30-13. Normal embryo at 8 weeks. Transvaginal sonogram shows vitelline duct (*arrow*), yolk sac *(ys)*, and embryo *(e)*.

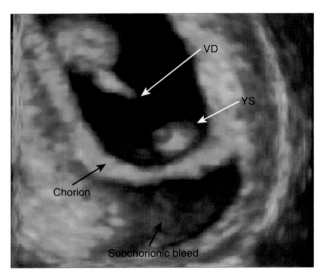

FIGURE 30-14. Vitelline duct. Three-dimensional (3-D) ultrasound image of an embryo at 8 weeks with the vitelline duct *(VD)* connecting to the yolk sac *(YS)*. There is also a subchorionic hemorrhage.

of yolk sacs and the number of amniotic sacs are the same. In a **monochorionic monoamniotic** (MCMA) twin gestation, there will be two embryos, one chorionic sac, one amniotic sac, and one yolk sac. Levi et al.[36] examined four MCMA twin pregnancies, all with a single yolk sac. One was a conjoined twin and one a twin ectopic, with both pregnancies terminated. The other two pregnancies delivered normally at 34 weeks. Of the four cases, two had a larger-than-normal yolk sac (>5.6 mm), and two had a normal sac. Therefore, in MCMA twins, a single, large, or normal-sized yolk sac with two live embryos can result in a normal twin delivery.

Visualization of the vitelline arteries and veins is possible on the vitelline duct and should be possible on the periphery of the yolk sac itself. A magnified 9 weeks sac shows irregularities in the wall of the yolk sac that correspond to the arteries (Fig. 30-16).

Embryo and Amnion

Yeh and Rabinowitz[37] described the **double-bleb sign** as the earliest demonstration of the amnion. The two blebs represent the amnion and yolk sac and can be identified as early as 5½ weeks when the **crown-rump length** (CRL) is 2 mm. At that point, the embryonic disk is situated between the yolk sac and amnion. However, although visualization of the tiny (<2 mm) bleb of amnion may occur before visualization of the embryo, this is a transient phenomenon. Visualization of the amnion in the absence of an embryo usually occurs in intrauterine embryonic death as a result of resorption of the embryo (Fig. 30-17).

Amniotic fluid initially is a colorless, fetal dermal transudate; as the skin cornifies and the kidneys begin to function, at about 11 weeks, it becomes pale yellow. Birnholz and Madanes[30] calculated the amniotic fluid volume after subtracting the estimated volume of the embryo.[30] The amnion becomes visible when the embryo has a CRL of 2 mm at 6 weeks. The cavity becomes almost spherical by about 7 weeks, likely a result of the more rapid increase in fluid volume relative to the growth of the sac membrane to accommodate it. The actual rate of fluid increase is more rapid after about 9 weeks, when fetal urine is produced. Fluid accumulates at about 5 mL (cc) per day at 12 weeks' MA. The amniotic cavity expands to fill the chorionic cavity completely by week 14 to 16. It is normal to identify the amnion as a separate membrane or sac within the chorionic cavity before 14 to 16 weeks (Fig. 30-18). Occasionally, the amnion and chorionic membranes may fail to fuse at week 16, and separation of these membranes may persist for a short time.[38]

Iatrogenic or spontaneous rupture of the amniotic membrane is a rare occurrence and even more rarely results in the **amniotic band sequence.** This rupture may result in retraction of the amnion in part or in whole, up to the base of the umbilical cord where the two membranes are adherent. More often, the floating amniotic membranes do not adhere to the fetus, and no fetal anomalies occur.

Embryonic Cardiac Activity

Using TVS, an embryo with a CRL as small as 1 to 2 mm may be identified immediately adjacent to the yolk sac (Fig. 30-19). In normal pregnancies the embryo can be identified in gestational sacs as small as 10 mm[4] and should always be identified when the MSD is 16 to 18 mm or larger with optimal scanning parameters and high-resolution TVS.

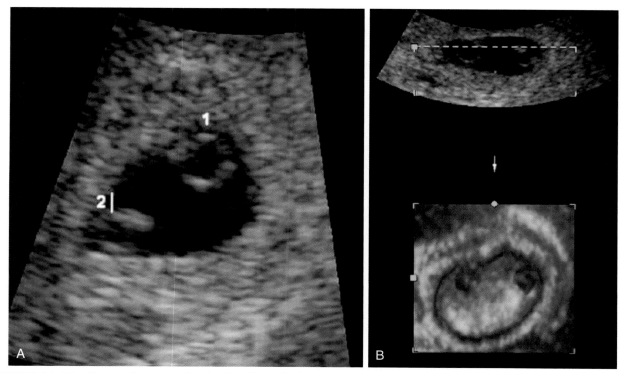

FIGURE 30-15. Six-week monochorionic diamniotic (MCDA) twins. Two separate yolk sacs are seen within a single gestational sac at 6 weeks on 2-D (**A**) and 3-D (**B**) images.

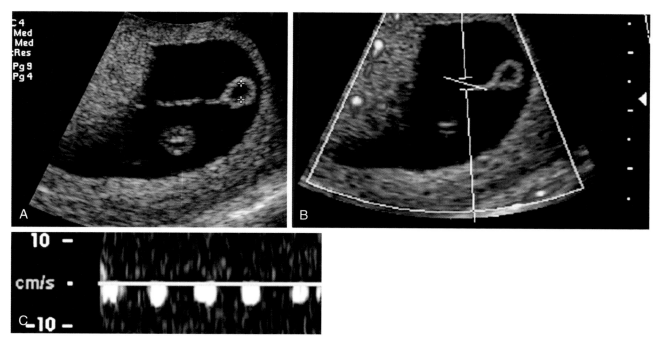

FIGURE 30-16. Normal yolk sac and vitelline duct. Transvaginal scans of 9-week pregnancy focusing on the yolk sac (**A**) and flow within the vitelline duct (**B** and **C**).

Embryologic data suggest the tubular heart begins to beat at 36 to 37 days' gestational age.[1] Cadkin and McAlpin[39] described cardiac activity adjacent to the yolk sac before visualization of the embryo at the end of the fifth week. Ragavendra et al.[40] placed a 12.5-MHz endoluminal catheter transducer into the endometrial canal adjacent to the gestational sac. They identified cardiac activity in an embryo with a CRL of 1.5 mm and resolved the two walls of the heart, seen only as a tube. Using TVS, absent cardiac activity may be normal in embryos of less than 4 to 5–mm CRL. In general, cardiac activity can be visualized in normal embryos of greater than 5-mm CRL. Normal embryonic cardiac activity is greater than 100 beats per minute (**Video 30-1**).

Umbilical Cord and Cord Cyst

The umbilical cord is formed at the end of the sixth week (CRL = 4.0 mm) as the amnion expands and envelops the connecting stalk, the yolk stalk, and the allantois. The cord contains two umbilical arteries, a single umbilical vein, the allantois, and yolk stalk (also called the **omphalomesenteric duct** or vitelline duct), all of which

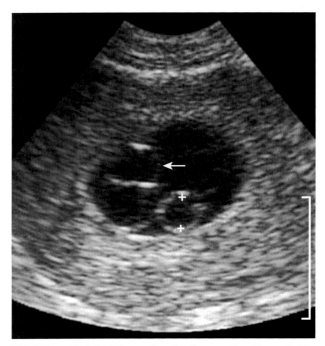

FIGURE 30-17. Monochorionic and diamniotic twins with one intrauterine embryonic death and one alive. Transvaginal sonogram at 10 weeks. On the left the arrow is pointing to one of two adjacent sacs, one is the amnion and the other the yolk sac. To the right is a single yolk sac *(calipers)* with the live embryo not in the scan plane. Both embryos went on to abort.

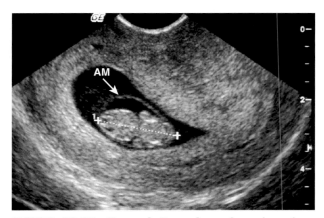

FIGURE 30-18. Normal 9-week embryo/amnion. Normal separation of amnion *(arrow)* and chorionic sacs at 9 weeks. Transvaginal sonography shows the embryo *(calipers)* and the amnion *(AM)*.

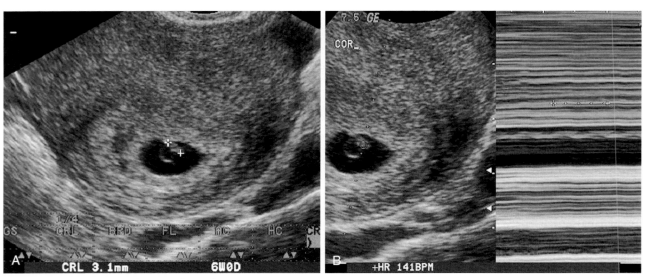

FIGURE 30-19. Normal 6-week embryo. A, Image shows 6-week embryo *(calipers)* adjacent to the yolk sac. **B,** M-mode ultrasound shows a heart rate of 141 beats/min.

are imbedded in **Wharton's jelly**. The **umbilical arteries** arise from the fetal internal iliac arteries and in the newborn become the superior vesical arteries and the medial umbilical ligaments. The **umbilical vein** carries oxygenated blood from the placenta to the fetus. The oxygenated blood is shunted through the ductus venosus into the inferior vena cava and the heart. The single left umbilical vein in the newborn becomes the ligamentum teres, which attaches to the left branch of the portal vein. The ductus venosus becomes the ligamentum venosum.

The **allantois** is associated with bladder development and becomes the urachus and the median umbilical ligament. It extends into the proximal portion of the umbilical cord. The **yolk stalk** connects the primitive gut to the yolk sac. The paired **vitelline arteries and veins** accompany the stalk to provide blood supply to the yolk sac. The arteries arise from the dorsal aorta to supply initially the yolk sac, then the primitive gut. The arteries remain as the celiac axis, superior and inferior mesenteric arteries supplying the foregut, midgut, and hindgut, respectively. The vitelline veins drain directly into the sinus venosus of the heart. The right vein is later incorporated into the right hepatic vein. The portal vein is also formed by an anastomotic network of vitelline veins.

The length of the umbilical cord has a close linear relationship with gestational age in normal pregnancies. Hill et al.[41] found they could reliably measure the cord lengths in 53 fetuses at 6 to 11 weeks' gestational age. Also, the cord lengths in 60% of dead fetuses were more than two standard deviations (2 SD) below the value for that expected gestational age.

The width of the umbilical cord has also been measured sonographically in first-trimester pregnancies, and Ghezzi et al.[42] found a steady increase from 8 to 15 weeks. There was a significant correlation between cord diameter and gestational age ($r = 0.78$; $p < 0.001$), CRL ($r = 0.75$; $p < 0.001$), and biparietal diameter ($r = 0.81$; $p < 0.001$), but no correlation with birth weight or placental weight. The cord diameter was significantly smaller by at least 2 SD in patients who developed preeclampsia or had a miscarriage.

Cysts and pseudocysts within the cord have been described in the first trimester.[43] Cysts are usually seen in the eighth week and disappear by the 12th week. They are singular, closer to the fetus than the placenta, with a mean size of 5.2 mm. Cysts may originate from remnants of the allantois or omphalomesenteric duct and characteristically have an epithelial lining[44] and usually resolve in utero. Although umbilical cord cysts have been associated with chromosomal abnormalities if seen in the second and third trimesters, those seen in the first trimester have been normal at delivery. It is hypothesized that the cyst is an **amnion inclusion cyst** that occurs as the amnion was enveloping the umbilical cord (Fig. 30-20). In a series of 1159 consecutive patients scanned between 7 and 14 weeks, Ghezzi et al.[45] found 24 cord cysts at a prevalence of 2.1%. Single cysts in the first

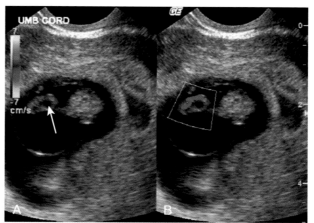

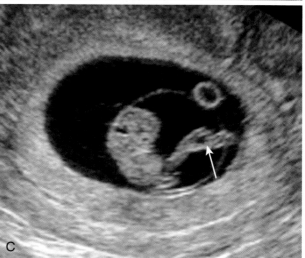

FIGURE 30-20. Umbilical cord cyst. A, Live embryo at 9 weeks' menstrual age with a cyst on the cord *(arrow)* close to the embryonic end. On subsequent examination (not shown) the cyst was no longer seen. **B,** Color Doppler image of the cord and cyst with flow in the vessels of the cord and no flow in the cyst. **C,** Another example of a 9-week cord cyst *(arrow)* in the midportion of the cord, with good visualization of the whole cord, embryo, and yolk sac.

trimester were associated with a normal outcome and a healthy infant, whereas multiple or complex cysts were associated with an increased risk of miscarriage or aneuploidy.

ESTIMATION OF GESTATIONAL AGE

During the first trimester, gestational age may be estimated sonographically with greater accuracy than at any other stage of pregnancy. As pregnancy progresses, biologic variation results in wider variation around the mean for all sonographic parameters at a given gestational age. In order of appearance, the following structures can be measured as indicators of gestational age: sac, CRL, and biparietal diameter.

Gestational Sac Size

It is possible to estimate gestational age from weeks 5 to 10 on the basis of gestational sac size. Dating of the gestational sac alone is important because it is the first structure seen before visualization of the yolk sac and then the embryo. The pregnancy should be followed, however, until the embryo with cardiac activity is identified as a reliable indicator of embryonic life. Most practitioners actually "eyeball" the sac; if MSD is very small, about 2 mm, gestational age is 4 to 4½ weeks (see Fig. 30-11), and MSD of about 5 mm is 5 weeks. At 5½ weeks, a yolk sac appears. At 6 weeks, an embryo first appears adjacent to the yolk sac.

The MSD is measured using the sum of three orthogonal dimensions of the fluid–sac wall interface divided by three. The measurements are most accurate when obtained by a high-frequency transvaginal probe in the sagittal and transverse planes at right angles to one another. Normally, a yolk sac will be present when the MSD is 8 mm or less, and an embryo will be seen at 16 mm or less. Gestational sacs larger than 8 mm without a yolk sac or larger than 16 mm without an embryo should be watched carefully for impending early pregnancy failure. Occasionally, a gestational sac up to 20 mm will be seen without an embryo, and the outcome will be a normal pregnancy. Although this is uncommon, the clinician must always give the pregnancy the benefit of the doubt and use not only the gestational sac measurements but clinical presentation as well.

Crown-Rump Length

Using TVS, the embryo can be visualized from the fifth week onward. Conventional CRL charts are available beginning from 6 weeks, 2 days. A well-performed CRL measurement in the first trimester of pregnancy is accurate to 5 to 7 days.

Biparietal Diameter

By the end of the first trimester, measurement of the biparietal diameter (BPD) becomes more accurate than the CRL, which by that time reflects errors associated with fetal flexion and extension.[46]

If the patient is to receive only **one ultrasound examination** during pregnancy, a first-trimester sonographic examination solely to assess gestational age is not recommended.[47] Although this is the most accurate time for estimation of gestational age, there is inadequate embryonic development to identify confidently anomalies that could be seen in the second trimester. Currently, late first trimester is considered the ideal time to screen for aneuploidy using a combination of maternal serum screening and nuchal translucency (see Chapter 31).

EARLY PREGNANCY FAILURE

One of the most important roles of ultrasound in the first trimester is to identify early pregnancies that have already failed or that are more likely to fail. Many clinical and sonographic terms are used to describe an early pregnancy failure. This term is descriptive of a **process** rather than of what one suspects based on the clinical or sonographic changes. The pregnancy shows sonographic evidence that the process of growth and development has stopped, ideally with supportive clinical findings. A large, empty gestational sac; a gestational sac and yolk sac only; a smaller-than-normal or even an appropriate-sized embryo with no cardiac activity; or only the remnants of a gestational sac all could be appropriately described as "early pregnancy failure." The clinical descriptors of "threatened" or "missed" or "incomplete" abortion or "blighted ovum" contribute little to the understanding of the findings. Early pregnancy failure indicates that whatever is in the endometrial cavity, it will never produce a live baby.

Studies have demonstrated a 20% to 31% rate of early pregnancy loss after implantation in normal healthy volunteers.[48,49] Overall, about 75% of all pregnancies will fail. About 15% of fertilized ova fail to divide, 15% are lost before implantation, 30% during implantation, 13% to 16% after implantation and before the first missed period,[49] and 9% to 10% after the first missed period. Wilcox et al.[48] found that the rate of unrecognized or preclinical pregnancy loss after implantation was 22%. Many pregnancies aborted before the time when a gestational sac would be demonstrable by TVS. The higher numbers of preclinical losses reported more recently likely reflect the use of more sensitive pregnancy tests. Cytogenetic abnormalities have also been documented in 20% of ostensibly normal in vitro fertilization embryos.[50] All these findings are consistent with the early pathologic studies of Hertig and Rock,[49] who showed a high frequency of morphologic abnormalities in preimplantation embryos. Loss rates are increased with increased maternal age and use of tobacco and alcohol.

Sorokin et al.[51] performed chorionic villous sampling (CVS) in 795 first-trimester pregnancies and found that 35 had a nonviable pregnancy before the procedure; 19 of the 35 women had subsequent CVS, and all were aneuploid. Ten cases had chromosomal abnormalities, virtually always lethal in the embryonic period, and nine had defects with moderate potential for fetal viability. Gestations with low viability potential had a larger discrepancy (23.4 ± 8.3 days) in estimated minus observed gestational age, which was significantly greater than that of gestations with moderate viability potential (8.9 ± 4.3 days; p <0.001). The absence of an embryonic pole was more common in the first group. This demonstrates that the more severe the anomaly, the more likely that very early embryonic demise or **intrauterine growth restriction** (IUGR) will occur.

The etiology of first-trimester pregnancy loss is still not fully understood, with many known and suspected causes. In a study of 232 first-trimester patients (normal, healthy women with good nutrition, good medical/prenatal care, positive urinary pregnancy test, and no vaginal bleeding) with TVS at the first visit, Goldstein[52] determined the incidence of subsequent pregnancy loss by following all to delivery or spontaneous abortion. This group had an overall pregnancy loss rate of 11.5% in the embryonic period, (i.e., <70 days from last menstrual period [LMP]). The loss rate diminished as the pregnancy progressed. The loss rate was 8.5% when a yolk sac was seen, 7.2% with an embryo of CRL less than 5 mm, 3.3% with CRL 6 to 10 mm, and 0.5% with CRL greater than 10 mm. The loss rate leveled off at 2% from 14 to 20 weeks, the fetal period. Therefore, under the best circumstances, the pregnancy loss rate will be 11.5% overall, from 5 weeks onward. Once the embryo reaches a CRL of 10 mm, there is about a 98% chance of a successful outcome.

Patients who present with bleeding have a much higher incidence of pregnancy loss. In patients who present with a closed cervical os and uterine bleeding in the first trimester, 50% will eventually abort. Using TVS, Falco et al.[53] studied 270 patients with first-trimester bleeding at 5 to 12 weeks' gestation; 45% were diagnosed initially as a nonviable pregnancy or anembryonic sac. Those with multiple gestations were excluded. Of the 149 remaining with demonstrable fetal cardiac activity, 15% (23/149) subsequently aborted.

Table 30-1 summarizes the rate of spontaneous abortion in a number of studies of women with and without bleeding in early pregnancy.[52-55]

Another cause of early pregnancy failure is **luteal phase defect,** thought to be failure of the corpus luteum to support the conceptus adequately once implantation has occurred. This may result from a shortened luteal phase in cases of ovulation induction and in vitro fertilization, or from luteal dysfunction, more frequently seen in obese women or women over 37 years of age.[56] Luteal phase defect has been defined as a delay of more than 2 days in histologic development of the endometrium relative to the day of the cycle. The underlying cause may be decreased hormone production by the corpus luteum, decreased levels of FSH or LH or abnormal patterns of secretion, or a decreased response of the endometrium to progesterone.

Angiogenesis of the corpus luteum may be needed for the regulation of progesterone production. Kupesic et al.[57] found that the resistive index (RI) in intraovarian arteries in normal nongravid women dropped below 0.47 in the luteal phase compared to a group with luteal phase defect who had a high resistance throughout the menstrual cycle, with RI always above 0.50. They suggest that Doppler sonography may predict functional capacity of the corpus luteum, at least in the nongravid state. Blumenfeld and Ruach[56] were successful in treating luteal phase defect in a group undergoing ovulation induction and in patients with previous abortions, using hCG administration twice weekly in the sixth and tenth weeks. This reduced the rate of miscarriage from 49% to 17.8% (p <0.01).

Currently, clinical management centers on whether or not the embryo is present and alive. Menstrual history may be unreliable, and sonographic diagnosis of embryonic demise based on the menstrual history may be incorrect. It is more appropriate to predict outcome by comparing sonographic findings to quantifiable parameters, including other sonographic measurements (MSD) or quantitative serum β-hCG. Menstrual age can be used if there is corroboration with a previous positive β-hCG test result. For example, if a patient had a positive serum β-hCG test result 5 weeks ago, the current gestational age must be at least 8 weeks.

Sonographic Diagnosis of Embryonic Demise

After the gestational sac becomes demonstrable on ultrasound, the diagnosis of early pregnancy failure can be made reliably using sonographic criteria.

TABLE 30-1. RATE OF SPONTANEOUS ABORTION IN EARLY PREGNANCY*

STUDY	AGE (WK)	NUMBER	INDICATION	ABORTION RATE (%)
Goldstein[52]	5-10	232	Routine	11.5
Pandya et al.[54]	10-13	17,870	Routine	2.8
Stabile et al.[55]	5-16	624	Bleeding	45
Falco et al.[53]	5-12	270	Bleeding	51.5
Falco et al.[53]	5-12	149	Bleeding + live fetus	15
Pandya et al.[54]	10-13	17,870	Bleeding	15.6

*In women with and without bleeding.

TABLE 30-2. PRESENCE OR ABSENCE OF CARDIAC ACTIVITY IN NORMAL EMBRYOS*

| CRL (MM) | Cardiac Activity at TVS | |
	PRESENT	ABSENT
0-0.9	0	0
1-1.9	0	3
2-2.9	12	0
3-3.9	11	2
4-4.9	12	0
TOTAL	**35**	**5**

From Levi CS, Lyons EA, Zheng XH, et al. Endovaginal ultrasound:
demonstration of cardiac activity in embryos of less than 5.0 mm in crown-rump
length. Radiology 1990;176:71-74.
*Based on crown-rump length (CRL) (N = 40); TVS, transvaginal sonography.

TABLE 30-4. PERCENTAGE OF EMBRYOS THAT ABORTED AFTER SONOGRAPHIC DEMONSTRATION OF CARDIAC ACTIVITY*

CRL (MM)	SPONTANEOUS ABORTIONS/TOTAL	PERCENTAGE ABORTED
0-0.9	0/0	0%
1-1.9	1/1	100%
2-2.9	1/1	38%
3-3.9	6/17	35%
4-4.9	3/15	20%
TOTAL	**11/46**	**24%**

From Levi CS, Lyons EA, Zheng XH, et al. Endovaginal ultrasound:
demonstration of cardiac activity in embryos of less than 5.0 mm in crown-rump
length. Radiology 1990;176:71-74.
*At specific crown-rump length (CRL).

TABLE 30-3. PRESENCE OR ABSENCE OF CARDIAC ACTIVITY IN EMBRYOS THAT SUBSEQUENTLY ABORTED IN FIRST TRIMESTER*

| CRL (MM) | Cardiac Activity at TVS | |
	PRESENT	ABSENT
0-0.9	0	0
1-1.9	1	0
2-2.9	1	8
3-3.9	6	6
4-4.9	3	6
TOTAL	**11**	**20**

From Levi CS, Lyons EA, Zheng XH, et al. Endovaginal ultrasound:
demonstration of cardiac activity in embryos of less than 5.0 mm in crown-rump
length. Radiology 1990;176:71-74.
*Based on crown-rump length (CRL) (N = 31); TVS, transvaginal sonography.

Embryonic Cardiac Activity

The most important feature for the confirmation of embryonic and fetal life is the identification of cardiac activity. The presence of cardiac activity indicates that the embryo is alive. The absence of cardiac activity does not necessarily indicate embryonic demise, however, because TVS can identify a normal early embryo without cardiac activity.

We reviewed a series of 96 patients with CRL of less than 5 mm to assess the predictive value of the presence or absence of cardiac activity using TVS[3] (Tables 30-2, 30-3, and 30-4). Of the 71 patients available for follow-up, 46 embryos had cardiac activity, 35 progressed to at least the late second trimester, and 11 ended as first-trimester demise. Of the 25 embryos without demonstrable cardiac activity, 5 (20%) were normal and 20 (80%) ended as first-trimester embryonic deaths. Of the

five normal embryos without demonstrable cardiac activity on initial TVS, three had initial CRL of less than 1.9 mm. Standard embryology texts indicate that the embryonic heart begins to beat at the beginning of the sixth week, when the CRL is 1.5 to 3 mm. Thus, it is not surprising that we were unable to identify cardiac activity in normal embryos with less than 2 mm CRL. Initial TVS assessment failed to identify cardiac activity in 2 of 25 normal embryos with CRL of 2 to 4 mm. TVS enabled correct identification of cardiac activity in 100% of normal embryos with CRL of 4 to 4.9 mm.

Pennell et al.[58] found that 16 of 18 embryos with CRL less than 5 mm had no cardiac activity on initial transvaginal assessment but demonstrated cardiac activity on follow-up TVS. Cardiac motion was seen on transvaginal scan in all pregnancies with CRL greater than 5 mm. As a result, in our practice, follow-up sonography is performed in patients with embryos of less than 5-mm CRL with no cardiac activity, unless the yolk sac is absent. We allow a few millimeters of leeway and follow up otherwise normal-appearing embryos with no cardiac activity on initial examination. The history and other sonographic findings must be considered before making the diagnosis of embryonic demise.

The combination of vaginal bleeding and absent cardiac activity in embryos of CRL less than 5 mm on TVS is associated with a very poor prognosis. Aziz et al.[59] reviewed outcomes in embryos of CRL 5 mm or less with absent cardiac activity on TVS, in women presenting with vaginal bleeding; all resulted in pregnancy failure.

Using TVS, the embryo and embryonic cardiac activity can be reliably and consistently identified earlier than with TAS. Before making a diagnosis of embryonic demise, it is critical to ensure that the examination is of high quality, performed with modern equipment and an appropriate transducer frequency, and that the entire embryo is visualized. A high frame rate must be used, and the frame-averaging mode must be turned off. If there is any doubt in the diagnosis, follow-up examination should be performed.

 In patients with a sonographically demonstrable embryo, absent cardiac activity is clearly the most important factor in predicting the pregnancy outcome (**Video 30-2**). It is also important to know the predictive value of the presence of cardiac activity in an embryo with respect to its ultimate viability. After 7 weeks' gestational age, the pregnancy loss rate is 2% to 2.3%,[60,61] and after 16 weeks, the rate is only 1%.[62] In our series of predominantly symptomatic patients with embryos of less than 5-mm CRL, identification of cardiac activity with TVS was associated with a 24% risk of spontaneous abortion.[3] Falco et al.[53] found a 15% abortion rate in pregnancies from 5 to 12 weeks with TVS-demonstrated cardiac activity.

Other secondary findings may also be helpful in predicting the outcome of a pregnancy. In our series, the combination of absent cardiac activity and vaginal bleeding was associated with 100% embryonic mortality.[3] Subchorionic hemorrhages and absent cardiac activity were associated with 88% embryonic mortality.

Gestational Sac Features

In many patients the embryo is not visualized on the initial sonogram, and the diagnosis of pregnancy failure cannot be made on the basis of abnormal cardiac activity. In these patients the diagnosis of pregnancy failure may be made based on gestational sac characteristics. The most reliable indicator of abnormal outcome based on gestational sac features is **abnormal size**.[2,33] In 1985 using TAS, Bernard and Cooperberg[63] observed that a gestational sac with MSD greater than 20 mm and no embryo had a poor outcome. In 1986, also using TAS, Nyberg et al.[33] refined the definition of an abnormal gestational sac as MSD of 25 mm or more without an embryo, or MSD of 20 mm or more without a yolk sac.

These criteria were reevaluated for TVS. MSD of 8 mm or more without a demonstrable yolk sac, or 16 mm with no demonstrable embryo, is abnormal and indicates pregnancy failure.[35] Most authors allow a few millimeters of leeway in MSD measurements as a margin of error, and many do not use the absent yolk sac as a sign of pregnancy failure. Furthermore, these parameters only apply to high-resolution TVS and cannot be used for examinations performed with a 5-MHz transvaginal probe. Rowling et al.[64] studied early pregnancies with lower-frequency transvaginal probes (5 MHz) as well as higher-frequency probes (9-5 MHz broadband). The gestational sac was first seen at 6.4 mm in size with the lower frequency but at 4.6 mm with higher frequencies. A yolk sac was always seen in normal pregnancies with a gestational sac greater than 5 mm, and an embryo was always seen with a sac of 13 mm, using frequencies above 5 MHz.

Our practice is to use the 8-mm and 16-mm sac size values and to repeat a suspicious or indeterminate study in 1 week. Normal gestational sac growth is 1.1 mm/day. Nyberg et al.[65] found that patients with early pregnancy failure had MSD growth rates of less than 0.7 mm/day. This growth rate is useful information in assessing the normal development in serial examinations. With an expected growth rate of 1.1 mm/day, one should see an appropriate increase in sac size and, if normal, the appearance of a yolk sac or an embryo. If the growth is less than expected, it gives one confidence in the diagnosis of early pregnancy failure. It is also important to view the pregnancy in light of the clinical condition. A patient who is in the process of a spontaneous abortion will often present with brownish spotting, a decrease in the symptoms of pregnancy (breast tenderness, nausea), and on examination, a uterus smaller than expected. The latter sign is subjective and not reliable in early gestation (Fig. 30-21).

In their study of early sac size from 4 to 6 weeks' MA, Oh et al.[15] found that MSD less than 6.5 mm was able to predict an abnormal outcome with a sensitivity of 89.3%, a specificity of 63.2%, and a negative and positive predictive value of 80%. In practical terms, this value is useful only if one is absolutely sure of the date of the LMP.

Other gestational sac criteria are less reliable alone, but together or with an abnormally large sac, these features provide additional support for the diagnosis of early pregnancy failure: distorted gestational sac **shape** (Fig. 30-22), thin **trophoblastic reaction** (<2 mm), weakly echogenic **trophoblast,** and **abnormally low position** of the gestational sac within the endometrial cavity[33] (Fig. 30-23).

A gestational sac greater than 16 mm without an embryo is a strong sign of early pregnancy failure. However, a sac of 16 mm or less without an embryo and with bleeding does *not* guarantee a positive outcome. In a prospective study of 50 patients with MSD of 16 mm or less, no embryo, and first-trimester bleeding, Falco et al.[66] found that 64% eventually miscarried; 13/18 (72%) of those who continued to delivery had a yolk sac seen; and 13/32 (40%) went on to fail even though a yolk sac was present. Advanced maternal age (>35) and low serum β-hCG (<1200 mIU/mL IRP) were associated with increased risk of pregnancy failure. The finding of a smaller-than-expected MSD (<1.34 SD) carried a risk of miscarriage of 93%.

The intact gestational or chorionic sac and embryo are not usually seen after abortion. Figure 30-24 demonstrates sonographic and pathologic correlation in a 7-week, 3-day embryo within an intact sac immediately after a spontaneous abortion.

Amnion and Yolk Sac Criteria

Visualization of the amnion in the absence of a sonographically demonstrable embryo after 7 weeks' MA is

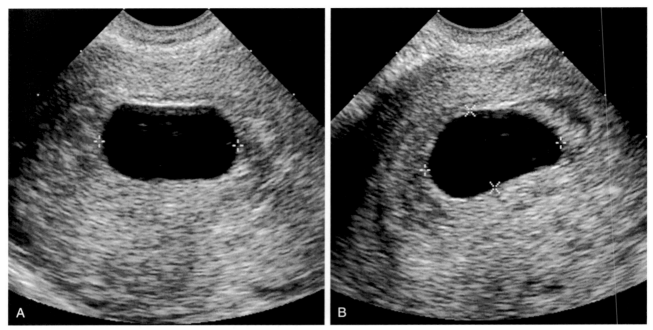

FIGURE 30-21. Early pregnancy failure with large, empty sac. A, Transvaginal coronal, and **B,** transvaginal sagittal, images of an empty gestational sac. Mean sac diameter *(calipers)* is 18 mm. No yolk sac is identified.

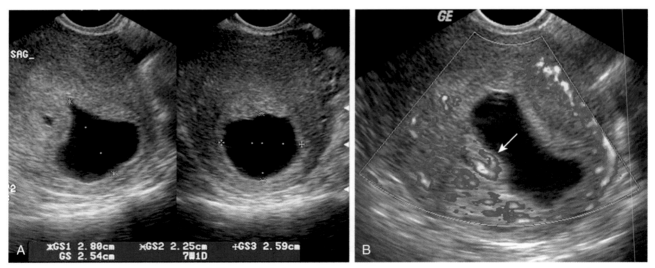

FIGURE 30-22. Early pregnancy failure with irregular sac. A, Transvaginal sagittal and transverse views of an irregular empty gestational sac in a 40-year-old woman with spotting at 11 weeks. Mean sac diameter *(calipers)* is 25 mm. No yolk sac or embryo is present, the sac is irregular, and the trophoblast is thin. **B,** Power Doppler ultrasound with a small area of vascularity at the implantation site *(arrow).*

abnormal and diagnostic of a nonviable pregnancy. The amnion is usually visualized *after* the embryo, so it should not be visualized in the absence of an embryo. The clinician may see two sacs within the gestational sac. Although it may be a monochorionic diamniotic pregnancy, it may also be a failed pregnancy with an empty amnion and a yolk sac. Other findings that may be useful in the diagnosis of embryonic demise include a collapsing, irregularly marginated amnion (Fig. 30-25) and yolk

sac calcification. In general, however, other signs of embryonic demise are present when these findings are positive.

Sonographic Predictors of Abnormal Outcome

Sonographic findings may be used to predict abnormal outcome in the presence of a live embryo, or before

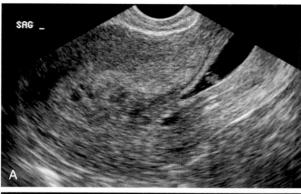

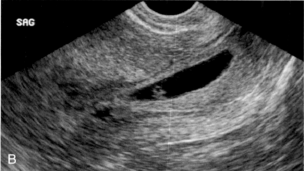

FIGURE 30-23. Aborting sac. A 23-year-old pregnant woman at 8 weeks' gestation presented with cramps and spotting. **A,** Transvaginal sagittal scan shows a gestational sac in the lower uterine segment extending into the cervix. **B,** Sagittal scan of the sac within the upper cervix. Note the small yolk sac and the adjacent small embryo. No cardiac activity was detected.

visualization of the embryo. These findings can be used to identify a high-risk subgroup of embryos at risk for embryonic demise or subsequent diagnosis of fetal anomaly that require close follow-up.

Embryonic Bradycardia

Although embryonic cardiac activity indicates that the embryo is alive at examination, an abnormally slow heart rate may predict impending demise. Doubilet and Benson[67] found that a heart rate less than 80 beats/min in embryos with a CRL less than 5 mm was universally associated with subsequent embryonic demise (Fig. 30-26). A rate of 80 to 90 beats/min was associated with a 64% risk of demise, 90 to 99 beats/min with a 32% risk, and 100 beats/min with an 11% risk. Heart rates above 100 beats/min are considered normal in embryos of CRL less than 5 mm. In embryos of CRL 5 to 9 mm, a heart rate less than 100 beats/min was always associated with abnormal outcome, with the normal rate 120 beats/min or more. In embryos of CRL 10 to 15 mm, a heart rate less than 110 beats/min appears to be associated with a very poor prognosis.

Arrhythmia is also an indicator of first-trimester loss.[68] In a group of 950 patients, Vaccaro et al.[68] found four arrhythmias, with three having ventricular brady-

cardia, all of which were dead on follow-up scan within 2 weeks.

Mean Sac Diameter and Crown-Rump Length

Bromley et al.[69] found that in 16 patients at 5½ to 9 weeks' gestational age with MSD less than 5 mm greater than the CRL (i.e., MSD − CRL = <5 mm), sometimes termed **early oligohydramnios**, 15 had spontaneous first-trimester abortion despite a normal heart rate for age (Figs. 30-27 and 30-28).

Yolk Sac Size and Shape

Perhaps the most important consideration is that yolk sac abnormalities may predict abnormal outcome in pregnancies that appear otherwise completely normal by all other ultrasound criteria.[70] Rat embryo experiments demonstrate defects in the yolk sac structure and ultrastructure in response to **hyperglycemia.** Human data indicate that yolk sac malformations occur in embryos of diabetic mothers in the first trimester of pregnancy before 9 weeks.[71]

Studies have attempted to characterize the normal sonographic appearance of the yolk sac and to identify abnormal morphologic features may predict poor fetal outcome. Green and Hobbins[72] found that in patients at 8 and 12 weeks' gestation, yolk sacs 2 mm or less in size were associated with a poor outcome. A solid, echodense yolk sac was associated with fetal death or an anomalous fetus. In our experience, an echogenic yolk sac is not always associated with anomalies or impending demise and may revert to a more normal appearance.

Lindsay et al.[35] compared yolk sac **internal diameter** to gestational age, CRL, and MSD (Fig. 30-29). A yolk sac diameter outside the 95% confidence limits for these other parameters is a relative indicator of increased risk of embryonic demise or fetal abnormality. However, the sensitivity of yolk sac size as a predictor of outcome is only 15.6%, because 50% of abnormal pregnancies have a sonographically normal yolk sac. Although the 5% and 95% confidence limits can be used to predict increased risk, a yolk sac diameter greater than 5.6 mm between 5 and 10 weeks is always associated with an abnormal outcome in singleton pregnancies (Fig. 30-30). A yolk sac greater than 5.6 mm may be seen normally in MCMA twins.[36] Furthermore, a thick, symmetrical yolk sac has a predictive value of 93.3% for normal outcome.[35] A thin yolk sac has a predictive value of 53.8% for abnormal outcome.

Yolk sac **shape** is not as predictive of outcome as size. Kucuk et al.[70] found that 10 of 219 normal pregnancies (4.5%) and 9 of 31 early pregnancy failures (29%) had an abnormal yolk sac shape. Shape alone had a sensitivity of 29% and specificity of 95% in predicting an abnormal outcome.

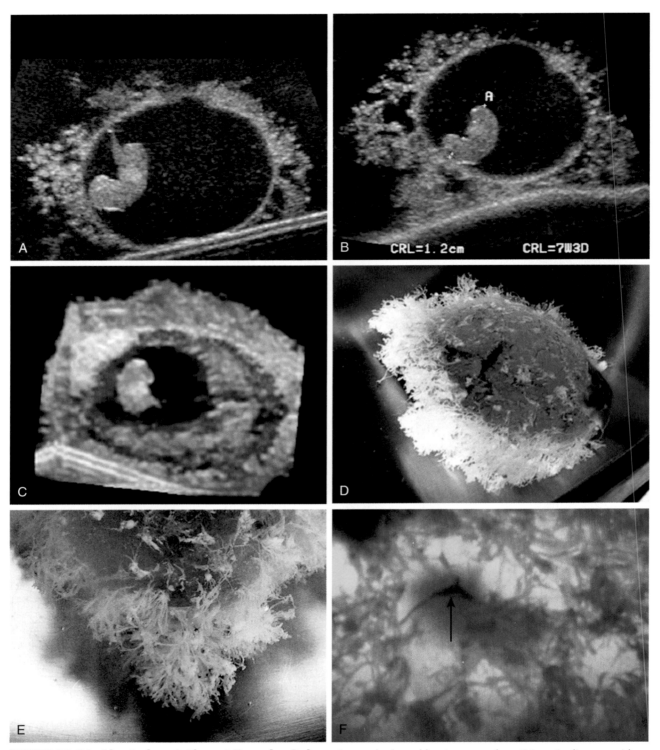

FIGURE 30-24. Aborted gestation at 7 weeks, 3 days. A recently aborted but intact sac about 2.8 cm in diameter with an embryo. The sac was scanned in a water bath so that the frondlike chorionic villi can be seen around the sac floating freely. **A** and **B,** Embryo with 12-mm crown-rump length is attached to the wall by a short umbilical cord. No yolk sac was seen; it likely regressed. **C,** 3-D view. **D,** Sac is floating in a water bath so that the white chorionic villi are seen extending outward. The villi only cover a portion of the sac. The villi normally degenerate over the area of the sac not at the implantation site. **E,** Magnified view of the villi, and **F,** a vessel within the sac *(arrow)*.

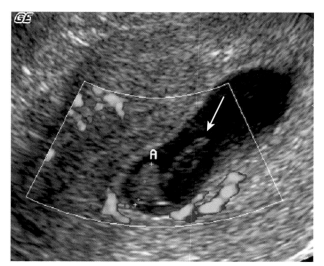

FIGURE 30-25. Collapsed amnion. Transvaginal power Doppler ultrasound scan of a gestational sac in a 39-year-old woman who presented with spotting at 9½ weeks. The embryo is small with a crown-rump length *(calipers)* of 7 mm, consistent with 7 weeks. No cardiac activity is seen. The amniotic membrane *(arrow)* is collapsed adjacent to the embryo.

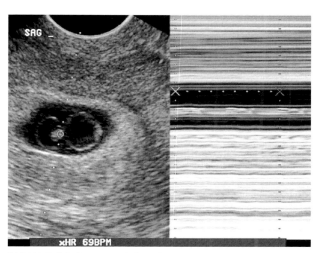

FIGURE 30-26. Fetal bradycardia. A small embryo in a 10-week gestation with a heart rate of 69 beats/min. This embryo died, and the pregnancy aborted within 1 week. The embryo is seen within a round amniotic sac on the left and lies beside a large yolk sac on the right.

An **abnormally large yolk sac** is often the first sonographic indicator of pathology and is invariably associated with subsequent embryonic demise (Fig. 30-30). Even if the pregnancy survives the first trimester, however, the fetus may still be abnormal. In our experience, although the number of cases is small, large yolk sacs have been associated with fetal pathologic states, including chromosomal abnormalities (trisomy 21, partial molar pregnancy[73]) and omphalocele. Yolk sac abnormalities should be used as a predictor of abnormal

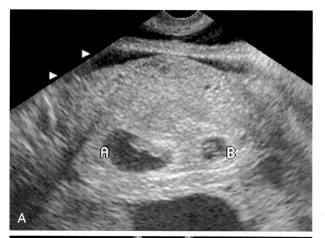

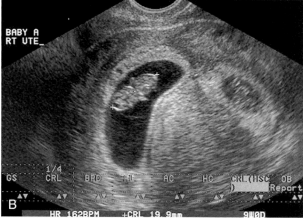

FIGURE 30-27. Twins: one normal, one with small sac. A, Transverse transvaginal scan at 8 weeks shows two sacs *(A, B),* with the left larger than the right sac. **B,** At 9 weeks the normal-sized embryo on the maternal right is of appropriate size, 19.9 mm *(calipers),* with a normal-sized gestational sac. The other twin did not grow normally.

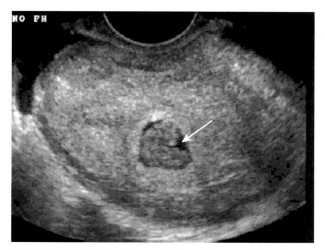

FIGURE 30-28. Small gestational sac and embryo. Sagittal transvaginal scan of a 21-year-old woman at 9 weeks' gestational age with spotting. There is a small gestational sac that is no larger than the embryo *(arrow).* The crown-rump length and mean sac diameter are about equal. No heartbeat was seen.

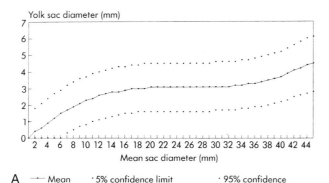

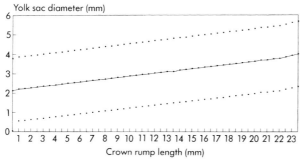

FIGURE 30-29. Normal obstetric data. A, Yolk sac versus mean sac diameter. B, Crown-rump length versus yolk sac. Yolk sac diameter and shape at endovaginal ultrasound are predictors of pregnancy outcome in the first trimester. *(From Lindsay DJ, Lovett IS, Lyons EA, et al. Yolk sac diameter and shape at endovaginal ultrasound: predictors of pregnancy outcome in the first trimester. Radiology 1992;183:115-118.)*

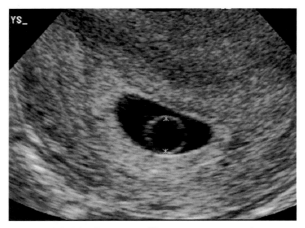

FIGURE 30-30. Large yolk sac. Transvaginal scan at 9 weeks shows gestational sac with a small embryo with bradycardia *(not shown)* and a large yolk sac *(calipers)* with mean internal diameter of 5.9 mm. On follow-up examination 7 days later (not shown), no cardiac activity was identified, indicating embryonic demise and the yolk sac had become smaller and more echogenic.

outcome, and patients with abnormal yolk sac size or shape should be followed closely. If the fetus survives the first trimester, follow-up examination should be performed at 18 to 20 weeks' MA to evaluate the fetus for anomalies. Genetic counseling should also be offered.

A **calcified yolk sac** appears as a shadowing echogenic mass in the absence of any other identifiable yolk sac. It has not been reported to be associated with a live embryo before 12 weeks' MA. In fact, a calcified yolk sac will only be seen with a dead embryo and may calcify within 36 hours after demise (Fig. 30-31; **Video 30-3**).

The yolk sac can be filled with **echogenic material** and is not the same as one that is calcified. This can be seen in live pregnancies (Fig. 30-32). Szabo et al.[74] followed such cases alone and in conjunction with **nuchal lucency** in 3620 first-trimester pregnancies. They found 39 cases (1.0%) of echogenic yolk sacs 1.8 to 4.0 mm in diameter in pregnancies at 9 to 11 weeks' MA; 19 of the 39 (49%) had both a nuchal lucency greater than 3 mm and an echogenic yolk sac, with all 19 chromosomally abnormal, and the other 20 (51%) had an echogenic yolk sac as the only unusual finding, with all delivered normally.

In our experience, in pregnancies less than 10 weeks' gestation, an embryo without a visible yolk sac is abnormal and associated with an abnormal outcome (assuming that careful TVS has been performed to look for the yolk sac). If the embryo is alive and a yolk sac is not visible, the index of suspicion for abnormal outcome should be increased and a follow-up examination performed.

Low Human Chorionic Gonadotropin

Nyberg et al.[20] found that 65% of abnormal pregnancies had a disproportionately low serum β-hCG for gestational sac size. This had a positive predictive value and specificity of 100%.

Subchorionic Hemorrhage

Subchorionic hemorrhage, or a hematoma resulting from abruption of the placental margin or marginal sinus rupture,[75] causes elevation of the chorionic membrane. This is an uncommon finding late in the first trimester and may be associated with vaginal bleeding. Ball et al.[76] found an overall incidence of 1.3%. The chorionic membrane is stripped from the endometrium (decidua vera) and elevated by the hematoma (Figs. 30-33 and 30-34). These hemorrhages are contiguous with the placental edge, but the predominant accumulation of blood products is often remote from the placenta.[77] **Acute hemorrhage** is usually hyperechoic or isoechoic relative to the placenta. The hemorrhage gradually becomes sonolucent in 1 to 2 weeks. Often the cause of membrane elevation is obvious because fluid is present deep to the membrane and is more echoic than the amniotic fluid, indicating a subchorionic hemorrhage.

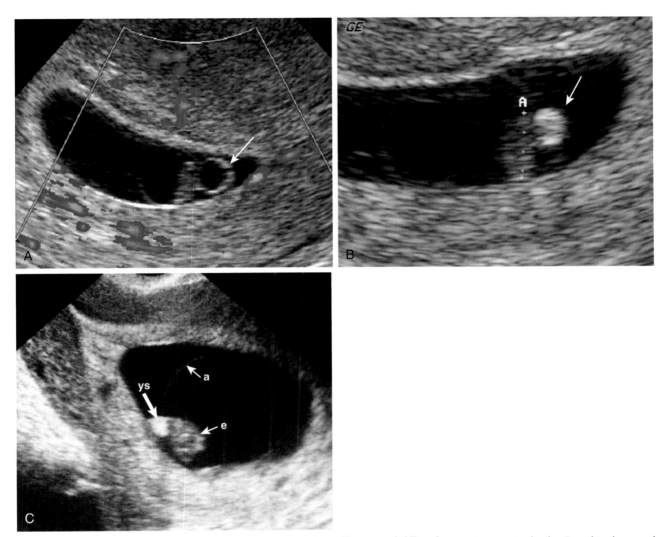

FIGURE 30-31. Intrauterine embryonic death with yolk sac calcification. A, Transvaginal color Doppler ultrasound scan of a pregnancy at 6½ weeks' menstrual age (CRL, 6.5 mm) shows an embryo with no cardiac activity (no color), and a normal-appearing yolk sac *(arrow).* **B,** Repeat scan 5 days later shows no change in the size of the embryo *(calipers)* and a dense yolk sac *(arrow)* with faint distal shadowing. **C,** In a different pregnancy, transvaginal sagittal scan shows calcified yolk sac *(ys).* No cardiac activity was identified in embryo with crown-rump length of 18 mm. *a,* Amnion; *e,* embryo.

In a group of patients with vaginal bleeding at 10 to 20 weeks' gestation, identification of a subchorionic hemorrhage was associated with a 50% fetal loss rate.[77] In a retrospective study of 516 patients with first-trimester bleeding, Bennett et al.[78] found an overall pregnancy loss rate of 9.3%. This increases with increasing maternal age and decreasing gestational age. For women over age 35, the rate is 13.8% (vs. 7.3 for those ≤35), and for those presenting at or before 8 weeks, it is 13.7% (vs. only 5.9% for those later in gestation). The most important predictor for pregnancy loss was the presence of a large subchorionic hemorrhage.[78] The small or medium-sized hemorrhages (i.e., ≤50% the sac circumference) had a miscarriage rate of 9%, versus 18.8% for the larger subchorionic hemorrhages.

Ball et al.[76] found an increased risk of miscarriage (odds ratio [OR], 2.8), stillbirth (OR, 4.5), abruptio placentae

(OR, 11.2), and preterm labor (OR, 2.6) when women with hemorrhaging were compared with controls without subchorionic hemorrhage or bleeding. The presence of bleeding alone also increased the risk of miscarriage.

Abu-Yousef et al.[79] followed 21 cases of subchorionic hematoma (8-19 weeks' gestation), and 17 had vaginal bleeding; 71% had an unfavorable outcome of spontaneous abortion or prematurity. They found significant correlation between pregnancy outcome and hematoma size, severity of bleeding, and presence of pain, but no correlation between outcome and elevation of the placental edge.

Pedersen and Mantoni[80] studied 342 pregnant women from 9 to 20 weeks' gestation presenting with vaginal bleeding and found subchorionic hematomas in 18%, averaging 20 cc (range, 2-150) in size. Although most studies show an association between subchorionic

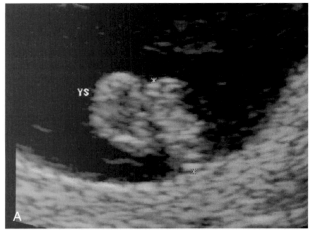

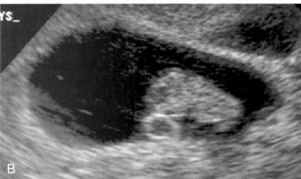

FIGURE 30-32. Echogenic material within yolk sac.
A, Single live embryo at 7 weeks' gestational age with echogenic material within the yolk sac *(ys)* next to a live embryo. **B,** One week later the yolk sac looks normal, and the pregnancy continued uneventfully.

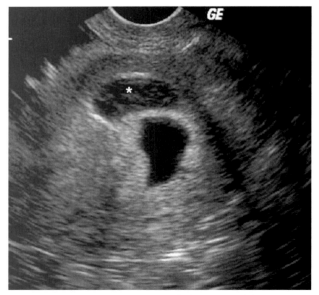

FIGURE 30-33. Moderate subchorionic bleed. Sagittal transvaginal scan of an 8-week gestation with no spotting. The moderate subchorionic bleed (*) is seen adjacent to the gestational sac. The live embryo was not in the field of view. The bleed resolved and pregnancy continued uneventfully.

hemorrhage and abnormal outcome, this study found no difference in the rate of miscarriage (10%) or premature delivery (11%) between the patients with and without subchorionic hematomas.

Doppler Ultrasound Assessment

In the normal pregnancy, maternal peripheral vascular resistance decreases as early as 5 weeks' gestation.[81] Uterine arterial flow resistance decreases progressively after implantation but increases in women with pre-eclampsia or IUGR.[82] Normally, before 12 weeks' gestation, no flow is detectable within the trophoblastic ring, consisting of the intervillous space, chorionic villi, and their fetal vessels.[83] As noted previously, low-resistance arterial flow is present normally in the decidual spiral arteries.[7]

Controversy surrounds whether Doppler sonography of the uterine or spiral arteries is useful in predicting pregnancy outcome. Extravillous trophoblastic cells invade the decidual spiral arteries. Inadequate trophoblastic invasion of the spiral arteries may be seen in early pregnancy failure and may be associated with increased resistance to flow in the spiral arteries. Jaffe et al.[83] suggest that an abnormal RI (>0.55) in the decidual spiral arteries and active arterial blood flow in the intervillous space may be associated with an increased incidence of early pregnancy failure. They speculate that abnormal, high-pressure blood flow in the spiral arteries may result in significantly increased pressure to the immature villi, causing detachment of the early villi and subsequent miscarriage. Others have not found Doppler ultrasound to be predictive of pregnancy outcome.[84,85]

Nakatsuka et al.[86] found that the **pulsatility index** (PI) of the uterine artery in two groups (N = 52) of women at 4 to 5 weeks' gestation was significantly higher in the group with recurrent pregnancy loss (≥2 consecutive losses), as well as in women with elevated antinuclear or antiphospholipid antibodies, compared to the control group. In the group with recurrent loss, uterine artery PI was significantly higher even in those without elevated antibodies. The authors strongly suggest that uterine artery PI is an independent index for recurrent pregnancy loss. The mean values of PI for the controls were 2.20 ± 0.52, and for the recurrent loss group, 2.5 ± 0.52. Those with elevated antibodies and recurrent loss had PI of 3.08 ± 0.61 or higher. The study outcome was not entirely clear because women with recurrent losses were treated with aspirin, heparin, or both in early pregnancy, a result of the current belief that coagulopathy and vascular dysfunction may impair uterine perfusion and result in pregnancy loss. Leible et al.[87] studied the uterine artery PI in 318 consecutive early pregnancies from 6 to 12 weeks and found that a significant difference between the two uterine arteries was strongly associated with pregnancy failure before 20 weeks, likely because of uterine ischemia.

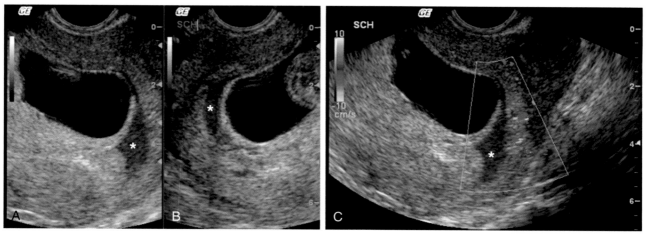

FIGURE 30-34. Small subchorionic bleed. A, Sagittal transvaginal scan of a 10-week gestation with a small subchorionic hemorrhage (*) elevating the posterior placental edge in the lower uterine segment. **B,** Transverse scan of the small bleed. **C,** Sagittal transvaginal color Doppler ultrasound showing no flow in the subchorionic bleed.

Amniotic Sac Abnormalities

A large amniotic sac compared to the CRL is predictive of abnormal outcome. Horrow[88] demonstrated that the difference between the CRL and the amniotic sac diameter is 1.1 ± 2.0 mm in normal embryos, but 8.6 ± 3.8 mm in abnormal pregnancies. In abnormal early pregnancies the chorionic cavity remained appropriate in size relative to the embryonic CRL, indicating that the increased difference in CRL compared to amnion diameter is caused by enlargement of the amnion rather than a small embryo. This finding is especially useful in early embryos before visualization of cardiac activity. As with other predictors of abnormal outcome, patients with abnormal amnion diameters should be considered at increased risk and should have a follow-up ultrasound examination.

Termination of Early Pregnancy Failure

Termination may be surgical, medical, or expectant management. **Surgical termination** is generally by suction dilation and curettage (D&C) of the intrauterine contents under local or light general anesthesia. **Medical termination,** using mifepristone (600 mg) then misoprostol (400 μg) orally 2 days later, was found to be more acceptable to women than surgical intervention; the majority would repeat this management or would recommend it to others.[89] Later regimens used misoprostol vaginally rather than orally with greater success. In 220 consecutive pregnancy failures using repeated doses of mifepristone and misoprostol, Wagaarachchi et al.[90] defined success as complete uterine evacuation within 3 days.[90] The overall success rate was 84%. Success in symptomatic women was 80%, versus 94% in asymptomatic women.

Expectant management of incomplete first-trimester miscarriage was tested by Luise et al.,[91] who found that 91% (201/221) miscarried within 9 days (range, 1-32); 54% were complete within 7 days, 83% within 14 days, and 89% within 21 days. There was no correlation between the presence or absence of a gestational sac and failed medical management. Twenty women required surgery, with 19 elective and uneventful and one emergent with excessive bleeding, pain, fever, and leukocytosis.

Retained Products of Conception

Retained products of conception (RPOC) can have a spectrum of sonographic appearances, from a seemingly empty uterus to a large, echogenic mass of tissue filling the endometrial canal. We have found that the presence of focal increased vascularity is of great importance in distinguishing between blood clots and RPOC. There can be a single vessel or a large group of vessels, either superficially in the myometrium or extending deep within it. The vascularity shows high-velocity flow up to 160 cm/sec with a mass of vessels. This can appear very dramatic on the scan and, because of the high flow, can raise concern about performing D&C. We have seen this as a common finding, however, with a surprising lack of any untoward bleeding during or after the surgery (Fig. 30-35).

ECTOPIC PREGNANCY

Ectopic pregnancy remains one of the leading causes of maternal death in the United States. It accounts for 1.4% of all pregnancies and approximately 15% of maternal deaths. Although the incidence of ectopic pregnancy is increasing, the mortality has declined to less than 1 in 1000 cases compared with 3.5 in 1000 in 1970.[92,93] The increased incidence is likely caused by

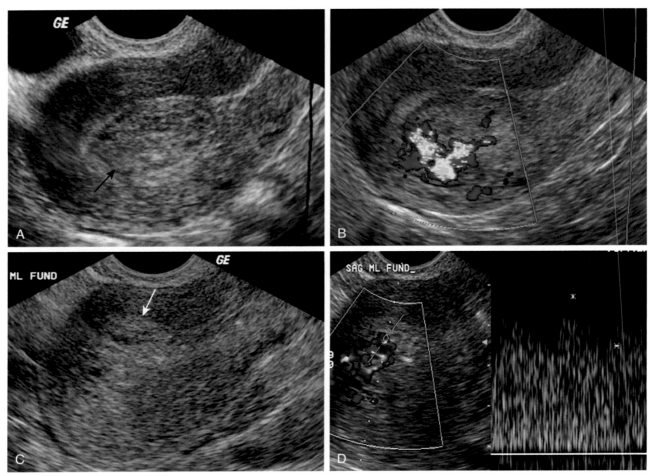

FIGURE 30-35. Retained products of conception. A, Sagittal transvaginal scan of a 22-year-old woman who presented 5 weeks after a suction dilation and curettage (D&C) therapeutic abortion with vaginal bleeding. The endometrial canal is distended with a 1.8 × 2.5–cm echogenic mass (*arrows*). **B,** Color Doppler ultrasound shows an area of marked increase in vascularity at the base of the mass at its attachment to the myometrium. **C,** Sagittal transvaginal scan of a 28-year-old woman who had suction D&C for a therapeutic abortion 6 weeks previously with vaginal bleeding. The myometrium in the body anteriorly was heterogeneous with increased echogenicity. **D,** Color spectral Doppler ultrasound shows increased vascularity with velocities of 1.3 m/sec.

increased prevalence of the risk factors as well as earlier diagnosis, whereas heightened awareness and improved diagnostic capabilities have decreased mortality.

Clinical Presentation

The classic clinical triad of pain, abnormal vaginal bleeding, and a palpable adnexal mass is only present in approximately 45% of patients with ectopic pregnancy.[94] In addition, the positive predictive value of this triad is only 14%. Other presenting signs and symptoms include any combination of the classic triad, as well as amenorrhea, adnexal tenderness, and cervical motion tenderness. Schwartz and DiPietro[94] found that only 9% of patients with clinically suspected ectopic pregnancy actually had an ectopic pregnancy, whereas 17% had symptomatic ovarian cysts, 13% had pelvic inflammatory disease, 8% had dysfunctional uterine bleeding, and 7% had spontaneous abortions. The clinical presentation is thus nonspecific.

Importantly, even in the early 1990s, 5% of proven ectopic pregnancies bypass all imaging and go directly to surgery. In addition, even in retrospect, 8.7% of proven ectopic pregnancies are sonographically normal.[95]

The **prevalence** of ectopic pregnancy varies according to the patient population and their inherent risk factors. Nevertheless, all patients in the reproductive age group are at risk. Factors that increase the **risk** of ectopic pregnancy include tubal abnormality preventing passage of the zygote or resulting in delayed transit; previous tubal pregnancy,[96,97] cesarean section, or tubal reconstructive surgery; pelvic inflammatory disease; chlamydial salpingitis;[98] intrauterine contraceptive devices; and increased age or parity.

There is a strong association between **infertility** and ectopic pregnancy, likely because of the shared tubal abnormalities in both conditions. The risk factors for ectopic pregnancy are therefore present in patients who undergo ovulation induction or in vitro fertilization (IVF) and embryo transfer. The increased incidence of

RISK OF ECTOPIC PREGNANCY

Any tubal abnormality that may prevent passage of
   zygote or result in delayed transit
Previous tubal pregnancy
History of tubal reconstructive surgery
Pelvic inflammatory disease
Intrauterine contraceptive device
Increased maternal age
Increased parity
Previous cesarean section

multiple pregnancies with ovulation induction and IVF further increases the risk for both ectopic and **hetero-topic** (coexistent intrauterine and ectopic) gestation. The hydrostatic forces generated during embryo transfer may also contribute to the increased risk.[99] The frequency of heterotopic pregnancy was originally estimated on a theoretic basis to be 1 in 30,000 pregnancies. More recent data indicate that the rate is approximately 1 in 7000 pregnancies.[100,101]

Sonographic Diagnosis

When women present with a positive pregnancy test or a history suggestive of ectopic pregnancy (missed period, pain, unprotected intercourse), it is critical to identify the presence and location of the gestational sac. Pelvic ultrasound and especially TVS must be the first line of imaging investigation. TVS allows for a more detailed evaluation of the endometrium, endometrial canal, and adnexa than TAS. The imaging component must be augmented by the clinical findings of tenderness elicited by the transvaginal probe. Uterine tenderness is uncommon, but adnexal tenderness may be important in leading to the ectopic site or less often to a ruptured or leaking corpus luteum cyst. Focal uterine tenderness may be seen with an IUP and a degenerating fibroid or in the nongravid female from adenomyosis. Endometritis and pelvic inflammatory disease are causes of a more generalized type of pelvic pain.

 We begin the examination with TAS through a full bladder, if possible, looking for a large or complex mass that may be outside the range of the transvaginal probe. The mass may be the extrauterine gestational sac or a large hematoma. At the end of TAS, we always look for free fluid in the hepatorenal space (Fig. 30-36; **Video 30-4**). This provides a sense of the degree of blood loss. Although hemodynamically stable with a large volume of fluid loss, the patient could decompensate rapidly. Fluid seen in the hepatorenal space should impart a greater sense of urgency to the surgeon.

We then perform a vaginal scan, assessing the uterus, ovaries, and adnexal regions. If the ovary and tube cannot be seen on one side, in a suspected ectopic pregnancy, a

helpful maneuver is to try and push the ovary down toward the transvaginal probe by pressing firmly on the anterior abdominal wall. The clinician must watch the screen carefully for an echogenic mass or ectopic sac as the adnexa is pushed downward and into the field of view.

In early IUP, early pregnancy failure, or ectopic pregnancy, it is not always possible to identify the gestational sac. Several nonspecific sonographic findings may help in localization of the gestational sac. However, ectopic pregnancy is generally excluded with the demonstration of an IUP (which reduces the risk of coexistent ectopic pregnancy to 1 in 7000) or is confirmed with demonstration of a live embryo in the adnexa.

Specific Findings

The earlier demonstration of an IUP is the most important contribution of TVS (vs. TAS) in the evaluation of patients presenting with suspected ectopic pregnancy. In a series of suspected ectopic pregnancies by Dashefsky et al.,[102] all 19 normal intrauterine pregnancies were identified by TVS, versus only 11 of 19 for TAS. In addition, TVS identified 7 of 16 abnormal IUPs, versus 3 of 16 for TAS.[102]

As described earlier, the intradecidual sign and the double-decidual sign can be used to identify an IUP before visualization of the yolk sac or embryo. The double-decidual sign must be distinguished from the **decidual cast** or **pseudogestational sac** of ectopic pregnancy. A **pseudosac** is an intrauterine fluid collection surrounded by a single decidual layer (Fig. 30-37), as opposed to the two concentric rings of the double-decidual sign. TVS allows for differentiation of the decidua, which produces the pseudogestational sac, from the choriodecidual reaction of the double-decidual sign of IUP.[103]

Doppler ultrasound and in particular color flow Doppler imaging may further help distinguish a gestational sac from pseudosac. **Peritrophoblastic flow** is high-velocity, low-resistance flow with low RI and PI. Dillon et al.[104] studied a series of 40 patients with an empty saclike structure in the uterus. They defined peritrophoblastic flow as a peak systolic frequency of 0.8 kHz or greater (corresponding to 21 cm/sec with no angle correction) and correctly classified 26 of 31 IUPs and 9 of 9 pseudogestational sacs.[104]

When there is no sonographic evidence of an IUP, the pregnant patient is more likely to harbor an extra-uterine gestation. Because TVS allows for the earlier identification of an IUP, it significantly increases the accuracy of diagnosis in patients with suspected ectopic gestation.[105]

The sonographic demonstration of a **live embryo in the adnexa** is specific for the diagnosis of ectopic pregnancy (Fig. 30-38). A live extrauterine embryo/fetus has been detected with TVS in 17% to 28% of patients

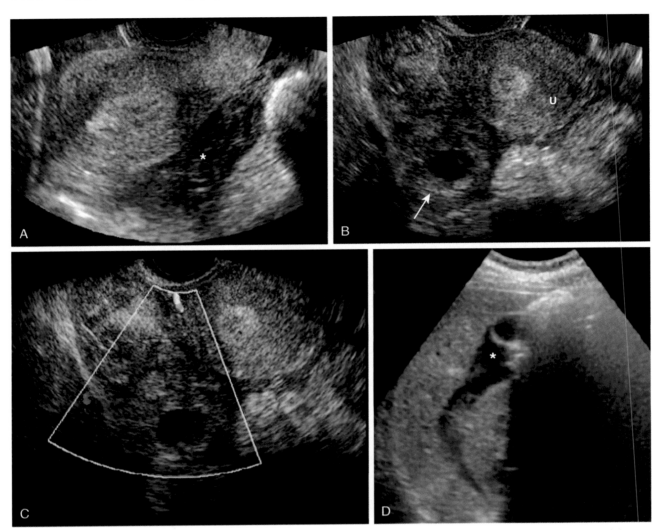

FIGURE 30-36. Ruptured ectopic pregnancy with hemoperitoneum. A 35-year-old woman presented at 6 weeks' gestation with right lower quadrant pain. **A,** Sagittal transvaginal scan shows echogenic material within the endometrial cavity but no gestational sac. Blood clot is (*) seen around the uterus. **B,** Coronal transvaginal scan of the uterus *(U)* and a complex right adnexal mass with a sac at its posterior aspect *(arrow)*. **C,** Coronal color Doppler sonogram with no vascularity seen. **D,** Sagittal scan of the left upper abdomen showing free fluid (*).

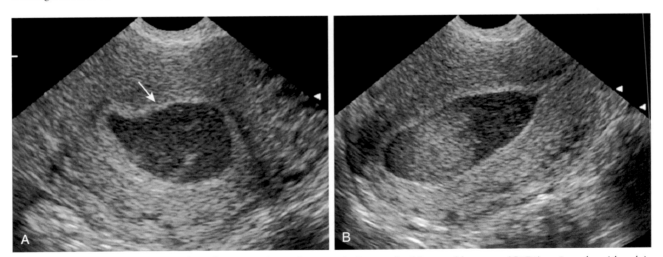

FIGURE 30-37. Pseudogestational sac. A, Coronal transvaginal scan of a 33-year-old woman (G2P1) at 8 weeks with pelvic pain. There is a rounded intrauterine sac filled with low-level echoes. No yolk sac or embryo is seen. There is a single echogenic ring around the fluid *(arrow)*. This is a fluid-filled endometrial canal, a decidual cast, or pseudogestational sac. **B,** Sagittal transvaginal scan shows a large pseudogestational sac with echogenic debris. Note the acute angle at the lower end, uncommon in a gestational sac.

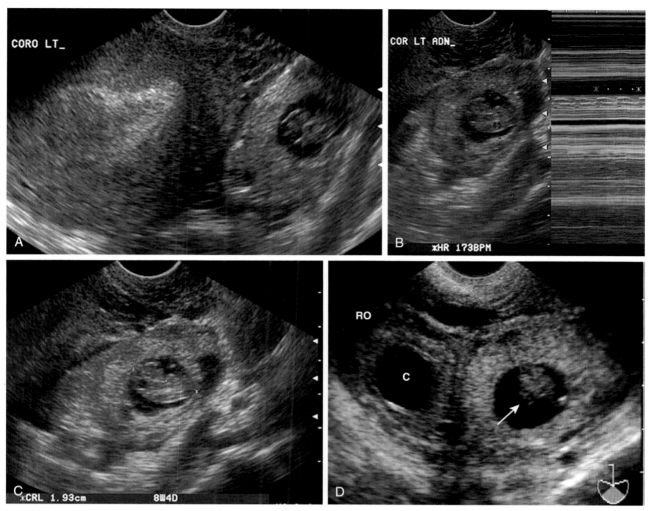

FIGURE 30-38. Live ectopic pregnancy. A 33-year-old woman presented with left lower quadrant pain at 9 weeks' gestation. **A,** Coronal transvaginal scan shows the empty endometrial cavity on the right and a gestational sac and embryo on the left. **B,** M-mode image demonstrates a live embryo with cardiac activity at a rate of 173 beats/min. **C,** The embryonic crown-rump length is 19 mm. **D,** In a different patient, coronal transvaginal scan of the right ovary with a corpus luteum cyst *(c)* and a gestational sac with a single live embryo immediately adjacent *(arrow).*

with ectopic pregnancy,[106,107] versus only 10% with TAS. Cardiac activity can be demonstrated with M-mode, color, or power Doppler sonography.

Nonspecific Findings

When the sonographic findings are nonspecific, correlation with serum β-hCG levels improves the ability of sonography to distinguish between intrauterine and ectopic pregnancy. **A negative β-hCG essentially excludes the presence of a live pregnancy.** The serum β-hCG test yields positive results at approximately 23 days of gestational age.[108] This is before a normal intrauterine gestational sac may be imaged with TVS. Different types of sonographic techniques and equipment have different hCG discriminatory levels above which gestational sacs are large enough to be imaged routinely. Nyberg et al.[109] identified a β-hCG threshold level of 1800 mIU/mL (Second IS), above which it was always

possible to identify a normal intrauterine gestational sac by TAS. Threshold levels of 500 to 1000 mIU/mL (Second IS) have been proposed for TVS (1000-2000 for IRP).[109] Some further refinement of a threshold level is recommended for the equipment and expertise in each individual institution. If the hCG level is above the threshold level, it should be possible to identify a normal intrauterine gestational sac. If an intrauterine gestational sac is not identified, an ectopic pregnancy becomes the diagnosis of exclusion. An early complete or incomplete abortion, however, may give a similar clinical and sonographic appearance. As noted earlier, published threshold levels do not take into consideration multifetal pregnancies or patients with an enlarged uterus from fibroids.[110]

If the β-hCG level is below the threshold level, the sonogram may still identify an ectopic pregnancy. The utility of the threshold level is to raise the index of suspicion for an ectopic pregnancy when no intrauterine gestational sac is identified. TVS should be performed even when the β-hCG levels are low because some patients may have suggestive or diagnostic findings. In indeterminate cases when the patient is clinically stable, serial quantitative serum hCG levels may be helpful in distinguishing ectopic pregnancy, early pregnancy failure, and early IUP. The β-hCG level in a normal pregnancy has a doubling time of approximately 2 days, whereas patients with a dead or dying gestation have a falling β-hCG level. Patients with ectopic pregnancy usually have a slower increase in hCG levels, although they occasionally show patterns similar to a normal pregnancy or spontaneous abortion.

The presence of nonspecific adnexal findings improves the ability of sonography to predict an ectopic pregnancy. An adnexal mass can be found in conditions other than ectopic pregnancy (hemorrhagic corpus luteum cyst, endometriosis, and abscess) and is therefore not diagnostic. However, the presence of an adnexal mass in patients without sonographic evidence of an IUP and a positive β-hCG test result strongly suggests an ectopic pregnancy. A suspected ectopic mass should be assessed during the transvaginal examination for local tenderness. The probe is used to apply light pressure on the mass. This pressure almost always elicits pain similar to the sensation that brought the patient to hospital initially. Pain can also be felt with other inflammatory or expanding masses, such as a hemorrhagic corpus luteum. Because the fallopian tube is the most common location for an ectopic pregnancy, scanning with the vaginal probe should allow for visualization of the ectopic pregnancy moving separate from the ovary as probe pressure is applied. This motion helps distinguish between a hemorrhagic corpus luteum cyst and an ectopic pregnancy.

Fleischer et al.[103] found an **ectopic tubal ring** in 49% of patients with ectopic pregnancy and in 68% of unruptured tubal pregnancies, using TVS (Fig. 30-39). The tubal ring can usually be differentiated from a corpus

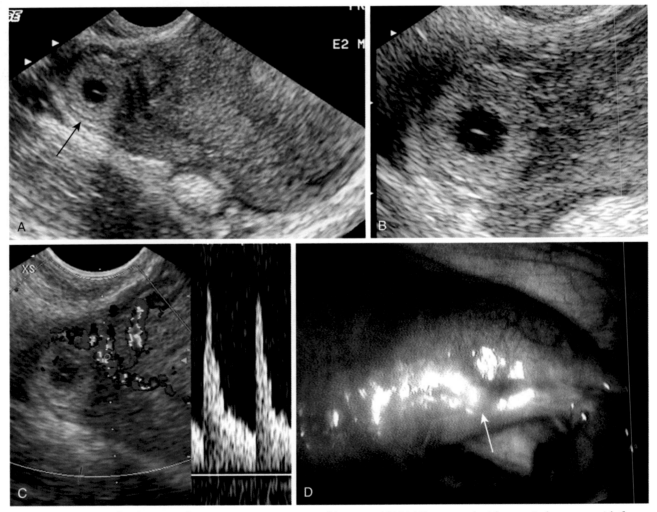

FIGURE 30-39. Isthmic ectopic pregnancy. A 35-year-old woman (G3P1A1) presented with no pain but was at risk for an ectopic pregnancy. **A,** Coronal transvaginal scan shows an empty uterus and a tubal ring (*arrow*) immediately adjacent to the uterus. **B,** Magnified view of the ring shows a gestational sac with a yolk sac, confirming an ectopic pregnancy. **C,** Color flow Doppler ultrasound shows increased vascularity around the sac with high-velocity flow. **D,** At laparoscopy, ectopic site can be seen bulging the isthmic portion of the tube (*arrow*). It was successfully removed by salpingostomy.

luteum cyst because the cyst is eccentrically located with a rim of ovarian tissue. A tubal ring is a concentric ring created by the trophoblast of the ectopic pregnancy surrounding the chorionic sac. This ring is often within a hematoma that may be confined to the fallopian tube or that may extend outside it. Frates et al.[111] found that an ectopic tubal ring was more echogenic than ovarian parenchyma, whether or not the sac was empty or had a yolk sac or embryo. The corpus luteum in a proven IUP was as or less echogenic than ovarian parenchyma in 93% of cases. The wall of the corpus luteum is usually less echogenic than the endometrium. Stein et al.[112] found that the tubal ring of an ectopic pregnancy was more echogenic than the endometrium in 32% of cases, a finding that can be helpful in distinguishing between a tubal ring and a corpus luteum cyst.

The ectopic tubal ring may be obscured or replaced by a mass that is often echogenic (Fig. 30-40) but may be of mixed echogenicity (Fig. 30-41). Easily overlooked or mistaken for fat or bowel, these masses will be found only with a high index of suspicion and careful TVS of the adnexa, looking for the tubal ring or mass that is focally tender.

Transvaginal ultrasound is extremely sensitive in detecting **free pelvic fluid.** The presence of echogenic free fluid (hemoperitoneum; Fig. 30-40, *B*) or blood clots in the posterior cul-de-sac in pregnant patients, without sonographic evidence of an IUP, should strongly suggest an ectopic pregnancy. The presence of small amounts of nonechogenic free fluid is nonspecific and is seen in normal patients.

In 132 consecutive patients with surgical confirmation, Frates et al.[113] found that the presence or the amount of intraperitoneal fluid was not a reliable indicator of rupture. Rupture was present in 21% of patients with no fluid and increasingly, up to 63%, with large amounts. Interestingly, 37% of patients with a large amount of fluid had intact tubes and no evidence of rupture. Intraperitoneal fluid is possible if the blood escapes through the fimbriated end of the intact fallopian tube.

Implantation Site

Ectopic pregnancy may occur in several sites. Approximately 95% of ectopic pregnancies occur in the ampul-

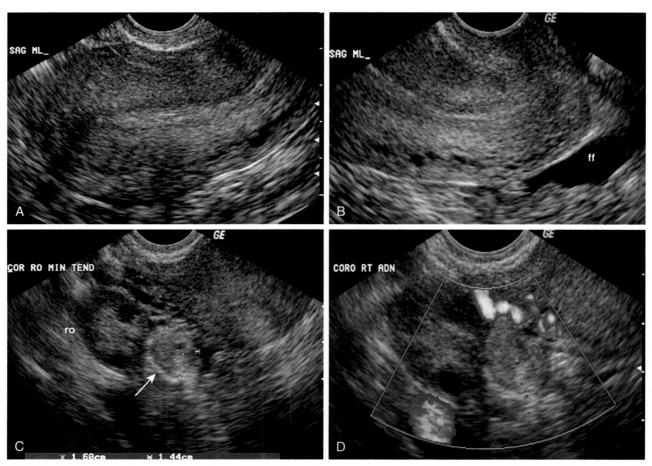

FIGURE 30-40. Ectopic pregnancy seen as echogenic mass. A 33-year-old woman presented at 7 weeks' gestation with right lower quadrant pain. **A,** Transvaginal scan shows an empty uterus. **B,** Free fluid *(ff)* in the cul-de-sac. **C,** In right adnexa there was a 1.4 × 1.6–cm echogenic mass *(arrow)* adjacent to a normal ovary *(ro).* The mass was focally tender to palpation with the vaginal probe. **D,** Power Doppler ultrasound shows minimal internal vascularity.

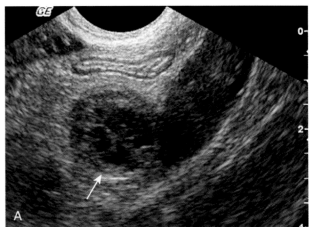

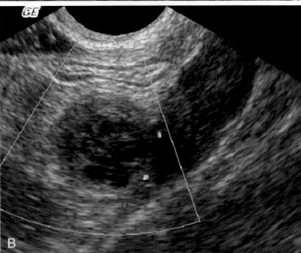

FIGURE 30-41. Ectopic pregnancy seen as mixed-echogenicity mass. A 30-year-old woman presented with left lower quadrant pain at 7 weeks' gestation and β-hCG of 500 mIU/mL and falling over a 3-day period. **A,** In the left adnexa, medial to the left ovary, there was a 2-cm mass *(arrow)* with mixed echogenicity, and **B,** only minimal peripheral vascularity. A left ectopic pregnancy was confirmed and based on a falling β-hCG was treated expectantly and resolved without complication.

lary or isthmic portions of the fallopian tube. The second most common site, about 2% to 3% of all ectopic pregnancies, is an interstitial pregnancy occurring in the intramural portion of the tube, where it traverses the wall of the uterus to enter the endometrial canal. Ovarian, cervical, and abdominal sites of ectopic pregnancy are extremely rare.

Implantation in the superior lateral portion of the endometrial canal *but not* within the intramural portion of the tube is normal and is *not* an ectopic pregnancy. This is often mistaken for an ectopic pregnancy, but echogenic endometrium can be seen around the sac (double-decidual sign), and if followed even for 1 week, the sac grows and usually extends into the endometrial canal.

Because of its intramural location, **interstitial ectopic pregnancies** (cornual) rupture later than other tubal gestations, often causing massive intraperitoneal hemorrhage from the dilated arcuate arteries and veins, which lie in the outer third of the myometrium between the thin outer myometrium and the thick intermediate layer. The mortality of interstitial pregnancy is twice that of other ectopic pregnancies. Ackerman et al.[114] found that the two currently used sonographic signs of myometrial thinning and sac eccentricity are unreliable and described the more useful **interstitial line sign** (Fig. 30-42). The interstitial line is a thin, echogenic line extending from the endometrial canal up to the center of the interstitial sac or hemorrhagic mass. It was seen in 92% of interstitial ectopic pregnancies. The line is the nondistended, empty endometrial canal. The interstitial ectopic pregnancy is usually surrounded by trophoblast but should not have a double-decidual sign. Thinning of the myometrial mantle was seen in three of four interstitial sacs; however, eight additional patients had only a mass, with no sac, and therefore no mantle thinning or eccentricity of the sac. All these sacs had an interstitial line. Treatment is usually laparotomy and cornual resection, although methotrexate therapy may be preferable, depending on the size of the interstitial ectopic pregnancy.

Cervical scar implantation appears to be increasing, with more cases appearing in the literature.[115] The patient may present with painless vaginal bleeding and a history of one or more cesarean sections. An early sonogram will show a sac implanted in the lower uterine segment, with local thinning of the myometrium (Fig. 30-43; **Video 30-5**). There is usually prominent vascularity at the implantation site. Catastrophic hemorrhage may result, with the need for complete hysterectomy and, if involved, major bladder reconstruction. Remember that an aborting gestational sac may present in the lower uterine segment on its way out of the uterus. Sonographically, the sac will be oblong, the embryo if present will be dead, and there will be *no* trophoblastic vascularity because it has detached from the uterine wall. Vascularity is an important distinguishing feature between a cervical scar implantation and an incomplete abortion. Clinically, both situations are associated with vaginal bleeding, but the abortion more likely with crampy pain as well. Treatment of a scar implantation is often protracted. A D&C is seldom advised because the thin lower segment may be perforated. Medical therapy is more common, with methotrexate taken systemically and often injected locally as well. Presence of a live embryo may require careful injection of potassium chloride (KCl) into the embryo to stop cardiac activity.

Cervical pregnancy is rare. As in scar pregnancy, vascularity is an important distinguishing feature between a cervical implantation and an incomplete abortion. Treatment is typically with injection of KCl. **Abdominal pregnancies** are also rare. When diagnosed in the first

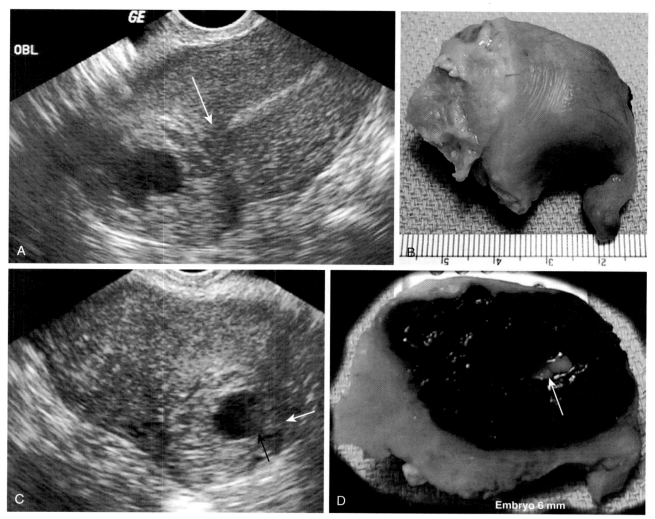

FIGURE 30-42. Interstitial ectopic pregnancy. An 18-year-old woman presented with mild pelvic discomfort with a bulging left cornua. **A,** Sagittal transvaginal sac just to the left of midline. The empty endometrial canal is seen in the body of the uterus with the thin echogenic "interstitial line" *(arrow)* leading to the interstitial ectopic pregnancy. **B,** Postoperative specimen of the wedge resection and removal of the left cornua. **C,** Coronal transvaginal scan of the expanded left cornua with a thin myometrial mantle *(white arrow),* the gestational sac, and the small embryo *(black arrow).* **D,** Bisected specimen shows the sac and the white embryo *(arrow)* that corresponds to the sonogram in **C.**

trimester, these are typically treated similar to tubal ectopic pregnancies. When diagnosed in the third trimester, abdominal pregnancies may result in a viable neonate.

Heterotopic Gestation

When the presence of an IUP is demonstrated with ultrasound, the extremely low frequency of heterotopic pregnancy effectively excludes the diagnosis of an ectopic gestation. However, heterotopic pregnancy should be suspected in the appropriate clinical setting, such as in patients undergoing ovulatory induction or IVF. In IVF patients the rate of heterotopic pregnancy can be as high as 1%. Clearly, if a live embryo is demonstrated in the adnexa in a patient with an intrauterine gestational sac, a specific diagnosis can be made (Fig. 30-44).

Doppler Confirmation

Achiron et al.[116] studied 76 patients with suspected ectopic pregnancy, 42 of whom had ectopic pregnancies, 19 had intrauterine gestations, and 9 had complete abortions. All were stable with a positive β-hCG. They compared standard 2-D imaging with Doppler ultrasound. Trophoblastic flow (high velocity, low impedance) seen outside the uterus had a sensitivity of only 48%, although trophoblastic flow within the uterus or its absence outside excluded an ectopic pregnancy (specificity, 89%). The positive predictive value for ectopic pregnancy was 91% and for 2-D imaging was 95%; negative predictive values were 89% for imaging and 44% for Doppler ultrasound. These data suggest that Doppler sonography has a significantly lower sensitivity and negative predictive value and does not provide more useful diagnostic information than 2-D imaging alone for a

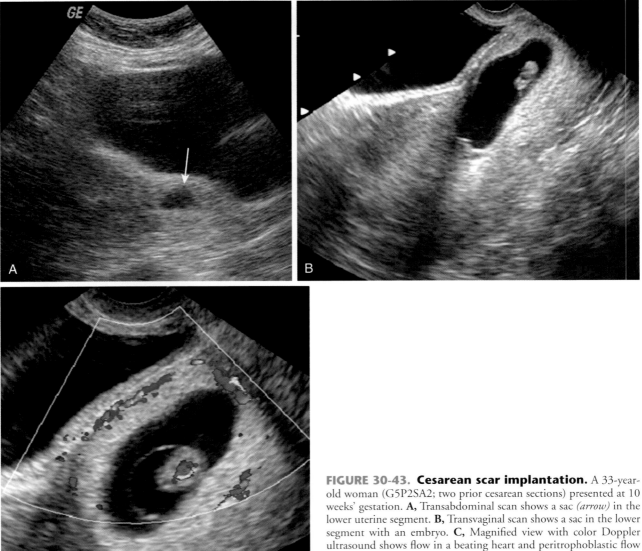

FIGURE 30-43. Cesarean scar implantation. A 33-year-old woman (G5P2SA2; two prior cesarean sections) presented at 10 weeks' gestation. **A,** Transabdominal scan shows a sac *(arrow)* in the lower uterine segment. **B,** Transvaginal scan shows a sac in the lower segment with an embryo. **C,** Magnified view with color Doppler ultrasound shows flow in a beating heart and peritrophoblastic flow anteriorly. Notice how close the echogenic trophoblast is to the anterior serosal surface of the uterus and to the bladder wall.

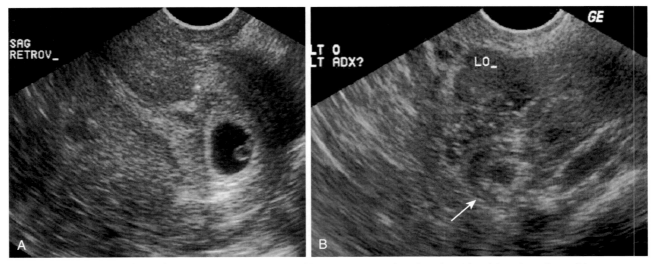

FIGURE 30-44. Heterotopic pregnancy. A 30-year-old woman presented at 6 weeks with pelvic pain and a positive pregnancy test. **A,** Sagittal scan shows a retroverted uterus with a normally positioned 6-week gestational sac with yolk sac. **B,** In the left adnexa, adjacent to the left ovary *(LO),* there is a tubal ring *(arrow)* that proved to be an ectopic sac at laparoscopy.

stable patient with a suspected ectopic pregnancy. In routine practice, Doppler ultrasound is of limited benefit in detecting an ectopic pregnancy but may help decide therapy. If there is good flow around the ectopic site, the tissue presumably is viable, and surgery or methotrexate would be the treatment of choice. If no vascularity is present, the tissue may be nonviable, and the ectopic pregnancy may be aborting spontaneously. Correlation with serial β-hCG levels is helpful, and falling levels provide further evidence that the tissue is being aborted. All these laboratory and sonographic findings must be interpreted in light of the clinical findings of pain and hemodynamic stability.

Pregnancy of Unknown Location

In first-trimester symptomatic patients, the initial TVS correctly identifies the site of implantation in most cases. In a series of unselected patients attending an early pregnancy clinic, the initial TVS examination accurately diagnosed pregnancy location in over 90% of patients and diagnosed 73.9% of ectopic pregnancies.[117] In the absence of a well-defined IUP, or in the absence of an ectopic pregnancy, other findings can suggest the location of the implantation but are nonspecific and can result in diagnostic error. Recently, patients in whom the site of implantation has not been identified with certainty have been categorized as having **pregnancy of unknown location** (PUL). The term refers to an empty endometrial cavity, with no evidence of an intrauterine gestational sac or RPOC, and no extrauterine pregnancy visualized.[118] In classifying a patient as PUL, the assumption is that the diagnostic criteria for ectopic pregnancy are "an empty endometrial cavity with (1) an inhomogeneous adnexal mass or (2) an extrauterine gestational sac with or without a yolk sac and/or embryonic pole." The differential diagnosis for PUL includes a very early IUP, an abnormal IUP, spontaneous miscarriage, and ectopic pregnancy.[119] The proportion of patients categorized as PUL depends on gestational age at examination.

In a series of 5318 unselected women, 456 (8.7%) were classified as PUL.[117] Of the 456 patients classified as PUL, 31 (6.8%) had ectopic pregnancies. The PUL group benefits from close follow-up because of their high incidence of ectopic pregnancy and because they represent 20% to 25% of all ectopic pregnancies. Using the diagnostic criteria just quoted for extrauterine (tubal) pregnancy, some women with an initial ultrasound diagnosis of ectopic pregnancy who are managed nonsurgically may be misdiagnosed. Kirk et al.[117] showed that a single TVS examination using these criteria correctly diagnosed ectopic pregnancy in 96.1% of patients undergoing surgical management. Therefore, using these criteria, 3.9% of patients diagnosed with ectopic pregnancy and treated nonsurgically could have normal or abnormal IUPs. Thus it is important to consider the clinical history and presentation before using nonspecific param-eters in the management of patients with ectopic pregnancy.

Management

The conventional management of ectopic pregnancy has been surgical, with resection of the diseased tube. Improved diagnostic capabilities, including TVS, allow for earlier diagnosis and the potential for a more conservative approach to treatment. The ultimate goal is to diagnose the ectopic pregnancy before tubal rupture and to treat it so as to minimize tubal scarring while maintaining tubal patency. Studying the vascular patterns and histology of tubal pregnancies, Kemp et al.[120] found that those implanted on the mesosalpingeal side of the tube had deeper trophoblastic invasion, more intense trophoblastic proliferation, and increased villous vascularization than those implanted on the anti-mesosalpingeal wall. They suggest conservative management for the anti-mesosalpingeal implantation, because it is more likely to abort spontaneously, and a surgical approach for the potentially more viable mesosalpingeal implantation.

Laparoscopy is often used for definitive diagnosis in ectopic pregnancy and for the more conservative surgical procedures such as salpingotomy.[121] The diseased tube is incised and microdissection used to remove the gestational sac. The incision is then left to heal by secondary intention. The rate of subsequent IUP in these surgical patients is 61.4%, with a 15% rate of recurrent ectopic pregnancy.[122]

Medical management has also been successful in the treatment of early ectopic pregnancy. Cell growth inhibitors such as methotrexate are injected systemically (IV/IM or oral administration) and the serum β-hCG levels followed closely. The methotrexate kills the rapidly dividing trophoblastic cells, which are then reabsorbed, resulting in falling β-hCG levels and, ideally, preservation of the tubal lumen.[123] Success rates range from 61% to 93% for local injection[124] and from 65% to 94% for intramuscular treatment.[125] The rate of side effects is 21% with parenteral administration and 2% with local injection under ultrasonic guidance. Success rate for conception was 58% for IUP, with a 9% recurrent ectopic rate.

Treatment is most successful in tubal pregnancies (vs. interstitial ectopic pregnancy or cervical ectopic pregnancy) and those without embryonic cardiac activity.

Barnhart et al.[126] reviewed studies of multidose and single-dose regimens of methotrexate and found an overall success rate of 89% (1181 of 1327 women). The single dose was used more often but was associated with a significantly greater chance of failure than multidose therapy, although it had fewer side effects. Hajenius et al.[124] compared treatment options of laparoscopy, laparotomy, methotrexate (local vs. systemic, single vs. multiple dose), and expectant management. Multidose IM methotrexate is most cost-effective in patients with low serum β-hCG than laparoscopic salpingostomy. In all cases, both therapies had similar results, with laparoscopy having a higher cost and longer hospital stay.

Nazac et al.[125] studied 137 women with an unruptured ectopic pregnancy and hematosalpinx seen on TVS. They found that in cases with an hCG level less than 1000 mIU/mL, local injection of methotrexate (1 mg/kg) directly into the sac after first aspirating the contents had a 92.5% success rate compared with 67% for IM administration. The local injection was performed vaginally using the same technique as for follicle aspiration during oocyte retrieval in IVF.

A common complication of methotrexate therapy is a rupture of the ectopic pregnancy, with increased pelvic pain and tenderness and the appearance of a hemorrhagic mass (Fig. 30-45). Usually these will resolve with conservative management but occasionally will require surgical intervention.

Conservative management is becoming more common for the stable patient with low or declining

levels of β-hCG. Success rates of up to 69.2% have been reported.[122]

EVALUATION OF THE EMBRYO

The diagnosis of specific fetal anomalies in the first trimester is discussed in the chapters pertaining to the involved organ system. Nuchal translucency screening is discussed in the Chapter 31. This discussion is limited to general principles of assessment of the embryo in the first trimester. Current trends in first-trimester diagnosis, including widespread acceptance of TVS, nuchal translucency screening, and a shift toward testing late in the first trimester, combined with improved equipment resolution, have resulted in the potential diagnosis of a wide range of fetal defects in the first trimester. As the resolution of ultrasound equipment improves, visualization of embryologic structures becomes possible. It is critical that incorrect decisions are not made on the basis

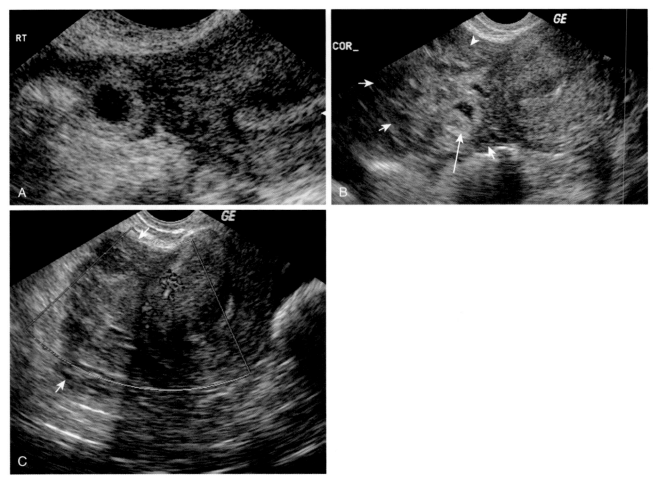

FIGURE 30-45. Ectopic pregnancy with hematoma after methotrexate injection. A, Transvaginal coronal scan through the uterine fundus shows an early isthmic ectopic pregnancy in the right adnexa. **B,** Three days after intramuscular methotrexate, the patient returned with increasing pelvic pain. Transverse scan of the fundus and right adnexa now shows an echogenic mass *(arrowheads)* surrounding the irregular gestational sac *(arrow).* **C,** Sagittal power Doppler ultrasound through the uterus shows vascularity in the myometrium but not in the hematoma superior to it *(short arrows).*

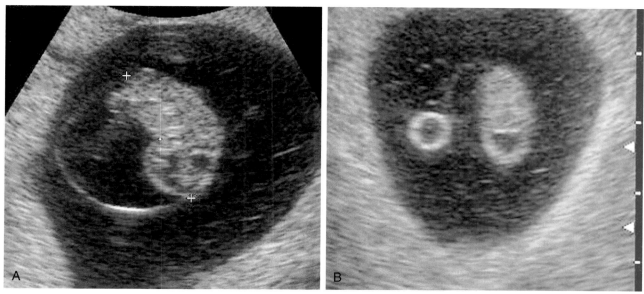

FIGURE 30-46. Normal embryonic intracranial anatomy. A and **B,** Sagittal, and coronal images of 9-week embryo (CRL, 19 mm) clearly show the cystic rhombencephalon.

of incomplete understanding of normal and abnormal embryonic and fetal anatomy in the first trimester. Therefore, if any uncertainty surrounds the findings in an early scan, a follow-up sonographic examination may be indicated for evaluation of fetal morphologic characteristics in the second trimester.

Three major points should be considered: normal embryologic/fetal development may mimic pathology; abnormal embryos/fetuses may appear normal early in pregnancy; and discrepancies between dates and embryo size may be the only visible manifestation of pathology in some first-trimester fetuses.

Normal Embryologic Development Mimicking Pathology

Normal embryologic development in the first trimester may mimic pathologic changes more often seen in the second and third trimesters.

Intracranial Cystic Structures in First Trimester

During the sixth week, three primary brain vesicles form: the **prosencephalon** (forebrain), the **mesencephalon** (midbrain), and the **rhombencephalon** (hindbrain).[1] Small cystic structures can be seen normally in the posterior aspect of the embryonic head. The earliest cystic structure seen at 6 to 8 weeks' gestation represents the normal embryonic rhombencephalon, which later forms the normal fourth ventricle and should not be mistaken for a posterior fossa cyst of pathologic importance[127] (Fig. 30-46; see also Fig. 30-20, *C*). The prosencephalon divides into an anterior portion known as the **telen-**

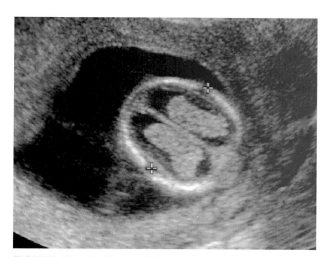

FIGURE 30-47. Normal lateral ventricles. Transverse scan of a 13-week fetus with choroid plexus filling most of the lateral ventricles.

cephalon and a posterior **diencephalon.** The telencephalic vesicles later form the lateral ventricles, and the diencephalon (and to a lesser degree the telencephalon) forms the third ventricle. After approximately 9 weeks, the lateral ventricles can be identified sonographically as two small cystic spaces in the embryonic head at 11 weeks and are more evident with the large choroid plexus almost filling them at 13 weeks (Fig. 30-47). By 12 weeks the lateral ventricles extend almost to the inner table of the skull, and on sonography, only a small rim of cerebral cortex can be demonstrated to surround them. The choroid plexus is echogenic and fills the lateral ventricles completely except for the frontal horns.

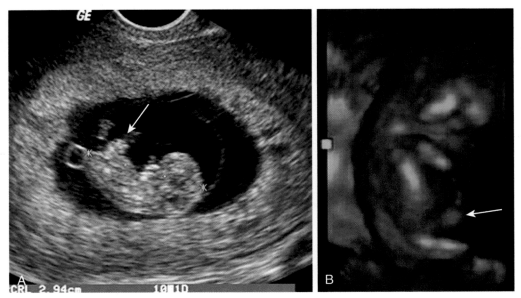

FIGURE 30-48. Physiologic midgut herniation. A, Ten-week embryo has the typical echogenic bowel herniated into the base of the umbilical cord (*arrow*). **B,** 3-D view of an 11-week embryo also shows midgut herniation (*arrow*).

Physiologic Anterior Abdominal Wall Herniation

During embryogenesis, the midgut normally herniates into the umbilical cord at the beginning of the eighth week of gestation. The midgut rotates 90 degrees counterclockwise and then returns to the abdomen during the 12th week. As the midgut returns to the abdomen, further rotation occurs, completing the normal rotation of the midgut.

Schmidt et al.[128] describe the normal physiologic appearance of the anterior abdominal wall during this period. The herniated bowel appears as a small, echogenic mass (6-9 mm) protruding into the cord at approximately 8 weeks (CRL, 17-20 mm). The echogenic mass decreases to 5 to 6 mm at 9 weeks (CRL, 23-26 mm). The size of the mass of herniated bowel varies. Follow-up examinations reveal reduction of the hernia between 10 and 12 weeks. In up to 20% of normal pregnancies, the herniated bowel may still be found outside the fetal abdomen at 12 weeks (Fig. 30-48).

Normal-Appearing Abnormal Embryos

Many grossly abnormal embryos may appear normal in the first trimester.

Anencephaly

Anencephaly results from failure of the rostral neuropore to close (normal closure occurs at approximately 42 days). The resultant abnormality is absence of the bony calvarium. The first-trimester sonographic appearances differ from those in the second trimester.[129] In the second trimester the sonographic diagnosis depends on the absence of the cranial vault superior to the level of the skull base and the orbits. In the first trimester a variable amount of neural tissue (usually grossly deformed) may be present superior to the orbital line, but with time it usually erodes away.

The presence of neural tissue above the orbital line, with failure to recognize absence of the cranial vault late in the first trimester, may result in a missed diagnosis of exencephaly/anencephaly. In a series by Goldstein and Filly,[130] one case of anencephaly was missed at 12½ weeks (Fig. 30-49). This can be a difficult diagnosis before ossification of the skull.

In a first-trimester fetus with exencephaly/anencephaly, in the coronal plane the cerebral lobes will appear as two semicircular structures above the orbits, floating in amniotic fluid.[129] This finding has been referred to as the "Mickey Mouse" sign and can be used for accurate diagnosis of anencephaly late in the first trimester.

Renal Agenesis

The fetal kidneys and adrenals can be demonstrated by approximately 9 weeks. By 12 weeks the bladder can be visualized routinely.[131] In the first trimester, amniotic fluid is predominantly a filtrate of fetal blood across the fetal skin. Fetal urine production begins at about 11 to 13 weeks' gestation. **Oligohydramnios** caused by absent renal function is often not identified before 16 weeks' gestation. In the first trimester, normal amniotic fluid volume cannot be used to predict the presence of

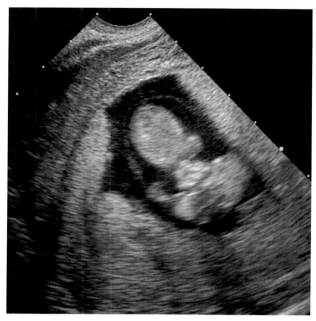

FIGURE 30-49. Anencephaly. Coronal scan of anencephalic fetus at 11 weeks' gestational age shows a large, irregular cranial end inferiorly with no visible echogenic calvarium.

functioning kidneys. Conversely, nonvisualization of the kidneys and bladder may suggest renal agenesis in the first trimester. However, it is not until the second trimester that associated oligohydramnios will demonstrate the lack of renal function.

Discrepancy between Dates and Embryo Size

Although discrepancy between the estimated gestational age by sonographic CRL and menstrual history is common, a major discrepancy in dates may result from growth restriction in the first trimester.[132] First-trimester IUGR is usually related to gross fetal abnormality, often genetic, or the result of viral infection.

FIRST-TRIMESTER MASSES

Ovarian Masses

The most common mass seen in the first trimester of pregnancy is the **corpus luteum cyst.** The corpus luteum cyst secretes progesterone to support the pregnancy until the placenta can take over its hormonal function. It forms in the secretory phase of the menstrual cycle and increases in size if a pregnancy occurs. The corpus luteum of pregnancy can be visualized in 98% of patients,[133] is usually less than 5 cm in diameter (mean diameter, ~1.9 cm), and most often appears as a thick-walled cyst with circumferential vascular flow, although its appearance may vary considerably. Corpus luteum cysts occasionally reach a size of greater than 10 cm. Internal

septation and echogenic debris may be present secondary to internal hemorrhage (Fig. 30-50). The cyst wall and septation may be extremely thick.[134]

Clearly, a functional hemorrhagic corpus luteum cyst may be impossible to differentiate from a pathologic cyst on the basis of a single ultrasound examination. Corpus luteum cysts usually regress or have decreased in size on follow-up sonographic examination at 16 to 18 weeks. Cystic masses that persist should be followed. Surgical intervention is often indicated in large cysts that do not regress by mid–second trimester. However, not all corpus luteum cysts regress, and differentiation from a pathologic cyst may be impossible on sonography.

Adnexal cystic masses less than 5 cm in diameter in the first trimester are usually follicular or corpus luteum cysts and almost always resolve spontaneously. In an asymptomatic patient with a simple or benign-appearing adnexal cyst measuring less than 5 cm, no further follow-up of the cyst is necessary.[135]

Other cystic masses may present in the first trimester of pregnancy because of displacement by the enlarged uterus. **Torsion, rupture,** and **dystocia** have all been described as complications of ovarian cystic masses associated with pregnancy. In a series of 38 episodes of surgically proven ovarian torsion,[136] 48.5% occurred in pregnancies conceived by ovulation induction or IVF. Most episodes of ovarian torsion occurred in the first trimester (55.3%). In 47.6% of first-trimester ovarian torsions, the ovary had a multicystic appearance, and in 23.5% the ovary appeared normal. Doppler ultrasound may be normal in patients with ovarian torsion.[137]

Malignant ovarian **neoplasm** associated with pregnancy is rare. When elective surgical intervention is

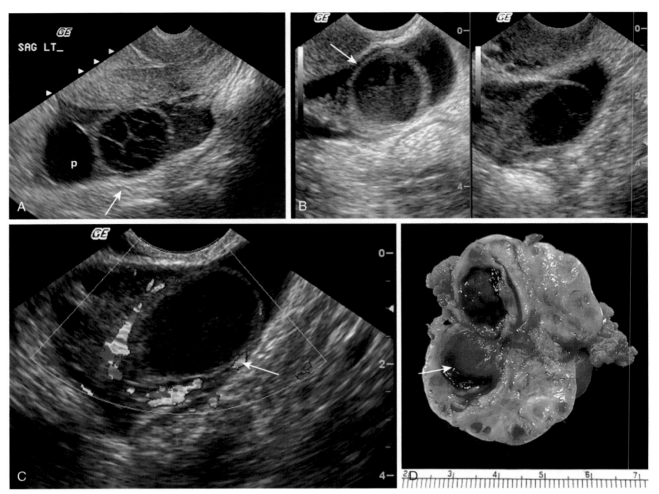

FIGURE 30-50. Hemorrhagic corpus luteum cyst (arrow) at 6 weeks. A, The filamentous bands within the cyst are consistent with hemorrhage. There is also a paraovarian cyst *(p)*, which is echolucent. **B,** Hemorrhaging corpus luteum with a small amount of adjacent free fluid. **C,** The vascularity is a typical **ring of fire** with flow in the wall around the cyst. **D,** Pathologic specimen of an ovary with a corpus luteum cyst *(arrow).*

indicated, it is usually performed in the second trimester, when risk of inducing premature labor is considered lowest. **Dermoid cysts** may present the characteristic appearance of a cystic mass with focal calcification and a fluid-fluid level. Other cystic masses may be more difficult to differentiate from corpus luteum cysts (Fig. 30-51). All cysts should be observed carefully to assess change in size.

Uterine Masses

Uterine **fibroids** are a common pelvic mass often identified during pregnancy and often associated with localized pain and tenderness. Most fibroids do not change in size during pregnancy, although some may enlarge rapidly as a result of estrogenic stimulation. **Infarction** and **necrosis** may occur because of rapid growth. These patients often experience pain. Sonographically, uterine fibroids appear as solid, often hypoechoic uterine masses. They may have areas of calcification and infrequently have cystic, avascular areas related to necrosis. Fibroids may

be differentiated from focal myometrial contractions by the transient nature of myometrial contractions. A repeat examination 20 to 30 minutes after the initial examination reveals disappearance of a focal myometrial contraction, whereas a fibroid will still be present. Fibroids also may distort the uterine contour (serosal surface), whereas focal myometrial contractions usually bulge into the amniotic cavity.

Fibroids are associated with almost twice the spontaneous loss rate in early singleton pregnancies with documented cardiac activity. Benson et al.[138] noted a loss rate of 14% in women with fibroids compared to 7.6% in a control group.[138] Multiple fibroids had a higher loss rate than did single masses (23.6% vs. 8%; $p < 0.05$), but there was no association with size or location.

CONCLUSION

First-trimester sonography plays an important role in establishing the location of a pregnancy and determining

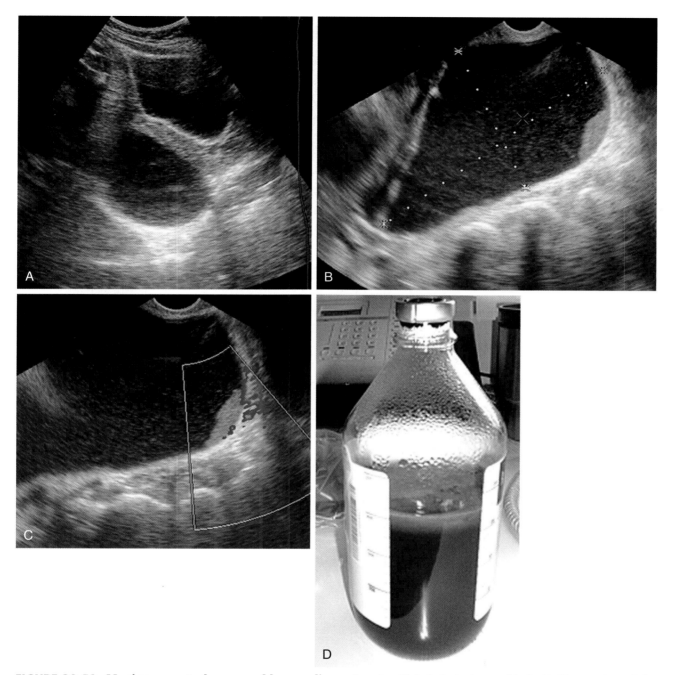

FIGURE 30-51. Mucinous cystadenoma of low malignant potential. A, Sagittal scan with the bladder anterior and the cystic mass posterior compressing the lower segment of the gravid uterus. **B,** Transvaginal scan shows low-level echoes within the mass and some debris at the lower end. **C,** Color Doppler ultrasound shows no flow in the debris. **D,** The fluid was aspirated before delivery and was old blood. The mass recurred and was removed at cesarean delivery.

if the pregnancy is potentially viable (cardiac activity seen). Knowledge of the landmarks with respect to the appearance of the gestational sac, yolk sac, and embryo are important in the appropriate triage of patients who present with pain and bleeding in the first trimester.

References

1. Moore KL, Persaud TVN, editors. The developing human: clinically oriented embryology. 6th ed. Philadelphia: Saunders; 1998.

2. Levi CS, Lyons EA, Lindsay DJ. Early diagnosis of nonviable pregnancy with endovaginal ultrasound. Radiology 1988;167: 383-385.

3. Levi CS, Lyons EA, Zheng XH, et al. Endovaginal ultrasound: demonstration of cardiac activity in embryos of less than 5.0 mm in crown-rump length. Radiology 1990;176:71-74.

4. Nyberg DA, Filly RA. Predicting pregnancy failure in "empty" gestational sacs. Ultrasound Obstet Gynecol 2003;21:9-12.

5. Levi CS. Prediction of early pregnancy failure on the basis of mean gestational sac size and absence of a sonographically demonstrable yolk sac. Radiology 1995;195:873.

6. Rowling SE, Langer JE, Coleman BG, et al. Sonography during early pregnancy: dependence of threshold and discriminatory values on

transvaginal transducer frequency. AJR Am J Roentgenol 1999;172: 983-988.

7. Taylor KJ, Ramos IM, Feyock AL, et al. Ectopic pregnancy: duplex Doppler evaluation. Radiology 1989;173:93-97.

Maternal Physiology and Embryology

8. Oehninger S, Hodgen GD. Hypothalamic-pituitary-ovarian uterine axis. In: Copeland LJ, editor. Textbook of gynecology. Philadelphia: Saunders; 1993.

9. Jones GS, Jones HW. Cyclical cytology and histology. In Jones GS, Jones HW, editors. Gynecology. 3rd ed. Baltimore: Williams & Wilkins; 1982, p. 46-68.

10. Settlage DS, Motoshima M, Tredway DR. Sperm transport from the external cervical os to the fallopian tubes in women: a time and quantitation study. Fertil Steril 1973;24:655-661.

11. Lyons EA, Taylor PJ, Zheng XH, et al. Characterization of subendometrial myometrial contractions throughout the menstrual cycle in normal fertile women. Fertil Steril 1991;55:771-774.

12. Hustin J. Vascular physiology and pathophysiology of early pregnancy. In: Bourne T, Jauniaux E, Jurkovic D, editors. Transvaginal color Doppler. Heidelberg: Springer-Verlag; 1995. p. 47-56.

13. Jauniaux E. Intervillous circulation in the first trimester: the phantom of the color Doppler obstetric opera. Ultrasound Obstet Gynecol 1996;8:73-76.

14. Hustin J, Jauniaux E, Schaaps JP. Histological study of the materno-embryonic interface in spontaneous abortion. Placenta 1990;11: 477-486.

15. Oh JS, Wright G, Coulam CB. Gestational sac diameter in very early pregnancy as a predictor of fetal outcome. Ultrasound Obstet Gynecol 2002;20:267-269.

16. Folkman J. Tumor angiogenesis: therapeutic implications. N Engl J Med 1971;285:1182-1186.

Sonographic Appearance of Normal Intrauterine Pregnancy

17. Kawakami Y, Andoh K, Mizunuma H, et al. Assessment of the implantation site by transvaginal ultrasonography. Fertil Steril 1993;59:1003-1006.

18. Magann EF, Roberts WE, McCurley S, et al. Dominant maternal sleep position influences site of placental implantation. Mil Med 2002;167:67-69.

19. Yeh HC, Goodman JD, Carr L, Rabinowitz JG. Intradecidual sign: an ultrasound criterion of early intrauterine pregnancy. Radiology 1986;161:463-467.

20. Nyberg DA, Filly RA, Filho DL, et al. Abnormal pregnancy: early diagnosis by ultrasound and serum chorionic gonadotropin levels. Radiology 1986;158:393-396.

21. Nyberg DA, Filly RA, Mahony BS, et al. Early gestation: correlation of hCG levels and sonographic identification. AJR Am J Roentgenol 1985;144:951-954.

22. Nyberg DA, Mack LA, Laing FC, Jeffrey RB. Early pregnancy complications: endovaginal sonographic findings correlated with human chorionic gonadotropin levels. Radiology 1988;167: 619-622.

23. Bree RL, Edwards M, Bohm-Velez M, et al. Transvaginal sonography in the evaluation of normal early pregnancy: correlation with hCG level. AJR Am J Roentgenol 1989;153:75-79.

24. Sengoku K, Tamate K, Ishikawa M, et al. [Transvaginal ultrasonographic findings and hCG levels in early intrauterine pregnancies]. Nippon Sanka Fujinka Gakkai Zasshi 1991;43:535-540.

25. Keith SC, London SN, Weitzman GA, et al. Serial transvaginal ultrasound scans and beta-human chorionic gonadotropin levels in early singleton and multiple pregnancies. Fertil Steril 1993;59: 1007-1010.

26. Pellicer A, Calatayud C, Miro F, et al. Comparison of implantation and early development of human embryos fertilized in vitro versus in vivo using transvaginal ultrasound. J Ultrasound Med 1991; 10:31-35.

27. Nyberg DA, Laing FC, Filly RA, et al. Ultrasonographic differentiation of the gestational sac of early intrauterine pregnancy from the pseudogestational sac of ectopic pregnancy. Radiology 1983;146: 755-759.

28. Parvey HR, Dubinsky TJ, Johnston DA, Maklad NF. The chorionic rim and low-impedance intrauterine arterial flow in the diagnosis of early intrauterine pregnancy: evaluation of efficacy. AJR Am J Roentgenol 1996;167:1479-1485.

29. Benacerraf BR, Shipp TD, Bromley B. Does the 10-MHz transvaginal transducer improve the diagnostic certainty that an intrauterine fluid collection is a true gestational sac? J Clin Ultrasound 1999;27:374-377.

30. Birnholz JC, Madanes AE. Amniotic fluid accumulation in the first trimester. J Ultrasound Med 1995;14:597-602.

31. Campbell J, Wathen N, Macintosh M, et al. Biochemical composition of amniotic fluid and extraembryonic coelomic fluid in the first trimester of pregnancy. Br J Obstet Gynaecol 1992;99:563-565.

32. Emerson DS, Cartier MS, Altieri LA, et al. Diagnostic efficacy of endovaginal color Doppler flow imaging in an ectopic pregnancy screening program. Radiology 1992;183:413-420.

33. Nyberg DA, Laing FC, Filly RA. Threatened abortion: sonographic distinction of normal and abnormal gestation sacs. Radiology 1986;158:397-400.

34. Nyberg DA, Mack LA, Harvey D, Wang K. Value of the yolk sac in evaluating early pregnancies. J Ultrasound Med 1988;7:129-135.

35. Lindsay DJ, Lovett IS, Lyons EA, et al. Yolk sac diameter and shape at endovaginal ultrasound: predictors of pregnancy outcome in the first trimester. Radiology 1992;183:115-118.

36. Levi CS, Lyons EA, Dashefsky SM, et al. Yolk sac number, size and morphologic features in monochorionic monoamniotic twin pregnancy. Can Assoc Radiol J 1996;47:98-100.

37. Yeh HC, Rabinowitz JG. Amniotic sac development: ultrasound features of early pregnancy: the double bleb sign. Radiology 1988;166:97-103.

38. Kaufman AJ, Fleischer AC, Thieme GA, et al. Separated chorioamnion and elevated chorion: sonographic features and clinical significance. J Ultrasound Med 1985;4:119-125.

39. Cadkin AV, McAlpin J. Detection of fetal cardiac activity between 41 and 43 days of gestation. J Ultrasound Med 1984;3:499-503.

40. Ragavendra N, McMahon JT, Perrella RR, et al. Endoluminal catheter-assisted transcervical ultrasound of the human embryo. Work in progress. Radiology 1991;181:779-781.

41. Hill LM, DiNofrio DM, Guzick D. Sonographic determination of first trimester umbilical cord length. J Clin Ultrasound 1994;22: 435-438.

42. Ghezzi F, Raio L, Di Naro E, et al. First-trimester sonographic umbilical cord diameter and the growth of the human embryo. Ultrasound Obstet Gynecol 2001;18:348-351.

43. Skibo LK, Lyons EA, Levi CS. First-trimester umbilical cord cysts. Radiology 1992;182:719-722.

44. Sepulveda W. Beware of the umbilical cord "cyst". Ultrasound Obstet Gynecol 2003;21:213-214.

45. Ghezzi F, Raio L, Di Naro E, et al. Single and multiple umbilical cord cysts in early gestation: two different entities. Ultrasound Obstet Gynecol 2003;21:215-219.

Estimation of Gestational Age

46. Hadlock FP, Deter RL, Harrist RB, Park SK. Estimating fetal age: computer-assisted analysis of multiple fetal growth parameters. Radiology 1984;152:497-501.

47. Filly RA. Appropriate use of ultrasound in early pregnancy. Radiology 1988;166:274-275.

Early Pregnancy Failure

48. Wilcox AJ, Weinberg CR, O'Connor JF, et al. Incidence of early loss of pregnancy. N Engl J Med 1988;319:189-194.

49. Hertig AT, Rock J. A series of potentially abortive ova recovered from fertile women prior to the first missed menstrual period. Am J Obstet Gynecol 1949;58:968-993, illust.

50. Bateman BG, Nunley WC, Kolp LA, et al. Vaginal sonography findings and hCG dynamics of early intrauterine and tubal pregnancies. Obstet Gynecol 1990;75:421-427.

51. Sorokin Y, Johnson MP, Uhlmann WR, et al. Postmortem chorionic villus sampling: correlation of cytogenetic and ultrasound findings. Am J Med Genet 1991;39:314-316.

52. Goldstein SR. Embryonic death in early pregnancy: a new look at the first trimester. Obstet Gynecol 1994;84:294-297.

53. Falco P, Milano V, Pilu G, et al. Sonography of pregnancies with first-trimester bleeding and a viable embryo: a study of prognostic indicators by logistic regression analysis. Ultrasound Obstet Gynecol 1996;7:165-169.

54. Pandya PP, Snijders RJ, Psara N, et al. The prevalence of non-viable pregnancy at 10-13 weeks of gestation. Ultrasound Obstet Gynecol 1996;7:170-173.

55. Stabile I, Campbell S, Grudzinskas JG. Ultrasonic assessment of complications during first trimester of pregnancy. Lancet 1987;2: 1237-1240.
56. Blumenfeld Z, Ruach M. Early pregnancy wastage: the role of repetitive human chorionic gonadotropin supplementation during the first 8 weeks of gestation. Fertil Steril 1992;58:19-23.
57. Kupesic S, Kurjak A, Vujisic S, Petrovic Z. Luteal phase defect: comparison between Doppler velocimetry, histological and hormonal markers. Ultrasound Obstet Gynecol 1997;9:105-112.
58. Pennell RG, Needleman L, Pajak T, et al. Prospective comparison of vaginal and abdominal sonography in normal early pregnancy. J Ultrasound Med 1991;10:63-67.
59. Aziz S, Cho RC, Baker DB, et al. Five-millimeter and smaller embryos without embryonic cardiac activity: outcomes in women with vaginal bleeding. J Ultrasound Med 2008;27:1559-1561.
60. Wilson RD, Kendrick V, Wittmann BK, McGillivray B. Spontaneous abortion and pregnancy outcome after normal first-trimester ultrasound examination. Obstet Gynecol 1986;67:352-355.
61. Cashner KA, Christopher CR, Dysert GA. Spontaneous fetal loss after demonstration of a live fetus in the first trimester. Obstet Gynecol 1987;70:827-830.
62. Simpson JL. Incidence and timing of pregnancy losses: relevance to evaluating safety of early prenatal diagnosis. Am J Med Genet 1990;35:165-173.
63. Bernard KG, Cooperberg PL. Sonographic differentiation between blighted ovum and early viable pregnancy. AJR Am J Roentgenol 1985;144:597-602.
64. Rowling SE, Coleman BG, Langer JE, et al. First-trimester ultrasound parameters of failed pregnancy. Radiology 1997;203: 211-217.
65. Nyberg DA, Mack LA, Laing FC, Patten RM. Distinguishing normal from abnormal gestational sac growth in early pregnancy. J Ultrasound Med 1987;6:23-27.
66. Falco P, Zagonari S, Gabrielli S, et al. Sonography of pregnancies with first-trimester bleeding and a small intrauterine gestational sac without a demonstrable embryo. Ultrasound Obstet Gynecol 2003;21:62-65.
67. Doubilet PM, Benson CB. Embryonic heart rate in the early first trimester: what rate is normal? J Ultrasound Med 1995;14:431-434.
68. Vaccaro H, Amor F, Leyton M, Sepulveda W. Arrhythmia in early pregnancy: a predictor of first-trimester pregnancy loss. Ultrasound Obstet Gynecol 1998;12:248-251.
69. Bromley B, Harlow BL, Laboda LA, Benacerraf BR. Small sac size in the first trimester: a predictor of poor fetal outcome. Radiology 1991;178:375-377.
70. Kucuk T, Duru NK, Yenen MC, et al. Yolk sac size and shape as predictors of poor pregnancy outcome. J Perinat Med 1999;27: 316-320.
71. Pedersen JF, Molsted-Pedersen L, Mortensen HB. Fetal growth delay and maternal hemoglobin A$_{1c}$ in early diabetic pregnancy. Obstet Gynecol 1984;64:351-352.
72. Green JJ, Hobbins JC. Abdominal ultrasound examination of the first-trimester fetus. Am J Obstet Gynecol 1988;159:165-175.
73. Gurel SA, Gurel H. A large yolk sac may be important in the early diagnosis of gestational trophoblastic disease: a case report. Eur J Obstet Gynecol Reprod Biol 2000;91:91-93.
74. Szabo J, Gellen J, Szemere G, Farago M. [Significance of hyperechogenic yolk sac in first-trimester screening for chromosome aneuploidy]. Orv Hetil 1996;137:2313-2315.
75. Sauerbrei EE, Pham DH. Placental abruption and subchorionic hemorrhage in the first half of pregnancy: ultrasound appearance and clinical outcome. Radiology 1986;160:109-112.
76. Ball RH, Ade CM, Schoenborn JA, Crane JP. The clinical significance of ultrasonographically detected subchorionic hemorrhages. Am J Obstet Gynecol 1996;174:996-1002.
77. Nyberg DA, Cyr DR, Mack LA, et al. Sonographic spectrum of placental abruption. AJR Am J Roentgenol 1987;148:161-164.
78. Bennett GL, Bromley B, Lieberman E, Benacerraf BR. Subchorionic hemorrhage in first-trimester pregnancies: prediction of pregnancy outcome with sonography. Radiology 1996;200:803-806.
79. Abu-Yousef MM, Bleicher JJ, Williamson RA, Weiner CP. Subchorionic hemorrhage: sonographic diagnosis and clinical significance. AJR Am J Roentgenol 1987;149:737-740.
80. Pedersen JF, Mantoni M. Prevalence and significance of subchorionic hemorrhage in threatened abortion: a sonographic study. AJR Am J Roentgenol 1990;154:535-537.

81. Robson SC, Hunter S, Boys RJ, Dunlop W. Serial study of factors influencing changes in cardiac output during human pregnancy. Am J Physiol 1989;256:H1060-H1065.
82. Steel SA, Pearce JM, McParland P, Chamberlain GV. Early Doppler ultrasound screening in prediction of hypertensive disorders of pregnancy. Lancet 1990;335:1548-1551.
83. Jaffe R, Dorgan A, Abramowicz JS. Color Doppler imaging of the uteroplacental circulation in the first trimester: value in predicting pregnancy failure or complication. AJR Am J Roentgenol 1995;164: 1255-1258.
84. Arduini D, Rizzo G, Romanini C. Doppler ultrasonography in early pregnancy does not predict adverse pregnancy outcome. Ultrasound Obstet Gynecol 1991;1:180-185.
85. Frates MC, Doubilet PM, Brown DL, et al. Role of Doppler ultrasonography in the prediction of pregnancy outcome in women with recurrent spontaneous abortion. J Ultrasound Med 1996;15: 557-562.
86. Nakatsuka M, Habara T, Noguchi S, et al. Impaired uterine arterial blood flow in pregnant women with recurrent pregnancy loss. J Ultrasound Med 2003;22:27-31.
87. Leible S, Cumsille F, Walton R, et al. Discordant uterine artery velocity waveforms as a predictor of subsequent miscarriage in early viable pregnancies. Am J Obstet Gynecol 1998;179:1587-1593.
88. Horrow MM. Enlarged amniotic cavity: a new sonographic sign of early embryonic death. AJR Am J Roentgenol 1992;158: 359-362.
89. Winikoff B, Ellertson C, Elul B, Sivin I. Acceptability and feasibility of early pregnancy termination by mifepristone-misoprostol: results of a large multicenter trial in the United States. Mifepristone Clinical Trials Group. Arch Fam Med 1998;7:360-366.
90. Wagaarachchi PT, Ashok PW, Narvekar N, et al. Medical management of early fetal demise using a combination of mifepristone and misoprostol. Hum Reprod 2001;16:1849-1853.
91. Luise C, Jermy K, Collons WP, Bourne TH. Expectant management of incomplete, spontaneous first-trimester miscarriage: outcome according to initial ultrasound criteria and value of follow-up visits. Ultrasound Obstet Gynecol 2002;19:580-582.

Ectopic Pregnancy
92. Atrash HK, Friede A, Hogue CJ. Ectopic pregnancy mortality in the United States, 1970-1983. Obstet Gynecol 1987;70:817-822.
93. Lawson HW, Atrash HK, Saftlas AF, et al. Ectopic pregnancy surveillance, United States, 1970-1985. MMWR CDC Surveill Summ 1988;37:9-18.
94. Schwartz RO, DiPietro DL. Beta-hCG as a diagnostic aid for suspected ectopic pregnancy. Obstet Gynecol 1980;56:197-203.
95. Ackerman TE, Levi CS, Lyons EA, et al. Decidual cyst: endovaginal sonographic sign of ectopic pregnancy. Radiology 1993;189: 727-731.
96. Nagamani M, London S, Amand PS. Factors influencing fertility after ectopic pregnancy. Am J Obstet Gynecol 1984;149:533-535.
97. Schoen JA, Nowak RJ. Repeat ectopic pregnancy: a 16-year clinical survey. Obstet Gynecol 1975;45:542-546.
98. Coupet E. Ectopic pregnancy: the surgical epidemic. J Natl Med Assoc 1989;81:567-572.
99. Rein MS, Di Salvo DN, Friedman AJ. Heterotopic pregnancy associated with in vitro fertilization and embryo transfer: a possible role for routine vaginal ultrasound. Fertil Steril 1989;51:1057-1058.
100. Hann LE, Bachman DB, McArdlock C. Coexistent intrauterine and ectopic pregnancy: a re-evaluation. Radiology 1984;152:812-813.
101. Wong WS, Mao K. Combined intrauterine and tubal ectopic pregnancy. Aust NZ J Obstet Gynaecol 1989;29:76-77.
102. Dashefsky SM, Lyons EA, Levi CS, Lindsay DJ. Suspected ectopic pregnancy: endovaginal and transvesical ultrasound. Radiology 1988;169:181-184.
103. Fleischer AC, Pennell RG, McKee MS, et al. Ectopic pregnancy: features at transvaginal sonography. Radiology 1990;174:375-378.
104. Dillon EH, Feyock AL, Taylor KJ. Pseudogestational sacs: Doppler ultrasound differentiation from normal or abnormal intrauterine pregnancies. Radiology 1990;176:359-364.
105. Timor-Tritsch IE, Yeh MN, Peisner DB, et al. The use of transvaginal ultrasonography in the diagnosis of ectopic pregnancy [see comments]. Am J Obstet Gynecol 1989;161:157-161.
106. Thorsen MK, Lawson TL, Aiman EJ, et al. Diagnosis of ectopic pregnancy: endovaginal vs transabdominal sonography. Am J Roentgenol 1990;155:307-310.

107. Cacciatore B, Stenman UH, Ylostalo P. Comparison of abdominal and vaginal sonography in suspected ectopic pregnancy. Obstet Gynecol 1989;73:770-774.
108. Golstein DP, Koaca TS. The subunit radioimmunoassay for hCG: clinical application. In: Taymar M, Green TH, editors. Progress in gynecology. New York: Grune & Stratton; 1975. p. 145-184.
109. Nyberg DA, Filly RA, Laing FC, et al. Ectopic pregnancy: diagnosis by sonography correlated with quantitative hCG levels. J Ultrasound Med 1987;6:145-150.
110. Mehta TS, Levine D, Beckwith B. Treatment of ectopic pregnancy: is a human chorionic gonadotropin level of 2,000 mIU/mL a reasonable threshold? Radiology 1997;205:569-573.
111. Frates MC, Visweswaran A, Laing FC. Comparison of tubal ring and corpus luteum echogenicities: a useful differentiating characteristic. J Ultrasound Med 2001;20:27-31.
112. Stein MW, Ricci ZJ, Novak L, et al. Sonographic comparison of the tubal ring of ectopic pregnancy with the corpus luteum. J Ultrasound Med 2004;23:57-62.
113. Frates MC, Brown DL, Doubilet PM, Hornstein MD. Tubal rupture in patients with ectopic pregnancy: diagnosis with transvaginal ultrasound. Radiology 1994;191:769-772.
114. Ackerman TE, Levi CS, Dashefsky SM, et al. Interstitial line: sonographic finding in interstitial (cornual) ectopic pregnancy. Radiology 1993;189:83-87.
115. Wang W, Long W, Yu Q. Complication of cesarean section: pregnancy on the cicatrix of a previous cesarean section. Chin Med J (Engl) 2002;115:242-246.
116. Achiron R, Goldenberg M, Lipitz S, et al. Transvaginal Doppler sonography for detecting ectopic pregnancy: is it really necessary. Isr J Med Sci 1994;30:820-825.
117. Kirk E, Papageorghiou AT, Condous G, et al. The diagnostic effectiveness of an initial transvaginal scan in detecting ectopic pregnancy. Hum Reprod 2007;22:2824-2828.
118. Bottomley C, Van Belle V, Mukri F, et al. The optimal timing of an ultrasound scan to assess the location and viability of an early pregnancy. Hum Reprod 2009;24:1811-1817.
119. Moschos E, Twickler DM. Endometrial thickness predicts intrauterine pregnancy in patients with pregnancy of unknown location. Ultrasound Obstet Gynecol 2008;32:929-934.
120. Kemp B, Kertschanska S, Handt S, et al. Different placentation patterns in viable compared with nonviable tubal pregnancy suggest a divergent clinical management. Am J Obstet Gynecol 1999;181:615-620.
121. Stangel JJ. Recent techniques for the conservative management of tubal pregnancy: surgery, laparoscopy and medicine. J Reprod Med 1986;31:98-101.
122. Yao M, Tulandi T. Current status of surgical and nonsurgical management of ectopic pregnancy. Fertil Steril 1997;67:421-433.
123. Ory SJ, Villanueva AL, Sand PK, Tamura RK. Conservative treatment of ectopic pregnancy with methotrexate. Am J Obstet Gynecol 1986;154:1299-1306.
124. Hajenius PJ, Mol BW, Bossuyt PM, et al. Interventions for tubal ectopic pregnancy. Cochrane Database Syst Rev 2000:CD000324.
125. Nazac A, Gervaise A, Bouyer J, et al. Predictors of success in methotrexate treatment of women with unruptured tubal pregnancies. Ultrasound Obstet Gynecol 2003;21:181-185.
126. Barnhart KT, Gosman G, Ashby R, Sammel M. The medical management of ectopic pregnancy: a meta-analysis comparing "ingle dose" and "multidose" regimens. Obstet Gynecol 2003;101:778-784.

Evaluation of the Embryo

127. Cyr DR, Mack LA, Nyberg DA, et al. Fetal rhombencephalon: normal ultrasound findings. Radiology 1988;166:691-692.
128. Schmidt W, Yarkoni S, Crelin ES, Hobbins JC. Sonographic visualization of physiologic anterior abdominal wall hernia in the first trimester. Obstet Gynecol 1987;69:911-915.
129. Chatzipapas IK, Whitlow BJ, Economides DL. The "Mickey Mouse" sign and the diagnosis of anencephaly in early pregnancy. Ultrasound Obstet Gynecol 1999;13:196-199.
130. Goldstein RB, Filly RA. Prenatal diagnosis of anencephaly: spectrum of sonographic appearances and distinction from the amniotic band syndrome. AJR Am J Roentgenol 1988;151:547-550.
131. Sebire NJ, Von Kaisenberg C, Rubio C, et al. Fetal megacystis at 10-14 weeks of gestation. Ultrasound Obstet Gynecol 1996;8:387-390.
132. Benacerraf BR. Intrauterine growth retardation in the first trimester associated with triploidy. J Ultrasound Med 1988;7:153-154.

First-Trimester Masses

133. Frates MC, Doubilet PM, Durfee SM, et al. Sonographic and Doppler characteristics of the corpus luteum: can they predict pregnancy outcome? J Ultrasound Med 2001;20:821-827.
134. Pennes DR, Bowerman RA, Silver TM. Echogenic adnexal masses associated with first-trimester pregnancy: sonographic appearance and clinical significance. J Clin Ultrasound 1985;13:391-396.
135. Glanc P, Salem S, Farine D. Adnexal masses in the pregnant patient: a diagnostic and management challenge. Ultrasound Q 2008;24:225-240.
136. Smorgick N, Maymon R, Mendelovic S, et al. Torsion of normal adnexa in postmenarcheal women: can ultrasound indicate an ischemic process? Ultrasound Obstet Gynecol 2008;31:338-341.
137. Pena JE, Ufberg D, Cooney N, Denis AL. Usefulness of Doppler sonography in the diagnosis of ovarian torsion. Fertil Steril 2000;73:1047-1050.
138. Benson CB, Chow JS, Chang-Lee W, et al. Outcome of pregnancies in women with uterine leiomyomas identified by sonography in the first trimester. J Clin Ultrasound 2001;29:261-264.

CHAPTER 31

Chromosomal Abnormalities

Bryann Bromley and Beryl Benacerraf

Chapter Outline

$\mathcal{T}$he current standard of obstetric care in the United States is to offer prenatal screening for aneuploidy to all women who present for care before 20 weeks' gestation.[1] If the woman chooses to have a prenatal risk assessment for aneuploidy, multiple sonographic markers and biochemical parameters are available in both the first and the second trimester. The choices available depend on the gestational age of the fetus at presentation for obstetric care and the availability of resources within the local demographic area. Many women who choose to undergo screening will terminate an affected pregnancy.[2] Those choosing to continue the pregnancy will have the opportunity to prepare for the birth of a child with potentially substantial medical needs.

Background risk for **aneuploidy** (deviation from exact multiple of haploid number of chromosomes) depends on maternal age, fetal gestational age, family history, and previously affected pregnancy. Whereas trisomies 13, 18, and 21 increase in frequency as maternal age increases, 45,X and triploidy remain at a constant rate (Fig. 31-1 and Table 31-1).

Trisomy 21 (Down syndrome) is the most common aneuploidy to result in a live birth and is the most frequently identifiable genetic cause of mental retardation. The estimated prevalence has increased over the last 20 years because of trends in advancing maternal age and is estimated to be 1 per 504 live births (1:504 or 1/504).[3]

Trisomies 18 and 13 are rarer, with a prevalence of 1/5000 and 1/10,000, respectively.[4] The prevalence of aneuploidy varies with the availability and use of prenatal screening.[5] In addition, the frequency of aneuploidy is higher earlier in gestation because of the high fetal loss rate with advancing gestation associated with chromosomal abnormalities. Fetal death with trisomy 21 between the first or second trimester and birth is 30% and 20%, respectively. Fetal death between the first trimester and birth with trisomies 18 and 13 is approximately 80%.[6,7]

FIRST-TRIMESTER SCREENING FOR ANEUPLOIDY

First-trimester screening for aneuploidy has the advantage of a patient-specific numeric risk estimate early in pregnancy. Most pregnancies are normal, so most women can be reassured early in gestation. Others may find that the risk estimate for aneuploidy is high enough that they may decide to undergo a diagnostic procedure such as a chorionic villus sampling (CVS) or amniocentesis to obtain a karyotype. If the karyotype is abnormal, the patient has some time to make a decision about continuing or terminating a pregnancy. The decision to terminate can be made with privacy and at a time in pregnancy when safer methods of pregnancy interruption are available.

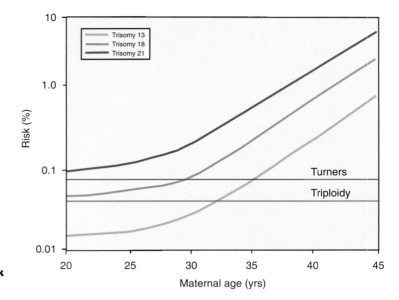

FIGURE 31-1. Maternal age–related risk for chromosomal abnormalities.

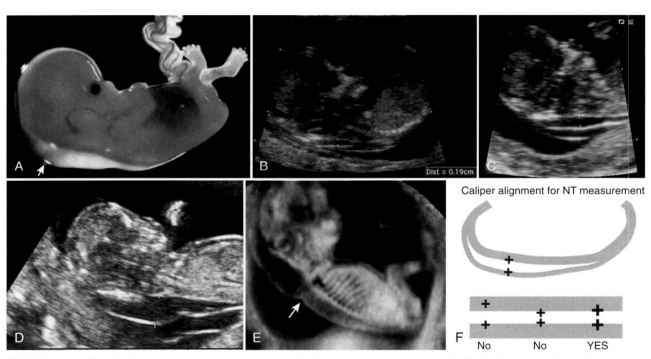

FIGURE 31-2. Nuchal translucency. A, Gross image of a fetus with trisomy 21 shows the fluid collection at the back of the neck known as the nuchal translucency (NT; *arrow*). **B,** Midsagittal view of an euploid fetus shows the correct method of NT measurement. The NT is in a normal range. **C,** Midsagittal view shows the correct method of NT measurement. Note that NT is prominent (measured 3.3 mm). **D,** Midsagittal view of a first-trimester fetus shows a very thick NT (measured 7.9 mm). A nasal bone is not seen. **E,** Increased nuchal fluid associated with generalized subcutaneous edema *(arrow)*. **F,** Schematic shows correct method of caliper placement. *(A courtesy Dr. Eva Pajkrt, University of Amsterdam; F courtesy Dr. Bernard Benoit, Princess Grace Hospital, Monaco.)*

Nuchal Translucency and Trisomy 21

In 1866, Langdon Down reported on the physical characteristics of individuals with developmental delay now known to be caused by **Down syndrome** (trisomy 21 syndrome). He described the skin as "deficient in elasticity, giving the appearance of being too large of the body."[8] Fetuses with trisomy 21 and other chromosomal anomalies often have excess fluid in the subcutaneous tissue behind the fetal neck (Fig. 31-2; **Video 31-1**). Sonographically, this appears as an echolucent fluid collection between the soft tissue over the cervical spine and an echogenic line representing the skin edge. This fluid space is called the **nuchal translucency** (NT).[9] The lucency is thought to represent mesenchymal edema and is often associated with distended jugular lymphatics.

TABLE 31-1. ESTIMATED RISK FOR TRISOMIES BASED ON MATERNAL AGE AND GESTATION

MATERNAL AGE (YR)	Gestational Age (wk)					
	10	12	14	16	20	40
Trisomy 21						
20	1/983	1/1068	1/1140	1/1200	1/1295	1/1527
25	1/870	1/946	1/1009	1/1062	1/1147	1/1352
30	1/576	1/626	1/668	1/703	1/759	1/895
31	1/500	1/543	1/580	1/610	1/658	1/776
32	1/424	1/461	1/492	1/518	1/559	1/659
33	1/352	1/383	1/409	1/430	1/464	1/547
34	1/287	1/312	1/333	1/350	1/378	1/446
35	1/229	1/249	1/266	1/280	1/302	1/356
36	1/180	1/196	1/209	1/220	1/238	1/280
37	1/140	1/152	1/163	1/171	1/185	1/218
38	1/108	1/117	1/125	1/131	1/142	1/167
39	1/82	1/89	1/95	1/100	1/108	1/128
40	1/62	1/68	1/72	1/76	1/82	1/97
41	1/47	1/51	1/54	1/57	1/62	1/73
42	1/35	1/38	1/43	1/43	1/46	1/55
43	1/26	1/29	1/30	1/32	1/35	1/41
44	1/20	1/21	1/23	1/24	1/26	1/30
45	1/15	1/16	1/17	1/18	1/19	1/23
Trisomy 18						
20	1/1993	1/2484	1/3015	1/3590	1/4897	1/18013
25	1/1765	1/2200	1/2670	1/3179	1/4336	1/15951
30	1/1168	1/1456	1/1766	1/2103	1/2869	1/10554
31	1/1014	1/1263	1/1533	1/1825	1/2490	1/9160
32	1/860	1/1072	1/1301	1/1549	1/2490	1/7775
33	1/715	1/891	1/1081	1/1287	1/1755	1/6458
34	1/582	1/725	1/880	1/1047	1/1429	1/5256
35	1/465	1/580	1/703	1/837	1/1142	1/4202
36	1/366	1/456	1/553	1/659	1/899	1/3307
37	1/284	1/354	1/430	1/512	1/698	1/2569
38	1/218	1/272	1/330	1/393	1/537	1/1974
39	1/167	1/208	1/252	1/300	1/409	1/1505
40	1/126	1/157	1/191	1/227	1/310	1/1139
41	1/95	1/118	1/144	1/171	1/233	1/858
42	1/71	1/89	1/108	1/128	1/175	1/644
43	1/53	1/66	1/81	1/96	1/131	1/481
44	1/40	1/50	1/60	1/72	1/98	1/359
Trisomy 13						
20	1/6347	1/7826	1/9389	1/11042	1/14656	1/42423
25	1/5621	1/6930	1/8314	1/9778	1/12978	1/37567
30	1/3719	1/4585	1/5501	1/6470	1/8587	1/24856
31	1/3228	1/3980	1/4774	1/5615	1/7453	1/21573
32	1/2740	1/3378	1/4052	1/4766	1/6326	1/18311
33	1/2274	1/2806	1/3366	1/3959	1/5254	1/15209
34	1/1852	1/2284	1/2740	1/3222	1/4277	1/12380
35	1/1481	1/1826	1/2190	1/2576	1/3419	1/9876
36	1/1165	1/1437	1/1724	1/2027	1/2691	1/7788
37	1/905	1/1116	1/1339	1/1575	1/2090	1/6050
38	1/696	1/858	1/1029	1/1210	1/1606	1/4650
39	1/530	1/654	1/784	1/922	1/1224	1/3544
40	1/401	1/495	1/594	1/698	1/927	1/2683
41	1/302	1/373	1/447	1/526	1/698	1/2020
42	1/227	1/280	1/335	1/395	1/524	1/1516
43	1/170	1/209	1/251	1/295	1/392	1/1134
44	1/127	1/156	1/187	1/220	1/292	1/846

From Snijders RJM, Sebire NJ, Nicolaides KH: Maternal age and gestational age-specific risk for chromosomal defects. Fetal Diagn Ther 1995;10:356-367.

The prevailing theory suggests an alteration in lymphangiogenesis and delayed lymphatic development. Other possible etiologies include cardiac failure and abnormal extracellular matrix, but these do not explain the localized and transient nature of the NT. Most likely, the etiology is a complex interaction of factors.[10] NT normally increases with advancing gestational age, and therefore the measurement is compared to **crown-rump length** (CRL). A thin NT is seen in most normal fetuses. An NT greater than 95% for CRL is considered thickened. An NT greater than 99% does not change significantly with CRL and is approximately 3.5 mm.[11]

In 1992, Nicolaides et al.[9] reported that an NT greater than 3 mm in the first trimester was associated with a 35% risk of chromosomal abnormality. The association between chromosome anomalies and a thickened NT was subsequently confirmed in a large, prospective multicenter trial of 20,804 pregnancies. In normal pregnancies, NT increased with advancing gestational age. The risk of trisomy 21 can be calculated by multiplying the *a priori* (presumptive) risk by **a likelihood ratio** (LR) derived from the degree of deviation in NT from the expected NT. This methodology, in conjunction with a risk cutoff of 1:300, resulted in the identification of 80% of fetuses with trisomy 21, with a **false-positive rate** (FPR) of 5%.[12] Later, Snijders et al.[13] evaluated the use of NT and maternal age to detect trisomy 21 in a multicenter trial that included 22 different sites and 306 trained sonographers. Using a threshold of 1/300, the sensitivity for the detection of trisomy 21 was 82% for an FPR of 8%. For other aneuploidies, the sensitivity was 78%. If the FPR was set at 5%, the sensitivity for the detection of trisomy 21 was 77%.

Serum Biochemical Markers

A variety of serum biochemical markers have different concentrations in pregnancies with trisomy 21 compared with euploid pregnancies. The maternal serum of women carrying fetuses with trisomy 21 has a higher concentration of **free beta human chorionic gonadotropin** (free β-hCG) and lower concentration of **pregnancy-associated plasma protein A** (PAPP-A) compared with the serum of women carrying euploid fetuses. The use of these serum markers, in conjunction with maternal age, results in identification of 62% of fetuses with trisomy 21 at FPR of 5%.[14]

Combined First-Trimester Screening

There is no association between NT measurement and serum levels of free β-hCG or PAPP-A in euploid fetuses or in those with trisomy 21. This independence allows the combination of NT screening and biochemical screening, resulting in a more effective method of risk assessment than either method individually.[15,16] Wald et al.[17] demonstrated that the combination of NT measurement with maternal serum PAPP-A and free β-hCG, known as the "combined" first-trimester screening test, results in the detection of 85% of trisomy 21 fetuses at FPR of 5%.

First-trimester screening using NT measurement and serum biochemical measurement has been further validated in four large studies. The One-Stop Clinic to Assess Risk (OSCAR) screening trial in the United Kingdom (UK) studied 12,339 women with singleton pregnancies between 10 and 14 weeks' gestation. First-trimester screening was accepted by 97.5% of the women, and if they screened positive (risk ≥1/300), 77% underwent invasive diagnostic testing. There were 25 cases of

trisomy 21, of which 23 (92%) were detected, with FPR of 5%. The detection rates of trisomy 13 and 18 were both 100%.[18]

A multicenter trial in North America (BUN study) similarly evaluated 8514 patients with singleton pregnancies between 74 and 97 days' gestation. A screening result was considered positive if the risk of trisomy 21 was 1/270 or higher, or the risk of trisomy 18 was 1/150 or higher. There were 61 cases of trisomy 21; detection rate was 79% with a 5% FPR. The detection rate of trisomy 18 was 90% with a 2% FPR.[19]

The Serum, Urine and Ultrasound Screening Study (SURUSS) evaluated the efficacy, safety, and cost-effectiveness of first- and second-trimester screening for trisomy 21. This prospective study was conducted primarily in the UK on 47,053 pregnancies between 9 and 13 weeks' gestation. In the first trimester the combined test had a sensitivity of 85% for the detection of trisomy 21 with FPR of 6%.[20]

The First and Second Trimester Evaluation of Risk (FASTER) was the largest trial based in the United States and was designed to determine how best to screen pregnant women for trisomy 21. This multicenter trial included 36,120 patients with complete first trimester data, of whom 92 fetuses had trisomy 21. The trial included NT measurements as well as serum biochemistry in both the first and the second trimester, revealing the results to patients only in the second trimester, after both serum screens. The detection rate of trisomy 21 was 87%, 85%, and 82% at 11, 12, and 13 weeks' gestation, respectively, at a 5% FPR. This study confirmed that the NT alone (without biochemical data) was not a reasonable option for screening. For a detection rate of 85%, NT alone had an unacceptably high FPR of 20%. If the FPR was set at the more acceptable level of 5%, the sensitivity for detection of trisomy 21 fell to 68%.[18,21]

The exception to this is in multiple pregnancies, for which NT is the most reliable method of screening for chromosomal anomalies.[7] Sebire et al.[22] studied a series of 448 twin pregnancies and identified 88% of trisomy 21 fetuses (FPR of 7%) using an NT greater than 95%. The prevalence of increased NT was higher in euploid monochorionic twins than in euploid dichorionic twins. Additionally, discordance in NT measurements may predict twin-to-twin transfusion syndrome in monochorionic twins.[23] Although Spencer and Nicolaides[24] identified 75% of trisomy 21 fetuses (FPR of 7%) using biochemical markers and NT measurement, the role of serum markers has not been clearly established in twin gestations. The authors caution that counseling on twins should be primarily based on NT measurements.

A major question is whether an NT measurement exists above which there is no benefit to additional biochemical screening. Results of the FASTER trial were evaluated with specific attention to this question. An NT of 4 mm or greater was identified in 32 patients (0.3%). In this group the lowest combined risk assessment for trisomy 21 in euploid fetuses was 1:8 and for fetuses with trisomy 21 was 7:8. There were 128 patients with NT of 3 mm or more. The lowest risk of trisomy 21 among euploid fetuses using combined screening was 1:1479, and the lowest risk among those with trisomy 21 was 1:2. Ten patients (8%) had the risk lowered below 1:200 and had normal outcome. These authors concluded that there is minimal benefit in waiting for combined screening in fetuses with NT of 3 mm or greater, and no benefit for those with NT of 4 mm or greater.[25]

Integrated and Sequential Screening

In 1999, Wald et al.[26] introduced the concept of **integrated screening,** in which first- and second-trimester evaluation is used to provide a single risk estimate for trisomy 21. The integrated test is a two-step protocol that initially begins with a first-trimester evaluation that includes NT and PAPP-A. The patient returns in the midtrimester for a serum test **quad screen** that includes alpha fetoprotein (AFP), unconjugated estriol (uE$_3$), β-hCG, and inhibin. The results of the first-trimester and second-trimester tests are integrated, and a final risk estimate is given to the patient when both components are complete. Using a 1/120 or greater risk estimate as a positive result, the detection rate of trisomy 21 was 85% with FPR of 0.9%.[26]

The FASTER trial compared screening strategies across the first and second trimesters. There were 33,546 patients with complete first- and second-trimester data available, including 87 fetuses with trisomy 21. The fully integrated screen that included first-trimester NT measurement along with PAPP-A and a second-trimester quad screen resulted in the detection of 95% of fetuses with trisomy 21 at a 5% FPR or 87% if the FPR was set at 1%.[21] The advantage of this protocol is the substantial decrease in FPR while maintaining the high sensitivity for the detection of trisomy 21.[26] A disadvantage of integrated screening is that the patient does not have any screening results in the first trimester, and fetuses at high risk of trisomy 21 are not identified until the midtrimester.[27] Compounding this, as many as 20% of patients may not comply with the second-trimester screen.[20,28]

Two alternative approaches to screening have been proposed in response to the criticism of late notification of patients at "high" risk of aneuploidy. Each of these alternatives is a type of sequential screening. Both protocols disclose first-trimester results to patients above a certain "cutoff" risk (e.g., ≥1/50).[27-29] Thus, women at substantial risk can be referred for genetic counseling and karyotypic evaluation early in gestation. In the step-wise alternative, those not identified in the high-risk group undergo a quad screen in the second trimester. In these patients, risk of both first- and second-trimester evaluations are integrated and reported as a single number. Those with a risk of 1/270 or higher are offered genetic

counseling and karyotypic evaluation. In the "contingent" alternative, those at high risk (e.g., ≥1/50) based on first-trimester testing are offered genetic counseling and karyotype (CVS) while those at very low risk (<1/1500) are not offered additional screening because they are unlikely to become screen positive. Only those women at intermediate risk (≥1/50 and <1/1500) go on to the second-trimester quad test. In this intermediate-risk group, the results of the first and second trimesters are integrated and a final risk estimate reported. Those with a risk of 1:270 or greater are offered genetic counseling and karyotypic evaluation.

In a recent study by Cuckle et al.,[28] midtrimester risks of trisomy 21 were retrospectively calculated from the FASTER trial data. First-trimester risk estimates were calculated using NT, PAPP-A, and free β-hCG. In this study, patients were categorized as high risk (>1/30), borderline risk (1/30-1/1500), and low risk (<1/1500) based on the results of the first-trimester evaluation. Only patients in the borderline category underwent recalculation of risk based on a second serum screen between 15 and 18 weeks, which included AFP, β-hCG, uE$_3$, and inhibin. The initial detection of trisomy 21 (>1/30) after first-trimester screening was 60% with FPR of 1.2%. Of the remaining population, 23% were at borderline risk and calculated as having additional screening. Contingent screening identified 91% of fetuses with trisomy 21, with a 4.5% FPR. Stepwise screening, in which all women other than those at highest risk had calculated first- and second-trimester testing, had a detection rate of 92% with FPR of 5.1%, Integrated screening, in which all women had both first-semester and second-trimester testing, had a detection rate of 88% with FPR of 4.9%. This study showed that **contingent screening,** in which only 23% of the population went on to the second-trimester serum screen, had a similar detection rate of trisomy 21 as the protocols in which most if not all patients had recalculation of risk with second-trimester biochemistry.[28]

It is critical that the results of first- and second-trimester screening are not evaluated independently because the FPR is unacceptably high.[1,30] In an analysis of the data from the BUN trial, the use of independent sequential screening resulted in a 98% detection rate of trisomy 21 but with a 17% FPR. Tables 31-2 and 31-3 compare the different screening strategies.

Standardization of Nuchal Translucency Measurement Technique

In order for nuchal translucency screening to be accurate, standardization of technique, training, and ongoing monitoring are crucial. This involves measurement of CRL and obtaining the appropriate NT measurement.

Primarily, two separate groups provide training, credentialing, and monitoring. The Fetal Medicine

TABLE 31-2. TYPES OF TRISOMY 21 SCREENING USING NUCHAL TRANSLUCENCY (NT)

SCREENING TEST	FIRST TRIMESTER	SECOND TRIMESTER	DISCLOSURE/FOLLOW-UP
NT alone	NT	—	**Not recommended for screening.**
Combined	NT, β-hCG, PAPP-A	—	Results disclosed in first trimester.
Fully integrated	NT, PAPP-A	Quad screen	Results integrated and disclosed as a single risk estimate at end of screening in second trimester.
Serum integrated	PAPP-A	Quad screen	Results integrated and disclosed as a single risk estimate at end of screening in second trimester.
Stepwise sequential	NT, β-hCG, PAPP-A	Quad screen	Results revealed after first part of test. Risk (high): offered karyotype. All others: quad screening.
Contingent sequential	NT, β-hCG, PAPP-A	Quad screen	Results revealed after first part of test. Risk (high): offered karyotype. Risk (borderline): quad screening. Risk (low): no further testing.
Quad screen		AFP, β-hCG	Results disclosed in second trimester.

β-hCG, Beta subunit of human chorionic gonadotropin; PAPP-A, pregnancy-associated plasma protein A.
Quad screen: alpha fetoprotein (AFP), unconjugated estriol (uE₃), β-hCG, and inhibin.
Threshold for what is considered high risk, borderline risk, and low risk varies and will influence the detection rate and false-positive rate.

TABLE 31-3. TRISOMY 21: DETECTION RATE AND FALSE-POSITIVE RATE (FPR) OF DIFFERENT STUDIES

TEST (+ MATERNAL AGE)	DETECTION RATE	FPR
First Trimester		
NT Alone (No Biochemistry)		
UK multicenter[13]	77%	5%
SURUSS[20]	85%	15%
FASTER[21]	68%	5%
FASTER[21]	85%	23%
Combined First		
OSCAR[18]	92%	5.2%
BUN[19]	79%	5%
BUN[19]	85%	9.4%
SURUSS[20]	85%	4.3%
FASTER[21]	85%	4.8%
Sequential Strategies		
Serum Integrated (No NT)		
SURUSS[20]	85%	3.9%
FASTER[21]	85%	4.4%
Fully Integrated		
SURUSS[20]	85%	0.9%
FASTER[21]	85%	0.8%
FASTER[21]	95%	5%
Stepwise Screening		
SURUSS[20]	94%	9%
FASTER[28]	92%	5.1%
Contingent Screening		
FASTER[28]	91%	4.5%
Quad Screen[4]		
FASTER[21]	85%	7.3%
FASTER[21]	81%	5%
SURUSS[20]	85%	6.2%

From Wald NJ, Rodeck C, Hackshaw AF et al. SURUSS in perspective. Semin Perinatol 2005;29:225-235.
NT, Nuchal translucency; UK, United Kingdom; SURUSS, Serum, Urine and Ultrasound Screening Study; FASTER, First and Second Trimester Evaluation of Risk; OSCAR, One-Stop Clinic to Assess Risk.

Foundation (FMF) in the UK was the first to describe the criteria for standardizing the NT measurement. The Nuchal Translucency Quality Review (NTQR) program is based in the United States. The initial criteria of the FMF were modified minimally, most notably by including a shorter CRL. The measurement of NT must be done on equipment that will allow the demarcation of a clear NT. The calipers must be able to be adjusted in increments of 0.1 mm. The examination is usually performed transabdominally, although transvaginal measurements can be used as necessary. Approximately 20 minutes should be allocated to obtain the required measurement. The criteria for properly measuring the nuchal translucency is illustrated in Figure 31-2. The specific details for credentialing can be found at www.ntqr.com or www.fetalmedicine.com.

Crown-rump length must be between 38 and 84 mm (some labs use 45-84 mm). This measurement is key because the NT measurement is converted into multiples of the median (MOM) based on the CRL. The CRL is measured as the longest straight line of the fetus while the head is in a neutral position. The CRL used for risk assessment should be the average of three good measurements. In the setting of a nuchal cord, the measurement above and below the cord should be averaged.

Haddow et al.[31] showed that accuracy is critical in obtaining an NT measurement and relates to the sensitivity of identifying affected fetuses. In 4412 women who underwent first-trimester screening with biochemistry and NT, measurements of NT varied considerably between centers and could not be reliably incorporated into risk calculations. No specific training in NT measurement was required for this study, although the method for measuring NT was a standard protocol. Furthermore, the center with the highest success rate in

FETAL NUCHAL TRANSLUCENCY (NT) MEASUREMENT TECHNIQUE

Clear NT margins
- Thin NT line
- Harmonics off for edge enhancement
- Angle of insonation perpendicular to NT space
- Fetus horizontal on image

Fetus in midsagittal plane
- Fetal spine midsagittal in thoracic and cervical region
- Tip of nose in profile
- Third and fourth ventricles in brain
- Ribs, stomach, and heart not visible

Fetus occupies majority of image
- Head, neck, and upper thorax fill image.
- Fetus occupies more than 50% of width and length of image.

Head in a neutral position
- Pocket of fluid should be visible between chin and neck.
- Angle of neck and chest is less than 90 degrees.

Fetus seen separate from the amnion

Calipers (cursors) must be + (plus/positive).

Measurement
- Calipers are placed at inner border of line that makes up lucency, *not in* lucency.
- Measurement is perpendicular to long axis of fetus.
- Lucency is measured in widest space.
- Measure three times.
- Report largest of three technically correct measurements.

obtaining an NT measurement (100%) had the lowest sensitivity (0%) for picking up trisomy 21. Results from the BUN trial revealed that after training, measurements were initially smaller than expected compared with normative values developed by FMF. With increasing experience, the measurements of the BUN trial were in concordance with published norms.[19,32]

A poorly done NT measurement has a negative impact on detection of aneuploidy, and inaccuracy of 0.5 mm decreases sensitivity by 18%.[33] Training an inexperienced examiner to obtain reliable reproducible NT measurements takes 80 to 100 scans.[34]

Screening using an NT measurement is not always possible because of limited availability of this specialized ultrasound in certain areas and a variety of maternal conditions, including large myomas and high maternal body mass index, which may hamper the ability to obtain a reliable measurement. Initial studies suggest that an NT value is obtainable in 99% of cases, but clinical studies report an 80% initial success rate.[35,36]

If a reliable NT measurement is not possible, a serum-only version of the integrated test can be offered. In this case, maternal serum PAPP-A is measured at 10 to 13 weeks' gestation, followed by the quad screen markers at 15 to 20 weeks. The performance of the serum integrated test with no ultrasound component is approximately 85% detection rate at a 5% FPR.[18,21,26]

Nuchal Translucency and Other Aneuploidies

A thickened NT has been used to detect fetuses with trisomy 18. These fetuses have an abnormal biochemical pattern with very low β-hCG and very low PAPP-A. The BUN trial of 8514 screened pregnancies, using a risk cutoff of 1/150, identified 91% of fetuses with trisomy 18 with a 2% FPR. Additionally, 4 in 5 fetuses with trisomy 13 were identified.[19] These trisomies result in fetuses that have multiple congenital malformations and rarely survive beyond the first year of life. The FASTER trial reported a detection rate of 78% for all non–trisomy 21 aneuploidies at FPR of 6% when first-trimester screening for cystic hygroma or combined screening. The detection rate for trisomy 18 was 82% at a 6% FPR.[37] Spencer and Nicolaides[38] developed an algorithm for the detection of trisomy 18 and 13 that included maternal age, NT, free β-hCG, and PAPP-A. Using a risk cutoff of 1/150, they predicted a 95% detection rate for these chromosomal defects with FPR of 0.3%.

Cystic Hygroma

The distinction between a first-trimester cystic hygroma and a thick NT is controversial. Historically, a cystic hygroma has been diagnosed when the hypoechoic space at the back of the neck extends down the fetal back and contains septations (Fig. 31-3; **Video 31-2**). Malone et al.[39] reported on 134 cases of cystic hygroma identified in the FASTER trial from 38,167 screened pregnancies, Chromosomal abnormalities were present in 51% of these patients, and major structural anomalies were identified in 34% of those without karyotypic anomaly. Survival with normal outcome was confirmed in 17% of cases. These investigators reported an increased risk of aneuploidy, cardiac malformations, and fetal death in fetuses with cystic hygroma compared with those who had a simple, thickened NT.[39] Other investigators have reported that septations are seen in all thickened NTs if examined in the transverse suboccipitobregmatic plane and that the incidence of adverse outcome is related to NT thickness versus appearance.[40,41]

Nasal Bone

Dr. Down, in his original essay describing the physical features of a category of developmentally delayed individuals, identified the nose as being small.[8] Not surprisingly, fetuses with trisomy 21 have small or absent nasal bone. The fetal nasal bone can be seen by ultrasound starting at approximately 11 weeks' gestation. The first-trimester nasal bone evaluation is technically difficult,

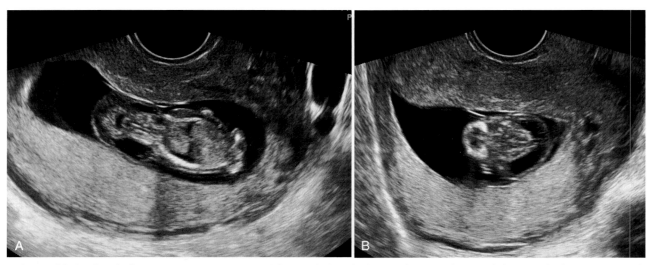

FIGURE 31-3. Cystic hygroma. A, First-trimester fetus with skin thickening that extends around the entire body, consistent with cystic hygroma, and bilateral distended jugular lymphatic sacs. Note the bilateral pleural effusions, indicating hydrops. **B,** Axial scan through the head of the same fetus shows septations within the nuchal thickening.

CRITERIA FOR GOOD NASAL BONE EVALUATION

Fetus in midsagittal plane
  Fetal spine midsagittal in thoracic and cervical region
  Tip of nose clearly seen in nasal profile
  Third and fourth ventricle in brain
  Ribs, stomach and heart not visible
Fetus occupies majority of image
  Head, neck, and upper thorax fill image
  Fetus occupies more than50% of width and length of image
Margins of fetal anatomy clear without ambiguity in nasal anatomy
Angle of insonation 45 degrees to fetal profile, perpendicular to nasal bone
Brightness of nasal bone same as for overlying skin or brighter, appearing as "=" sign

---

and competency in assessing nasal bone reportedly takes on average 80 scans.[42] The criteria for a nasal bone evaluation are shown in Figure 31-4. Initial first-trimester screening studies report that the nasal bone is absent in 73% of fetuses with trisomy 21 and 0.5% of euploid fetuses.[43] Since that initial study, an absent nasal bone was shown to be related to ethnicity. Cicero et al.[44] studied 5918 fetuses between 11 and 14 weeks and obtained a fetal profile in 99%. An absent fetal nasal bone in euploid fetuses varied by ethnicity. A nasal bone was not identified in 2.2% of Caucasian fetuses, 9% of African-Caribbean fetuses, and 5% of Asian fetuses. Younger fetuses also have a higher incidence of non-visualization of the nasal bone. Absence of the nasal bone was seen in 4.7%, 3.4%, 1.4%, and 1% of euploid

fetuses with CRL of 45 to 54 mm, 55 to 64 mm, 65 to 74 mm, and 75 to 84 mm, respectively.

Similarly, nonvisualization of the nasal bone increases with thickening NT. In fetuses with an NT below 95th centile, 1.6% had a nonvisualized nasal bone, compared with 2.7% for NT above 95th percentile of 3.4 mm, 5.4% for NT 3.5 to 4.4 mm, 6% for NT 4.5 to 5.4 mm, and 15% for NT of 5.5 mm or greater. In this same study, an absent nasal bone was seen in 69% of trisomy 21 fetuses and in 32% of fetuses with other chromosomal defects.[44]

No significant association exists between the biochemical markers free β-hCG and PAPP-A and the fetal nasal bone; therefore these can be combined to refine the first-trimester risk assessment for trisomy 21.[45] Cicero et al.[46] prospectively evaluated 20,418 singleton fetuses between 11 and 14 weeks. The fetal nasal bone was absent in 238 (1.2%), was present in 19,937 (97.6%), and could not be evaluated in 243 (1.2%). A fetal nasal bone was absent in 113/20,165 (0.6%) of chromosomally normal fetuses and in 87/140 (62.1%) of fetuses with trisomy 21. The combination of NT and biochemical markers in the first trimester (combined first-trimester screening) resulted in the identification of 90% of fetuses with trisomy 21 at FPR of 5%. Inclusion of the nasal bone resulted in the same rate of detection of trisomy 21 but with FPR decreasing to 2.5%. These statistics held true if all fetuses underwent screening with a nasal bone evaluation as well as in a two-stage approach in which only those at intermediate risk based on NT and biochemistry underwent nasal bone evaluation.

Not all investigators have been as successful using the fetal nasal bone to assess for aneuploidy. Sepulveda et al.[47] reported on a series of 1287 consecutive fetuses being evaluated for NT and presence or absence of a

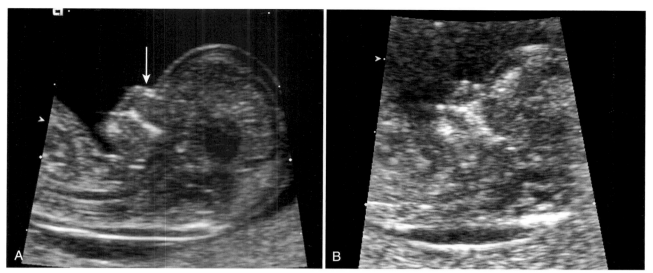

FIGURE 31-4. **First-trimester nasal bone assessment.** **A,** Midsagittal profile of a fetus shows the correct method of assessing the nasal bone. Note that the nasal bone and the overlying skin form an "=" sign *(arrow).* **B,** Midsagittal profile of a fetus with trisomy 21 shows the echogenic overlying skin but absent nasal bone.

nasal bone. Overall, 110 fetuses (8.5%) had an NT detection rate of 95% or greater, and 25 (1.9%) had an absent nasal bone. Of the 31 trisomy 21 fetuses, 28 had NT above 95% and 13 had an absent nasal bone. The detection rate of trisomy 21 was 90.3% using NT and 41.9% using an absent nasal bone. All but one fetus with an absent nasal bone had a thickened NT, and only two normal fetuses had an absent nasal bone. These authors concluded that although an absent nasal bone is highly predictive of trisomy 21, it is less useful as a sonographic marker than the NT. Malone et al.[48] reported that the nasal bone evaluation was not a useful test for population screening.

It is evident that the issues surrounding nasal bone (NB) screening in the first trimester are complex. The identification of the nasal bone as present or absent is a specialized skill that is attained with experience, even for competent imagers. It has been recommended that the nasal bone be considered a contingency marker in patients whose first-trimester risk based on NT and biochemistry is in an intermediate-risk category between 1/101 and 1/1000.[46,49,50]

Other Markers for Aneuploidy

Flattened Facies

Individuals with trisomy 21 are known to have flattened facies. Recently, the frontomaxillofacial angle of the fetus has been studied to determine whether this might be a useful marker for trisomy 21. On a midsagittal view of the face, the angle between the upper surface of the maxilla and the frontal bone is measured. Early data have shown that the angle is greater than 85 degrees in 69% of fetuses with trisomy 21, compared with 5% of euploid fetuses. Importantly, there was no association between

the angle and NT or serum biochemistries, suggesting that this may ultimately prove to be a useful adjunct in screening for trisomy 21.[51]

Reversed Flow in Ductus Venosus

The ductus venosus directs well-oxygenated blood from the umbilical vein to the coronary and cerebral circulation. Abnormal blood flow demonstrated as a reversed *a* wave in the ductus venosus is seen in 80% of fetuses with trisomy 21 and in 5% of euploid fetuses[7,52] (Fig. 31-5).

Tricuspid Regurgitation

Tricuspid regurgitation has also been proposed as a method of risk assessment. Falcon et al.[53] compared 77 fetuses with trisomy 21 and 232 chromosomally normal fetuses from singleton pregnancies at 11 to 14 weeks of gestation. Tricuspid regurgitation was identified in 57 (74%) of trisomy 21 fetuses and in 16 (7%) of euploid fetuses. No relationship between tricuspid regurgitation and the levels of maternal serum free β-hCG and PAPP-A was identified. The authors concluded that an integrated sonographic and biochemical test can identify about 90% of trisomy 21 fetuses for a 2% to 3% FPR.

Thickened Nuchal Translucency with Normal Karyotype

A thickened NT is associated with an increased risk of **congenital heart defects** (CHDs). In a study of 29,154 euploid fetuses at 10 to 14 weeks' gestation, Hyett et al.[54] identified 50 with CHDs; 56% of the fetuses were from a group of 1822 with an NT thickness greater than 95%. In a meta-analysis evaluating the screening

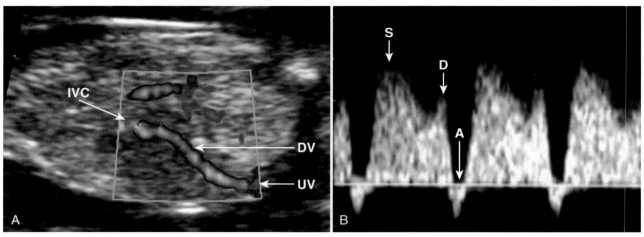

FIGURE 31-5. Reversed flow in ductus venosus. A, Color Doppler anatomy of vessels at oblique sagittal view of fetal trunk; *UV,* umbilical vein; *DV,* ductus venosus; *IVC,* inferior vena cava. **B,** Abnormal ductus venosus sonogram shows a reverse *a* wave. Absent or reversed a-wave flow can occur in cardiac failure, with or without cardiac defects, and in chromosomally abnormal fetuses.

performance of increased first-trimester NT for the detection of major CHDs, eight independent studies with 58,492 patients were reviewed. An NT above 99% had a sensitivity of 30% for the detection of CHDs. If an NT above 99% is used as an indication for a fetal echocardiogram, 1 in 16 referred cases would have CHDs. If the threshold was lowered to fetuses with an NT above 95%, 1 in 33 referred cases would have a major CHD.[55] Data from the FASTER trial confirmed that the incidence of major CHD increased with increasing NT, although the sensitivity for CHD detection was only 9.6%. These investigators concluded that NT lacked the qualities of a good screening test for heart disease; however, an NT of 2.5 MOM (99%) or greater is considered an indication for fetal echocardiography.[56]

Fetuses with a thick NT are at increased risk for a variety of major congenital abnormalities[11] (Fig. 31-6). A **major abnormality** is one that is defined as requiring medical or surgical treatment or is associated with developmental delay. These include not only cardiac defects but also **diaphragmatic hernia, body stalk anomalies,** and **abdominal wall defects,** among a multitude of other syndromes and anomalies. In combined data of 28 studies of 6153 euploid fetuses with thick NT, the prevalence of major anomalies was 7.3% (range, 3% to 50%). The prevalence of major anomalies increased from 1.6% in those with an NT less than 95 percentile to 2.5% for 95 to 99 percentile, 10% with an NT of 3.5 to 4.4 mm, and increasing dramatically thereafter to 46% in those with an NT greater than 6.5 mm.[11] Similarly, a thickened NT has been associated with a myriad of genetic disorders.[7,11]

In chromosomally normal fetuses, the risk of intrauterine demise increases with increasing NT. In a study of 6650 pregnancies undergoing NT screening, the prevalence of miscarriage, fetal death, or termination for an anomaly was 1.5% in euploid fetuses with an NT below 95 percentile compared with 18% in those with an NT above 99 percentile.[57]

Not all fetuses with a thick NT have an abnormal outcome. In 2001, Souka et al.[58] reported on 1320 euploid singleton pregnancies with an NT of 3.5 mm or greater. These fetuses underwent sonographic evaluation at 14 to 16 weeks and 20 to 22 weeks. The chance of a live birth with no defect was 86% in the group with an NT of 3.5 to 4.4 mm, 77% for NT of 4.5 to 5.4 mm, and 67% for NT of 5.5 to 6.4 mm. In fetuses with an NT of 6.5 mm or greater, the chance of normal outcome was 31%. In total, there were 200 fetuses (15.5%) with abnormalities, 80% of which were diagnosed prenatally. There were 1080 (82%) survivors, 60 (6%) of whom had abnormalities requiring medical or surgical care or were developmentally delayed. In a group of 82 fetuses with persistent nuchal thickening but an otherwise normal scan, 19% had an adverse outcome. In the group of 980 euploid fetuses with a normal second-trimester scan, there were 22 (2%) with adverse outcome. Severe developmental delay was seen in 1 of 82 (1%) with isolated persistent nuchal thickening, compared with 4 of 980 (0.4%) with a normal scan.[58]

Bilardo et al.[59] reviewed the outcome of 675 pregnancies with an increased NT, known karyotype, and known pregnancy outcome. Of the study group, 451 (67%) had a normal karyotype, and 19% of these euploid pregnancies had an adverse outcome. The range of abnormal outcome varied with the degree of NT thickening, from 8% with NT between the 95% and 3.4 mm to 80% with NT of 6.5 mm or greater. Second-trimester sonography was performed on 425 euploid fetuses, and an abnormality was identified in 50 fetuses (12%). Of fetuses with a suspicious or abnormal scan, 86% had an adverse outcome. A normal second-trimester ultrasound was reported on 375 (88%) of fetuses, and 96% of those are

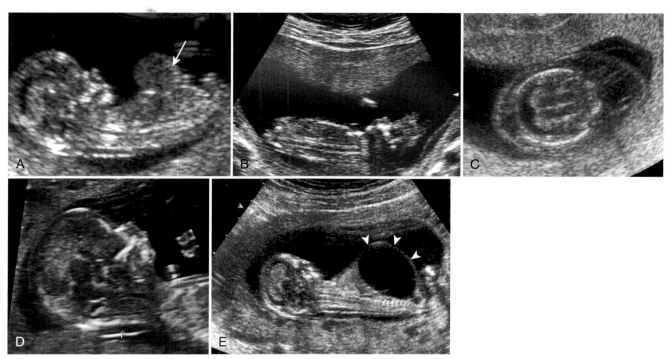

FIGURE 31-6. Structural abnormalities seen at nuchal translucency screening. A, Omphalocele; B, anencephaly; C, holoprosencephaly; D, micrognathia; E, megacystis.

alive and well. Of fetuses with a thickened NT in the first trimester, normal karyotype, and normal second-trimester scan, 4% had an adverse outcome, which included intrauterine demise, structural defects, and genetic syndromes. The most frequently missed anomalies on ultrasound were cardiac defects, underscoring the need for detailed fetal echocardiography in fetuses with a thick NT. Westin et al.[60] reported on 16,260 euploid fetuses from an unselected population to determine how well NT measurements predicted adverse outcome. The overall rate of adverse outcome was 2.7%. The risk of adverse outcome increased with thickening NT values. An NT of 3 mm or greater was associated with a 6-fold increase in adverse outcome, 3.5 mm or greater with a 15-fold increased risk, and 4.5 mm or greater with a 30-fold increased risk. These authors concluded that likelihood ratios could be used to calculate an individual's risk of adverse outcome but could not reliably diatinguish between normal and adverse outcome.

Senat et al.[61] prospectively evaluated long-term outcome in children with a normal karyotype and a nuchal translucency at or greater than the 99%. An external control group was utilized for comparison. The study population consisted of 179 fetuses that underwent midtrimester sonography as well as fetal echocardiography. There were 17 fetal losses, including 10 malformations, 5 intrauterine demises, 1 miscarriage, and 1 termination. One hundred and sixty two liveborns were evaluated with serial pediatric examinations and formal developmental testing. At 2 years of age, 89% of

children had no malformations and normal developmental testing. Eleven percent of children had a structural abnormality noted after birth. Two children (1.2%) had neurologic delay. In one child, the delay was isolated, and in the other it was associated with an unidentified syndrome. These authors concluded that when the karyotype is normal and the sonogram is normal with resolution of the NT, the outcome is not adversely affected at 2 years of age.

SECOND-TRIMESTER SCREENING FOR TRISOMY 21

Although first-trimester risk assessment allows a patient the benefit of **time** in using the information to make decisions regarding pregnancy, not all women present for prenatal care early enough in gestation to take advantage of this benefit. In addition, first-trimester screening may not be readily available in all areas. Until about the last decade, the only method of prenatal risk assessment for aneuploidy was multiple marker serum screening and midtrimester genetic sonography. Serum screening, which now includes four biochemical markers and is known as the quad screen, is performed in the second trimester and has a sensitivity of approximately 80% for the detection of trisomy 21 with an FPR of 5%.[1]

Ultrasound is an integral part of risk assessment for aneuploidy in the middle trimester.[62-70] Approximately 25% of fetuses with trisomy 21 have a major congenital

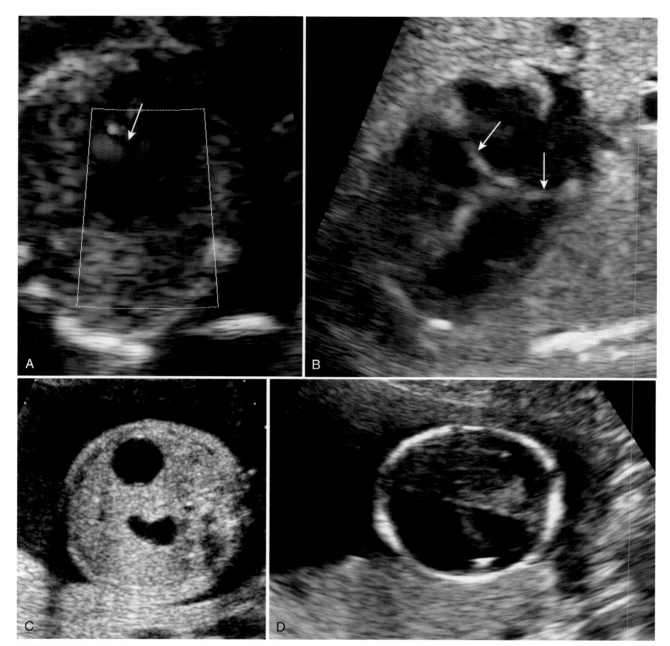

FIGURE 31-7. Major congenital anomalies in trisomy 21. A, Ventriculoseptal defect (VSD). Four chamber view of the heart with a ventriculoseptal defect (arrow) demonstrated with color flow Doppler. **B, Atrioventricular (A-V) canal.** Four-chamber view of the fetal heart demonstrates a complete A-V canal. Note the abnormal "flattening" of the mitral and tricuspid valves into a common A-V valve (arrows). **C, Duodenal atresia.** Axial scan through the fetal abdomen shows a double bubble. **D, Ventriculomegaly.** Axial scan through the cranium of a fetus with trisomy 21 shows dangling choroid in fetus with ventriculomegaly.

anomaly, such as cardiac defect, duodenal atresia, or ventriculomegaly[66,67] (Fig. 31-7). The cornerstone to identifying fetuses with trisomy 21 has been the recognition of sonographic "markers." Some of these markers are well known physical entities that were first described by Dr. Down in 1866, such as the thickened nuchal fold and the small nasal bone.[8] Others are findings specific to prenatal sonography, such as echogenic bowel, echogenic intracardiac focus, pyelectasis, and short femoral and humeral length.

Nuchal Fold

Early studies showed that the presence of a thickened nuchal fold identified 40% of fetuses with trisomy 21 with FPR of 0.1%.[71-74] This measurement is obtained using an axial view through the fetal head, across the thalami and angled posteriorly to include the cerebral peduncles, cerebellar hemispheres, and cisterna magna as well as the occipital bone. The measurement is made from the surface of the occipital bone to the surface

TRISOMY 21: SONOGRAPHIC MARKERS

Nuchal fold
Absent/hypoplastic nasal bone
Short femur
Short humerus
Echogenic bowel
Echogenic intracardiac focus
Pyelectasis
Heart defect
Mild ventriculomegaly
Hypoplasia of fifth digit
Wide iliac angle
Ear length
Frontothalamic distance

Nasal Bone

The fetal nasal bone is a recent sonographic marker included in second-trimester genetic sonography[85] (Fig. 31-9). The technique for visualizing the nasal bone in the midtrimester involves obtaining a midsagittal fetal profile. The angle of insonation should be 90 degrees to the longitudinal axis of nasal bone. If the nasal bone is viewed "on end" (0 or 180 degrees), it will appear erroneously as absent. A slightly oblique angle (45 or 135 degrees) helps to define the edges of the nasal bone more sharply.[86] In 239 fetuses referred for amniocentesis due to a risk of trisomy 21 of 1/270 or greater, Bromley et al.[87] reported that 6/16 (37%) fetuses with trisomy 21 did not have a detectable nasal bone. Of the fetuses with a detectable nasal bone, the mean length was shorter in those with trisomy 21 than in euploid fetuses. A

of the skin edge (Fig. 31-8). Care must be taken not to angle below the occiput because this will lead to spuriously large measurements. Initially, a measurement of 6 mm or greater was considered abnormal; however, 5 mm was later determined to be a more sensitive threshold, with little change in the specificity.[75] Interobserver variability for this measurement is small (1 mm), establishing the nuchal fold as a highly reproducible measurement.[76] Many investigators have subsequently reported that a thickened nuchal skin fold is an important marker for detecting trisomy 21, and after more than 20 years, it remains one of the most specific second-trimester markers.[77-82] More recently, some have suggested that because the nuchal fold measurement fits a log gaussian distribution, it should be evaluated as a continuous variable and interpreted in the context of gestation-specific norms, to allow a more refined method of risk analysis.[83,84]

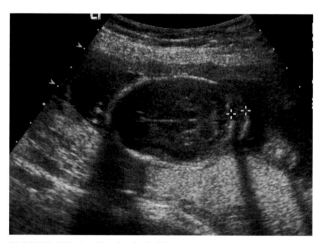

FIGURE 31-8. Nuchal fold. Axial scan through the fetal head of a midtrimester fetus shows a thickened nuchal fold, measuring 6 mm.

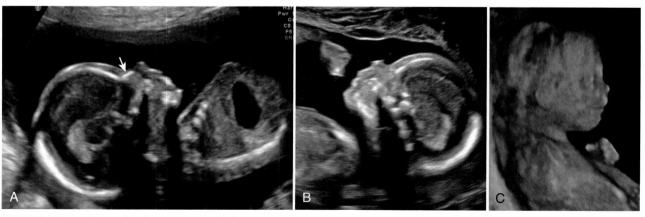

FIGURE 31-9. Second-trimester nasal bone assessment. A, Midsagittal profile of an 18-week fetus shows a normal nasal bone *(arrow).* **B,** Midsagittal profile of a second-trimester fetus demonstrates an absent nasal bone. **C,** 3-D image of a midtrimester fetus with trisomy 21 shows a flat profile.

receiver-operator characteristic curve for the prediction of trisomy 21 based on biparietal diameter (BPD)/nasal bone length reveals that a cutoff of 11 or greater identifies 69% of trisomy 21 fetuses with a 5% FPR.

Vintzileos et al.[88] retrospectively evaluated the significance of the nasal bone ossification in fetuses referred for genetic sonogram; 29 fetuses with trisomy 21 were compared to 102 euploid fetuses. Absence of the nasal bone was seen in 41% of fetuses with trisomy 21 and none of the euploid fetuses. Other authors recommend measurement of less than 5 percentile or an absolute measurement as thresholds to predict aneuploidy.[89-92]

More recently, several groups have suggested that evaluating the nasal bone length as a multiple of the median is the optimal method of using this marker. Odibo et al.[93] evaluated 3634 women at increased risk for aneuploidy. Nasal bone assessment was possible in 3197 women (88%), of whom 23 had fetuses with trisomy 21. A nasal bone length of less than 0.75 MOM provided the best definition of nasal bone hypoplasia and had a sensitivity and specificity of 49% and 92%, respectively, compared with 61% and 84% for BPD/nasal bone length greater than 11. These investigators favor the incorporation of absent nasal bone as a major marker for trisomy 21 in the second-trimester genetic sonographic screening because of its ease of identification and better specificity compared with MOM of less than 0.75. The absence of the fetal nasal bone can be as powerful a marker for trisomy 21 as the thickened nuchal fold.[94]

Of note, there is variation in the prevalence of a hypoplastic or absent nasal bone depending on ethnicity. Cicero et al.[91] reported that 8.8% of patients of African-Caribbean ancestry had an absent or hypoplastic nasal bone, compared with 0.5% of Caucasian fetuses, thus limiting the utility of this marker in patients of African-Caribbean heritage.

Three-dimensional (3-D) ultrasound has been used to evaluate the presence or absence of the fetal nasal bone. In 20 fetuses with trisomy 21, Benoit and Chaoui[95] found nine had either an absent or a hypoplastic nasal bone on 2-D ultrasound. The 3-D evaluation showed bilateral nasal bone absence in six fetuses and unilateral nasal bone absence in three.

Femur Length

A short femur was one of the earliest recognized features in the sonographic detection of trisomy 21.[96] The expected femoral length (FL = −9.645 + 0.9338 × BPD) accounts for 94% of variation in normal length.[97] Based on BPD, a measured-to-expected femur length ratio of 0.91 or less identifies 40% of fetuses with trisomy 21, with a 5% FPR.[98] Although all agree that fetuses with trisomy 21 have shorter femurs than euploid fetuses, the difference is quite small, and the clinical utility of this finding remains controversial.[99] Additionally, femur length varies among fetuses of different ethnicity. Asian fetuses tend to have shorter femurs and black fetuses longer femurs compared with white fetuses.[100] Such differences may be sufficient to question the usefulness of the femur as a marker in many populations.

Humeral Length

The length of the humerus is a more sensitive and specific marker for trisomy 21 than the femoral length.[101] Benacerraf et al.[102] found that the measured humeral length was shorter than the expected humeral length in fetuses with trisomy 21, with a measured/expected humeral length ratio of less than 0.90 the optimal criterion for detecting affected fetuses (expected humeral length = −7.9404 + 0.8492 × BPD). The use of this ratio identified 50% of the fetuses with trisomy 21, with a 6.2% FPR.[102]

Mild Pyelectasis

In the second trimester, mild pyelectasis is considered present if the anteroposterior diameter of the renal pelvis 4 mm or greater[103] (Fig. 31-10, A). Among fetuses with trisomy 21, 17% to 25% have mild pyelectasis, compared with 2% to 3% of euploid fetuses.[103,104]

Echogenic Bowel

Echogenic bowel is seen in 0.2% to 0.8% of midtrimester fetuses.[105-107] To be considered echogenic, the bowel must appear as a well-delineated homogeneous area that is as bright as the adjacent bone using a transducer with a frequency of 5 MHz or less (Fig. 31-10, B; **Video 31-3**). The incidence of chromosomal abnormalities in the setting of echogenic bowel ranges from 3% to 27%.[105-110] The etiology of echogenic bowel seen in association with aneuploidy may be related to poor bowel motility and decreased water content of meconium.[110] In addition to aneuploidy, echogenic bowel is associated with cystic fibrosis, infectious etiologies such as cytomegalovirus, primary bowel abnormalities, and severe growth restriction. It has also been associated with fetal ingestion of blood and impending fetal demise.[105-110]

Echogenic Intracardiac Focus

An echogenic intracardiac focus (EIF) is a discrete, bright white dot, seen in the region of the papillary muscle of the heart (Fig. 31-10, C). Echogenic intracardiac foci are usually located within the left ventricle but can be seen in both sides of the heart. Most also are seen as a single focus but may occur as multiple foci. This sonographic finding is caused by mineralization of the papillary muscle and is seen in 16% of fetuses with trisomy 21.[111] However, EIF is also present in up to 5% of fetuses without trisomy 21.[112]

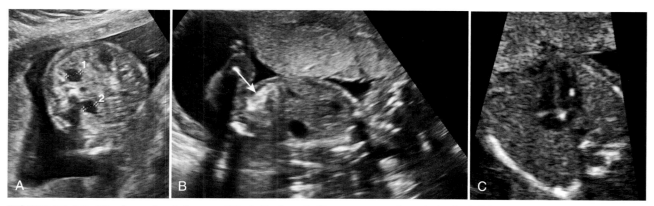

FIGURE 31-10. Markers for trisomy 21. A, Pyelectasis. Transverse scan through the fetal abdomen at 18 weeks shows bilateral pyelectasis. **B, Echogenic bowel.** Sagittal scan through the fetal abdomen in the midtrimester reveals echogenic bowel *(arrow)*. Note that the bowel is as bright as bone. **C, Echogenic intracardiac focus** (EIF). Axial scan through the fetal chest showing the four chamber view of the heart demonstrates an EIF in the left ventricle.

An EIF is the most common marker to occur as an isolated entity both in fetuses with trisomy 21 and in euploid fetuses.[66,67] This finding carries a twofold to fourfold increased risk of trisomy 21.[66,67,70,112,113] Importantly, this marker cannot be used reliably in patients of Asian ancestry because of the high prevalence of the EIF in the euploid Asian population.[114]

The identification of an EIF is confounded by technical considerations such as cardiac position. When the interventricular septum is pointing directly toward or away from the transducer beam in an apical or basal view, an EIF is detected more often than when the septum is imaged perpendicular to the transducer beam in a lateral view. To be convinced that an EIF is present, it must be as bright as bone and seen in several planes. Other normal specular reflectors in the fetal heart, such as the moderator band in the right ventricle, can be mistaken for an EIF. Winn et al.[115] evaluated 200 patients scanned between 18 and 22 weeks' gestation. The rate of "true" echogenic intracardiac foci was 11/200 (5.5%). The rate of "false" echogenic foci was 34/200 (17%). The most common locations for a false EIF were the moderator band, endocardial cushion, and tricuspid valve annulus.

Structural Anomalies

Approximately 25% of fetuses with trisomy 21 are identified as having a structural anomaly, including cardiac defects, duodenal atresia, ventriculomegaly, and hydrops.[66,67,105,116] Cardiac defects are seen in approximately 50% of newborns with trisomy 21 and include atrioventricular septal defects and ventriculoseptal defects. With meticulous technique, these can be found prenatally in 80% to 90% of fetuses with trisomy 21.[117] However, the detection rate of most practitioners is not this high.

Adjunct Features of Trisomy 21

Adjunctive features of trisomy 21 that can be sought sonographically include iliac angle measurements, ear length, clinodactyly, hypoplasia of the middle phalanx of the fifth digit, and frontothalamic distance. Many of these features are difficult to standardize, and there is substantial overlap between those with and without trisomy 21. This limits the utility or these adjunct characteristics in identifying fetuses with trisomy 21.[118-124]

The fetal **iliac length and angle** measurements have been addressed as a potential sonographic marker for trisomy 21. Abuhamad et al.[118] reported that the iliac length measurement is increased in fetuses with trisomy 21. These investigators derived a linear regression of iliac length measurement (cm) = −0.2723 + 0.0333 BPD (mm) and found that a ratio of observed/expected iliac length measurement of 1.21 or greater had a sensitivity of 40% and specificity of 98% for the detection of trisomy 21. The angle between the two iliac bones measured on a cross section of the fetal pelvis is wider in fetuses with trisomy 21. Using an iliac angle of 90 degrees or greater as abnormal, Shipp et al.[119] identified 37% of fetuses with trisomy 21 with FPR of 4.3%. The angle measurement varies considerably depending on the level at which the image is obtained, and the ideal level of angle determination has not been established.

Frontal lobe dimensions are smaller in fetuses with trisomy 21. Bahado-Singh et al.[120] reported that 52% of trisomy 21 fetuses between 16-21 weeks' gestation had a frontothalamic distance of less than the 10th percentile. These investigators found that an observed/expected frontothalamic distance ratio of 0.84 or less had a sensitivity and specificity of 21.2% and 95.2%, respectively, for the detection of trisomy 21.

About 60% of neonates with trisomy 21 have hypoplasia of the middle phalanx of the fifth digit.

Benacerraf et al.[121] reported that the ratio of the middle phalanx of the fifth digit over the middle phalanx of the fourth digit differed between euploid and trisomy 21 fetuses. The median ratio for normal fetuses was 0.85 and for trisomy 21 fetuses, 0.59. Using a cutoff of 0.70, 75% of trisomy 21 fetuses were identified; however, this finding was also present in 18% of normal fetuses. The sonographic appearance of the fetal digits was not suggested as a screening tool for trisomy 21, but rather as an adjunct to other signs.

Short fetal ear length has been reported as a potential marker for trisomy 21.[122,123] Gill et al.[124] demonstrated a significant difference between the ear sizes of normal and trisomy 21 abortuses, but the wide range seen within each gestational age window makes this finding not diagnostically useful.

Cases of trisomy 21 have been reported in fetuses with choroid plexus cysts.[125] However, this is believed to result from the population incidence of choroid plexus cysts rather than from trisomy 21.[126]

Combined Markers

The finding of individual sonographic markers can be used to estimate a risk of aneuploidy.[127-133] In 1992, our laboratory developed a scoring index that rated the markers previously described as "major" (score of 2 for thickened nuchal fold or major anomaly) and "minor" (score of 1 for each finding, such as short femur, short humerus, pyelectasis, echogenic bowel, and EIF).[127,128] A cumulative score of 2 or more identified 73% of fetuses with trisomy 21, with an FPR of 4%. Nyberg et al.[66,132] suggested integrating these markers into risk assessment by using Bayes theorem and likelihood ratios. He showed that likelihood ratios could be calculated for each isolated marker, then applied to the patient's *a priori* (presumptive) risk using Bayes theorem. This resulted in a revised risk of aneuploidy based on the presence or absence of specific markers. Table 31-4 shows a comparison of four studies that computed likelihood ratios for trisomy 21 using isolated markers.[66,67,70,132]

Clusters of markers, even minor ones, confer more risk than individual markers alone[66,67] (Table 31-5).

TRISOMY 21: REVISED RISK RATIO

Revised risk = A priori risk × Likelihood ratio (LR)

Example 1
A 25-year-old woman with a priori risk of trisomy 21 of 1/500 based on quad screen.
Detailed ultrasound shows an isolated EIF (LR ~2).

$$\text{Revised risk} = 1/500 \times 2 = 1/250$$

Example 2
A 39-year-old woman with a priori risk of trisomy 21 of 1/1000 based on quad screen.
Detailed ultrasound shows EIF and mild pyelectasis (LR ≈ 6 from two markers).

$$\text{Revised risk} = 1/1000 \times 6 = 1/166$$

EIF, Echogenic intracardiac focus.

Winter et al.[65] demonstrated that the genetic sonogram scoring index and the method of ultrasound risk assessment using likelihood ratios were essentially equivalent in the detection rate of trisomy 21. The advantage of using likelihood ratios is that a patient's specific risk of aneuploidy can be calculated and balanced against the risk of pregnancy loss associated with an invasive procedure.

Genetic sonography is best used in conjunction with a priori risk estimates based on serum screening.[133-138] Souter et al.[136] demonstrated that serum biochemical marker analytes and sonography are independent and therefore can be used in conjunction with each other to modify the risk of aneuploidy. Several investigators have shown that patients of advanced maternal age who had a normal genetic sonogram and reassuring serum screen are at low risk for trisomy 21.[66,67,135,138]

The use of genetic sonography in risk assessment after a variety of screening protocols has recently been assessed. Adding the genetic sonogram to the results of the screening tests within the FASTER trial substantially increased

---

TABLE 31-4. LIKELIHOOD RATIOS (LR) OF MARKERS FOR TRISOMY 21

MARKER	ISOLATED LR[66]	ISOLATED LR[67]	ISOLATED LR[70]
Nuchal fold	11	—	17
Short humerus	5.1	5.8	7.5
Short femur	1.5	1.2	2.7
Echogenic bowel	6.7	—	6.1
EIF*	1.8	1.4	2.8
Pyelectasis	1.5	1.5	1.9
Structural anomaly	—	3.3	—

* Echogenic intracardiac focus.

TABLE 31-5. TRISOMY 21: LIKELIHOOD RATIOS (LR) OF CLUSTER OF MARKERS

MARKERS (#)	LR[66]	LR[67]
0	0.36	0.2
1	2	1.9
2	9.7	6.2
3	115.2	80

the detection rate of Down syndrome for some protocols. At an FPR of 5%, adding genetic sonography increased the detection rate of Down syndrome from 81% to 90% for the combined test and the quad screen. Furthermore, adding genetic sonography to the integrated test increased the detection from 93% to 98%. A smaller increase in detection rate from 97% to 98% was observed for the stepwise test, and detection rate for the contingent protocol increased from 95% to 97%.[139]

Rozenberg et al.[140] performed a multicenter interventional study in an unselected population to evaluate the performance of first-trimester combined screening followed by second-trimester ultrasound. First-trimester combined screening identified 80% of fetuses with trisomy 21 at a screen-positive rate of 2.7%. Using a thickened nuchal fold or the presence of a major anomaly on a second-trimester ultrasound increased the detection rate to 90%, with a screen-positive rate of 4.2%.

Krantz et al.[141] performed a simulation study to assess genetic sonography as a sequential screen for trisomy 21 after first-trimester risk assessment. First-trimester combined screening resulted in a detection rate of 88.5% with a 4.2% FPR. A follow-up with genetic sonography using individual marker likelihood ratios to modify the first-trimester risk for screen-negative patients detected an additional 6.1% of trisomy 21 cases for an additional 1.2% FPR, giving a total detection rate of 94.6% and a total FPR of 5.4%. If a contingent protocol were adopted in which only patients with a first-trimester risk between 1/300 and 1/2500 were evaluated, the additional detection rate would be 4.8% with FPR of 0.7%, giving a total detection rate of 93% and a total FPR of 4.9%. These authors concluded that second-trimester genetic sonography, if used properly, can be an effective sequential screen after first-trimester risk assessment.

TRISOMY 18 (EDWARDS SYNDROME)

Trisomy 18 is the second most common multiple-malformation syndrome after trisomy 21, with an incidence of 6.4 per 10,000 in the second trimester and 1.6 per 10,000 live births.[142] Individuals with this disorder have a limited capacity for survival, with 44% of those identi-

fied in utero dying before birth.[143] About 50% of affected newborns die within the first week, and only 5% to 10% survive beyond the first year of life. Those who survive are severely mentally and physically handicapped.[144]

Fetuses with trisomy 18 have a plethora of anomalies. Sonographically, 77% to 97% of fetuses with trisomy 18 can be identified by the presence of these structural malformations.[145-149] The more common structural anomalies in fetuses with trisomy 18 include congenital heart defects, neural tube defects, hydrocephalus, diaphragmatic hernia, omphalocele, and abnormally clenched and fisted hands[145-149] (Fig. 31-11). In our experience, cases of trisomy 18 not identified by prenatal ultrasound have been scanned early in the second trimester, when a complete structural survey was not feasible or when other factors such as surgical scarring or maternal body habitus precluded optimal visualization of the fetus.[127,128]

TRISOMY 18: COMMON SONOGRAPHIC ABNORMALITIES

Choroid plexus cyst
Strawberry-shaped skull
Abnormal cerebellum
Abnormal cisterna magna
Neural tube defects
Cystic hygroma
Micrognathia
Cardiac defects
Omphalocele
Diaphragmatic hernia
Clenched hands
Radial ray anomalies
Clubfeet
Rocker-bottom feet
Intrauterine growth restriction (especially with polyhydramnios)

The sonographic findings observed in fetuses with trisomy 18 vary with gestational age. As expected, anomalies such as cystic hygromas are seen more frequently in the early midtrimester, whereas cardiac defects and growth restriction tend to be later findings. In a review of 47 fetuses with trisomy 18, Nyberg et al.[148] identified cardiac defects in 14% before 24 weeks' gestation and in 78% scanned after 24 weeks. **Intrauterine growth restriction** (IUGR) was seen in 28% of affected fetuses scanned at less than 24 weeks and in 89% of those evaluated in the third trimester. IUGR, in combination with **polyhydramnios,** is an ominous observation highly predictive of Edwards syndrome.[148,150] Central nervous system (CNS) anomalies are reported in 34% of affected fetuses.[146,149] Fetuses with trisomy 18 often have omphaloceles, 70% of which only contain bowel.[151] Abnormalities of the extremities, such as clenched hands with overlapping index fingers, are characteristic of trisomy 18. Other findings, such as radial ray defects, rocker-

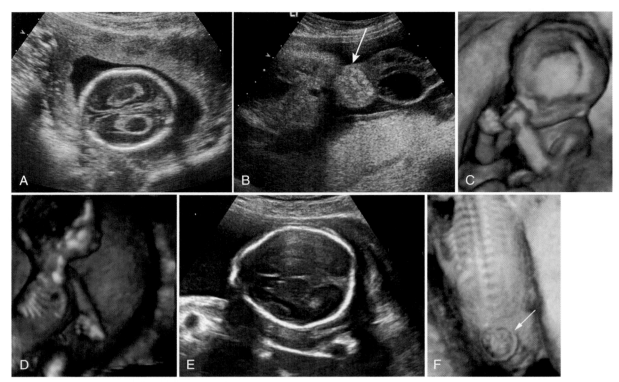

FIGURE 31-11. Sonographic findings in trisomy 18. A, Choroid plexus cyst. Scan through the fetal head at 18 weeks shows bilateral choroid plexus cysts. **B, Omphalocele.** Scan of the fetal lower abdomen shows a bowel-containing omphalocele *(arrow)* as well as an umbilical cord cyst. **C, Clenched fists.** 3-D scan of a midtrimester fetus shows characteristic clenching of the hands and overlapping fingers. **D, Radial ray anomaly.** 3-D scan demonstrates a radial ray anomaly. Note the micrognathia as well. **E,** Strawberry-shaped skull. **F,** 3D scan of the fetal spine at 18 weeks demonstrating a **neural tube defect** *(arrow)*.

bottom feet, clubfeet, strawberry-shaped skull (flattening of occiput with pointing of frontal bones), and abnormal-appearing cerebellum and cisterna magna, have been reported.[144-155]

Choroid Plexus Cysts

Choroid plexus cysts (CPCs) are discrete echolucencies within the choroid plexus that result from the folding of the neuroepithelium, trapping secretory products and desquamated cells[156] (Fig. 31-11, *A*). CPCs are seen in 1% to 2% of the normal fetuses and are most common in the second trimester, usually resolving by 28 weeks' gestation.[145-147] About 30% of fetuses with trisomy 18 have CPCs.[147,148] The majority of fetuses with trisomy 18 also have other structural anomalies to suggest aneuploidy; therefore, karyotyping is recommended for the fetus with a CPC and another finding.[145-148] Cyst number, size, and laterality are not useful in distinguishing affected fetuses from normals.[157-159] Additionally, resolution of CPCs does not necessarily reflect a normal karyotype.[160]

The predictive value of isolated CPCs for aneuploidy is low when no other abnormalities are seen.[125,147] Therefore, after a CPC is seen, there should be a detailed ultrasound assessment, as well as correlation with a priori risk assessment based on an accepted screening protocol is recommended,[125,161] but invasive testing is not necessarily warranted.[150,158,159,162-166] Cheng et al.[167] reported on the significance of isolated CPCs in a population previously screened with NT and found that the likelihood ratio for trisomy 18 was not increased in those with normal NT measurements.

TRISOMY 13 (PATAU SYNDROME)

The incidence of trisomy 13 in live-born infants is approximately 1:12,000.[168] Individuals with trisomy 13 have numerous structural abnormalities and are severely malformed and retarded. Anomalies often seen include forebrain defects, ocular malformations, facial clefts, and heart defects, as well abnormal extremities. About 45% of those born alive die in the first month, and 90% do not survive beyond 6 months of age. Rarely, survival is more long term.[169] Sonographic detection of fetuses with trisomy 13 is 90% to 100% (Fig. 31-12).[127,128,170-174]

Cardiac and CNS defects are the most frequently identified anomalies. The most common CNS malformations identified in trisomy 13 are holoprosencephaly, ventriculomegaly, microcephaly, Dandy-Walker malfor-

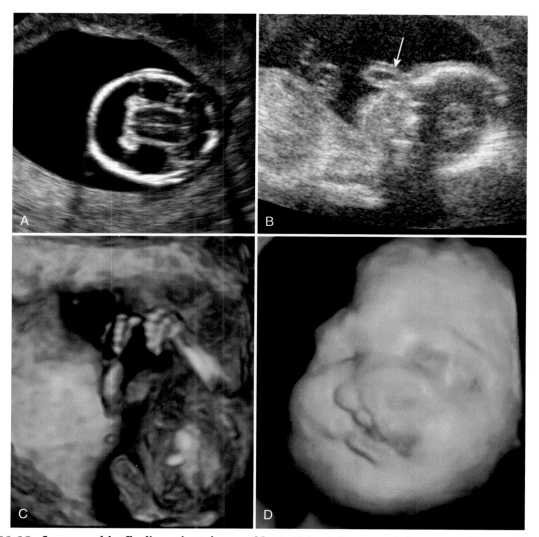

FIGURE 31-12. Sonographic findings in trisomy 13. A, Alobar holoprosencephaly at 11 weeks. **B,** Proboscis *(arrow).* **C,** Postaxial polydactyly on 3-D image at 14 weeks. **D,** 3-D scan of a third-trimester fetus shows a large, midline facial cleft.

TRISOMY 13: SONOGRAPHIC FINDINGS

Holoprosencephaly
Microcephaly
Neural tube defects
Facial clefts
Ocular anomalies
Cardiac defects
Echogenic intracardiac focus
Cystic hygroma
Postaxial polydactyly
Echogenic kidneys
Intrauterine growth restriction

mation, and other abnormalities of the posterior fossa. **Alobar holoprosencephaly** is often associated with severe midline facial defects, including hypotelorism, microphthalmia, and cyclopia. In addition, fetuses with trisomy 13 often have postaxial polydactyly, abnormal hand configuration, echogenic kidneys (30%), atypical calcifications,[170-174] and IUGR.[172]

TRIPLOIDY

Triploidy is the result of a complete extra set of chromosomes (69 chromosomes) and is not related to maternal age.[175] The extra set of chromosomes is often paternally

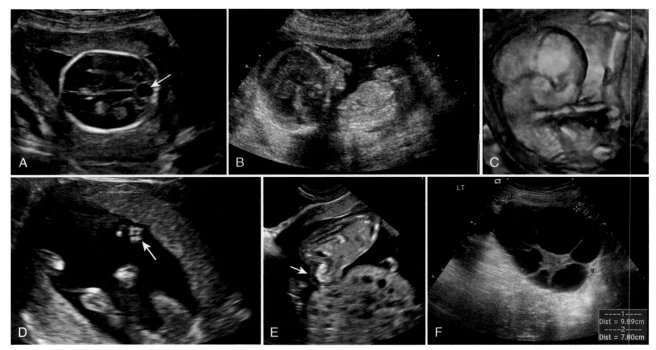

FIGURE 31-13. Sonographic findings in triploidy. A, Dandy-Walker malformation *(arrow).* **B** and **C,** Asymmetrical growth restriction. Note the discrepancy in size of the head and body. **D,** Syndactyly of the fingers. **E,** Scan through the placenta showing multiple lucencies as well as an omphalocele *(arrow).* **F,** Maternal ovaries with multiple cysts.

derived (73%) and usually occurs from a double fertilization. Less often, triploidy results from fertilization of a diploid egg.[176] Triploidy occurs in 1% to 3% of conceptions, and most are spontaneously aborted.[177,178] The prevalence of triploidy between 16 and 20 weeks is 1:5000 pregnancies, and survival of a fetus with triploidy beyond 20 weeks' gestation is unusual.[175] Fetuses with triploidy surviving into the midtrimester have a multitude of structural malformations, most often involving the CNS, heart, and hands, as well as marked asymmetrical growth restriction[178,179] (Fig. 31-13).

TRIPLOIDY: SONOGRAPHIC FINDINGS

3-4 Syndactyly
Cardiac defects
Neural tube defects
Posterior fossa anomalies
Heart defects
Cystic hygroma
Asymmetric growth restriction
Abnormal placenta
Oligohydramnios
Renal anomalies
Omphalocele

Paternal triploid origin is associated with a large placenta filled with cystic spaces. Triploidy on the basis of an extra maternal chromosomal complement is usually associated with a small placenta and IUGR.[176,177] Triploidy can be associated with maternal complications, including early-onset preeclampsia, bilateral multicystic ovaries, hyperemesis gravidarum, and persistent trophoblastic disease.[180,181]

Jauniaux et al.[178] described 70 cases of triploidy scanned between 13 and 29 weeks' gestation. Anatomic defects were found in 93% of cases, with abnormalities of the hands (predominantly 3-4 syndactyly) the most frequent finding (52%). Cerebral ventriculomegaly was identified in 37%. Cardiac defects were detected in 34% of fetuses, primarily atrioventricular septal defects. Micrognathia affected 26% of fetuses. Placental molar changes were seen in 29%, and amniotic fluid volume was decreased in 44%. Asymmetrical growth restriction was noted in 72% of cases, and each of these fetuses had a sonographically normal–appearing placenta.[178]

TURNER (45,X) SYNDROME

Turner syndrome is the result of a 45,X chromosomal complement, usually caused by loss of the paternal X chromosome, and is unrelated to maternal age. About 95% of conceptuses are spontaneously aborted. Turner syndrome occurs in 1:2000 to 1:5000 live births.[182-185] The lethal type of Turner syndrome seen in the midtrimester of pregnancy generally presents with large septated cystic hygromas, total body lymphedema, pleural effusions, ascites, and cardiac defects[182,183] (Fig. 31-14).

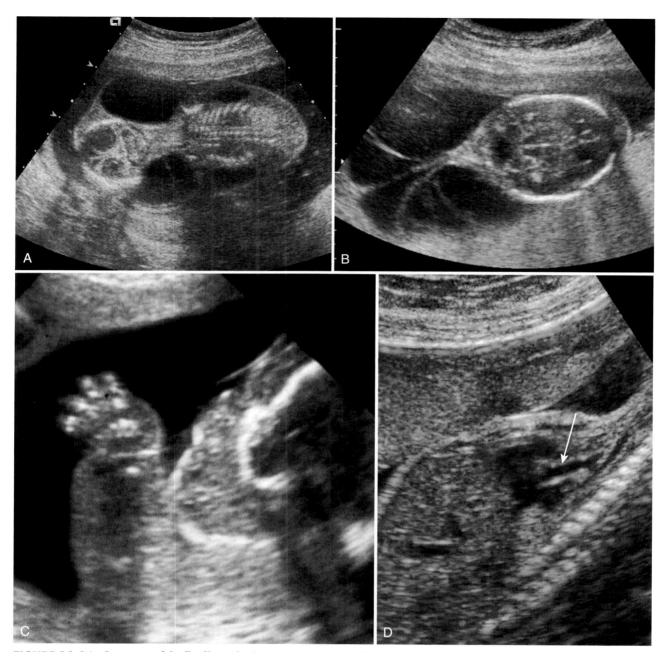

FIGURE 31-14. Sonographic findings in Turner (45,X) syndrome. A and **B,** Large septated cystic hygromas. **C,** Hydropic fetal arm in a fetus with severe lymphangiectasia. **D,** Small aorta *(arrow)* in fetus with interrupted aortic arch.

Cystic hygromas are malformations of the lymphatic system and appear as saccular septated fluid collections, most often surrounding the back of the fetal head and neck. Azar et al.[184] reported that 75% of fetuses with bilateral dorsal septated nuchal cervical cystic hygromas had chromosomal anomalies, the most common being Turner syndrome (94%). Although many second-trimester fetuses with cystic hygromas have Turner syndrome, other karyotypic abnormalities, including trisomies 21, 18, and 13 and triploidy, have also been reported. In general, cystic hygromas in fetuses with Turner syndrome are larger than those seen with other karyotypic abnormalities, and Turner fetuses may also have generalized lymphedema extending down the torso and extremities.

Cardiac abnormalities, most often left-sided defects such as coarctation of the aorta, may be identified in 10% to 48% of fetuses with Turner syndrome. However, this may be an underestimation because many fetuses are identified late in the first semester or early in the second trimester, when optimal cardiac evaluation is not likely.[182-185] Baena et al.[182] reported on 125 cases of Turner syndrome from an unselected population and noted that 67% were identified prenatally. The most common sonographic findings were cystic hygromas (59%) and hydrops (19%).

CONCLUSION

Over the last two decades, risk assessment for aneuploidy has been refined to the point that maternal age alone is no longer considered adequate in determining the risk of having a chromosomally abnormal offspring. Obstetric sonography, in conjunction with serum analysis, has become a powerful tool in the assessment of risk for aneuploidy, in both the first and the second trimester. In the midtrimester the diverse sonographic patterns seen in the different aneuploidies allows clinicians to guide patients to a presumptive diagnosis. The information obtained noninvasively helps the expectant couple to weigh the risks of invasive testing against the probability of having a child with an abnormality. The goal of screening is the detection of a greater number of karyotypically abnormal fetuses with fewer invasive procedures and subsequently the loss of fewer normal fetuses.

References

1. ACOG Practice Bulletin No. 77. Screening for fetal chromosomal abnormalities. Obstet Gynecol 2007;109:217-227.
2. Peller AJ, Westgate MN, Holmes LB. Trends in congenital malformations, 1974-1999: effect of prenatal diagnosis and elective termination. Obstet Gynecol 2004;104:957-964.
3. Egan JF, Benn P, Borgida AF, et al. Efficacy of screening for fetal Down syndrome in the United States from 1974 to 1997. Obstet Gynecol 2000;96:979-985.
4. Schreinemachers DM, Cross PK, Hook EB. Rates of trisomies 21, 18, 13 and other chromosome abnormalities in about 20,000 prenatal studies compared with estimated rates in live births. Hum Genet 1982;61:318-324.
5. Resta RG. Changing demographics of advanced maternal age (AMA) and the impact on the predicted incidence of Down syndrome in the United States: implications for prenatal screening and genetic counseling. Am J Med Genet A 2005;133A:31-36.
6. Snijders RJ, Sebire NJ, Nicolaides KH. Maternal age and gestational age–specific risk for chromosomal defects. Fetal Diagn Ther 1995;10:356-367.
7. Nicolaides KH. Nuchal translucency and other first-trimester sonographic markers of chromosomal abnormalities. Am J Obstet Gynecol 2004;191:45-67.

First-Trimester Screening for Aneuploidy
8. Langdon JLH. Observations on an ethnic classification of idiots. In Clinical Lectures and Reports; 1866:259.
9. Nicolaides KH, Azar G, Byrne D, et al. Fetal nuchal translucency: ultrasound screening for chromosomal defects in first trimester of pregnancy. BMJ 1992;304:867-869.
10. Bekker MN, Haak MC, Rekoert-Hollander M, et al. Increased nuchal translucency and distended jugular lymphatic sacs on first-trimester ultrasound. Ultrasound Obstet Gynecol 2005;25:239-245.
11. Souka AP, von Kaisenberg CS, Hyett JA, et al. Increased nuchal translucency with normal karyotype. Am J Obstet Gynecol 2005;192:1005-1021.
12. Pandya PP, Snijders RJ, Johnson SP, et al. Screening for fetal trisomies by maternal age and fetal nuchal translucency thickness at 10 to 14 weeks of gestation. Br J Obstet Gynaecol 1995;102:957-962.

13. Snijders RJ, Noble P, Sebire N, et al. UK multicentre project on assessment of risk of trisomy 21 by maternal age and fetal nuchal-translucency thickness at 10-14 weeks of gestation. Fetal Medicine Foundation First Trimester Screening Group. Lancet 1998;352:343-346.
14. Wald NJ, Kennard A, Hackshaw AK. First trimester serum screening for Down's syndrome. Prenat Diagn 1995;15:1227-1240.
15. Brizot ML, Snijders RJ, Bersinger NA, et al. Maternal serum pregnancy-associated plasma protein A and fetal nuchal translucency thickness for the prediction of fetal trisomies in early pregnancy. Obstet Gynecol 1994;84:918-922.
16. Brizot ML, Snijders RJ, Butler J, et al. Maternal serum hCG and fetal nuchal translucency thickness for the prediction of fetal trisomies in the first trimester of pregnancy. Br J Obstet Gynaecol 1995;102:127-132.
17. Wald NJ, Kennard A, Hackshaw A, McGuire A. Antenatal screening for Down's syndrome. J Med Screen 1997;4:181-246.
18. Spencer K, Spencer CE, Power M, et al. Screening for chromosomal abnormalities in the first trimester using ultrasound and maternal serum biochemistry in a one-stop clinic: a review of three years prospective experience. BJOG 2003;110:281-286.
19. Wapner R, Thom E, Simpson JL, et al. First-trimester screening for trisomies 21 and 18. N Engl J Med 2003;349:1405-1413.
20. Wald NJ, Rodeck C, Hackshaw AK, et al. First and second trimester antenatal screening for Down's syndrome: the results of the Serum, Urine and Ultrasound Screening Study (SURUSS). J Med Screen 2003;10:56-104.
21. Malone FD, Canick JA, Ball RH, et al. First-trimester or second-trimester screening, or both, for Down's syndrome. N Engl J Med 2005;353:2001-2011.
22. Sebire NJ, Snijders RJ, Hughes K, et al. Screening for trisomy 21 in twin pregnancies by maternal age and fetal nuchal translucency thickness at 10-14 weeks of gestation. Br J Obstet Gynaecol 1996;103:999-1003.
23. Kagan KO, Gazzoni A, Sepulveda-Gonzalez G, et al. Discordance in nuchal translucency thickness in the prediction of severe twin-to-twin transfusion syndrome. Ultrasound Obstet Gynecol 2007;29:527-532.
24. Spencer K, Nicolaides KH. Screening for trisomy 21 in twins using first trimester ultrasound and maternal serum biochemistry in a one-stop clinic: a review of three years experience. BJOG 2003;110:276-280.
25. Comstock CH, Malone FD, Ball RH, et al. Is there a nuchal translucency millimeter measurement above which there is no added benefit from first trimester serum screening? Am J Obstet Gynecol 2006;195:843-847.
26. Wald NJ, Watt HC, Hackshaw AK. Integrated screening for Down's syndrome on the basis of tests performed during the first and second trimesters. N Engl J Med 1999;341:461-467.
27. Palomaki GE, Steinort K, Knight GJ, Haddow JE. Comparing three screening strategies for combining first- and second-trimester Down syndrome markers. Obstet Gynecol 2006;107:367-375.
28. Cuckle HS, Malone FD, Wright D, et al. Contingent screening for Down syndrome: results from the FASTER trial. Prenat Diagn 2008;28:89-94.
29. Ball RH, Caughey AB, Malone FD, et al. First- and second-trimester evaluation of risk for Down syndrome. Obstet Gynecol 2007;110:10-17.
30. Platt LD, Greene N, Johnson A, et al. Sequential pathways of testing after first-trimester screening for trisomy 21. Obstet Gynecol 2004;104:661-666.
31. Haddow JE, Palomaki GE, Knight GJ, et al. Screening of maternal serum for fetal Down's syndrome in the first trimester. N Engl J Med 1998;338:955-961.
32. Snijders RJ, Thom EA, Zachary JM, et al. First-trimester trisomy screening: nuchal translucency measurement training and quality assurance to correct and unify technique. Ultrasound Obstet Gynecol 2002;19:353-359.
33. Evans MI, van Decruyes H, Nicolaides KH. Nuchal translucency measurements for first-trimester screening: the 'price' of inaccuracy. Fetal Diagn Ther 2007;22:401-404.
34. Braithwaite JM, Kadir RA, Pepera TA, et al. Nuchal translucency measurement: training of potential examiners. Ultrasound Obstet Gynecol 1996;8:192-195.
35. Nicolaides KH. The 11-13+6 weeks scan. London: Fetal Medicine Foundation; 2004.

36. Wax JR, Pinette MG, Cartin A, Blackstone J. The value of repeated evaluation after initial failed nuchal translucency measurement. J Ultrasound Med 2007;26:825-828; quiz 829-830.

37. Breathnach FM, Malone FD, Lambert-Messerlian G, et al. First- and second-trimester screening: detection of aneuploidies other than Down syndrome. Obstet Gynecol 2007;110:651-657.

38. Spencer K, Nicolaides KH. A first trimester trisomy 13/trisomy 18 risk algorithm combining fetal nuchal translucency thickness, maternal serum free beta-hCG and PAPP-A. Prenat Diagn 2002;22:877-879.

39. Malone FD, Ball RH, Nyberg DA, et al. First-trimester septated cystic hygroma: prevalence, natural history, and pediatric outcome. Obstet Gynecol 2005;106:288-294.

40. Molina FS, Avgidou K, Kagan KO, et al. Cystic hygromas, nuchal edema, and nuchal translucency at 11-14 weeks of gestation. Obstet Gynecol 2006;107:678-683.

41. Sonek J, Croom C, McKenna D, Neiger R. First-trimester septated cystic hygroma: prevalence, natural history, and pediatric outcome. Obstet Gynecol 2006;107:424; author reply 425.

42. Cicero S, Dezerega V, Andrade E, et al. Learning curve for sonographic examination of the fetal nasal bone at 11-14 weeks. Ultrasound Obstet Gynecol 2003;22:135-137.

43. Cicero S, Curcio P, Papageorghiou A, et al. Absence of nasal bone in fetuses with trisomy 21 at 11-14 weeks of gestation: an observational study. Lancet 2001;358:1665-1667.

44. Cicero S, Rembouskos G, Vandecruys H, et al. Likelihood ratio for trisomy 21 in fetuses with absent nasal bone at the 11-14–week scan. Ultrasound Obstet Gynecol 2004;23:218-223.

45. Cicero S, Bindra R, Rembouskos G, et al. Integrated ultrasound and biochemical screening for trisomy 21 using fetal nuchal translucency, absent fetal nasal bone, free beta-hCG and PAPP-A at 11 to 14 weeks. Prenat Diagn 2003;23:306-310.

46. Cicero S, Avgidou K, Rembouskos G, et al. Nasal bone in first-trimester screening for trisomy 21. Am J Obstet Gynecol 2006;195:109.

47. Sepulveda W, Wong AE, Dezerega V. First-trimester ultrasonographic screening for trisomy 21 using fetal nuchal translucency and nasal bone. Obstet Gynecol 2007;109:1040-1045.

48. Malone FD, Ball RH, Nyberg DA, et al. First-trimester nasal bone evaluation for aneuploidy in the general population. Obstet Gynecol 2004;104:1222-1228.

49. Rosen T, D'Alton ME, Platt LD, Wapner R. First-trimester ultrasound assessment of the nasal bone to screen for aneuploidy. Obstet Gynecol 2007;110:399-404.

50. Ville Y. What is the role of fetal nasal bone examination in the assessment of risk for trisomy 21 in clinical practice? Am J Obstet Gynecol 2006;195:1-3.

51. Sonek J, Borenstein M, Dagklis T, et al. Frontomaxillary facial angle in fetuses with trisomy 21 at 11-13(6) weeks. Am J Obstet Gynecol 2007;196:271 e1-e4.

52. Borrell A, Gonce A, Martinez JM, et al. First-trimester screening for Down syndrome with ductus venosus Doppler studies in addition to nuchal translucency and serum markers. Prenat Diagn 2005;25:901-905.

53. Falcon O, Auer M, Gerovassili A, et al. Screening for trisomy 21 by fetal tricuspid regurgitation, nuchal translucency and maternal serum free beta-hCG and PAPP-A at 11 + 0 to 13 + 6 weeks. Ultrasound Obstet Gynecol 2006;27:151-155.

54. Hyett J, Perdu M, Sharland G, et al. Using fetal nuchal translucency to screen for major congenital cardiac defects at 10-14 weeks of gestation: population based cohort study. BMJ 1999;318:81-85.

55. Makrydimas G, Sotiriadis A, Ioannidis JP. Screening performance of first-trimester nuchal translucency for major cardiac defects: a meta-analysis. Am J Obstet Gynecol 2003;189:1330-1335.

56. Simpson LL, Malone FD, Bianchi DW, et al. Nuchal translucency and the risk of congenital heart disease. Obstet Gynecol 2007;109:376-383.

57. Michailidis GD, Economides DL. Nuchal translucency measurement and pregnancy outcome in karyotypically normal fetuses. Ultrasound Obstet Gynecol 2001;17:102-105.

58. Souka AP, Krampl E, Bakalis S, et al. Outcome of pregnancy in chromosomally normal fetuses with increased nuchal translucency in the first trimester. Ultrasound Obstet Gynecol 2001;18:9-17.

59. Bilardo CM, Muller MA, Pajkrt E, et al. Increased nuchal translucency thickness and normal karyotype: time for parental reassurance. Ultrasound Obstet Gynecol 2007;30:11-18.

60. Westin M, Saltvedt S, Almstrom H, et al. By how much does increased nuchal translucency increase the risk of adverse pregnancy outcome in chromosomally normal fetuses? A study of 16,260 fetuses derived from an unselected pregnant population. Ultrasound Obstet Gynecol 2007;29:150-158.

61. Senat MV, Bussieres L, Couderc S, et al. Long-term outcome of children born after a first-trimester measurement of nuchal translucency at the 99th percentile or greater with normal karyotype: a prospective study. Am J Obstet Gynecol 2007;196:53 e1-e6.

Second-Trimester Screening for Trisomy 21

62. Vintzileos AM, Egan JF. Adjusting the risk for trisomy 21 on the basis of second-trimester ultrasonography. Am J Obstet Gynecol 1995;172:837-844.

63. Bromley B, Lieberman E, Benacerraf BR. The incorporation of maternal age into the sonographic scoring index for the detection at 14-20 weeks of fetuses with Down's syndrome. Ultrasound Obstet Gynecol 1997;10:321-324.

64. Bromley B, Shipp T, Benacerraf BR. Genetic sonogram scoring index: accuracy and clinical utility. J Ultrasound Med 1999;18:523-528; quiz 529-530.

65. Winter TC, Uhrich SB, Souter VL, Nyberg DA. The "genetic sonogram": comparison of the index scoring system with the age-adjusted ultrasound risk assessment. Radiology 2000;215:775-782.

66. Nyberg DA, Souter VL, El-Bastawissi A, et al. Isolated sonographic markers for detection of fetal Down syndrome in the second trimester of pregnancy. J Ultrasound Med 2001;20:1053-1063.

67. Bromley B, Lieberman E, Shipp TD, Benacerraf BR. The genetic sonogram: a method of risk assessment for Down syndrome in the second trimester. J Ultrasound Med 2002;21:1087-1096; quiz 1097-1098.

68. Vintzileos AM, Guzman ER, Smulian JC, et al. Second-trimester genetic sonography in patients with advanced maternal age and normal triple screen. Obstet Gynecol 2002;99:993-995.

69. Hobbins JC, Lezotte DC, Persutte WH, et al. An 8-center study to evaluate the utility of mid-term genetic sonograms among high-risk pregnancies. J Ultrasound Med 2003;22:33-38.

70. Smith-Bindman R, Hosmer W, Feldstein VA, et al. Second-trimester ultrasound to detect fetuses with Down syndrome: a meta-analysis. JAMA 2001;285:1044-1055.

71. Benacerraf BR, Barss VA, Laboda LA. A sonographic sign for the detection in the second trimester of the fetus with Down's syndrome. Am J Obstet Gynecol 1985;151:1078-1079.

72. Benacerraf BR, Frigoletto Jr FD. Soft tissue nuchal fold in the second-trimester fetus: standards for normal measurements compared with those in Down syndrome. Am J Obstet Gynecol 1987;157:1146-1149.

73. Benacerraf BR, Laboda LA, Frigoletto FD. Thickened nuchal fold in fetuses not at risk for aneuploidy. Radiology 1992;184:239-242.

74. Benacerraf BR, Frigoletto Jr FD, Cramer DW. Down syndrome: sonographic sign for diagnosis in the second-trimester fetus. Radiology 1987;163:811-813.

75. Crane JP, Gray DL. Sonographically measured nuchal skinfold thickness as a screening tool for Down syndrome: results of a prospective clinical trial. Obstet Gynecol 1991;77:533-536.

76. Donnenfeld AE, Meister D, Allison J, et al. Interobserver variability of sonographically determined second-trimester nuchal skinfold thickness measurements. Ultrasound Obstet Gynecol 1995;5:119-122.

77. Gray DL, Crane JP. Optimal nuchal skin-fold thresholds based on gestational age for prenatal detection of Down syndrome. Am J Obstet Gynecol 1994;171:1282-1286.

78. Grandjean H, Sarramon MF. Sonographic measurement of nuchal skinfold thickness for detection of Down syndrome in the second-trimester fetus: a multicenter prospective study. The AFDPHE Study Group. Association Francaise pour le Depistage et la Prevention des Handicaps de l'Enfant. Obstet Gynecol 1995;85:103-106.

79. Watson WJ, Miller RC, Menard MK, et al. Ultrasonographic measurement of fetal nuchal skin to screen for chromosomal abnormalities. Am J Obstet Gynecol 1994;170:583-586.

80. Landwehr Jr JB, Johnson MP, Hume RF, et al. Abnormal nuchal findings on screening ultrasonography: aneuploidy stratification on the basis of ultrasonographic anomaly and gestational age at detection. Am J Obstet Gynecol 1996;175:995-999.

81. Lynch L, Berkowitz GS, Chitkara U, et al. Ultrasound detection of Down syndrome: is it really possible? Obstet Gynecol 1989;73:267-270.

82. Smith-Bindman R, Chu P, Goldberg JD. Second trimester prenatal ultrasound for the detection of pregnancies at increased risk of Down syndrome. Prenat Diagn 2007;27:535-544.

83. Borrell A, Costa D, Martinez JM, et al. Criteria for fetal nuchal thickness cut-off: a re-evaluation. Prenat Diagn 1997;17:23-29.

84. Wapner RJ. Nuchal fold and nasal bone: how should we use them in Down syndrome screening? Am J Obstet Gynecol 2008;199:213-214.

85. Sonek JD, Nicolaides KH. Prenatal ultrasonographic diagnosis of nasal bone abnormalities in three fetuses with Down syndrome. Am J Obstet Gynecol 2002;186:139-141.

86. Sonek JD, Cicero S, Neiger R, Nicolaides KH. Nasal bone assessment in prenatal screening for trisomy 21. Am J Obstet Gynecol 2006;195:1219-1230.

87. Bromley B, Lieberman E, Shipp TD, Benacerraf BR. Fetal nose bone length: a marker for Down syndrome in the second trimester. J Ultrasound Med 2002;21:1387-1394.

88. Vintzileos A, Walters C, Yeo L. Absent nasal bone in the prenatal detection of fetuses with trisomy 21 in a high-risk population. Obstet Gynecol 2003;101:905-908.

89. Odibo AO, Sehdev HM, Dunn L, et al. The association between fetal nasal bone hypoplasia and aneuploidy. Obstet Gynecol 2004;104:1229-1233.

90. Bunduki V, Ruano R, Miguelez J, et al. Fetal nasal bone length: reference range and clinical application in ultrasound screening for trisomy 21. Ultrasound Obstet Gynecol 2003;21:156-160.

91. Cicero S, Sonek JD, McKenna DS, et al. Nasal bone hypoplasia in trisomy 21 at 15-22 weeks' gestation. Ultrasound Obstet Gynecol 2003;21:15-18.

92. Cusick W, Provenzano J, Sullivan CA, et al. Fetal nasal bone length in euploid and aneuploid fetuses between 11 and 20 weeks' gestation: a prospective study. J Ultrasound Med 2004;23:1327-1333.

93. Odibo AO, Sehdev HM, Stamilio DM, et al. Defining nasal bone hypoplasia in second-trimester Down syndrome screening: does the use of multiples of the median improve screening efficacy? Am J Obstet Gynecol 2007;197:361e1-e4.

94. Odibo AO, Sehdev HM, Gerkowicz S, et al. Comparison of the efficiency of second-trimester nasal bone hypoplasia and increased nuchal fold in Down syndrome screening. Am J Obstet Gynecol 2008;199:281e1-e5.

95. Benoit B, Chaoui R. Three-dimensional ultrasound with maximal mode rendering: a novel technique for the diagnosis of bilateral or unilateral absence or hypoplasia of nasal bones in second-trimester screening for Down syndrome. Ultrasound Obstet Gynecol 2005;25:19-24.

96. Lockwood C, Benacerraf B, Krinsky A, et al. A sonographic screening method for Down syndrome. Am J Obstet Gynecol 1987;157:803-808.

97. Benacerraf BR, Gelman R, Frigoletto Jr FD. Sonographic identification of second-trimester fetuses with Down's syndrome. N Engl J Med 1987;317:1371-1376.

98. Benacerraf BR, Cnann A, Gelman R, et al. Can sonographers reliably identify anatomic features associated with Down syndrome in fetuses? Radiology 1989;173:377-380.

99. Nyberg DA, Resta RG, Hickok DE, et al. Femur length shortening in the detection of Down syndrome: is prenatal screening feasible? Am J Obstet Gynecol 1990;162:1247-1252.

100. Shipp TD, Bromley B, Mascola M, Benacerraf B. Variation in fetal femur length with respect to maternal race. J Ultrasound Med 2001;20:141-144.

101. FitzSimmons J, Droste S, Shepard TH, et al. Long-bone growth in fetuses with Down syndrome. Am J Obstet Gynecol 1989;161:1174-1177.

102. Benacerraf BR, Neuberg D, Frigoletto Jr FD. Humeral shortening in second-trimester fetuses with Down syndrome. Obstet Gynecol 1991;77:223-227.

103. Benacerraf BR, Mandell J, Estroff JA, et al. Fetal pyelectasis: a possible association with Down syndrome. Obstet Gynecol 1990;76:58-60.

104. Corteville JE, Dicke JM, Crane JP. Fetal pyelectasis and Down syndrome: is genetic amniocentesis warranted? Obstet Gynecol 1992;79:770-772.

105. Nyberg DA, Resta RG, Luthy DA, et al. Prenatal sonographic findings of Down syndrome: review of 94 cases. Obstet Gynecol 1990;76:370-377.

106. Bromley B, Doubilet P, Frigoletto Jr FD, et al. Is fetal hyperechoic bowel on second-trimester sonogram an indication for amniocentesis? Obstet Gynecol 1994;83:647-651.

107. Dicke JM, Crane JP. Sonographically detected hyperechoic fetal bowel: significance and implications for pregnancy management. Obstet Gynecol 1992;80:778-782.

108. Nyberg DA, Resta RG, Mahony BS, et al. Fetal hyperechogenic bowel and Down's syndrome. Ultrasound Obstet Gynecol 1993;3:330-333.

109. Scioscia AL, Pretorius DH, Budorick NE, et al. Second-trimester echogenic bowel and chromosomal abnormalities. Am J Obstet Gynecol 1992;167:889-894.

110. Sepulveda W, Sebire NJ. Fetal echogenic bowel: a complex scenario. Ultrasound Obstet Gynecol 2000;16:510-514.

111. Roberts DJ, Genest D. Cardiac histologic pathology characteristic of trisomies 13 and 21. Hum Pathol 1992;23:1130-1140.

112. Bromley B, Lieberman E, Laboda L, Benacerraf BR. Echogenic intracardiac focus: a sonographic sign for fetal Down syndrome. Obstet Gynecol 1995;86:998-1001.

113. Winter TC, Anderson AM, Cheng EY, et al. Echogenic intracardiac focus in 2nd-trimester fetuses with trisomy 21: usefulness as a US marker. Radiology 2000;216:450-456.

114. Shipp TD, Bromley B, Lieberman E, Benacerraf BR. The frequency of the detection of fetal echogenic intracardiac foci with respect to maternal race. Ultrasound Obstet Gynecol 2000;15:460-462.

115. Winn VD, Sonson J, Filly RA. Echogenic intracardiac focus: potential for misdiagnosis. J Ultrasound Med 2003;22:1207-1214; quiz 1216-1217.

116. Rotmensch S, Liberati M, Bronshtein M, et al. Prenatal sonographic findings in 187 fetuses with Down syndrome. Prenat Diagn 1997;17:1001-1009.

117. DeVore GR, Alfi O. The use of color Doppler ultrasound to identify fetuses at increased risk for trisomy 21: an alternative for high-risk patients who decline genetic amniocentesis. Obstet Gynecol 1997;90:187.

118. Abuhamad AZ, Kolm P, Mari G, et al. Ultrasonographic fetal iliac length measurement in the screening for Down syndrome. Am J Obstet Gynecol 1994;171:1063-1067.

119. Shipp TD, Bromley B, Lieberman E, Benacerraf BR. The iliac angle as a sonographic marker for Down syndrome in second-trimester fetuses. Obstet Gynecol 1997;89:446-450.

120. Bahado-Singh RO, Wyse L, Dorr MA, et al. Fetuses with Down syndrome have disproportionately shortened frontal lobe dimensions on ultrasonographic examination. Am J Obstet Gynecol 1992;167:1009-1014.

121. Benacerraf BR, Harlow BL, Frigoletto Jr FD. Hypoplasia of the middle phalanx of the fifth digit: a feature of the second trimester fetus with Down's syndrome. J Ultrasound Med 1990;9:389-394.

122. Shimizu T, Salvador L, Hughes-Benzie R, et al. The role of reduced ear size in the prenatal detection of chromosomal abnormalities. Prenat Diagn 1997;17:545-549.

123. Lettieri L, Rodis JF, Vintzileos AM, et al. Ear length in second-trimester aneuploid fetuses. Obstet Gynecol 1993;81:57-60.

124. Gill P, Vanhook J, Fitzsimmons J, et al. Fetal ear measurements in the prenatal detection of trisomy 21. Prenat Diagn 1994;14:739-743.

125. Gupta JK, Cave M, Lilford RJ, et al. Clinical significance of fetal choroid plexus cysts. Lancet 1995;346:724-729.

126. Bromley B, Lieberman R, Benacerraf BR. Choroid plexus cysts: not associated with Down syndrome. Ultrasound Obstet Gynecol 1996;8:232-235.

127. Benacerraf BR, Neuberg D, Bromley B, Frigoletto Jr FD. Sonographic scoring index for prenatal detection of chromosomal abnormalities. J Ultrasound Med 1992;11:449-458.

128. Benacerraf BR, Nadel A, Bromley B. Identification of second-trimester fetuses with autosomal trisomy by use of a sonographic scoring index. Radiology 1994;193:135-140.

129. Vintzileos AM, Campbell WA, Guzman ER, et al. Second-trimester ultrasound markers for detection of trisomy 21: which markers are best? Obstet Gynecol 1997;89:941-944.

130. Bahado-Singh RO, Oz AU, Kovanci E, et al. New Down syndrome screening algorithm: ultrasonographic biometry and multiple serum

markers combined with maternal age. Am J Obstet Gynecol 1998;179:1627-1631.

131. Bahado-Singh RO, Deren O, Tan A, et al. Ultrasonographically adjusted midtrimester risk of trisomy 21 and significant chromosomal defects in advanced maternal age. Am J Obstet Gynecol 1996;175:1563-1568.

132. Nyberg DA, Luthy DA, Resta RG, et al. Age-adjusted ultrasound risk assessment for fetal Down's syndrome during the second trimester: description of the method and analysis of 142 cases. Ultrasound Obstet Gynecol 1998;12:8-14.

133. Vintzileos AM, Campbell WA, Rodis JF, et al. The use of second-trimester genetic sonogram in guiding clinical management of patients at increased risk for fetal trisomy 21. Obstet Gynecol 1996;87:948-952.

134. Nyberg DA, Luthy DA, Cheng EY, et al. Role of prenatal ultrasonography in women with positive screen for Down syndrome on the basis of maternal serum markers. Am J Obstet Gynecol 1995;173:1030-1035.

135. Vintzileos AM, Guzman ER, Smulian JC, et al. Choice of second-trimester genetic sonogram for detection of trisomy 21. Obstet Gynecol 1997;90:187-190.

136. Souter VL, Nyberg DA, Benn PA, et al. Correlation of second-trimester sonographic and biochemical markers. J Ultrasound Med 2004;23:505-511.

137. Pinette MG, Egan JF, Wax JR, et al. Combined sonographic and biochemical markers for Down syndrome screening. J Ultrasound Med 2003;22:1185-1190.

138. DeVore GR, Romero R. Genetic sonography: an option for women of advanced maternal age with negative triple-marker maternal serum screening results. J Ultrasound Med 2003;22:1191-1199.

139. Aagaard-Tillery KM, Malone FD, Nyberg DA, et al. Role of second-trimester genetic sonography after Down syndrome screening. Obstet Gynecol 2009;114:1189-1196.

140. Rozenberg P, Bussieres L, Chevret S, et al. Screening for Down syndrome using first-trimester combined screening followed by second-trimester ultrasound examination in an unselected population. Am J Obstet Gynecol 2006;195:1379-1387.

141. Krantz DA, Hallahan TW, Macri VJ, Macri JN. Genetic sonography after first-trimester Down syndrome screening. Ultrasound Obstet Gynecol 2007;29:666-670.

Trisomy 18 (Edwards Syndrome)

142. Hook EB, Woodbury DF, Albright SG. Rates of trisomy 18 in livebirths, stillbirths, and at amniocentesis. Birth Defects Orig Artic Ser 1979;15:81-93.

143. Yamanaka M, Setoyama T, Igarashi Y, et al. Pregnancy outcome of fetuses with trisomy 18 identified by prenatal sonography and chromosomal analysis in a perinatal center. Am J Med Genet A 2006;140:1177-1182.

144. Jones KL. Smith's recognizable patterns of human malformation, 5th ed. Philadelphia: Saunders; 1997.

145. Papp C, Ban Z, Szigeti Z, et al. Role of second trimester sonography in detecting trisomy 18: a review of 70 cases. J Clin Ultrasound 2007;35:68-72.

146. Watson WJ, Miller RC, Wax JR, et al. Sonographic findings of trisomy 18 in the second trimester of pregnancy. J Ultrasound Med 2008;27:1033-1038; quiz 1039-1040.

147. Benacerraf BR, Harlow B, Frigoletto Jr FD. Are choroid plexus cysts an indication for second-trimester amniocentesis? Am J Obstet Gynecol 1990;162:1001-1006.

148. Nyberg DA, Kramer D, Resta RG, et al. Prenatal sonographic findings of trisomy 18: review of 47 cases. J Ultrasound Med 1993;12:103-113.

149. Goetzinger KR, Stamilio DM, Dicke JM, et al. Evaluating the incidence and likelihood ratios for chromosomal abnormalities in fetuses with common central nervous system malformations. Am J Obstet Gynecol 2008;199:285e1-e6.

150. Carlson DE, Platt LD, Medearis AL. The ultrasound triad of fetal hydramnios, abnormal hand posturing, and any other anomaly predicts autosomal trisomy. Obstet Gynecol 1992;79:731-734.

151. Benacerraf BR, Saltzman DH, Estroff JA, Frigoletto Jr FD. Abnormal karyotype of fetuses with omphalocele: prediction based on omphalocele contents. Obstet Gynecol 1990;75:317-319.

152. Nicolaides KH, Salvesen DR, Snijders RJ, Gosden CM. Strawberry-shaped skull in fetal trisomy 18. Fetal Diagn Ther 1992;7:132-137.

153. Nyberg DA, Mahony BS, Hegge FN, et al. Enlarged cisterna magna and the Dandy-Walker malformation: factors associated with chromosome abnormalities. Obstet Gynecol 1991;77:436-442.

154. Hill LM, Marchese S, Peterson C, Fries J. The effect of trisomy 18 on transverse cerebellar diameter. Am J Obstet Gynecol 1991;165:72-75.

155. Thurmond AS, Nelson DW, Lowensohn RI, et al. Enlarged cisterna magna in trisomy 18: prenatal ultrasonographic diagnosis. Am J Obstet Gynecol 1989;161:83-85.

156. Shuangshoti S, Roberts MP, Netsky MG. Neuroepithelial (colloid) cysts: pathogenesis and relation to choroid plexus and ependyma. Arch Pathol 1965;80:214-224.

157. Achiron R, Barkai G, Katznelson MB, Mashiach S. Fetal lateral ventricle choroid plexus cysts: the dilemma of amniocentesis. Obstet Gynecol 1991;78:815-818.

158. Benacerraf BR, Laboda LA. Cyst of the fetal choroid plexus: a normal variant? Am J Obstet Gynecol 1989;160:319-321.

159. Nadel AS, Bromley BS, Frigoletto Jr FD, et al. Isolated choroid plexus cysts in the second-trimester fetus: is amniocentesis really indicated? Radiology 1992;185:545-548.

160. Platt LD, Carlson DE, Medearis AL, Walla CA. Fetal choroid plexus cysts in the second trimester of pregnancy: a cause for concern. Am J Obstet Gynecol 1991;164:1652-1655; discussion 1655-1656.

161. Leonardi MR, Wolfe HM, Lanouette JM, et al. The apparently isolated choroid plexus cyst: importance of minor abnormalities in predicting the risk for aneuploidy. Fetal Diagn Ther 1998;13:49-52.

162. Reinsch RC. Choroid plexus cysts: association with trisomy: prospective review of 16,059 patients. Am J Obstet Gynecol 1997;176:1381-1383.

163. Coco C, Jeanty P. Karyotyping of fetuses with isolated choroid plexus cysts is not justified in an unselected population. J Ultrasound Med 2004;23:899-906.

164. Bronsteen R, Lee W, Vettraino IM, et al. Second-trimester sonography and trisomy 18: the significance of isolated choroid plexus cysts after an examination that includes the fetal hands. J Ultrasound Med 2004;23:241-245.

165. Bethune M. Time to reconsider our approach to echogenic intracardiac focus and choroid plexus cysts. Aust NZ J Obstet Gynaecol 2008;48:137-141.

166. Ouzounian JG, Ludington C, Chan S. Isolated choroid plexus cyst or echogenic cardiac focus on prenatal ultrasound: is genetic amniocentesis indicated? Am J Obstet Gynecol 2007;196:595e1-e3; discussion e3.

167. Cheng PJ, Shaw SW, Soong YK. Association of fetal choroid plexus cysts with trisomy 18 in a population previously screened by nuchal translucency thickness measurement. J Soc Gynecol Investig 2006;13:280-284.

Trisomy 13 (Patau Syndrome)

168. Hook EB. Rates of 47, + 13 and 46 translocation D/13 Patau syndrome in live births and comparison with rates in fetal deaths and at amniocentesis. Am J Hum Genet 1980;32:849-858.

169. Redheendran R, Neu RL, Bannerman RM. Long survival in trisomy-13-syndrome: 21 cases including prolonged survival in two patients 11 and 19 years old. Am J Med Genet 1981;8:167-172.

170. Benacerraf BR, Frigoletto Jr FD, Greene MF. Abnormal facial features and extremities in human trisomy syndromes: prenatal ultrasound appearance. Radiology 1986;159:243-246.

171. Benacerraf BR, Miller WA, Frigoletto Jr FD. Sonographic detection of fetuses with trisomies 13 and 18: accuracy and limitations. Am J Obstet Gynecol 1988;158:404-409.

172. Watson WJ, Miller RC, Wax JR, et al. Sonographic detection of trisomy 13 in the first and second trimesters of pregnancy. J Ultrasound Med 2007;26:1209-1214.

173. Papp C, Beke A, Ban Z, et al. Prenatal diagnosis of trisomy 13: analysis of 28 cases. J Ultrasound Med 2006;25:429-435.

174. Lehman CD, Nyberg DA, Winter 3rd TC, et al. Trisomy 13 syndrome: prenatal ultrasound findings in a review of 33 cases. Radiology 1995;194:217-222.

Triploidy

175. Ferguson-Smith MA, Yates JR. Maternal age specific rates for chromosome aberrations and factors influencing them: report of a collaborative European study on 52,965 amniocenteses. Prenat Diagn 1984;4 Spec No:5-44.

176. Jacobs PA, Szulman AE, Funkhouser J, et al. Human triploidy: relationship between parental origin of the additional haploid complement and development of partial hydatidiform mole. Ann Hum Genet 1982;46:223-231.

177. McFadden DE, Robinson WP. Phenotype of triploid embryos. J Med Genet 2006;43:609-612.

178. Jauniaux E, Brown R, Rodeck C, Nicolaides KH. Prenatal diagnosis of triploidy during the second trimester of pregnancy. Obstet Gynecol 1996;88:983-989.

179. Jauniaux E, Brown R, Snijders RJ, et al. Early prenatal diagnosis of triploidy. Am J Obstet Gynecol 1997;176:550-554.

180. Rijhsinghani A, Yankowitz J, Strauss RA, et al. Risk of preeclampsia in second-trimester triploid pregnancies. Obstet Gynecol 1997;90:884-888.

181. Goldstein DP, Berkowitz RS. Current management of complete and partial molar pregnancy. J Reprod Med 1994;39:139-146.

Turner (45,X) Syndrome

182. Baena N, De Vigan C, Cariati E, et al. Turner syndrome: evaluation of prenatal diagnosis in 19 European registries. Am J Med Genet A 2004;129A:16-20.

183. Wax JR, Blakemore KJ, Baser I, Stetten G. Isolated fetal ascites detected by sonography: an unusual presentation of Turner syndrome. Obstet Gynecol 1992;79:862-863.

184. Azar GB, Snijders RJ, Gosden C, Nicolaides KH. Fetal nuchal cystic hygromata: associated malformations and chromosomal defects. Fetal Diagn Ther 1991;6:46-57.

185. Papp C, Beke A, Mezei G, et al. Prenatal diagnosis of Turner syndrome: report on 69 cases. J Ultrasound Med 2006;25:711-717; quiz 718-720.

CHAPTER 32

Multifetal Pregnancy

Tejas S. Mehta

Chapter Outline

*M*ultiple gestations have become more common in the United States and are associated with increased morbidity and mortality compared with singleton births. The higher the number of fetuses the greater the number of risks associated with the pregnancy. Fetuses with a shared placenta have certain risks that fetuses with their own placenta do not have. When assessing a pregnant patient, it is important not only to identify if multiple gestations are present, but also to determine the number and placentation of the fetuses early in gestation. This will enable the physician to counsel the patient accurately about potential risks associated with the pregnancy, to screen for these risks appropriately, and to care for the patient as needed.

INCIDENCE

The number of multiple births in the United States has risen dramatically over the past 3 decades. Twins account for 3.2% of all live births[1] and 94% of all multiple births.[2] In the United States in 2005, twins and higher-order multiple gestations accounted for 31.1 and 1.8 per 1000 live births, respectively.[3] The two most important factors contributing to this change are the use of assisted reproductive technology (ART) and delaying childbearing to a later age. Other influential factors include race

and geography, family history, parity, and body habitus. Higher education level and socioeconomic status of the woman have been reported as factors, although these are thought to be linked to use of ART.[2]

RISK FACTORS FOR MULTIFETAL PREGNANCY

Assisted reproductive therapy
Increased maternal age
Race/geography
Family history
Increased parity
Obesity

Assisted Reproductive Technology

A common type of ART is **in vitro fertilization** (IVF). In the early practice of IVF, multiple embryos were transferred to obtain a higher rate of achieving and maintaining pregnancy. More recent studies have shown that transfer of fewer embryos can still yield a successful pregnancy. With as few as two embryos transferred, the rate of dizygotic twins is as high as 28%.[4,5] Even when only one embryo is transferred, that embryo can cleave into monozygotic twins.[6]

Maternal Age

Dizygotic twinning occurs more frequently in older women, even without fertility therapy. The incidence of naturally conceived twins increases fourfold between ages 15 and 35 years,[7] with peak age at 37, when there is maximum hormonal stimulation and increased rate of double ovulation.[8] The trend toward delaying child-bearing to a later age, without factoring in use of ART, accounts for up to 33% of the increase in multiple births.[2]

Race and Geography

Some black populations of Africa have the highest rate of naturally conceived twins, at 1 in 30, whereas some Asian populations have much lower rates of less than 1 in 100. The incidence in Caucasians falls between these two groups at 1 in 80.[9,10] In the United States, more twins and higher-order gestations occur in whites than in Hispanics or blacks.[2]

Family History

The genetic component for twins can be inherited by either parent but is thought to be expressed in women.[11] If a woman is a dizygotic twin, the rate of giving birth to twins is 1 in 58. If the husband is a twin and the woman is not, the rate of twinning is 1 in 116.[12]

Parity and Body Habitus

Increase in parity is associated with increased rate of twinning, even when controlling for maternal age.[7,13] Women who are obese (body mass index [BMI] ≥30 kg/m²) and women who are tall (≥65 inches [162 cm]) are more likely to have dizygotic twins than women who are underweight (BMI <20 kg/m²) and women who are short (<61 inches [152 cm]).[14,15]

ZYGOSITY AND PLACENTATION

Zygosity refers to the type of conception. If twins arise from fertilization of two sperm and two ova, they are **dizygotic twins** or **fraternal twins.** In this situation, there are two blastocysts that form, resulting in two placentas, and subsequently two chorions, amnions, and fetuses. **Monozygotic twins** or **"identical" twins** result when there is fertilization of one sperm and one ovum into one zygote, which then undergoes **cleavage** to result in twins. For spontaneous conception, dizygotic twins are more common than monozygotic twins, at a 70:30 ratio.[16] The frequency of dizygotic twins compared to monozygotic twins in the setting of ART with multiple embryo transfers is much higher, at a 95:5 ratio.[17]

Chorionicity refers to type of placentation. In a dizygotic gestation, each zygote forms its own placenta, and thus each fetus has its own chorion and amnion, a **diamniotic dichorionic** twin gestation.

In a monozygotic gestation, the chorionicity and amnionicity are determined by when cleavage occurs. When there is **early cleavage** of a zygote before blastocyst formation, which is before day 4 after fertilization, the result is two blastocysts. The blastocyst implants in the endometrial cavity and eventually forms the placenta, chorion, amnion, and fetus. Thus, with early cleavage, two blastocysts result in two placentas and two fetuses, each with its own chorion. As the chorion forms before the amnion, if there are two chorions, there must be two amnions (diamniotic dichorionic twin gestation).

If **late cleavage** occurs between days 4 and 8 after fertilization, the blastocyst has already formed, and thus there is only one placenta. What cleaves at this point is the inner cell mass. The amnion has not yet formed, and thus cleavage during this time results in a gestation with one chorion and two amnions, a **diamniotic monochorionic** pregnancy.

If cleavage occurs 8 days after fertilization, at a time after both the chorion and the amnion have formed, what cleaves is the **embryonic disc;** this results in a **monoamniotic** (and thus **monochorionic**) twin pregnancy. A **conjoined twin** results if there is incomplete cleavage of the embryonic disc by day 13 (Table 32-1).[18]

All dizygotic twins and one third of monozygotic twins are dichorionic, resulting in 80% of all natural twins. Almost two thirds of monozygotic twins are monochorionic diamniotic. Monoamniotic twins are rare, representing less than 1% of monozygotic twins (Fig. 32-1).

TABLE 32-1. EVENTS INVOLVING PLACENTATION IN A MONOZYGOTIC GESTATION

DAYS AFTER FERTILIZATION	UNIT THAT CLEAVES	CHORIONICITY	AMNIONICITY
Before 4 days	Zygote	Dichorionic	Diamniotic
4-8 days	Inner cell mass	Monochorionic	Diamniotic
8-12 days*	Embryonic disc	Monochorionic	Monoamniotic

*Incomplete cleavage of embryonic disc by day 13 results in conjoined twins.

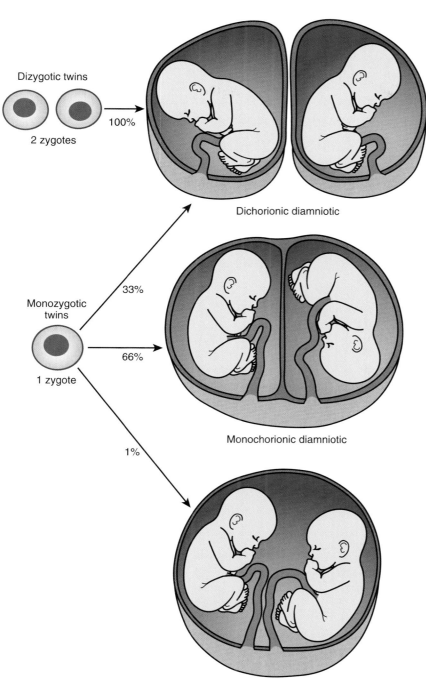

Dizygotic twins

2 zygotes

100%

Dichorionic diamniotic

Monozygotic twins

1 zygote

33%

66%

1%

Monochorionic diamniotic

Monochorionic monoamniotic

FIGURE 32-1. Diagram illustrating zygosity and placentation in twins. Of all twins, 70% are dizygotic (from 2 sperm and 2 eggs) and 30% of twins are monozygotic (from 1 sperm and 1 egg). From all dizygotic twins, 100% form dichorionic diamniotic placenta. From all monozygotic twins, 33% are dichorionic diamniotic, 66% are monochorionic diamniotic, and 1% are monochorionic monoamniotic.

SONOGRAPHIC DETERMINATION OF CHORIONICITY AND AMNIONICITY

Chorionicity can be determined with high reliability in the first trimester with accuracy of 98% to 100%.[19-21] Very early in gestation, between 6 and 9 weeks, the membrane thickness can be used to determine **chorionicity** and the number of yolk sacs used to determine **amnionicity.** If a thick membrane (>2 mm) is seen, it

is a dichorionic gestation. If there is a thin or no perceptible membrane seen this early in gestation, it is a monochorionic gestation. In a monochorionic diamniotic gestation, a thin membrane is usually seen surrounding the individual embryos if the gestational age is sufficient for a visible amnion to be present (about 8 weeks). If a membrane is not seen, assessing the number of yolk sacs is helpful. A monoamniotic gestation is present when there is one yolk sac with two embryos.[22-25] If there are two yolk sacs with two embryos, even if an intervening membrane is not seen, it still has to be a diamniotic gestation (Fig. 32-2; **Videos 32-1, 32-2,** and **32-3**). Follow-up later in gestation will demonstrate the two amniotic sacs in these cases.

As the gestation progresses, other factors can be used to determine chorionicity and amnionicity.

Membrane Thickness

Membrane thickness, in experienced hands, has 100% intraobserver concordance and 91% interobserver concordance,[26] making it a reliable tool to assess chorionicity (Fig. 32-3). Problems can arise late in gestation when a "thick" membrane becomes perceptibly "thin."[27] Technical factors such as assessing the membrane close to the placental attachment site, or having the membrane perpendicular to the ultrasound beam, can have the opposite effect and cause a "thin" membrane to appear "thick."[16]

In a study of twins between 10 and 14 weeks' gestation, a membrane thickness cutoff of 1.5 mm or greater was 100% specific and 92.6% sensitive for dichorionicity, with a positive predictive value (PPV) of 100% and negative predictive value (NPV) of 80%.[20] Another study examined twins later in gestation, at 20 to 35 weeks, and assessed membrane thickness using two-dimensional (2-D) and three-dimensional (3-D) ultrasound. Using a cutoff of 1.8 mm, the sensitivity and specificity for dichorionicity were 97% and 94%, respectively, for 3-D and 83% and 83%, respectively, for 2-D sonography.[28]

Fetal Gender

In the second and third trimesters, if different genders are seen, by definition the twins have to be dizygotic and thus dichorionic. The only exception to this rule is a rare case of **postzygotic nondysjunction,** in which one twin appears male, with an XY karyotype. However, the Y chromosome becomes lost in the second twin, resulting in a 45 XO female fetus with Turner syndrome. If the fetuses are of the same gender, zygosity cannot be determined using this criterion, and thus chorionicity cannot be based on gender alone.

Placenta

If two clearly separate placentas are present, one for each twin, dichorionicity can be stated with certainty[29] (Fig. 32-4, *A;* **Video 32-4**). The only exception to this rule is a **succenturiate lobe** in a monochorionic twin. Therefore, attention must be paid to the size of the placentas being about equal, and each fetus having a separate placenta. In some cases, because of the sites of implantation, two placentas are located adjacent to each other, making it difficult to determine if there are indeed two "fused" placentas or only a single placenta. The former would imply dichorionicity and the later monochorionicity.

The **"twin peak" sign** can be used to distinguish between these two entities.[30] This finding, also called the **lambda sign,** is produced by proliferating chorionic villi growing into the potential space between the two layers of chorion in the intertwin membrane[31,32] (Figs. 32-4, *B* and *C*). The presence of twin-peak sign indicates dichorionicity, but its absence does not indicate monochorionicity.[20,33,34] This is especially true in the second and third trimesters, as the sign regresses in conspicuity with progression of gestation.[33]

In a **monochorionic gestation**, there is a single placenta and a single chorion, and thus the potential space for the twin-peak sign does not exist. The two layers of amnion extend to the placenta, referred to as the **"T" sign** (Fig. 32-4, *D;* **Video 32-5**). This sign predicts monochorionicity with sensitivity of 100% and specificity of 98.2%.[20]

Umbilical Cord

Sometimes it can be difficult to identify an intervening membrane to distinguish diamnionicity from monoamnionicity. In general, the **insertion sites** of the umbilical cords into the placenta are closer to each other in monoamniotic twins than in diamniotic twins (Fig. 32-5, *A*). However, the only way to diagnose monoamnionicity with certainty is to identify one twin's cord either around the other twin or entangled with the cord of the other twin[35] (Fig. 32-5, *B*).

Accuracy

Using the tools just described, chorionicity, even later in gestation, can be determined quite reliably. One study of 410 twins (≤24 weeks' gestation) accurately identified chorionicity in 392 (95.6%).[36] Another study of 150 twins earlier in gestation (10-14 weeks) used a combination of membrane thickness, number of placental sites, and lambda and T signs and accurately predicted chorionicity in all but one.[20] Another study of 100 twins with scans in the second trimester used fetal gender, placental number, twin-peak sign, and dividing-membrane thickness and predicted chorionicity, amnionicity, and zygosity with 91% or higher sensitivity and specificity.[37]

MORBIDITY AND MORTALITY

Infant mortality of twins is five times that for singletons (37 vs. 7 per 1000 live births).[38] Twins account for 12% to 15% of neonatal deaths.[39] When assessing morbidity and mortality, gestational age at delivery, chorionicity, and sonographic findings are each independent, statistically significant, prognostic factors.[19] The risk of preterm delivery is higher for multiples than singletons and increases with increasing number of gestations. However, when controlling for gestational age, outcomes of

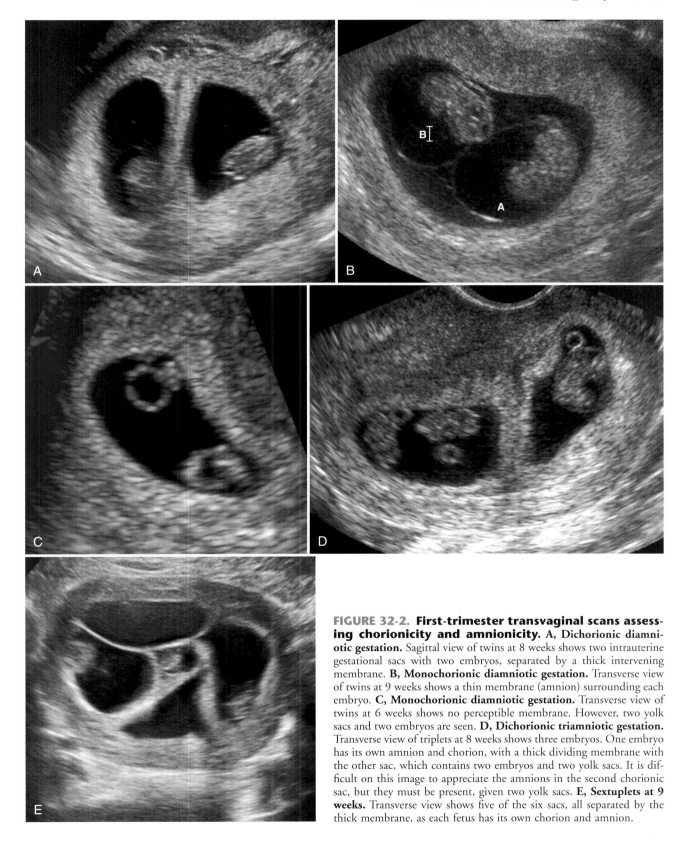

FIGURE 32-2. **First-trimester transvaginal scans assessing chorionicity and amnionicity.** **A,** Dichorionic diamniotic gestation. Sagittal view of twins at 8 weeks shows two intrauterine gestational sacs with two embryos, separated by a thick intervening membrane. **B, Monochorionic diamniotic gestation.** Transverse view of twins at 9 weeks shows a thin membrane (amnion) surrounding each embryo. **C, Monochorionic diamniotic gestation.** Transverse view of twins at 6 weeks shows no perceptible membrane. However, two yolk sacs and two embryos are seen. **D, Dichorionic triamniotic gestation.** Transverse view of triplets at 8 weeks shows three embryos. One embryo has its own amnion and chorion, with a thick dividing membrane with the other sac, which contains two embryos and two yolk sacs. It is difficult on this image to appreciate the amnions in the second chorionic sac, but they must be present, given two yolk sacs. **E, Sextuplets at 9 weeks.** Transverse view shows five of the six sacs, all separated by the thick membrane, as each fetus has its own chorion and amnion.

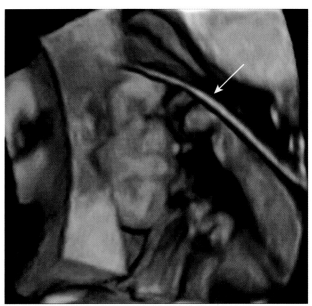

FIGURE 32-3. Three-dimensional membrane. Dichorionic diamniotic gestation. 3-D image of a 17-week gestation shows a thick, intervening membrane *(arrow)* separating twins.

SONOGRAPHIC FINDINGS FOR DETERMINING CHORIONICITY AND AMNIONICITY

Different fetal genders = dizygotic and thus dichorionic
Two separate placentas = dichorionic but can be monozygotic or dizygotic
Lambda or twin-peak sign = dichorionic, but if absent does not mean monochorionic
T sign with 1 placenta = monochorionic diamniotic
1 yolk sac with 2 embryos very early in gestation = monoamniotic
Entangled cords or cord of one fetus around other fetus = monoamniotic

otherwise normal multiples are similar to singletons.[40] This suggests that **prematurity** and **intrauterine growth restriction** (IUGR) are the main issues that increase neonatal morbidity and mortality in multiple gestations.

Although most twin gestations are dichorionic, the monochorionic pregnancies account for up to 50% of the mortalities of twin pregnancies.[41] Monochorionic gestations have a higher rates of fetal loss before 24 weeks, stillbirth after 28 weeks, preterm delivery, IUGR and discordant growth, and neurologic morbidity compared to dichorionic twins.[42-46] Of the monochorionic twins, the monoamniotic gestations have the highest mortality, up to 50%, primarily from cord accidents.[47]

Intrauterine Fetal Demise

The incidence of twins is higher than actually documented because early pregnancies with subsequent loss of a fetus are not diagnosed as multiple gestations. In one study of 1000 first-trimester scans, twins were seen in 3.3%. Of these 21.2% "vanished" later in the first trimester.[48] Thus, depending on if and when a first-trimester scan is performed, a twin gestation with early demise may be classified as a singleton pregnancy.

Higher rates of at least one embryonic loss have been reported in multiple gestations conceived with ART, with rates of 35% to 36% in twins, 53% to 59% in triplets, and 47% to 65% in quadruplets.[49,50] Some of this increase could be caused by an earlier onset and increased frequency of performing first-trimester scans.

In general, single fetal death occurs in 2.6% to 9% of twins.[19,51,52] This is twice as common in monochorionic twins than dichorionic twins.[53] The chance of survival of the other fetus depends on the chorionicity and is inversely related to the time of death of the twin fetus.[52] When loss of a twin occurs before 16 weeks, outcome is much better than when loss of a twin occurs after 16 weeks, when there is up to 50% chance of prematurity, 22% risk of IUGR, and 13% perinatal mortality[54] (Fig. 32-6). In monochorionic twins with loss of a twin after the first trimester, the "twin embolization" syndrome can occur, as discussed later.

Structural Anomalies

Major malformations are twice as common and **minor** malformations 1.5 times more common in twins than singletons.[55] Triplets have up to a threefold increase in major malformations compared with twins, and higher-order gestations have a more than sixfold increase.[56] The later in gestation the cleavage into twins occurs, the higher the incidence of structural abnormalities. Monozygotic twins have more structural defects compared with dizygotic twins and singletons,[57] with rates of 3.1% to 3.7% versus 1.9% to 2.5%, respectively.[58] Of the monozygotic twins, the monochorionic gestations have increased risk of malformations compared to the dizygotic gestations. Even though monozygotic twins have the same chromosomal makeup, they can have **discordant anomalies.** The extreme example of late cleavage is conjoined twins, which all have structural abnormalities.

Of all anomalies, those involving the central nervous system (CNS) are most common (Fig. 32-7). **Cerebral palsy** is more likely to occur in twins than singleton pregnancies.[59] The prevalence of cerebral palsy in twins is 7.3 to 12.6 per 1000 infants, increasing in triplets up to 28 to 44.8 per 1000, compared to singletons with rates of 1.6 to 2.3 per 1000.[60,61] Antenatal necrosis of the cerebral white matter is more common in monochorionic twins, likely from the presence of vascular connections in the placenta.[44]

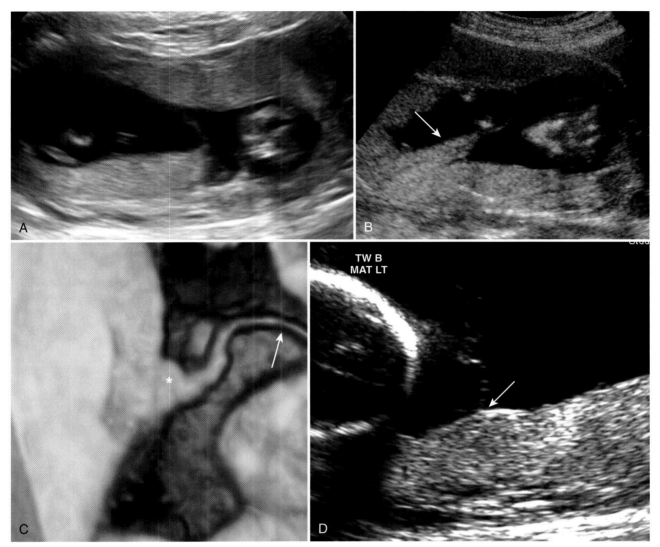

FIGURE 32-4. Placental findings to determine chorionicity. A, Dichorionic gestation. Transverse view of twins at 12 weeks' gestation shows two separate placentas, one anterior and one posterior. **B, Dichorionic gestation.** Sagittal view of twins at 14 weeks' gestation shows two "fused" posterior placentas, with a "twin peak" sign *(arrow)*. **C, Dichorionic gestation.** 3-D image shows the "twin peak" sign with placental tissue extending into the potential space between the two layers of chorion (*), and a thick membrane *(arrow)*. **D, Monochorionic diamniotic gestation.** Transverse view of twins at 22 weeks shows a thin membrane perpendicular to a single posterior placenta, forming the "T" sign *(arrow)*.

Other Screening Tests for Anomalies

There are multiple tests used to screen for anomalies with twins. **Maternal serum alpha fetoprotein** (MS-AFP) is increased in all twins (because more than one fetus is present). However, when the MS-AFP in twins is greater than 4.5 multiples of the median (MOM), there is an increase in perinatal mortality, especially when it is a monochorionic diamniotic gestation.[47]

Screening for trisomy by **nuchal translucency** (NT) is performed in twins in a similar manner as performed in singletons. The detection rates are similar, but the false-positive rates in normal monochorionic twins are higher, at 8%.[62] NT, combined with serum human

chorionic gonadotropin and pregnancy-associated plasma protein A, identifies 90% of trisomy 21 in singletons, and 80% in twins.[63]

Chorionic villus sampling (CVS) and amniocentesis can safely be performed in twins, without associated increase in fetal loss rate.[64-67] For CVS, the sample error rate is 1.2% to 1.5%.[64,68] In some cases, CVS of one twin is performed at the same time as fetal reduction of the other twin. This same-day dual procedure does not increase the rate of fetal loss.[68] Some have proposed delaying the reduction to slightly later in gestation (13-14 weeks), after CVS results are confirmed. This allows for increase in detection rate of abnormal findings, including abnormal NT, **growth discordance, cystic hygroma**, and CNS anomalies, but

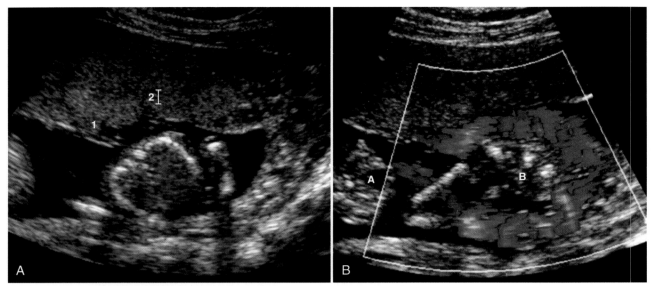

FIGURE 32-5. Monoamniotic twins at 16 weeks' gestation. A, Transverse view shows a single anterior placenta with the cord insertion sites *(1, 2)* of the twins in proximity to each other. **B,** Color Doppler image shows the cord of the fetus on the right *(A)* wrapped around the fetus on the left *(B)*, confirming that the twins are in the same sac and are monoamniotic.

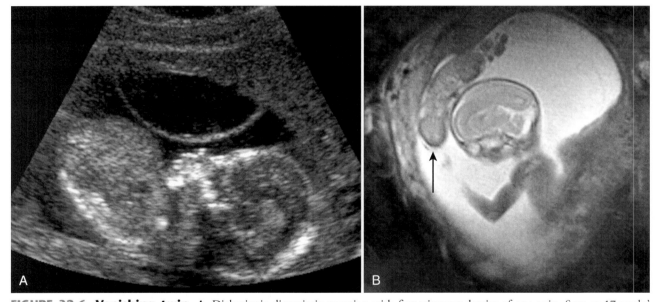

FIGURE 32-6. Vanishing twin. A, Dichorionic diamniotic gestation with first-trimester demise of one twin. Scan at 17 weeks' gestation shows the live fetus and an empty sac anterior to the fetal head. There has been resorption of the embryonic tissue, although a small sac from demised twin remains. **B,** In a different gestation after demise of co-twin, note the small compressed twin *(arrow)* against the wall of the uterus.

does not increase the risk of pregnancy loss caused by reduction.[69]

When performing **amniocentesis,** indigo carmine or Evan's blue dye is often instilled into one sac after removal of fluid, to ensure that the second sample is obtained from the correct sac. Methylene blue is not used in pregnancy due to risks of fetal hemolytic anemia, intestinal atresia, and fetal demise.[70-72] Amniocentesis of both sacs is performed in dichorionic twins because the majority of these are chromosomally different. Amnio-

centesis of both sacs is also often performed in monozygotic twins because even though they are "identical," they can have varied karyotypes, including mosaicism and small-scale mutations.[73]

Growth Restriction and Discordant Growth

Abnormal fetal growth is defined in two ways: (1) the estimated fetal weight is below the 10th centile on a

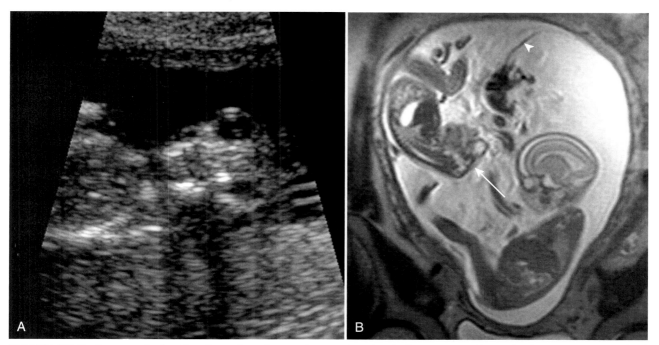

FIGURE 32-7. Anencephaly. One fetus of a twin gestation at 19 weeks. **A,** Sonogram. **B,** T2-weighted MR image. Arrowhead shows the dividing membrane. Arrow indicates anencephalic twin. Structural anomalies are more common in twins than in singletons, especially anomalies of the central nervous system.

singleton curve; or (2) there is a 20% or more discordance in estimated weight between twins.

Birth weight discordance complicates more than 15% of twin pregnancies.[74] There is a higher rate of IUGR in twins compared to singletons, probably caused by uteroplacental insufficiency resulting from increased metabolic demand or an abnormality involving placental implantation. Triplets are even more likely to have discordant growth compared to twins.[75] The neonatal mortality rate increases with increasing growth discordancy. In a large twin study, with no discordance the mortality rate was 3.8:1000 live births; with 15% to 19% discordance, 5.6:1000 live births; with 20% to 24% discordance, 8.4:1000 live births; with 25% to 30% discordance, 18.4:1000 live births; and with 30% or more discordance, 43.4:1000 live births. In this series, fetal weight of less than 10th percentile was more common in discordant twins (60%) compared to non-discordant twins (5%).[76]

Growth discordance can be detected as early as the first trimester. A difference of 3 mm or less in mean sac diameter or crown-rump length (CRL) between twin gestations has up to a 50% embryo loss rate, much greater than when the difference is 1 mm or less. A recent study found 45% discordance at birth when first-trimester CRL was greater than 3 days discrepant, versus 9% discordance at birth with CRL 3 days discrepant or earlier. Discordance seen in the first trimester increases the risk of congenital anomalies[77] and IUGR later in gestation.[78]

Doppler waveforms, fetal biometry (especially abdominal circumference), and estimated fetal weight are all helpful in assessing for discordance in the second and third trimesters.

Premature Delivery

The risk of preterm delivery is higher for multiple pregnancies compared to singletons.[79] There is an inverse relationship between the number of fetuses and the gestational age at delivery.[3] The rate of premature delivery is increased up to five times in twins and nine times in triplets compared to singleton gestations.[80] Preterm delivery accounts for much of the increase in morbidity and mortality in multiple gestations.[40]

Cervical Incompetence

Cervical length on transvaginal scan in the middle of the second trimester is inversely related to risk of preterm delivery[81] (Fig. 32-8). Women with twins or higher-order multiple gestations are more likely to have a shorter cervix than women with singleton pregnancy.[82] One study of twins found that a cervical length of 2.5 cm or less at 24 weeks was the most powerful predictor of preterm delivery.[83] Another study using 2.0 cm as the cutoff for cervical length found a NPV of 99%, 98%, 95%, and 93% for delivery at <28, <30, <32, and <34 weeks' gestation, respectively.[84] Prophylactic cerclage in patients with twins has not

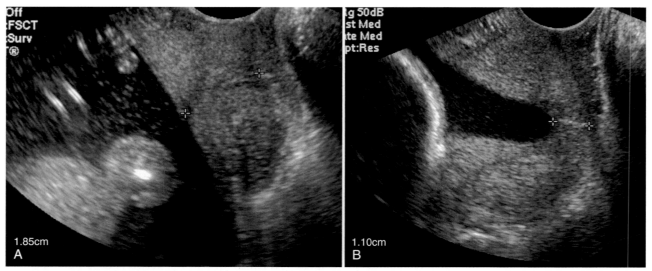

FIGURE 32-8. Transvaginal imaging of the cervix. A, Short cervix *(calipers)* measuring 1.8 cm. Transvaginal scan of cervix in a twin pregnancy at 19 weeks. **B,** Funneling with closed cervical length of 1.0 cm *(calipers)*. Transvaginal scan of the cervix in a different patient with twins at 30 weeks' gestation.

been shown to be effective in preventing preterm delivery.[85-87]

Placental Abnormalities: Marginal and Velamentous Insertion

When the umbilical cord, instead of inserting directly into the placenta, inserts into the membrane with blood vessels traversing to the placenta, it is termed **velamentous insertion.**[88] An umbilical cord that inserts at the periphery of the placenta, rather than centrally, is referred to as **marginal insertion.** Abnormal insertion sites of the cord into the placenta are associated with increased perinatal morbidity and mortality[89,90] and are more common in multiple gestations than singletons.[47,91] Up to one third of monoamniotic pregnancies have either a marginal or a velamentous insertion.[92] Velamentous and marginal cord insertion sites are associated with IUGR and growth discordance, twin-twin transfusion syndrome (TTTS), and preterm labor.[93-96]

Umbilical Cord Doppler Ultrasound

Doppler sonography is helpful in assessing the well being of a fetus, and can help in the assessment of intrauterine IUGR, TTTS, and discordant growth of twins. The systolic-to-diastolic (S/D) ratio is often used to assess level of resistance of blood flow in the umbilical artery. As the pregnancy progresses, there is a decrease in the peripheral resistance of blood flow because of an increase in arterioles in the placenta.[97] Thus, normally the S/D ratio decreases after 20 weeks' gestation. The low-resistive system results from the presence of end diastolic flow. The normal S/D ratio in the third trimester ranges from 1.7 to 2.4. When obtaining Doppler waveforms, it is important to sample at a free-floating loop of cord; falsely elevated ratios can be obtained if sampling is from the fetal end at the cord insertion site.[98]

An elevated S/D ratio is associated with increase in morbidity and mortality in twins.[99] Differences in S/D ratios of twin pairs are predictive of discordant growth[100,101] (Fig. 32-9). An elevated S/D ratio occurs when approximately 30% of the fetal villous vasculature is abnormal. When this increases to 60% to 70% abnormal vessels, there is absent or reversed flow.[102,103]

COMPLICATIONS

Monochorionic Twins

Complications unique to monochorionic twins are caused by the single shared placenta. Vascular communications are almost always found in monochorionic gestations. The communication can be arterial-arterial, venous-venous, or arterial-venous. The **arterial-arterial** and **venous-venous** connections are end-to-end anastomoses that occur at the placental surface. Arterial-arterial communications are much more common than venous-venous communications.[104] In contrast, the **arterial-venous** anastomosis, which has a feeding artery, enters the placenta to the capillary bed of a cotyledon, where it drains into the venous system of the other twin. Depending on the imbalances in the types of communications, various complications can arise.

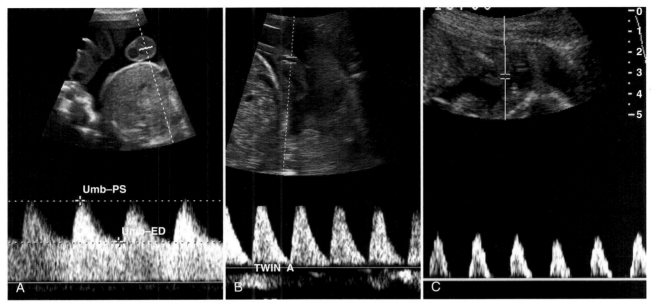

FIGURE 32-9. Umbilical artery Doppler in twins at 28 weeks' gestation. A, Normal arterial waveforms. Doppler image of one twin shows normal arterial waveforms with normal S/D ratio and presence of diastolic flow. **B,** Elevated S/D ratio with absent end diastolic flow. Doppler image of the other twin. Biometry (not shown) revealed this fetus to be in the 3rd percentile for weight. Note that the spectral Doppler scale is too low, cutting off peak systole of the waveform. **C,** Absent diastolic flow on Doppler ultrasound of a twin at 23 weeks' gestation by dates and 19 weeks' gestation by ultrasound.

Twin-Twin Transfusion Syndrome

Twin-twin transfusion syndrome occurs in up to 15% of monochorionic twins.[105] One hypothesis on the etiology of TTTS is an imbalance in the formation of the arterial and venous connections of both fetuses with a single placenta.[106] The presence of one-way arterial-venous connections, without the presence of other connections that can compensate for this unidirectional flow, can cause TTTS.[107-110] One study examining placentas found that those from pregnancies with TTTS had significantly fewer anastomoses than those without TTTS, although in those with TTTS the anastomoses present were more likely to be deep rather than superficial (80% vs. 36% in control).[107] The superficial anastomoses, especially arterial-arterial, are believed to be protective against TTTS, decreasing its incidence by ninefold.[109] Another study of monochorionic twins found TTTS in 58% pregnancies with no arterial-arterial anastomoses, compared to 5% when arterial-arterial anastomoses were present.[111] In pregnancies where TTTS develops despite the presence of arterial-arterial anastomoses, there is improved outcome.[109]

In TTTS, one twin is referred to as the "donor" and the other the "recipient." The donor has blood shunted away from it, thus causing anemia, hypovolemia, IUGR, and oligohydramnios. The recipient of this excess blood is the larger twin, with hypervolemia, cardiac overload, polyhydramnios and possibly hydrops.

The criteria to diagnose TTTS include documentation of a monochorionic gestation, with significant weight discrepancy of the fetuses (difference >20%) and polyhydramnios in the larger twin and oligohydramnios in the smaller twin. When TTTS is severe, it may be difficult to see the membrane around the donor twin due to severe oligohydramnios. The membrane appears "stuck" to the fetus, and the fetus has limited motion, being adherent to the uterine wall. In severe cases the donor twin may not have fluid visible in the stomach or bladder. In contrast, the recipient, who has polyhydramnios, may have a large bladder (Fig. 32-10; **Videos 32-6** and **32-7**).

Other disorders that should be considered when there is discordance in the amount of amniotic fluid around twins, or discrepancy in twin size, are **placental insufficiency**, **umbilical cord abnormalities**, **intrauterine infection**, **congenital anomaly** (e.g., renal agenesis in one twin), and **premature rupture of membranes** (Fig. 32-11).

Quintero et al.[112] proposed a staging system to help determine severity and predict outcome. The overall perinatal survival rate for TTTS is 65%; however, it is higher for stage I-II at 76% and lower for higher stages at 52% (Table 32-2).

Options for treatment of TTTS include serial amnioreduction, laser photocoagulation of communicating vessels, septostomy, and termination.[113-116] One study of 173 cases of TTTS, in which 78 were treated with amnioreduction and 95 with laser therapy, reported at least one surviving infant in 67% of cases with amnioreduction and in 83% with laser therapy. The neurologic morbidity was lower with laser, 4% versus 24% with

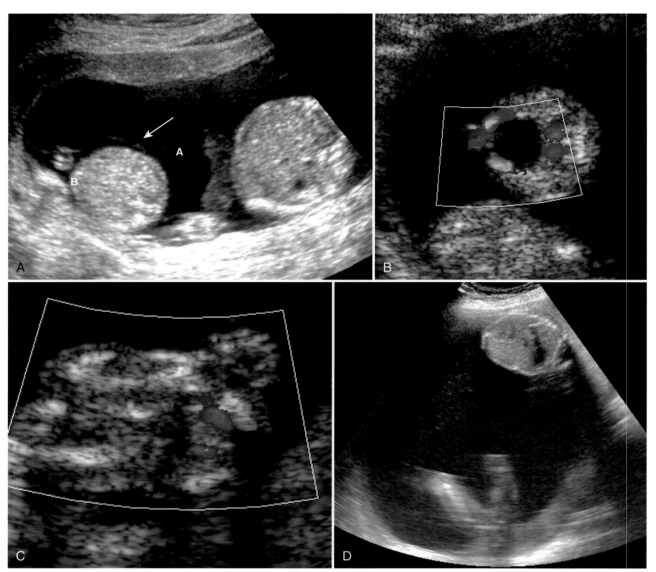

FIGURE 32-10. Twin-twin transfusion syndrome. A, Twins at 18 weeks' gestation. Note the discrepancy in abdominal size of the fetuses, with fetus B being smaller than fetus A. A separating membrane is seen *(arrow),* with the membrane close to fetus B due to oligohydramnios. A stomach bubble was not seen in this fetus. **B** and **C,** Different twin gestation at 17 weeks. **B,** "Recipient" twin shows polyhydramnios and a distended bladder. **C,** "Donor" twin had oligohydramnios and no visible fluid in the bladder. **D,** Severe polyhydramnios of a recipient twin with the donor twin "stuck" anteriorly in a different case of twins at 21 weeks' gestation.

amnioreduction.[112] Other studies report survival rates with amnioreduction of 60% to 65%,[117] and for laser therapy, 70%, with at least one fetus surviving in 81%.[118] Another study performing septostomy in a small group of patients with TTTS reported 83% survival.[115]

Twin Embolization Syndrome

Demise of one twin in a monochorionic pregnancy occurs in up to 20% of cases, the majority occurring in the first trimester.[119] A major complication of TTTS with the death of one twin is twin embolization syndrome. One theory for this occurrence is that thromboplastin-rich blood from the dead twin travels via placental anastomoses to the live twin.[120] The more accepted current theory proposes that the injuries are not caused by emboli, but by changes in perfusion with blood loss from the survivor to the more relaxed circulation of the dead twin. This **hypoperfusion** can affect many organs, especially those that typically are well perfused.[121] The result is structural defects resulting from ischemia.

The brain is extremely susceptible to the effects of twin embolization syndrome[122] (Fig. 32-12). The gastrointestinal tract can also be affected, with splenic and hepatic infarcts, as well as atresias of the small bowel, colon, and appendix. Other anomalies include renal cortical necrosis, pulmonary infarctions, limb anomalies, and aplasia cutis.[123]

The prognosis for twin embolization syndrome is poor, with only 21% of the surviving twins being developmentally normal.[124] The effects occur soon after the death of one twin, before any detectable abnormality on ultrasound. By the time the ultrasound shows an abnormality, the damage is generally severe and irreversible. Fetal magnetic resonance imaging (MRI) can be helpful for earlier recognition of brain abnormalities, before they become apparent on ultrasound.[125]

Twin Reversed Arterial Perfusion Sequence

The syndrome known as the twin reversed arterial perfusion (TRAP) sequence is rare, affecting 1 in 35,000 births.[126] The findings are that of a fetus that does not have a cardiac pump but that continues to grow. Thus, this is also referred to as an **acardiac parabiotic twin.** There must be at least one arterial-arterial and one venous-venous placental anastomosis. The physiology is that arterial blood flows in a retrograde fashion from one twin (known as the "pump" twin) to the affected "acardiac" twin.[127] Thus, arterial flow in the acardiac twin is

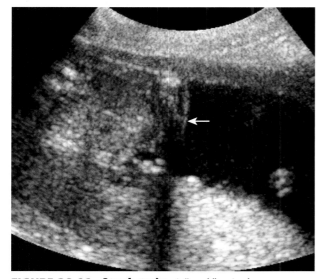

FIGURE 32-11. Stuck twin. A "stuck" twin does not necessarily imply monochorionicity. This is a dichorionic 19-week gestation in which one twin is "stuck" because of renal agenesis. The membrane *(arrow)* is seen abutting the fetus, with no measurable fluid in that sac.

TABLE 32-2. QUINTERO STAGING OF TWIN-TWIN TRANSFUSION SYNDROME

STAGE	FINDINGS
I	Oligohydramnios in one sac, polyhydramnios in other sac
II	Anuria of donor twin (not visualized fetal bladder)
III	Abnormal Doppler waveforms
IV	Hydrops
V	Intrauterine death of a single fetus

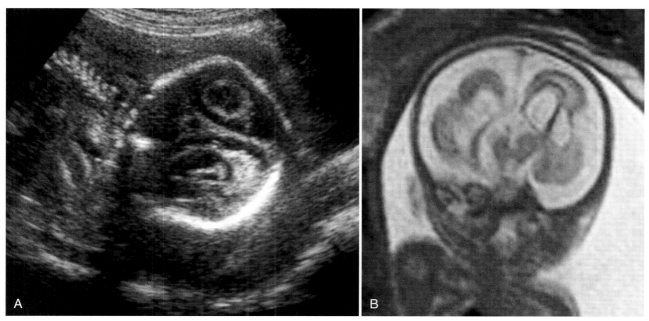

FIGURE 32-12. Twin embolization syndrome in live fetus after demise of monochorionic co-twin. A, Image through brain shows ventriculomegaly with abnormal, increased echogenicity of the surrounding parenchyma. **B,** Coronal T2-weighted MR image shows parenchymal atrophy and porencephaly. (Current theory: caused by hypoperfusion.)

reversed. The poorly oxygenated and nutrient-depleted blood, rather than going from the pump twin into the placenta, goes directly to the acardiac twin. It enters the umbilical arteries and preferentially perfuses the lower structures.

These acardiac fetuses are classified based on morphology.[128] **Acardius acephalus** is the most common type, with well-developed pelvis and lower limbs and no head, and no or rudimentary thoracic region and upper limbs. The least differentiated form is **acardius amorphous,** where there is a mass of tissue.

Two theories explain the etiology of TRAP sequence. The first, more accepted, theory is that a primary abnormality of the vasculature exists, with secondary alteration of the cardiac development.[127] The second theory is that a primary abnormality in cardiac embryogenesis causes secondary alterations in vasculature and flow patterns.[129] Thus, ultrasound will show either no heart or a poorly functioning heart in the acardiac twin.

The diagnosis should be considered on ultrasound when there is a monochorionic twin gestation, with a fetus that continues to grow despite lack of cardiac activity. Because the acardiac twin is perfused through the umbilical arteries, the lower extremities are more developed than the upper extremities or head. The diagnosis is certain when arterial flow is seen entering the umbilical artery of the anomalous acardiac fetus (Fig. 32-13). The pump twin may appear normal or may have polyhydramnios and signs of cardiac failure, including hydrops.

The perinatal mortality of the pump twin is 35% to 55%.[130,131] Three factors increase the mortality rate. First, continued growth of the acardiac twin can result in increase in intrauterine volume, resulting in preterm delivery. Second, the shunting of blood to the acardiac twin increases the demands on the pump twin. This shunting in turn may lead to heart failure and polyhydramnios. Third, the blood that exits the acardiac twin is further deoxygenated and circulates back to the pump twin through a venous-venous anastomosis. This "double used" blood can cause hypoxia and IUGR as well as high output cardiac failure. The larger the ratio of weight of acardiac twin to weight of pump twin, the higher is the incidence of preterm delivery, polyhydramnios, and pump twin cardiac failure.[131]

Attempts to treat TRAP sequence with minimally invasive techniques include cord occlusion and intrafetal ablation, typically using laser coagulation. The latter is more successful in terms of lower rate of technical failure and preterm delivery and higher rate of clinical success (survival of pump twin).[132,133] Unlike most cases of monochorionic twins, in which death of one twin increases the risk of twin embolization syndrome, in the case of TRAP sequence, because all the blood is already shared, there is no risk of changes in perfusion with blood loss from the survivor to the more relaxed circulation of the dead twin.

Monoamniotic Twins

Monoamniotic twins have the highest mortality of all twins.[134] They are at risk for all the complications previously mentioned with twins. However, TTTS is infrequent in monoamniotic twins,[110] presumably because of differences in the pattern of vascular anastomoses. Arterial-venous anastomoses are much less common and arterial-arterial anastomoses much more frequent in monoamniotic twins compared to monochorionic diamniotic twins.[110] The presence of arterial-arterial anastomoses is thought to be protective against development of TTTS.[108] Amniotic fluid is shared, so no oligohydramnios-polyhydramnios combination can occur.

Cord Entanglement

The main factor contributing to the increased mortality in monoamniotic twins is cord entanglement. There is no intervening membrane between the fetuses, so the two umbilical cords can intertwine, constricting blood flow to one or both fetuses. Cord entanglement is visualized on ultrasound in 34% to 42% of cases of monoamniotic twins[135,136] (Fig. 32-14). This can be identified either by tracing out the route of the cord from each fetus or by widening the Doppler gate and showing different heart rates in entwined loops of cord. Intermittent compression of the cord can result in neurologic abnormalities.[137,138]

Conjoined Twin

A rare type of monoamniotic twin is a conjoined twin, accounting for 1:100,000 births.[139] This type of twinning results from incomplete division of the embryonic disc. There is a 3:1 female predominance.[140] Conjoined twins are not associated with maternal age or parity and do not have a genetic predisposition.[141] The diagnosis can be suspected as early as 7 weeks' gestation.[142] To confirm this diagnosis, the clinician must first ensure that the placentation is of a monoamniotic gestation. As the name implies, conjoined twins are connected at various parts of the body, and thus separate bodies or skin contours cannot be detected at the site of connection. In addition, as the twins are connected, there is no change in relationship of body positions.[141,143] A single cord with more than three vessels can also confirm diagnosis.[141]

Conjoined twins are classified by whether fusion is **dorsal** (13%) or **ventral** (87%).[143] The classification is further subdivided by location of fusion. **Thoracopagus** (ventral fusion at or near the sternum) is the most common type, followed by **omphalopagus** (ventral fusion from the xyphoid process to the umbilicus)[144] (Fig. 32-15). In thoracopagus twins, the fetuses are continuously facing each other and may have hyperextension of the cervical spine. Other structural anomalies are also present, not

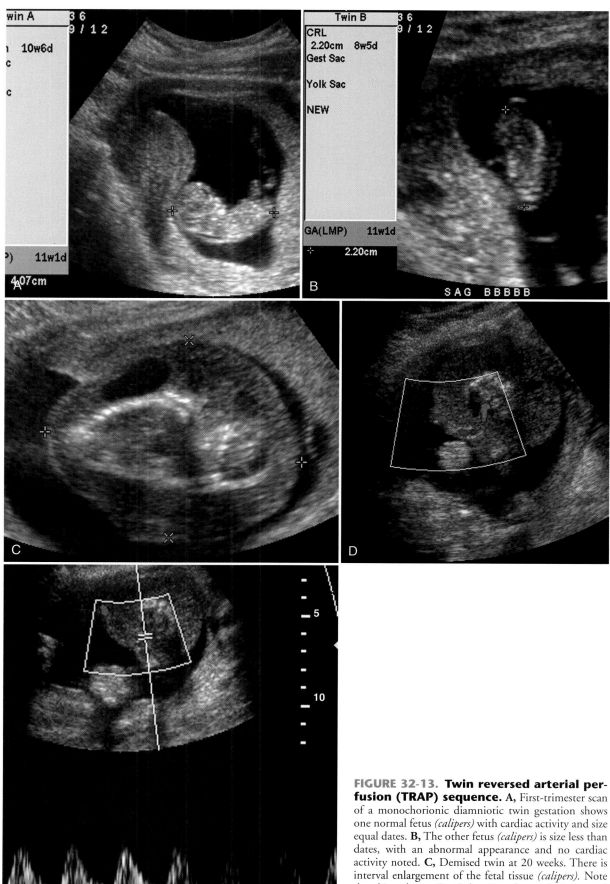

FIGURE 32-13. Twin reversed arterial perfusion (TRAP) sequence. A, First-trimester scan of a monochorionic diamniotic twin gestation shows one normal fetus *(calipers)* with cardiac activity and size equal dates. **B,** The other fetus *(calipers)* is size less than dates, with an abnormal appearance and no cardiac activity noted. **C,** Demised twin at 20 weeks. There is interval enlargement of the fetal tissue *(calipers)*. Note the skin edema. **D,** Color Doppler, and **E,** spectral Doppler with ultrasound show arterial flow entering the acardiac twin from an umbilical artery.

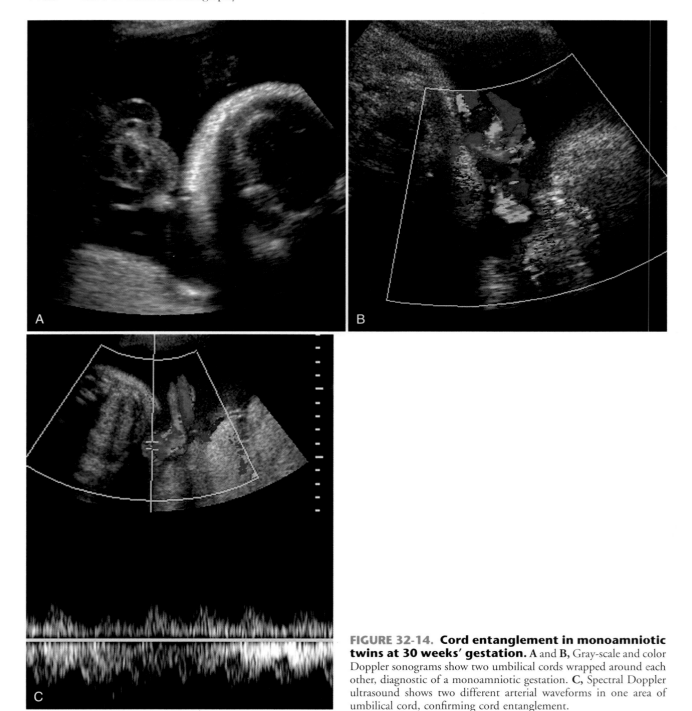

FIGURE 32-14. Cord entanglement in monoamniotic twins at 30 weeks' gestation. A and **B,** Gray-scale and color Doppler sonograms show two umbilical cords wrapped around each other, diagnostic of a monoamniotic gestation. **C,** Spectral Doppler ultrasound shows two different arterial waveforms in one area of umbilical cord, confirming cord entanglement.

 necessarily at the site of fusion, with cardiac abnormalities predominating[145] (Fig. 32-16; **Video 32-8**).

SELECTIVE MULTIFETAL REDUCTION

Fetal reduction is performed when high-order multiple gestations are present, in hopes to improve pregnancy outcome. Selective reduction can also be performed in the setting of multiples when there is one anomalous fetus. When selective termination of a twin in a dichorionic gestation is performed, the pregnancy loss rate is 2.4% to 2.5%.[146,147] This increases with an increasing number of fetuses. Elective reduction of triplets to twins increases the risk of miscarriage by 4%, but this is offset by decreasing the rate of preterm birth.[148] Despite improved outcomes with reduction to twins, when com-

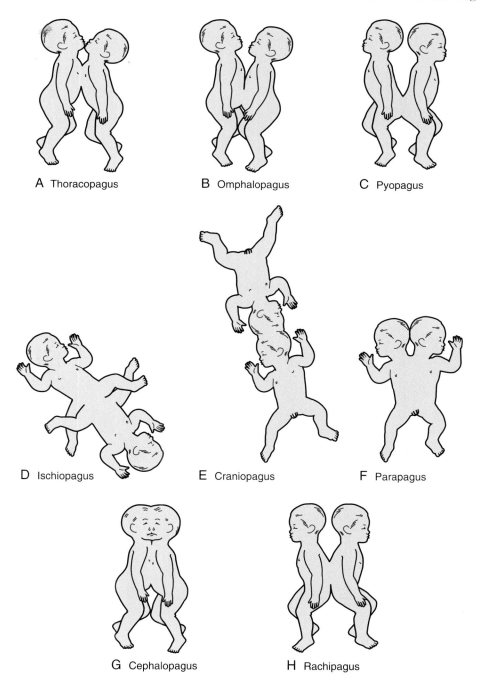

FIGURE 32-15. Classification of conjoined twins. A, Joined at or near sternal region. **B,** Joined from xyphoid to umbilicus. **C,** Joined dorsally at sacral and perineal regions. **D,** Joined in pelvic region; usually with separate spinal columns and varied number of legs (2-4). **E,** Joined at any part of the skull, usually ventral or parietal; otherwise separate. **F,** Lying side by side and joined at ventral and lateral regions (with 2-4 arms, 2-3 legs). **G,** Joined from vertex to umbilicus and usually have one face. **H,** Joined dorsally with fusion above sacrum.

paring reduced twins to nonreduced twins, the incidence of growth discordance and IUGR remains high.[149] In one study the incidence of IUGR in nonreduced twins was 19.4%, versus 36.3% in triplets reduced to twins, 41.6% in quadruplets reduced to twins, and 50% in higher multiples reduced to twins.[150]

If a patient has a higher-order multiple gestation and one of the multiples is a monochorionic twin, both twins should be reduced. If there is an anomalous fetus that threatens the well-being of a monochorionic co-twin, selective reduction can be performed by cord ligation.

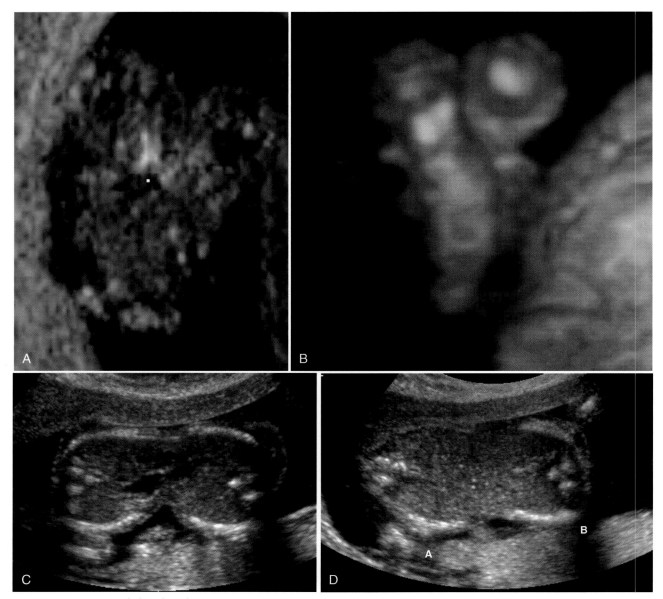

FIGURE 32-16. Conjoined twins. Thoraco-omphalopagus twins. **A** and **B,** 2-D and 3-D images at 10 weeks' gestation show two embryonic heads, with connection at the thorax and abdomen. **C** and **D,** Transverse views of a different pregnancy at 18 weeks' gestation show thoraco-omphalopagus twins with shared heart and shared liver.

CONCLUSION

Evaluation of twins and higher-order multiple pregnancies can be challenging. An understanding of the embryology will facilitate determining the placentation and the chorionicity and amnionicity of the fetuses. This categorization is of utmost importance to identify fetuses at risk for TTTS, twin embolization syndrome, TRAP sequence, and other conditions unique to monochorionic gestations. Monoamniotic gestations have added risk of cord entanglement and conjoined twins. In addition, multiple gestations have overall increased morbidity and mortality, regardless of zygosity and chorionicity, compared to singleton gestations. Knowledge of these specific and general conditions will allow the clinician to provide better care and counsel for these patients. In some pregnancies, early identification of a problem can improve outcome.

References

Incidence
1. Martin JA, Hamilton BE, Sutton PD, et al. Births: final data for 2005. Natl Vital Stat Rep 2007;56:1-103.
2. Luke B, Martin JA. The rise in multiple births in the United States: who, what, when, where, and why. Clin Obstet Gynecol 2004;47:118-133.
3. Hamilton BE, Martin JA, Ventura SJ. Births: preliminary data for 2005. Natl Vital Stat Rep 2006;55:1-18.
4. Martikainen H, Tiitinen A, Tomas C, et al. One versus two embryo transfer after IVF and ICSI: a randomized study. Hum Reprod 2001;16:1900-1903.

5. Vilska S, Tiitinen A, Hyden-Granskog C, Hovatta O. Elective transfer of one embryo results in an acceptable pregnancy rate and eliminates the risk of multiple birth. Hum Reprod 1999;14:2392-2395.
6. Moayeri SE, Behr B, Lathi RB, et al. Risk of monozygotic twinning with blastocyst transfer decreases over time: an 8-year experience. Fertil Steril 2007;87:1028-1032.
7. Bulmer MG. The biology of twinning in man. Oxford, UK: Clarendon Press; 1970.
8. Bulmer MG. The effect of parental age, parity and duration of marriage on the twinning rate. Ann Hum Genet 1959;23:454-458.
9. MacGillivray I. Epidemiology of twin pregnancy. Semin Perinatol 1986;10:4-8.
10. Nylander PP. The factors that influence twinning rates. Acta Genet Med Gemellol (Roma) 1981;30:189-202.
11. Hoekstra C, Zhao ZZ, Lambalk CB, et al. Dizygotic twinning. Hum Reprod Update 2008;14:37-47.
12. White C, Wyshak G. Inheritance in human dizygotic twinning. N Engl J Med 1964;271:1003-1005.
13. Pettersson F, Smedby B, Lindmark G. Outcome of twin birth: review of 1,636 children born in twin birth. Acta Paediatr Scand 1976;65:473-479.
14. Basso O, Nohr EA, Christensen K, Olsen J. Risk of twinning as a function of maternal height and body mass index. JAMA 2004; 291:1564-1566.
15. Reddy UM, Branum AM, Klebanoff MA. Relationship of maternal body mass index and height to twinning. Obstet Gynecol 2005;105: 593-597.

Zygosity and Placentation
16. Filly RA, Goldstein RB, Callen PW. Monochorionic twinning: sonographic assessment. AJR Am J Roentgenol 1990;154:459-469.
17. Verstraelen H, Goetgeluk S, Derom C, et al. Preterm birth in twins after subfertility treatment: population based cohort study. BMJ 2005;331:1173.
18. Moore K. The developing human: clinically oriented embryology. 4th ed. Philadelphia: Saunders; 1988.

Sonographic Determination of Chorionicity and Amnionicity
19. Benson CB, Doubilet PM, David V. Prognosis of first-trimester twin pregnancies: polychotomous logistic regression analysis. Radiology 1994;192:765-768.
20. Carroll SG, Soothill PW, Abdel-Fattah SA, et al. Prediction of chorionicity in twin pregnancies at 10-14 weeks of gestation. BJOG 2002;109:182-186.
21. Menon DK. A retrospective study of the accuracy of sonographic chorionicity determination in twin pregnancies. Twin Res Hum Genet 2005;8:259-261.
22. Babinszki A, Mukherjee T, Kerenyi T, et al. Diagnosing amnionicity at 6 weeks of pregnancy with transvaginal three-dimensional ultrasonography: case report. Fertil Steril 1999;71:1161-1164.
23. Bromley B, Benacerraf B. Using the number of yolk sacs to determine amnionicity in early first trimester monochorionic twins. J Ultrasound Med 1995;14:415-419.
24. Hill LM, Chenevey P, Hecker J, Martin JG. Sonographic determination of first trimester twin chorionicity and amnionicity. J Clin Ultrasound 1996;24:305-308.
25. Levi CS, Lyons EA, Dashefsky SM, et al. Yolk sac number, size and morphologic features in monochorionic monoamniotic twin pregnancy. Can Assoc Radiol J 1996;47:98-100.
26. Townsend RR, Simpson GF, Filly RA. Membrane thickness in ultrasound prediction of chorionicity of twin gestations. J Ultrasound Med 1988;7:327-332.
27. Hertzberg BS, Kurtz AB, Choi HY, et al. Significance of membrane thickness in the sonographic evaluation of twin gestations. AJR Am J Roentgenol 1987;148:151-153.
28. Senat MV, Quarello E, Levaillant JM, et al. Determining chorionicity in twin gestations: three-dimensional (3D) multiplanar sonographic measurement of intra-amniotic membrane thickness. Ultrasound Obstet Gynecol 2006;28:665-669.
29. Mahony BS, Filly RA, Callen PW. Amnionicity and chorionicity in twin pregnancies: prediction using ultrasound. Radiology 1985;155: 205-209.
30. Finberg HJ. The "twin peak" sign: reliable evidence of dichorionic twinning. J Ultrasound Med. 1992;11:571-577.
31. Bessis R, Papiernik E. Echographic imagery of amniotic membranes in twin pregnancies. Prog Clin Biol Res 1981;69A:183-187.
32. Sepulveda W, Sebire NJ, Hughes K, et al. The lambda sign at 10-14 weeks of gestation as a predictor of chorionicity in twin pregnancies. Ultrasound Obstet Gynecol 1996;7:421-423.
33. Sepulveda W, Sebire NJ, Hughes K, et al. Evolution of the lambda or twin-chorionic peak sign in dichorionic twin pregnancies. Obstet Gynecol 1997;89:439-441.
34. Wood SL, St Onge R, Connors G, Elliot PD. Evaluation of the twin peak or lambda sign in determining chorionicity in multiple pregnancy. Obstet Gynecol 1996;88:6-9.
35. Nyberg DA, Filly RA, Golbus MS, Stephens JD. Entangled umbilical cords: a sign of monoamniotic twins. J Ultrasound Med 1984;3: 29-32.
36. Lee YM, Cleary-Goldman J, Thaker HM, Simpson LL. Antenatal sonographic prediction of twin chorionicity. Am J Obstet Gynecol 2006;195:863-867.
37. Scardo JA, Ellings JM, Newman RB. Prospective determination of chorionicity, amnionicity, and zygosity in twin gestations. Am J Obstet Gynecol 1995;173:1376-1380.

Morbidity and Mortality
38. Misra DP, Ananth CV. Infant mortality among singletons and twins in the United States during 2 decades: effects of maternal age. Pediatrics 2002;110:1163-1168.
39. Taylor MJ. The management of multiple pregnancy. Early Hum Dev 2006;82:365-370.
40. Garite TJ, Clark RH, Elliott JP, Thorp JA. Twins and triplets: the effect of plurality and growth on neonatal outcome compared with singleton infants. Am J Obstet Gynecol 2004;191:700-707.
41. Sebire NJ, D'Ercole C, Hughes K, et al. Dichorionic twins discordant for intrauterine growth retardation. Arch Dis Child Fetal Neonatal Ed 1997;77:F235-F236.
42. Adegbite AL, Castille S, Ward S, Bajoria R. Neuromorbidity in preterm twins in relation to chorionicity and discordant birth weight. Am J Obstet Gynecol 2004;190:156-163.
43. Bajoria R, Wee LY, Anwar S, Ward S. Outcome of twin pregnancies complicated by single intrauterine death in relation to vascular anatomy of the monochorionic placenta. Hum Reprod 1999;14: 2124-2130.
44. Bejar R, Vigliocco G, Gramajo H, et al. Antenatal origin of neurologic damage in newborn infants. II. Multiple gestations. Am J Obstet Gynecol 1990;162:1230-1236.
45. Lee YM, Wylie BJ, Simpson LL, D'Alton ME. Twin chorionicity and the risk of stillbirth. Obstet Gynecol 2008;111:301-308.
46. Sebire NJ, Snijders RJ, Hughes K, et al. The hidden mortality of monochorionic twin pregnancies. Br J Obstet Gynaecol 1997;104: 1203-1207.
47. Pretorius DH, Budorick NE, Scioscia AL, et al. Twin pregnancies in the second trimester in women in an alpha-fetoprotein screening program: sonographic evaluation and outcome. AJR Am J Roentgenol 1993;161:1007-1013.
48. Landy HJ, Weiner S, Corson SL, et al. The "vanishing twin": ultrasonographic assessment of fetal disappearance in the first trimester. Am J Obstet Gynecol 1986;155:14-19.
49. Dickey RP, Taylor SN, Lu PY, et al. Spontaneous reduction of multiple pregnancy: incidence and effect on outcome. Am J Obstet Gynecol 2002;186:77-83.
50. La Sala GB, Nucera G, Gallinelli A, et al. Spontaneous embryonic loss following in vitro fertilization: incidence and effect on outcomes. Am J Obstet Gynecol 2004;191:741-746.
51. Gaucherand P, Rudigoz RC, Piacenza JM. Monofetal death in multiple pregnancies: risks for the co-twin, risk factors and obstetrical management. Eur J Obstet Gynecol Reprod Biol 1994;55:111-115.
52. Johnson CD, Zhang J. Survival of other fetuses after a fetal death in twin or triplet pregnancies. Obstet Gynecol 2002;99:698-703.
53. Saito K, Ohtsu Y, Amano K, Nishijima M. Perinatal outcome and management of single fetal death in twin pregnancy: a case series and review. J Perinat Med. 1999;27:473-477.
54. Prompeler HJ, Madjar H, Klosa W, et al. Twin pregnancies with single fetal death. Acta Obstet Gynecol Scand 1994;73:205-208.
55. Kohl SG, Casey G. Twin gestation. Mt Sinai J Med 1975;42: 523-539.
56. Yokoyama Y, Shimizu T, Hayakawa K. Incidence of handicaps in multiple births and associated factors. Acta Genet Med Gemellol (Roma) 1995;44:81-91.

57. Schinzel AA, Smith DW, Miller JR. Monozygotic twinning and structural defects. J Pediatr 1979;95:921-930.

58. Cameron AH, Edwards JH, Derom R, et al. The value of twin surveys in the study of malformations. Eur J Obstet Gynecol Reprod Biol 1983;14:347-356.

59. Grether JK, Nelson KB, Cummins SK. Twinning and cerebral palsy: experience in four northern California counties, births 1983 through 1985. Pediatrics 1993;92:854-858.

60. Petterson B, Nelson KB, Watson L, Stanley F. Twins, triplets, and cerebral palsy in births in Western Australia in the 1980s. BMJ 1993;307:1239-1243.

61. Pharoah PO, Cooke T. Cerebral palsy and multiple births. Arch Dis Child Fetal Neonatal Ed 1996;75:F174-F177.

62. Sebire NJ, Snijders RJ, Hughes K, et al. Screening for trisomy 21 in twin pregnancies by maternal age and fetal nuchal translucency thickness at 10-14 weeks of gestation. Br J Obstet Gynaecol 1996;103:999-1003.

63. Spencer K, Nicolaides KH. Screening for trisomy 21 in twins using first trimester ultrasound and maternal serum biochemistry in a one-stop clinic: a review of three years experience. BJOG 2003;110:276-280.

64. Brambati B, Tului L, Baldi M, Guercilena S. Genetic analysis prior to selective fetal reduction in multiple pregnancy: technical aspects and clinical outcome. Hum Reprod 1995;10:818-825.

65. Ghidini A, Lynch L, Hicks C, et al. The risk of second-trimester amniocentesis in twin gestations: a case-control study. Am J Obstet Gynecol 1993;169:1013-1016.

66. Stephen JA, Timor-Tritsch IE, Lerner JP, et al. Amniocentesis after multifetal pregnancy reduction: is it safe? Am J Obstet Gynecol 2000;182:962-965.

67. Wapner RJ, Johnson A, Davis G, et al. Prenatal diagnosis in twin gestations: a comparison between second-trimester amniocentesis and first-trimester chorionic villus sampling. Obstet Gynecol 1993;82:49-56.

68. Eddleman KA, Stone JL, Lynch L, Berkowitz RL. Chorionic villus sampling before multifetal pregnancy reduction. Am J Obstet Gynecol 2000;183:1078-1081.

69. Lipitz S, Shulman A, Achiron R, et al. A comparative study of multifetal pregnancy reduction from triplets to twins in the first versus early second trimesters after detailed fetal screening. Ultrasound Obstet Gynecol 2001;18:35-38.

70. Cragan JD. Teratogen update: methylene blue. Teratology 1999;60:42-48.

71. Nicolini U, Monni G. Intestinal obstruction in babies exposed in utero to methylene blue. Lancet 1990;336:1258-1259.

72. Van der Pol JG, Wolf H, Boer K, et al. Jejunal atresia related to the use of methylene blue in genetic amniocentesis in twins. Br J Obstet Gynaecol 1992;99:141-143.

73. Machin GA. Some causes of genotypic and phenotypic discordance in monozygotic twin pairs. Am J Med Genet 1996;61:216-228.

74. Rodis JF, Vintzileos AM, Campbell WA, Nochimson DJ. Intrauterine fetal growth in discordant twin gestations. J Ultrasound Med 1990;9:443-448.

75. Mordel N, Benshushan A, Zajicek G, et al. Discordancy in triplets. Am J Perinatol 1993;10:224-225.

76. Branum AM, Schoendorf KC. The effect of birth weight discordance on twin neonatal mortality. Obstet Gynecol 2003;101:570-574.

77. Weissman A, Achiron R, Lipitz S, et al. The first-trimester growth-discordant twin: an ominous prenatal finding. Obstet Gynecol 1994;84:110-114.

78. Kalish RB, Chasen ST, Gupta M, et al. First trimester prediction of growth discordance in twin gestations. Am J Obstet Gynecol 2003;189:706-709.

79. Rydhstroem H, Heraib F. Gestational duration, and fetal and infant mortality for twins vs singletons. Twin Res 2001;4:227-231.

80. Martin JA, Hamilton BE, Ventura SJ, et al. Births: final data for 2001. Natl Vital Stat Rep 2002;51:1-102.

81. Iams JD, Goldenberg RL, Meis PJ, et al. The length of the cervix and the risk of spontaneous premature delivery. National Institute of Child Health and Human Development Maternal Fetal Medicine Unit Network. N Engl J Med 1996;334:567-572.

82. Kushnir O, Izquierdo LA, Smith JF, et al. Transvaginal sonographic measurement of cervical length: evaluation of twin pregnancies. J Reprod Med 1995;40:380-382.

83. Goldenberg RL, Iams JD, Miodovnik M, et al. The preterm prediction study: risk factors in twin gestations. National Institute of Child Health and Human Development Maternal-Fetal Medicine Units Network. Am J Obstet Gynecol 1996;175:1047-1053.

84. Guzman ER, Walters C, O'Reilly-Green C, et al. Use of cervical ultrasonography in prediction of spontaneous preterm birth in twin gestations. Am J Obstet Gynecol 2000;183:1103-1107.

85. Dor J, Shalev J, Mashiach S, et al. Elective cervical suture of twin pregnancies diagnosed ultrasonically in the first trimester following induced ovulation. Gynecol Obstet Invest 1982;13:55-60.

86. Newman RB, Krombach RS, Myers MC, McGee DL. Effect of cerclage on obstetrical outcome in twin gestations with a shortened cervical length. Am J Obstet Gynecol 2002;186:634-640.

87. Weekes AR, Menzies DN, de Boer CH. The relative efficacy of bed rest, cervical suture, and no treatment in the management of twin pregnancy. Br J Obstet Gynaecol 1977;84:161-164.

88. Wilson RL, Cetrulo CL, Shaub MS. The prepartum diagnosis of conjoined twins by the use of diagnostic ultrasound. Am J Obstet Gynecol 1976;126:737.

89. Kouyoumdjian A. Velamentous insertion of the umbilical cord. Obstet Gynecol 1980;56:737-742.

90. Paavonen J, Jouttunpaa K, Kangasluoma P, et al. Velamentous insertion of the umbilical cord and vasa previa. Int J Gynaecol Obstet 1984;22:207-211.

91. Robinson LK, Jones KL, Benirschke K. The nature of structural defects associated with velamentous and marginal insertion of the umbilical cord. Am J Obstet Gynecol 1983;146:191-193.

92. Baldwin V. Twinning mechanisms and zygosity determination. In: Pathology of multiple gestation. New York: Springer-Verlag; 1994.

93. Brody S, Frenkel DA. Marginal insertion of the cord and premature labor. Am J Obstet Gynecol. 1953;65:1305-1312.

94. Bruner JP, Rosemond RL. Twin-to-twin transfusion syndrome: a subset of the twin oligohydramnios-polyhydramnios sequence. Am J Obstet Gynecol 1993;169:925-930.

95. Fries MH, Goldstein RB, Kilpatrick SJ, et al. The role of velamentous cord insertion in the etiology of twin-twin transfusion syndrome. Obstet Gynecol 1993;81:569-574.

96. Hanley ML, Ananth CV, Shen-Schwarz S, et al. Placental cord insertion and birth weight discordancy in twin gestations. Obstet Gynecol 2002;99:477-482.

97. Giles WB, Trudinger BJ, Baird PJ. Fetal umbilical artery flow velocity waveforms and placental resistance: pathological correlation. Br J Obstet Gynaecol 1985;92:31-38.

98. Abramowicz JS, Warsof SL, Arrington J, Levy DL. Doppler analysis of the umbilical artery: the importance of choosing the placental end of the cord. J Ultrasound Med 1989;8:219-221.

99. Kochenour NK. Doppler velocimetry in pregnancy. Semin Ultrasound CT MR 1993;14:249-266.

100. Divon MY, Girz BA, Sklar A, et al. Discordant twins: a prospective study of the diagnostic value of real-time ultrasonography combined with umbilical artery velocimetry. Am J Obstet Gynecol. 1989;161:757-760.

101. Farmakides G, Schulman H, Saldana LR, et al. Surveillance of twin pregnancy with umbilical arterial velocimetry. Am J Obstet Gynecol 1985;153:789-792.

102. Morrow RJ, Adamson SL, Bull SB, Ritchie JW. Effect of placental embolization on the umbilical arterial velocity waveform in fetal sheep. Am J Obstet Gynecol 1989;161:1055-1060.

103. Wilcox GR, Trudinger BJ, Cook CM, et al. Reduced fetal platelet counts in pregnancies with abnormal Doppler umbilical flow waveforms. Obstet Gynecol 1989;73:639-643.

Complications

104. Robertson EG, Neer KJ. Placental injection studies in twin gestation. Am J Obstet Gynecol 1983;147:170-174.

105. Galea P, Jain V, Fisk NM. Insights into the pathophysiology of twin-twin transfusion syndrome. Prenat Diagn 2005;25:777-785.

106. Sebire NJ, Talbert D, Fisk NM. Twin-to-twin transfusion syndrome results from dynamic asymmetrical reduction in placental anastomoses: a hypothesis. Placenta 2001;22:383-391.

107. Bajoria R, Wigglesworth J, Fisk NM. Angioarchitecture of monochorionic placentas in relation to the twin-twin transfusion syndrome. Am J Obstet Gynecol 1995;172:856-863.

108. Denbow ML, Cox P, Taylor M, et al. Placental angioarchitecture in monochorionic twin pregnancies: relationship to fetal growth,

fetofetal transfusion syndrome, and pregnancy outcome. Am J Obstet Gynecol 2000;182:417-426.

109. Taylor MJ, Denbow ML, Duncan KR, et al. Antenatal factors at diagnosis that predict outcome in twin-twin transfusion syndrome. Am J Obstet Gynecol 2000;183:1023-1028.

110. Umur A, van Gemert MJ, Nikkels PG. Monoamniotic-versus diamniotic-monochorionic twin placentas: anastomoses and twin-twin transfusion syndrome. Am J Obstet Gynecol 2003;189:1325-1329.

111. Denbow ML, Cox P, Talbert D, Fisk NM. Colour Doppler energy insonation of placental vasculature in monochorionic twins: absent arterio-arterial anastomoses in association with twin-twin transfusion syndrome. Br J Obstet Gynaecol 1998;105:760-765.

112. Quintero RA, Dickinson JE, Morales WJ, et al. Stage-based treatment of twin-twin transfusion syndrome. Am J Obstet Gynecol 2003;188:1333-1340.

113. Mahony BS, Petty CN, Nyberg DA, et al. The "stuck twin" phenomenon: ultrasonographic findings, pregnancy outcome, and management with serial amniocenteses. Am J Obstet Gynecol 1990;163:1513-1522.

114. Pinette MG, Pan Y, Pinette SG, Stubblefield PG. Treatment of twin-twin transfusion syndrome. Obstet Gynecol 1993;82:841-846.

115. Saade GR, Belfort MA, Berry DL, et al. Amniotic septostomy for the treatment of twin oligohydramnios-polyhydramnios sequence. Fetal Diagn Ther 1998;13:86-93.

116. Senat MV, Deprest J, Boulvain M, et al. Endoscopic laser surgery versus serial amnioreduction for severe twin-to-twin transfusion syndrome. N Engl J Med 2004;351:136-144.

117. Mari G, Roberts A, Detti L, et al. Perinatal morbidity and mortality rates in severe twin-twin transfusion syndrome: results of the International Amnioreduction Registry. Am J Obstet Gynecol 2001;185:708-715.

118. Hecher K, Plath H, Bregenzer T, et al. Endoscopic laser surgery versus serial amniocenteses in the treatment of severe twin-twin transfusion syndrome. Am J Obstet Gynecol 1999;180:717-724.

119. Barth RCH. Ultrasound evaluation of multifetal gestations. 4th ed. Philadelphia: Saunders; 2000.

120. Hoyme HE, Higginbottom MC, Jones KL. Vascular etiology of disruptive structural defects in monozygotic twins. Pediatrics 1981;67:288-291.

121. Benirschke K. Intrauterine death of a twin: mechanisms, implications for surviving twin, and placental pathology. Semin Diagn Pathol 1993;10:222-231.

122. Hughes HE, Miskin M. Congenital microcephaly due to vascular disruption: in utero documentation. Pediatrics. 1986;78:85-87.

123. Szymonowicz W, Preston H, Yu VY. The surviving monozygotic twin. Arch Dis Child 1986;61:454-458.

124. Melnick M. Brain damage in survivor after in-utero death of monozygous co-twin. Lancet 1977;2:1287.

125. Levine D. Fetal magnetic resonance imaging. Top Magn Reson Imaging 2001;12:1-2.

126. Coulam CB, Wright G. First trimester diagnosis of acardiac twins. Early Pregnancy 2000;4:261-270.

127. Van Allen MI, Smith DW, Shepard TH. Twin reversed arterial perfusion (TRAP) sequence: a study of 14 twin pregnancies with acardius. Semin Perinatol 1983;7:285-293.

128. Napolitani FD, Schreiber I. The acardiac monster: a review of the world literature and presentation of 2 cases. Am J Obstet Gynecol 1960;80:582-589.

129. Severn CB, Holyoke EA. Human acardiac anomalies. Am J Obstet Gynecol 1973;116:358-365.

130. Healey MG. Acardia: predictive risk factors for the co-twin's survival. Teratology 1994;50:205-213.

131. Moore TR, Gale S, Benirschke K. Perinatal outcome of forty-nine pregnancies complicated by acardiac twinning. Am J Obstet Gynecol 1990;163:907-912.

132. Lee H, Wagner AJ, Sy E, et al. Efficacy of radiofrequency ablation for twin-reversed arterial perfusion sequence. Am J Obstet Gynecol. 2007;196:459 e1-e4.

133. Tan TY, Sepulveda W. Acardiac twin: a systematic review of minimally invasive treatment modalities. Ultrasound Obstet Gynecol. 2003;22:409-419.

134. Benirschke K, Kim CK. Multiple pregnancy. 1. N Engl J Med 1973;288:1276-1284.

135. Roque H, Gillen-Goldstein J, Funai E, et al. Perinatal outcomes in monoamniotic gestations. J Matern Fetal Neonatal Med 2003;13:414-421.

136. Cordero L, Franco A, Joy SD. Monochorionic monoamniotic twins: neonatal outcome. J Perinatol 2006;26:170-175.

137. Gaffney G, Squier MV, Johnson A, et al. Clinical associations of prenatal ischaemic white matter injury. Arch Dis Child Fetal Neonatal Ed 1994;70:F101-F106.

138. MacLennan A. A template for defining a causal relation between acute intrapartum events and cerebral palsy: international consensus statement. BMJ 1999;319:1054-1059.

139. Edmonds LD, Layde PM. Conjoined twins in the United States, 1970-1977. Teratology 1982;25:301-308.

140. Keith LG, Machin GA, Bamforth F. An atlas of multiple pregnancy: biology and pathology. New York: CRC Press; 1999.

141. Barth RA, Filly RA, Goldberg JD, et al. Conjoined twins: prenatal diagnosis and assessment of associated malformations. Radiology 1990;177:201-207.

142. Hill LM. The sonographic detection of early first-trimester conjoined twins. Prenat Diagn 1997;17:961-963.

143. Spitz L, Kiely EM. Conjoined twins. JAMA 2003;289:1307-1310.

144. Angtuaco TL, Angtuaco EJ, Quirk Jr JG. Ultrasound case of the day. Complete brain duplication with fusion at the posterior fossa (diprosopus tetraophthalmos). Radiographics 1999;19:260-263.

145. O'Neill Jr JA, Holcomb 3rd GW, Schnaufer L, et al. Surgical experience with thirteen conjoined twins. Ann Surg 1988;208:299-312.

Selective Multifetal Reduction

146. Eddleman KA, Stone JL, Lynch L, Berkowitz RL. Selective termination of anomalous fetuses in multifetal pregnancies: two hundred cases at a single center. Am J Obstet Gynecol 2002;187:1168-1172.

147. Stone J, Eddleman K, Lynch L, Berkowitz RL. A single center experience with 1000 consecutive cases of multifetal pregnancy reduction. Am J Obstet Gynecol 2002;187:1163-1167.

148. Papageorghiou AT, Avgidou K, Bakoulas V, et al. Risks of miscarriage and early preterm birth in trichorionic triplet pregnancies with embryo reduction versus expectant management: new data and systematic review. Hum Reprod 2006;21:1912-1917.

149. Silver RK, Helfand BT, Russell TL, et al. Multifetal reduction increases the risk of preterm delivery and fetal growth restriction in twins: a case-control study. Fertil Steril 1997;67:30-33.

150. Depp R, Macones GA, Rosenn MF, et al. Multifetal pregnancy reduction: evaluation of fetal growth in the remaining twins. Am J Obstet Gynecol 1996;174:1233-1238.

CHAPTER 33

The Fetal Face and Neck

Ana Lourenco and Judy Estroff

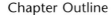

Chapter Outline

With technical advances in gray-scale and three-dimensional imaging, sonographic evaluation of the fetal face and neck has become a routine part of the second-trimester fetal anatomic survey.[1] Also, an increasing number of anomalies have become detectable in the first trimester. Abnormalities of the fetal face are particularly important because they may be markers for syndromes and chromosomal anomalies. This chapter reviews the embryology and normal development of the fetal face and neck and describes anomalies that can be detected sonographically.

EMBRYOLOGY AND DEVELOPMENT

Face

Fetal face development begins at approximately 4 weeks' gestation and rapidly progresses, with the completion of major events by 8 weeks' gestation (Fig. 33-1). In this complex process, ectoderm, mesoderm, endoderm, and neural crest cells all interact to develop the classic human facial features. Ectoderm surrounds the **stomodeum** (primitive mouth). The paired pharyngeal arches, or **branchial arches,** composed of central mesenchyme with outer ectoderm and inner endoderm coverings, progress to fuse in the midline. **Neural crest cells** give rise to connective tissues of the face (cartilage, bone, ligaments).

Five main tissue buds (called **prominences**) form the fetal face. The **frontonasal** prominence forms the forehead and dorsum apex of the nose. The **lateral nasal** prominences form the nasal ala. The **medial nasal** prominences form the nasal septum. **Maxillary** prominences form the upper cheeks and most of the upper lip. **Mandibular** prominences form the lower cheeks, lower lip, and chin. The maxillary and mandibular processes are derived from the first branchial arch. The remaining branchial arches go on to form the oropharynx.

During the fourth week of gestation, the frontal prominence forms at the cephalic end of the embryo. The two nasal **placodes** are present on the frontal prominence, and the optic discs are present posterolaterally. In the stomodeum, the buccopharyngeal membrane becomes fenestrated.

The fifth week brings development of nasal pits in the nasal placodes and differentiation of medial and lateral nasal prominences. The lens vesicles invaginate within the optic discs, and the caudal end of the medial nasal prominences begins to fuse with the maxillary prominences.

During the sixth week, six **auricular hillocks** (mesenchymal swellings) form and will become the pinna of the ears. Auricular pits may arise when these nodules do not fuse completely. Medial and lateral nasal

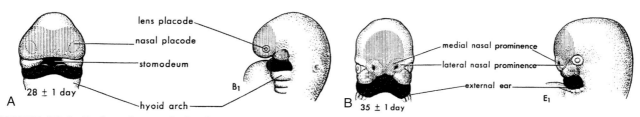

FIGURE 33-1. Embryology of the face. Stages of development of the fetal face. Note the initial wide separation of the eyes, high wide separation of the nostrils (nasal placodes), and low position of the ears. *(From Moore KL: Essentials of human embryology. Toronto, 1988, BC Decker.)*

prominences fuse, and the maxillary prominences begin to form the upper jaw. The nasal septum forms as the medial nasal prominences join in the midline. The edges of the optic fissures fuse, and the hyaloid vessels are present in the center of the optic stalk. These vessels will eventually form the retinal artery and vein.

By the seventh week, the tip of the nose is visible in profile, and the pinna of the ears is taking shape. The central axis of the nose and philtrum are formed as fusion of the medial nasal prominences is completed. Eyelids become prominent.[2-5] By the end of the eighth week, the developing eye is up to 2 mm in diameter.[6]

Neck

Development of the fetal neck is similarly complex, with extensive embryologic events contributing to development of vascular, neurologic, musculoskeletal, lymphatic, and endocrine systems. The laryngotracheal groove forms during the fourth week of gestation along the floor of the primitive mouth. After evagination of this groove, the laryngotracheal diverticulum forms. The distal end forms the lung bud. The endoderm of this diverticulum forms the epithelium of the larynx and trachea. The endothelium of the larynx proliferates and temporarily occludes its lumen. Recanalization occurs by the tenth gestational week, with formation of the laryngeal ventricle, vocal folds, and vestibular folds. The fourth and sixth pharyngeal arches form the surrounding cartilage and muscles.[2-4]

At 4 to 6 weeks' gestation, right and left jugular lymph sacs develop as diverticula of the subclavian veins. Lymphatic capillaries permeate the body and drain into these sacs. Abnormal connections between the lymphatic sacs and venous system are thought to contribute to lymphatic malformation and thickened nuchal translucency in the first trimester, as well as thickened nuchal fold in the second trimester.[7]

SONOGRAPHY OF THE NORMAL FETAL FACE

Sonographic evaluation of the fetal face is part of the routine anatomic survey in midpregnancy, but little is actually required. According to the American Institute of Ultrasound in Medicine 2007 practice guidelines, only visualization of the fetal upper lip is mandatory during an anatomic survey.[1] Although not required, it is possible to obtain exquisite multiplanar two-, three-, and four-dimensional (2-D, 3-D, 4-D) views of the fetal face with state-of-the-art equipment.[8] Profile and 3-D[9] views are helpful, especially when a true coronal view cannot be obtained because of fetal position. Sagittal 3-D volumes of the fetal face can often be obtained in these situations, and the image can then be rotated to show the upper lip and palate clearly. Coronal and axial views of the fetal nose and lips are obligatory in screening for fetal cleft lip (Fig. 33-2, *A* and *B*).

The sagittal **facial profile** view is acquired whenever possible and should demonstrate the presence and normal configuration of the nasal bone, lips, chin, and forehead. Axial views of the orbits can be obtained to verify that both globes are present, of normal size, and at a normal distance apart (Fig. 33-2, *C*). Axial images of the maxilla and alveolar ridge can be obtained to determine if a cleft primary palate is present (Fig. 33-2, *D*). The palate separates the nasal cavity from the oral cavity. The **secondary palate** is difficult to visualize on 2-D sonography but may be evaluated with special 3-D sonographic views[10-12] and is often readily visible on midline sagittal and coronal fetal magnetic resonance imaging (MRI; Fig. 33-2, *H*).

Images of the **fetal neck** are obtained in sagittal, axial, and coronal planes to evaluate the cervical spine, airway, and to assess for masses (Fig. 33-3). The neck should also be evaluated for abnormal positioning, such as hyperextension, which can be present with anterior neck masses such as an enlarged thyroid or cervical teratoma. Thickening of the nuchal fold should be evaluated at the second-trimester survey and is measured in the suboccipital bregmatic plane, where notable landmarks include the cavum septum pellucidum, cerebral peduncles, cerebellar hemispheres, and cisterna magna.

ABNORMALITIES OF THE HEAD

Abnormal Size

The fetal head is typically oval in configuration, and in this case, measurements of biparietal diameter (BPD)

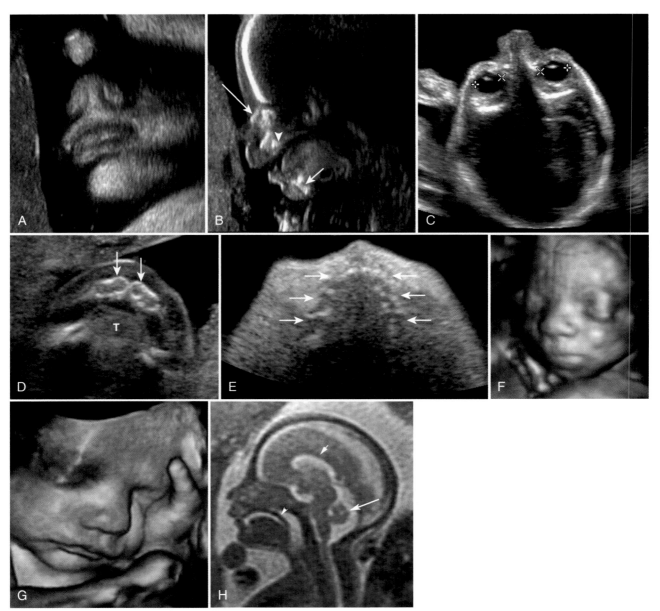

FIGURE 33-2. Normal fetal face. A, Nose and lips. Coronal sonogram at 36 weeks' gestation. **B,** Profile of the face of a 17-week fetus shows a normal nasal bone *(long arrow)*, maxilla *(short arrow)*, and mandible *(arrowhead)*. **C, N**ormal orbits in axial view *(cursors: +, outer orbital distance; x, inner orbital distance)*. **D, Normal maxilla.** Axial view of anterior aspect of the maxilla in a 17-week fetus shows tooth buds in the alveolus *(arrows)* and tongue *(T)*. **E, Normal mandible.** Axial view shows multiple tooth buds. **F,** 3-D sonogram of a normal 23-week fetus. **G,** 3-D sonogram of a normal 30-week fetus in **F. H,** Sagittal T2-weighted MR image of a normal fetal face at 27 weeks' gestation shows normal midline structures, such as corpus callosum *(thick arrow)*, cerebellar vermis *(V)*, and secondary palate *(thin arrow)*.

and head circumference will give similar estimates of gestational age. If sonographic head measurements are three standard deviations (3 SD) below the mean, microcephaly is diagnosed.[13] If the measurements are greater than 2 SD above the mean, macrocephaly is suggested.[5] Abnormalities of head size are important. **Microcephaly** may be associated with abnormalities of brain development and often leads to poor neurologic outcome. **Macrocephaly** may have a benign cause, such as a family history of a large head, or pathologic causes such as underlying brain maldevelopment or injury or rarely, a

space-occupying lesion. If the fetal head is sufficiently large, cephalopelvic disproportion can occur at delivery, leading to failure of labor to progress and the need for cesarean delivery.

Abnormal Shape

Abnormal head shape takes many forms. An abnormally long and narrow (oblong) cranium is described as **dolichocephaly** and is more frequently seen in fetuses in breech position and in the setting of oligohydramnios.

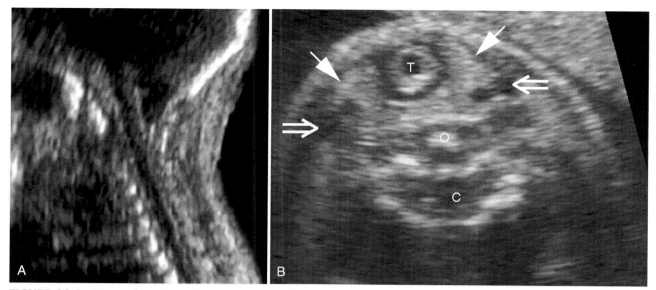

FIGURE 33-3. Normal neck. A, Sagittal view. Cervical spine and the soft tissues of the posterior neck can be evaluated along with the degree of flexion or extension of the neck. **B,** Axial view shows **thyroid** *(arrows)*. The carotids medially and the jugular veins laterally can be seen *(open arrows)* posterior to the thyroid. The trachea *(T)* is seen in the midline behind the isthmus and behind it a vertebral body with a small central developing ossification center *(O)*. The spinal cord *(C)* is cradled within the vertebral arch.

An abnormally round head is termed **brachycephaly,** which may be caused by premature fusion of the coronal sutures. A **lemon-shaped skull,** with indentation of the frontal bones, is often seen in association with open neural tube defects and the Chiari II malformation of the hindbrain, but it may also be seen in normal fetuses[14,15] (Fig. 33-4). A **strawberry-shaped skull,** presenting as flattening of the occiput and narrowing of the bifrontal portion of the cranium, may be seen in association with trisomy 18.[16] A **cloverleaf-shaped skull** is seen with some dwarfs, especially **thanatophoric dysplasia,** and in some fetuses with craniosynostosis.

Craniosynostosis

Craniosynostosis describes a heterogeneous group of disorders in which there is premature fusion of one or several of the cranial sutures. Although abnormal head shape may be diagnosed in utero, this diagnosis often does not become evident until after birth. It occurs in about 1 in 2500 births. Recent research suggests the pathophysiology of craniosynostosis is related to abnormal molecular signaling by fibroblast growth factors (FGFs),[17-19] leading to premature closure of cranial sutures (Fig. 33-5). About 85% of cases are isolated and about 15% syndromic. Craniosynostosis is associated with multiple syndromes, including **Apert, Crouzon, Pfeiffer, Antley-Bixler, Beare-Stevenson, Fetter,** and **Carpenter**, as well as **thanatophoric dysplasia.** The abnormal head shapes resulting from craniosynostosis can lead to facial abnormalities, including **hypertelorism, hypotelorism, exorbitism,** and **midface hypoplasia.**

Dolichocephaly **(oblong head)** is the most common craniosynostosis condition and results from premature fusion of the sagittal suture. Asymmetrical heads are termed **plagiocephalic.**[20]

When fetal position is favorable, it is possible to trace the sutures sonographically and to evaluate their patency using high-frequency linear array probes.

CLASSIFICATION OF SKULL DEFORMITIES BASED ON SUTURES INVOLVED

Dolichocephaly/scaphocephaly: sagittal suture; most common synostosis
Anterior plagiocephaly: 1 coronal suture
Posterior plagiocephaly: 1 lambdoid suture
Brachycephaly: bilateral coronal suture; second most common synostosis
Trigonocephaly: metopic suture
Oxycephaly/turricephaly: all skull sutures and sutures at base of skull
Cloverleaf (kleeblattschädel): all but squamous (squamosal) suture

Prenatal diagnosis can be difficult; fetuses can appear normal in midtrimester but show changes in late pregnancy, when normal physiologic molding can be a confounder. In at-risk cases, head shape changes have been seen as early as 12 weeks. The fused sutures can be detected as absence of the sonolucent space normally seen between skull bones. The loss of hypoechoic suture appearance lags shape changes by 4 to 16 weeks.

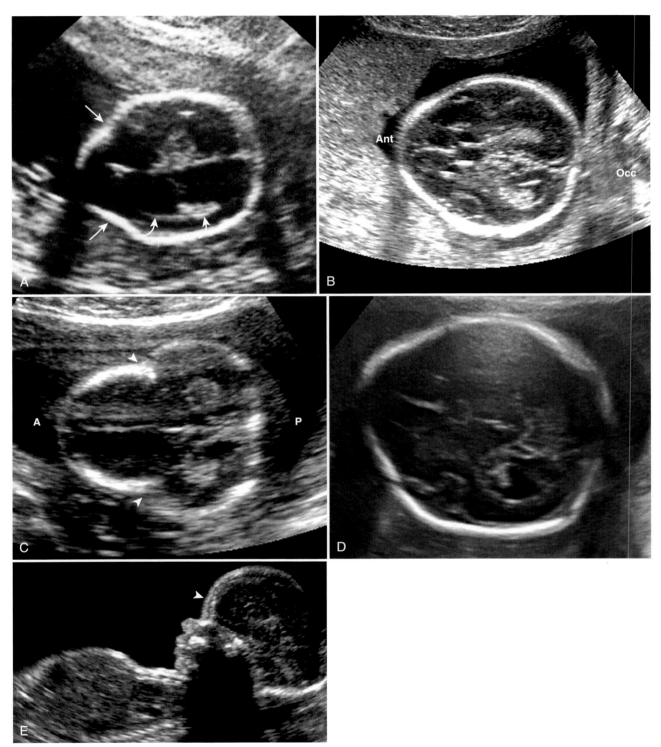

FIGURE 33-4. Variety of abnormal head shapes. A, Lemon-shaped skull in association with neural tube defect. Axial sonograms shows concave deformity of the frontal bone *(straight arrows)* as well as ventriculomegaly *(curved arrows)* at 22 weeks' gestation. **B, Brachycephaly and strawberry shape** (pointing anteriorly, flat occiput) at 20 weeks in a fetus with trisomy 18. Cephalic index is 96% (normal, 80%); *Occ,* occiput; *Ant,* forehead. **C, Craniosynostosis with cloverleaf skull.** Note the trilobite shape seen with craniosynostosis of the coronal *(arrowheads)* and other sutures except the squamosal in this fetus with **thanatophoric dysplasia;** *A,* anterior; *P,* posterior. **D, Metopic craniosynostosis.** Axial sonogram of a 27-week fetus with a pointed anterior skull secondary to metopic synostosis. **E, Frontal bossing** in a fetus with hypochondroplasia. Also note a "saddle nose," with the nasal bone meeting the frontal bone at an abnormal 90 degrees. There is a small thorax and a protuberant abdomen. *(A, B, and C courtesy Ants Toi, MD).*

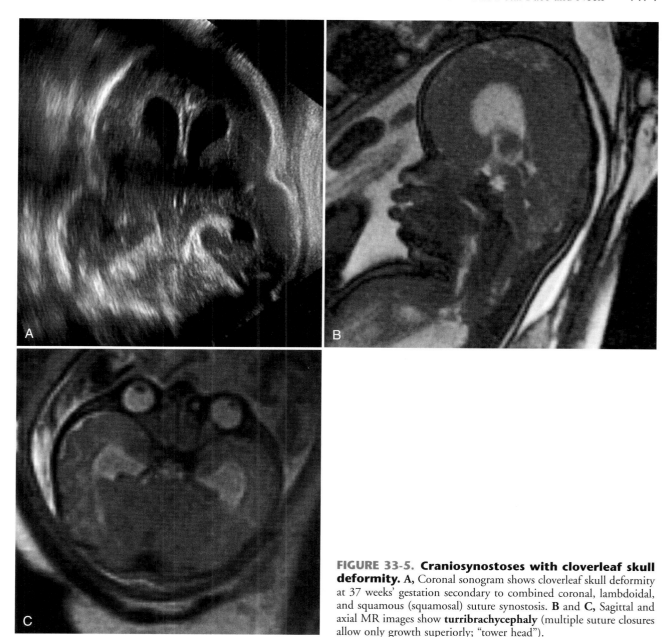

FIGURE 33-5. Craniosynostoses with cloverleaf skull deformity. A, Coronal sonogram shows cloverleaf skull deformity at 37 weeks' gestation secondary to combined coronal, lambdoidal, and squamous (squamosal) suture synostosis. **B** and **C,** Sagittal and axial MR images show **turribrachycephaly** (multiple suture closures allow only growth superiorly; "tower head").

Three-dimensional multiplanar and surface rendering are helpful. Associated anomalies can allow differentiation between types.[21-23]

Additional problems can arise from the cranial deformity, including intracranial hypertension, obstructive apnea, proptosis, visual loss, dental malocclusion, and intellectual impairment. Learning disorders have been observed in 47% of school-age children.[22]

Fetuses prenatally suspected to have craniosynostosis should undergo detailed neurologic and anatomic sonography. MRI may be helpful. Postnatally, computed tomography (CT) surface rendering helps confirm the diagnosis and is needed for surgical treatment planning. Family history and molecular analysis for FGFR and TWIST mutations can help. Multidisciplinary counseling, including craniofacial and neurosurgical specialists, is important because therapy can involve molding helmets and surgery.[22,24,25]

Wormian Bones

Wormian bones are ossicles located in the sutures or fontanelles and may be associated with multiple conditions, such as **pyknodysostosis, osteogenesis imperfecta, cleidocranial dysplasia, hypothyroidism,** and **trisomy 21.** Three-dimensional views are particularly useful in the assessment of wormian bones (Fig. 33-6).

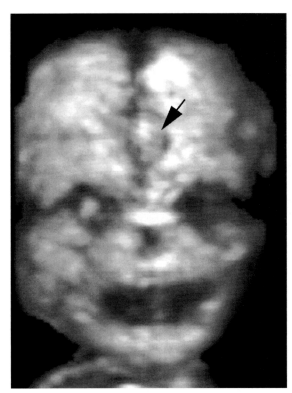

FIGURE 33-6. Wormian bone. An extra ossification center (*arrow*) is identified between the frontal bones of a fetus with trisomy 18.

DIFFERENTIAL DIAGNOSIS OF WORMIAN BONES

Cleidocranial dysplasia
Congenital hypothyroidism
Hypophosphatasia
Osteogenesis imperfecta
Trisomy 21
Menkes' kinky-hair syndrome
Progeria
Pyknodysostosis

Forehead Abnormalities

The forehead is best evaluated in the sagittal profile view, where the angle between the frontal and nasal bone can be assessed. **Frontal bossing** is abnormal prominence of the frontal bones and is a rare finding on fetal sonography. However, it has been reported in a variety of bony dysplasias and syndromes, including achondroplasia and thanatophoric dysplasia, and in syndromes with associated craniosynostosis.

Wolf-Hirschhorn (4p−) syndrome has an abnormally sloped forehead, the "Greek warrior facies" (Fig. 33-7). The forehead can also be sloped in the settings of **microcephaly** and **encephalocele,** in which the forebrain is underdeveloped (Fig. 33-8).

DIFFERENTIAL DIAGNOSIS OF FRONTAL BOSSING

Achondroplasia
Acromegaly
Basal cell nevus
Cleidocranial dysostosis
Congenital syphilis
Crouzon syndrome
Fetal trimethadione
Pfeiffer syndrome
Russell-Silver syndrome
Thanatophoric dysplasia

Encephaloceles

An encephalocele or **cephalocele** is an abnormal protrusion of the brain and/or meninges through a defect in the skull and is considered a form of **spinal dysraphism.** In the United States and Western Europe, the occiput is the most common location for encephaloceles. Frontoethmoidal encephaloceles are more often found in Southeast Asia. Many encephaloceles are diagnosed at fetal sonography, where they present as abnormal defects in the calvarium with herniation of brain tissue or meninges. Fetal MRI is excellent for evaluating contents of the encephalocele and in assessing the appearance of the intracranial brain parenchyma. Frontal encephaloceles can present during sonographic evaluation of the fetal face and are often associated with hypertelorism and midline facial clefting[26] (see Chapter 34).

ORBIT ABNORMALITIES

Sonographic evaluation of the fetal orbits is best obtained in axial or coronal views, where one can confirm the presence of both orbits, evaluating their sizes, shapes, and the distance between them. The sagittal view may help to evaluate abnormal anterior displacement of the globes (**proptosis** or **exorbitism**). The orbits should be symmetrical in size and the outer and inner interorbital distances within a normal range. Detailed nomograms are available for reference[27,28] (Table 33-1).

Hypotelorism

Hypotelorism is defined as an abnormally small distance between the orbits and is often associated with other anomalies[29,30] (Fig. 33-9). In particular, **alobar holoprosencephaly** can be associated with **cyclopia** (single midline eye with failed development of nose with or without a proboscis; Fig. 33-10), **ethmocephaly** (hypotelorism with failed development of nose and a proboscis), or **cebocephaly** (hypotelorism and poorly developed nose with a single nostril).

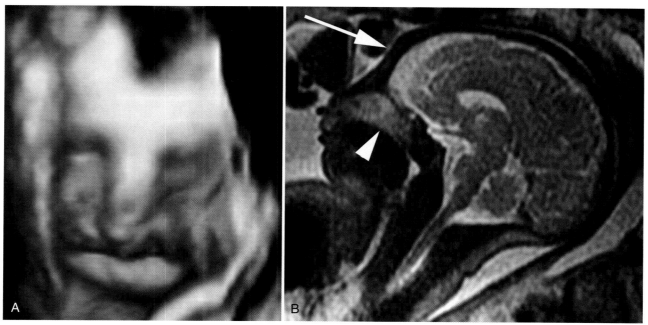

FIGURE 33-7. Sloped forehead in fetus with Wolf-Hirschhorn syndrome and cleft palate. A, Coronal 3-D, and **B,** sagittal MR, images show a broad, flat nasal bridge and forehead at 34 weeks' gestation, the so-called "Greek warrior helmet" facies. Note sloped forehead (*arrow* in **B**) and absence of the secondary palate (*arrowhead* in **B**, showing nasopharynx communicating with oropharynx).

CONDITIONS ASSOCIATED WITH HYPOTELORISM
Abnormalities of the brain 　Holoprosencephaly 　Microcephaly Chromosomal abnormalities 　Trisomies 13, 18, and 21 　Chromosome 5p deletion Head shape abnormalities 　Trigonocephaly Syndromes 　Langer-Giedion syndrome 　Oculodentodigital dysplasia 　Nasal maxillary dysostosis (Binder syndrome) 　Myotonic dystrophy 　Meckel-Gruber syndrome 　Williams syndrome

CONDITIONS ASSOCIATED WITH HYPERTELORISM
Chromosomal abnormalities 　Trisomy 9p 　45,XO Single-gene disorders 　Apert syndrome 　Crouzon syndrome 　Noonan syndrome Developmental abnormalities 　Craniosynostosis 　Anterior encephalocele 　Median facial cleft 　Megalencephaly 　Agenesis of the corpus callosum 　Orbital teratoma 　Cleft lip Teratogens 　Dilantin 　Valproate

Hypertelorism

Hypertelorism is defined as widely spaced eyes (Figs. 33-11 and 33-12; see also Fig. 33-17, *E* and *F*). Given the embryologic development of the eyes and their migration from a lateral position to midline, hypertelorism may result from abnormalities that interfere with this normal migration. Large orbits can result in abnormal orbital measurements; tables provide normal diameter of the globes.[31]

Microphthalmia and Anophthalmia

Abnormally small (microphthalmia) or absent (anophthalmia) orbits are rarely diagnosed on fetal sonography, but, when present, are frequently associated with chromosomal abnormalities or syndromes[32,33] (Fig. 33-13). Fetal karyotype analysis should be considered and a careful search for additional fetal abnormalities undertaken.

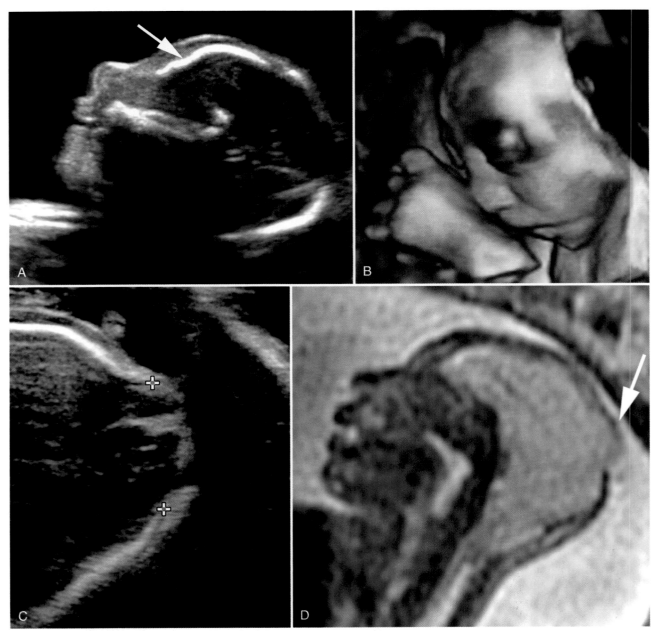

FIGURE 33-8. Sloped forehead in fetus with posterior encephalocele. **A** and **B,** 2-D and 3-D sonographic profiles of a 28-week fetus with microcephaly and a small posterior encephalocele. The sloping forehead *(arrow)* is caused by a lack of forebrain development. **C,** Axial sonogram shows high occipital defect *(calipers)* through which a small amount of dysplastic brain protrudes. **D,** Sagittal MR image shows microcephaly and the high occipital defect in the skull *(arrow).*

Coloboma

Coloboma results from incomplete closure of the optic fissure and most often affects the **iris** inferiorly[6] (Fig. 33-14). However, it can affect any structure from the eyelid to the optic nerve or retina. Vision may or may not be affected, depending on the structures affected and the severity of the abnormality. Diagnosis in utero depends on visualization of a focal bulge in the posterior aspect of the globe. In cases where bones cause artifacts in this region and this assessment is crucial, 3-D ultrasound[34] or

MRI[35] can be helpful. Coloboma is a rare diagnosis (0.26:1000)[36] and may be associated with other anomalies and syndromes, such as **CHARGE syndrome** (**c**oloboma, **h**eart defects, choanal **a**tresia, **r**estriction of growth and development, **g**enital and **e**ar anomalies).

Dacryocystocele

Dacryocystoceles result from obstruction of the **nasolacrimal ducts** (Fig. 33-15). These present as cystic masses that may contain low-level internal echoes, located

TABLE 33-1. NORMAL ORBITAL DIAMETERS IN THE FETUS

GESTATIONAL AGE (wk)	Inner Diameters (mm)			Outer Diameters (mm)		
	5th %ile	50th %ile	95th %ile	5th %ile	50th %ile	95th %ile
13	4	7	10	12	16	20
14	5	8	11	14	18	22
15	5	8	11	17	21	25
16	6	9	12	19	23	27
17	7	10	13	21	25	29
18	8	11	14	24	27	31
19	8	11	14	26	30	34
20	9	12	15	28	32	36
21	10	13	16	30	34	38
22	10	13	16	32	36	40
23	11	14	17	33	37	41
24	12	14	17	35	39	43
25	12	15	18	37	41	45
26	13	16	19	39	43	47
27	13	16	19	40	44	48
28	14	17	20	42	46	50
29	14	17	20	43	47	51
30	15	18	21	45	49	52
31	15	18	21	46	50	54
32	16	19	22	47	51	55
33	17	20	23	48	52	56
34	17	20	23	49	53	57
35	18	21	24	50	54	58

From Trout T, Budorick NE, Pretorius DH, McGahan JP. Significance of orbital measurements in the fetus. J Ultrasound Med 1994;13:937-943.
  Table generated from raw data using two separate quadratic regression models:

$$\text{Outer diameter} = -2.17 + 3.36\,(\text{Age}) - 0.03\,(\text{Age}^2)$$

$$R^2 = 0.96,\ p < 0.001$$

$$\text{Inner Diameter} = -4.14 + 0.94\,(\text{Age}) - 0.007\,(\text{Age}^2)$$

$$R^2 = 0.84;\ p < 0.001$$

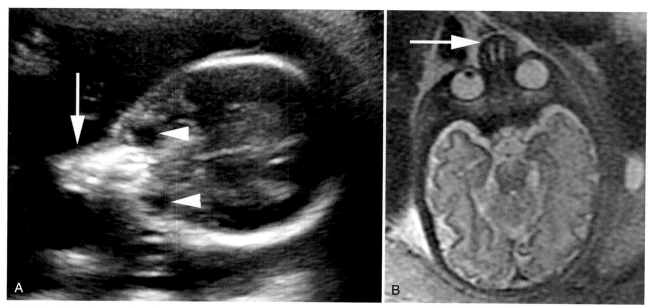

FIGURE 33-9. Hypotelorism. A, Microtia and **hypotelorism.** Axial sonogram shows small orbits *(arrowheads)*, close together in the face, and the protuberant maxilla *(arrow)*. The fetus also had agnathia and low-set ears (see Figs. 33-16, *A,* and 33-25). **B, Hypotelorism** and abnormal nose *(arrow)* at 35 weeks' gestation. Axial MR image of a 35-week fetus shows the relatively small intraorbital distance and an abnormal nose. The fetus was in deep vertex prone position, and the face could not be seen on fetal sonography before MRI. This fetus was diagnosed postnatally with a complex Tessier cleft.

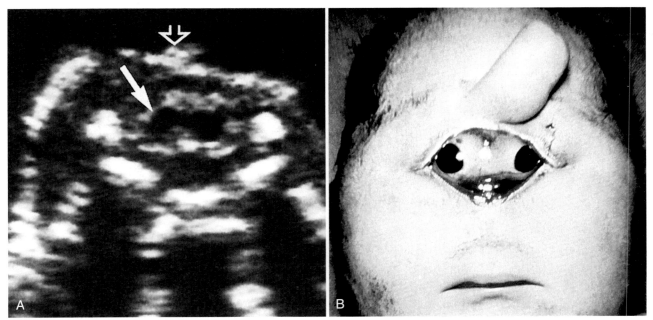

FIGURE 33-10. Cyclops and proboscis at 18 weeks' gestation. A, Transverse scan through the orbit shows fused, dumbbell-shaped globe *(arrow)* and small supraorbital nubbin of tissue, the proboscis *(open arrow).* Only the outer orbital bony margin is present, and the medial bony walls are absent. **B,** Cyclops with fused globes, supraorbital proboscis, and absent nose. *(Courtesy Margot Van Allan, MD, Hospital for Sick Children, Toronto.)*

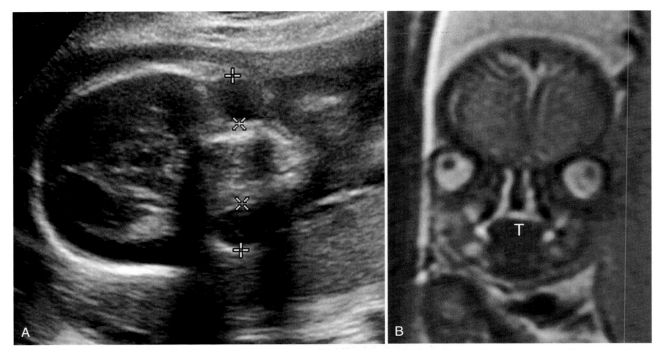

FIGURE 33-11. Hypertelorism in fetus at 25 weeks with bilateral cleft lip and palate. A, Axial sonogram shows hypertelorism *(cursors:* +, outer orbital diameter; *x,* inner orbital diameter). **B,** Coronal MR image shows hypertelorism and bilaterally absent palatal shelves. Note the absent secondary palate above the tongue *(T)* with communication of the amniotic fluid between the oropharynx and nasopharynx.

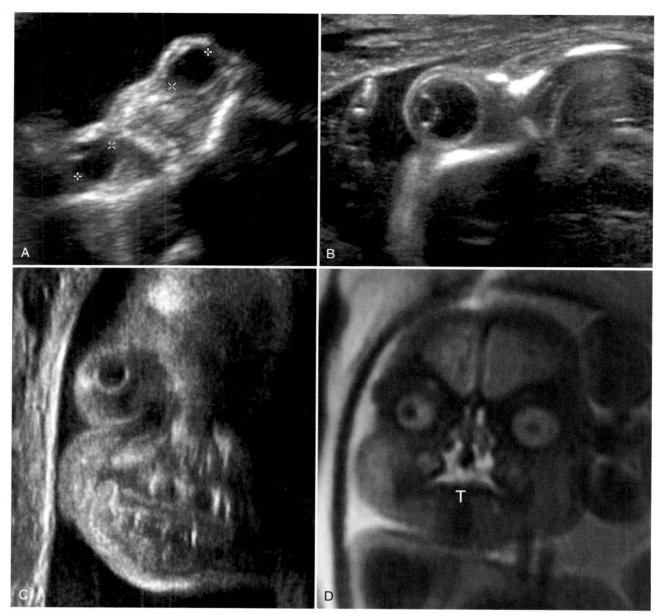

FIGURE 33-12. Hypertelorism with exorbitism in fetus with Pfeiffer syndrome. A, Axial sonogram demonstrates hypertelorism (*cursors: +,* outer orbital diameter; *x,* inner orbital diameter) at 22 weeks' gestation. The outer orbital diameter was consistent with 25 weeks and 3 days (3 weeks greater than age by dates). **B** and **C,** Axial and coronal sonograms show abnormally protuberant globe (exorbitism, *arrow*). **D,** Coronal MR image shows hypertelorism and bilateral cleft palate. Note the communication of the oropharynx with the nasopharynx, caused by defect in the palate above the tongue *(T).*

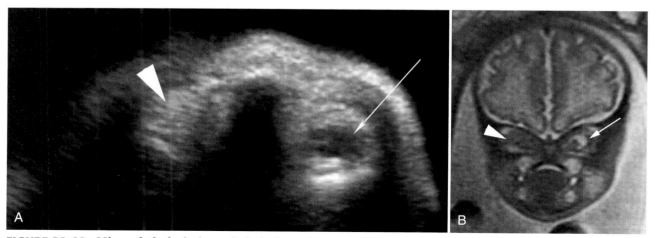

FIGURE 33-13. Microphthalmia/anophthalmia at 34 weeks' gestation. A, Axial sonogram, and **B,** coronal MR image, show right anophthalmia *(arrowhead)* and left microphthalmia *(arrow).*

ASSOCIATIONS WITH MICROPHTHALMOS

Single-gene disorders
  Walker-Warburg syndrome
  Fraser (cryptophthalmos) syndrome
  Meckel Gruber syndrome
Chromosomal abnormalities
  Trisomy 13
  Trisomy 18
Drugs/irradiation
  Ionizing radiation (4-11 weeks)
  Ethanol
  Thalidomide
  Isotretinoin (retinoic acid)
Maternal disease
  Diabetes
  Cytomegalovirus
  Rubella
  Toxoplasmosis
Other
  Encephalocele
  Orbital tumors
  CHARGE syndrome
  VATER association

CHARGE, Coloboma, heart defects, choanal atresia, growth/development restriction, genital/ear anomalies; *VATER*, vertebral defect, imperforate anus, tracheoesophageal fistula, radial and renal dysplasia.

DIFFERENTIAL DIAGNOSIS OF CONGENITAL CATARACTS

Arthrogryposis
Chondrodysplasia punctata
Congenital aniridia
Congenital ichthyosis
Chromosomal abnormalities (21, 18, 13)
C6PD deficiency
Homocystinuria
Hypochondroplasia
Microphthalmia
Infection
  Rubella
  Toxoplasmosis
Syndromes
  Marfan
  Neu-Laxova
  Smith-Lemli-Opitz
  Walker-Warburg
X-linked cataract (Hutterite)

G6PD, Glucose-6-phosphate dehydrogenase.

inferomedial to the orbit in the expected location of the nasolacrimal duct. There is usually no mass effect on the globe, and there is no increased vascular flow in or around these masses. Diagnosis is usually made after 30 weeks' gestation; the nasolacrimal ducts do not complete canalization until the third trimester.[37] The characteristic appearance and location of dacryocystoceles should allow differentiation from other facial masses, such as **teratomas** (often solid or mixed cystic and solid, and may contain calcifications) or **hemangiomas** (solid, echogenic sonographic appearance, with increased vascular flow). The natural history of dacryocystoceles is variable, with some resolving in utero, or postnatally with conservative measures such as massage and application of warm compresses, and others requiring probing or surgical intervention after birth.[38]

Congenital Cataracts

Congenital cataracts may be diagnosed on prenatal sonography, which will show a rounded echogenic mass in the anterior portion of the globe. Causes of congenital cataracts include genetic disorders, infection, syndromes, and microphthalmia.[5] Some cases are inherited by either autosomal dominant or autosomal recessive transmission. This is a rare disorder, with a reported incidence of approximately 3:10,000 births.[39]

EAR ABNORMALITIES

Abnormalities of the ears can be very difficult to diagnose on fetal sonography, but **low-set ears** are associated with multiple syndromes, including **Noonan syndrome** and certain trisomies. Low-set ears are described as the helix joining the cranium at a level below a horizontal plane through the inner canthi of the eyes. Ear anomalies may be more easily detected on 3-D sonography than on 2-D studies[40] (Fig. 33-16).

Microtia, or small ears, is a rare anomaly with an incidence of approximately 1:10,000 live births[41] and is often associated with syndromes and aneuploidy. Of 96 aneuploid fetuses, Yeo et al.[42] reported that 66% had small (<10th percentile) ears on sonography.

Otocephaly is a condition with union of the ears on the front of the neck and is caused by failure of ascent of the auricles during embryologic development. This is generally a fatal anomaly, often associated with agnathia or micrognathia, as well as holoprosencephaly. The most severe form of otocephaly may be associated with absence of the eyes, forebrain, and mouth.

MIDFACE ABNORMALITIES

Hypoplasia

The midface is the area between the upper lip and forehead. Midface hypoplasia can arise from a variety of causes, including syndromes such as **Apert, Crouzon, Treacher Collins,**[43] **Wolf-Hirschhorn,**[44] **Pfeiffer** (see Fig. 33-11), **Turner,** and **trisomy 21**. Midface hypoplasia may also result from facial clefts, craniosynostosis, and

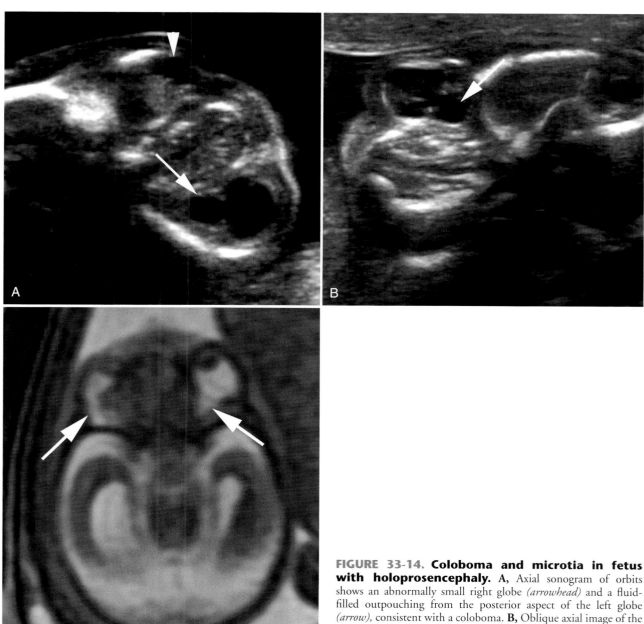

FIGURE 33-14. Coloboma and microtia in fetus with holoprosencephaly. A, Axial sonogram of orbits shows an abnormally small right globe *(arrowhead)* and a fluid-filled outpouching from the posterior aspect of the left globe *(arrow),* consistent with a coloboma. **B,** Oblique axial image of the left globe shows the coloboma. **C,** Axial MR image of the globes demonstrates bilateral colobomas *(arrows)* and right microtia. Note also the brain abnormality with a monoventricle, in the holoprosencephaly spectrum.

skeletal dysplasias. Midface hypoplasia is best demonstrated on sagittal midline views of the face, where one can see abnormal concavity of the midface, between the lower margin of the orbits and the upper jaw (Fig. 33-17).

Absent Nasal Bone

Hypoplastic or absent nasal bone is seen with increased incidence in fetuses with **trisomy 21** and can be evaluated sonographically in the first trimester as part of early risk assessment. The fetal nasal bone is best evaluated in a midsagittal plane at sonography (Fig. 33-18). Some have found that combining data regarding the presence or absence of the fetal nasal bone with nuchal translucency measurements improves the accuracy of detection of trisomy 21 at first-trimester screening.[45] Cicero's initial study on evaluation of the nasal bone in first-trimester examinations found that 73% of fetuses with trisomy 21 had an absent nasal bone.[45] Other studies have reported absent nasal bone in 50% to 67% of fetuses with trisomy 21.[46,47] The absence of a nasal bone at second-trimester sonography, or abnormally short nasal bone measurements in combination with other markers of aneuploidy, increases detection of aneuploidy.[48,49]

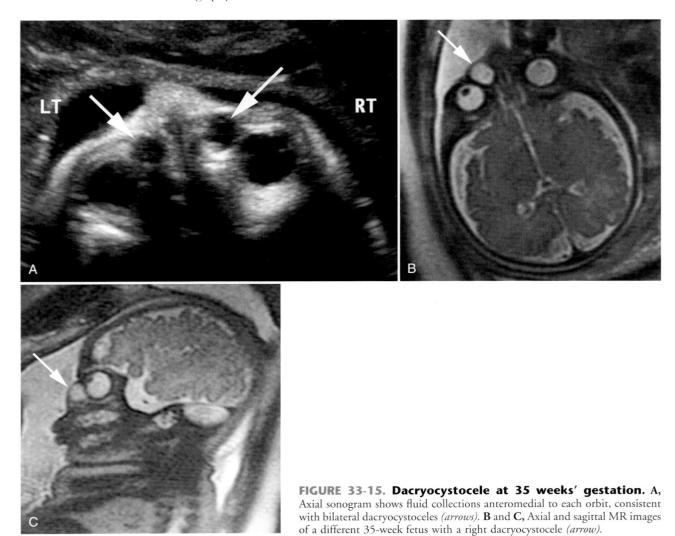

FIGURE 33-15. Dacryocystocele at 35 weeks' gestation. A, Axial sonogram shows fluid collections anteromedial to each orbit, consistent with bilateral dacryocystoceles *(arrows).* **B** and **C,** Axial and sagittal MR images of a different 35-week fetus with a right dacryocystocele *(arrow).*

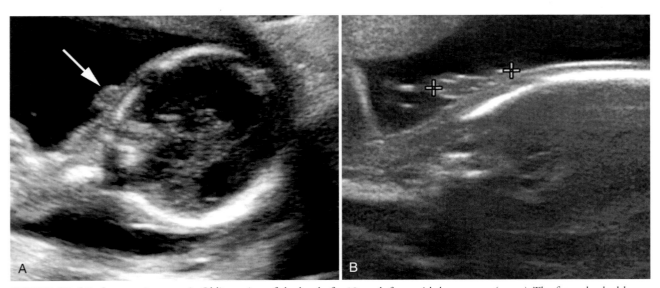

FIGURE 33-16. Low-set ears. A, Oblique view of the head of a 19-week fetus with low-set ear *(arrow).* The fetus also had hypotelorism and agnathia (see Figs. 33-9, *A,* and 33-25). **B,** Low-set ear *(cursors)* in a different fetus, at 20 weeks, who had Pierre-Robin sequence.

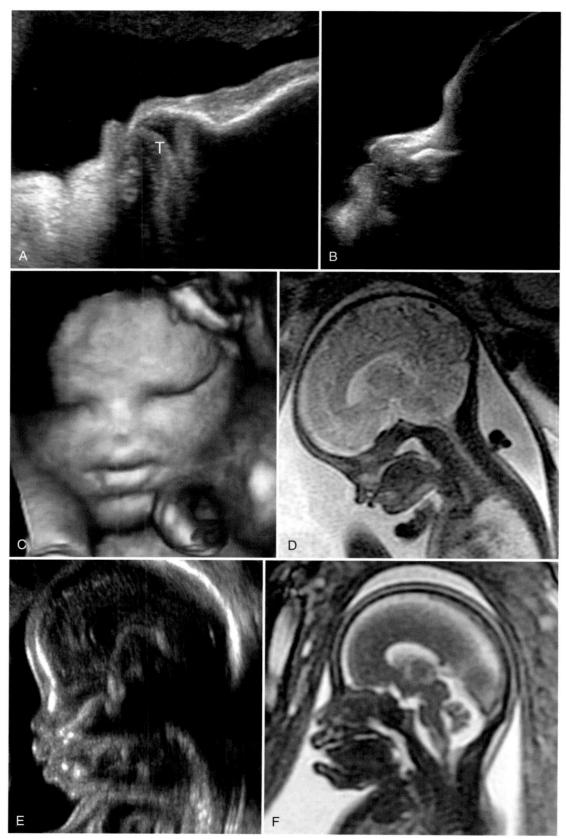

FIGURE 33-17. Midface hypoplasia. A, Midface hypoplasia in association with **cleft lip and palate.** Sagittal view of the face shows midface retrusion in a 34-week fetus with unilateral complete left cleft lip and palate. Note the absent palate above the tongue *(T).* **B, C,** and **D,** Midface hypoplasia in association with **microphthalmia** seen with sagittal ultrasound, 3-D ultrasound, and MRI, respectively. **E** and **F,** Midface hypoplasia in a fetus with **hypertelorism** *(not shown).* **E,** Sagittal sonogram, and **F,** MR image, show an abnormally shaped skull and midface hypoplasia. This is the same fetus as in Fig. 33-12.

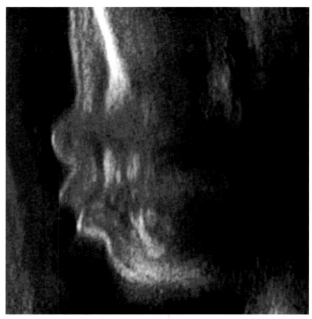

FIGURE 33-18. Absent nasal bone. Profile of third-trimester fetus with absent nasal bone.

It is important to note, however, that accurate sonographic evaluation of the fetal nasal bone can be technically challenging. There are specific guidelines for nasal bone imaging.[50] Studies have shown that even experienced sonographers need to perform at least 80 supervised examinations that conform to specified standards before they are proficient in sonographic nasal bone evaluation.[51]

Cleft Lip and Palate

Worldwide incidence of cleft lip, with or without cleft palate, is approximately 1 in 700 live births,[52] with incidence in Caucasians in approximately 1:1000 live births. The incidence of facial clefting is lower in the African-American population (0.3:1000), higher among Asians (2:1000) and highest in Native Americans (3.6:1000 live births). It is more common in males than females.[53] These abnormalities usually result from failure of fusion of the medial nasal prominences and maxillary prominences. Although facial clefts may occur as an isolated finding, they are present with increased frequency in chromosomal anomalies, including **trisomies 13 and 18,** and in other structural anomalies, especially those involving the heart and central nervous system.[54-56] Reports vary, with aneuploidy rates between 5% and 30% in association with facial clefts.[57-59] Thus, identification of a facial cleft should prompt a detailed and complete evaluation of the fetus for additional anomalies. Some isolated facial clefts are familial, with the recurrence risk dependent on number of affected parents and siblings.[60]

Reported accuracy in the sonographic detection of fetal cleft lip/palate ranges from 16% to 93%.[61-66] Robinson et al.[65] found that sonography performed after

---

DIFFERENTIAL DIAGNOSIS OF CLEFT LIP AND PALATE

Teratogens
  Diphenylhydantoin (phenytoin)
  Valproic acid
  Retinoic acid
  Carbamazepine
  Diazepam
Amniotic band syndrome
Holoprosencephaly
Ectodermal dysplasia
Frontonasal dysplasia
Robert syndrome
Miller syndrome
Trisomies 13, 18, and 21
Triploidy

---

20 weeks' gestation had a significantly higher detection rate for cleft lip than those studies performed before 20 weeks, and they subsequently recommended that fetuses at high risk for cleft lip be evaluated after 20 weeks' gestation. Using state-of-the-art equipment, high-frequency probes, and endovaginal sonography, detection is possible at earlier gestational ages. Some question the efficiency and utility of 3-D sonography in evaluating clefts,[67] but many have found 3-D applications to be extremely helpful.[8,68,69]

Fetal facial clefts should be described as completely as possible, using standard craniofacial terminology and should include accurate description and classification of the cleft in relation to the lip, nostril, alveolus (maxillary tooth bearing arc), and secondary palate (Fig. 33-19). The secondary palate has an anterior, bony segment and a posterior, soft tissue segment. Both cleft lip and cleft palate may be unilateral or bilateral.

Information important to the surgeons for accurate parental counseling, postnatal repair planning, and prognosis includes whether the cleft is unilateral or bilateral and complete or incomplete. A **complete cleft lip** is defined as a cleft that fully divides the lip and extends completely through the base of the ala of the nose and that usually is associated with a cleft of the underlying tooth-bearing alveolus as well. An **incomplete cleft lip** involves a portion of the lip, but at least a band of soft tissue spans the cleft. Incomplete cleft lip does not involve the ipsilateral underlying bony tooth-bearing alveolus (Fig. 33-20).

Associated sonographic signs of a cleft palate include an abnormally high position of the fetal tongue, hypertelorism, deviation of the **vomer** (a triangular bone in the nasal septum forming the posterior and inferior portion of the septum), and micrognathia.[59,70,71] To describe the type of cleft, two embryonic structures are considered: (1) the primary palate, formed by the prolabium, premaxilla, and columella, which includes the lip, nares, and alveolus, and (2) the secondary palate, which begins at the incisive foramen and is formed by a horizontal portion of the maxilla, the horizontal portion of the palatine bones, and the soft palate.

Cleft palate may interfere with fetal swallowing and result in polyhydramnios. Infants with cleft palate have difficulty with feeding, are at increased risk of otitis media, and may have difficulty with hearing and speech.[53]

ASSOCIATED SIGNS OF CLEFT PALATE WITH CLEFT LIP

Axial/Coronal Views
Lips: cleft
Nares: flattened or deformed
Vomer: deviated away from side of cleft; often midline if bilateral cleft lip/palate
Maxilla: interrupted alveolus, wide gap
Orbits: hypertelorism

Sagittal Views
Profile: midface retrusion
Tongue: high position in oropharynx

Unilateral Cleft Lip/Palate

Unilateral clefts occur more often on the left side. In a unilateral cleft lip and palate, there is often an offset between the two sides of the cleft, which are described as the "greater segment" on the side opposite the cleft, and the "lesser segment" on the side of the cleft (Fig. 33-21).

Bilateral Cleft Lip/Palate

Only about 10% of facial clefts are bilateral. In bilateral cleft lip/palate, the midsagittal view will often show an abnormal premaxillary protrusion of soft tissue anterior to and above the normal position of the upper lip (Fig. 33-22). Bilateral cleft lip/palate may be symmetrical or asymmetrical.

Median Cleft Lip/Palate

Median cleft lip is a classic finding in **alobar holoprosencephaly.** In these cases, head size is small for

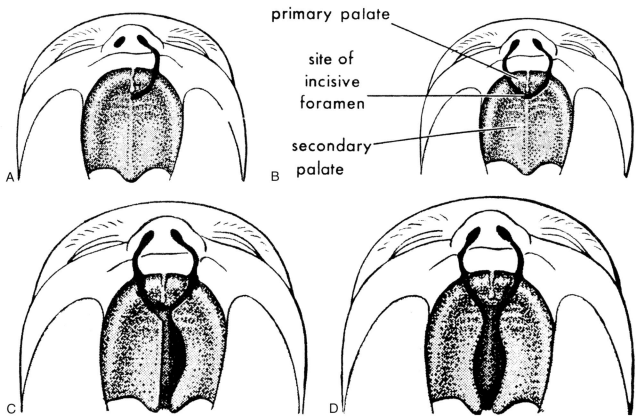

FIGURE 33-19. Patterns of clefting of lip and palate. A, Isolated complete cleft lip/palate. This involves the lip and nose and the primary palate. **B,** Bilateral cleft lip and palate. The medial part of the lip and alveolar ridge, the premaxilla, which usually protrudes anteriorly, can be recognized as a mass below the nose. **C** and **D,** Bilateral cleft lip and palate. The lip clefting extends to involve one or both sides of the secondary hard palate in continuity. *(Modified from Moore KL: Essentials of human embryology. Toronto, 1988, BC Decker.)*

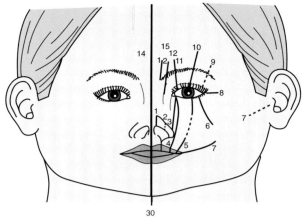

Soft tissue clefts of the face

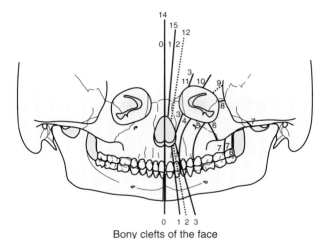

Bony clefts of the face

FIGURE 33-20. Classification of Tessier clefts. These clefts are classified by the relationship of the cleft to the mouth, nose, and eye sockets and are numbered from 1 to 14 with the midline designated as 0. Knowledge of these types of clefts is important for prenatal imaging, so that when unusual clefts are seen, they can be recognized as part of this spectrum. *(Modified from Tessier P. Anatomical classification: facial, cranio-facial and latero-facial clefts. J Maxillofac Surg 1976;4:69-92.)*

menstrual dates and there is hypotelorism.[72] However, median cleft lip and palate can also be seen without holoprosencephaly. In these cases, head size and ocular diameters are normal.[72]

Unusual Facial (Tessier) Clefts

Asymmetrical clefts in unusual locations may be the result of **amniotic band syndrome** or may fall into the **Tessier cleft** category (see Fig. 33-20). Tessier clefts are rare, occurring in between 1 and 5 per 100,000 live births.[73] These clefts are classified by the relationship of the cleft to the mouth, nose, and eye sockets and are numbered from 1 to 14, with the midline designated as 0. Tessier clefts can involve either the soft tissues (e.g., hairline, eyebrows, eyelids, nostrils, lips, ears) or the skeleton.[74]

Isolated Cleft of Secondary Palate

Isolated clefts of the secondary palate are embryologically distinct from cleft lip/palate and are less common, occurring in approximately 1 in 2500 live births.[52] This abnormality is infrequently identified on prenatal sonography because of shadowing from overlying bony structures. Sonographic diagnosis is based on secondary signs, such as abnormal oropharyngeal fluid flow with color Doppler imaging[59] and high position of the tongue.[62,64,75] Cleft soft palate without cleft lip is more strongly associated with syndromes and chromosomal anomalies than cleft palate in concert with cleft lip.[64]

Syndromes associated with clefts of the secondary palate (without cleft lip) include **Goldenhar syndrome, Pierre-Robin sequence, Treacher Collins syndrome, Stickler syndrome,** and **velocardiofacial syndrome**. Three-dimensional sonography is often helpful in assessing the secondary palate, given a favorable fetal position, gestational age, and adequate amniotic fluid.[10-12,76-79] Sagittal fetal MRI is helpful in delineating the normal soft tissues of the palate and in accurately characterizing palatal clefting, even when isolated to the posterior secondary (soft) palate.[70,71,80]

LOWER FACE ABNORMALITIES

Macroglossia and Oral Masses

Macroglossia, an abnormally enlarged tongue, has a variety of etiologies and can, at times, be identified on fetal sonography, visualized as the tongue protruding outside the oral cavity, typically on sagittal or axial views (Fig. 33-23). Etiologies of macroglossia include Beckwith-Wiedemann syndrome, Trisomy 21, and vascular malformations such as lymphatic malformation or hemangioma.[81] If macroglossia is identified, a careful evaluation for the associated findings of **Beckwith-Wiedemann syndrome** and for markers of **trisomy 21** should follow.

CONDITIONS ASSOCIATED WITH MACROGLOSSIA

Beckwith-Wiedemann syndrome
Trisomy 21
Congenital hypothyroidism
Lymphangioma
Hemangioma
Inborn error of metabolism
Isolated autosomal dominant trait
Lingual thyroid
Neurofibroma
Epignathus

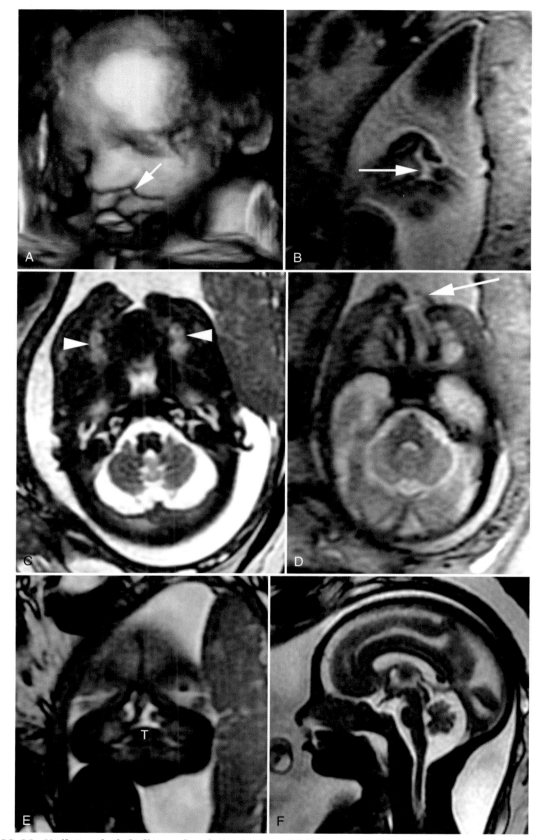

FIGURE 33-21. Unilateral cleft lip and palate. A, Coronal 3-D sonogram of the fetal lip and nose shows a normal right nostril and lip, cleft left lip *(arrow),* and a downward-sloping left nostril at 29 weeks' gestation. **B,** Coronal MR image shows complete left cleft lip, with deformation of left nostril *(arrow).* **C,** Axial MR image shows complete cleft left alveolus and lip *(arrowheads* indicate lateral margins of bony tooth-bearing alveolus), with greater segment on the right and lesser segment on the left. **D,** Axial MR image shows deviation of the tip of the bony nasal septum (vomer) away from the side of the cleft *(arrow).* **E,** Coronal MR image shows an intact right horizontal palatal shelf and absence of the left palatal shelf above the tongue *(T).* Note how a small amount of amniotic fluid in the oral cavity is helpful in making this determination. **F,** Sagittal MR image shows an abnormally high position of the tongue, in keeping with a complete left cleft lip and palate.

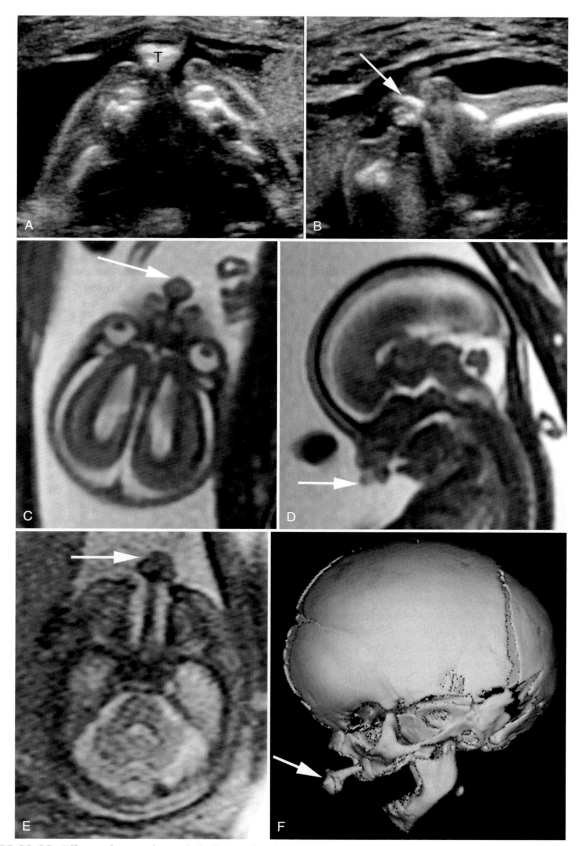

FIGURE 33-22. Bilateral complete cleft lip and palate. A, Axial sonogram of 18-week fetus with bilateral complete cleft lip/palate shows bilateral clefts in the tooth-bearing alveolus of the maxilla, with two tooth buds *(T)* displaced anteriorly in the intermaxillary segment. **B,** Sagittal sonogram shows protrusion of the intermaxillary segment of the maxilla *(arrow)*. **C** and **D,** Coronal and sagittal MR images show bilateral cleft lip and the anteriorly displaced intermaxillary segment of the maxilla *(arrow)*. **E,** In a different fetus at 22 weeks with **Pfeiffer syndrome,** axial MR shows bilateral cleft palate with displaced intermaxillary segment of the maxilla *(arrow)* (see also Fig. 33-12). **F,** Postnatal 3-D CT reconstruction shows coronal craniosynostosis and the marked anterior position of the intermaxillary segment *(arrow)*.

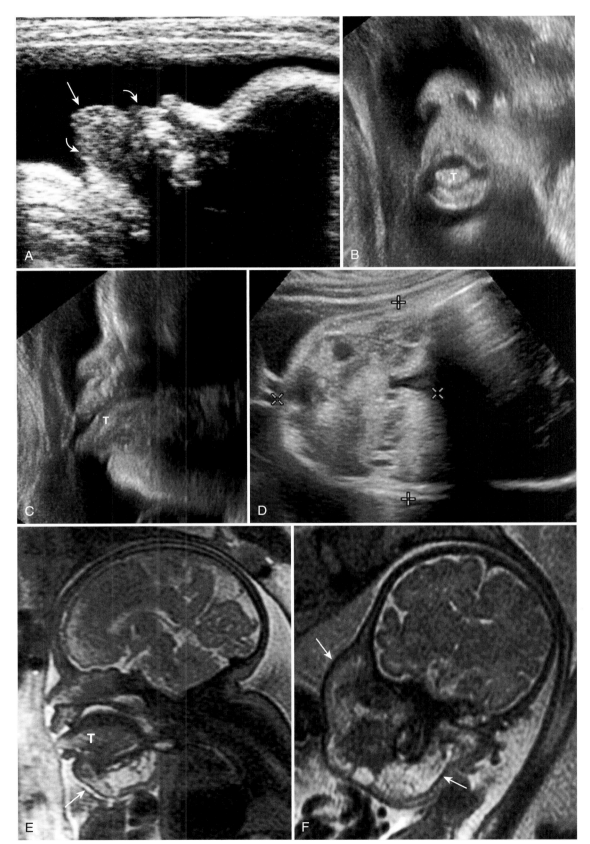

FIGURE 33-23. Macroglossia. A, Macroglossia with **Beckwith-Wiedemann** syndrome at 33 weeks' gestation. Note the enlarged tongue *(arrow)* protruding from the mouth *(curved arrows,* lips). **B** to **F,** Macroglossia in association with **lymphatic malformation** at 35 weeks' gestation. **B** and **C,** Coronal and sagittal sonograms show tongue protrusion *(T)* secondary to a lymphatic malformation involving both sides of the face and infiltrating the base of the tongue. **D,** Coronal sonogram shows the complex facial mass *(cursors).* **E** and **F,** Sagittal and coronal MR images show macroglossia *(T)* and the lymphatic malformation *(arrows)* infiltrating the deep facial structures.

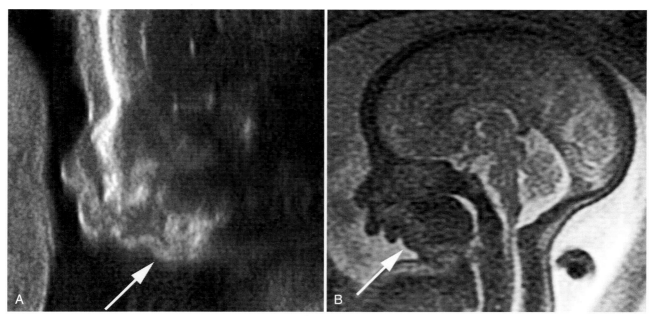

FIGURE 33-24. Micrognathia with Pierre-Robin sequence. A, Sonographic, and **B,** MR, profiles of a 20-week fetus with Pierre-Robin sequence show severe micrognathia/retrognathia *(arrow).* At follow-up at age 5 (not shown), the child is tracheostomy dependent secondary to airway issues.

Micrognathia and Retrognathia

Micrognathia is a small chin, and retrognathia (retrognathism) is a posteriorly displaced chin. These are distinct abnormalities that frequently occur together. **Pierre-Robin sequence** is the term used to describe an abnormally small and often posteriorly displaced lower jaw with associated cleft soft palate (Fig. 33-24). This finding is associated with syndromes (e.g., Stickler, velocardiofacial, Miller-Diecker, Beckwith-Wiedemann, Treacher Collins, Pfeiffer), chromosomal anomalies (typically trisomy 18 or 13), and skeletal dysplasias (e.g., diastrophic, spondyloepiphyseal, congenital, camptomelic). If the abnormality is severe enough to interfere with fetal swallowing in utero, polyhydramnios may result. Micrognathia can lead to substantial feeding difficulties and problems with airway management after birth.

Micrognathia is best seen on midsagittal views of the fetal face and is identified by subjective assessment by the sonologist. Although there have been attempts to standardize fetal jaw measurements[82-84] to identify micrognathia more objectively, there is no consensus on methodology. Three-dimensional sonography offers an additional method for the evaluation of micrognathia, because 2-D data can be manipulated to obtain a true sagittal view of the fetal face, which might otherwise not be possible.[85] Many fetuses with micrognathia have additional abnormalities,[86] so the physician should carefully search for associated anomalies, and fetal karyotyping is recommended.

Agnathia is total or partial absence of the lower jaw and is often associated with holoprosencephaly (Fig. 33-25). **Microstomia** is a small mouth, often associated with agnathia and otocephaly.[5]

SOFT TISSUE TUMORS

Soft tissue or bony tumors can cause alterations in head size or shape. A relatively common soft tissue lesion involving the face is a **hemangioma** (Fig. 33-26). Vascular anomalies such as hemangiomas are the most common tumors of infancy, and most are medically insignificant. On fetal sonography, hemangiomas often present as echogenic, predominantly solid masses. These masses may contain detectable vascular channels with flow on Doppler ultrasound evaluation. Hemangiomas often increase in size during fetal life and can be infiltrative, affecting large areas. Classically, hemangiomas do not infiltrate bony structures. Hemangiomas can occur in any location and can involve the fetal face or neck. The adjacent skull may be thinner and may be associated with brain anomalies as in **Sturge-Weber syndrome**.[87-90]

NECK ABNORMALITIES

Nuchal Translucency and Thickening

The **nuchal translucency** (NT) is the fluid collection that forms posterior to the fetal neck during early development. Studies have shown that thickened-NT measurements in the first trimester are associated with

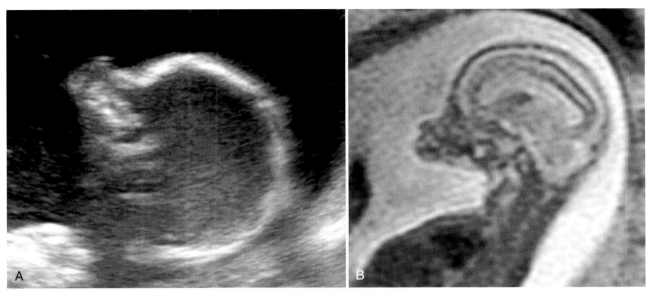

FIGURE 33-25. Agnathia microstomia. A, Sagittal sonogram, and **B,** MR image, show the absent mandible. This is the same fetus as in Figs. 33-9, *A,* and 33-16, *A.*

fetal aneuploidy, cardiac defects, other major malformations, and adverse pregnancy outcome.[91-95] In the second trimester, the **nuchal fold thickness** is measured in the suboccipital bregmatic plane. A measurement of 6 mm or greater from 15 to 22 weeks is associated with an increased risk of trisomy 21.[96,97] The measurement is taken in the midline from outer edge of the occipital bone to the outer edge of the skin (see Chapter 31).

Lymphatic Malformation (Cystic Hygroma)

Lymphatic malformation, known historically as cystic hygroma, is a septated fluid collection behind the fetal neck, thought to result from early maldevelopment of the lymphatic system. This abnormality is highly associated with **Turner syndrome** (XO), other chromosomal anomalies, and cardiac structural abnormalities. When associated with hydrops, fetal mortality is very high. As with an increased NT, if a lymphatic malformation is diagnosed and chromosomes are found to be normal, the fetus should still be carefully evaluated for cardiac abnormalities.

Lymphatic malformations can occur elsewhere in the head and neck and may be microcystic or macrocystic. They are presumed to result from obstructed lymphatic sacs that do not communicate with main lymphatic channels. Although benign, morbidity is associated with mass effect on the fetal airway when such masses arise in the face and neck (Fig. 33-27). In this setting, fetal MRI is often useful for evaluation of the fetal airway and for delivery planning. Fluid-filled lymphatic malformations, even when large, are much more malleable than solid

teratomas of the head and neck and are less likely to compromise the airway. When these malformations involve the tongue, cystic hygromas may interfere with swallowing and feeding after birth.

Cervical Teratoma

Teratoma is the most common tumor in neonates, with the majority located at the sacrum and coccyx. Approximately 5% of teratomas arise in the neck or oropharynx. Cervical teratomas occur equally in males and females.[98] Sonographically, teratomas are usually complex masses composed of both cystic and solid elements and are often associated with regions of calcification. There is usually vascular flow within the solid portions of the mass. In the neck, they are usually anterolateral in location and can become quite large, often involving the thyroid gland. When they arise in the neck, teratomas may impinge on the airway, interfere with fetal swallowing, and result in polyhydramnios. Evaluation of the fetal airway is particularly important to delivery planning and is often best accomplished with fetal MRI (Fig. 33-28).

When teratomas arise in the neck, there can be hyperextension of the fetal neck, best seen in sagittal views. Teratomas of the oropharynx (**epignathus**) often protrude from the mouth. Although most teratomas are histologically benign, prognosis depends on the degree of mass effect on the trachea and the ability to secure the infant's airway at delivery. If there is substantial mass effect on the airway, the **ex utero intrapartum treatment** (EXIT) **procedure** may be necessary. This complex procedure requires a team of specialists for the mother and fetus and involves cesarean delivery, with

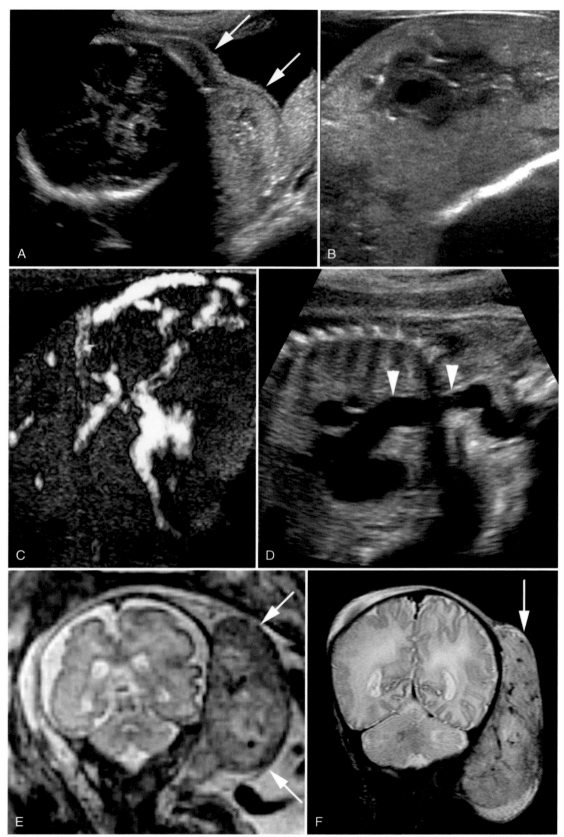

FIGURE 33-26. Hemangioma at 30 weeks' gestation. A, Axial sonogram shows a large, lateral and posterior soft tissue scalp mass *(arrows)*. **B,** High-frequency coned-down view illustrates the heterogeneous echogenicity of the mass. **C,** Power Doppler view demonstrates the vascularity of the mass. **D,** Oblique sonogram of the fetal chest and neck show a greatly enlarged superior vena cava *(arrowheads)*. The heart was also enlarged, and the fetus was in heart failure from the volume of blood circulating through the scalp mass. **E,** Coronal prenatal, and **F,** postnatal, MR images show the left scalp mass *(arrows)*.

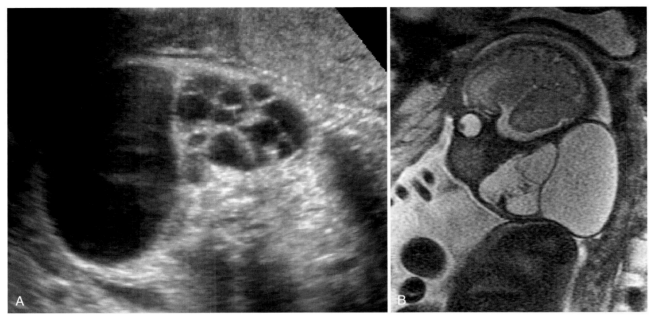

FIGURE 33-27. Cervical lymphatic malformation at 29 weeks' gestation (cystic hygroma). A, Axial sonogram, and **B,** sagittal MR image, of a 29-week fetus with a septated cystic mass in the neck, consistent with a lymphatic malformation.

preservation of the maternal-fetal circulation through the placenta until the neonatal airway can be secured.[99-103]

Thyromegaly and Goiter

Fetal goiter is rare (1 : 30,000-50,000 live births)[104] and most often related to maternal thyroid disease, such as **Graves' disease** or **Hashimoto's thyroiditis,** with antibodies that cross the placenta and lead to fetal thyroid dysfunction. Maternal use of **thyroid blocking agents** (e.g., propylthiouracil) may also result in fetal goiter. Primary fetal thyroid dysfunction may also cause goiter.

Fetal goiter presents as a midline homogeneous solid mass in the anterior neck surrounding the trachea (Fig. 33-29). There may be increased blood flow to the goiter. When large, fetal goiters cause hyperextension of the neck, leading to interference with fetal swallowing and resultant polyhydramnios. Neck hyperextension can lead to fetal malpresentation and can cause difficulties at delivery. Cordocentesis may be necessary to determine if there is fetal hypothyroidism or hyperthyroidism. In the setting of fetal **hypothyroidism,** treatment with intra-amniotic thyroid hormone will often lead to a decrease in size of the fetal goiter.[105] Following treatment with intrauterine thyroxine, fetal goiter may decrease in size,

and hyperextension of the fetal neck may resolve. In cases of fetal **hyperthyroidism,** it is important to evaluate for fetal tachycardia and high-output cardiac failure.

CONCLUSION

Prenatal sonographic evaluation of the fetal face and neck offers an opportunity to identify many abnormalities. These observations are often essential to prenatal counseling and prognosis because of the association of many of these abnormalities with syndromes and chromosomal anomalies. Appropriate diagnosis of abnormalities allows for planning of the appropriate mode of delivery and therapy when the fetal airway is potentially compromised.

Acknowledgments

We would like to acknowledge with gratitude the assistance of librarians Alison Clapp and Miriam Geller and the administrative assistance of Susan Ivey, Department of Radiology, at Children's Hospital Boston. Special thanks also to Ants Toi, MD, for the discussion on craniosynostosis.

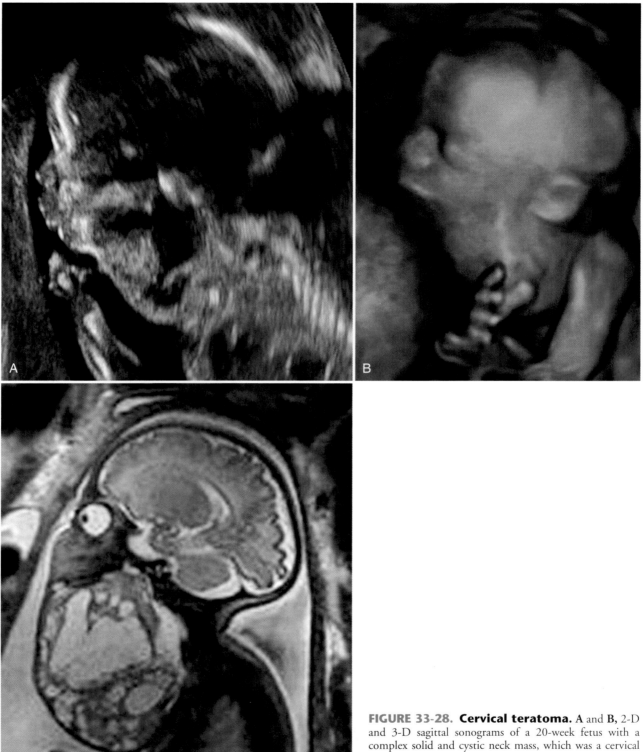

FIGURE 33-28. Cervical teratoma. A and B, 2-D and 3-D sagittal sonograms of a 20-week fetus with a complex solid and cystic neck mass, which was a cervical teratoma. **C,** Sagittal MR image of same fetus at 34 weeks' gestation.

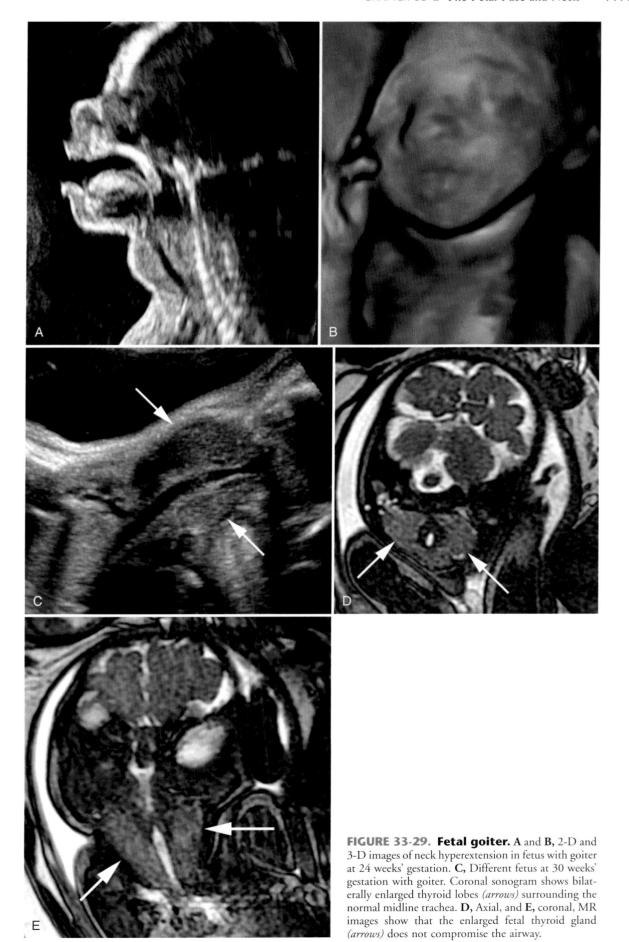

FIGURE 33-29. Fetal goiter. A and **B,** 2-D and 3-D images of neck hyperextension in fetus with goiter at 24 weeks' gestation. **C,** Different fetus at 30 weeks' gestation with goiter. Coronal sonogram shows bilaterally enlarged thyroid lobes *(arrows)* surrounding the normal midline trachea. **D,** Axial, and **E,** coronal, MR images show that the enlarged fetal thyroid gland *(arrows)* does not compromise the airway.

References

1. American Institute of Ultrasound in Medicine. AIUM practice guidelines for the performance of obstetric ultrasound examinations, 2007.

Embryology and Development

2. Moore KL, Persaud T. The developing human: clinically oriented embryology. Philadelphia: Saunders; 2002.
3. Van de Water TR, Staecker H. Otolaryngology: basic science and clinical review. Stuttgart: Thieme; 2006.
4. Brookes M, Zietman A. Clinical embryology: a color atlas and text. Boca Raton, Fla: CRC Press; 2008.
5. Nyberg DA, McGahan JP, Pretorius DH, Pilu G. Diagnostic imaging of fetal anomalies. Philadelphia: Lippincott–Williams & Williams; 2002.
6. Forrester JV, Dick AD, McMenamin PG, Lee WR. The eye: basic sciences in practice. St Louis: Elsevier Health Sciences; 2002.
7. Haak MC, Bartelings MM, Jackson DG, et al. Increased nuchal translucency is associated with jugular lymphatic distension. Hum Reprod 2002;17:1086-1092.

Sonography of the Normal Fetal Face

8. Kurjak A, Azumendi G, Andonotopo W, et al. Three- and four-dimensional ultrasonography for the structural and functional evaluation of the fetal face. Am J Obstet Gynecol 2007;196:16-28.
9. Johnson DD, Pretorius DH, Budorick NE, et al. Fetal lip and primary palate: three-dimensional versus two-dimensional ultrasound. Radiology 2000;217:236-239.
10. Campbell S, Lees C, Moscoso G, Hall P. Ultrasound antenatal diagnosis of cleft palate by a new technique: the 3D "reverse face" view. Ultrasound Obstet Gynecol 2005;25:12-18.
11. Chen ML, Chang CH, Yu CH, et al. Prenatal diagnosis of cleft palate by three-dimensional ultrasound. Ultrasound Med Biol 2001;27:1017-1023.
12. Lee W, Kirk JS, Shaheen KW, et al. Fetal cleft lip and palate detection by three-dimensional ultrasonography. Ultrasound Obstet Gynecol 2000;16:314-320.

Abnormalities of the Head

13. Chervenak FA, Jeanty P, Cantraine F, et al. The diagnosis of fetal microcephaly. Am J Obstet Gynecol 1984;149:512-517.
14. Thomas M. The lemon sign. Radiology 2003;228:206-207.
15. Nyberg DA, Mack LA, Hirsch J, Mahony BS. Abnormalities of fetal cranial contour in sonographic detection of spina bifida: evaluation of the "lemon" sign. Radiology 1988;167:387-392.
16. Nicolaides K, Salvesen D, Snijders R, Gosden C. Strawberry-shaped skull in fetal trisomy 18. Fetal Diagn Ther 1992;7:132-137.
17. Slater BJ, Lenton KA, Kwan MD, et al. Cranial sutures: a brief review. Plast Reconstr Surg 2008;121:170e-178e.
18. Hajihosseini MK. Fibroblast growth factor signaling in cranial suture development and pathogenesis. Front Oral Biol 2008;12:160-177.
19. Rawlins JT, Opperman LA. TGF-beta regulation of suture morphogenesis and growth. Front Oral Biol 2008;12:178-196.
20. Hukki J, Saarinen P, Kangasniemi M. Single suture craniosynostosis: diagnosis and imaging. Front Oral Biol 2008;12:79-90.
21. Delahaye S, Bernard JP, Renier D, Ville Y. Prenatal ultrasound diagnosis of fetal craniosynostosis. Ultrasound Obstet Gynecol 2003;21:347-353.
22. Flores-Sarnat L. New insights into craniosynostosis. Semin Pediatr Neurol 2002;9:274-291.
23. Gorincour G, Rypens F, Grignon A, et al. Prenatal diagnosis of cloverleaf skull: watch the hands! Fetal Diagn Ther 2005;20:296-300.
24. Dover MS. Abnormal skull shape: clinical management. Pediatr Radiol 2008;38(Suppl 3):484-487.
25. Renier D, Lajeunie E, Arnaud E, Marchac D. Management of craniosynostoses. Child Nerv Syst 2000;16:645-658.
26. Brunelle F, Baraton J, Renier D. Intracranial venous anomalies associated with atretic cephalocoeles. Pediatr Radiol 2000;30:743-747.

Orbit Abnormalities

27. Robinson AJ, Blaser S, Toi A, et al. MRI of the fetal eyes: morphologic and biometric assessment for abnormal development with ultrasonographic and clinicopathologic correlation. Pediatr Radiol 2008;38:971-981.
28. Trout T, Budorick NE, Pretorius DH, McGahan JP. Significance of orbital measurements in the fetus. J Ultrasound Med 1994;13:937-943.
29. Tan ST, Mulliken JB. Hypertelorism: nosologic analysis of 90 patients. Plast Reconstr Surg 1997;99:317-327.
30. Bianchi DW, Crombleholme TM, D'Alton ME. Fetology: diagnosis and management of the fetal patient. New York: McGraw-Hill; 2000.
31. Dilmen G, Koktener A, Turhan NO, Tez S. Growth of the fetal lens and orbit. Int J Gynaecol Obstet 2002;76:267-271.
32. Verma AS, Fitzpatrick DR. Anophthalmia and microphthalmia. Orphanet J Rare Dis 2007;2:47.
33. Warburg M. Classification of microphthalmos and coloboma. J Med Genet 1993;30:664-669.
34. Bault JP, Quarello E. Retinal coloboma: prenatal diagnosis using a new technique, the "virtual fetal eyeground." Ultrasound Obstet Gynecol 2009;33:495-496.
35. Righini A, Avagliano L, Doneda C, et al. Prenatal magnetic resonance imaging of optic nerve head coloboma. Prenat Diagn 2008;28:242-246.
36. Bateman JB. Microphthalmos. Int Ophthalmol Clin 1984;24:87-107.
37. Cohen AJ, Mercandetti M, Brazzo BG. The lacrimal system. New York: Springer; 2006.
38. Wong RK, VanderVeen DK. Presentation and management of congenital dacryocystocele. Pediatrics 2008;122:e1108-e1112.
39. Rahi JS, Dezateux C. Measuring and interpreting the incidence of congenital ocular anomalies: lessons from a national study of congenital cataract in the UK. Invest Ophthalmol Vis Sci 2001;42:1444-1448.

Ear Abnormalities

40. Shih JC, Shyu MK, Lee CN, et al. Antenatal depiction of the fetal ear with three-dimensional ultrasonography. Obstet Gynecol 1998;91:500-505.
41. Eavey RD. Microtia and significant auricular malformation: ninety-two pediatric patients. Arch Otolaryngol Head Neck Surg 1995;121:57-62.
42. Yeo L, Guzman ER, Ananth CV, et al. Prenatal detection of fetal aneuploidy by sonographic ear length. J Ultrasound Med 2003;22:565-576.

Midface Abnormalities

43. Lowe LH, Booth TN, Joglar JM, Rollins NK. Midface anomalies in children. Radiographics 2000;20:907-922; quiz 1106-1107, 1112.
44. Dietze I, Fritz B, Huhle D, et al. Clinical, cytogenetic and molecular investigation in a fetus with Wolf-Hirschhorn syndrome with paternally derived 4p deletion: case report and review of the literature. Fetal Diagn Ther 2004;19:251-260.
45. Cicero S, Curcio P, Papageorghiou A, et al. Absence of nasal bone in fetuses with trisomy 21 at 11-14 weeks of gestation: an observational study. Lancet 2001;358:1665-1667.
46. Orlandi F, Bilardo CM, Campogrande M, et al. Measurement of nasal bone length at 11-14 weeks of pregnancy and its potential role in Down syndrome risk assessment. Ultrasound Obstet Gynecol 2003;22:36-39.
47. Otano L, Aiello H, Igarzabal L, et al. Association between first trimester absence of fetal nasal bone on ultrasound and Down syndrome. Prenat Diagn 2002;22:930-932.
48. Vintzileos A, Walters C, Yeo L. Absent nasal bone in the prenatal detection of fetuses with trisomy 21 in a high-risk population. Obstet Gynecol 2003;101:905-908.
49. Cusick W, Provenzano J, Sullivan CA, et al. Fetal nasal bone length in euploid and aneuploid fetuses between 11 and 20 weeks' gestation: a prospective study. J Ultrasound Med 2004;23:1327-1333.
50. Rosen T, D'Alton ME, Platt LD, Wapner R. First-trimester ultrasound assessment of the nasal bone to screen for aneuploidy. Obstet Gynecol 2007;110:399-404.
51. Cicero S, Dezerega V, Andrade E, et al. Learning curve for sonographic examination of the fetal nasal bone at 11-14 weeks. Ultrasound Obstet Gynecol 2003;22:135-137.
52. Sadler T. Langman's medical embryology. Philadelphia: Lippincott–Williams & Wilkins; 2000.

53. Kirschner RE, LaRossa D. Cleft lip and palate. Otolaryngol Clin North Am 2000;33:1191-1215, v-vi.

54. Berge SJ, Plath H, van de Vondel PT, et al. Fetal cleft lip and palate: sonographic diagnosis, chromosomal abnormalities, associated anomalies and postnatal outcome in 70 fetuses. Ultrasound Obstet Gynecol 2001;18:422-431.

55. Chmait R, Pretorius D, Moore T, et al. Prenatal detection of associated anomalies in fetuses diagnosed with cleft lip with or without cleft palate in utero. Ultrasound Obstet Gynecol 2006;27:173-176.

56. Calzolari E, Pierini A, Astolfi G, et al. Associated anomalies in multi-malformed infants with cleft lip and palate: an epidemiologic study of nearly 6 million births in 23 EuroCat registries. Am J Med Genet A 2007;143:528-537.

57. Nyberg DA, Sickler GK, Hegge FN, et al. Fetal cleft lip with and without cleft palate: ultrasound classification and correlation with outcome. Radiology 1995;195:677-684.

58. Walker SJ, Ball RH, Babcook CJ, Feldkamp MM. Prevalence of aneuploidy and additional anatomic abnormalities in fetuses and neonates with cleft lip with or without cleft palate: a population-based study in Utah. J Ultrasound Med 2001;20:1175-1180; quiz 1181-1182.

59. Perrotin F, de Poncheville LM, Marret H, et al. Chromosomal defects and associated malformations in fetal cleft lip with or without cleft palate. Eur J Obstet Gynecol Reprod Biol 2001;99:19-24.

60. Benacerraf BR. Ultrasound of fetal syndromes. St Louis: Elsevier Health Sciences; 2007.

61. Stoll C, Clementi M. Prenatal diagnosis of dysmorphic syndromes by routine fetal ultrasound examination across Europe. Ultrasound Obstet Gynecol 2003;21:543-551.

62. Shaikh D, Mercer NS, Sohan K, et al. Prenatal diagnosis of cleft lip and palate. Br J Plast Surg 2001;54:288-289.

63. Cash C, Set P, Coleman N. The accuracy of antenatal ultrasound in the detection of facial clefts in a low-risk screening population. Ultrasound Obstet Gynecol 2001;18:432-436.

64. Clementi M, Tenconi R, Bianchi F, Stoll C. Evaluation of prenatal diagnosis of cleft lip with or without cleft palate and cleft palate by ultrasound: experience from 20 European registries. EuroScan study group. Prenat Diagn 2000;20:870-875.

65. Robinson JN, McElrath TF, Benson CB, et al. Prenatal ultrasonography and the diagnosis of fetal cleft lip. J Ultrasound Med 2001; 20:1165-1170; quiz 1172-1173.

66. Hanikeri M, Savundra J, Gillett D, et al. Antenatal transabdominal ultrasound detection of cleft lip and palate in Western Australia from 1996 to 2003. Cleft Palate Craniofac J 2006;43:61-66.

67. Ghi T, Perolo A, Banzi C, et al. Two-dimensional ultrasound is accurate in the diagnosis of fetal craniofacial malformation. Ultrasound Obstet Gynecol 2002;19:543-551.

68. Wang LM, Leung KY, Tang M. Prenatal evaluation of facial clefts by three-dimensional extended imaging. Prenat Diagn 2007;27: 722-729.

69. McGahan MC, Ramos GA, Landry C, et al. Multislice display of the fetal face using 3-dimensional ultrasonography. J Ultrasound Med 2008;27:1573-1581.

70. Ghi T, Tani G, Savelli L, et al. Prenatal imaging of facial clefts by magnetic resonance imaging with emphasis on the posterior palate. Prenat Diagn 2003;23:970-975.

71. Stroustrup Smith A, Estroff JA, Barnewolt CE, et al. Prenatal diagnosis of cleft lip and cleft palate using MRI. AJR Am J Roentgenol 2004;183:229-235.

72. Cohen Jr MM. Holoprosencephaly: clinical, anatomic, and molecular dimensions. Birth Defects Res A Clin Mol Teratol 2006;76: 658-673.

73. Longaker MT, Lipshutz GS, Kawamoto Jr HK. Reconstruction of Tessier no. 4 clefts revisited. Plast Reconstr Surg 1997;99:1501-1507.

74. Tessier P. Anatomical classification: facial, cranio-facial and latero-facial clefts. J Maxillofac Surg 1976;4:69-92.

75. Benacerraf BR, Sadow PM, Barnewolt CE, et al. Cleft of the secondary palate without cleft lip diagnosed with three-dimensional ultrasound and magnetic resonance imaging in a fetus with Fryns' syndrome. Ultrasound Obstet Gynecol 2006;27:566-570.

76. Pilu G, Segata M. A novel technique for visualization of the normal and cleft fetal secondary palate: angled insonation and three-dimensional ultrasound. Ultrasound Obstet Gynecol 2007;29: 166-169.

77. Faure JM, Baumler M, Boulot P, et al. Prenatal assessment of the normal fetal soft palate by three-dimensional ultrasound examination: is there an objective technique? Ultrasound Obstet Gynecol 2008;31:652-656.

78. Faure JM, Captier G, Baumler M, Boulot P. Sonographic assessment of normal fetal palate using three-dimensional imaging: a new technique. Ultrasound Obstet Gynecol 2007;29:159-165.

79. Wong HS, Tait J, Pringle KC. Viewing of the soft and the hard palate on routine 3-D ultrasound sweep of the fetal face: a feasibility study. Fetal Diagn Ther 2008;24:146-154.

80. Levine D, Cavazos C, Kazan-Tannus JF, et al. Evaluation of real-time single-shot fast spin-echo MRI for visualization of the fetal midline corpus callosum and secondary palate. AJR Am J Roentgenol 2006;187:1505-1511.

Lower Face Abnormalities

81. Neville B, Damm D, Allen C, Bouquot J. Oral and maxillofacial pathology. St Louis: Elsevier Health Sciences; 2008.

82. Otto C, Platt LD. The fetal mandible measurement: an objective determination of fetal jaw size. Ultrasound Obstet Gynecol 1991; 1:12-17.

83. Chitty LS, Campbell S, Altman DG. Measurement of the fetal mandible: feasibility and construction of a centile chart. Prenat Diagn 1993;13:749-756.

84. Paladini D, Morra T, Teodoro A, et al. Objective diagnosis of micrognathia in the fetus: the jaw index. Obstet Gynecol 1999;93: 382-386.

85. Lee W, McNie B, Chaiworapongsa T, et al. Three-dimensional ultrasonographic presentation of micrognathia. J Ultrasound Med 2002;21:775-781.

86. Vettraino IM, Lee W, Bronsteen RA, et al. Clinical outcome of fetuses with sonographic diagnosis of isolated micrognathia. Obstet Gynecol 2003;102:801-805.

Soft Tissue Tumors

87. Mulliken JB, Glowacki J. Hemangiomas and vascular malformations in infants and children: a classification based on endothelial characteristics. Plast Reconstr Surg 1982;69:412-422.

88. Enjolras O, Mulliken JB. Vascular tumors and vascular malformations (new issues). Adv Dermatol 1997;13:375-423.

89. Mulliken JB, Anupindi S, Ezekowitz RA, Mihm Jr MC. Case records of the Massachusetts General Hospital. Weekly clinicopathological exercises. Case 13-2004. A newborn girl with a large cutaneous lesion, thrombocytopenia, and anemia. N Engl J Med 2004; 350:1764-1775.

90. Legiehn GM, Heran MK. Venous malformations: classification, development, diagnosis, and interventional radiologic management. Radiol Clin North Am 2008;46:545-597, vi.

Neck Abnormalities

91. Hyett J, Perdu M, Sharland G, et al. Using fetal nuchal translucency to screen for major congenital cardiac defects at 10-14 weeks of gestation: population based cohort study. BMJ 1999;318:81-85.

92. Souka AP, Krampl E, Bakalis S, et al. Outcome of pregnancy in chromosomally normal fetuses with increased nuchal translucency in the first trimester. Ultrasound Obstet Gynecol 2001;18:9-17.

93. Michailidis GD, Economides DL. Nuchal translucency measurement and pregnancy outcome in karyotypically normal fetuses. Ultrasound Obstet Gynecol 2001;17:102-105.

94. Makrydimas G, Sotiriadis A, Ioannidis JP. Screening performance of first-trimester nuchal translucency for major cardiac defects: a meta-analysis. Am J Obstet Gynecol 2003;189:1330-1335.

95. Tanriverdi HA, Ertan AK, Hendrik HJ, et al. Outcome of cystic hygroma in fetuses with normal karyotypes depends on associated findings. Eur J Obstet Gynecol Reprod Biol 2005;118:40-46.

96. Benacerraf BR, Frigoletto Jr FD. Soft tissue nuchal fold in the second-trimester fetus: standards for normal measurements compared with those in Down syndrome. Am J Obstet Gynecol 1987;157: 1146-1149.

97. Benacerraf BR, Gelman R, Frigoletto Jr FD. Sonographic identification of second-trimester fetuses with Down's syndrome. N Engl J Med 1987;317:1371-1376.

98. Woodward PJ, Sohaey R, Kennedy A, Koeller KK. From the archives of the AFIP: a comprehensive review of fetal tumors with pathologic correlation. Radiographics 2005;25:215-242.

99. Hirose S, Farmer DL, Lee H, et al. The ex utero intrapartum treatment procedure: looking back at the EXIT. J Pediatr Surg 2004; 39:375-380, discussion.

100. Otteson TD, Hackam DJ, Mandell DL. The ex utero intrapartum treatment (EXIT) procedure: new challenges. Arch Otolaryngol Head Neck Surg 2006;132:686-689.

101. Bouchard S, Johnson MP, Flake AW, et al. The EXIT procedure: experience and outcome in 31 cases. J Pediatr Surg 2002;37:418-426.

102. Wagner W, Harrison MR. Fetal operations in the head and neck area: current state. Head Neck 2002;24:482-490.

103. Leva E, Pansini L, Fava G, et al. The role of the surgeon in the case of a giant neck mass in the EXIT procedure. J Pediatr Surg 2005;40:748-750.

104. Fisher DA, Klein AH. Thyroid development and disorders of thyroid function in the newborn. N Engl J Med 1981;304:702-712.

105. Morine M, Takeda T, Minekawa R, et al. Antenatal diagnosis and treatment of a case of fetal goitrous hypothyroidism associated with high-output cardiac failure. Ultrasound Obstet Gynecol 2002;19:506-509.

CHAPTER 34

The Fetal Brain

Ants Toi and Deborah Levine

Chapter Outline

*A*nomalies of the central nervous system (CNS) are the most common cause of referral for prenatal diagnosis and result in great anxiety for parents. CNS anomalies occur with a frequency of about 1.4 to 1.6 per 1000 live births but are seen in about 3% to 6% of stillbirths.[1] The increased use of maternal serum alpha-fetoprotein (MS-AFP) screening has resulted in increased numbers of pregnancies being referred for evaluation of the CNS and suspected anomalies. Fortunately, protocol-based ultrasound carefully performed by a knowledgeable and experienced examiner following established guidelines is very sensitive in evaluating the CNS.[2-4] Routine scanning is currently recommended at 18 to 20 weeks of gestation. Although many cerebral anomalies are detectable in the first semester and early in the second trimester, others develop or only become apparent later in pregnancy.[5]

Magnetic resonance imaging (MRI) is increasingly used to supplement ultrasound evaluation. Currently, in vivo MRI has less spatial resolution but higher contrast resolution than ultrasound. MRI is multiplanar and can evaluate many tissue properties beyond morphology using techniques such as diffusion weighted imaging (DWI), diffusion tensor imaging, and magnetic resonance spectroscopy (MRS).[6-8] This provides new insights into ischemia, tumor characteristics, bleeding, and brain metabolism and allows unprecedented clarification of suspected disorders. There is debate regarding the role of ultrasound versus MRI in evaluating the fetal CNS.[9] We believe that ultrasound will continue to be the initial screening modality and that MRI will increasingly be used to clarify findings. The important issues for the examiner are familiarity with the strengths and limitations of these imaging modalities, expertise in their use, and collaboration with other specialties.[10,11]

DEVELOPMENTAL ANATOMY

Embryology

Knowledge of fetal gestational age is particularly important when evaluating anatomy in early pregnancy. In this chapter we use **menstrual age** and **gestational age** to mean "age from last menses," as typically used clinically and with ultrasound studies. We convert published ages to menstrual age by adding 2 weeks to the conceptual age.

Central nervous system development starts at about the fifth menstrual week, when cells destined to form the notochord infiltrate into the embryonic disc. This notochord tissue induces overlying embryonic tissue to thicken and ultimately fold over and fuse as the neural tube. The fusion starts in the midtrunk of the embryo and subsequently extends to the cranial and caudal ends

TABLE 34-1. DIFFERENTIATION OF BRAIN REGIONS FROM PRIMARY VESICLES

PRIMARY VESICLE	SECONDARY VESICLE	MATURE STRUCTURE
Forebrain	Telencephalon	Cerebral hemispheres
		Basal ganglia
		Olfactory system
	Diencephalon	Thalamus
		Hypothalamus
Midbrain	Mesencephalon	Midbrain
Hindbrain	Metencephalon	Pons
		Cerebellum
	Myelencephalon	Medulla

Modified from Moore KL. *Essentials of human embryology.* Toronto, 1988, BC Decker.

(Table 34-1). The anterior end, the **rostral neuropore,** closes by about $5\frac{1}{2}$ menstrual weeks, and the caudal end closes about $\frac{1}{2}$ week later. By the sixth week, the cephalic end enlarges and flexes to become the brain.[12,13] By 12 to 15 menstrual weeks, almost all structures are in their final form. Exceptions are the **corpus callosum, cerebellar vermis, neuronal migration** from the periventricular germinal matrix, development of the **sulci** and **gyri,** and **myelination.** These latter structures and processes start developing from about 15 weeks onward. The corpus callosum is formed by 20 weeks. As it develops, the corpus callosum induces the formation of the two septi pellucidi and the intervening space, which is the **cavum septi pellucidi** and **cavum vergae** (after Andrea Verga in 1851).

The **cerebellum** and **vermis** develop as proliferations into the cephalic part of a thin dorsal membrane (area membranacea) that forms the dorsal aspect of the **rhombencephalic neural tube.** The enclosed part of the hindbrain neural tube is the rhombencephalic cavity. This cavity enlarges rapidly in early pregnancy, forming a conspicuous dorsal cystlike space that should not be mistaken for abnormality[14] (Fig. 34-1, *A*). The cerebellar hemispheres grow into this membrane from the sides, and the vermis arises from its cephalic aspect.[15] The lower part of the rhombencephalic membrane below the vermis eventually fenestrates to form the foramina of Magendie and Luschka. This membranous part can bulge to a variable extent, forming **Blake's pouch.** With high-resolution equipment, Blake's pouch can be seen in most fetuses, where it is often mistaken for arachnoid strands.[15-17] The cerebellum and vermis are essentially formed by 22 weeks. Care must be taken to avoid mistaking the incompletely developed vermis for vermian dysplasia/hypoplasia.[18] Midsagittal views with ultrasound, especially 3D midsagittal scans, and MRI can show the normal development of the vermis, the fourth ventricle with pointed fastigial point (dorsal pointed apex of fourth ventricle), and the vermian fissures, as well as overall size of vermis and the normal brainstem-vermis angle of less than 10 degrees. All these elements are used to evaluate normal vermian development.[19,20]

The **cortex** also undergoes complex development at the neuronal cellular level. The cells that will become the brain cells (**neurons**) at the outer surface of the cortex undergo complex development in three overlapping phases: proliferation, migration, and organization. In general, neuron development starts at about 5 weeks and is largely finished by 28 weeks. Neurons derive and proliferate from stem cells located in the germinal matrix by the ependyma-lined ventricles. These stem cells proliferate and differentiate into glial cells and neurons. The glial cells send processes to the cortical surface, creating a scaffold along which the neurons then migrate to the cortex. To accommodate the accumulating neurons, the cortex undergoes folding into gyri and sulci. Failure of normal migration results in **heterotopia** (collections of neurons in abnormal locations) and abnormal or absent cortical convolutions (**pachygyria** or **type 1 lissencephaly**). A normally functioning outermost layer of the cortex serves to stop neuron migration and prevents overmigration of neurons into the meninges. Failure of this stopping function results in neurons migrating beyond the normal limits of the cortex into the meninges and subarachnoid space. This gives the brain surface a finely granular texture called **cobblestone lissencephaly.** Once the neurons arrive at the cortex, they organize local connections and send axons remotely, thereby forming large tracts or **commissures** such as the corpus callosum to connect the hemispheres. All these elements require the normal function of many genes working together, and the process is easily disrupted by intrinsic and extrinsic insults, such as fetal and maternal metabolic disorders, hypoxia, infections, and teratogens.[21]

Sonographic Anatomy

The early embryo is best examined transvaginally. The cephalic end is identifiable by about 8 weeks (see Fig. 34-1). By 10 to 11 weeks, bones of the vault show mineralization. At this age, the brain mantle is very thin. The ventricles are large and filled with choroid, which provides nourishment for the developing brain.[22] A large, echo-free space behind the hindbrain represents the **rhombencephalic cavity,** which decreases in size as the cerebellum begins to form. This normal echo-free space appears especially large and prominent in first-trimester scanning and should not be mistaken for abnormality.[14]

After about 13 to 14 weeks, most of the cerebral structures can be identified ultrasonographically. Three standard transaxial planes or views (thalamic, ventricular, cerebellar) can lead to the detection of more than 95% of sonographically detectable cerebral anomalies.[2,4] These three views form a useful starting point, but the examination should not be limited to these views alone. The entire brain should be examined, using whatever

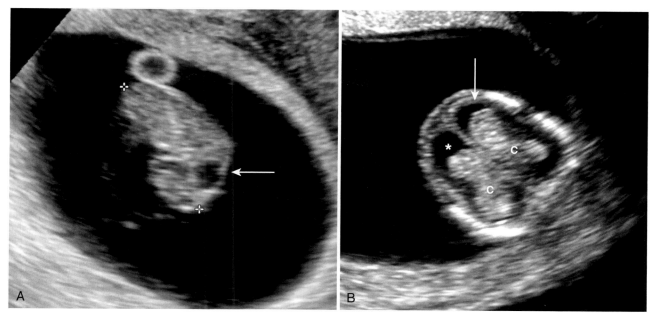

FIGURE 34-1. Early normal fetal head images obtained with transvaginal probe. A, At 9 menstrual weeks the head is clearly differentiated from the trunk and limb buds. The intracranial cystic structure is the fetal rhombencephalic cavity *(arrow)*, a normal space that eventually becomes the fourth ventricle. **B, Scan at 12½ weeks.** Note that the cerebral cortex is very thin *(at tip of arrow)*. The choroid plexuses *(C)* are very large and fill the ventricles (*) from side to side. Ossification is already visible in the skull bones.

projections are needed to show all the structures (Fig. 34-2; **Videos 34-1, 34-2,** and **34-3**). The transvaginal approach can be employed when the head is deep in the pelvis and allows a better view of the brain.[4,23]

The **thalamic view** used to measure the biparietal and occipitofrontal diameters (BPD and OFD) (see Fig. 34-2). It displays the **thalamus, third ventricle, fornices, basal ganglia, insula,** and **ambient cistern.** The **ventricular view** is slightly higher than the thalamic view and shows the bodies and, more importantly, the **atrium of the lateral ventricle** as well as the **interhemispheric fissure.** The atrium of the lateral ventricle is at the base of the occipital horn, where it joins with the temporal horn and the body of the ventricle. The atrium is an important landmark at which ventricular size is measured. The **cerebellar view** is obtained by rotating the transducer into a suboccipitobregmatic plane centered on the thalamus to show the **cerebellar hemispheres.** This view shows the cerebellum, cisterna magna, **cavum septi pellucidi** (CSP), and frequently the anterior horns of the lateral ventricles. Cerebellar measurements may be used to determine gestational age if the head has undergone molding.[24] The **cisterna magna** is the cerebrospinal fluid space between the cerebellum and the occipital bone. It is the distance between the cerebellar vermis and inner surface of the occipital bone measured on an axial plane that includes the anterior end of the CSP and the midplane of the cerebellum posteriorly. The cisterna magna should be noted at every study and normally measures 2 to 10 mm.[4] Its obliteration suggests a **Chiari II malformation,** a common finding in spina bifida. Its excessive enlargement is termed

CRANIAL STRUCTURES TO NOTE AT ROUTINE ANATOMIC SCAN

Measurement of biparietal diameter and head circumference
Head shape
Bone density
Ventricle size and appearance
Cavum septi pellucidi
Thalamus
Cerebellum and vermis
Cisterna magna
Nuchal fold

mega–cisterna magna, which may be normal if found in isolation,[25] but also increases risks of abnormalities such as **trisomy 18** and cerebral dysfunction.[26]

Additional sonographic views and projections that exploit the normal windows provided by the fontanelles and sutures can be helpful in clarifying brain anatomy and development. The **median (midsagittal) view** through the metopic suture–anterior fontanelle–sagittal suture shows midline structures such as the corpus callosum and occasionally the cerebellar vermis and brainstem. The posterolateral mastoid fontanelles provide effective access to the cerebellum and occipital lobes and ventricles. The sulci and gyri undergo predictable development patterns that can be assessed as early as 18 weeks. Special views to optimize sulcal development can be helpful in detecting abnormal development such as lissencephaly[27,28] (Fig. 34-3).

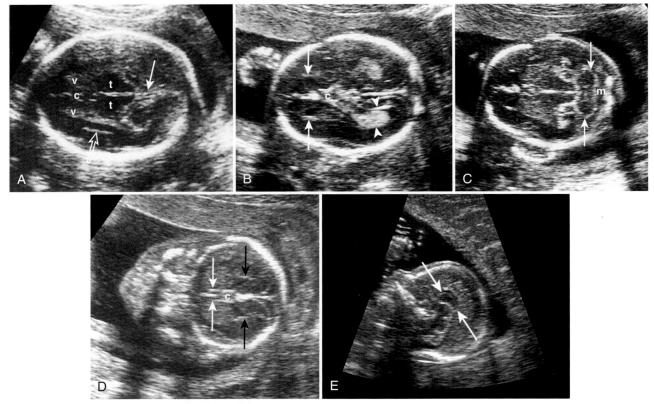

FIGURE 34-2. Standard planes for viewing cerebral structures. A, Thalamic view at 20 menstrual weeks. This transverse view at the level of the diamond-shaped thalamus-hypothalamus complex *(t)* contains the slitlike midline third ventricle. The echogenic triangular area behind the thalamus and between the occipital lobes is the ambient cistern *(arrow),* which contains cerebrospinal fluid (CSF) but is rendered echogenic because of strands of meninges supporting the brain structures. The insula is a short, brightly echogenic line *(open arrow)* containing the pulsating middle cerebral artery branches. It is surrounded by normal white matter that is very hypoechoic and should not be mistaken for fluid. The echogenic band between thalamus and insula is the basal ganglia. Anteriorly are the tips of the anterior frontal horns of the lateral ventricles *(v)* and between them is the boxlike cavum septi pellucidi *(c).* **B, Ventricular view at 18 weeks.** The atrium of the occipital horn is filled with echogenic choroid, and the ventricle measurement is indicated *(arrowheads).* Note that the choroid fills more than 60% of atrium width. The measurement between the medial ventricle wall and the choroid is less than 3 mm. The tips of the anterior frontal horns are visible *(arrows); c,* cavum septi pellucidi. **C, Cerebellar view at 18 menstrual weeks** is obtained by rotating the transducer from the thalamic view so that the cerebellar hemispheres *(arrows)* in the posterior fossa come into view, connected in the midline by the slightly more echogenic vermis. The cisterna magna *(m)* is visible between the cerebellum and the occipital bone. Also visible in this view are the thalamus, third ventricle, anterior horns, and cavum septi pellucidi. **D, Coronal view at 19 weeks through the coronal suture** shows anterior frontal horns *(black arrows)* and large nerve trunks; the fornices *(white arrows)* are clearly visible below the cavum septi pellucidi *(c).* **E, Midsagittal view through metopic suture at 19 weeks** shows normal corpus callosum *(arrows)* containing the cavum septi pellucidi in its arc below the corpus callosum. The echogenic cerebellar vermis is visible posteriorly.

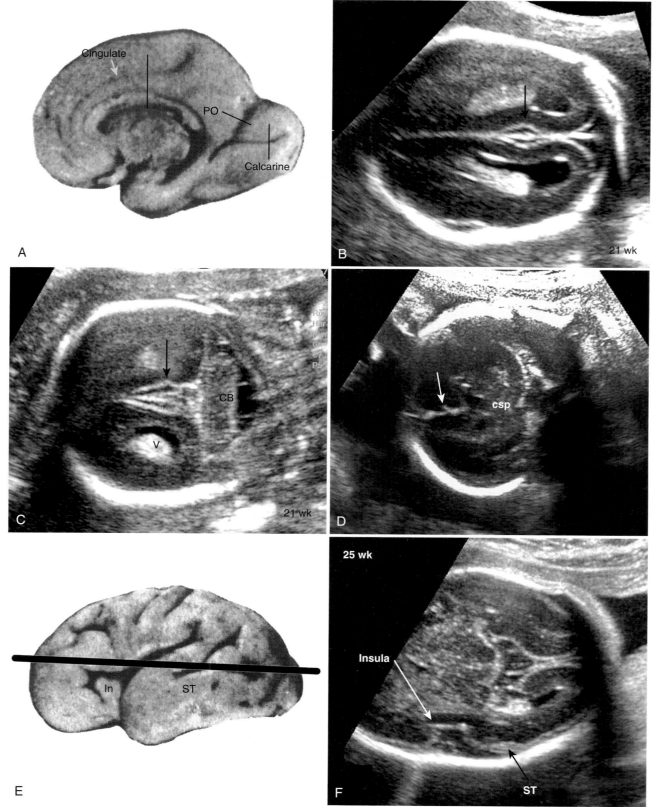

FIGURE 34-3. Scan planes (*dark lines*) used to assess early-appearing sulci. Note that the scan planes are perpendicular to the direction of the sulcus being evaluated. **A, Medial hemispheric surface at 26 weeks.** Coronal scan plane (CP) is best for cingulate sulcus (*yellow arrow*) and calcarine sulcus. Semi-axial plane is best for parieto-occipital sulcus (*PO*). **B, Axial view at 21 weeks** shows the diamond shape formed by the normal parieto-occipital sulci (*arrow*). **C, Coronal view through the occipital lobes at 21 weeks** shows the calcarine sulcus (*arrow*) of the upper occipital lobe; the lower calcarine sulcus has not developed as far yet. This slight side-to-side variation is normal. *CB,* Cerebellum. **D,** Coronal view shows the notch of the cingulate sulcus above the bodies of the lateral ventricles and cavum septi pellucidi (*csp*). **E,** Lateral view of brain surface at **26 weeks** shows the scan plane used to evaluate the insula (*In*) and superior temporal sulcus (*ST*) behind it. **F,** Axial view shows the angular plateau of the insula and behind it the subtle indentation of the superior temporal sulcus (*arrow with ST*). (*Anatomic images modified from Dorovini-Zis K, Dolman CL. Gestational development of brain. Arch Pathol Lab Med 1977;101:192-195. Ultrasound images from Toi A, Chitayat D, Blaser S. Abnormalities of the foetal cerebral cortex. Prenat Diagn 2009;29:355-371.*)

Multiplanar three-dimensional (3-D) imaging can be utilized to reconstruct axial and median views to assess the brain from any perspective. Midsagittal reconstructions are especially helpful in evaluating abnormalities of the corpus callosum and cerebellum.[23] Head shape and ossification should be noted at all these views (see Chapter 33).

Although ultrasound is the mainstay of a prenatal examination, MRI is useful as a problem-solving technique when questions remain after the ultrasound scan. Currently, MRI provides excellent anatomic images after about 22 weeks' gestation and is superior in evaluating the character of brain tissue and the periphery of the brain, where ultrasound visibility is limited (Fig. 34-4). However, MRI has limitations in showing cerebral calcifications and small cysts.[10,29,30]

Variants (Usually Normal)

Choroid Plexus Cysts

Choroid plexus cysts (CPCs) are cystlike spaces in the choroid plexus (Fig. 34-5; **Video 34-4**). They are common, seen in 1% to 6% of fetuses between 14 and 24 weeks' gestation. Most are small and disappear without consequence by about 28 weeks. CPCs are thought to represent entrapment of cerebrospinal fluid within an infolding of neuroepithelium. Many suggest that only CPCs over 3 mm should be considered substantial enough to be termed "choroid plexus cyst." Although frequently found in normal fetuses, CPC are associated with trisomy 18.

The incidence of CPCs in trisomy 18 is about 50%, and in about 10% of trisomy 18 fetuses, CPC is the only ultrasonographic findings. Likelihood ratios of trisomy 18 with isolated CPC are about 7 (range 4-12) times the mother's background risk.[31] Size and bilaterality of the cysts do not impact incidence of aneuploidy.

Fetuses with trisomy 18 almost always have other detectable abnormalities. Therefore, when a CPC is found, there should be a detailed search for features of trisomy 18, especially the hands, heart, and CNS. Maternal age should be taken into account because the risk of trisomy 18 increases with age. Maternal serum and first-trimester nuchal translucency can be helpful as independent screens for trisomy 18.[31,32]

Blake's Pouch Cyst

Blake's pouch cyst describes a thin-walled cystic structure normally seen in the posterior fossa behind the lower portion of the cerebellar vermis (Fig. 34-6, A). It should not be mistaken for abnormality. Its walls appear as lines or strands that were previously thought to represent "suspensory ligaments of the cerebellum." In fact, these are most likely remnants of the extremely thin-walled posterior roof of the rhombencephalon. The

cephalad part of the rhombencephalic roof forms the cerebellum and vermis; the inferior part remains thin and eventually fenestrates to form the foramina of Magendie and Luschka. The lower part of this membrane often bulges into the posterior fossa as a "cyst" described by Robert Blake over 100 years ago. Because it contains cerebrospinal fluid, this cyst is echo free, unlike the adjacent subarachnoid fluid, which is rendered slightly echogenic due to fine strands in the subarachnoid space. With careful scanning, the Blake's pouch cyst is visible in almost every fetus, varying in size from tiny to large and conspicuous. If large, the cyst can elevate and rotate the vermis, creating an appearance that mimics **vermian dysplasia,** but in these cases, midsagittal scans show that the vermis is intact (Fig. 34-6, B and C). Some think that mega–cisterna magna is simply a large Blake's pouch, possibly resulting from delayed fenestration of the foramina.[15,17]

Cavum Veli Interpositi

Cavum veli interpositi describes a small cystic collection in the midline, usually seen below the splenium of the corpus callosum, behind the upper brainstem and above the region of the pineal gland (Fig. 34-7). It represents fluid in the potential space in the telea choroidea above the third ventricle. Most collections are seen below the splenium, but can extend anteriorly above the third ventricle to the foramina of Monroe.[33] Although infrequently described in the prenatal ultrasound literature, we have found small cysts, less than 8 mm, to be very common on scans at 18 to 20 weeks. A cavum veli interpositi incidence of 5.5% to 34% is reported in the pediatric literature.[34] Most cysts are of no clinical consequence; many recede spontaneously, and long-term neurologic outcome is normal.[34-36] Occasionally, however, the cyst is large and can distort the brainstem and adjacent brain, causing obstructive hydrocephalus, and requires treatment by unroofing. There is no known genetic association.

Cavum veli interpositi cysts are readily seen at axial scanning when specifically sought and can be confirmed with coronal and midsagittal views and multiplanar 3-D images (Fig. 34-7). The remaining brain should be scanned to confirm normal anatomy, especially with respect to corpus callosum and ventricle size. Color Doppler ultrasound is used to exclude vascular dilations, such as vein of Galen aneurysms. Cavum veli interpositi cysts usually are seen at 18 weeks, but the larger cysts may present in the first trimester.[34]

The physiologic cavum veli interpositi cysts tend to be isolated, unilocular, and small (<10 mm) and remain stable or recede over time. The differential diagnosis includes cysts and cystlike conditions that occur in the midline, such as **dilated cavum vergae, glioependymal cysts, arachnoid cysts, cystic tumors** (mainly cystic teratomas), **vein of Galen aneurysm, pineal**

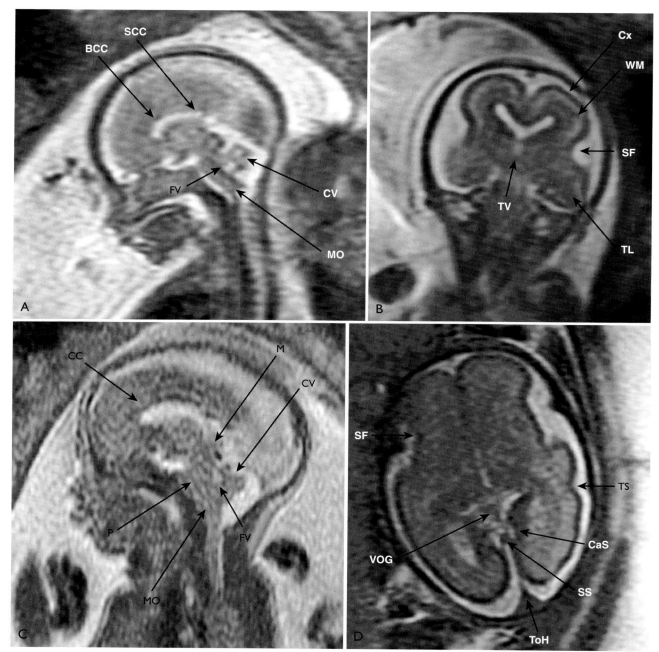

FIGURE 34-4. Normal brain appearance on MRI. T2-weighted images at 20 weeks (**A** and **B**), 22 weeks (**C**), 26 weeks (**D** and **E**), 27 weeks (**F, G,** and **H**), and 34 weeks (**I**); in sagittal midline (**A, C, G, I**), parasagittal (**F**), coronal (**B, H**), and axial (**D, E**) planes. Note developing body *(BCC)* and splenium of the corpus callosum *(SCC),* fourth ventricle *(FV),* cerebellar vermis *(CV),* medulla oblongata *(MO),* cerebral cortex *(Cx),* white matter *(WM),* sylvian fissure *(SF),* temporal lobe *(TL),* third ventricle *(TV),* pons *(P),* midbrain *(M),* ethmoid bone *(E),* extra-axial space *(EAS),* sphenoid bone *(S),* middle cerebellar peduncle *(MCP),* cerebellar hemispheres *(CH),* vein of Galen *(VOG),* straight sinus *(SS),* calcarine sulcus *(CaS),* torcular Herophili *(ToH),* temporal sulcus *(TS),* precentral sulcus *(PreCS),* central sulcus *(CeS),* post–central sulcus *(PostCS),* cingulate sulcus *(CiS),* cingulate gyrus *(CG),* parieto-occipital sulcus *(POS),* tectum *(Te),* interhemispheric fissure *(IHF),* superior sagittal sinus *(SSS),* and choroid plexus *(CP). (From Levine D, Robson C. MR imaging of normal brain in the second and third trimesters. In Levine D, editor.* Atlas of fetal MRI. *Bristol, Pa, Taylor & Francis, 2005.)*

Continued

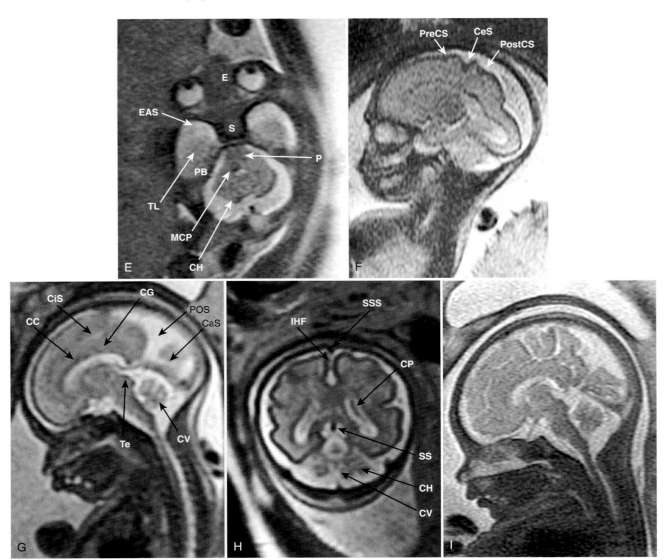

FIGURE 34-4, cont'd. Normal brain appearance on MRI. T2-weighted images at 20 weeks (**A** and **B**), 22 weeks (**C**), 26 weeks (**D** and **E**), 27 weeks (**F, G,** and **H**), and 34 weeks (**I**); in sagittal midline (**A, C, G, I**), parasagittal (**F**), coronal (**B, H**), and axial (**D, E**) planes. Note developing body *(BCC)* and splenium of the corpus callosum *(SCC),* fourth ventricle *(FV),* cerebellar vermis *(CV),* medulla oblongata *(MO),* cerebral cortex *(Cx),* white matter *(WM),* sylvian fissure *(SF),* temporal lobe *(TL),* third ventricle *(TV),* pons *(P),* midbrain *(M),* ethmoid bone *(E),* extra-axial space *(EAS),* sphenoid bone *(S),* middle cerebellar peduncle *(MCP),* cerebellar hemispheres *(CH),* vein of Galen *(VOG),* straight sinus *(SS),* calcarine sulcus *(CaS),* torcular Herophili *(ToH),* temporal sulcus *(TS),* precentral sulcus *(PreCS),* central sulcus *(CeS),* post–central sulcus *(PostCS),* cingulate sulcus *(CiS),* cingulate gyrus *(CG),* parieto-occipital sulcus *(POS),* tectum *(Te),* interhemispheric fissure *(IHF),* superior sagittal sinus *(SSS),* and choroid plexus *(CP). (From Levine D, Robson C. MR imaging of normal brain in the second and third trimesters. In Levine D, editor.* Atlas of fetal MRI. *Bristol, Pa, Taylor & Francis, 2005.)*

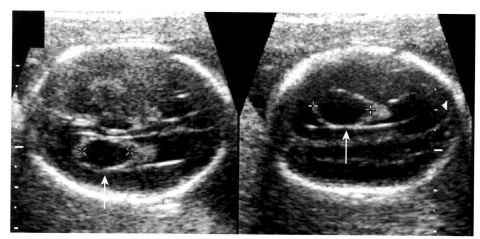

FIGURE 34-5. **Bilateral choroid plexus cysts** *(arrows)* on transverse ventricular view.

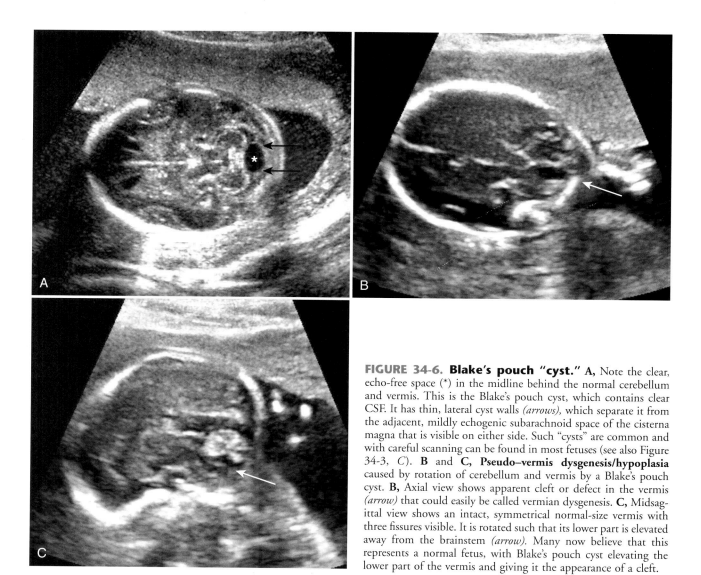

FIGURE 34-6. Blake's pouch "cyst." A, Note the clear, echo-free space (*) in the midline behind the normal cerebellum and vermis. This is the Blake's pouch cyst, which contains clear CSF. It has thin, lateral cyst walls *(arrows),* which separate it from the adjacent, mildly echogenic subarachnoid space of the cisterna magna that is visible on either side. Such "cysts" are common and with careful scanning can be found in most fetuses (see also Figure 34-3, *C*). **B and C, Pseudo–vermis dysgenesis/hypoplasia** caused by rotation of cerebellum and vermis by a Blake's pouch cyst. **B,** Axial view shows apparent cleft or defect in the vermis *(arrow)* that could easily be called vermian dysgenesis. **C,** Midsagittal view shows an intact, symmetrical normal-size vermis with three fissures visible. It is rotated such that its lower part is elevated away from the brainstem *(arrow).* Many now believe that this represents a normal fetus, with Blake's pouch cyst elevating the lower part of the vermis and giving it the appearance of a cleft.

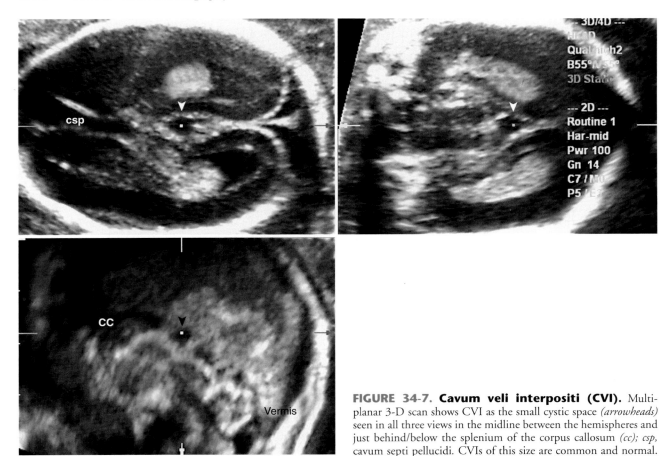

FIGURE 34-7. Cavum veli interpositi (CVI). Multiplanar 3-D scan shows CVI as the small cystic space *(arrowheads)* seen in all three views in the midline between the hemispheres and just behind/below the splenium of the corpus callosum *(cc); csp,* cavum septi pellucidi. CVIs of this size are common and normal.

cyst, and **hemorrhage.** Pathologic cystic collections are generally larger, enlarge over time, and have associated abnormalities, such as corpus callosum dysgenesis, ventriculomegaly, or solid masses.[33,34,36]

Fetuses with suspected cavum veli interpositi cysts should undergo detailed neurosonography and anatomic scan. If there are any atypical features or associated findings, MRI can be helpful in further investigation. We no longer monitor incidentally discovered small (<8 mm) isolated cysts but perform follow-up scans if the cysts are especially conspicuous or if there is parental concern.

VENTRICULOMEGALY AND HYDROCEPHALUS

The term **ventriculomegaly** (VM) describes large ventricles. The head itself may be normal, large, or even smaller than expected for menstrual age. **Hydrocephalus** (HC) refers to enlarged ventricles associated with increased intracranial pressure and thus is typically associated with head enlargement. Ventriculomegaly is the most commonly encountered cranial abnormality at prenatal ultrasound, with incidence ranging from 0.3 to 1.5 in 1000 births.[37-40]

Enlargement of the lateral cerebral ventricles is not the primary problem. Although VM may be an isolated finding, it is usually the sonographically conspicuous finding of numerous disorders and syndromes.[37,39] The underlying changes in the brain are clinically important, not only the size and appearance of the ventricles. Cerebral functional alterations are only variably predicted by ventricular size, cortical thinning, and appearance.[41-43]

Pathogenesis

Cerebrospinal fluid (CSF) is secreted by the choroid plexus of the lateral, third, and fourth ventricles, as well as by the cerebral capillaries.[44] CSF flows from the lateral ventricles through the foramina of Monro, third ventricle, aqueduct of Sylvius, and fourth ventricle and out the foramina of Magendie and Luschka, into the subarachnoid space of the posterior fossa. CSF then courses over the surface of the brain to the **pacchionian** or **arachnoid granulations,** which are distributed at the top of the head adjacent to the superior sagittal sinus and absorb CSF. Ventricular enlargement generally results from obstruction of CSF flow in the brain (**intraventricular obstructive hydrocephalus**). Alternatively, the site of blockage may be outside the ventricular system,

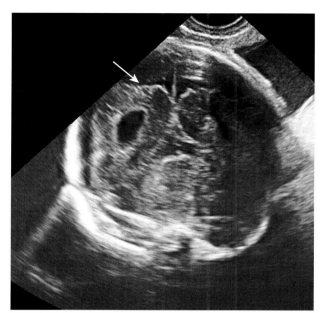

FIGURE 34-8. Ventriculomegaly at 30 weeks and polymicrogyria. The ventricles are large. The shrunken brain has fallen away from the skull, leaving a wide, CSF-filled subarachnoid space **(hydrocephalus ex vacuo).** Note also the fine nodularity of the surface of the brain *(arrow),* characteristic of polymicrogyria.

ABNORMALITIES COMMONLY ASSOCIATED WITH VENTRICULOMEGALY

Obstructive hydrocephalus
Aqueductal stenosis (idiopathic, infections, bleeding, X-linked, masses)
Spina bifida with Chiari II malformation
Excess cerebrospinal fluid (CSF) production
Choroid plexus cyst
Cerebral malformations
Agenesis of corpus callosum
Vermian dysgenesis and Dandy-Walker malformation
Holoprosencephaly
Neuronal migration abnormalities
Microcephaly
Macrocephaly
Lissencephaly
Schizencephaly
Destructive processes (encephaloclasis)
Vascular insults, infections, porencephaly
Aneuploidy (trisomies 21, 18, 13)
Many syndromes

or there may be failure of absorption (**extraventricular obstructive hydrocephalus,** or **communicating hydrocephalus**). Less often, VM results from excess CSF secretion with **choroid plexus papillomas** or follows cerebral destruction and shrinkage (**hydrocephalus ex vacuo**) as a result of diverse insults (Fig. 34-8).

Associated CNS and somatic malformations are common and seen in about 70% to 83% of cases. Chromosomal abnormalities are more common with non-isolated (25%-36%) than isolated (3%-6%) VM and include the **trisomies** and **X-linked hydrocephalus** in males. D'Addario et al.[37] reports that the main associations with VM are **aqueductal stenosis** (30%-40%), **Chiari II malformation** with spina bifida (25%-30%), **Dandy-Walker complex** (7%-10%), **agenesis of the corpus callosum**, and other, less common conditions.

Ultrasound Examination

Ventricles

Determining the cause of VM can be difficult. Several approaches to measuring ventricular size have been described: atrial width, choroid separation, ventricle/hemisphere ratio, combined anterior horn width, and visual anatomic appearance. Of these, the universally accepted method is the **transverse measurement of the atrium of the occipital horn** (see Figs. 34-2, *B;* 34-9, *A;* 34-10, *B;* and 34-11). The detection of ventricular enlargement is the clue to the detection of most cerebral

anomalies.[2] The size of the head is not helpful in detecting VM, and frequently the BPD remains normal even with severe ventricular enlargement.[45] Nomograms of other ventricular dimensions are available but not in common use.[46]

In the first trimester the choroid plexus should fill the prominent-appearing lateral ventricle, except for the conspicuous anterior frontal horn of the lateral ventricle, which should not be mistaken for abnormality (see Fig. 34-1, *B*). VM manifests as a small-appearing choroid plexus with excess surrounding fluid.[14]

Atrial Width (Occipital Horn Width). This is the most useful and accepted measurement of the ventricles.[4] The atrium of the lateral ventricles is the site of confluence of the bodies, occipital horns, and temporal horns. This measurement is easily obtained during routine obstetric scanning, but the measurement must be taken on true axial views of the head, and calipers are placed in the widest part of the ventricle, just touching inner ventricle walls (see Figs. 34-2, *B*, and 34-11, *A*). Fortuitously, this is the part of the ventricle that undergoes the earliest and most marked enlargement.

There are pitfalls to ventricular measurement. Errors arise if the plane of view is not axial or if there is an improper choice of ventricle boundary.[47] The insula, the extreme capsule of the basal ganglia, the supraventricular veins, and reverberation echoes of the proximal skull all can appear as lines, which should not be mistaken for ventricular walls (see Fig. 34-2, *A*). In the second trimester the normal white matter is so homogeneous that it has been mistaken for abnormal intracranial fluid.

Usually, only the ventricular atrium farther from the transducer is measured, because the near ventricle is obscured by artifact created by the skull bone. The ventricles are presumed to be symmetrical. It is possible, however, to measure the near ventricle directly by exploiting access provided by the squamosal and lambdoid sutures and the posterolateral (mastoid) fontanelles and on 3-D multiplanar reconstructions[48] (Fig. 34-9). Visualization of the near ventricle should be performed whenever VM is suspected.

Between 14 and 38 menstrual weeks, the transverse atrial measurement is reportedly constant at 7.6 mm (standard deviation [SD] 0.6 mm).[2] Measurements of 10 mm or larger suggest VM with a low false-positive rate.[2,49] Generally, 10 to 12 mm is termed **mild** or **borderline**; 12 to 15 is **moderate** (although some authors consider up to 15 mm in the mild range); and greater than 15 mm is **marked** VM.[41] Although 10.0 mm has been considered the upper limit of normal, there are reports of normal outcomes with ventricles larger than 10 mm,[49] and some have suggested raising the upper limit of normal to 11 or 12 mm. Ten millimeters is already about 4 SD above the mean, and we agree with others that 10 mm should remain the criterion above which counseling and investigation should occur[4,38,49] (Fig. 34-10).

Mild ventricular asymmetry is common, with the left being larger than the right. The 2-SD range is 2.4 mm.[48] Differences of more than 3 mm should be viewed with caution.[50] Further assessment of symmetry is possible by evaluating the anterior frontal horns in a coronal direction through the anterior fontanelle, either transabdominally or transvaginally (Fig. 34-9, C). Some suggest that male fetuses have larger measurements than female fetuses, 6.8 (±1.3) mm versus 6.4 (±1.3) mm, respectively.[51,52] Others have found no difference.[53]

Choroid Separation from Medial Ventricle Wall. Mahoney et al.[54] reported that the distance between the medial atrial wall and the choroid is 1 to 2 mm in normal fetuses after 15 weeks' gestation. Measurements of 3 mm and greater were associated with abnormal outcomes when combined with other fetal abnormalities, even if the ventricle measurement is normal. Hertzberg et al.[55] found that 20% of such fetuses had abnormal outcomes. However, many believe that this approach is too sensitive and unnecessarily creates anxiety in parents.

Anatomic Appearance. Qualitative appearances suggesting ventricular enlargement include **convexity** (outward bulge) to the lateral wall of the lateral ventricle and **asymmetry** of the left and right choroids, which fall with gravity when unsupported by ventricular walls as the choroids are denser than CSF ("droopy" or "dangling" choroids) (Fig. 34-11, B; **Video 34-5**). With massive ventricular enlargement, the interhemispheric structures, particularly the septum pellucidum, undulate and can become disrupted (fenestrate) allowing the left and right lateral ventricles to communicate. The upper choroid can fall across the midline through this hole and into the lower ventricle (Fig. 34-11, C).

Ventriculomegaly

Once ventricular enlargement is suspected, attention turns to etiology and associated abnormalities. Investigations include history, detailed ultrasound, karyotype, search for infections (TORCH screen: toxoplasmosis, other/syphilis, rubella, cytomegalovirus, herpes), search for causes of bleeding (e.g., platelet antibodies), and MRI. Associated brain abnormalities may be subtle and not readily appreciated on standard axial scanning. Coronal and sagittal views both transabdominally and transvaginally and use of 3-D multiplanar scans can be especially helpful to detect abnormalities of the cerebellar vermis and corpus callosum.[37] MRI adds additional information in 5% to 50% of cases, especially with respect to parenchymal injury, migrational disorders, ischemia, hemorrhage, and brainstem abnormalities.[7,39,40,56-59]

Prognosis. Prognosis relates to the degree of VM and especially the presence of associated abnormalities. In cases of VM associated with chromosomal or CNS and somatic abnormalities, the prognosis and recurrence risk relate to underlying conditions.[40] When VM is truly isolated, neurodevelopmental outcome relates to the degree of enlargement. Normal functional outcome is reported in about 85-96% of mild (10-12 mm), 76% of moderate (12-15 mm) and 28% of severe (>15 mm) cases. Outcome is better if VM is stable or decreases, and worse with enlarging ventricles.[39,60,61] Unilateral cases behave similarly.[61,62]

Counseling of parents remains difficult. Postpartum abnormalities were found in 10% to 20% of fetuses where VM appeared isolated and all prenatal testing was negative. Long-term outcome remains guarded. Laskin et al.[60] reported that initially, 85% of children had a favorable outcome, but this decreased to 79% by 20 months.

SPECIFIC ABNORMALITIES

Congenital CNS abnormalities often reflect the *time* of insult in prenatal life rather than the specific cause. Etiologic classification is not as useful for counseling as are specific malformation *patterns*. Many brain structures form at the same time, and thus the timing of the insult may affect final outcome more than its nature. Classification can be difficult. Even identical twins who sustain the same insult to development may be born with differing phenotypes.[63]

Increasingly, CNS abnormalities are being associated with **gene abnormalities** at the molecular level. The abnormal genes give rise to abnormal proteins that prevent normal cortical development and neuron migration. Understanding the **molecular mechanisms** of disease and maldevelopment will change the understanding of developmental disorders. Specific malformations are starting to be categorized based on their underlying

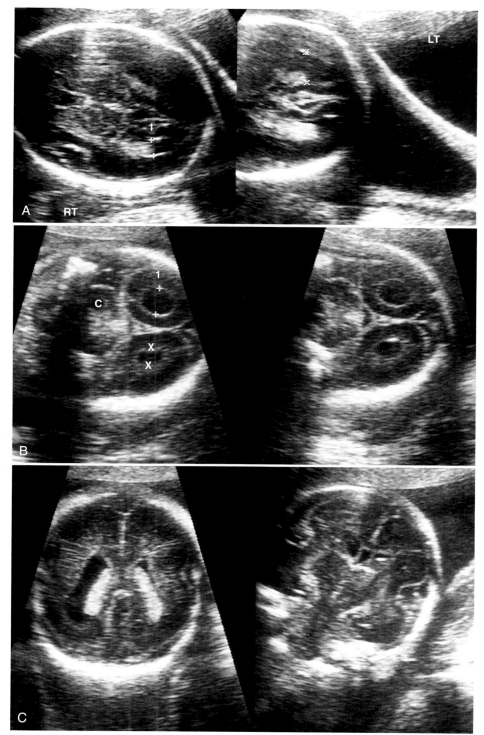

FIGURE 34-9. Assessment of ventricles at 23 weeks shows normal, mild asymmetry. A, Axial view at left shows the usually measured lower ventricle (*calipers* +). On the right image, by viewing through the posterior squamous (squamosal) suture, one can visualize the upper ventricle in the oblique axial plane (*calipers* x). Oblique image planes can increase the ventricular measurement; thus attempts should be made to obtain a true axial view for measurement if the upper ventricle appears enlarged. **B,** Coronal "owl's eye" view through the lambdoid suture shows asymmetry of the occipital horns *(calipers)*. Mild asymmetry less than 2 to 3 mm is common and normal; *c,* cerebellum. **C,** Views taken through the anterior fontanelle analogous to neonatal head ultrasound. Left image shows the occipital horns, and right image shows the anterior horns and confirms slight ventricular asymmetry.

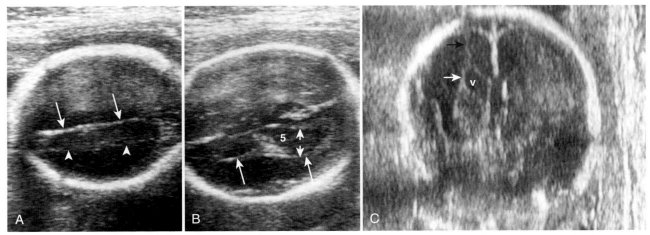

FIGURE 34-10. Supraventricular marginal venous echoes at 26 menstrual weeks versus ventricular walls. **A,** Transverse view above the level of the ventricles shows echoes from the marginal veins, which form a finely dotted line *(arrowheads)* parallel to the interhemispheric fissure *(long arrows).* **B,** Transverse view at the ventricular plane shows mild ventricular enlargement, with the occipital horn measuring over 10 mm *(short white arrows)* and the choroid separated from the medial wall of the occipital horn by 5 mm *(5).* The margin of the lateral ventricle *(long white arrows)* is curved and diverges from the midline, unlike the venous "line," which is straight and parallels the midline. **C,** Coronal view through the region of the thalamus. The lateral ventricle wall echo *(white arrow)* is lateral to the supraventricular venous echo *(black arrow),* which goes from the top of the ventricle *(v)* to the surface of the hemisphere.

genetic and molecular abnormalities rather than on morphologic appearances.[63-65] Even if the genes are normal, their functions can be variably disturbed by external influences, such as anoxia, infections, and teratogens. Again, the final outcomes will typically reflect the *timing* of the insults rather than their specific nature.[40,63,66]

To reach an accurate diagnosis and help with investigation, counseling, and treatment, the clinician should evaluate not only the obvious changes, but also look for additional, subtle findings. Clues can be found in pregnancy history, family history, course of current pregnancy (including maternal conditions such as diabetes), medications, illnesses, occupations and exposures, and evaluation of parents and close relatives. If there is a known risk of specific conditions, online resources such as Online Mendelian Inheritance in Man (OMIM, http://www.ncbi.nlm.nih.gov/omim) and other sites can be helpful in providing a list of findings to target at ultrasound.

Errors of Dorsal Induction

Errors of induction and development of the dorsal neural plate and canal **(neurulation)** result in defects of closure, including anencephaly, encephaloceles, spinal dysraphism, and Chiari malformations.

Acrania, Anencephaly, Exencephaly

Acrania, or absence of the cranial vault bones of the calvarium, is common to all these lesions. However, it should be understood that acrania can occur with a normal underlying brain, and therefore this term should not be used when the appropriate diagnosis is anencephaly or exencephaly. **Anencephaly** occurs in about 1 in 1000 births and is characterized by the absence of the cranial vault, cerebral hemispheres, and diencephalic structures. These are replaced by a flattened, amorphous vascular-neural mass (area cerebrovasculosa) (Fig. 34-12, *A*). The amorphous mass may resemble brain structures uncovered by bone **(exencephaly),** but in all cases, there is absence of normally formed skin, cranial bones, and brain superior to the orbits.[67,68] Facial structures and orbits are present. Associated spinal and non-CNS abnormalities and polyhydramnios are common.[69] On occasion, the dysraphic abnormality involves the head and entire spine **(craniorachischisis).** The outcome of anencephaly is invariably fatal, and pregnancy termination is offered at any gestational age.

Detection of anencephaly prior to 14 weeks can be difficult, although the diagnosis has been suggested as early as $10\frac{1}{2}$ weeks. Before 10 weeks, apparently normal-appearing brain structures are present. Unless the examiner specifically looks for ossified cranial bones, the diagnosis can be missed.[70,71] Using transvaginal probes, ultrasonically visible ossification of frontal bones may not be apparent until 10 weeks, and anencephaly should not be diagnosed before this gestational age. It has been suggested that exencephaly may be an early phase of anencephaly. In early pregnancy, the **area cerebrovasculosa** can be prominent and resemble brain structures without overlying ossified cranium (exencephaly), sometimes forming an appearance resembling "Mickey Mouse ears."[72] It is postulated that the brain becomes destroyed as pregnancy continues and assumes the characteristic flattened, disrupted appearance of anencephaly.[68,71] An

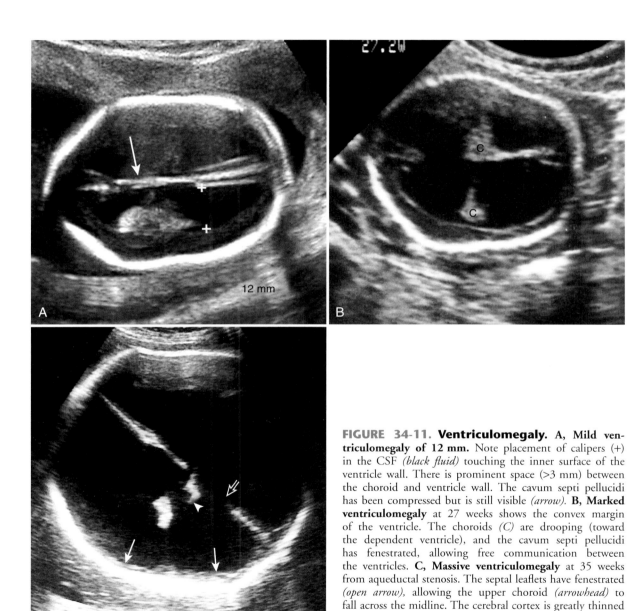

FIGURE 34-11. Ventriculomegaly. A, Mild ventriculomegaly of 12 mm. Note placement of calipers (+) in the CSF *(black fluid)* touching the inner surface of the ventricle wall. There is prominent space (>3 mm) between the choroid and ventricle wall. The cavum septi pellucidi has been compressed but is still visible *(arrow).* **B, Marked ventriculomegaly** at 27 weeks shows the convex margin of the ventricle. The choroids *(C)* are drooping (toward the dependent ventricle), and the cavum septi pellucidi has fenestrated, allowing free communication between the ventricles. **C, Massive ventriculomegaly** at 35 weeks from aqueductal stenosis. The septal leaflets have fenestrated *(open arrow),* allowing the upper choroid *(arrowhead)* to fall across the midline. The cerebral cortex is greatly thinned but present *(small arrows),* allowing differentiation from hydranencephaly.

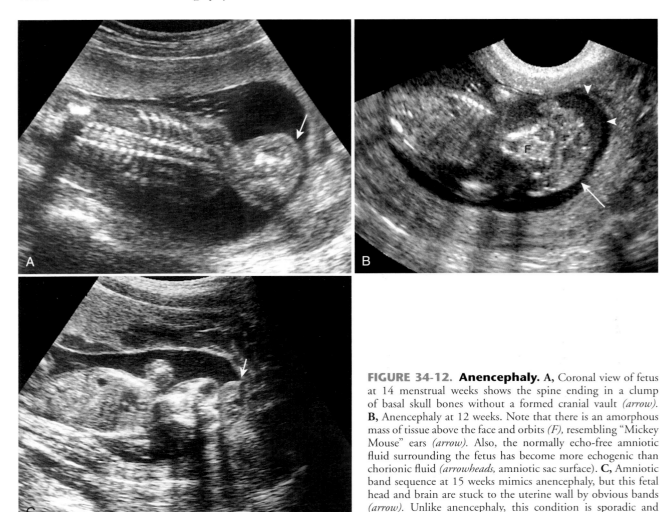

FIGURE 34-12. Anencephaly. A, Coronal view of fetus at 14 menstrual weeks shows the spine ending in a clump of basal skull bones without a formed cranial vault *(arrow).* **B,** Anencephaly at 12 weeks. Note that there is an amorphous mass of tissue above the face and orbits *(F),* resembling "Mickey Mouse" ears *(arrow).* Also, the normally echo-free amniotic fluid surrounding the fetus has become more echogenic than chorionic fluid *(arrowheads,* amniotic sac surface). **C,** Amniotic band sequence at 15 weeks mimics anencephaly, but this fetal head and brain are stuck to the uterine wall by obvious bands *(arrow).* Unlike anencephaly, this condition is sporadic and unlikely to recur.

additional clue to diagnosis is the identification of echogenic amniotic fluid caused by debris shed from the uncovered brain or other unprotected fetal parts[73] (Fig. 34-12, *B*).

Chromosomal abnormality is seen in 2% of fetuses with anencephaly and additional abnormalities seen in 4% to 8%.[74,75] Differential diagnosis includes other conditions in which the cranial bones are absent or lack mineralization, such as **amniotic band sequence**, large **encephaloceles, osteogenesis imperfecta** and **hypophosphatasia** (Fig. 34-4, *D*). With amniotic band sequence **(early amnion rupture sequence)** the fetuses generally have an asymmetrical defect accompanied by body wall defects and/or amputation of body parts and occasional oligohydramnios. Membranes may be visible in amniotic fluid, or the fetus may be stuck to the side of the uterus or placenta. Unlike anencephaly and open spina bifida, early amnion rupture sequence is sporadic and without increased recurrence risk.[69,76] Large encephaloceles generally have more calvarial development than seen with anencephaly, but occasionally the two can appear similar. In either case, the prognosis remains hopeless.

Cephalocele and Encephalocele

A **cephalocele** is a herniation of intracranial structures through a defect in the cranium. A cranial **meningocele** contains only meninges and CSF, whereas when the defect contains brain tissue, it is termed an **encephalocele.** Most encephaloceles occur in the midline in the occipital (75%) or frontal (13%) region, although some are parietal (12%) (Fig. 34-13). Encephaloceles can extend into the mouth, nasal, and sphenoid areas, where their identification can be difficult.[77-81] They can occur as isolated lesions or may be associated with other anomalies or syndromes, involving the head, spine, face, skeleton, or kidneys. Chromosomal abnormality is seen in about 14% to 18%, especially trisomies 18 and 13.[75]

Ultrasonographically, an encephalocele manifests as a cystic mass at the surface of the skull, typically in the midline. Brain tissue with a visible bony defect confirms

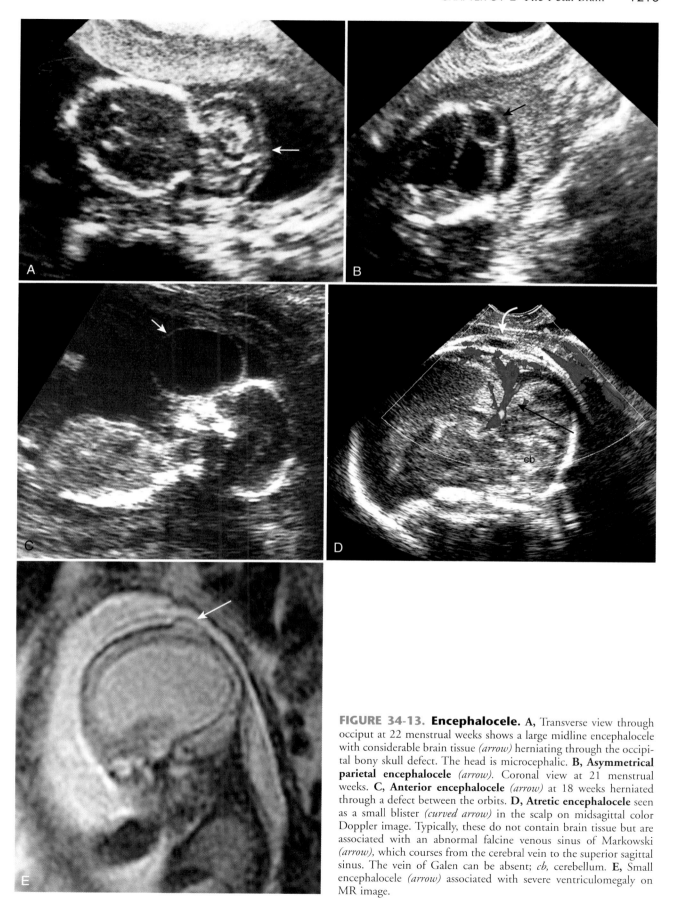

FIGURE 34-13. Encephalocele. A, Transverse view through occiput at 22 menstrual weeks shows a large midline encephalocele with considerable brain tissue *(arrow)* herniating through the occipital bony skull defect. The head is microcephalic. **B, Asymmetrical parietal encephalocele** *(arrow).* Coronal view at 21 menstrual weeks. **C, Anterior encephalocele** *(arrow)* at 18 weeks herniated through a defect between the orbits. **D, Atretic encephalocele** seen as a small blister *(curved arrow)* in the scalp on midsagittal color Doppler image. Typically, these do not contain brain tissue but are associated with an abnormal falcine venous sinus of Markowski *(arrow),* which courses from the cerebral vein to the superior sagittal sinus. The vein of Galen can be absent; *cb,* cerebellum. **E,** Small encephalocele *(arrow)* associated with severe ventriculomegaly on MR image.

the diagnosis, but the bony defect may be small and difficult to detect. Other lesions that should be considered in the differential diagnosis when a scalp lesion is visualized include **cystic hygroma, hemangioma, scalp edema** or **cephalohematoma, epidermal scalp cyst, branchial cleft cyst, dermoid cyst, dacryocystocele, epignathus,** and **cervical teratoma.**[80]

A variant that is infrequently recognized prenatally is the **atretic encephalocele** (Fig. 34-13, *D*), which usually manifests as small, blisterlike subcutaneous collection in the skin in the midline near the vertex, external to a seemingly intact skull. Diagnostic clues are abnormalities of the superior sagittal sinus, which can have multiple channels, and the persistence of the prosencephalic vein of Markowski, which runs in the falx (falcine sinus) from the region of the start of the vein of Galen to the sagittal sinus underlying the encephalocele. These children generally do well.[81,82]

Meckel-Gruber syndrome is a rare, lethal autosomal recessive condition characterized by encephalocele, cystic renal dysplasia, and polydactyly.[83] The detection of either cystic kidneys or an encephalocele should lead to a search for the other components of this syndrome, which has been detected as early as 14 weeks.[84]

The prognosis of encephalocele depends on the location of the lesion, the amount of brain herniation, the formation of the underlying brain, and associated anomalies. Mortality is up to 44%, and in survivors, intellectual impairment ranges from 40% to 91%. If discovered before viability, pregnancy termination is considered. Later in pregnancy, management depends on the size and location of the encephalocele and associated anomalies.[85]

Amniotic Band Sequence, Limb–Body Wall Complex

This variable collection of disruptive abnormalities is associated with anomalies of the amnion, often loosely referred to as "amniotic band sequence." Fetuses with these conditions have variable and complex abnormalities, such as asymmetrical encephaloceles and facial disruptions. Three overlapping types of processes are described: constrictive amniotic bands, amniotic adhesions, and limb–body wall complex. The literature on the etiology of these sporadic conditions is confusing and controversial regarding etiology and pathogenesis. There is a common theme of combinations of amniotic abnormality and asymmetrical fetal disruptions. **Constrictive amniotic bands** result in annular constrictions or amputations of limb parts. **Amniotic adhesions** result in severe defects that are covered by amnion. These often affect the craniofacial region and present as asymmetrical encephaloceles and facial clefts. They may be the result of disrupted fetal parts that are initially disrupted and then secondarily adhere to the amnion. **Limb–body wall complex** terminology is used if there is a more severe

malformation consisting of encephalocele with facial clefts, thoraco/abdominoschisis, and limb defects and generally associated with internal abnormalities that cannot be explained by amniotic bands, such as congenital heart disease, renal agenesis, and intestinal atresias. Some suggest that limb–body wall complex follows early vascular disruptions, with secondary involvement of amniotic membranes, or possibly represents general disordered morphogenesis.[86,87]

The findings at ultrasound vary with affected areas. With adhesions and limb–body wall complex, fetal anatomy can be disrupted and almost unrecognizable. This massive disruption is often the clue to the diagnosis, because the associated amniotic bands and adhesions may not be visible[88] (Fig. 34-12, *C*).

The incidence ranges from 1 in 1200 to 15,000 births, but is about five times more common in stillbirths. The major disruptions are lethal. 3-D ultrasound and MRI can be helpful in clarifying the extent of the lesions. Prognosis, counseling, and management depend on the nature and degree of disruptions. Fortunately, these anomalies are sporadic, with negligible recurrence risk.[88,89]

Cranial Changes in Spina Bifida

Spina bifida is classified as open or closed, depending on whether the spinal lesion is skin covered (closed) or not (open). Virtually all fetuses with **open spina bifida** have cerebral changes typical of a **Chiari II malformation** (Fig. 34-14; **Video 34-6**). However, those with closed, skin-covered lesions can have normal-appearing heads and brains (Fig. 34-15). The open spinal lesions are more readily detected prenatally and account for about 80% of spina bifida. Maternal serum alpha-fetoprotein (MS-AFP) is elevated in about 80% of fetuses with open spina bifida. In contrast, most fetuses with closed lesions, even if large, have no intracranial changes and normal MS-AFP levels.[90] It is important to examine the spine even if the head appears normal, to avoid missing an obvious deformity of closed spina bifida.

The characteristic head changes of open spina bifida include VM,[91] the "lemon" sign (bifrontal scalloping or indentation)[91-93] (see Fig. 34-4, *A*), the "banana" sign (Chiari II malformation)[94,95] (see Fig. 34-14), cisterna magna effacement,[96] "pointing" of the tips of the occipital ventricles,[97,98] and BPD and trunk measurements that are typically slightly small for gestational age. MRI often shows additional brain abnormalities, including cerebral hypoplasia, polymicrogyria, heterotopia, and callosal abnormality.[99]

Ventriculomegaly is common with open spina bifida but usually occurs in later pregnancy. Babcook et al.[91] found VM in 44% of fetuses under 24 weeks' gestation and in 94% after 24 weeks. It was often associated with severe posterior fossa deformities. After delivery and after repair of the skin lesion, virtually all infants

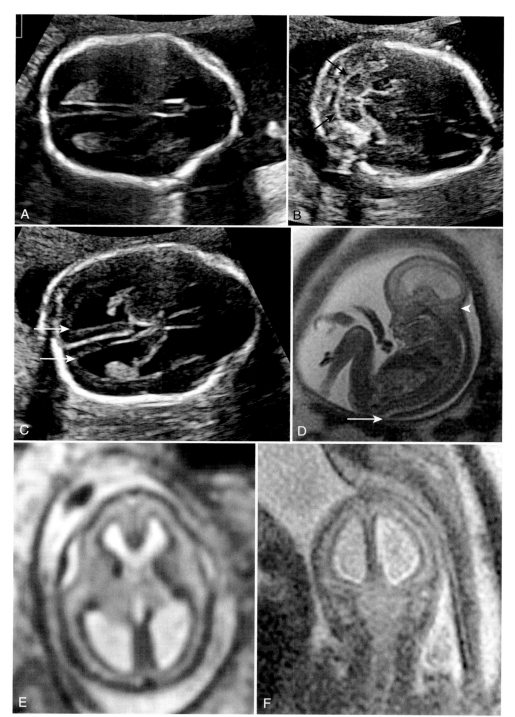

FIGURE 34-14. Cranial findings of Chiari II malformation typical (98%) with open spina bifida. A, Lemon **sign** with indentation of frontal bones. **B, Banana sign** of compressed cerebellum *(arrows)* viewed from the occipital direction. The cerebellum is tightly compressed against the occipital bone and obliterates the cisterna magna. **C,** Axial view of head shows the pointed appearance of the ventricles. **D,** Sagittal T2-weighted MR image shows inferior displacement of the cerebellum typical of the Chiari II malformation *(arrowhead)* and inferiorly, the spinal defect *(arrow)*. **E,** Axial MR image shows the pointed appearance of the ventricles. **F,** Coronal MR image shows ventriculomegaly and obliteration of the cisterna magna.

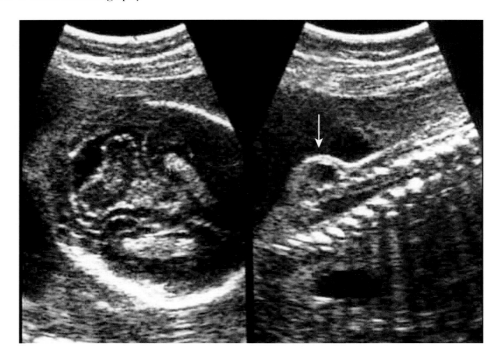

FIGURE 34-15. Closed, skin-covered spina bifida at 21 weeks. The right image shows an obvious meningomyelocele *(arrow)*. On the left image, note the normal ventricles, cerebellum, and cisterna magna. Fetuses with closed, skin-covered spina bifida do not have a Chiari II malformation and thus lack the typical intracranial signs. The MS-AFP is normal because the skin covers the defect.

FINDINGS ASSOCIATED WITH OPEN SPINA BIFIDA

Chiari II malformation
   Lemon sign
   Ventriculomegaly
   Banana sign: cerebellar tonsillar herniation into
     foramen magnum
   Effacement of cisterna magna
Slightly small fetal measurements
Spinal defects
Clubfoot (talipes)
Family history
Elevated maternal serum alpha-fetoprotein
   (MS-AFP)

develop progressive enlargement of ventricles and head (hydrocephalus) and require shunting.

The **lemon sign** or bifrontal indentation is seen in 89% to 98% of spina bifida fetuses under 24 weeks' gestation but becomes less obvious later.[92,93] It can also be seen in normal fetuses and others with diverse abnormalities, including encephalocele, Dandy-Walker malformation, and thanatophoric dysplasia.[100]

The **banana sign** and **effacement of the cisterna magna** are the result of fluid leakage from the open spinal defect and hypoplasia of the posterior fossa (see Fig. 34-14). This allows the cerebellum to be compressed into the lower posterior fossa and where it conforms to the remaining available space. The fluid in the cisterna magna is displaced (cisterna magna effacement) by the cerebellum. The cerebellar tonsils and vermis typically herniate inferiorly through the foramen magnum. The cerebellar hemispheres wrap around the lateral aspect of the brainstem, and the cerebellum assumes a C shape, the banana sign. These findings constitute the sonographic Chiari II malformation. On occasion, the cerebellum may be displaced so far inferiorly into the bony base of the skull that it cannot be imaged with ultrasound. This absence is generally artifactual due to shadowing by bone. It is rare for the cerebellar compression in Chiari II actually to result in cerebellar atrophy, but it can occur and may be associated with neurologic disturbances.[101] Fluid leak as the cause of cerebellar changes is supported by observations that after in utero repair of the open spinal defect, the cerebellum may migrate upward, and the cerebellum and posterior fossa may assume a more normal appearance.[102]

Remember, even large, closed, skin-covered spina bifida cases typically have no cranial findings, so a normal cranial examination cannot exclude spinal abnormality (Fig. 34-15). The MS-AFP will also be normal with skin-covered lesions.[103] Fetuses with isolated neural tube defect (NTD) have an increased incidence of chromosomal abnormality ranging from 7% to 16%, and antenatal genetic evaluation should be considered.[75,104,105]

The intracranial changes are similar for all levels of spinal abnormality. Functional prognosis depends primarily on the level of the spinal lesion.[106] Randomized trials of in utero spina bifida closure are currently underway. Initial experience suggests that cerebellar changes appear to reverse, and there is less need for postnatal ventricular shunting. However, there is mortality associated with the procedure, and it is not clear if there is long-term functional improvement.[90]

The accuracy of diagnosis of spina bifida depends on operator experience. Experienced referral centers have close to 100% detection. The RADIUS trial, which used MS-AFP and ultrasound reported 80% detection. MS-AFP screening may be marginally more sensitive than routine ultrasound.[107] Folic acid supplementation has greatly decreased the incidence of open NTDs. Attention to cerebral findings should allow a very high detection rate of open spina bifida. Closed spina bifida remains a problem for ultrasound diagnosis because MS-AFP is normal and there is no Chiari malformation.

The **iniencephaly** sequence is a rare and special case of dysraphism involving the back of the cranium and the contiguous upper spine; "inion" refers to the nape of the neck. It is associated with segmentation errors of the upper spine and has been suspected as early as 9 weeks.[108] The resulting deformity greatly shortens the neck, and the head is dorsiflexed (star-gazing position). Associated anomalies are common; the outcome is fatal. Iniencephaly may be associated with **anencephaly** or **Klippel-Feil syndrome;** in the latter there is segmentation error and shortening in the cervical vertebrae, but no dysraphism. Marked hyperextension can also be seen with anterior neck masses (teratoma, goiter), anencephaly and distortions of uterine cavity (e.g., from oligohydramnios, fibroids, uterine synechiae, or twins).

Errors of Ventral Induction: Holoprosencephaly

Errors of ventral induction occur in the rostral end of the embryo and result in brain abnormalities and usually affect facial development. These are in the holoprosencephaly spectrum. **Holoprosencephaly** is a complex brain malformation resulting from various degrees of incomplete cleavage of the prosencephalon. It is the most common abnormality of brain development and is seen in about 1 in 250 conceptuses but only 1 in 16,000 live births, because most affected fetuses die in utero.[40,109,110]

Normally, at about 5 weeks' gestational age, prechordal mesoderm migrates into the area anterior to the

---

FACTORS ASSOCIATED WITH HOLOPROSENCEPHALY

Environmental teratogens: alcohol, smoking, retinoic acid, salicylates, anticonvulsants
Metabolic: insulin-dependent diabetes (1% risk)
Infections: cytomegalovirus, toxoplasmosis, rubella
Syndromes with normal karyotype (about 25% of holoprosencephaly)
   Smith-Lemle-Opitz
   Pallister-Hall
   Velocardiofacial
Chromosomal abnormalities
   Trisomy 13 (70% have holoprosencephaly)
   Trisomy 18
   Triploidy
Gene mutations
   Sonic hedgehog (expressed in notochord and floor plate of neural tube)
   ZIC2 (has role in neurulation in dorsal midline)

---

notochord, where it participates in midface development and induces forebrain development. This fails in holoprosencephaly. As result, anterior midline cerebral structures fail to form, and the more lateral dorsal structures fuse in the midline to varying degrees. In severe cases the abnormality extends to involve midline facial structures. The severity of facial dysmorphism correlates with cerebral abnormalities in about 80% of cases ("the face predicts the brain").[63,110] Additional abnormalities involving any part of the body are found in about 70% of cases.[40,109]

Etiology and phenotype are heterogeneous, possibly resulting from multiple, varied genetic and environmental "hits" to the development process. Holoprosencephaly is part of many different syndromes and many chromosomal and gene abnormalities.[40,109-111]

Isolated holoprosencephaly can have autosomal dominant inheritance with incomplete penetrance and variable expression. Parents of affected children should be examined for mild manifestations such as single central incisor and absent nasal cartilage.[40,111,112]

Prognosis is variable and depends on holoprosencephaly severity, associated abnormalities, and medical and neurologic complications. Severely affected fetuses die in utero or do poorly. Mildly affected children may exhibit few symptoms and may live a normal life. About 75% need shunting.[110] In general, the severity of clinical problems and neurologic dysfunction correlates with the degree of hemispheric and hypothalamic failure of separation. Abnormal functions can manifest as endocrinopathy (especially diabetes insipidus), temperature dysregulation, motor and movement abnormalities, and developmental delay.[111,113]

Holoprosencephaly is a continuum of malformations that is classically divided into three ranges of increasing severity: **alobar** (only one hemisphere), **semilobar** (partial attempt to form two hemispheres), **lobar** (two hemispheres form, but midline structures are abnormal). Severe cases often have a dorsal cyst, thought to result from obstruction to CSF flow by fused thalami. Prenatal distribution is alobar 75%, semilobar and lobar about 10% each, and the remainder consisting of atypical forms[109,111] (Fig. 34-16). However, the range of abnormalities is much larger than these simple categorizations suggest and involve not only the cerebrum but also basal ganglia and other lower areas. Affected fetuses and children may have microforms with mild manifestations such as single midline incisor tooth or absence of olfactory lobes. Diagnosis may be difficult even after delivery. Also, some holoprosencephaly manifests as anencephaly with associated facial abnormality.[109-111]

Recently, a fourth variant has been described, **middle interhemispheric form** of holoprosencephaly, also called **syntelencephaly,** in which there is separation of the anterior and posterior parts of the hemispheres, but fusion is present in the central region of the brain between parietal hemispheres[111,114,115] (Fig. 34-16, E). Those with the middle interhemispheric form tend to do better, and they have functional disabilities similar to those with lobar holoprosencephaly, but their endocrine functions are normal because the hypothalamus tends to be spared.[114]

Prenatal diagnosis is based mainly on imaging findings. The diagnostic features of the alobar and semilobar types are absence of the falx and fusion of the thalami. **Alobar holoprosencephaly** has three variants: pancake, cup, and ball. The **pancake** type has a small, flattened plate of cerebrum anteriorly, with a large dorsal cyst posteriorly. The **cup** type has more anterior cerebrum, forming an anterior cuplike mantle and a dorsal cyst. The **ball** type has a single, featureless, monoventricle surrounded by a mantle of ventricle of varying thickness.[111,116] With **semilobar holoprosencephaly** a rudimentary attempt at cerebral cleavage of occipital horns may be seen (Fig. 34-16, D). Because it forms lobes, **lobar holoprosencephaly** may be difficult if not impossible to diagnose prenatally. Features that suggest lobar holoprosencephaly include absence of septi pellucidi, fusion and squaring of the frontal horns, and an abnormal appearance of two large nerve trunks, the **fornices,** which are rudimentary and appear fused into a single tract above the third ventricle.[117,118] With color Doppler sonography, the anterior cerebral artery may have an azygous (wandering) course "crawling" under the skull. Fusion of the fornices in holoprosencephaly can help differentiate holoprosencephaly from septo-optic dysplasia.[119]

Many authors emphasize detection of associated facial abnormalities in making the diagnosis (Fig. 34-16, B). Facial changes are seen more frequently with more severe holoprosencephaly. The facial changes have been categorized into four main groups, with severity approximating degree of brain abnormality.[109,111]

GENERAL ANATOMIC CLASSIFICATION OF HOLOPROSENCEPHALY*

ALOBAR
Single forebrain ventricle
No interhemispheric division
Absent olfactory tracts
Absent corpus callosum
Nonseparation of deep gray nuclei (fusion)
Dorsal cyst

SEMILOBAR
Rudimentary cerebral lobes
Incomplete anterior hemisphere division
Absent/small olfactory tracts
Absent corpus callosum
Variable nonseparation of deep gray nuclei

LOBAR
Fully developed cerebral lobes
Distinct interhemispheric division
Midline continuous frontal neocortex
Corpus callosum absent, hypoplastic, or normal
Separation of deep gray nuclei
Fused fornices[117]
Azygous "wandering" anterior cerebral artery

MIDLINE INTERHEMISPHERIC FORM (Syntelencephaly)
Failed separation of parietal hemispheres
Anterior and posterior corpus callosum formed
Absent/abnormal central corpus callosum
Normal separation of hypothalamus and lentiform nuclei
Gray matter heterotopia

Modified from Dubourg C, Bendavid C, Pasquier L, et al. Holoprosencephaly. Orphanet J Rare Dis 2007;2:8.
*There is considerable overlap and variation.

Middle hemispheric holoprosencephaly (syntelencephaly) can be a difficult prenatal ultrasound diagnosis because the anterior and posterior parts of the interhemispheric fissure are present, the thalami are normally separated, and the face is generally normal. Middle hemispheric holoprosencephaly can resemble VM with secondary septal fenestration. Cases generally show mild VM, absence of parts of the septi pellucidi, abnormality of the midpart of the corpus callosum, and dorsal cysts (Fig. 34-16, E). Coronal scanning may show fusion of the central parts of the hemispheres. MRI helps confirm this appearance and typically shows sylvian fissures connecting abnormally across the midline.[115,120-122]

Alobar holoprosencephaly has been diagnosed as early as 9 weeks through demonstration of a single ventricle, single orbit, and proboscis.[109] In such early cases, it is important not to mistake the normal rhombencephalic cavity, which represents the developing fourth ventricle, for holoprosencephaly. The presence of facial changes is important in this regard.

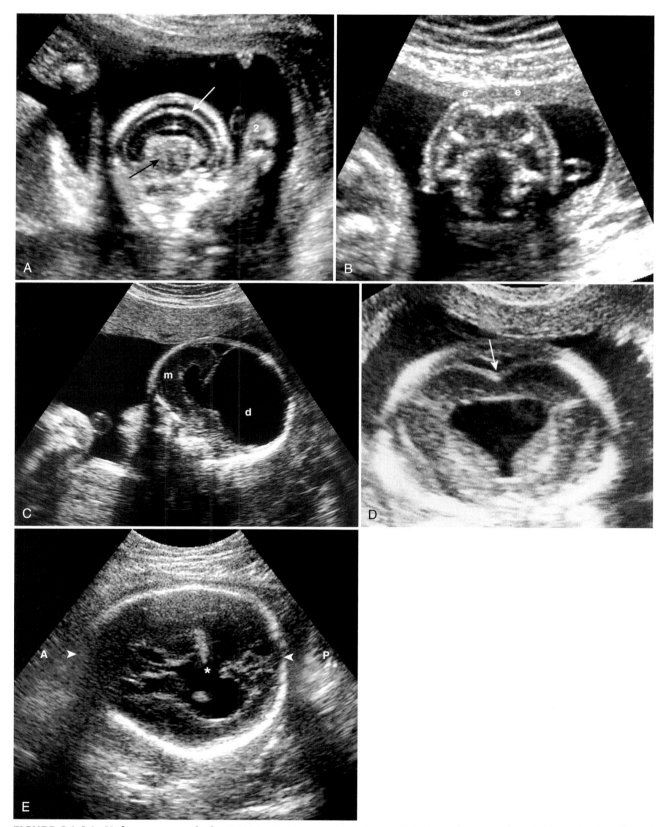

FIGURE 34-16. Holoprosencephaly. A, Alobar holoprosencephaly (coronal view) at 13 menstrual weeks shows fused nubbin of thalamus *(black arrow)* capped by a single hemisphere *(white arrow)* and underlying monoventricle. There is no falx or interhemispheric fissure. Also note the **two-vessel umbilical cord** in this fetus, which has **trisomy 13. B, Hypotelorism.** Axial view across face shows the eyes *(e)* in very close approximation. This is an example of the facial abnormalities that are common with severe alobar holoprosencephaly. **C, Cup type of alobar holoprosencephaly.** Midsagittal view shows the anterior "cup" of brain mantle *(m)* and a large dorsal cyst. **D, Semilobar holoprosencephaly** at 20 weeks. There is a single monoventricle but also rudimentary development of falx and interhemispheric fissure *(arrow).* **E, Syntelencephaly,** or middle hemispheric variant of holoprosencephaly. There is a communication between the ventricles centrally (*), but the anterior *(A arrowhead)* and posterior *(P arrowhead)* interhemispheric fissures have formed.

FACIAL CHANGES ASSOCIATED WITH HOLOPROSENCEPHALY

1. Cyclopia with single eye, with or without proboscis
2. Ethmocephaly (hypotelorism and proboscis between the eyes)
3. Cebocephaly (hypotelorism, nose with single nostril)
4. Median cleft lip/palate and hypotelorism

Differential diagnosis includes severe **hydrocephalus, septo-optic dysplasia, schizencephaly, hydranencephaly,** and **porencephaly.**[120,121] For counseling purposes, it is important to determine the degree of cerebral malformation and whether it is isolated or part of a syndrome or associated with additional abnormalities.[110,111] MRI and chromosome and microarray analysis can be helpful. Pregnancy termination is generally considered after prenatal diagnosis.

Posterior Fossa and Cerebellum

Counseling about fetuses with posterior fossa abnormalities is difficult because fetuses with different conditions are variously grouped together.[123-125] Frustratingly, prenatal appearances often do not correlate with findings at pathology.[126] Abnormal genes have been described with many posterior fossa disorders, and many have autosomal recessive inheritance.[124] If posterior abnormalities are suspected, expert imaging opinion and interdisciplinary consultation should be considered.[127]

Cerebellar development starts at about 6 to 7 weeks' gestation, and the final gross form is achieved by about 18 to 20 weeks. Cerebellar components continue to develop to about 7 months after birth, and final neuronal organization continues to about 20 months after delivery.[124] The cerebellum develops as thickenings of lateral rhombic lips, which enlarge posteriorly and are joined in the midline by the vermis, which develops from the rostral aspect. These thickenings grow into the thin-membranous dorsal aspect of the neural tube, the **area membranacea,** which is the rhombencephalic "cyst" that is prominent in early pregnancy (see Fig. 34-1) and later becomes the fourth ventricle and fenestrates, forming the foramina of Magendie and Luschka.[17,128] As the posterior fossa develops, the brainstem initially becomes flexed or kinked (mesencephalic, pontine, and cervical flexures) but again straightens out by about 14 to 16 weeks as the spinal cord expands with developing spinal nerve tracts.[19] The genetic and molecular mechanisms involved in cerebellar development play roles in other CNS regions. Consequently, abnormal cerebellar

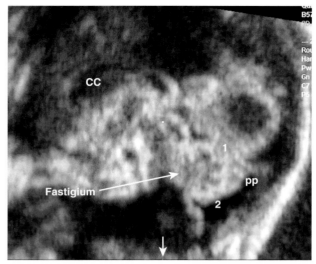

FIGURE 34-17. Normal midsagittal view of brain at 21 weeks with 3-D scan and volume contrast imaging (VCI). This is basically a thick-slice scan that increases contrast and decreases noise. Note the triangular shape of the cerebellar vermis behind the brainstem. This is the best view to evaluate the corpus callosum and vermis. Arrow indicates apex of the fourth ventricle and fastigial point. Normally, the upper and lower parts of the cerebellum touch the brainstem. A line connecting the fastigium and declive (the most posterior bulging part of the vermis) normally divides the vermis into approximately equal upper and lower portions. Also, at about 20 to 21 weeks, three vermian fissures can usually be identified as white septa invaginating into the darker cerebellum. They are the primary *(1)*, the prepyramidal *(pp)*, and the secondary *(2)* fissures.

development is often accompanied by developmental and functional changes in the cerebral cortex and other parts of the body.[63]

Functionally, the cerebellum not only controls voluntary movements but is also involved in nonmotor and cognitive functions. Many children with cerebellar malformations come to medical attention because of developmental and behavioral issues.[129-131]

The cerebellum is routinely examined with standard axial views, focusing on transverse diameter,[132] the intactness and size of the vermis, and the depth of the cisterna magna, which should measure less than 10 mm.[4] When an abnormality is suspected, midsagittal views are important to evaluate the integrity, size, rotation, and fissures of the vermis[127,133-136] (Fig. 34-17), as well as the appearance of the fourth ventricle. Transvaginal scanning, 3-D ultrasound, and MRI are especially effective in this regard and also allow assessment of the brainstem.[20,59,137-140] Practical diagnostic approaches have been suggested to evaluate suspected abnormalities of the posterior fossa, starting with initial determination of posterior fossa fluid and cerebellar size and anatomy.[127,138,139]

A large spectrum of abnormalities involves the cerebellum and posterior fossa, including malformations (e.g.,

Dandy-Walker complex, rhombencephalosynapsis, Joubert syndrome) and disruptions to normal development (e.g., infections, hemorrhage, hypoxia, toxins, intrauterine growth restriction [IUGR], metabolic abnormalities) and abnormal fluid collections. Resultant defects can be global, unihemispheric, or focal[127,141] and may be associated with many conditions.[124]

In a series of symptomatic children presenting postnatally, the relative frequency of specific common abnormalities were Dandy-Walker malformation 27%, molar-tooth (Joubert syndrome) 17%, congenital muscular dystrophy (Walker-Warburg phenotype) 14%, rhombencephalosynapsis 11%, cytomegalovirus (CMV) infection 9%, hypoplasia 4%, lissencephaly 4%, focal dysplasias 3%, and miscellaneous conditions 6%.[125] At a prenatal MRI referral center examining fetuses with sonographically suspected problems, the distribution of abnormalities was inferior vermian hypoplasia 37% (82% of these were isolated), Dandy-Walker malformation 25%, mega–cisterna magna 15%, cerebellar hypoplasia 7%, hemorrhage 7%, and rhombencephalosynapsis 2%.[142] The differences between the postnatal and prenatal series highlight the difficulties of precise and complete prenatal diagnosis, possible late manifestation or development of some disorders, and possible in utero lethality of conditions diagnosed during pregnancy, including iatrogenic pregnancy termination.

Dandy-Walker Malformation

The classic Dandy-Walker malformation (DWM) consists of four elements. At ultrasound, a large, abnormal fluid collection in the posterior fossa is associated with a small cerebellum and elevated tentorium and torcula (Fig. 34-18). Midsagittal imaging is important because prognosis is associated with the degree of vermian abnormality as well as the presence of additional abnormalities.[133] Additional CNS anomalies occur in 50% to 70%, especially VM,[129] brainstem dysgenesis, dysgenesis of the corpus callosum, migrational disorders, encephaloceles, and spina bifida. Somatic abnormalities occur in 20% to 30%, including cystic kidneys, congenital heart disease, and facial clefts.

Classic DWM is uncommon and occurs in about 1 in 30,000 pregnancies.[133] It was initially believed that the DWM resulted from simple failure of fenestration of the foramina of Magendie and Luschka. Now it is believed to represent a more generalized abnormality following developmental arrest of the rhombencephalon at about 7 to 10 weeks, with lack of fusion of the cerebellum in the midline and enlargement of the fluid spaces.[128] It has a multifactorial etiology, and most cases are seen in association with genetic and nongenetic syndromes. Molecular genetic abnormalities have been found in some cases.[124,143]

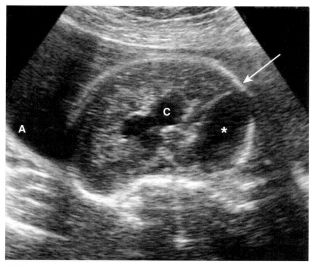

FIGURE 34-18. Dandy-Walker malformation (DWM) at 22 weeks. Midsagittal view shows a large cyst in the posterior fossa (*). The tentorium is elevated *(arrow)*, and the cerebellum is virtually not visible. Fetuses with DWM usually have other midline abnormalities; this fetus has agenesis of the corpus callosum associated with an interhemispheric cyst *(C); A,* anterior.

DANDY-WALKER MALFORMATION

1. Cystic dilation of the fourth ventricle communicating with a posterior fossa fluid space
2. Elevated tentorium and high position of the torcula (confluence of the superior sagittal and lateral venous sinuses)
3. Small, rotated, raised, or absent vermis
4. Anterolateral displacement of seemingly normal cerebellar hemispheres

The prognosis of DWM depends on associated abnormalities. Those with isolated findings do better, but outcomes are poor in those with associated CNS or somatic abnormalities. Neonatal mortality ranges from 12% to 55%.[129] Karyotype abnormalities occur in about 15%, mainly in cases with associated abnormalities. In liveborn children, intelligence is normal in about 40%, borderline in 20%, and subnormal in 40%.[129,133]

The differential diagnosis includes other **vermian dysplasias, Blake's pouch cyst,** and **posterior fossa subarachnoid cysts.** Arachnoid cysts displace an otherwise normally formed cerebellum and frequently lie behind or above the cerebellum, and do not communicate with the fourth ventricle. Investigation can include fetal MRI, assessment for maternal TORCH infection, chromosome analysis, microarray analysis, and consideration of syndromic forms, including **Walker-Warburg syndrome.**

Vermis Hypoplasia or Dysplasia

Vermis hypoplasia or dysplasia describes a conspicuous cleft separating the inferior parts of the cerebellar hemispheres due to deficiency or absence of the lower part of the vermis. Controversy surrounds this appearance, which has been variously termed **Dandy Walker variant, Dandy Walker continuum, vermian hypoplasia/dysgenesis/ agenesis,** and **Blake's pouch cyst.**[127] The currently accepted term is **vermian hypoplasia or dysplasia.**

The vermis develops superiorly to inferiorly. Hypoplasia or developmental arrest results in varying-size deficits of the inferior portion, leaving a relatively square defect that communicates with the fourth ventricle and separates the lower cerebellar hemispheres. Generally, the posterior fossa is not enlarged. Midsagittal scans, 3-D imaging, and MRI are important to evaluate the size and shape of the vermis, the shape of the fourth ventricle, and determine if the early fissures have developed[20,138] (see Fig. 34-17).

There are multiple diagnostic pitfalls. Hypoplasia or dysplasia should not be diagnosed prior to 18 weeks, before vermian development is complete.[18] An abnormally steep scanning angle may mimic a prominent cleft between the lower portions of the cerebellar hemispheres.[18,144] Axial scans may show a conspicuous notch, but when scanned in the midsagittal plane, the cerebellar vermis may be normal in size and appearance but may be simply rotated upward by a prominent Blake's pouch cyst[16] (see Fig. 34-6).

True cases of vermian dysplasia are usually associated with additional abnormalities similar to those seen with Dandy-Walker malformation, and these help confirm the diagnosis (Fig. 34-19). Vermian hypoplasia can be associated with several syndromes, including **Joubert syndrome, Walker-Warburg syndrome, cerebro-oculo-muscular syndrome,** and **pontocerebellar syndrome.**[124,127,128]

Counseling is difficult. In one series, up to 50% of fetuses with the characteristic ultrasound findings of vermian dysplasia were functionally normal after delivery.[107] In another series, autopsy did not confirm 55% of prenatally diagnosed cases. Ultrasound findings more likely to predict true abnormality were **trapezoidal vermian defect,** cisterna magna larger than 10 mm, and complete aplasia of the vermis. In contrast, normal cases tended to have a **keyhole-shaped defect.**[126] Prenatal MRI is helpful but also has limitations. In one study, postnatal MRI failed to confirm prenatal MRI findings in 6 of 42 cases (5 vermian hypoplasia, 1 mega–cisterna magna) but found additional, mainly cerebral abnormalities in 10 of 42 cases (heterotopias, brainstem hypoplasia, lissencephaly, hemorrhage).[131,142] Because of the diagnostic uncertainties, whenever vermian abnormality is suspected, additional anomalies should be sought and expert referral and MRI considered. Additional investigation includes history, assessment for maternal TORCH infection, MRI, fetal chromosome analysis, and fetal molecular DNA analysis (microarray) if the chromosomes are normal.

Rhombencephalosynapsis

Rhombencephalosynapsis is a rare hypoplasia of the cerebellum characterized by complete or partial absence of the vermis and fusion of the cerebellar hemispheres and dentate nuclei. Most cases are sporadic, although familial cases are described. Most die in childhood, but some survive into adulthood. Most survivors are neurologically delayed and have movement disorders.[134,145,146]

Rhombencephalosynapsis typically presents as hydrocephalus as early as 14 weeks, and VM may be the only

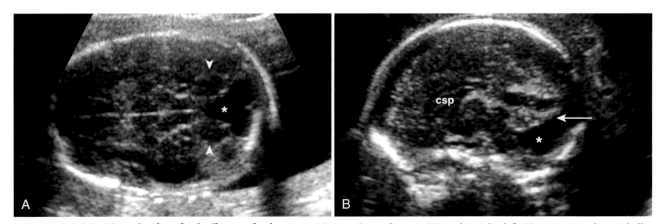

FIGURE 34-19. Vermis dysplasia/hypoplasia. A, Axial view shows fetus at 20 weeks with cleft (*) separating the cerebellar hemispheres *(arrowheads).* **B,** Sagittal view shows the cerebellar vermis to be deficient in its inferior portion, with a fluid space in the expected region of the lower vermis; corpus callosum and cavum septi pellucidi *(csp).*

prenatally evident ultrasound finding. Cerebellar findings may not be initially conspicuous on the usual axial views. The defining findings at ultrasound are a small, bean-shaped cerebellum that lacks the typical echogenic narrowing or "waisting" at the vermis and cerebellar hemispheric fissures, which are continuous from side to side without midline interruption. Midsagittal views show absence of the typical vermian fissures and may show an abnormally shaped fourth ventricle. These findings are more readily seen on MRI.[134,145,146]

Additional cerebral and somatic abnormalities are common. Cerebral findings primarily involve midline structures and include **aqueductal stenosis** (thus hydrocephalus), **agenesis of the corpus callosum**, **absent septum pellucidum**, and **septo-optic dysplasia.** Somatic abnormalities include segmentation errors of the spine, phalangeal and radial ray defects, and occasional defects of the cardiovascular, respiratory, and urinary tract. Some have the VACTERL-hydrocephalus association.[145,146]

Vertebral abnormalities, anal atresia, cardiac abnormalities, tracheoesophageal fistula, renal agenesis, and limb defects.

The differential diagnosis of small vermis includes molar-tooth abnormalities (**Joubert syndrome**), **Dandy-Walker malformation,** and **vermian hypogenesis,** but in these conditions there is a gap in the region of the vermis.[145] Pregnancy termination is considered in prenatally diagnosed cases; newborns generally receive supportive care.

Mega–Cisterna Magna

Mega–cisterna magna refers to an enlargement of the cisterna magna beyond 10 mm with intact vermis (Fig. 34-20). When this is an isolated finding, almost all

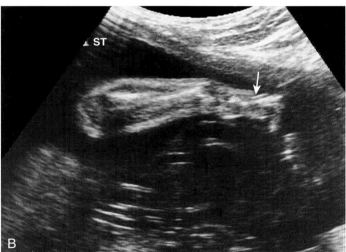

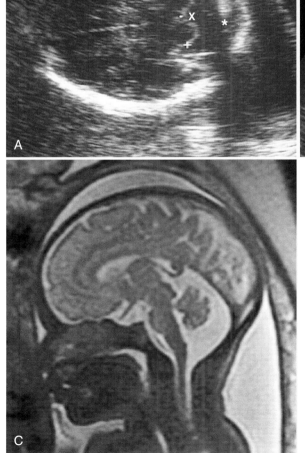

FIGURE 34-20. Mega–cisterna magna with and without associated anomalies. A, Mega–cisterna magna and cerebellar hypoplasia at 25 weeks. The cisterna magna measured 11 mm (*calipers* x). The cerebellum (*calipers* +) is small and under the tenth percentile. This fetus has cerebellar hypoplasia associated with olivopontocerebellar (OPC) dysplasia. **B,** Abnormal hand position caused by neurologic deficit with OPC dysplasia. The metacarpophalangeal joints were in fixed hyperextension (*arrow*) and fingers in fixed flexion. All fetal limb movements were abnormal. **C,** In a different fetus, mega–cisterna magna and otherwise normal-appearing brain on sagittal T2-weighted MR image.

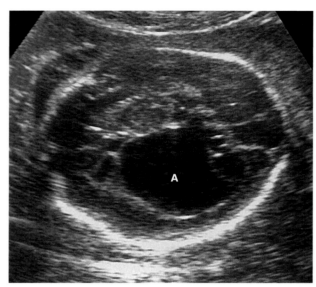

FIGURE 34-21. **Arachnoid cyst** (A) in the supratentorial, interhemispheric position at 25 weeks.

children (97%-100%) are normal.[25] However, if not isolated, only 11% have normal outcome. The majority of nonisolated cases have VM, congenital infection, or karyotype abnormalities, especially trisomy 18.[147,148] With aneuploidy, the ventricles are often of normal size.[149] When a large cisterna magna is found, there should be a careful search for other abnormalities.

Other Posterior Fossa Abnormalities

The vermis receives a disproportionate degree of discussion because vermian abnormalities are relatively easily seen at routine second-trimester ultrasound. Numerous other, difficult-to-detect or late-appearing abnormalities also involve the posterior fossa. These include hypoplasia, clefts, changes related to ischemia, bleed and infarct, cortical migration disorders (type II cobblestone lissencephaly), metabolic disorders, and miscellaneous neurodegenerative disorders.[123,124,130,141]

Arachnoid Cysts

Arachnoid cysts are benign, noncommunicating fluid collections within arachnoid membranes. Most appear stable and require no surgical treatment. They can occur intracranially and in the spinal canal. Locations by order of frequency are the sylvian fissure or temporal fossa, posterior fossa, over the cerebral convexity, and midline supratentorial, including suprasellar (Fig. 34-21). Even if very large, arachnoid cysts rarely cause symptoms. Occasionally they interfere with CSF circulation and require decompression. Arachnoid cysts in the suprasellar region may be associated with pituitary dysfunction. The differential diagnosis depends on the location. Arachnoid cysts in the posterior fossa can be confused with **Dandy-**

Walker malformation, **inferior vermian hypoplasia**, **mega–cisterna magna**, and **Blake's pouch cysts**. The differential diagnosis of supratentorial cysts includes **cavum veli interpositi**, **aneurysm of vein of Galen**, **hemorrhage**, and **cystic tumors**. Pediatric neurosurgical opinion is important in evaluating and counseling these patients, many of whom require no treatment. Midline cysts can accompany dysgenesis of the corpus callosum. Therefore, when a supratentorial cyst is seen, it is important to evaluate the entire corpus callosum.[15,36,128,150,151]

Malformations of Cortical Development

Malformations of cortical development are a heterogeneous collection of conditions involving disturbances in the normal proliferation, migration, and organization of neurons. Etiologies include intrinsic abnormalities in the genes controlling brain development or extrinsic causes that affect normal gene functions, such as maternal diseases (phenylketonuria), teratogens (anoxia, drugs, x-rays), and fetal infections. Often, etiology cannot be determined.[21,152-155] The final brain appearance and functional outcome relate to both the gene abnormality and the time of the insult. The responsible genes often function in many different body structures apart from the brain. As a result, abnormalities may be found in seemingly unrelated organs, as in **thanatophoric skeletal dysplasia,** where abnormal function of the FGFR3 gene causes both cortical brain malformations and skeletal abnormalities.[156] The detection of malformations of cortical development requires familiarity with normal developmental appearances and examination targeted to suspected changes. MRI is helpful, and multidisciplinary consultation is important for optimal prenatal assessment and counseling.

Barkovich et al.[152] have classified malformations of cortical development based on the stage of development (cell proliferation, neuronal migration, cortical organization) at which cortical development was first affected. The categories are based on known developmental steps, known pathologic features, known genetics (when possible), and neuroimaging features. All the conditions share variable degrees of thickened, disorganized cortical neuronal layers and alterations in sulcal and gyral patterns. The current classification is acknowledged to be neither perfect nor complete and is subject to updating; new genes and gene functions are regularly being discovered.

Microcephaly

Microcephaly implies a disproportionately small head for fetal age and body size. Precise diagnostic definition is difficult, but generally, microcephaly is diagnosed if the head circumference less than 3 SD below the mean for age and gender. Some suggest using 2 SD, but this will

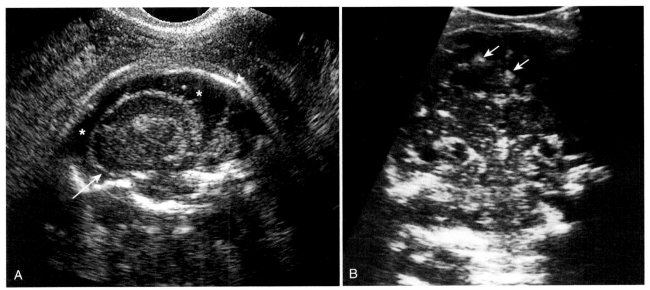

FIGURE 34-22. Microcephaly. A, Parasagittal view at 20 weeks shows the cerebrum to be very small and smooth *(arrow)*. The subarachnoid fluid is increased (*). Tentorium is visible *(arrowhead)*. Biparietal diameter (BPD) was only slightly smaller than expected for dates, but the scan clearly shows the small brain (micrencephaly). **B,** Coronal view of a different fetus with a small head shows abnormal brain texture and multiple calcifications *(arrows)* initially thought to indicate infection, but infection tests were negative, and ultimately a mitochondrial abnormality was diagnosed.

CLASSIFICATION OF MALFORMATIONS OF CORTICAL DEVELOPMENT (MCD)

ABNORMAL NEURONAL PROLIFERATION OR APOPTOSIS
Abnormal brain size
  Microcephaly
  Macrocephaly
  Hemimegalencephaly
Tumorlike conditions

ABNORMAL NEURONAL MIGRATION
Type 1: lissencephaly and subcortical band
  heterotopia
Type 2: cobblestone lissencephaly and complex or
  congenital muscular dystrophy

HETEROTOPIA

ABNORMAL CORTICAL ORGANIZATION
Polymicrogyria
Schizencephaly

MCD NOT OTHERWISE CLASSIFIED
Secondary to inborn errors of metabolism
Other

Modified from Barkovich AJ, Kuzniecky RI, Jackson GD, et al. A developmental and genetic classification for malformations of cortical development. Neurology 2005;65:1873-1887.

include many normal individuals. Incidence at birth ranges from 1 in 6250 to 8500.[157] Small head size can be associated with subnormal mental ability; the smaller the head circumference, the lower the performance level. The diagnosis implies failure of brain development (**micrencephaly**) following a great variety of prenatal causes, including genetic, environmental, asphyxia, infectious (CMV), maternal **phenylketonuria**, drugs (e.g., fetal alcohol syndrome), syndromes (e.g., **Smith-Lemli-Opitz, Cornelia de Lange**), and **irradiation**.[21,152,158,159] At pathologic examination, the brain may be small but normal in appearance, or it may have diverse findings, including porencephaly, abnormal gyri, absent corpus callosum, and VM. Associated CNS and non-CNS abnormalities are common.[158]

Microcephaly must be suspected if the hydrocephalus is more than 3 SD below the mean for gestational age. Other findings include abnormal head/abdomen circumference ratio, sloping forehead, and small frontal lobe size[157,160-162] (Fig. 34-22). Measurements alone have only a limited ability to diagnose microcephaly. In one study, only 4 of 24 fetuses with small measurements had the diagnosis confirmed at delivery.[161]

When a smaller-than-expected fetal head is encountered, there should be a careful search for cerebral and other anomalies that would help to confirm clinical importance. Examination of the brain often is difficult because the cranial bones become closely approximated and hinder visibility. MRI is helpful to depict the cerebral parenchyma and associated abnormalities. The diagnosis has been made as early as 15 weeks in pregnancies known to be at risk, but microcephaly may not be evident until late in pregnancy when the head size fails to grow normally.[5,163,164] Prenatally suspected cases should be thoroughly evaluated, including MRI, and counseled by a multidisciplinary team.[165] Additional investigation can include assessment for maternal TORCH infection, fetal chromosome analysis for mutation in chromosome 17.3, and if the chromosomes are normal, then microarray analysis may be considered.

Macrocephaly and Megalencephaly

Macrocephaly implies a large head with the occipito-frontal circumference above the 98th centile for gestational age. **Megalencephaly** refers to cerebral gigantism, or enlarged brain, and is rare. It can be isolated or seen with many conditions, such as overgrowth syndromes (**Beckwith-Wiedemann, Sotos, Weaver**), skeletal dysplasias (**thanatophoric dysplasia, achondroplasia**), and neurocutaneous syndromes (**neurofibromatosis type 1**).[21,165-168]

Benign familial macrocephaly (external hydrocephalus) accounts for about 50% of cases of macrocephaly. It is an autosomal dominant condition with increased subarachnoid fluid (Fig. 34-23). It typically presents late in pregnancy or even after delivery, but has been seen as early as 18 weeks when there is a history of other family

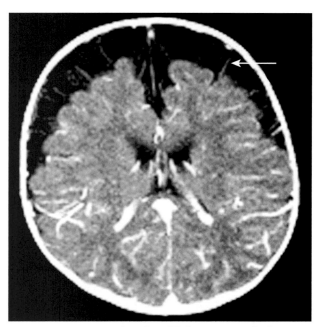

FIGURE 34-23. Benign familial macrocephaly. These cases often present at term or postnatally. Postnatal CT scan shows the subarachnoid fluid to be increased and traversed by normal arachnoid vessels *(arrow)*. These vessels help to differentiate this generally benign condition from subdural bleeds. *(Courtesy Dr. Charles Raybaud, Hospital for Sick Children, Toronto.)*

members who had large heads.[169-172] Most children are functionally normal.[173]

When the head measurements are larger than expected (macrocephaly), there should be a careful search for intracranial abnormalities.[5] Prenatal diagnosis of true megalencephaly (bilateral cerebral giantism with otherwise normal-appearing brain) would only be possible if dates have been established in early pregnancy, and asymmetrical IUGR thus can be excluded.[21] Prenatally suspected cases should be thoroughly evaluated, including MRI, and counseled by a multidisciplinary team.[165]

Hemimegalencephaly

Hemimegalencephaly is a malformation of cortical development with hamartomatous enlargement of one hemisphere. Most cases are sporadic and of unknown etiology. It may be isolated or associated with neurocutaneous and somatic hemihypertrophy syndromes. The affected hemisphere and ventricle are enlarged and have abnormal texture and sulcation. The unaffected hemisphere is generally normal but distorted due to compression. Functional deficiency and seizures are common, the latter on occasion requiring hemispherectomy.[174-176]

Lissencephaly

Lissencephaly describes a brain surface that is smooth and lacks the normal sulci and gyri. It follows a global disturbance in neuronal migration.[27,40,177] The most severe manifestation is a completely smooth cortex lacking gyri (**agyria**), but some cases show large, malformed gyri (**pachygyria**). There are two types, caused by fundamentally different mechanisms. In **type 1** lissencephaly, neurons fail to migrate to the cortex. In **type 2** lissencephaly, the neurons do not stop at the cortical surface and overmigrate into the subarachnoid membranes, resulting in "cobblestone cortex." Both types are etiologically heterogeneous and related to many gene mutations, with additional CNS and somatic abnormalities.[40,152,178,179] Previously it was thought that diagnosis was not possible before 28 weeks, but familiarity with the stages of sulcal development has allowed diagnosis of type 1 (**Miller-Dieker syndrome**) by 23 weeks.[27,177] Severe cases of type 2 (**Walker-Warburg syndrome**) may be evident even earlier, and an at-risk fetus has been suspected at 12 weeks.[180]

Type 1, or **classical lissencephaly,** manifests as a smooth cortex and hourglass-shaped brain with mild VM, a primitive insula and delayed or absent sulcation and sparing of the cerebellar vermis, and abnormal cortical vascularity (Fig. 34-24). There are several variants. The more common Miller-Dieker syndrome with gene abnormality at 17p13.3 (LIS1) typically has **congenital heart disease, omphalocele, genitourinary abnormalities, IUGR,** and **dystrophic facies.** In the **X-linked** type 1 lissencephaly, the girls may function

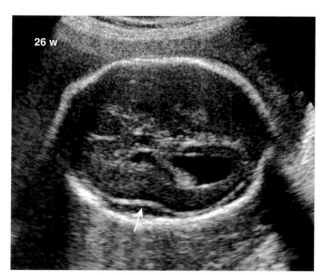

FIGURE 34-24. Type 1 lissencephaly (Miller-Dieker syndrome) in 23-week fetus. Note the mild ventriculomegaly and lack of sulcal formation. The insula is very smooth and shallow *(arrow)* and lacks the angular plateau appearance expected at this age.

normally despite "double cortex" cerebral changes that can be seen with MRI, but boys do poorly.[27,152,177,181]

Type 2, or **cobblestone lissencephaly,** is associated with malfunction of genes that also function in muscle development (e.g., POMT1/2, FKRP, FKTN). The conditions are grouped with **congenital muscular dystrophy.** These infants typically have additional CNS and somatic abnormalities and lack muscle tone at birth. The most severe phenotype, Walker-Warburg syndrome, is also called **HARD-E** for hydrocephalus, agyria, retinal dysplasia, and/or encephalocele. Less severe phenotypes include **Fukuyama syndrome** and **muscle-eye-brain disease.**[11,40] Ultrasound changes may be evident by 20 weeks and include VM and absent, delayed, or abnormal sulcal development; cerebellar vermian dysplasia; eye abnormalities; small encephalocele; and abnormal brainstem[27] (Fig. 34-25). Fetal MRI and gene mutation analysis can help confirm the diagnosis. Postnatal outcome is poor.[10,40,152,155,182]

Focal Cortical Changes

Focal cortical changes typically manifest late and are difficult to detect with ultrasound.[181] They are typically found at MRI in fetuses referred for evaluation of other abnormalities initially detected by ultrasound.

Polymicrogyria is characterized by numerous small, abnormal gyri with variable distribution. It is the most common cortical malformation in children presenting with epilepsy. Polymicrogyria may be isolated or associated with many genetic and acquired conditions. Presentation typically is in late pregnancy but can be seen in the midtrimester (Fig. 34-26; see also Fig. 34-8).

Heterotopia describes localized clusters of disorganized neurons in abnormal locations anywhere in the brain. It is very common and has heterogeneous etiology. Cases can be isolated or associated with many different syndromes. Intraparenchymal nodules can be difficult to recognize by ultrasound. Subependymal periventricular heterotopia manifests as nodular ventricular contours[181,183-185] (Fig. 34-27). Affected children may be normal or may have variable deficits and epilepsy.

Pachygyria describes large, abnormal disordered sulci and gyri that can accompany different syndromes.

Schizencephaly (split brain) is a rare structural malformation of the cerebrum characterized by congenital clefts or defects that are usually symmetrical and involve the parietal or temporal brain. The clefts are lined by cortical gray matter, unlike porencephaly, where white matter lines the clefts. Etiology can be destructive **(encephaloclastic)** or developmental. Destructive etiologies include vascular injury, teratogen exposure (e.g., cocaine), infections (especially CMV), and trauma, and appearances can be similar to porencephaly or hydranencephaly. Developmental cases arise from disordered neuronal migration and organization and are considered to be related to polymicrogyria. The tracts may be open **(open lip),** allowing CSF communication between the ventricle and subarachnoid space, or may be solid **(closed lip,** consisting of an abnormal, solid gray matter tract between the ventricle and brain surface).[152,186-188] Most cases are found in late pregnancy during investigation of VM, but a case was reported at 23 weeks.[188] The diagnosis rests on detection of the cerebral clefts or abnormal gray matter traversing from ventricle to cortex (Fig. 34-28). Midline brain defects may occur, including septo-optic dysplasia, dysgenesis of the corpus callosum, and absence of the septi pellucidi. Fetal MRI allows superior delineation of upper cortex and gray matter.[11,152,187,188] Neurodevelopmental delay and seizures are common. Prognosis relates to the size of the defect. Suspected cases benefit from multidisciplinary consultation and counseling.[187,189,190]

Other Malformations of Cortical Development

Cortical malformations can accompany infections, inborn errors of metabolism (e.g., peroxisomal disorders), mitochondrial disease, and conditions with unknown etiology.[21,152] Many metabolic conditions are associated with abnormal brain development.[191-193] All these are rarely encountered prenatally. The most common is **Zellweger (cerebrohepatorenal) syndrome,** which is lethal and has multiple abnormalities, including neuronal impairment, hepatic disorders, cystic renal malformations, and **chondrodysplasia punctata.** It may manifest in the first trimester as nuchal thickening[194] and in the second trimester as VM, cortical renal cysts, and hepatomegaly. Third-trimester changes include

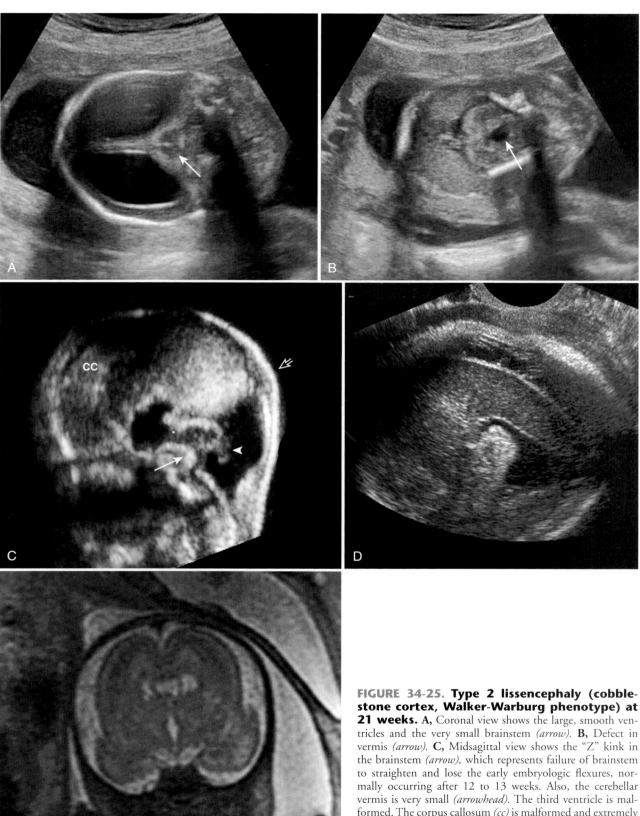

FIGURE 34-25. Type 2 lissencephaly (cobble-stone cortex, Walker-Warburg phenotype) at 21 weeks. A, Coronal view shows the large, smooth ventricles and the very small brainstem *(arrow)*. **B,** Defect in vermis *(arrow)*. **C,** Midsagittal view shows the "Z" kink in the brainstem *(arrow),* which represents failure of brainstem to straighten and lose the early embryologic flexures, normally occurring after 12 to 13 weeks. Also, the cerebellar vermis is very small *(arrowhead).* The third ventricle is malformed. The corpus callosum *(cc)* is malformed and extremely elevated. There is a minute occipital encephalocele *(open arrowhead).* This fetus also had eye abnormalities. **D,** In a different fetus at 36 weeks, transvaginal scan shows smooth cortex, abnormal for this gestational age. **E,** Coronal T2-weighted MR image shows the smooth cortex and abnormal bands of high signal intensity in the parenchyma. Note the prominent extra-axial CSF spaces.

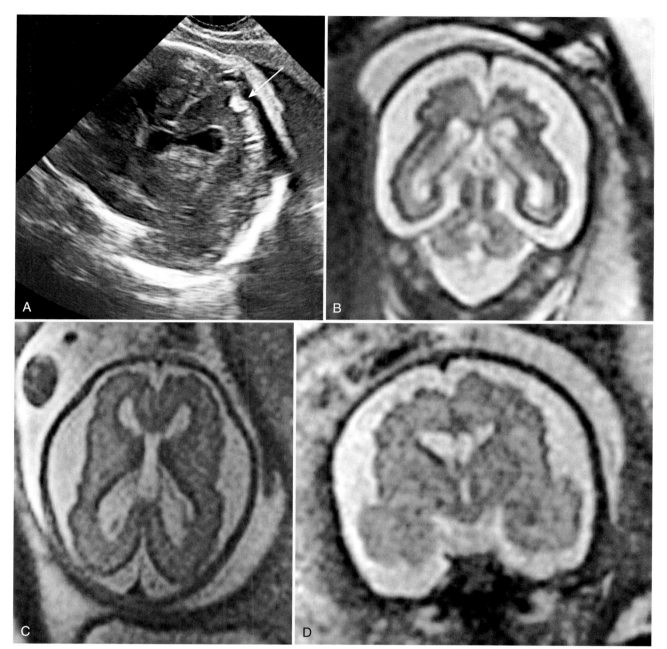

FIGURE 34-26. Polymicrogyria. A, Irregular appearance to the cortex and cortical calcification *(arrow)* on coronal transvaginal sonogram at 25 weeks. **B** and **C,** Coronal and axial T2-weighted MR images show sawtooth appearance to the cortex at 25 weeks. Note how the calcifications were better visualized on the sonogram than on MRI. **D,** Polymicrogyria at 30 weeks' gestational age. Note prominent extra-axial CSF.

abnormal gyration, periventricular leukodystrophy, and subependymal pseudocysts.[195] The diagnosis can be confirmed by DNA and biochemical testing of fetal cells obtained by chorionic villus sampling (CVS).[194]

Tuberous sclerosis (TSC) is a multisystem, hamartomatous condition with abnormal proliferation of anomalous cerebral cell types. There is notable involvement of the brain, skin, heart, and kidneys. It is autosomal dominant, and two genes have been discovered to date, TSC1 and TSC2. However, about 70% of cases represent a new

(de novo) mutation. Epilepsy and neurologic impairment are common. Morbidity and mortality predominantly relate to CNS and renal disease. The diagnosis is made clinically based on a list of findings, including tubers, subependymal nodules, giant cell astrocytomas, cardiac rhabdomyomas, and renal angiomyolipomas.[196]

Prenatal diagnosis generally is made in late pregnancy after discovery of echogenic cardiac rhabdomyomas and demonstration of subependymal nodule or cortical tubers on neurosonography or MRI (Fig. 34-29). In

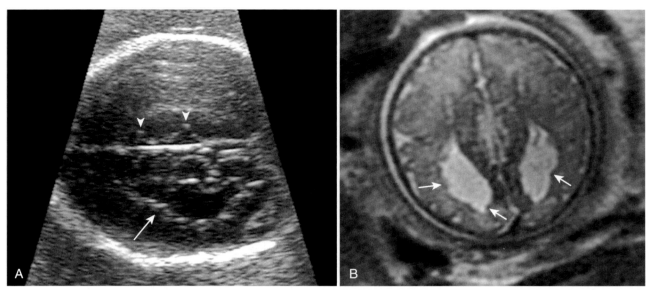

FIGURE 34-27. Periventricular nodular heterotopia and agenesis of the corpus callosum ACC). A, In fetus with ACC at 31 weeks, note the very nodular lining of the ventricle wall *(arrow)*. This represents accumulations of neurons that have failed to migrate to the cortex. Note the separation of the hemispheres and abnormal alignment of interhemispheric sulci *(arrowheads)*. **B,** Transverse T2-weighted MR image in a different fetus at 35 weeks shows ACC and nodular heterotopias *(arrows)*.

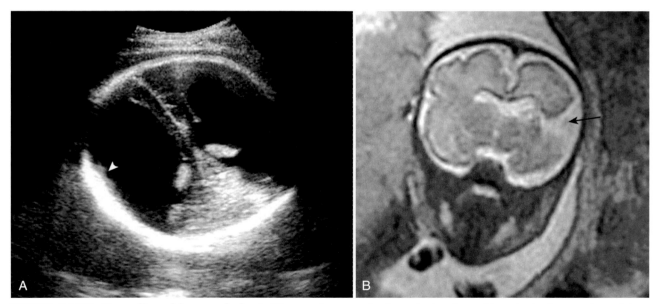

FIGURE 34-28. Open-lip schizencephaly. A, There are large gaps in the parietal regions with no brain tissue at the periphery *(arrowhead)*. There is partial sparing of the frontal and occipital regions. **B,** Coronal T2-weighted MR image in a different fetus with absent septal leaflets (absent septum pellucidum) shows region of schizencephaly *(arrow)*.

at-risk fetuses, MRI has shown lesions as early as 21 weeks.[197] In at-risk families, if the abnormal gene is known, diagnosis is possible using CVS or amniocentesis. Diagnosis in other suspected cases may be aided by looking for subtle manifestations of TSC in the parents.

Agenesis/Dysgenesis of Corpus Callosum

These disorders describe abnormalities of the development of the corpus callosum, which is the largest of the neural commissures connecting the cerebral hemispheres. The corpus callosum starts to develop at about 12 weeks from the lamina terminalis near the anterior end of the third ventricle, as a bundle of fibers connecting the left to the right hemisphere, and becomes detectable by about 15 weeks and complete by 20 weeks. It develops in an anteroposterior manner, beginning anteriorly with the rostrum and then forming the genu, body, and finally the splenium posteriorly.[14,23,111,198] The normal corpus callosum measures 17 mm at 18 weeks and grows to 44 mm by term. There is no gender difference in

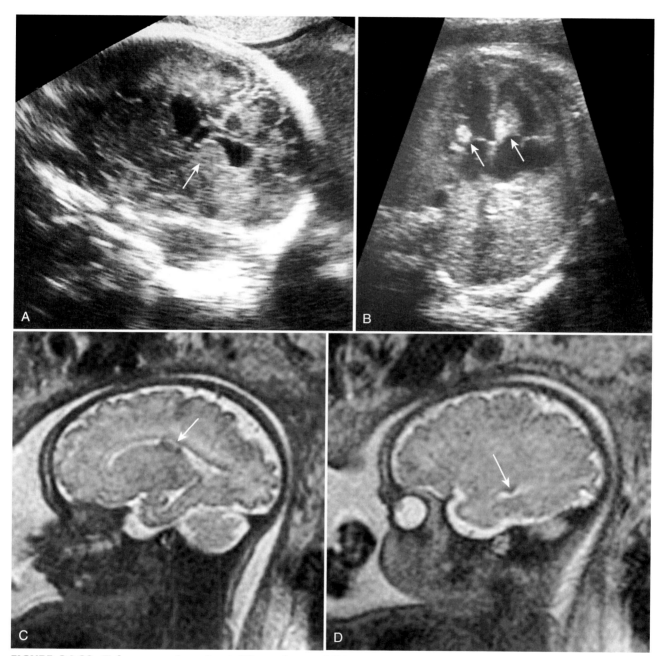

FIGURE 34-29. Tuberous sclerosis at 30 weeks on MRI. A, Typical hamartoma, or **giant-cell tumor,** is visible at the foramen of Monro indenting the anterior frontal horn of the lateral ventricle *(arrow).* Both ventricles are dilated. **B, Rhabdomyomas** involving the heart are visible as echogenic cardiac masses in the left and right ventricles *(arrows).* **C** and **D,** Subependymal hamartomas in a different fetus with cardiac rhabdomyomas. Sagittal views demonstrate low-signal-intensity lesions projecting into the body and temporal horn of the lateral ventricles. These subependymal tubers were not identified sonographically. *(C and D from Levine D. MR imaging of fetal brain and spine. In Magnetic resonance imaging of the brain and spine. Philadelphia, Lippincott 2008.)*

length, but the corpus callosum is thicker in girls.[199-201] Corpus callosum development is associated with the development of the leaflets of the cavum septi pellucidi (CSP).[23] When the septal leaflets are present, at least the anterior portion of the corpus callosum has formed.

Agenesis of the corpus callosum (ACC) may be complete or partial, developmental or acquired.[111,198] The prevalence of ACC in neonates is about 3:1000 to 7:1000, but is higher in developmentally disabled individuals. It may be an isolated abnormality with very little functional disturbance, but most cases have additional problems. Additional CNS abnormalities occur in up to 80%, especially Dandy-Walker malformation, inferior vermian hypoplasia, and abnormal neuronal migration. Somatic and metabolic abnormalities are seen in up to 60%, including face, congenital heart disease, and skeletal and genitourinary abnormalities. The high incidence of associated malformations suggests that ACC is part of a widespread developmental disturbance.[111,198,202]

Developmental disturbances after the corpus callosum has started to form usually interrupt the formation of the more posterior parts of the corpus callosum, but insults after callosal development is complete can cause secondary atrophy of previously developed central portions. Because callosal development is not complete until 20 weeks, early diagnosis of ACC may be difficult.[111,198,203] The key to early diagnosis is the cavum septi pellucidi (CSP), which is generally seen by 17 weeks.[2] If the cavum of the septum pellucidum is absent or has an abnormal shape, ACC and other malformations should be suspected. In the second trimester, however, ACC can easily be missed.[29,204] Ultrasonic appearances are subtle on axial scans (Fig. 34-30; see also Fig. 34-27; **Videos 34-7** and **34-8**).

Once the diagnosis is suspected, coronal and parasagittal views and 3-D ultrasound help to confirm the diagnosis. On coronal views the third ventricle is elevated; the medial walls of the anterior horns are indented from their medial aspect by the bundles of Probst (buildup of fibers that failed to cross midline; Viking horn configuration). As a result, on the coronal view the anterior horns configuration changes from V to U (Viking horn appearance), and an interhemispheric cyst may be present. On parasagittal views the corpus callosum is absent, and in the third trimester the sulci on the interhemispheric brain surface show a "sunburst" orientation radiating from the thalamus.[111,198] Before about 24 weeks, the metopic suture of the frontal bone and anterior fontanelle offer a clear window for visualizing the corpus callosum. Multiplanar 3-D ultrasound scanning is helpful to obtain midsagittal views, but attention should be paid to identifying the actual corpus callosum, not only the pericallosal sulcus.[205,206] If the head is deep in the pelvis, transvaginal scans can provide especially clear views. Color flow Doppler scans can be used to demonstrate an abnormal course of the cingulate and pericallosal arteries. Normally these vessels follow the contour of the calloso-marginal sulcus, but with ACC they assume a more radial course. Occasionally, fetuses with callosal abnormalities develop interhemispheric cysts or a midline **lipoma.** MRI is helpful to confirm the diagnosis and search for additional, subtle abnormalities, such as migrational disorders.[111,183,198,204]

Pitfalls in sonographic interpretation include mistaking the high position of the third ventricle, other fluid spaces, and the fornices for the cavum of the septum pellucidum. If the axial head views do not show the normal appearance of the septal leaflets, additional views can be obtained to evaluate the corpus callosum.[207] Also, the corpus callosum is hypoechoic, but the surrounding pericallosal sulcus is echogenic. On 3-D reconstructions, some authors have incorrectly labeled the echogenic pericallosal sulcus as the corpus callosum. Lipomas associated with callosal dysgenesis are echogenic and can parallel the superior margin of the corpus callosum. Care must be taken to correctly identify structures on 3-D reconstructions.[184,205]

Investigation of suspected cases includes detailed ultrasound, karyotype (chromosomal abnormalities occur in about 10%), microarray, screen for TORCH infections, and MRI. Prognosis relates to the associated anomalies. The prognosis for isolated ACC can be good, but up to 15% to 36% will develop problems that may not become apparent until later in life. If other anomalies are detected, outcome is poor.[183,198,202,208,209]

Absence of Septi Pellucidi and Septo-Optic Dysplasia

Septal agenesis is rare and occurs in about 2 to 3 per 100,000 pregnancies. It may be isolated but more often is seen in association with other developmental abnormalities, such as septo-optic dysplasia, ACC, holoprosencephaly, and malformations of cortical development.[111] **Septo-optic dysplasia** (SOD; **De Morisier syndrome**) is heterogeneous in etiology and appearance. It manifests as variable degrees of hypoplasia of the optic nerves, absence of septi pellucidi, pituitary hypoplasia, and endocrine defects. The prognosis is variable and includes disturbed vision and hypothalamic-pituitary insufficiency, including growth deficit and diabetes insipidus.[111,210] At ultrasound, there is absence of the septi pellucidi. On coronal views the frontal horns are squared with inferior pointing. Differentiation from mild degrees of holoprosencephaly can be difficult. In holoprosencephaly the fornices are more likely to be fused. Multiplanar 3-D and MRI are helpful.

Intracranial Calcifications

Fetal intracranial calcifications are rare. They usually occur late in gestation (see Figs. 34-22, *B;* 34-26, *A;* and 34-31, *A*), are often associated with fetal infections, and

---

> ### ULTRASOUND FINDINGS OF ABSENCE OF CORPUS CALLOSUM
>
> Mild ventriculomegaly (VM) with very thin anterior horns and pointing (teardrop shape = colpocephaly).
> Ventricles are parallel.
> Too many lines between hemispheres on axial views (3 lines = falx + medial surface of each hemisphere).
> Cavum septi pellucidi is absent.
> Too many sulci perpendicular to the interhemispheric fissure (hairy midline).
> Third-trimester midsagittal view shows radial orientation of sulci from the thalamus (sunburst appearance).

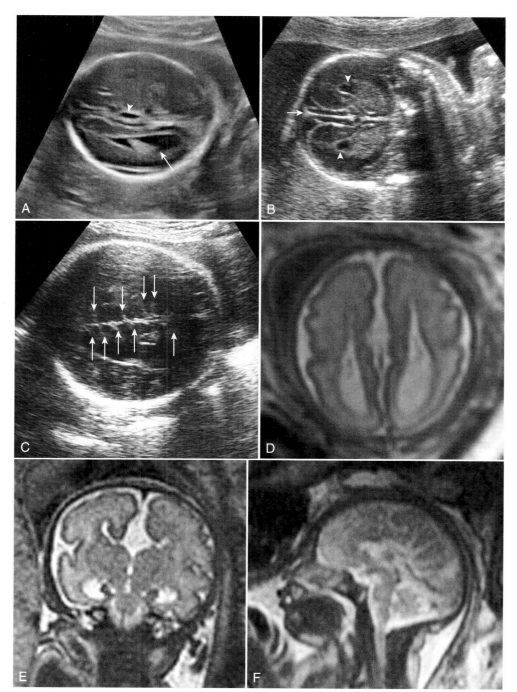

FIGURE 34-30. Agenesis of corpus callosum (ACC). A, Ventricular view at 21 menstrual weeks shows characteristic borderline dilation of occipital ventricle *(arrow)* and pointed, slightly spread anterior horns. This "teardrop" ventricle configuration is called **colpocephaly.** The midline fluid space *(arrowhead)* is the elevated dilated third ventricle, which should not be mistaken for the cavum septi pellucidi, which should be more rectangular and is absent in fetuses with ACC. **B,** Coronal view through the anterior ventricles *(arrows)* shows that the frontal horns have a U or "Viking horn" configuration instead of the normal V orientation. The hemispheres are excessively separated from the falx *(arrow),* and the septal leaflets are absent. **C,** Axial ventricular view at 33 weeks demonstrates ventriculomegaly and too many sulci perpendicular to the interhemispheric fissure *(arrows),* the axial correlate of the "sunburst" sign. **D,** Transverse T2-weighted MR image at 29 weeks shows colpocephaly with teardrop-shaped ventricles and parallel orientation of the frontal horns. **E,** Coronal MR image in a different fetus at 30 weeks shows the vertical orientation of the frontal horns and lack of crossing fibers of the corpus callosum. **F,** Sagittal view from fetus at 31 weeks with **partial ACC** shows the sunburst pattern posteriorly, where interhemispheric sulci extend farther inferiorly than normal due to lack of corpus callosum.

suggest a poor prognosis. Anatomically, calcifications occur in areas of cell necrosis and may line ventricles or occur in the parenchyma. Associated severe CNS changes are common, including microcephaly, VM, intracranial hemorrhage, and porencephalic cysts. Differential diagnosis includes intrauterine infections (especially CMV and toxoplasmosis), teratoma, tuberous sclerosis, Sturge-Weber syndrome, and venous sinus thrombosis.[211,212]

Branching linear densities are described in the thalami and basal ganglia. These represent **mineralization of the thalamostriate vessels** (Fig. 34-31). Some believe these relate to calcification, whereas others suggest mineral deposits such as iron.[213] These mineralized densities may be seen in normal fetuses but also occur in association with many conditions, including infection (CMV, rubella, syphilis), aneuploidy (especially trisomy 13), alcohol, asphyxia, twin-twin transfusion, dysmorphism, and congenital disorders.[211,213-215]

Infections

A variety of organisms can cross the placenta and infect the fetus causing encephalitis, variably followed by microcephaly, VM, calcifications, and malformations of cortical development. The TORCH group is seen most often, but other organisms include **varicella, congenital lymphocytic choriomeningitis, parvovirus B19, echovirus,** and **parasites.** About 5% of VM has been attributed to infections. CMV is the most common infection, followed by **toxoplasmosis** (*Toxoplasma gondii* is a protozoan parasite acquired through contact with uncooked

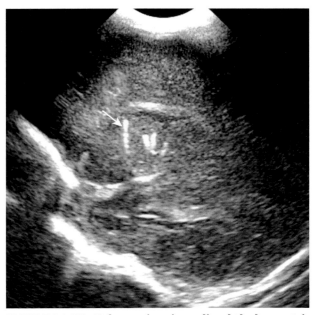

FIGURE 34-31. Echogenic mineralized thalamostriate vessels (arrow). These form an echogenic arborizing (branching) pattern in the thalamus and may be seen in normal fetuses but can be associated with many fetal conditions.

meat and animals, particularly cats and cat litter) and **herpes simplex.**[63, 216] The severity of injury often relates more to the age when infection first occurred and affected brain development than to the specific organism.[63]

Cytomegalovirus, the most common infection, affects about 0.2% to 2.0% of live births. CMV is typically acquired through contact with people, especially children, because CMV is prevalent in the population. After maternal infection, transmission to the fetus ranges from 25% to 70%. Even supposedly immune mothers may still infect their fetus. Fetal infection varies from mild to severe. About 60% of infected fetuses are symptomatic to varying degree. Of these, 20% die. Among survivors, 90% develop neurologic sequelae of possibly late onset.[217]

Early-onset infections before 20 weeks can result in malformations of cortical development, striking periventricular echoes and cysts, calcifications, schizencephaly, thalamostriate vessel echogenicity, and abnormalities of the corpus callosum and cerebellum (Fig. 34-32). Infections acquired in later pregnancy generally have normal cortical appearances but may also develop periventricular and parenchymal echogenicity, as well as **IUGR, hydrops, hepatosplenomegaly,** and large or small placenta.

The general consensus is that ultrasound plays a limited role in the prenatal diagnosis of CMV because it is only about 20% sensitive. However, positive ultrasound findings predict infection in about 80%, and major findings such as microcephaly, cortical malformations, and parenchymal lesions strongly predict a poor prognosis.[212,218,219] Investigation of fetuses with suggestive cerebral findings includes maternal history, TORCH screen, and amniocentesis (for CMV and parvovirus B19), although these tests are not completely accurate.[218,220] Treatment depends on the etiology of the infection. For example, with toxoplasmosis, successful antimicrobial treatment postnatally can decrease the size of the calcifications and improve neurologic status.[221]

Vascular Malformations

A variety of vascular abnormalities involve the fetal brain. The most common is **aneurysm of vein of Galen,** which describes dilation of the vein in association with a spectrum of arteriovenous malformations, some of which may be pial.[216,222,223] Typically, prenatal ultrasound shows an elongated anechoic structure behind the thalamus in the expected region of the vein of Galen, with flow on color Doppler (Fig. 34-33). Findings of high-output cardiac failure may include prominent neck veins, edema, and hydrops.[216,223,224]

The dilated vein may be the vein of Galen but often is a persistent dilated prosencephalic vein of Markowski or falcine sinus, the course of which is not into the straight sinus but rather cephalad in the falx to the

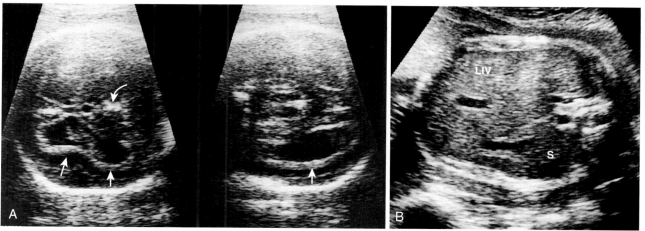

FIGURE 34-32. Fetal cytomegalovirus (CMV) infection at 28 weeks. A, CMV infection shows enlarged ventricles with thick, calcified walls *(straight arrows)*. There is also calcification in the brainstem *(curved arrow)*. **B,** Hepatosplenomegaly compressing the fetal stomach helps confirm fetal infection; *LIV,* liver; *S,* spleen.

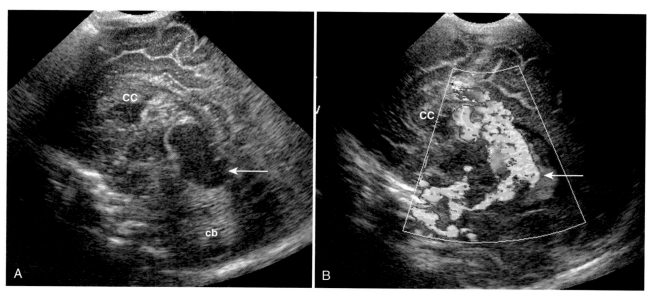

FIGURE 34-33. Vein of Galen aneurysm. A, Midsagittal view shows a hypoechoic "cyst" *(arrow)* behind the brainstem and under the splenium of the corpus callosum *(cc); cb,* cerebellum. At first glance it could be mistaken to be a cavum veli interpositi. **B,** Color Doppler examination shows the extensive vascularity due to the arteriovenous malformation associated with this dilated vein.

superior sagittal sinus.[225] The differential diagnosis includes cystic lesions such as arachnoid cyst, cavum veli interpositi, hematoma, and pineal tumor. Doppler examination establishes the diagnosis.[216,224]

Arteriovenous malformations frequently result in cardiac overload and heart failure in utero and postnatally.[216] Of prenatally diagnosed cases, 50% die prenatally or in early childhood, generally from progressive heart failure. Variable neurodevelopmental sequelae were found in 10%, and about 25% had normal development. Prognosis of prenatally detected cases is poor if additional findings are present, including hydrops and cerebral changes such as VM, edema, and porenceph-

aly.[223] Postnatal treatment includes hemodynamic stabilization and angiographic embolization as needed.[216,224]

Thrombosis of Dural Sinuses

Thrombosis in dural sinuses can be idiopathic (40%), but cases can be seen with hypercoagulable states such as **trauma, infection, polycythemia,** and **deficiency of physiologic anticoagulants** (e.g., antithrombin protein C, protein S, factor V Leiden). Ultrasound typically reveals an echogenic mass (the thrombus) surrounded by a hypoechogenic area in the region of the venous sinuses, generally near the torcula and associated with absence of

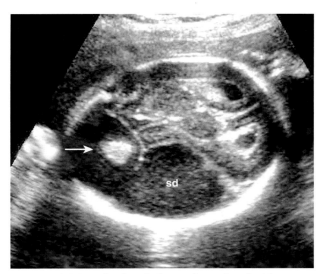

FIGURE 34-34. Sagittal sinus thrombosis. There is an echogenic mass *(arrow)* in a fluidlike space in the midline anteriorly. This represents thrombus in a dilated sagittal sinus. There is also a subdural collection *(sd). (Courtesy Dr. Katherine Fong, Mt. Sinai Hospital, Toronto).*

flow (Fig. 34-34). The more proximal sinuses may be dilated and the brain compressed. Many dural thromboses are initially misdiagnosed as tumors or subdural bleeds. Most cases are found in the second and third trimesters and can be confirmed with MRI. The prognosis is variable and may be favorable if no other abnormalities are found and the brain appears normal.[216,226]

Hemorrhagic Lesions

Intracranial hemorrhage describes bleeding in and around the brain. The incidence is about 1 in 10,000 live births.[227] The most common sites are similar to those seen in premature neonates. In a series of 109 cranial bleeds, 89 were intracerebral (79 intraventricular, 10 infratentorial), and 20 were subdural.[228] As in neonates, cerebral bleeds are graded from 1 to 4 and may be followed by **chemical ventriculitis** (thick echogenic ventricular lining), hydrocephalus, porencephalic cysts, white matter injury, and periventricular leukomalacia. About half are idiopathic. Predisposing factors include hypoxia, fetal coagulation disorders (including **alloimmune thrombocytopenia** and maternal anticoagulation), death of a monochromic co-twin, seizures, viral or bacterial infection, febrile disease, drugs (cocaine), maternal-fetal hemorrhage, and trauma.[216,227-230]

At ultrasound, the bleed appears as an echogenic collection in the ventricles and surrounding brain (Fig. 34-35). This hemorrhage later organizes and condenses into clots and may be associated with VM and echogenic thickening of ventricular walls (chemical ventriculitis). The findings may resolve or progress to hydrocephalus, porencephaly, cerebral clefts, and cortical malformations. Those with ischemia may also develop cystic

leukomalacia. Subdural hemorrhages appear as an echogenic collection underlying the skull and compressing the adjacent brain.[227,228]

The prognosis varies greatly and depends largely on fetal age, extent of injury, and underlying factors. About 50% die in utero or shortly after birth, and about half the survivors have deficits. As expected, some with mild changes may resolve completely, and more severe (grade 3-4) changes and cerebral changes predict a poor outcome. Ultrasound can accurately diagnose bleeds, but MRI can more accurately define the extent of the lesion and may demonstrate additional ischemic changes in white matter.[227,228] Investigation of suspected cases includes trauma and drug history, as well as maternal screen for antiplatelet antibodies and thrombophilia.[227,228]

Hydranencephaly

Hydranencephaly is a rare disorder in which almost all the cerebral hemispheres in the approximate distribution of the supraclinoid middle cerebral artery are absent and replaced by CSF and debris covered by a thin, membranous sac. There is partial sparing in the distribution of the anterior and posterior cerebral arteries, including portions of the frontal, temporal, and occipital lobes. The basal ganglia and thalami are hypoplastic, but the brainstem and cerebellum are intact. Cases are sporadic, with an incidence of about 1 in 5000 pregnancies. Many consider hydranencephaly as the most severe form of porencephaly following occlusion of the internal carotid artery or middle cerebral artery. The exact predisposing cause is unknown but may be associated with infections, toxins, hypoxic conditions, and trauma and may be a complication of twin-twin transfusion syndrome.[231-233]

At ultrasound, the cerebrum is replaced by mildly echogenic fluid, and the parietal cerebral cortex is absent. Partial sparing is evident in the frontal and occipital lobes (Fig. 34-36). The falx is present but may be hypoplastic. Posterior fossa structures appear normal. Most cases are found in late pregnancy, but cases have been described as early as 11 weeks.[234] Findings start with cerebral echogenicity, thought to result form ischemia or hemorrhage, followed by characteristic fluid replacement of the cerebrum.[235] The differential diagnosis includes other conditions causing large, fluid-filled cranial spaces, such as severe hydrocephalus, alobar holoprosencephaly, bilateral subdural collections, and schizencephaly. With **hydrocephalus,** there is generally uniform ventricular enlargement and a peripheral thin cerebral mantle, and color Doppler ultrasound may show flow in the middle cerebral arteries. In **holoprosencephaly** there is thalamic fusion and absence of the falx. **Subdural collections** compress the brain into the midline.[232,233] Large **schizencephalic clefts** can appear similar to hydranencephaly, but in schizencephaly the lips of the clefts are lined by gray matter, which may be identifiable on MRI.

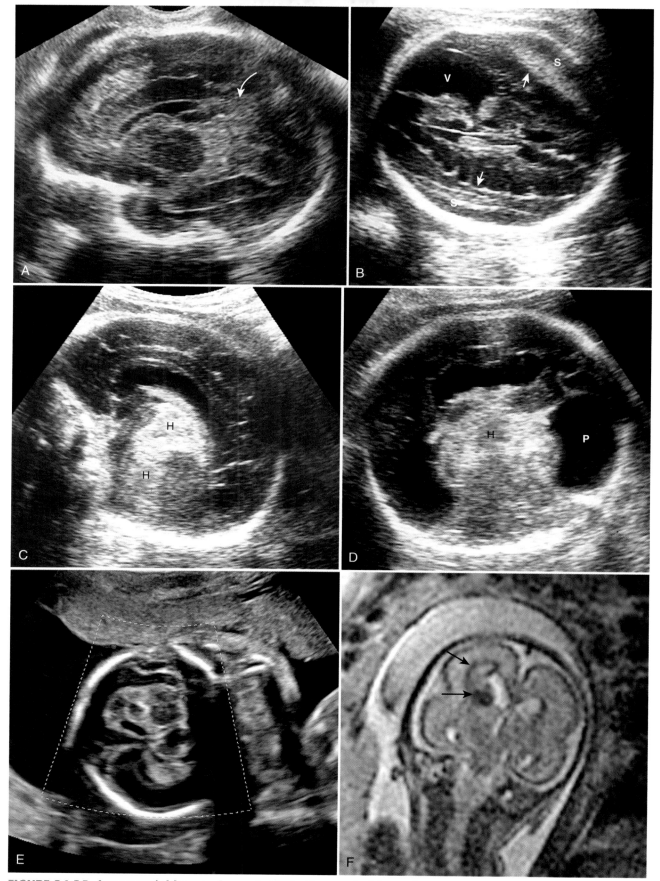

FIGURE 34-35. Intracranial hemorrhage. A, Grade 4 intracerebral hemorrhage with clot *(arrow)* extending into the occipital cortex on parasagittal view. **B, Bilateral subdural hemorrhages** *(S)* compressing the brain *(arrows)* and associated with slight asymmetrical ventricular enlargement *(V)*. These hemorrhages resolved spontaneously in this case, and the child did well. No cause was found. Most children with this finding do poorly. **C,** Parasagittal, and **D,** coronal, views of thalamic and brainstem hemorrhage *(H)* at 38 weeks. The posthemorrhagic porencephalic cyst *(P)* helps to differentiate this from tumor such as teratoma. Hypoxia was the likely etiology. This fetus died shortly after the examination. **E,** Coronal view at 23 weeks shows a grade 4 hemorrhage with clot extending into the parenchyma. **F,** T2-weighted MR image shows the low signal intensity of blood products in the parenchyma *(arrows)*. The relatively high signal intensity in the surrounding parenchyma suggests edema and venous infarction.

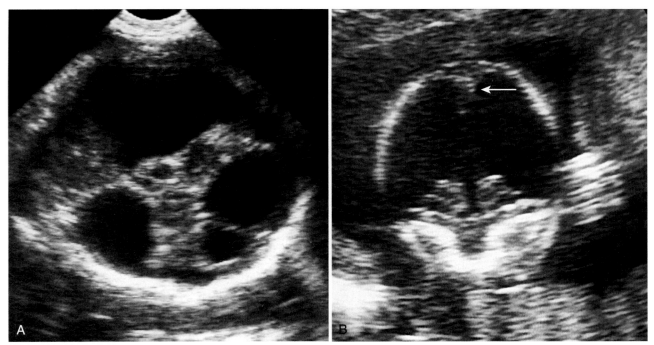

FIGURE 34-36. Hydranencephaly. A, Transverse thalamic view at 38 weeks shows asymmetrical cerebral destruction with preserved interhemispheric fissure. **B,** Hydranencephaly at 17 weeks shows cranium filled with fluid. At first, the appearance suggests alobar holoprosencephaly, but the presence of the falx *(arrow)* and lack of thalamic fusion as seen by the large third ventricle help confirm hydranencephaly. (*A from Toi A, Chitayat D, Blaser S. Abnormalities of the foetal cerebral cortex. Prenat Diagn 2009;29:355-371.*)

Many affected fetuses die in utero. Survivors may appear and initially behave normal at birth, even though they lack a cerebral cortex. The diagnosis can be readily made clinically by cerebral transillumination[236] and confirmed with ultrasound or MRI. Most die in the first year, but survival to 32 years has been described in a vegetative state.[237]

Tumors

Prenatal intracranial solid tumors are rare, occurring in about 1.4 to 4.1 per 100,000 pregnancies. Most are sporadic. A few are associated with familial syndromes that have genetic abnormalities, such as **neurofibromatosis, tuberous sclerosis, von Hippel–Lindau,** and **Li-Fraumeni syndrome**.[238,239] Fetal brain tumors tend to be supratentorial in location, unlike tumors in older children, which are more likely to involve posterior fossa structures. Brain tumors account for about 10% of all perinatal tumors. Approximate frequencies of tumors described include **teratomas** 45%, **neuroepithelial tumors** (astrocytomas, medulloblastoma, choroid plexus papilloma, gliomas) 43%, **craniopharyngioma** 7%, **mesenchymal tumors** (meningioma, sarcoma) 5%, and **hemangioblastoma** 0.4%.[238-240]

The prenatal sonographic finding is a complex intracranial mass, occasionally with calcifications, macrocephaly, and hydrocephalus (Fig. 34-37). The tumors grow quickly and can erode into the orbit, oral cavity, or neck. Associated findings include polyhydramnios and intracranial hemorrhage. Diagnosis is generally made in the third trimester at ultrasound, triggered by excessive uterine growth,[238] although teratomas have been discovered as early as 17 weeks.[240] The differential diagnosis includes intracranial hemorrhage, vascular malformations, and dural sinus thrombosis.

Outcomes are poor, especially if tumors appear early. Overall survival is about 28%. Survival and outcome relate to size and location of tumor, its histology, surgical resectability, response to chemotherapy and condition of the fetus at diagnosis. From 40% to 100% of survivors have long-term neurologic deficits. Slightly better survival is seen with choroid plexus papilloma (73%) and meningeal tumors (36%).[238,239]

Choroid plexus papillomas are large, finely nodular masses that grow into the lateral ventricle and produce excessive CSF, resulting in severe dilation of the entire ventricular system and macrocephaly. They are described in association with **Aicardi syndrome** and **giant pigmented nevi.** Surgical resection can be curative but is technically difficult, and the vascular nature of choroid plexus papillomas can result in fatal hemorrhage. Overall survival is about 73%.[238]

Fetuses suspected to have brain tumors should undergo detailed ultrasound examination to look for associated abnormalities, which can occur in about 12.5% of cases, especially involving the face. Karyotype is generally of limited value because chromosomal abnormalities are uncommon. MRI is helpful in characterizing the mass and helping differentiate tumors from other conditions

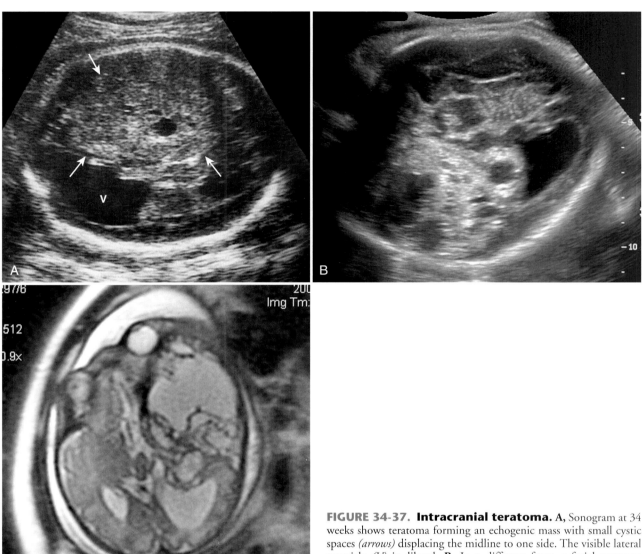

FIGURE 34-37. Intracranial teratoma. A, Sonogram at 34 weeks shows teratoma forming an echogenic mass with small cystic spaces *(arrows)* displacing the midline to one side. The visible lateral ventricle *(V)* is dilated. **B,** In a different fetus, a facial teratoma invades the brain. **C,** MR image of same fetus in **B** shows the intracranial extent of the tumor.

such as hemorrhage and sinus thrombosis. The large head size can interfere with delivery and require cephalocentesis to allow vaginal delivery.[238,239,241]

Intracranial lipomas are not "neoplasms" but rather represent abnormal differentiation of the meninx primitiva, which normally forms the subarachnoid space. Instead of resorbing at 8 to 10 weeks, the meninx persists and develops into mature adipose tissue. The incidence is 4 to 40 per 100,000 autopsies. Most occur in the interhemispheric region close to the corpus callosum and are usually associated with dysgenesis of the corpus callosum. At ultrasound, intracranial lipomas appear as an echogenic mass in the midline in the region of the corpus callosum (Fig. 34-38). MRI is helpful to confirm the fatty nature of the mass and further evaluate changes in the corpus callosum. Most do not grow. Many patients are asymptomatic, but associated abnormalities may cause

symptoms.[242,243] Surgical treatment of the lipoma is generally not indicated. Surgery can be dangerous because of the strong attachment of the lipoma to surrounding structures and the nerves and vessels within the mass.[244]

CONCLUSION

Until recently, the assessment of the fetal central nervous system was the domain of those performing prenatal ultrasound, radiologists and obstetricians. The introduction of MRI to prenatal neurologic diagnosis has introduced many other experts to the diagnosis, investigation, and management of fetal conditions, including pediatric neuroradiologists, neurologists, and neurosurgeons. Our understanding of the genetic basis of many syndromes and CNS findings as well as the nature of fetal CNS

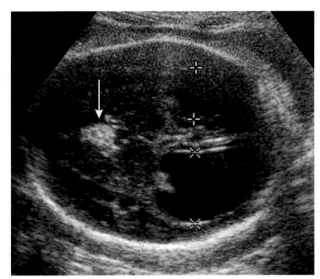

FIGURE 34-38. Lipoma. Midline lipoma forming an echogenic mass near the foramina of Monro at the expected anterior end of the corpus callosum *(arrow)*. These are not neoplasms and represent abnormal differentiation of meninges into fat. Midline lipomas are often associated with dysgenesis of the corpus callosum, as in this fetus, where the cavum septi pellucidi is absent and the ventricles are dilated.

abnormalities has also increased in recent years as a result of cross-fertilization among specialties. Those performing ultrasound are increasingly learning the complexities and large spectrum of neonatal diseases. Those in pediatrics are discovering that conditions affecting the fetus are often very different from conditions affecting neonates who survive pregnancy and are born alive.

Acknowledgments

The advice and support of my colleagues Drs. Susan Blaser, David Chitayat, Katherine Fong, Charles Raybaud, and Patrick Shannon is acknowledged and appreciated.

References

1. Chitty LS, Pilu G. The challenge of imaging the fetal central nervous system: an aid to prenatal diagnosis, management and prognosis. Prenat Diagn 2009;29:301-302.
2. Filly RA, Cardoza JD, Goldstein RB, Barkovich AJ. Detection of fetal central nervous system anomalies: a practical level of effort for a routine sonogram. Radiology 1989;172:403-408.
3. Grandjean H, Larroque D, Levi S. The performance of routine ultrasonographic screening of pregnancies in the Eurofetus Study. Am J Obstet Gynecol 1999;181:446-454.
4. Malinger G, Monteagudo A, Pilu G, et al. Sonographic examination of the fetal central nervous system: guidelines for performing the "basic examination" and the "fetal neurosonogram." Ultrasound Obstet Gynecol 2007;29:109-116.
5. Malinger G, Lerman-Sagie T, Watemberg N, et al. A normal second-trimester ultrasound does not exclude intracranial structural pathology. Ultrasound Obstet Gynecol 2002;20:51-56.
6. Garel C. New advances in fetal MR neuroimaging. Pediatr Radiol 2006;36:621-625.
7. Garel C. Fetal MRI: what is the future? Ultrasound Obstet Gynecol 2008;31:123-128.
8. Salomon LJ, Garel C. Magnetic resonance imaging examination of the fetal brain. Ultrasound Obstet Gynecol 2007;30:1019-1032.
9. Timor-Tritsch IE, Monteagudo A. Magnetic resonance imaging versus ultrasound for fetal central nervous system abnormalities. Am J Obstet Gynecol 2003;189:1210-1211; author reply 1211-1212.
10. Guibaud L. Contribution of fetal cerebral MRI for diagnosis of structural anomalies. Prenat Diagn 2009;29:420-433.
11. Hagmann CF, Robertson NJ, Leung WC, et al. Foetal brain imaging: ultrasound or MRI: a comparison between magnetic resonance imaging and a dedicated multidisciplinary neurosonographic opinion. Acta Paediatr 2008;97:414-419.

Developmental Anatomy

12. Greene ND, Copp AJ. Development of the vertebrate central nervous system: formation of the neural tube. Prenat Diagn 2009;29:303-311.
13. O'Rahilly R, Müller R, editors. Human embryology and teratology. 2nd ed. New York: Wiley-Liss; 1996.
14. Blaas HG, Eik-Nes SH. Sonoembryology and early prenatal diagnosis of neural anomalies. Prenat Diagn 2009;29:312-325.
15. Nelson Jr MD, Maher K, Gilles FH. A different approach to cysts of the posterior fossa. Pediatr Radiol 2004;34:720-732.
16. Calabro F, Arcuri T, Jinkins JR. Blake's pouch cyst: an entity within the Dandy-Walker continuum. Neuroradiology 2000;42:290-295.
17. Robinson AJ, Goldstein R. The cisterna magna septa: vestigial remnants of Blake's pouch and a potential new marker for normal development of the rhombencephalon. J Ultrasound Med 2007;26:83-95.
18. Bromley B, Nadel AS, Pauker S, et al. Closure of the cerebellar vermis: evaluation with second trimester US. Radiology 1994;193:761-763.
19. Nakayama T, Yamada R. MR imaging of the posterior fossa structures of human embryos and fetuses. Radiat Med Med Imaging Radiat Oncol 1999;17:105-114.
20. Robinson AJ, Blaser S, Toi A, et al. The fetal cerebellar vermis: assessment for abnormal development by ultrasonography and magnetic resonance imaging. Ultrasound Q 2007;23:211-223.
21. Toi A, Chitayat D, Blaser S. Abnormalities of the foetal cerebral cortex. Prenat Diagn 2009;29:355-371.
22. Crade M, Patel J, McQuown D. Sonographic imaging of the glycogen stage of the fetal choroid plexus. AJR Am J Roentgenol 1981;137:489-491.
23. Monteagudo A, Timor-Tritsch IE. Normal sonographic development of the central nervous system from the second trimester onwards using 2D, 3D and transvaginal sonography. Prenat Diagn 2009;29:326-339.
24. McLeary RD, Kuhns LR, Barr Jr M. Ultrasonography of the fetal cerebellum. Radiology 1984;151:439-442.
25. Haimovici JA, Doubilet PM, Benson CB, Frates MC. Clinical significance of isolated enlargement of the cisterna magna (>10 mm) on prenatal sonography. J Ultrasound Med 1997;16:731-734; quiz 735-736.
26. Zimmer EZ, Lowenstein L, Bronshtein M, et al. Clinical significance of isolated mega cisterna magna. Arch Gynecol Obstet 2007;276:487-490.
27. Ghai S, Fong KW, Toi A, et al. Prenatal ultrasound and MR imaging findings of lissencephaly: review of fetal cerebral sulcal development. Radiographics 2006;26:389-405.
28. Toi A, Lister WS, Fong KW. How early are fetal cerebral sulci visible at prenatal ultrasound and what is the normal pattern of early fetal sulcal development? Ultrasound Obstet Gynecol 2004;24:706-715.
29. Levine D, Barnes PD, Madsen JR, et al. Central nervous system abnormalities assessed with prenatal magnetic resonance imaging. Obstet Gynecol 1999;94:1011-1019.
30. Pooh RK, Nagao Y, Pooh K. Fetal neuroimaging by transvaginal 3D ultrasound and MRI. Ultrasound Rev Obstet Gynecol 2006;6:123-134.
31. Van den Hof MC, Wilson RD. Fetal soft markers in obstetric ultrasound. J Obstet Gynaecol Can 2005;27:592-636.
32. Sepulveda W, Lopez-Tenorio J. The value of minor ultrasound markers for fetal aneuploidy. Curr Opin Obstet Gynecol 2001;13:183-191.
33. Chen CY, Chen FH, Lee CC, et al. Sonographic characteristics of the cavum velum interpositum. AJNR Am J Neuroradiol 1998;19:1631-1635.

34. Shah PS, Blaser S, Toi A, et al. Cavum veli interpositi: prenatal diagnosis and postnatal outcome. Prenat Diagn 2005;25:539-542.
35. Eisenberg VH, Zalel Y, Hoffmann C, et al. Prenatal diagnosis of cavum velum interpositum cysts: significance and outcome. Prenat Diagn 2003;23:779-783.
36. Vergani P, Locatelli A, Piccoli MG, et al. Ultrasonographic differential diagnosis of fetal intracranial interhemispheric cysts. Am J Obstet Gynecol 1999;180:423-428.

Ventriculomegaly and Hydrocephalus
37. D'Addario V, Pinto V, Di Cagno L, Pintucci A. Sonographic diagnosis of fetal cerebral ventriculomegaly: an update. J Matern Fetal Neonatal Med 2007;20:7-14.
38. Filly RA, Goldstein RB, Callen PW. Fetal ventricle: importance in routine obstetric sonography. Radiology 1991;181:1-7.
39. Gaglioti P, Danelon D, Bontempo S, et al. Fetal cerebral ventriculomegaly: outcome in 176 cases. Ultrasound Obstet Gynecol 2005;25:372-377.
40. Jeng LB, Tarvin R, Robin NH. Genetic advances in central nervous system malformations in the fetus and neonate. Semin Pediatr Neurol 2001;8:89-99.
41. Gaglioti P, Oberto M, Todros T. The significance of fetal ventriculomegaly: etiology, short- and long-term outcomes. Prenat Diagn 2009;29:381-388.
42. Pilu G, Perolo A, Falco P, et al. Ultrasound of the fetal central nervous system. Curr Opin Obstet Gynecol 2000;12:93-103.
43. Young HF, Nulsen FE, Weiss MH, Thomas P. The relationship of intelligence and cerebral mantle in treated infantile hydrocephalus (IQ potential in hydrocephalic children). Pediatrics 1973;52:38-44.
44. Vintzileos AM, Ingardia CJ, Nochimson DJ. Congenital hydrocephalus: a review and protocol for perinatal management. Obstet Gynecol 1983;62:539-549.
45. Callen PW, Chooljian D. The effect of ventricular dilatation upon biometry of the fetal head. J Ultrasound Med 1986;5:17-19.
46. Monteagudo A, Timor-Tritsch IE, Moomjy M. Nomograms of the fetal lateral ventricles using transvaginal sonography. J Ultrasound Med 1993;12:265-269.
47. Heiserman J, Filly RA, Goldstein RB. Effect of measurement errors on sonographic evaluation of ventriculomegaly. J Ultrasound Med 1991;10:121-124.
48. Achiron R, Yagel S, Rotstein Z, et al. Cerebral lateral ventricular asymmetry: is this a normal ultrasonographic finding in the fetal brain? Obstet Gynecol 1997;89:233-237.
49. Farrell TA, Hertzberg BS, Kliewer MA, et al. Fetal lateral ventricles: reassessment of normal values for atrial diameter at ultrasound. Radiology 1994;193:409-411.
50. Toi A, Brown A. Measurement of the upper (proximal) cerebral ventricle. Ultrasound Obstet Gynecol 1996;8(Suppl):75.
51. Nadel AS, Benacerraf BR. Lateral ventricular atrium: larger in male than female fetuses. Int J Gynaecol Obstet 1995;51:123-126.
52. Patel MD, Goldstein RB, Tung S, Filly RA. Fetal cerebral ventricular atrium: difference in size according to sex. Radiology 1995;194:713-715.
53. Haddad S, Peleg D, Matilsky M, Ben-Ami M. Cerebral lateral ventricular atrial diameter of male and female fetuses at 20-24 weeks' gestation. Ultrasound Obstet Gynecol 2001;18:155-156.
54. Mahoney BS, Nyberg DA, Hirsch JH, et al. Mild idiopathic lateral cerebral ventricular dilatation in utero: sonographic evaluation. Radiology 1988;169:715-721.
55. Hertzberg BS, Lile R, Foosaner DE, et al. Choroid plexus–ventricular wall separation in fetuses with normal-sized cerebral ventricles at sonography: postnatal outcome. AJR Am J Roentgenol 1994;163:405-410.
56. Levine D, Barnes PD, Madsen JR, et al. Fetal CNS anomalies revealed on ultrafast MR imaging. AJR Am J Roentgenol 1999;172:813-818.
57. Levine D, Barnes PD, Robertson RR, et al. Fast MR imaging of fetal central nervous system abnormalities. Radiology 2003;229:51-61.
58. Morris JE, Rickard S, Paley MN, et al. The value of in utero magnetic resonance imaging in ultrasound diagnosed foetal isolated cerebral ventriculomegaly. Clin Radiol 2007;62:140-144.
59. Stroustrup Smith A, Levine D, Barnes PD, Robertson RL. Magnetic resonance imaging of the kinked fetal brain stem: a sign of severe dysgenesis. J Ultrasound Med 2005;24:1697-1709.
60. Laskin MD, Kingdom J, Toi A, et al. Perinatal and neurodevelopmental outcome with isolated fetal ventriculomegaly: a systematic review. J Matern Fetal Neonatal Med 2005;18:289-298.
61. Sadan S, Malinger G, Schweiger A, et al. Neuropsychological outcome of children with asymmetric ventricles or unilateral mild ventriculomegaly identified in utero. BJOG 2007;114:596-602.
62. Senat MV, Bernard JP, Schwarzler P, et al. Prenatal diagnosis and follow-up of 14 cases of unilateral ventriculomegaly. Ultrasound Obstet Gynecol 1999;14:327-332.

Specific Abnormalities
63. Barkovich AJ. Pediatric neuroimaging. 4th ed. Philadelphia: Lippincott–Williams & Wilkins; 2005.
64. Sarnat HB, Flores-Sarnat L. Integrative classification of morphology and molecular genetics in central nervous system malformations. Am J Med Genet 2004;126A:386-392.
65. Uher BF, Golden JA. Neuronal migration defects of the cerebral cortex: a destination debacle. Clin Genet 2000;58:16-24.
66. Itabashi HH. Forensic neuropathology: a practical review of the fundamentals. Boston: Academic Press–Elsevier; 2007.
67. Cox GG, Rosenthal SJ, Holsapple JW. Exencephaly: sonographic findings and radiologic-pathologic correlation. Radiology 1985;155:755-756.
68. Hendricks SK, Cyr DR, Nyberg DA, et al. Exencephaly: clinical and ultrasonic correlation to anencephaly. Obstet Gynecol 1988;72:898-901.
69. Goldstein RB, Filly RA. Prenatal diagnosis of anencephaly: spectrum of sonographic appearances and distinction from the amniotic band syndrome. AJR Am J Roentgenol 1988;151:547-550.
70. Goldstein RB, Filly RA, Callen PW. Sonography of anencephaly: pitfalls in early diagnosis. J Clin Ultrasound 1989;17:397-402.
71. Wilkins-Haug L, Freedman W. Progression of exencephaly to anencephaly in the human fetus: an ultrasound perspective. Prenat Diagn 1991;11:227-323.
72. Chatzipapas IK, Whitlow BJ, Economides DL. The "Mickey Mouse" sign and the diagnosis of anencephaly in early pregnancy. Ultrasound Obstet Gynecol 1999;13:196-199.
73. Cafici D, Sepulveda W. First-trimester echogenic amniotic fluid in the acrania-anencephaly sequence. J Ultrasound Med 2003;22:1075-1079; quiz 1080-1081.
74. David TJ, Nixon A. Congenital malformations associated with anencephaly and iniencephaly. J Med Genet 1976;13:263-265.
75. Sepulveda W, Corral E, Ayala C, et al. Chromosomal abnormalities in fetuses with open neural tube defects: prenatal identification with ultrasound. Ultrasound Obstet Gynecol 2004;23:352-356.
76. Chen CP, Chang TY, Lin YH, Wang W. Prenatal sonographic diagnosis of acrania associated with amniotic bands. J Clin Ultrasound 2004;32:256-260.
77. Carlan SJ, Angel JL, Leo J, Feeney J. Cephalocele involving the oral cavity. Obstet Gynecol 1990;75:494-496.
78. Cullen MT, Athanassiadis AP, Romero R. Prenatal diagnosis of anterior parietal encephalocele with transvaginal sonography. Obstet Gynecol 1990;75:489-491.
79. Hoving EW. Nasal encephaloceles. Childs Nerv Syst 2000;16:702-706.
80. Lowe LH, Booth TN, Joglar JM, Rollins NK. Midface anomalies in children. Radiographics 2000;20:907-922; quiz 1106-1107, 1112.
81. Moron FE, Morriss MC, Jones JJ, Hunter JV. Lumps and bumps on the head in children: use of CT and MR imaging in solving the clinical diagnostic dilemma. Radiographics 2004;24:1655-1674.
82. Patterson RJ, Egelhoff JC, Crone KR, Ball Jr WS. Atretic parietal cephaloceles revisited: an enlarging clinical and imaging spectrum? AJNR Am J Neuroradiol 1998;19:791-795.
83. Jones KL, Smith DW. Smith's recognizable patterns of human malformation. 6th ed. Philadelphia: Saunders-Elsevier; 2006.
84. Chen CP. Meckel syndrome: genetics, perinatal findings, and differential diagnosis. Taiwan J Obstet Gynecol 2007;46:9-14.
85. Bannister CM, Russell SA, Rimmer S, et al. Can prognostic indicators be identified in a fetus with an encephalocele? Eur J Pediatr Surg Suppl 2000;10:20-23.
86. Bamforth JS. Amniotic band sequence: Streeter's hypothesis reexamined. Am J Med Genet 1992;44:280-287.
87. Moerman P, Fryns JP, Vandenberghe K, Lauweryns JM. Constrictive amniotic bands, amniotic adhesions, and limb–body wall complex: discrete disruption sequences with pathogenetic overlap. Am J Med Genet 1992;42:470-479.
88. Daltro P, Fricke BL, Kline-Fath BM, et al. Prenatal MRI of congenital abdominal and chest wall defects. AJR Am J Roentgenol 2005;184:1010-1016.

89. Paladini D, Foglia S, Sglavo G, Martinelli P. Congenital constriction band of the upper arm: the role of three-dimensional ultrasound in diagnosis, counseling and multidisciplinary consultation. Ultrasound Obstet Gynecol 2004;23:520-522.

90. Chen CP. Prenatal diagnosis, fetal surgery, recurrence risk and differential diagnosis of neural tube defects. Taiwan J Obstet Gynecol 2008;47:283-290.

91. Babcook CJ, Goldstein RB, Barth RA, et al. Prevalence of ventriculomegaly in association with myelomeningocele: correlation with gestational age and severity of posterior fossa deformity. Radiology 1994;190:703-707.

92. Nyberg DA, Mack LA, Hirsch J, Mahony BS. Abnormalities of fetal cranial contour in sonographic detection of spina bifida: evaluation of the "lemon" sign. Radiology 1988;167:387-392.

93. Van den Hof MC, Nicolaides KH, Campbell J, Campbell S. Evaluation of the lemon and banana signs in one hundred thirty fetuses with open spina bifida. Am J Obstet Gynecol 1990;162:322-327.

94. Benacerraf BR, Stryker J, Frigoletto Jr FD. Abnormal ultrasound appearance of the cerebellum (banana sign): indirect sign of spina bifida. Radiology 1989;171:151-153.

95. Campbell J, Gilbert WM, Nicolaides KH, Campbell S. Ultrasound screening for spina bifida: cranial and cerebellar signs in a high-risk population. Obstet Gynecol 1987;70:247-250.

96. Goldstein RB, Podrasky AE, Filly RA, Callen PW. Effacement of the fetal cisterna magna in association with myelomeningocele. Radiology 1989;172:409-413.

97. Levine D, Trop I, Mehta TS, Barnes PD. MR imaging appearance of fetal cerebral ventricular morphology. Radiology 2002;223:652-660.

98. Callen AL, Filly RA. Supratentorial abnormalities in the Chiari II malformation. I. The ventricular "point." J Ultrasound Med 2008;27:33-38.

99. Kawamura T, Morioka T, Nishio S, et al. Cerebral abnormalities in lumbosacral neural tube closure defect: MR imaging evaluation. Childs Nerv Syst 2001;17:405-410.

100. Ball RH, Filly RA, Goldstein RB, Callen PW. The lemon sign: not a specific indicator of meningomyelocele. J Ultrasound Med 1993;12:131-134.

101. Boltshauser E, Schneider J, Kollias S, et al. Vanishing cerebellum in myelomeningocoele. Eur J Paediatr Neurol 2002;6:109-113.

102. Sutton LN. Fetal surgery for neural tube defects. Best Pract Res Clin Obstet Gynaecol 2008;22:175-188.

103. Cameron M, Moran P. Prenatal screening and diagnosis of neural tube defects. Prenat Diagn 2009;29:402-411.

104. Harmon JP, Hiett AK, Palmer CG, Golichowski AM. Prenatal ultrasound detection of isolated neural tube defects: is cytogenetic evaluation warranted? Obstet Gynecol 1995;86:595-599.

105. Kennedy D, Chitayat D, Winsor EJ, et al. Prenatally diagnosed neural tube defects: ultrasound, chromosome, and autopsy or postnatal findings in 212 cases. Am J Med Genet 1998;77:317-321.

106. Cochrane DD, Wilson RD, Steinbok P, et al. Prenatal spinal evaluation and functional outcome of patients born with myelomeningocele: information for improved prenatal counselling and outcome prediction. Fetal Diagn Ther 1996;11:159-168.

107. Pilu G, Hobbins JC. Sonography of fetal cerebrospinal anomalies. Prenat Diagn 2002;22:321-330

108. Cuillier F, Koenig P, Lagarde L, Cartault JF. Transvaginal sonographic diagnosis of iniencephaly apertus and craniorachischisis at 9 weeks' gestation. Ultrasound Obstet Gynecol 2003;22:657-658.

109. Blaas HG, Eriksson AG, Salvesen KA, et al. Brains and faces in holoprosencephaly: pre- and postnatal description of 30 cases. Ultrasound Obstet Gynecol 2002;19:24-38.

110. Dubourg C, Bendavid C, Pasquier L, et al. Holoprosencephaly. Orphanet J Rare Dis 2007;2:8.

111. Volpe P, Campobasso G, De Robertis V, Rembouskos G. Disorders of prosencephalic development. Prenat Diagn 2009;29:340-354.

112. Ming JE, Muenke M. Holoprosencephaly: from Homer to Hedgehog. Clin Genet 1998;53:155-163.

113. Plawner LL, Delgado MR, Miller VS, et al. Neuroanatomy of holoprosencephaly as predictor of function: beyond the face predicting the brain. Neurology 2002;59:1058-1066.

114. Lewis AJ, Simon EM, Barkovich AJ, et al. Middle interhemispheric variant of holoprosencephaly: a distinct cliniconeuroradiologic subtype. Neurology 2002;59:1860-1865.

115. Simon EM, Hevner RF, Pinter JD, et al. The middle interhemispheric variant of holoprosencephaly. AJNR Am J Neuroradiol 2002;23:15115-15116.

116. Nyberg DA, Mack LA, Bronstein A, et al. Holoprosencephaly: prenatal sonographic diagnosis. AJR Am J Roentgenol 1987;149:1051-1058.

117. Pilu G, Ambrosetto P, Sandri F, et al. Intraventricular fused fornices: a specific sign of fetal lobar holoprosencephaly. Ultrasound Obstet Gynecol 1994;4:65-67.

118. Pilu G, Sandri F, Perolo A, et al. Prenatal diagnosis of lobar holoprosencephaly. Ultrasound Obstet Gynecol 1992;2:88-94.

119. Bernard JP, Drummond CL, Zaarour P, et al. A new clue to the prenatal diagnosis of lobar holoprosencephaly: the abnormal pathway of the anterior cerebral artery crawling under the skull. Ultrasound Obstet Gynecol 2002;19:605-607.

120. Malinger G, Lev D, Kidron D, et al. Differential diagnosis in fetuses with absent septum pellucidum. Ultrasound Obstet Gynecol 2005;25:42-49.

121. Picone O, Hirt R, Suarez B, et al. Prenatal diagnosis of a possible new middle interhemispheric variant of holoprosencephaly using sonographic and magnetic resonance imaging. Ultrasound Obstet Gynecol 2006;28:229-231.

122. Pulitzer SB, Simon EM, Crombleholme TM, Golden JA. Prenatal MR findings of the middle interhemispheric variant of holoprosencephaly. AJNR Am J Neuroradiol 2004;25:1034-1036.

123. Adamsbaum C, Moutard ML, Andre C, et al. MRI of the fetal posterior fossa. Pediatr Radiol 2005;35:124-140.

124. Parisi MA, Dobyns WB. Human malformations of the midbrain and hindbrain: review and proposed classification scheme. Mol Genet Metab 2003;80:36-53.

125. Patel S, Barkovich AJ. Analysis and classification of cerebellar malformations. AJNR Am J Neuroradiol 2002;23:1074-1087.

126. Phillips JJ, Mahony BS, Siebert JR, et al. Dandy-Walker malformation complex: correlation between ultrasonographic diagnosis and postmortem neuropathology. Obstet Gynecol 2006;107:685-693.

127. Malinger G, Lev D, Lerman-Sagie T. The fetal cerebellum: pitfalls in diagnosis and management. Prenat Diagn 2009;29:372-380.

128. Kollias SS, Ball Jr WS, Prenger EC. Cystic malformations of the posterior fossa: differential diagnosis clarified through embryologic analysis. Radiographics 1993;13:1211-1231.

129. Aletebi FA, Fung KF. Neurodevelopmental outcome after antenatal diagnosis of posterior fossa abnormalities. J Ultrasound Med 1999;18:683-689.

130. Boltshauser E. Cerebellar imaging-an important signpost in paediatric neurology. Childs Nerv Syst 2001;17:211-216.

131. Limperopoulos C, Robertson RL, Estroff JA, et al. Diagnosis of inferior vermian hypoplasia by fetal magnetic resonance imaging: potential pitfalls and neurodevelopmental outcome. Am J Obstet Gynecol 2006;194:1070-1076.

132. Goldstein I, Reece EA, Pilu G, et al. Cerebellar measurements with ultrasonography in the evaluation of fetal growth and development. Am J Obstet Gynecol 1987;156:1065-1069.

133. Klein O, Pierre-Kahn A, Boddaert N, et al. Dandy-Walker malformation: prenatal diagnosis and prognosis. Childs Nerv Syst 2003;19:484-489.

134. Malinger G, Ginath S, Lerman-Sagie T, et al. The fetal cerebellar vermis: normal development as shown by transvaginal ultrasound. Prenat Diagn 2001;21:687-692.

135. Paladini D, Volpe P. Posterior fossa and vermian morphometry in the characterization of fetal cerebellar abnormalities: a prospective three-dimensional ultrasound study. Ultrasound Obstet Gynecol 2006;27:482-489.

136. Vinals F, Munoz M, Naveas R, et al. The fetal cerebellar vermis: anatomy and biometric assessment using volume contrast imaging in the C-plane (VCI-C). Ultrasound Obstet Gynecol 2005;26:622-627.

137. Achiron R, Kivilevitch Z, Lipitz S, et al. Development of the human fetal pons: in utero ultrasonographic study. Ultrasound Obstet Gynecol 2004;24:506-510.

138. Guibaud L. Practical approach to prenatal posterior fossa abnormalities using MRI. Pediatr Radiol 2004;34:700-711.

139. Guibaud L, des Portes V. Plea for an anatomical approach to abnormalities of the posterior fossa in prenatal diagnosis. Ultrasound Obstet Gynecol 2006;27:477-481.

140. Pilu G, Segata M, Ghi T, et al. Diagnosis of midline anomalies of the fetal brain with the three-dimensional median view. Ultrasound Obstet Gynecol 2006;27:522-529.

141. Poretti A, Leventer RJ, Cowan FM, et al. Cerebellar cleft: a form of prenatal cerebellar disruption. Neuropediatrics 2008;39:106-112.

142. Limperopoulos C, Robertson Jr RL, Khwaja OS, et al. How accurately does current fetal imaging identify posterior fossa anomalies? AJR Am J Roentgenol 2008;190:1637-1643.

143. Goetzinger KR, Stamilio DM, Dicke JM, et al. Evaluating the incidence and likelihood ratios for chromosomal abnormalities in fetuses with common central nervous system malformations. Am J Obstet Gynecol 2008;199:285 e1-e6.

144. Babcook CJ, Chong BW, Salamat MS, et al. Sonographic anatomy of the developing cerebellum: normal embryology can resemble pathology. AJR Am J Roentgenol 1996;166:427-433.

145. McAuliffe F, Chitayat D, Halliday W, et al. Rhombencephalosynapsis: prenatal imaging and autopsy findings. Ultrasound Obstet Gynecol 2008;31:542-548.

146. Pasquier L, Marcorelles P, Loget P, et al. Rhombencephalosynapsis and related anomalies: a neuropathological study of 40 fetal cases. Acta Neuropathol 2009;117:185-200.

147. Forzano F, Mansour S, Ierullo A, et al. Posterior fossa malformation in fetuses: a report of 56 further cases and a review of the literature. Prenat Diagn 2007;27:495-501.

148. Malinger G, Dror R, Ber-Sira L, et al. Developmental outcome of children with a large cisterna magna diagnosed in-utero. Ultrasound Obstet Gynecol 2008;32:253.

149. Nyberg DA, Mahony BS, Hegge FN, et al. Enlarged cisterna magna and the Dandy-Walker malformation: factors associated with chromosome abnormalities. Obstet Gynecol 1991;77:436-442.

150. Boltshauser E, Martin F, Altermatt S. Outcome in children with space-occupying posterior fossa arachnoid cysts. Neuropediatrics 2002;33:118-121.

151. Hayward R. Postnatal management and outcome for fetal-diagnosed intra-cerebral cystic masses and tumours. Prenat Diagn 2009;29: 396-401.

152. Barkovich AJ, Kuzniecky RI, Jackson GD, et al. A developmental and genetic classification for malformations of cortical development. Neurology 2005;65:1873-1887.

153. De Wit MC, Lequin MH, de Coo IF, et al. Cortical brain malformations: effect of clinical, neuroradiological, and modern genetic classification. Arch Neurol 2008;65:358-366.

154. Montenegro MA, Guerreiro MM, Lopes-Cendes I, et al. Interrelationship of genetics and prenatal injury in the genesis of malformations of cortical development. Arch Neurol 2002;59:1147-1153.

155. Sarnat HB. CNS malformations: gene locations of known human mutations. Eur J Paediatr Neurol 2005;9:427-431.

156. Miller E, Blaser S, Shannon P, Widjaja E. Brain and bone abnormalities of thanatophoric dwarfism. AJR Am J Roentgenol 2009; 192:48-51.

157. Chervenak FA, Jeanty P, Cantraine F, et al. The diagnosis of fetal microcephaly. Am J Obstet Gynecol 1984;149:512-517.

158. Abuelo D. Microcephaly syndromes. Semin Pediatr Neurol 2007;14:118-127.

159. Tang BL. Molecular genetic determinants of human brain size. Biochem Biophys Res Commun 2006;345:911-916.

160. Chervenak FA, Rosenberg J, Brightman RC, et al. A prospective study of the accuracy of ultrasound in predicting fetal microcephaly. Obstet Gynecol 1987;69:908-910.

161. Goldstein I, Reece EA, Pilu G, et al. Sonographic assessment of the fetal frontal lobe: a potential tool for prenatal diagnosis of microcephaly. Am J Obstet Gynecol 1988;158:1057-1062.

162. Kurtz AB, Wapner RJ, Rubin CS, et al. Ultrasound criteria for in utero diagnosis of microcephaly. J Clin Ultrasound 1980;8:11-16.

163. Bromley B, Benacerraf BR. Difficulties in the prenatal diagnosis of microcephaly. J Ultrasound Med 1995;14:303-306.

164. Schwarzler P, Homfray T, Bernard JP, et al. Late onset microcephaly: failure of prenatal diagnosis. Ultrasound Obstet Gynecol 2003;22:640-642.

165. Malinger G, Lev D, Lerman-Sagie T. Assessment of fetal intracranial pathologies first demonstrated late in pregnancy: cell proliferation disorders. Reprod Biol Endocrinol 2003;1:110.

166. Almgren M, Schalling M, Lavebratt C. Idiopathic megalencephaly-possible cause and treatment opportunities: from patient to lab. Eur J Paediatr Neurol 2008;12:438-445.

167. McEwing RL, Joelle R, Mohlo M, et al. Prenatal diagnosis of neurofibromatosis type 1: sonographic and MRI findings. Prenat Diagn 2006;26:1110-1114.

168. Olney AH. Macrocephaly syndromes. Semin Pediatr Neurol 2007;14:128-135.

169. Kumar R. External hydrocephalus in small children. Childs Nerv Syst 2006;22:1237-1241.

170. Malinger G, Lerman-Sagie T, Achiron R, Lipitz S. The subarachnoid space: normal fetal development as demonstrated by transvaginal ultrasound. Prenat Diagn 2000;20:890-893.

171. Maytal J, Alvarez LA, Elkin CM, Shinnar S. External hydrocephalus: radiologic spectrum and differentiation from cerebral atrophy. AJR Am J Roentgenol 1987;148:1223-1230.

172. Saleh-Gargari S. Prenatal diagnosis of benign familial macrocephaly. Ultrasound Obstet Gynecol 2007;30:593.

173. Muenchberger H, Assaad N, Joy P, et al. Idiopathic macrocephaly in the infant: long-term neurological and neuropsychological outcome. Childs Nerv Syst 2006;22:1242-1248.

174. Flores-Sarnat L. Hemimegalencephaly. Part 1. Genetic, clinical, and imaging aspects. J Child Neurol 2002;17:373-384; discussion 384.

175. Flores-Sarnat L. Hemimegalencephaly syndrome. Handb Clin Neurol 2007;87:153-176.

176. Tinkle BT, Schorry EK, Franz DN, et al. Epidemiology of hemimegalencephaly: a case series and review. Am J Med Genet A 2005;139:204-211.

177. Fong KW, Ghai S, Toi A, et al. Prenatal ultrasound findings of lissencephaly associated with Miller-Dieker syndrome and comparison with pre- and postnatal magnetic resonance imaging. Ultrasound Obstet Gynecol 2004;24:716-723.

178. Kato M, Dobyns WB. Lissencephaly and the molecular basis of neuronal migration. Hum Mol Genet 2003;12 Spec No 1: R89-R96.

179. Malinger G, Lev D, Lerman-Sagie T. Normal and abnormal fetal brain development during the third trimester as demonstrated by neurosonography. Eur J Radiol 2006;57:226-232.

180. Blin G, Rabbe A, Ansquer Y, et al. First-trimester ultrasound diagnosis in a recurrent case of Walker-Warburg syndrome. Ultrasound Obstet Gynecol 2005;26:297-299.

181. Pellicer A, Cabanas F, Perez-Higueras A, et al. Neural migration disorders studied by cerebral ultrasound and colour Doppler flow imaging. Arch Dis Child Fetal Neonatal Ed 1995;73:F55-F61.

182. Fogliarini C, Chaumoitre K, Chapon F, et al. Assessment of cortical maturation with prenatal MRI. Part II. Abnormalities of cortical maturation. Eur Radiol 2005;15:1781-1789.

183. Glenn OA, Goldstein RB, Li KC, et al. Fetal magnetic resonance imaging in the evaluation of fetuses referred for sonographically suspected abnormalities of the corpus callosum. J Ultrasound Med 2005;24:791-804.

184. Malinger G, Kidron D, Schreiber L, et al. Prenatal diagnosis of malformations of cortical development by dedicated neurosonography. Ultrasound Obstet Gynecol 2007;29:178-191.

185. Wieck G, Leventer RJ, Squier WM, et al. Periventricular nodular heterotopia with overlying polymicrogyria. Brain 2005;128:2811-2821.

186. Curry CJ, Lammer EJ, Nelson V, Shaw GM. Schizencephaly: heterogeneous etiologies in a population of 4 million California births. Am J Med Genet A 2005;137:181-189.

187. Denis D, Chateil JF, Brun M, et al. Schizencephaly: clinical and imaging features in 30 infantile cases. Brain Dev 2000;22:475-483.

188. Denis D, Maugey-Laulom B, Carles D, et al. Prenatal diagnosis of schizencephaly by fetal magnetic resonance imaging. Fetal Diagn Ther 2001;16:354-359.

189. Barkovich AJ, Gressens P, Evrard P. Formation, maturation, and disorders of brain neocortex. AJNR Am J Neuroradiol 1992;13: 423-446.

190. Packard AM, Miller VS, Delgado MR. Schizencephaly: correlations of clinical and radiologic features. Neurology 1997;48:1427-1434.

191. Nissenkorn A, Michelson M, Ben-Zeev B, Lerman-Sagie T. Inborn errors of metabolism: a cause of abnormal brain development. Neurology 2001;56:1265-1272.

192. Sponsen FJ, Smit GP, Erwich JJ. Inherited metabolic diseases and pregnancy. BJOG 2005;112:2-11.

193. Wanders RJ. Metabolic and molecular basis of peroxisomal disorders: a review. Am J Med Genet A 2004;126A:355-375.

194. Strenge S, Froster UG, Wanders RJ, et al. First-trimester increased nuchal translucency as a prenatal sign of Zellweger syndrome. Prenat Diagn 2004;24:151-153.

195. Mochel F, Grebille AG, Benachi A, et al. Contribution of fetal MR imaging in the prenatal diagnosis of Zellweger syndrome. AJNR Am J Neuroradiol 2006;27:333-336.

196. Wortmann SB, Reimer A, Creemers JW, Mullaart RA. Prenatal diagnosis of cerebral lesions in tuberous sclerosis complex (TSC): case report and review of the literature. Eur J Paediatr Neurol 2008;12:123-126.

197. Levine D, Barnes P, Korf B, Edelman R. Tuberous sclerosis in the fetus: second-trimester diagnosis of subependymal tubers with ultra-fast MR imaging. AJR Am J Roentgenol 2000;175:1067-1069.

198. Volpe P, Paladini D, Resta M, et al. Characteristics, associations and outcome of partial agenesis of the corpus callosum in the fetus. Ultrasound Obstet Gynecol 2006;27:509-516.

199. Achiron R, Achiron A. Development of the human fetal corpus callosum: a high-resolution, cross-sectional sonographic study. Ultrasound Obstet Gynecol 2001;18:343-347.

200. Achiron R, Lipitz S, Achiron A. Sex-related differences in the development of the human fetal corpus callosum: in utero ultrasonographic study. Prenat Diagn 2001;21:116-120.

201. Malinger G, Zakut H. The corpus callosum: normal fetal development as shown by transvaginal sonography. AJR Am J Roentgenol 1993;161:1041-1043.

202. Fratelli N, Papageorghiou AT, Prefumo F, et al. Outcome of prenatally diagnosed agenesis of the corpus callosum. Prenat Diagn 2007;27:512-517.

203. Bennett GL, Bromley B, Benacerraf BR. Agenesis of the corpus callosum: prenatal detection usually is not possible before 22 weeks of gestation. Radiology 1996;199:447-450.

204. d'Ercole C, Girard N, Cravello L, et al. Prenatal diagnosis of fetal corpus callosum agenesis by ultrasonography and magnetic resonance imaging. Prenat Diagn 1998;18:247-253.

205. Malinger G, Lerman-Sagie T, Vinals F. Three-dimensional sagittal reconstruction of the corpus callosum: fact or artifact? Ultrasound Obstet Gynecol 2006;28:742-743.

206. Malinger G, Lev D, Lerman-Sagie T. The fetal corpus callosum: "the truth is out there." Ultrasound Obstet Gynecol 2007;30:140-141.

207. Callen PW, Callen AL, Glenn OA, Toi A. Columns of the fornix, not to be mistaken for the cavum septi pellucidi on prenatal sonography. J Ultrasound Med 2008;27:25-31.

208. Gupta JK, Lilford RJ. Assessment and management of fetal agenesis of the corpus callosum. Prenat Diagn 1995;15:301-312.

209. Moutard ML, Kieffer V, Feingold J, et al. Agenesis of corpus callosum: prenatal diagnosis and prognosis. Childs Nerv Syst 2003;19:471-476.

210. Willnow S, Kiess W, Butenandt O, et al. Endocrine disorders in septo-optic dysplasia (De Morsier syndrome): evaluation and follow-up of 18 patients. Eur J Pediatr 1996;155:179-184.

211. Ghidini A, Sirtori M, Vergani P, et al. Fetal intracranial calcifications. Am J Obstet Gynecol 1989;160:86-87.

212. Malinger G, Lev D, Zahalka N, et al. Fetal cytomegalovirus infection of the brain: the spectrum of sonographic findings. AJNR Am J Neuroradiol 2003;24:28-32.

213. Mittendorf R, Covert R, Pryde PG, et al. Association between lenticulostriate vasculopathy (LSV) and neonatal intraventricular hemorrhage (IVH). J Perinatol 2004;24:700-705.

214. Cabanas F, Pellicer A, Morales C, et al. New pattern of hyperechogenicity in thalamus and basal ganglia studied by color Doppler flow imaging. Pediatr Neurol 1994;10:109-116.

215. Kriss VM, Kriss TC. Doppler sonographic confirmation of thalamic and basal ganglia vasculopathy in three infants with trisomy 13. J Ultrasound Med 1996;15:523-526.

216. Carletti A, Colleoni GG, Perolo A, et al. Prenatal diagnosis of cerebral lesions acquired in utero and with a late appearance. Prenat Diagn 2009;29:389-395.

217. Enders G, Bader U, Lindemann L, et al. Prenatal diagnosis of congenital cytomegalovirus infection in 189 pregnancies with known outcome. Prenat Diagn 2001;21:362-377.

218. Benoist G, Salomon LJ, Jacquemard F, et al. The prognostic value of ultrasound abnormalities and biological parameters in blood of fetuses infected with cytomegalovirus. BJOG 2008;115:823-829.

219. Guerra B, Simonazzi G, Puccetti C, et al. Ultrasound prediction of symptomatic congenital cytomegalovirus infection. Am J Obstet Gynecol 2008;198:380 e1-e7.

220. Newton ER. Diagnosis of perinatal TORCH infections. Clin Obstet Gynecol 1999;42:59-70; quiz 174-175.

221. Patel DV, Holfels EM, Vogel NP, et al. Resolution of intracranial calcifications in infants with treated congenital toxoplasmosis. Radiology 1996;199:433-440.

222. Garel C, Azarian M, Lasjaunias P, Luton D. Pial arteriovenous fistulas: dilemmas in prenatal diagnosis, counseling and postnatal treatment—report of three cases. Ultrasound Obstet Gynecol 2005;26:293-296.

223. Sepulveda W, Platt CC, Fisk NM. Prenatal diagnosis of cerebral arteriovenous malformation using color Doppler ultrasonography: case report and review of the literature. Ultrasound Obstet Gynecol 1995;6:282-286.

224. Rodesch G, Hui F, Alvarez H, et al. Prognosis of antenatally diagnosed vein of Galen aneurysmal malformations. Child Nerv Syst 1994;10:79-83.

225. Raybaud CA, Strother CM, Hald JK. Aneurysms of the vein of Galen: embryonic considerations and anatomical features relating to the pathogenesis of the malformation. Neuroradiology 1989;31:109-128.

226. Laurichesse Delmas H, Winer N, Gallot D, et al. Prenatal diagnosis of thrombosis of the dural sinuses: report of six cases, review of the literature and suggested management. Ultrasound Obstet Gynecol 2008;32:188-198.

227. Elchalal U, Yagel S, Gomori JM, et al. Fetal intracranial hemorrhage (fetal stroke): does grade matter? Ultrasound Obstet Gynecol 2005;26:233-243.

228. Ghi T, Simonazzi G, Perolo A, et al. Outcome of antenatally diagnosed intracranial hemorrhage: case series and review of the literature. Ultrasound Obstet Gynecol 2003;22:121-130.

229. Simonazzi G, Segata M, Ghi T, et al. Accurate neurosonographic prediction of brain injury in the surviving fetus after the death of a monochorionic cotwin. Ultrasound Obstet Gynecol 2006;27:517-521.

230. Vergani P, Strobelt N, Locatelli A, et al. Clinical significance of fetal intracranial hemorrhage. Am J Obstet Gynecol 1996;175:536-543.

231. Mittelbronn M, Beschorner R, Schittenhelm J, et al. Multiple thromboembolic events in fetofetal transfusion syndrome in triplets contributing to the understanding of pathogenesis of hydranencephaly in combination with polymicrogyria. Hum Pathol 2006;37:1503-1507.

232. Quek YW, Su PH, Tsao TF, et al. Hydranencephaly associated with interruption of bilateral internal carotid arteries. Pediatr Neonatol 2008;49:43-47.

233. Tsai JD, Kuo HT, Chou IC. Hydranencephaly in neonates. Pediatr Neonatol 2008;49:154-157.

234. Lam YH, Tang MH. Serial sonographic features of a fetus with hydranencephaly from 11 weeks to term. Ultrasound Obstet Gynecol 2000;16:77-79.

235. Greene MF, Benacerraf B, Crawford JM. Hydranencephaly: ultrasound appearance during in utero evolution. Radiology 1985;156:779-780.

236. Barozzino T, Sgro M. Transillumination of the neonatal skull: seeing the light. CMAJ 2002;167:1271-1272.

237. Merker B. Life expectancy in hydranencephaly. Clin Neurol Neurosurg 2008;110:213-214.

238. Isaacs Jr H. Perinatal brain tumors: a review of 250 cases. II. Pediatr Neurol 2002;27:333-342.

239. Isaacs Jr H. Perinatal brain tumors: a review of 250 cases. I. Pediatr Neurol 2002;27:249-261.

240. Rickert CH. Neuropathology and prognosis of foetal brain tumours. Acta Neuropathol 1999;98:567-576.

241. Schlembach D, Bornemann A, Rupprecht T, Beinder E. Fetal intracranial tumors detected by ultrasound: a report of two cases and review of the literature. Ultrasound Obstet Gynecol 1999;14:407-418.

242. Demaerel P, van de Gaer P, Wilms G, Baert AL. Interhemispheric lipoma with variable callosal dysgenesis: relationship between embryology, morphology, and symptomatology. Eur Radiol 1996;6:904-909.

243. Ickowitz V, Eurin D, Rypens F, et al. Prenatal diagnosis and postnatal follow-up of pericallosal lipoma: report of seven new cases. AJNR Am J Neuroradiol 2001;22:767-772.

244. Yildiz H, Hakyemez B, Koroglu M, et al. Intracranial lipomas: importance of localization. Neuroradiology 2006;48:1-7.

CHAPTER 35

The Fetal Spine

Eric E. Sauerbrei

Chapter Outline

*A*bnormalities of the spine are some of the most common congenital abnormalities. In the United States, overall incidence of neural tube defects (NTDs) was approximately 1 to 2 per 1000 births[1] before 2000, but it is now 0.5 to 1.0 per 1000 pregnancies since the widespread use of folic acid before conception[2,3] and the addition of folic acid to enriched grain products.[4] Currently, 42 nations practice mandatory folic acid fortification to combat neural tube defects.[5-9]

Neural tube defects are associated with substantial morbidity and mortality. Many survivors have severe long-term morbidity that has a profound impact on the family—emotionally, physically, and fiscally. Fortunately, the birth incidence of spina bifida and anencephaly is decreasing in many areas of the world as a result of maternal screening programs (maternal serum tests and antenatal ultrasound) and more recently, the administration of folic acid to women of childbearing age.

In prenatal imaging, **three-dimensional** (3-D) **ultrasound** and **fetal magnetic resonance imaging** (MRI) are newer techniques that are making a positive impact, especially for precise localization of spina bifida and complete delineation of associated abnormalities. This precise information is useful for prognosis and possibly for prenatal surgery. Prenatal surgery for closure of myelomeningoceles is a relatively new procedure that is practiced in only a few centers at this time.

DEVELOPMENTAL ANATOMY

Embryology of the Spine

The precursors of the spinal cord and surrounding spinal column develop in the third and fourth week after conception (fifth and sixth menstrual weeks). During the third conceptual week, the bilaminar germ disc evolves into the trilaminar germ disc, which consists of the **ectoderm** layer (part of the amniotic cavity), the middle **mesoderm** layer, and the **endoderm** layer (part of the yolk sac cavity) (Fig. 35-1, *A*). The mesoderm layer develops a midline central tube, the **notochordal process,** which runs along the long axis of the embryonic disc. The mesoderm lateral to the notochordal process has three components: paraxial mesoderm, intermediate mesoderm, and lateral plate mesoderm. By day 21 conceptual age, the hollow-tube notochordal process has evolved into a solid cord called the **notochord,** and the paraxial mesoderm has developed multiple discrete bumps called **somites,** of which there are 37 pairs when finally developed (Fig. 35-1, *B*).

The notochord and rest of the intraembryonic mesoderm induce the development of the **neural plate** in the ectoderm layer (amniotic cavity side of germ disc), starting on conceptual day 18. The neural plate grows in length and breadth until conceptual day 21, when neurulation begins. **Neurulation** is the process of folding of the neural plate into the **neural tube,** probably induced by the adjacent notochord. The lateral edges of the neural folds begin to fuse dorsally into a closed neural tube in the occipito-cervical region, leaving an opening at the cranial end **(cranial neuropore)** and the caudal end **(caudal neuropore).** The hollow center of the neural tube is called the **neural canal,** which will become the central canal of the spinal cord and ventricular system of the brain. By day 24 conceptual age, the cranial neuropore closes, and by day 25 the caudal neuropore closes (Table 35-1).

The cranial end of the neural tube becomes the brain, and the caudal end becomes the spinal cord. In week 4

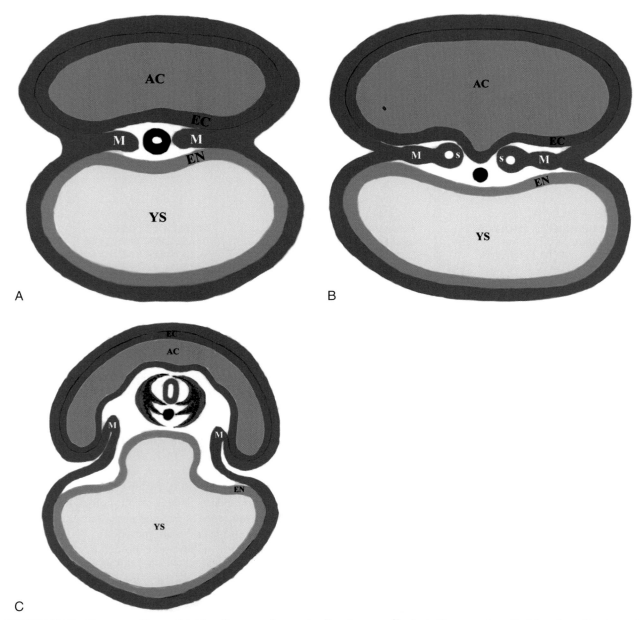

FIGURE 35-1. Cross section of trilaminar embryonic disc (germ disc). A, Cross section of midportion of embryonic disc 17 days after conception. The notochordal process is a hollow tube *(black circle)* that lies between the ectoderm *(EC) (red)* and endoderm *(EN) (green)* and is flanked by the mesoderm plate *(M) (blue)*. **B, Cross section of midportion of embryo 21 days after conception.** The medial portions of the mesoderm plate *(M) (blue)* are organizing into somites *(s)*. The ectoderm *(EC) (red)* is folding at the midline into the neural fold, which will soon become the neural tube. This folding is induced by the neighboring notochord *(solid black circle)*. Note that the notochord is now a solid cord that has evolved from the hollow process of day 17. **C, Cross section of embryo midportion at 28 days after conception.** The neural fold has evolved into a closed neural tube *(hollow red ovoid structure)* that has separated from its ectoderm layer *(EC) (red)*. The somites have ruptured along the medial sides. Migrating cells from the somites (the sclerotome) envelop the neural tube *(red ovoid)* and become the vertebral arches. The sclerotome surrounding the notochord *(black circle)* becomes the vertebral bodies and intervertebral discs. The notochordal remnants differentiate later to become the nucleus pulposus of the discs. The rest of the notochordal cells degenerate and disappear. *AC,* Amniotic cavity; *EN,* endoderm; *M,* mesoderm; *YS,* yolk sac. *(Illustrations by Karen Sauerbrei, RT, BA.)*

conceptual age, after the neural tube has formed, the adjacent 37 pairs of somites in the intraembryonic mesoderm give rise to the vertebral bodies and vertebral arches that will surround the spinal cord. A group of cells, (the **sclerotome,** migrates from the somites and surrounds

the adjacent neural tube and the notochord. The ventral portion of the sclerotome surrounds the notochord and forms the rudiment of the vertebral body. The dorsal portion of the sclerotome surrounds the neural tube and forms the precursors to the vertebral arch (Fig. 35-1, *C*).

TABLE 35-1. SPINE EMBRYOLOGY DURING THIRD AND FOURTH WEEKS AFTER CONCEPTION

MENSTRUAL AGE (DAYS)	CONCEPTUAL AGE (DAYS)	EMBRYO LENGTH (MM)	SAC DIAMETER (MM)	LANDMARKS
31	17	0.5	2	Trilaminar disc Notochordal process Paraxial mesoderm (Fig. 35-1, A)
35	21	2	4	Notochord Neural plate Somites (Fig. 35-1, B)
42	28	5	10	Neural tube Notochord Sclerotome (Fig. 35-1, C)

In the fetus the **notochordal remnant** corresponds to the nucleus pulposus of the intervertebral discs.[10]

Abnormalities of neural tube closure not only affect the spinal cord and brain, but also interfere with normal development of surrounding vertebral arches, which are derived from adjacent mesodermal somites. Disturbances of neural tube closure underlie **spina bifida** and **anencephaly** defects.

Caudal regression defects may be related to defective development of the mesoderm layer in week 3 conceptual age, during transformation of the germ disc from two layers (bilaminar) to three layers (trilaminar). Various degrees of abnormal mesoderm development account for the wide spectrum of abnormalities found in caudal regression.

A failure of part of the neural tube to close, called **spinal dysraphism,** disrupts development of the nervous system and disrupts the induction of the overlying vertebral arches. The resulting open vertebral canal is called **spina bifida.** If dura and arachnoid protrude from the spinal canal, the result is a **meningocele.** If neural tissue and meninges protrude, the result is a **myelomeningocele.** In the most severe NTDs, the neural tube fails to form and fails to separate from the overlying ectoderm. In the spine the condition is called **rachischisis** or **myeloschisis;** the opened spinal cord is exposed along the dorsal surface of the fetus. If the defect involves the cranial neural tube, the brain is represented by an exposed dorsal mass of undifferentiated neural tissue, called **exencephaly, anencephaly,** or **craniorachischisis.** Differentiated brain and meninges may bulge from a nonossified gap in the skull (**meningoencephalocele),** but this is not related to failure of neural tube closure.

In animals, certain teratogens can induce NTDs: **retinoic acid, insulin,** and **high plasma glucose levels.** In humans, implicated factors include **valproic acid** (antiepileptic), **maternal diabetes,** and **hyperthermia.** Valproic acid may interfere with folate metabolism.

Ossification of the Fetal Spine

Prenatal sonography readily portrays the ossified portions of the fetal spine, whereas the nonossified cartilage is more difficult to delineate. It is therefore important for sonographers and sonologists to understand the temporal and spatial ossification patterns during fetal development in order to optimize spinal evaluation.

Each vertebra will develop three ossification centers: the centrum, right neural process, and left neural process.[11] The **centrum** will form the central part of the vertebral body, and the **neural process** will form the posterolateral parts of the vertebral body and pedicles, the transverse processes, the laminae, and the articular processes.

Ossification begins in the lower thoracic fetal spine at approximately 10 weeks' gestation (menstrual age).[12] Ossification of the **centra** progresses in cranial and caudal directions simultaneously. **Neural arch** ossification proceeds caudally from the lower thoracic (T) spine to the lumbar (L) spine. It proceeds sequentially from L1 through L5 and then into the sacral (S) spine. By 13 weeks' menstrual age, there are three ossification centers in vertebrae C1 through L3[13] (Fig. 35-2). Neural arch ossification begins as a small focus at the base of the transverse process and extends simultaneously into the pedicle anteriorly and into the lamina posteriorly (Fig. 35-3).

Ultrasound evaluation for spina bifida usually occurs between 16 and 22 weeks' gestation. By 16 weeks, there is enough ossification in the neural arches to assess for spina bifida to level L5,[14] by 19 weeks to level S1, and by 22 weeks to level S2 (Figs. 35-4 and 35-5). In some fetuses, there may be enough neural arch ossification to assess for spina bifida before these gestational ages. Braithwaite et al.[15] assessed the fetal anatomy at 12 to 13 weeks' gestation by a combination of transabdominal and transvaginal sonography and reported successful

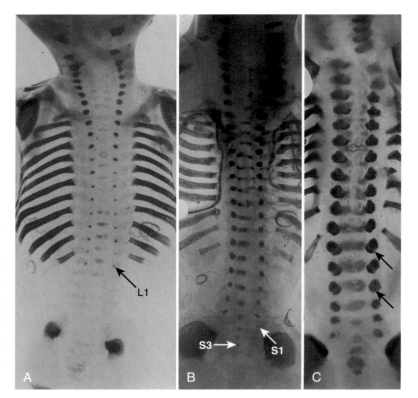

FIGURE 35-2. Spine ossification at 11 weeks + 4 days menstrual age. A, Ossification of neural processes extends from C1 to L1 *(arrow).* The neural process ossification starts at the base of the transverse process, which lies at the junction of the pedicle and the lamina. **B, Spine ossification at 13 weeks' menstrual age.** Ossification extends to level S1 neural process *(S1 arrow)* and S3 vertebral body *(S3 arrow).* **C, Spine ossification at 15 weeks + 2 days' menstrual age.** Ossification now extends into the laminae of the vertebral arches in the thoracic and lumbar spine. Arrows demonstrate ossification of the laminae at levels L1 and L3. Ossification of the laminae is negligible at S1.

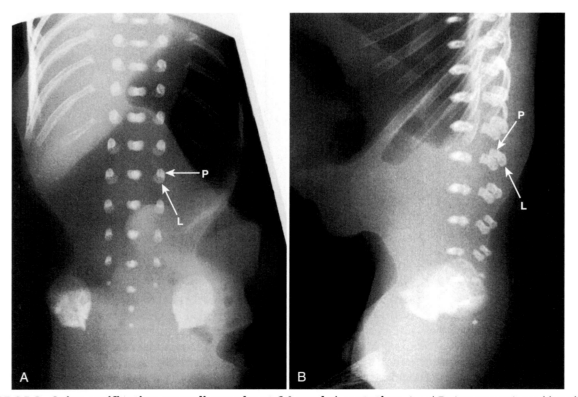

FIGURE 35-3. Spine ossification on radiographs at 14 weeks' gestation. A and **B,** Anteroposterior and lateral radiographs. Well-developed ossification in the centra now extends down to level S3. Ossification in the lumbar neural processes extends into the lamina *(L)* and pedicles *(P).* The neural process ossification starts to resemble the shape of the cartilaginous neural process rather than the focal dotlike ossification at 13 weeks' gestation.

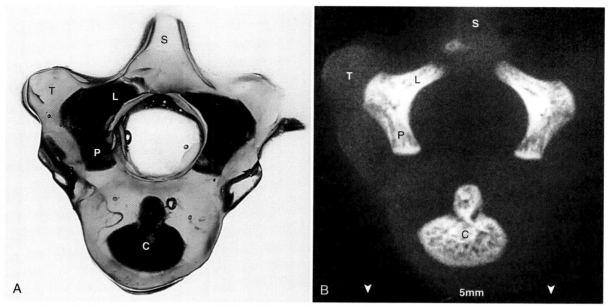

FIGURE 35-4. Vertebral ossification of T9 at 16 weeks' gestation. A, Specimen; **B,** radiograph. Ossification extends quite far into the pedicles *(P)* and laminae *(L)*. Note the early ossification in the base of the transverse processes *(T)*. The width of the vertebra is about 5 mm. Ossification within the centrum *(C)*. *S,* Spinous process (cartilage); *T,* transverse process (cartilage).

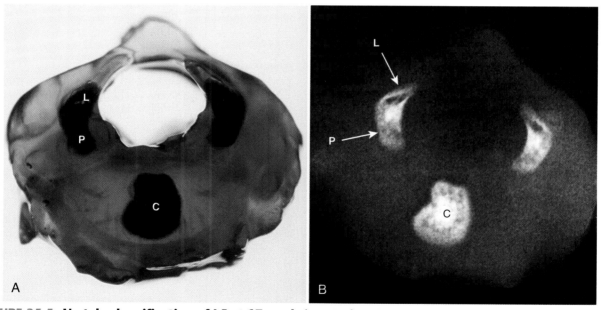

FIGURE 35-5. Vertebral ossification of L5 at 17 weeks' gestation. A, Specimen; **B,** radiograph. There is usually enough ossification at this gestation in the pedicles *(P)* and laminae *(L)* to determine the true course of these structures in radiographs and sonograms. The width of the vertebra is about 5 mm. *C,* Ossification within the centrum.

examination of the vertebrae and overlying skin in both the transverse and the coronal plane in all cases. Others have reported successful prenatal diagnosis of spina bifida at 12 to 14 weeks' gestation on the basis of abnormal cranial findings.[16-18] They caution that although the characteristic cranial findings may be present at 11 to 14 weeks, the prevalence of these findings in the first trimester remains to be determined (Table 35-2).

Normal Position of the Spinal Cord

For fetuses at 19 to 33 weeks' gestation, the **conus medullaris** is normally situated at level L2-L3 or higher (Fig 35-6). Level L3 is taken to be *indeterminate* and L3-L4 or lower as *abnormal.*[19] For those fetuses with tethered cord, the position of the conus medullaris is usually lower than normal. For earlier pregnancy (13-18 weeks' gestation), the conus medullaris may be normally as low as L4. At term, the conus is normally above L2.[20]

SCANNING TECHNIQUES

In clinical practice, the most useful scan planes to assess the posterior neural arches are posterior transaxial (Fig. 35-7), lateral transaxial (Fig. 35-8), lateral longitudinal (coronal) (Fig. 35-9), posterior longitudinal (sagittal) (Fig. 35-10), and posterior angled transaxial (Fig. 35-11). The posterior angled transaxial is useful to visualize the pedicles and laminae simultaneously. Because the laminae course caudal to the transaxial plane, which contains the centrum and pedicles, only the angled scan plane can depict the pedicles and laminae simultaneously in their entirety

The detection rate of spina bifida at 18 to 20 weeks' gestation may be 80% or less during routine screening ultrasound,[21] because the accuracy of ultrasound depends on the skill and experience of the operator. The accuracy of referral centers performing detailed targeted imaging because of a suspected NTD or high **maternal serum alpha-fetoprotein** (MS-AFP) is close to 100%.

A detailed sonogram of the fetal spine may be requested for several reasons: previous suspicious ultrasound; family history of NTD; and raised serum or amniotic fluid AFP. To enhance detection of spina bifida, a detailed protocol should be consistently followed. The first step in assessing for spina bifida is scanning the head, because most fetuses with spina bifida have signs of a **Chiari II malformation** in the brain at 16 to 22 weeks' gestation. These signs include obliterated cisterna magna **(banana sign)**, concave frontal bones **(lemon sign)**, and dilated lateral cerebral ventricles.[22,23] The sensitivity of the banana sign for open spina bifida is close to 99%, and false-positive diagnoses are rare, although the lemon sign may occur in 1% to 2% of normal fetuses.

The next step is to determine the position of the fetal spine. The scan plane is placed perpendicular to the long axis of the fetal spine, either posterior transaxial or lateral transaxial (see Figs. 35-7 and 35-8). The sonographer should scan from one end of the spine to the other while maintaining the scan plane perpendicular to the spine. This is repeated several times. In the process, one builds

TABLE 35-2. TIMING AND PATTERN OF FETAL SPINE OSSIFICATION (10-22 WEEKS' MENSTRUAL/ GESTATIONAL AGE)

AGE (WK)	EVENTS
10	Ossification appears in lower thoracic spine vertebral bodies.
13	Some ossification is present from C1 to L5 vertebral bodies and arches.
13-22	Neural arch ossification simultaneously extends anteriorly into the pedicles and posteriorly into the laminae.
16	Enough neural arch ossification appears to assess for spina bifida to level L5.
19	Enough neural arch ossification appears to assess for spina bifida to level S1.
22	Enough neural arch ossification appears to assess for spina bifida to level S2.

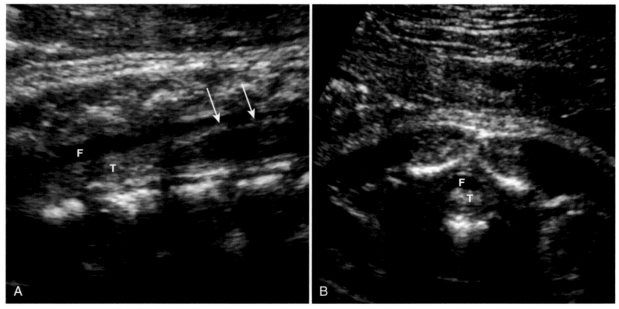

FIGURE 35-6. Normal spinal cord. A, Posterior longitudinal, and **B**, posterior transaxial (transverse), sonograms of a normal spinal cord. Note the normal position of the cord *(arrows)* and filum terminale *(T)* in the dependent portion of the spinal canal. Cerebrospinal fluid *(F)* between the anterior aspect of the spinal cord and the anterior wall of the spinal canal.

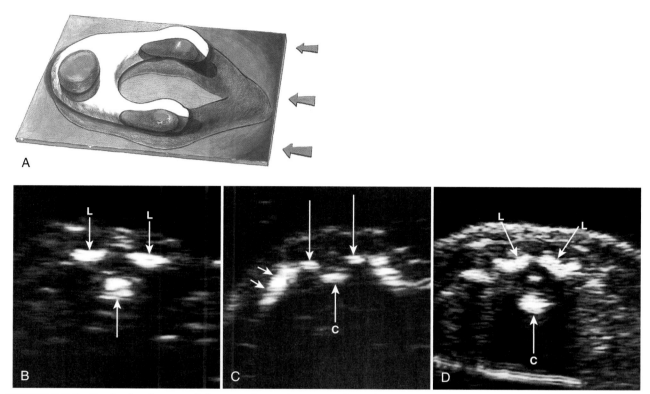

FIGURE 35-7. Posterior transaxial scan plane. A, Diagram shows the incident sound beam *(arrows)* reflecting off the posterior surfaces, clearly demonstrating the **laminae** and **centrum,** but not the pedicles. The red structures represent the ossified portions of the vertebra. **B,** The L3 vertebra at 17 weeks' gestation demonstrates the ossified laminae *(L)* and the ossified centrum *(bottom arrow)* but not the pedicles. **C,** Scan of S1 vertebra at 17 weeks shows early ossification at the lamina-pedicle junction on each side *(long thin arrows).* With this amount of ossification, determine the course of the laminae is not possible, and thus exclude spina bifida is difficult. *C,* Ossified centrum; *short arrows,* iliac wing. **D,** Scan of T10 at 24 weeks' gestation shows advanced ossification in the laminae *(L, arrows)* almost reaching midline. Despite their advanced ossification, the pedicles are not visualized in this scan plane. *C,* Ossified centrum.

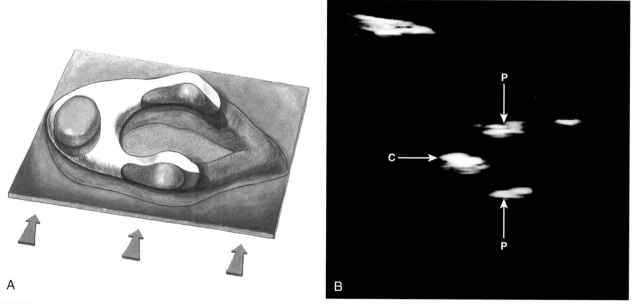

FIGURE 35-8. Lateral transaxial (transverse) scan plane. A, Diagram shows the incident sound beam *(arrows)* reflecting off the lateral surfaces of the centrum and the near pedicle and off the medial surface of the far pedicle, demonstrating the **centrum** and **pedicles,** but not the laminae. The laminae course toward midline (thus sound beam is not perpendicular to laminar surface) and caudally (thus out of the plane of sound beam). The red structures are ossified portions of the vertebra. **B,** Scan of vertebra L3 at 17 weeks' gestation shows the ossified pedicles *(P)* and the ossified centrum *(C),* but not the laminae.

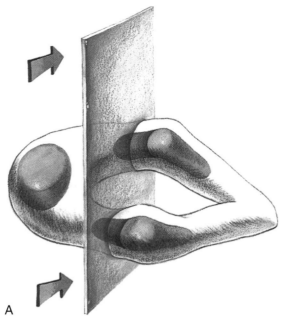

A

FIGURE 35-9. **Lateral longitudinal scan plane. A,** Diagram shows the incident sound beam *(arrows)* reflecting off the lateral surface of the near pedicle and the medial surface of the far pedicle. Therefore this scan plane will show the **cross section of the pedicles** of each vertebra, but not the centrum and laminae. The red structures are ossified portions of the vertebra. **B,** Lateral longitudinal scan of the lumbar spine at 16 weeks shows the **ossified pedicles** *(small arrows).* The lumbar pedicles usually form a series of parallel echogenic foci, although they may normally diverge by 1 to 2 mm. Note the faint echogenic structures between the pedicles; these represent echoes from the **centra** that intercept the edge of the insonating beam. *(large arrow,* iliac wing). **C,** When the tomographic scan plane is thick or is placed closer to the centrum, the **pedicles** and **centra** may be visualized simultaneously. The centra will appear as an extra set of echogenic dots *(arrows)* between the series of pedicles. **D,** 3-D scan of a 19-week fetus shows the **ossified spinal elements** from the cervical area to the lumbosacral level, as viewed from the posterior aspect of the fetus. The 12 ribs are visualized. L1 vertebra is immediately caudal to the 12th rib level *(arrows).* (**D** *courtesy Siemens Ultrasound.)*

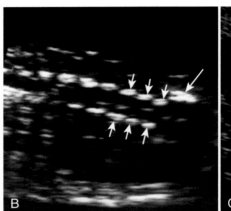

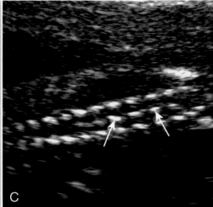

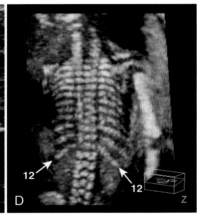

up an impression of the three-dimensional structures of the spine. The scan plane should then be repositioned parallel to the long axis of the fetal spine to obtain posterior longitudinal and lateral longitudinal views. The sonographer then examines all levels of the spine in posterior transaxial, lateral transaxial, lateral longitudinal, and posterior longitudinal scan planes. This may not be possible in a short time because of fetal position, but this usually changes enough in 30 to 45 minutes at 16 to 22 weeks to obtain all scan planes. If the spine cannot be visualized optimally, a repeat scan can be performed at a later gestational age.

Three-Dimensional Ultrasound

Three-dimensional ultrasound imaging has shown promise in evaluating normal fetal structures and in providing additional information in abnormalities of many fetal structures including the spine, hand, foot, and face.[24-33] Bony structures can be visualized with maximum-intensity projection methods (see Fig. 35-9, *D*). In evaluation of spinal abnormalities, 3-D ultrasound is most helpful in localizing spinal defects accurately by using simultaneous multiplanar imaging and referencing to the volume-rendered image.[24,27] For determination of spinal level, T12 is taken to be the most caudal vertebra with a corresponding rib.

SPINA BIFIDA

Spina bifida implies a physical defect in the structure of the spinal canal that may result in a protrusion of its contents (meninges, cerebrospinal fluid, and neural tissue) (Table 35-3). These defects usually occur along the dorsal midline (most often in the lumbosacral area) but rarely may occur anteriorly.

Open NTDs occur in 0.5 to 2 per 1000 births in North America and with higher frequencies in other geographic areas. In one area of China, the overall

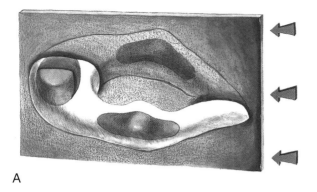

A

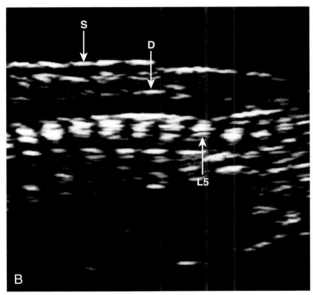

B

FIGURE 35-10. Posterior longitudinal scan plane.
A, Diagram shows the incident sound beam *(arrows)* reflecting off the posterior surface of the **centrum.** If there is no ossification in the laminae near the midline, the laminae will not be visible on the scan; only the centra will be seen. If the laminar ossification is present near the midline, the centra and laminae will be seen as echogenic foci. The red structures are ossified portions of the vertebra. **B,** Posterior longitudinal scan of the lumbosacral spine at 15 weeks shows **ossification in the centra** of the lower thoracic, lumbar, and sacral spine *(L5,* centrum of vertebra). In this midline scan, no ossification is present posterior to the posterior surface of the dural sac *(D). S,* Skin surface.

PROTOCOL TO EVALUATE SPINA BIFIDA WITH 3-D VOLUME DATA

Volume data are acquired from sagittal and transverse sweeps through the spine.
Volume data are reformatted to display standardized multiplanar views of the fetal spine.
3-D reconstruction of the fetal spine (with maximum-intensity projection filter) visualizes the ossified spinal elements.
To determine spinal level, the 12th thoracic (T12) is taken to be the most caudal vertebra with a corresponding rib.

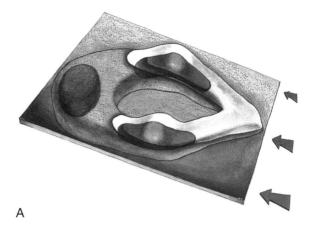

A

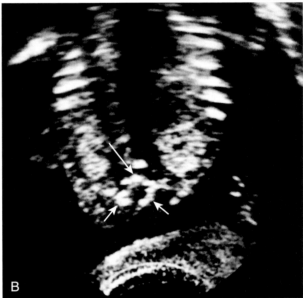

B

FIGURE 35-11. Posterior angled transaxial (transverse) scan plane. A, Diagram shows the incident sound beam *(arrows)* reflecting off the posterior aspects of the **laminae** and portions of the **pedicles.** The beam may also reflect off the ossified centrum. This scan plane can depict the **entire ring of ossification** of the spinal canal. The red structures are ossified portions of the vertebra. **B,** Endovaginal scan at 18 weeks in the midlumbar spine outlines the curvilinear structure of each neural arch *(short arrows,* lamina plus pedicle) and the ossified centrum *(long arrow).* Together these structures form the **ossified ring of the spinal canal.**

prevalence of NTDs in 2003 was 13.9 per 1000 live births.[34] In recent years, however, there has been a decline in the incidence of NTD. Some of this decline may be attributed to screening programs, which include measurement of MS-AFP and performance of second-trimester ultrasound.[35,36]

Folic Acid Fortification

Another major factor in the decline of the incidence of NTDs is the use of folic acid to prevent NTDs. Several

TABLE 35-3. DEFINITION OF TERMS FOR SPINAL ABNORMALITIES

TERM	DEFINITION	COMMENT
Spinal dysraphism (neural tube defect, NTD)	Failure of part of neural tube to close.	This disrupts both differentiation of central nervous system and induction of vertebral arches.
Spina bifida	Defect in posterior midline neural arch.	Arches fail to fuse along dorsal midline and fail to enclose vertebral canal.
Spina bifida occulta	Vertebral arches of a single vertebra fail to fuse.	Underlying neural tube differentiates normally; does not protrude from vertebral canal.
Meningocele	Dura and arachnoid protrude from vertebral canal through spina bifida defect in posterior midline neural arches	
Myelomeningocele	Dura, arachnoid, and neural tissue protrude from vertebral canal through spina bifida defect in posterior midline neural arches.	
Rachischisis (e.g., myeloschisis)	Neural folds corresponding to future spinal cord fail to fuse and fail to differentiate (myeloschisis), invaginate, and separate from surface ectoderm.	The deformed underdeveloped spinal cord is exposed dorsally. This is the most severe form of spinal neural tube defect.
Cranioschisis (e.g., exencephaly, anencephaly)	Neural folds corresponding to future brain fail to fuse and fail to differentiate, invaginate (exencephaly, anencephaly), and separate from surface ectoderm.	The brain is represented by an exposed dorsal mass of undifferentiated neural tissue.
Inionschisis	Failure of neural tube to differentiate properly and close in occipital and upper spinal region.	

clinical trials have demonstrated a decreased risk of NTD by at least 60% with the use of periconceptual folic acid supplements.[37-41] The reduction occurs in mothers with previously affected pregnancies and in mothers without this risk. In 1992 the U.S. Department of Health and Human Services[42] and the Expert Advisory Group in the United Kingdom[43] recommended supplementation of 0.4 mg of folic acid for women in the general population while trying to conceive. Women who are at high risk because of a previously affected fetus should take 4 mg of folic acid daily.[1] Routine folic acid supplementation around the time of conception confers a 72% to 87% decrease in probability of NTD.[3,38] However, this knowledge and these recommendations have not translated into a reduction of the incidence of NTD in the general population,[44,45] largely because only a minority take folic acid routinely in the reproductive years, and in those who do, supplementation may not be taken at the proper time. Studies in the 1990s demonstrated that less than 45% of pregnant women took folic acid before conception.[46-48] In 2007, 40% of all U.S. women of reproductive age (15-45 years) took daily supplements of folic acid. Daily supplements could be one serving of breakfast cereal fortified with 100% of the recommended daily value of folic acid or a supplement with 0.4 mg of folic acid daily.[4]

Another strategy to increase folic acid levels is the systematic fortification of food stuffs with folic acid. In March 1996 the U.S. Food and Drug Administration (FDA) ordered that fortification with folate of all enriched grain products be started no later than January 1, 1998 (0.14 mg per 100 grams of grain). Honein et al.[49] demonstrated a 19% reduction in NTDs in the United States as an effect of folic acid fortification of grains. This study did not take into account the large percentage of NTDs that are prenatally diagnosed and electively terminated. A study in Nova Scotia demonstrated a decrease of annual incidence of NTDs by 54% after implementation of folic acid fortification, from 2.58:1000 births from 1991 to 1997 to 1.17:1000 from 1998 to 2000.[50] This study included terminated pregnancies, which is important because more than 50% of all pregnancies affected with NTD in Nova Scotia result in elective termination. A failure to include these terminated pregnancies may underestimate the benefit of folic acid–fortified grains. In Canada, folic acid fortification of grain products was legislated to begin in November 1998, at levels similar to U.S. levels. Since then in Canada, the prevalence of NTDs nationally has decreased from 1.58:1000 before fortification to 0.86:1000 births during the full-fortification period, a 46% reduction.[6] Geographic differences almost disappeared after fortification began. The observed reduction rate was greater for spina bifida (53%) than for anencephaly and encephalocele (38% and 31%, respectively).

Lipomyelomeningocele (LMMC) is a type of NTD similar to myelomeningocele, with a prevalence of about 0.5 per 10,000 births. However, studies in Hawaii and Canada have shown that LMMC rates are not affected by folic acid fortification, unlike the significant rate reduction in myelomeningoceles. LMMC seems to be pathogenetically distinct from myelomengocele.[51,52]

The risk of NTD rises to 20 to 30 per 1000 live births for women with a previous infant with NTD. This

RISK FACTORS FOR NEURAL TUBE DEFECT (NTD)

Folic acid deficiency
Previous sibling with NTD
Maternal anticonvulsants
    Valproic acid
    Carbamazepine
Maternal warfarin
Maternal vitamin A
Pregestational diabetes
Obesity
Parent with spina bifida
Low maternal vitamin B_{12}

constitutes about a tenfold increase in risk over the general population.[53] A meta-analysis of randomized trials of folic acid for the prevention of recurrent NTDs demonstrated an 87% reduction in NTDs in women who took supplements before the start of pregnancy.[3] Other factors that increase the risk of NTD include anticonvulsant therapy with valproic acid or carbamazepine (10-20:1000), warfarin and vitamin A use, pregestational diabetes, obesity, parent with spina bifida (11:1000), and sibling of fetus with multiple vertebral defects and scoliosis (15-30:1000).[54] Low maternal vitamin B_{12} status may also be a risk factor for NTDs. In Ontario, Ray et al.[55] demonstrated a tripling of the risk for NTD in the presence of low maternal B_{12} status, as measured by serum holotranscobalamin at 15 to 20 weeks' gestation.

Pathogenesis and Pathology

Most cases of spina bifida result from failure of closure of the embryologic neural tube, although some may be caused by rupture of the neural tube after primary closure. Most NTDs occur as isolated malformations in chromosomally normal individuals, although 9% to 17% of fetuses with spina bifida have chromosomal abnormalities (mostly trisomy 18 and trisomy 13).[56,57] Typically, chromosomally abnormal fetuses have other sonographic abnormalities detected in addition to the spinal abnormality. Some NTDs are part of a genetic condition. Autosomal dominant conditions include **Lehman syndrome.** Autosomal recessive conditions include **Meckel-Gruber syndrome** and **VATER syndrome** (vertebral defect, imperforate anus, tracheoesophageal fistula, radial and renal dysplasia). Two X-linked conditions are the **Mathias laterality sequence** and **X-linked neural tube defects**.[2]

A number of studies have found the incidence of NTD to be about 10 times higher in spontaneously aborted pregnancies than in term births, indicating an in utero selection against embryos with such defects.[58]

In the most severe form of NTD, the embryologic neural tube (the precursor to the spinal cord) remains open in addition to the overlying mesodermal structures, which include the neural arch, muscles, and skin. The resultant pathology is **myeloschisis;** the open, flattened spinal cord is exposed posteriorly through a wide defect in the posterior neural arch and associated musculature and skin.

In less severe cases of NTD, the major anatomic defect is in the structures derived from the mesodermal tissues overlying the embryologic neural tube. Although the spinal cord often is anatomically intact, the embryologic neural tube has failed to induce closure of the overlying neural arches, muscles, and skin. The result is a **myelomeningocele,** a cystic mass protruding from the spinal canal. The cystic mass wall is composed of thin arachnoid membrane without skin covering, and the contents are cerebrospinal fluid (CSF) and neural elements. Occasionally, a myelomeningocele is covered with skin. A skin-covered myelomeningocele is considered a **closed defect,** and a myelomeningocele without skin covering is considered an **open defect.** An open defect allows AFP to escape into the surrounding amniotic fluid; a closed defect does not. Thus, a closed or skin-covered defect is not usually associated with raised levels of AFP in the amniotic fluid or maternal serum. Infrequently, the protruding cystic mass contains only CSF and no neural elements, a **meningocele.**

Spina bifida occulta is restricted to involvement of the mesoderm of the posterior vertebral arch and rarely exhibits intrinsic maldevelopment of the spinal cord. This may result from an insult occurring at the end of the fourth embryologic week (sixth menstrual week), causing failure of complete formation of the posterior midline structures. The prevalence of spina bifida occulta, excluding cases that later disappear (i.e., delayed ossification of preexisting intact cartilage), is approximately 17%.[59] The lumbosacral spine is most often involved. About 66% of spina bifida occulta cases have skin manifestations: nevi, lumbosacral lipomas, dermal sinus, hypertrichosis (tuft of hair, "horse's tail or fawn's tail"), or scarred area. A sacral pit or dimple is not highly correlated with spina bifida occulta. Although infrequently associated with other abnormalities, spina bifida occulta may be associated with urologic dysfunction and tethered cord syndrome, foot deformity, increased incidence of spondylolisthesis, and intervertebral disc herniation. Spina bifida occulta is difficult to detect with prenatal ultrasound unless it is associated with a **lipoma,** a simple **meningocele,** or **tethered cord.** A history of familial spina bifida occulta is not known to be a risk factor for an open neural tube defect.[2]

Alpha-Fetoprotein and Ultrasound Screening

Because most NTDs occur in families with no history of such abnormalities, prenatal detection relies on routine screening measures, including ultrasound and MS-AFP measurement.

Alpha-fetoprotein is a glycoprotein (molecular weight, 70,000) produced by fetal liver. Some of it enters the amniotic fluid through fetal urine, and a small amount crosses the placenta to maternal serum. Normal AFP levels in amniotic fluid and maternal serum vary with gestational age. MS-AFP and amniotic fluid AFP are elevated in NTDs that are not skin covered. If the upper limit of normal MS-AFP is taken to be 2.5 multiples of the median (MOM) for a given gestational age, MS-AFP will be elevated in approximately 90% of open NTDs. About 2% of normal pregnancies have an elevated MS-AFP; that is, of all the elevated test results for MS-AFP, most fetuses will be normal (Fig. 35-12). At this stage, a detailed ultrasound examination is required to determine which fetuses actually have an NTD.

Norem at al.[60] found that MS-AFP testing was normal in 25% of NTDs (25 of 102 cases). These included 15 of the 40 (38%) spina bifida cases screened, 6 of the 9 (67%) encephalocele cases screened, and 4 of the 53 (8%) anencephaly cases screened. Of the 186 NTD cases diagnosed prenatally, 115 (62%) were initially detected by routine sonography during the second trimester without knowledge of MS-AFP values. Sixty-nine (37%) were diagnosed by targeted sonography after MS-AFP screening indicated a higher risk for NTD. Two (1%) were diagnosed by pathology examination after miscarriage.

Maternal serum AFP is also elevated in **multifetal pregnancy, fetal death, fetomaternal transfusion,** and in other fetal anomalies associated with a defect in the skin, such as **omphalocele** and **gastroschisis** (50%-60% of cases), **congenital nephrosis** (Finnish type, 100% of cases), and infrequently in esophageal or duodenal atresia, polycystic kidney disease, renal agenesis, urinary obstruction, epidermolysis bullosa, sacrococcygeal

teratoma, cystic hygroma, osteogenesis imperfecta, cloacal exstrophy, and cyclopia.

Because of the high sensitivity of the cerebellar signs associated with open spina bifida, some centers rely almost exclusively on ultrasound to diagnose NTDs. For women with elevated MS-AFP and no sonographic explanation for the abnormal test result (e.g., wrong dates, multiple fetuses, dead fetus, anencephaly, spina bifida, abdominal wall defect, other fetal abnormality causing elevated AFP), or when there is poor visualization of the spine, **amniocentesis** may be offered. If the amniotic fluid AFP is normal and there is no **acetylcholinesterase** (AChE) present, the likelihood of an open NTD is very low. If the amniotic fluid AFP is elevated and AChE is present, an open NTD or abdominal wall defect may be present but undetected by sonography.

Between 1989 and 1990, 1.1 million women in California had MS-AFP tests in early pregnancy.[61] From these tests, 1390 fetal abnormalities were found (1.3 fetal anomalies per 1000 pregnancies), consisting of 710 NTDs (417 cases of anencephaly, 247 cases of spina bifida, and 46 cases of encephalocele) and 680 nonneural abnormalities (286 anterior abdominal wall defects, 163 cases of trisomy 21, and 231 other chromosomal abnormalities).

Sonographic Findings in the Spine

Spina bifida may occur anywhere in the fetal spine but is most common in the **lumbosacral** area.[62] Ultrasound findings in the spine consist of abnormalities of the ossified posterior elements and related soft tissues.

In spina bifida the **laminae** fail to converge toward midline, and this is best visualized with the posterior transaxial scan plane (Fig. 35-13, *A* and *B;* **Video 35-1**). If the **pedicles** are normally positioned and there is no myelomeningocele, the posterior transaxial scan plane is the only view that will depict the abnormality with reliability. When the pedicles are displaced more laterally than usual, the lateral transaxial and lateral longitudinal scan planes will also demonstrate the bony abnormalities of spina bifida (Fig. 35-13, *C* and *D*). All these scan planes will usually demonstrate the meningocele or myelomeningocele if it is present (Figs. 35-14, 35-15, and 35-16). The posterior longitudinal scan best demonstrates a myelomeningocele and the soft tissue defect when no cystic mass is present.

In most cases of spina bifida, there is abnormal divergence or splaying of the pedicles over several vertebral levels. This is best appreciated in 3-D images and in lateral longitudinal views, where multiple interpedicular distances can be evaluated simultaneously (Fig. 35-13). However, there is normally mild divergence of the pedicles in the cervical spine compared to the thoracic spine (Fig. 35-14), and there may be slight divergence (by 1 to 2 mm) in the lumbar spine compared with the thoracic spine in normal fetuses (see Fig. 35-2).

CAUSES OF ELEVATED MATERNAL SERUM ALPHA-FETOPROTEIN

Multifetal pregnancy
Fetal death
Fetomaternal transfusion
Omphalocele and gastroschisis
Congenital nephrosis
Esophageal or duodenal atresia
Polycystic kidney disease
Renal agenesis
Urinary obstruction
Epidermolysis bullosa
Sacrococcygeal teratoma
Cystic hygroma
Osteogenesis imperfecta
Cloacal exstrophy
Cyclopia
Normal (2% of pregnancies)

Sonography can also be used to determine the level and extent of the spinal abnormality. The level of the defect is taken to be the top or most cephalic end of the bone malformation.[63] Fetal MRI and fetal ultrasound are equally effective in determining the lesion level in a fetus with myelomeningocele,[64] although each modality may misdiagnose the upper level by two or more segments in 20% of cases. Fetal MRI is more sensitive in evaluation of the spinal cord itself, yielding additional information in about 10% of cases.[65]

The prognosis is influenced by the defect level, the NTD type, the presence or absence of associated anomalies, the presence or absence of chromosomal abnormalities, and the presence or absence of cranial abnormalities, such as Chiari II malformation and ventriculomegaly. Biggio et al.[66] described the outcome in 33 infants with isolated open spina bifida. Lower lesion levels and smaller ventricular size were associated with ambulatory status. All infants with L4-sacral NTD were ambulatory. Of patients with L1-L3 NTD, 50% were ambulatory. No infant with thoracic NTD was ambulatory. No infant with myeloschisis was ambulatory.

Associated Cranial Abnormalities

The biparietal diameter (BPD) may be less than expected (even when the lateral ventricles are enlarged).[67,68] Four other cranial findings are particularly useful in raising suspicion of an NTD: nonvisualization of the cisterna magna, deformation of the cerebellar shape (banana sign), concave frontal bones (lemon sign), and dilation of the lateral cerebral ventricles.

Chiari II malformation is highly associated with open spina bifida (>97% of cases). This cranial lesion consists of variable degrees of displacement of the cerebellar vermis, fourth ventricle, and medulla oblongata through the foramen magnum into the upper cervical canal and is usually easier to identify than the spinal lesion between 16 and 24 weeks' gestation. In transaxial scans through the posterior fossa, Chiari II malformation is manifest as a deformation of the cerebellar shape ("banana" sign) and nonvisualization of the cisterna magna. Cranial malformations may signal the sonographer that a detailed study of the spine is required to search for spina bifida.

Spinal dysraphism allows a leak of CSF from the spinal canal into the amniotic fluid, which causes low intracranial pressure (ICP) early in pregnancy. Low ICP induces a smaller-than-normal posterior fossa compartment. The cerebellum then grows into this abnormally small space, which leads to obliteration of the cisterna magna, compression of the cerebellar hemispheres, herniation of the cerebellar tonsils into the cervical spinal canal, and related abnormalities such as **ventriculomegaly.** Ventriculomegaly is usually mild in the second trimester and worsens postpartum after repair of the spinal defect. Ventriculomegaly is seen in 44% to 86% of fetuses with spina bifida.[69,70] The most common single cause of ventriculomegaly is spina bifida, although only 30% to 40% of fetuses with enlarged ventricles actually have spina bifida. On ultrasound, the Chiari II malformation manifests as obliteration of the cisterna magna.[71,72] The compression of the cerebellum changes its shape, giving the **banana sign.**[69,73] In two different series, obliteration of the cisterna magna was noted in 22 of 23 cases with spina bifida at 16 to 27 weeks' gestation[72] and in 18 of 20 cases at 24 weeks and earlier.[72]

Concave deformity of the fetal frontal bones in the second trimester is called the **lemon sign.**[74] Various authors have shown that 85% of fetuses with spina bifida before 24 weeks gestation have the lemon sign.[70,75-77] In practice, the lemon sign can be difficult to portray unequivocally. The lemon sign spontaneously resolves in the third trimester.[76] In addition, it is seen in 1% of normal fetuses.[75,76] The lemon sign should prompt detailed examination of the posterior fossa, to search for obliteration of the cisterna magna and for the banana sign, and the fetal spine, for direct evidence of spina bifida.

Associated Noncranial Abnormalities

Foot deformities, primarily **clubfoot,** and **dislocation of the hips** are frequently associated with spina bifida.[78] These are caused by imbalanced muscular actions

---

ANATOMIC LANDMARKS* USED TO ESTABLISH LEVEL OF BONY DEFECT

- T12 corresponds to the medial ends of the most caudal ribs.
- L5-S1 lies at the superior margin of the iliac wing.[27]
- S4 is the most caudal vertebral body ossification center in the second trimester.[63]
- S5 is the most caudal vertebral body ossification center in the third trimester.[63]

* Thoracic (T), lumbar (L), and sacral (S) vertebrae.

SONOGRAPHIC SIGNS OF SPINA BIFIDA

Nonvisualization of cisterna magna
Deformation of cerebellum (banana sign)
Concave frontal bones (lemon sign)
Dilation of the lateral ventricles
Chiari II malformation (97%)
Biparietal diameter lower than expected

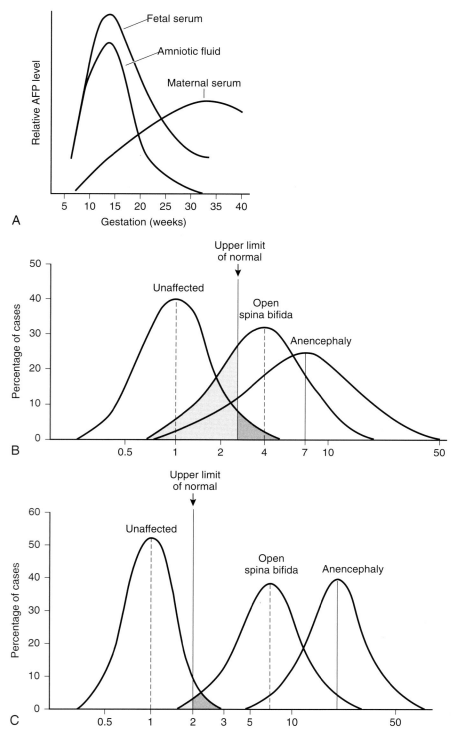

FIGURE 35-12. Alpha-fetoprotein (AFP) levels versus gestational (menstrual) age. A, Normal AFP levels in fetal serum, amniotic fluid, and maternal serum (MS) vary with gestational age. It is imperative to have accurate dating to evaluate AFP results properly. **B,** MS-AFP at 16 to 18 weeks' gestation. (Percentage of cases vs. AFP levels, expressed as multiples of the median [MOM] along horizontal axis.) There is considerable overlap in the values of MS-AFP between normal pregnancies and those with fetuses affected with open spina bifida and anencephaly. This illustration demonstrates the overlap (*shaded areas* under the curves) when 2.5 MOM are taken to be upper normal. A cutoff of 2.0 MOM would detect more affected pregnancies but increase the rate of amniocentesis in normal pregnancies. *Lighter-shaded area,* False negatives (i.e., test negative, but NTD present); *darker-shaded area,* false positives (i.e., test positive, but fetus normal). **C,** Amniotic fluid AFP at 16 to 18 weeks' gestation. (Percentage of cases vs. AFP levels, expressed as MOM along horizontal axis.) There is significantly less overlap between normal pregnancies and pregnancies with open NTDs. The shaded area under the curves to the left of 2 represents the false negatives, and the shaded area to the right of 2 represents the false positives. In practice, the false positives can be largely excluded by normal acetylcholinesterase levels in the amniotic fluid.

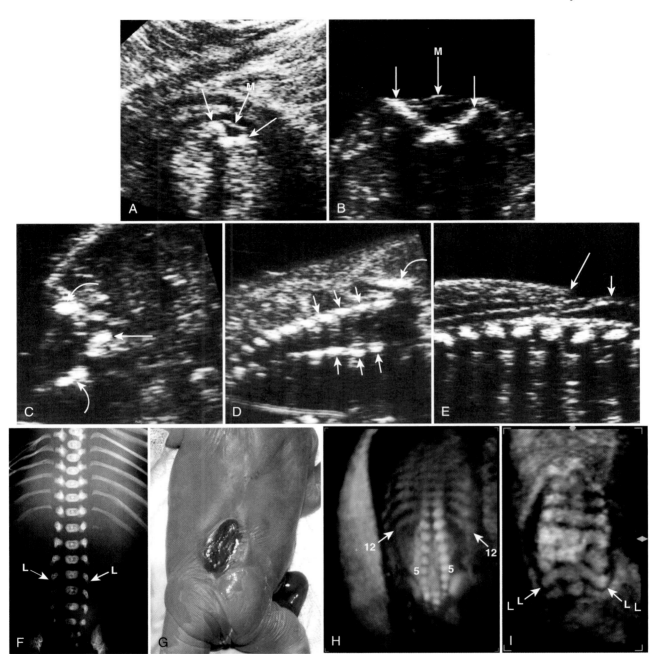

FIGURE 35-13. Myeloschisis. A, Posterior transaxial scan shows splaying of the lumbar laminae *(arrows)* away from midline. Only a thin membrane *(M)* overlies the spinal defect posteriorly. **B,** Posterior transaxial scan of the specimen after delivery shows in more detail the splaying of the laminae *(arrows)* away from midline and the membrane *(M)* covering the defect. **C,** Lateral transaxial scan of specimen shows increased distance between the pedicles *(curved arrows)* and mild lateral angulation of the pedicles away from their expected positions *(straight arrow,* ossified centrum). **D,** Lateral longitudinal scan of specimen shows the progressive enlargement of the interpedicular distances in the lumbar spine, indicative of spina bifida. Ossified pedicles *(straight arrows);* iliac wing *(curved arrow).* **E,** Posterior longitudinal scan of specimen shows abrupt truncation of the soft tissues of the fetal back *(long arrow)* at the site of the open neural tube defect (NTD); *short arrow,* spinal cord. **F,** Radiograph of specimen shows divergence of the laminae *(L)* away from midline instead of the normal course, which is toward midline. **G,** Photograph of myeloschisis defect of the thoracolumbar spine shows exposed, disorganized neural tissue within the defect. **H,** 3-D scan of another fetus at 19 weeks, as viewed from the posterior aspect of the fetus. Note the abnormal divergence of the pedicles in the lumbar spine *(arrows,* 12th rib level; *5,* level 5). **I,** 3-D scan of a different fetus at 21 weeks, as viewed from the posterior aspect of the fetus. Note the divergence of the lumbar pedicles and the splaying of the laminae *(L)* away from the midline. *(**I** courtesy Siemens Ultrasound.)*

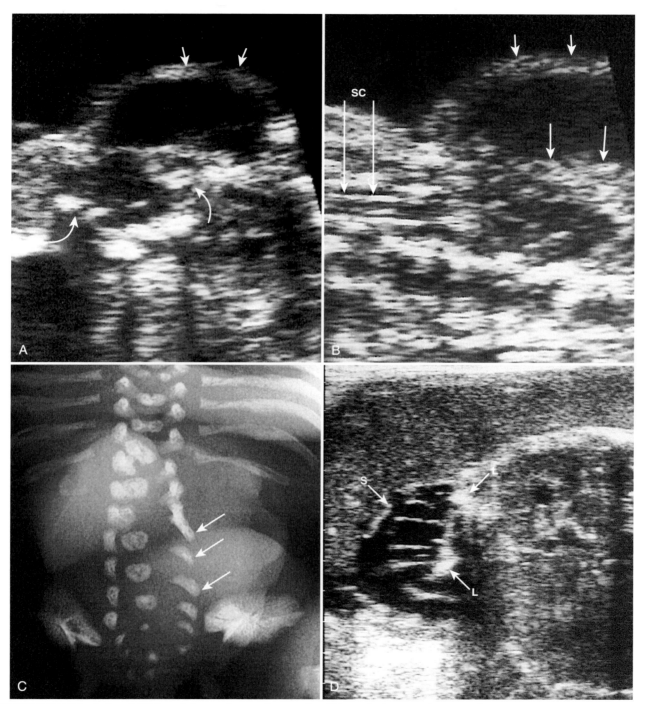

FIGURE 35-14. Spina bifida with myelomeningocele, 17 weeks' gestation specimen. A, Posterior transaxial scan of the midlumbar spine shows the splaying of the laminae *(curved arrows)* and the myelomeningocele sac *(short arrows)*. **B,** Posterior longitudinal scan of the thoracolumbar area shows the myelomeningocele sac *(short arrows)* and disorganized neural tissue *(long arrows)* within it; *SC,* spinal cord. **C,** Radiograph shows the interpedicular distances in the lumbar spine are widened and the laminae are splayed laterally *(arrows).* **D,** Lateral transaxial scan in a different fetus shows the myelomeningocele sac *(S)* containing linear echoes representing neural tissue and the splayed laminae/pedicles complex *(L, arrows).*

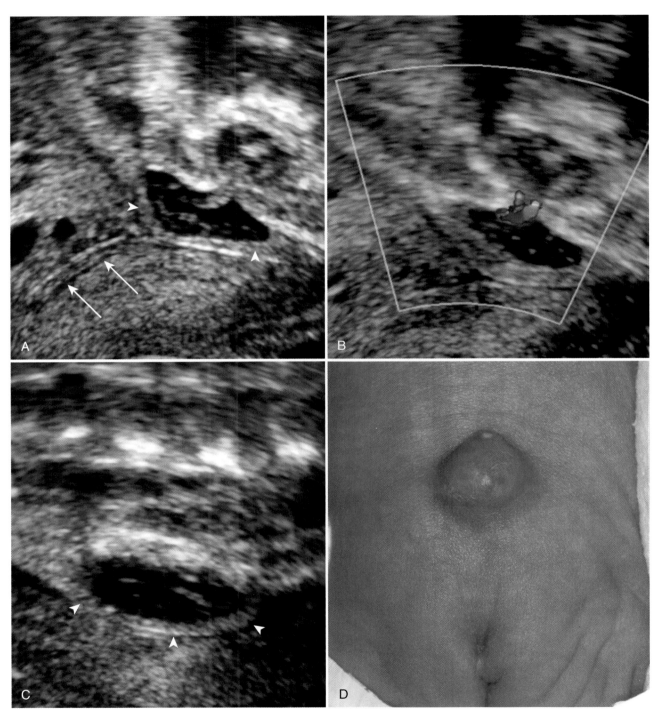

FIGURE 35-15. Skin-covered myelomeningocele. A, Endovaginal posterior transaxial scan shows a myelomeningocele sac covered by a thick wall *(arrowheads)*. Echogenic material passes through the spina bifida defect into the myelomeningocele sac. Endocervical canal *(arrows)*. **B,** Endovaginal color Doppler posterior transaxial scan demonstrates a blood vessel protruding from the spinal canal into the myelomeningocele sac. **C,** Endovaginal posterior longitudinal scan shows the myelomeningocele sac covered by a thick wall *(arrowheads)*. **D,** Neonatal picture shows the focal skin-covered lumbar myelomeningocele. The bluish tinge within the sac is a blood vessel detected by endovaginal color Doppler in **B.**

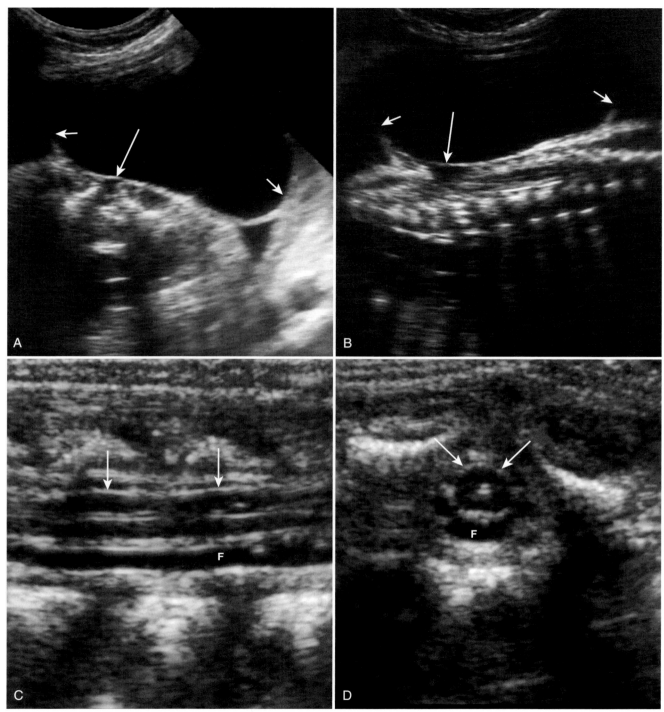

FIGURE 35-16. Lumbar meningocele, 34 weeks' gestation. A, Posterior transaxial sonogram demonstrates a fluid-filled sac *(small arrows)* along the fetal back. There is a small defect in the neural arch *(large arrow).* **B,** Posterior longitudinal sonogram shows the wall of the meningocele *(small arrows)* and the focal spina bifida defect in the posterior neural arch *(large arrow).* **C,** Posterior longitudinal and **D,** posterior transaxial sonograms demonstrate abnormally posterior thoracic spinal cord *(arrows)* in the nondependent portion of the spinal canal. Cerebrospinal fluid *(f)* is between the anterior aspect of the spinal cord and the anterior wall of the spinal canal.

resulting from peripheral nerve involvement with the NTD. In fetuses with open spina bifida, 24% demonstrate additional morphologic abnormalities on second-trimester sonography, such as renal abnormalities, **choroid plexus cysts, cardiac ventricular septal defect, omphalocele,** and **intrauterine growth restriction** (IUGR).[56]

Prognosis

It is difficult to predict the long-term prognosis in a fetus with an identified myelomeningocele. However, the outcome is better for low lesions (lower lumbar or sacral), closed defects, and those with minimal or no hydrocephalus and no compression of the hindbrain from Chiari II malformation.[53,64,73,79] In more than 880 patients[80] of live deliveries with spina bifida, about 85% survived past age 10, and 2% died in the neonatal period. Of the survivors, about 50% had some type of learning disability. About 25% of survivors had an IQ (intelligence quotient) above 100, with about 75% above 80. About 33% of survivors developed symptoms and signs related to pressure on the hindbrain and brainstem (e.g., pain, weakness, and spasticity in arms), and some required cervical laminectomy to relieve the pressure. Wong and Paulozzi[81] found 5-year survival rates of 82.7% for 1979-1983, 88.5% for 1984-1988, and 91.0% for 1989-1994. Determining prognosis for survival for current newborns is more difficult because of medical and surgical advances since studies describing patients born in the 1960s, 1970s, and 1980s.[2]

Beyond survival, multiple impairments may affect the individual, including **motor function, bladder and bowel dysfunction,** and **intellectual impairment.**[2] Degree of muscle dysfunction is defined by the highest level of the open NTD, not by the number of involved vertebrae or the size of the overlying sac. When the lesion is thoracic, the **legs** are without muscle function, and when it is upper lumbar (L1-L2), useful leg function is minimal. When the upper level is L3-L5, the prognosis for long-term walking and the need for assistive devices are difficult to predict. Those with sacral defects will usually be able to walk well but with imperfect gait. Almost all people with spina bifida, including those with sacral defects, will have some degree of bowel and bladder dysfunction.

It is very difficult to predict the ultimate level of **intellectual functioning.** In general, those who do not require ventricular shunting have much better outcomes for intellectual functioning. In those requiring shunts, the average IQ is approximately 80, which is low-normal range.[82] The rate of profound intellectual impairment (IQ <20) in those with shunts is 5%, usually related to medical complications such as shunt infections and Chiari II effects (e.g., apnea, hypoxia).

Fetal Surgery for Myelomeningocele

Fetal surgery for repair of myelomeningocele is regarded as an experimental procedure. Parents and others must evaluate the potential for improved function for the child against the risks of fetal death during or after surgery and fetal/maternal surgical morbidity. Fetal myelomeningocele is a nonlethal entity; in utero surgery for repair of myelomeningocele is potentially lethal.[83]

Although myelomeningocele is a primary embryologic disorder, neurologic damage is also secondary to progressive in utero damage to the exposed spinal cord. The development of techniques to close open NTDs before birth has generated great interest and hope for fetal interventions and outcomes. To date, preliminary observations from two centers suggest that improvements may occur not in spinal cord function as originally postulated,[84] but in the extent of the hindbrain herniation and the frequency that shunting is required to control hydrocephalus. In a report of 25 patients who underwent intrauterine myelomeningocele repair at Vanderbilt University, no improvement in leg function resulted from the surgery, but there was a substantially reduced incidence of moderate to severe hindbrain herniation (4% vs. 50%) and a moderate reduction in the incidence of shunt-dependent hydrocephalus (58% vs. 92%).[85] The hope for improved long-term neurologic improvement have not been realized. The number of U.S. centers is limited to three to prevent the uncontrolled proliferation of new centers offering this procedure.[86] Prospective parents electing surgery in the hope of mitigating possible damage to their child's mental life, through the potential benefits of reduced hydrocephalus and hindbrain herniation,[87] should be cautioned to carefully weigh the potential benefits of surgery against the potential risks of prematurity.[87-90]

MYELOCYSTOCELE

Myelocystocele is an uncommon form of spinal dysraphism. There is dilation of the central canal of the spinal cord. The central canal herniates posteriorly through the spinal cord and through the posterior neural arch to form an exterior sac. There may be no associated spina bifida lesion.

The sac is composed of three layers, from inner to outer: the **hydromyelia sac,** which is lined by spinal canal ependyma; the **meningeal layer,** which is contiguous with the meninges around the spinal cord; and the **skin.** The fluid within the inner sac is continuous with the fluid of the central canal of the spinal cord; the fluid between the hydromyelia sac and the meningeal layer is continuous with the subarachnoid fluid.

Myelocystocele may occur at any level of the spine and is often associated with Chiari II malformation.[91-93]

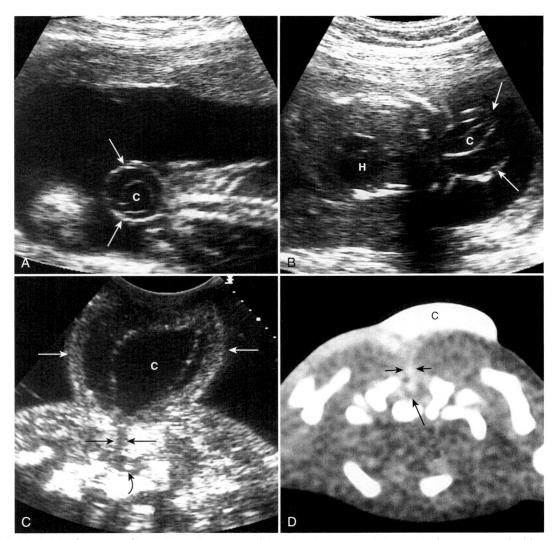

FIGURE 35-17. Myelocystocele. A, Coronal sonogram of thoracic spine at 18 weeks' gestation demonstrates a double-walled cystic mass *(arrows)* with inner cystic component *(c)* arising from the upper thoracic area. **B,** Axial sonogram of the fetal chest 1 week later demonstrates a double-walled cystic mass *(arrows)* arising along the posterior aspect of the fetal chest; *H,* fetal heart. The inner cystic component *(C)* is slightly smaller and flattened compared to the first scan. No abnormality was noted in the ossified neural arch. **C,** Sonogram of the specimen demonstrates the double-walled cystic mass *(white arrows)* arising from the posterior thorax with a hypoechoic tract *(black arrows)* extending from the posterior aspect of the spinal cord *(curved arrow)* toward the central cystic component *(C)* of the posterior mass. **D,** CT scan of the specimen after injection of water-soluble contrast material into the cyst demonstrates contrast within the cyst *(C)* and within a sinus tract *(small arrows),* leading to the spinal cord *(large arrow).*

Prenatal and postnatal sonography demonstrates a "cyst within a cyst" appearance (Fig. 35-17). Splaying of the laminae and pedicles may or may not be present. The prognosis for a myelocystocele is worse than for a simple meningocele; infants with a simple meningocele may remain normal neurologically after surgical repair. The prognosis with myelocystocele is worse because there is usually some degree of associated myelodysplasia (i.e., dysplasia of spinal cord). Although neurologic function is normal in the immediate postoperative period, neurologic deficits often become apparent later in life.

A **terminal myelocystocele** occurs at the spinal cord termination. The central canal of the spinal cord herniates with overlying arachnoid and cerebrospinal fluid

through a defect in posterior spinal elements and presents as a skin-covered mass along the posterior aspect of the lumbosacral area. There may be associated maldevelopment of the lower spine, pelvis, genitalia, bowel, bladder, kidneys, and abdominal wall. MRI provides the best imaging evaluation of the morphologic abnormalities after birth.[94-96]

DIASTEMATOMYELIA

Diastematomyelia, also termed **split-cord malformation,** is a partial or complete sagittal cleft in the spinal cord,

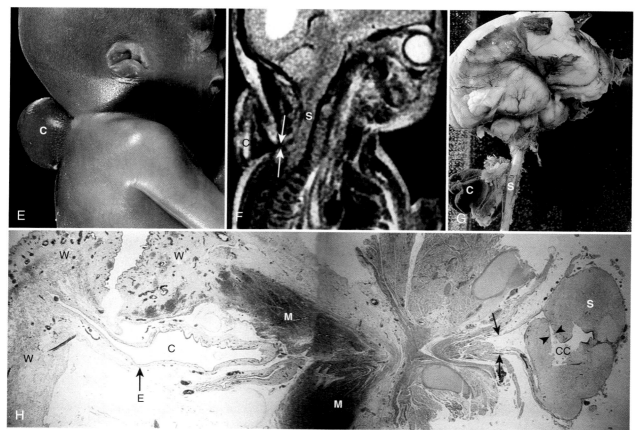

FIGURE 35-17, cont'd. E, Lateral view of the posterior cystic thoracic mass *(C).* **F,** Sagittal MR scan demonstrates the cystic mass along the upper thoracic area, with the small sinus tract *(arrows)* extending from the posterior aspect of the spinal cord *(S)* toward the cystic mass *(C).* **G,** Gross pathologic specimen demonstrates the collapsed cyst *(C)* in contiguity with the cervical portion of the spinal cord *(S).* **H,** Histologic section shows abnormal channel *(arrows)* communicating with the posterior aspect of the spinal cord *(S),* as well as defect in the posterior spinal cord *(arrowheads)* communicating with the central canal *(CC)* of the spinal cord; *C,* central cystic component of posterior mass *(M); E,* ependymal lining of central cyst, which communicates with central canal of spinal cord; *W,* outer wall of cystic mass.

the distal conus of the cord, or filum terminale. Diastema-tomyelia is characterized by a sagittal osseous or fibrous septum in the spinal cord.[97,98] This may be associated with a spina bifida defect and hydromyelia (dilation of central canal of spinal cord) but may occur in the absence of overt spina bifida.[99] Diastematomyelia may also be associated with segmental anomalies of the vertebral bodies or visceral malformations such as horseshoe or ectopic kidney, utero-ovarian malformation, and anorectal malformation. If the spinal canal is traversed by a **bony septum** or **spur,** the septum will appear as an abnormal hyperechoic focus,[100-102] which is best demonstrated in the posterior transaxial and lateral longitudinal scan planes (Fig. 35-18). When diastematomyelia is not associated with other spinal anomalies, the prognosis is favorable. In seven of eight cases reported by Has et al.,[103] the defects had normal amniotic AFP and AChE levels and were considered isolated. Their review of the literature showed 26 cases diagnosed prenatally, 12 of which had no associated abnormality and had a favorable prognosis.

SCOLIOSIS AND KYPHOSIS

Kyphosis is exaggerated curvature of the spine in the sagittal plane. **Scoliosis** is lateral curvature of the spine. Kyphosis and scoliosis may be positional and nonpathologic or permanent based on an underlying structural abnormality, such as **hemivertebrae, butterfly vertebrae,** and **block vertebrae.** Pathologic kyphosis and scoliosis are often associated with **spina bifida** or **ventral abdominal wall defects.**[104] Less common associations include limb–body wall complex, amniotic band syndrome, arthrogryposis, skeletal dysplasias, VACTERL association,[105,106] and caudal regression syndrome. Mild scoliosis may be caused by a **hemivertebra.**[103,106]

The posterior longitudinal scan is the best view to assess for kyphosis; the lateral longitudinal plane is the best to assess for scoliosis (Fig. 35-19). Because oligohydramnios can cause positional curvature in the fetal spine, a confident diagnosis of pathologic kyphosis or scoliosis should be made only if the curvature is severe.

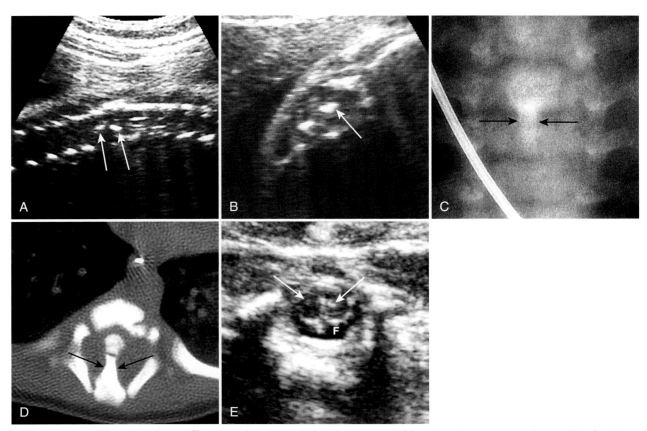

FIGURE 35-18. Diastematomyelia. A and **B,** Coronal and axial sonograms of the spine demonstrate two hyperechoic foci *(arrow)* caused by the bony septum within the spinal canal with intact skin along the fetal back. **C,** Anteroposterior radiograph, and **D,** CT scan, demonstrate a bony septum *(arrows)* within the central portion of the spinal canal. **E, Diplomyelia** and **tethered cord.** Posterior transaxial sonogram of another fetus shows cord in the nondependent portion of the spinal canal with fluid *(F)* interposed between the cord and anterior margin of the spinal canal. The anterior aspect of the cord has a bilobed shape instead of a smooth, circular arc with bilateral central canal echoes *(arrows).*

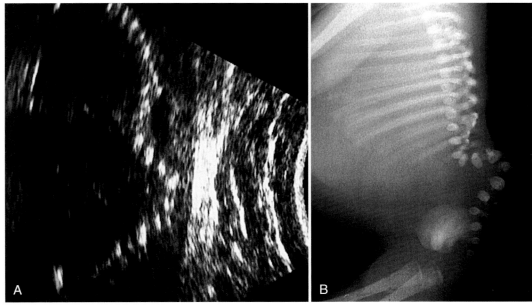

FIGURE 35-19. Kyphosis. A, Sagittal scan (turned to match radiograph) of the fetus demonstrates an S-shaped curvature to the thoracolumbar spine. **B,** Lateral radiograph of the neonate demonstrates the severe S-shaped curvature of the thoracolumbar spine.

CAUSES OF SCOLIOSIS OR KYPHOSIS

Hemivertebrae
Butterfly vertebrae
Block vertebrae
Spina bifida
Ventral abdominal wall defects
Limb–body wall complex
Amniotic band syndrome
Arthrogryposis
Skeletal dysplasias
VACTERL* association
Caudal regression syndrome

*Vertebral abnormalities, anal atresia, cardiac abnormalities, tracheoesophageal fistula, renal agenesis, and limb defects.

Possible associated anomalies must then be sought because prognosis depends on the coexistent anomalies.

A **hemivertebra** represents underdevelopment or nondevelopment of one half of a vertebral body; that is, one of the two early chondrification centers is deficient. The remaining ossification center is displaced laterally with respect to the vertebrae above and below it, leading to a short-segment mild scoliosis. The abnormalities can be detected prenatally and may be best portrayed with 3-D ultrasound.[30-33] Fetuses with an isolated hemivertebra have an excellent prognosis, whereas those with other fetal anomalies (e.g., Potter's syndrome; cardiac, intestinal, intracranial, and limb anomalies) have a poor prognosis.[107] The presence of associated anomalies reduces survival to approximately 50%. If oligohydramnios is also present, the mortality approaches 100%.[108]

SACRAL AGENESIS

Sacral agenesis is an uncommon fetal abnormality that may be present in conditions such as **caudal regression sequence**, **sirenomelia sequence**, **cloacal exstrophy sequence**, and the **VACTERL association** (vertebral abnormalities, anal atresia, tracheoesophageal fistula, renal dysplasia, and limb defects). The caudal regression sequence (caudal regression syndrome) and the sirenomelia sequence are thought to be separate pathologic entities.[109,110]

CAUDAL REGRESSION

In caudal regression or dysplasia, abnormalities of the lower spine and limbs occur, including **sacral agenesis, lumbar spine deficiency,** and leg anomalies such as **femoral hypoplasia** (Fig. 35-20). Defects of the neural tube and the genitourinary, gastrointestinal, and cardiac

systems are common. Occurrence is sporadic; caudal regression is more common in infants of mothers with diabetes mellitus. The etiology is not established. Sonography can demonstrate absence of the sacrum and shortened femurs. The legs can be flexed and abducted at the hips, and there may be clubfoot. Sonography may detect associated urinary anomalies (renal agenesis, cystic dysplasia, caliectasis) and gastrointestinal abnormalities (e.g., duodenal atresia).[111] The prognosis depends on the severity and extent of the skeletal abnormalities and associated anomalies. In sacral agenesis with no internal organ involvement, there are usually deficits in the legs and deficient control of bladder and bowel functions. In infants with internal organ involvement, the prognosis is related to these defects.

SIRENOMELIA

Sirenomelia sequence is a rare disorder in which the legs are fused and the feet are deformed or absent[112] (Fig. 35-21). The cause is probably an **aberrant fetal artery** that branches from the upper abdominal aorta and passes into the umbilical cord to the placenta.[113] Arterial blood flow bypasses the lower fetal body. The distal abdominal aorta, the aorta's distal branches, and subtended structures are small and underdeveloped. This leads to malformations of spine, legs, kidneys, gut, and genitalia. Normally the umbilical arteries, which arise from the fetal iliac arteries, carry blood from the fetus into the umbilical cord and then into the placenta.

At sonography, there is advanced **oligohydramnios** because of reduced or absent renal function. The legs are fused, or there is a single leg. The feet are absent, or there may be a single foot. There may be sacral agenesis, deficiency of the lower lumbar spine, and thoracic anomalies. These findings may be difficult to appreciate because of the advanced oligohydramnios or anhydramnios.[109] The prolonged anhydramnios causes pulmonary hypoplasia, which is usually fatal. The risk of recurrence is the same as in the general population.

SACROCOCCYGEAL TERATOMA

Fetal teratomas may arise from the sacrum or coccyx, from other midline structures from the level of the brain to the coccyx, or from the gonads.[114] Sacrococcygeal teratomas arise from the pluripotent cells of Hensen's node located anterior to the coccyx. Sacrococcygeal teratomas contain all three germ layers (ectoderm, mesoderm, and endoderm) and thus may contain elements of many tissues, including neural, respiratory, and gastrointestinal. Sacrococcygeal tumor is rare (1:35,000 births)[115] but the most common tumor of neonates. Females are affected four times more frequently than males. Sacrococcygeal teratomas are classified into four

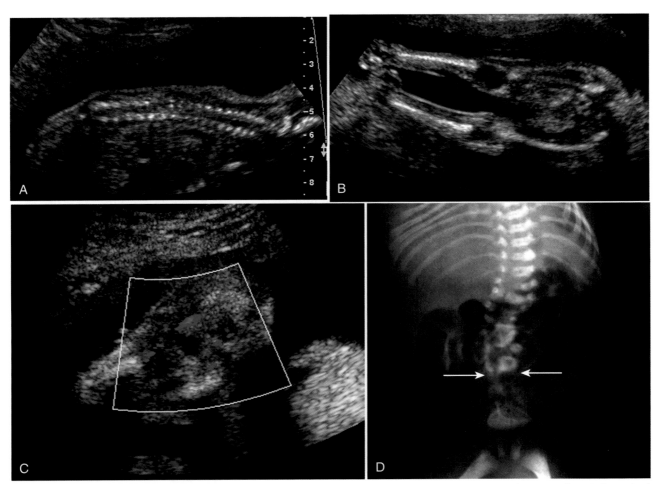

FIGURE 35-20. Caudal regression. A, Sagittal sonogram of spine at 21 weeks shows abrupt termination of ossified vertebral bodies. **B,** Transverse view of pelvis with legs in long axis shows lack of ossified pelvic bones and atrophic musculature about the lower extremities. **C,** Transverse color Doppler image at level of bladder shows lack of ossified pelvic bones. **D,** In a different fetal specimen, radiograph shows abrupt termination *(arrows)* of the lumbar spine and absence of the sacrum. The pelvic bones are small and deformed.

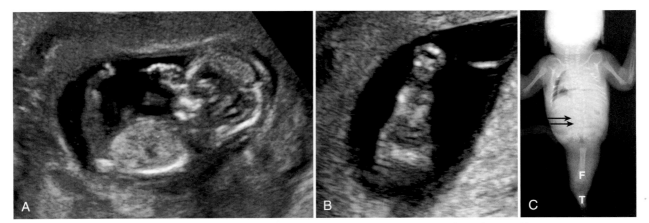

FIGURE 35-21 Sirenomelia. A, Sagittal view of fetus at 12 weeks' gestation shows unusual angulation of lower extremity. **B,** Long-axis view of a single lower extremity. **C,** In a different fetus, radiograph shows single femur *(F)* and single tibia *(T)*. Note the segmented defects in the vertebrae of the thoracic and lumbar spine *(arrows)*.

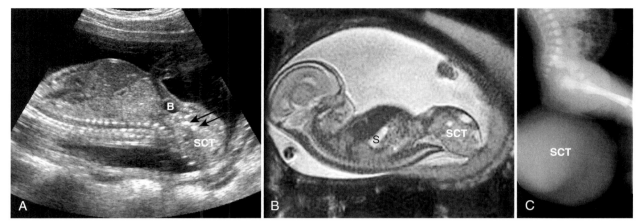

FIGURE 35-22. Sacrococcygeal teratoma. A, Sagittal sonogram shows type II sacrococcygeal teratoma *(SCT)* that is predominantly external but has a substantial intrapelvic component. The tumor extends up to level L5 and displaces the fetal urinary bladder *(B)* anteriorly. Note the calcifications *(arrows)* within the tumor. **B,** T2-weighted sagittal MR image demonstrates the extent and internal structure of the sacrococcygeal tumor *(SCT); S,* stomach. **C,** Lateral radiograph in a different neonate. *(A and B courtesy Drs. Fong, Pantazi, and Toi, Mt. Sinai Hospital, Toronto.)*

TYPES OF SACROCOCCYGEAL TERATOMAS

Type I (47%): external mass predominant
Type II (34%): external mass with significant internal component
Type III (9%): internal mass predominant, with smaller external component
Type IV (10%): presacral mass only

PRESACRAL MASSES

Sacrococcygeal teratoma
Chordoma
Anterior myelomeningocele
Neurenteric cyst
Neuroblastoma
Sarcoma
Lipoma
Bone tumor
Lymphoma
Rectal duplication

types:[115] **type I,** tumor predominantly external with only minimal presacral involvement; **type II,** tumor presenting externally but with significant intrapelvic extension; **type III,** tumor apparent externally but with predominant pelvic mass and extension into the abdomen; **type IV,** tumor presacral with no external presentation (Fig. 35-22).[114]

At birth, 75% of sacrococcygeal teratomas are benign, 12% are immature, and 13% are malignant. Because malignant potential increases with the age of the infant, surgery must be performed shortly after birth.

 Sonography usually demonstrates a mass in the rump or buttocks area adjacent to the spine[116] **(Video 35-2).** Most teratomas (85%) are either solid or mixed (solid + cystic); 15% are mostly cystic, which is a benign sign. Calcifications are frequently present. Large masses may displace and distort neighboring structures, such as the rectum and urinary bladder (see Fig. 35-21). Compression of the distal ureters may cause hydronephrosis. Larger solid tumors may develop substantial **arteriovenous shunting** causing **fetal cardiac failure** and **hydrops.**[117] The development of hydrops in the presence of a sacrococcygeal teratoma carries a poor prognosis,

and these findings should precipitate a cesarean section for fetal salvage.[117-121]

PRESACRAL FETAL MASS

The differential diagnosis of a presacral fetal mass also includes chordoma, anterior myelomeningocele, neurenteric cyst, neuroblastoma, sarcoma, lipoma, bone tumor, lymphoma, and rectal duplication. Amniotic fluid AFP is often elevated in sacrococcygeal tumor, and AChE is often present in the amniotic fluid. These results exclude most other etiologies, except a myelomeningocele.

If a fetal sacrococcygeal teratoma is suspected from prenatal sonograms, serial sonograms should be arranged to monitor the pregnancy to assess for complications, especially signs of fetal cardiac failure. Complete fetal assessment should also include the internal characteristics of the tumor, the size of the tumor, and associated fetal anomalies.

For masses less than 4.5 cm diameter, without associated abnormalities, elective vaginal delivery is recommended. For masses greater than 4.5 cm diameter, elective cesarean section may be advisable because of the risk of dystocia and hemorrhage during vaginal delivery. In utero surgery for arteriovenous shunting has been described for treatment of fetal hydrops from congestive heart failure in early pregnancy (<30 weeks), but this should be considered only in experienced hands.[117,118]

References

1. Fishman MA. Birth defects and supplemental vitamins. Curr Treat Options Neurol 2000;2:117-122.
2. Shaer CM, Chescheir N, Schulkin J. Myelomeningocele: a review of the epidemiology, genetics, risk factors for conception, prenatal diagnosis, and prognosis for affected individuals. Obstet Gynecol Surv 2007;62:471-479.
3. Grosse SD, Collins JS. Folic acid supplementation and neural tube defect recurrence prevention. Birth Defects Res A Clin Mol Teratol 2007;79:737-742.
4. Centers for Disease Control and Prevention: Trends in folic acid supplement intake among women of reproductive age—California, 2002-2006. MMWR 2007;56:1106-1109.
5. Solomons NW. Food fortification with folic acid: has the other shoe dropped? Nutr Rev 2007;65:512-515.
6. De Wals P, Tairou F, van Allen MI, et al. Reduction in neural-tube defects after folic acid fortification in Canada. N Engl J Med 2007;357:135-142.
7. Safdar OY, Al-Dabbagh AA, Abuelieneen WA, Kari JA. Decline in the incidence of neural tube defects after the national fortification of flour (1997-2005). Saudi Med J 2007;28:1227-1229.
8. Sayed AR, Bourne D, Pattinson R, et al. Decline in the prevalence of neural tube defects following folic acid fortification and its cost-benefit in South Africa. Birth Defects Res A Clin Mol Teratol 2008;82:211-216.
9. Jentink J, van de Vrie-Hoekstra NW, de Jong-van den Berg LT, Postma MJ. Economic evaluation of folic acid food fortification in The Netherlands. Eur J Public Health 2008;18:270-274.

Developmental Anatomy
10. Larsen WJ. Human embryology. 2nd ed. New York: Churchill Livingstone; 1997.
11. O'Rahilly R, Muller F, Meyer DB. The human vertebral column at the end of the embryonic period proper. 1. The column as a whole. J Anat 1980;131:565-575.
12. Bagnall KM, Harris PF, Jones PR. A radiographic study of the human fetal spine. 2. The sequence of development of ossification centres in the vertebral column. J Anat 1977;124:791-802.
13. Ford DM, McFadden KD, Bagnall KM. Sequence of ossification in human vertebral neural arch centers. Anat Rec 1982;203:175-178.
14. Budorick NE, Pretorius DH, Grafe MR, Lou KV. Ossification of the fetal spine. Radiology 1991;181:561-565.
15. Braithwaite JM, Armstrong MA, Economides DL. Assessment of fetal anatomy at 12 to 13 weeks of gestation by transabdominal and transvaginal sonography. Br J Obstet Gynaecol 1996;103:82-85.
16. Blumenfeld Z, Siegler E, Bronshtein M. The early diagnosis of neural tube defects. Prenat Diagn 1993;13:863-871.
17. Sebire NJ, Noble PL, Thorpe-Beeston JG, et al. Presence of the "lemon" sign in fetuses with spina bifida at the 10-14–week scan. Ultrasound Obstet Gynecol 1997;10:403-405.
18. Bernard JP, Suarez B, Rambaud C, et al. Prenatal diagnosis of neural tube defect before 12 weeks' gestation: direct and indirect ultrasonographic semeiology. Ultrasound Obstet Gynecol 1997;10:406-409.
19. Robbin ML, Filly RA, Goldstein RB. The normal location of the fetal conus medullaris. J Ultrasound Med 1994;13:541-546.
20. Zalel Y, Lehavi O, Aizenstein O, Achiron R. Development of the fetal spinal cord: time of ascendance of the normal conus medullaris as detected by sonography. J Ultrasound Med 2006;25:1397-1401; quiz 1402-1403.

Scanning Techniques
21. Thiagarajah S, Henke J, Hogge WA, et al. Early diagnosis of spina bifida: the value of cranial ultrasound markers. Obstet Gynecol 1990;76:54-57.
22. Babcook CJ, Goldstein RB, Barth RA, et al. Prevalence of ventriculomegaly in association with myelomeningocele: correlation with gestational age and severity of posterior fossa deformity. Radiology 1994;190:703-707.
23. Watson WJ, Chescheir NC, Katz VL, Seeds JW. The role of ultrasound in evaluation of patients with elevated maternal serum alpha-fetoprotein: a review. Obstet Gynecol 1991;78:123-128.
24. Dyson RL, Pretorius DH, Budorick NE, et al. Three-dimensional ultrasound in the evaluation of fetal anomalies. Ultrasound Obstet Gynecol 2000;16:321-328.
25. Riccabona M, Johnson D, Pretorius DH, Nelson TR. Three-dimensional ultrasound: display modalities in the fetal spine and thorax. Eur J Radiol 1996;22:141-145.
26. Bonilla-Musoles F, Machado LE, Osborne NG, et al. Two- and three-dimensional ultrasound in malformations of the medullary canal: report of four cases. Prenat Diagn 2001;21:622-626.
27. Lee W, Chaiworapongsa T, Romero R, et al. A diagnostic approach for the evaluation of spina bifida by three-dimensional ultrasonography. J Ultrasound Med 2002;21:619-626.
28. Schild RL, Wallny T, Fimmers R, Hansmann M. The size of the fetal thoracolumbar spine: a three-dimensional ultrasound study. Ultrasound Obstet Gynecol 2000;16:468-472.
29. Johnson DD, Pretorius DH, Riccabona M, et al. Three-dimensional ultrasound of the fetal spine. Obstet Gynecol 1997;89:434-438.
30. Wax JR, Watson WJ, Miller RC, et al. Prenatal sonographic diagnosis of hemivertebrae: associations and outcomes. J Ultrasound Med 2008;27:1023-1027.
31. Kalache KD, Bamberg C, Proquitte H, et al. Three-dimensional multi-slice view: new prospects for evaluation of congenital anomalies in the fetus. J Ultrasound Med 2006;25:1041-1049.
32. Merce LT, Barco MJ, Bau S. Three-dimensional volume sonographic study of fetal anatomy: intraobserver reproducibility and effect of examiner experience. J Ultrasound Med 2008;27:1053-1063.
33. Gindes L, Benoit B, Pretorius DH, Achiron R. Abnormal number of fetal ribs on 3-dimensional ultrasonography: associated anomalies and outcomes in 75 fetuses. J Ultrasound Med 2008;27:1263-1271.

Spina Bifida
34. Li Z, Ren A, Zhang L, et al. Extremely high prevalence of neural tube defects in a 4-county area in Shanxi Province, China. Birth Defects Res A Clin Mol Teratol 2006;76:237-240.
35. Cragan JD, Roberts HE, Edmonds LD, et al. Surveillance for anencephaly and spina bifida and the impact of prenatal diagnosis—United States, 1985-1994. MMWR CDC Surveill Summ 1995;44:1-13.
36. EuroCat Working Group. Prevalence of neural tube defects in 20 regions of Europe and the impact of prenatal diagnosis, 1980-1986. J Epidemiol Community Health 1991;45:52-58.
37. Laurence KM, James N, Miller MH, et al. Double-blind randomised controlled trial of folate treatment before conception to prevent recurrence of neural-tube defects. Br Med J Clin Res Ed 1981;282:1509-1511.
38. Prevention of neural tube defects: results of the Medical Research Council Vitamin Study. MRC Vitamin Study Research Group. Lancet 1991;338:131-137.
39. Werler MM, Shapiro S, Mitchell AA. Periconceptional folic acid exposure and risk of occurrent neural tube defects. JAMA 1993;269:1257-1261.
40. Czeizel AE. Prevention of congenital abnormalities by periconceptional multivitamin supplementation. BMJ 1993;306:1645-1648.
41. Lumley J, Watson L, Watson M, Bower C. Periconceptional supplementation with folate and/or multivitamins for preventing neural tube defects. Cochrane Database Syst Rev 2000:CD001056.
42. US Department of Health and Human Services. Recommendations for the use of folic acid to reduce the number of cases of spina bifida and other neural tube defects. MMWR 1992;41:1-7.
43. Expert Advisory Group: Folic acid and the prevention of neural tube defects. London: UK Department of Health; 1992.
44. Kadir RA, Sabin C, Whitlow B, et al. Neural tube defects and periconceptional folic acid in England and Wales: retrospective study. BMJ 1999;319:92-93.
45. Rosano A, Smithells D, Cacciani L, et al. Time trends in neural tube defects prevalence in relation to preventive strategies: an international study. J Epidemiol Community Health 1999;53:630-635.

46. Sharpe G, Young G. Folic acid and the prevention of neural tube defects: most pregnant women do not take folic acid. BMJ 1995; 311:256.

47. Wild J, Sutcliffe M, Schorah CJ, Levene MI. Prevention of neural-tube defects. Lancet 1997;350:30-31.

48. Huttly WJ, Wald NJ, Walters JC. Folic acid supplementation before pregnancy remains inadequate. BMJ 1999;319:1499.

49. Honein MA, Paulozzi LJ, Mathews TJ, et al. Impact of folic acid fortification of the U.S. food supply on the occurrence of neural tube defects. JAMA 2001;285:2981-2986.

50. Persad VL, van den Hof MC, Dube JM, Zimmer P. Incidence of open neural tube defects in Nova Scotia after folic acid fortification. CMAJ 2002;167:241-245.

51. Forrester MB, Merz RD. Descriptive epidemiology of lipomyelo-meningocele, Hawaii, 1986-2001. Birth Defects Res A Clin Mol Teratol 2004;70:953-956.

52. De Wals P, van Allen MI, Lowry RB, et al. Impact of folic acid food fortification on the birth prevalence of lipomyelomeningocele in Canada. Birth Defects Res A Clin Mol Teratol 2008;82:106-109.

53. Main DM, Mennuti MT. Neural tube defects: issues in prenatal diagnosis and counselling. Obstet Gynecol 1986;67:1-16.

54. Lescale KB, Eddleman KA, Chervenak FA. The fetal neck and spine. In: McGahan JP, Porto M, editors. Diagnostic obstetrical ultrasound. Philadelphia: Lippincott; 1994. p. 195.

55. Ray JG, Wyatt PR, Thompson MD, et al. Vitamin B_{12} and the risk of neural tube defects in a folic-acid-fortified population. Epidemiology 2007;18:362-366.

56. Babcook CJ, Goldstein RB, Filly RA. Prenatally detected fetal myelomeningocele: is karyotype analysis warranted? Radiology 1995;194:491-494.

57. Sepulveda W, Corral E, Ayala C, et al. Chromosomal abnormalities in fetuses with open neural tube defects: prenatal identification with ultrasound. Ultrasound Obstet Gynecol 2004;23:352-356.

58. Byrne J, Warburton D. Neural tube defects in spontaneous abortions. Am J Med Genet 1986;25:327-333.

59. Gregerson DM. Clinical consequences of spina bifida occulta. J Manipulative Physiol Ther 1997;20:546-550.

60. Norem CT, Schoen EJ, Walton DL, et al. Routine ultrasonography compared with maternal serum alpha-fetoprotein for neural tube defect screening. Obstet Gynecol 2005;106:747-752.

61. Filly RA, Callen PW, Goldstein RB. Alpha-fetoprotein screening programs: what every obstetric sonologist should know. Radiology 1993;188:1-9.

62. Ames MD, Schut L. Results of treatment of 171 consecutive myelo-meningoceles, 1963 to 1968. Pediatrics 1972;50:466-470.

63. Kollias SS, Goldstein RB, Cogen PH, Filly RA. Prenatally detected myelomeningoceles: sonographic accuracy in estimation of the spinal level. Radiology 1992;185:109-112.

64. Aaronson OS, Hernanz-Schulman M, Bruner JP, et al. Myelo-meningocele: prenatal evaluation–comparison between transabdominal ultrasound and MR imaging. Radiology 2003;227:839-843.

65. Von Koch CS, Glenn OA, Goldstein RB, Barkovich AJ. Fetal magnetic resonance imaging enhances detection of spinal cord anomalies in patients with sonographically detected bony anomalies of the spine. J Ultrasound Med 2005;24:781-789.

66. Biggio Jr JR, Owen J, Wenstrom KD, Oakes WJ. Can prenatal ultrasound findings predict ambulatory status in fetuses with open spina bifida? Am J Obstet Gynecol 2001;185:1016-1020.

67. Roberts AB, Campbell H, Boreham J, et al. Fetal head measurements in spina bifida. Br J Obstet Gynaecol 1980;87:927-928.

68. Wald N, Cuckle H, Boreham J, Stirrat G. Small biparietal diameter of fetuses with spina bifida: implications for antenatal screening. Br J Obstet Gynaecol 1980;87:219-221.

69. Nyberg DA, Mack LA, Hirsch J, et al. Fetal hydrocephalus: sonographic detection and clinical significance of associated anomalies. Radiology 1987;163:187-191.

70. Nicolaides KH, Campbell S, Gabbe SG, Guidetti R. Ultrasound screening for spina bifida: cranial and cerebellar signs. Lancet 1986; 2:72-74.

71. Pilu G, Romero R, Reece EA, et al. Subnormal cerebellum in fetuses with spina bifida. Am J Obstet Gynecol 1988;158:1052-1056.

72. Goldstein RB, Podrasky AE, Filly RA, Callen PW. Effacement of the fetal cisterna magna in association with myelomeningocele. Radiology 1989;172:409-413.

73. Benacerraf BR, Stryker J, Frigoletto Jr FD. Abnormal ultrasound appearance of the cerebellum (banana sign): indirect sign of spina bifida. Radiology 1989;171:151-153.

74. Furness ME, Barbary JE, Verco PW. A pointer to spina bifida: fetal head shape in the second trimester. In: Gill RW, Dadd MJ, editors. WFUMB (World Federation of Ultrasound in Medicine and Biology). Sidney: Pergamon Press; 1985. p. 296.

75. Campbell J, Gilbert WM, Nicolaides KH, Campbell S. Ultrasound screening for spina bifida: cranial and cerebellar signs in a high-risk population. Obstet Gynecol 1987;70:247-250.

76. Nyberg DA, Mack LA, Hirsch J, Mahony BS. Abnormalities of fetal cranial contour in sonographic detection of spina bifida: evaluation of the "lemon" sign. Radiology 1988;167:387-392.

77. Penso C, Redline RW, Benacerraf BR. A sonographic sign that predicts which fetuses with hydrocephalus have an associated neural tube defect. J Ultrasound Med 1987;6:307-311.

78. Sharrard WJ. The mechanism of paralytic deformity in spina bifida. Dev Med Child Neuri 1962;4:310-313.

79. Lorber J. Results of treatment of myelomeningocele: an analysis of 524 unselected cases, with special reference to possible selection for treatment. Dev Med Child Neurol 1971;13:279-303.

80. Nelson Jr MD, Bracchi M, Naidich TP, McLone DG. The natural history of repaired myelomeningocele. Radiographics 1988;8:695-706.

81. Wong LY, Paulozzi LJ. Survival of infants with spina bifida: a population study, 1979-94. Paediatr Perinat Epidemiol 2001;15:374-378.

82. Oakeshott P, Hunt GM. Long-term outcome in open spina bifida. Br J Gen Pract 2003;53:632-636.

83. Bliton MJ, Zaner RM. Over the cutting edge: how ethics consultation illuminates the moral complexity of open-uterine fetal repair of spina bifida and patients' decision making. J Clin Ethics 2001;12: 346-360.

84. Walsh DS, Adzick NS, Sutton LN, Johnson MP. The rationale for in utero repair of myelomeningocele. Fetal Diagn Ther 2001;16: 312-322.

85. Tulipan N, Bruner JP, Hernanz-Schulman M, et al. Effect of intrauterine myelomeningocele repair on central nervous system structure and function. Pediatr Neurosurg 1999;31:183-188.

86. Fichter MA, Dornseifer U, Henke J, et al. Fetal spina bifida repair: current trends and prospects of intrauterine neurosurgery. Fetal Diagn Ther 2008;23:271-286.

87. Bruner JP, Tulipan N, Paschall RL, et al. Fetal surgery for myelomeningocele and the incidence of shunt-dependent hydrocephalus. JAMA 1999;282:1819-1825.

88. Holmes NM, Nguyen HT, Harrison MR, et al. Fetal intervention for myelomeningocele: effect on postnatal bladder function. J Urol 2001;166:2383-2386.

89. Holzbeierlein J, Pope JI, Adams MC, et al. The urodynamic profile of myelodysplasia in childhood with spinal closure during gestation. J Urol 2000;164:1336-1339.

90. Sutton LN, Adzick NS, Bilaniuk LT, et al. Improvement in hindbrain herniation demonstrated by serial fetal magnetic resonance imaging following fetal surgery for myelomeningocele. JAMA 1999;282:1826-1831.

91. Steinbok P, Cochrane DD. The nature of congenital posterior cervical or cervicothoracic midline cutaneous mass lesions: report of eight cases. J Neurosurg 1991;75:206-212.

Myelocystocele

92. Bhargava R, Hammond DI, Benzie RJ, et al. Prenatal demonstration of a cervical myelocystocele. Prenat Diagn 1992;12:653-659.

93. Steinbok P. Dysraphic lesions of the cervical spinal cord. Neurosurg Clin North Am 1995;6:367-376.

94. Byrd SE, Harvey C, McLone DG, Darling CF. Imaging of terminal myelocystoceles. J Natl Med Assoc 1996;88:510-516.

95. Choi S, McComb JG. Long-term outcome of terminal myelocystocele patients. Pediatr Neurosurg 2000;32:86-91.

96. Muthukumar N. Terminal and nonterminal myelocystoceles. J Neurosurg 2007;107:87-97.

97. Allen LM, Silverman RK. Prenatal ultrasound evaluation of fetal diastematomyelia: two cases of type I split cord malformation. Ultrasound Obstet Gynecol 2000;15:78-82.

Diastematomyelia

98. Sonigo-Cohen P, Schmit P, Zerah M, et al. Prenatal diagnosis of diastematomyelia. Childs Nerv Syst 2003;19:555-560.
99. Dabra A, Gupta R, Sidhu R, et al. Sonographic diagnosis of diastematomyelia in utero: a case report and literature review. Australas Radiol 2001;45:222-224.
100. Raghavendra BN, Epstein FJ, Pinto RS, et al. Sonographic diagnosis of diastematomyelia. J Ultrasound Med 1988;7:111-113.
101. Anderson NG, Jordan S, MacFarlane MR, Lovell-Smith M. Diastematomyelia: diagnosis by prenatal sonography. AJR Am J Roentgenol 1994;163:911-914.
102. Korsvik HE, Keller MS. Sonography of occult dysraphism in neonates and infants with MR imaging correlation. Radiographics 1992;12:297-306; discussion 307-308.
103. Has R, Yuksel A, Buyukkurt S, et al. Prenatal diagnosis of diastematomyelia: presentation of eight cases and review of the literature. Ultrasound Obstet Gynecol 2007;30:845-849.
104. Harrison LA, Pretorius DH, Budorick NE. Abnormal spinal curvature in the fetus. J Ultrasound Med 1992;11:473-479.

Scoliosis and Kyphosis

105. Patten RM, van Allen M, Mack LA, et al. Limb–body wall complex: in utero sonographic diagnosis of a complicated fetal malformation. AJR Am J Roentgenol 1986;146:1019-1024.
106. Van Allen MI, Curry C, Walden CE, et al. Limb–body wall complex: II. Limb and spine defects. Am J Med Genet 1987;28:549-565.
107. Benacerraf BR, Greene MF, Barss VA. Prenatal sonographic diagnosis of congenital hemivertebra. J Ultrasound Med 1986;5:257-259.
108. Zelop CM, Pretorius DH, Benacerraf BR. Fetal hemivertebrae: associated anomalies, significance, and outcome. Obstet Gynecol 1993;81:412-416.
109. Twickler D, Budorick N, Pretorius D, et al. Caudal regression versus sirenomelia: sonographic clues. J Ultrasound Med 1993;12:323-330.

Sacral Agenesis

110. Sepulveda W, Corral E, Sanchez J, et al. Sirenomelia sequence versus renal agenesis: prenatal differentiation with power Doppler ultrasound. Ultrasound Obstet Gynecol 1998;11:445-449.

111. Baxi L, Warren W, Collins MH, Timor-Tritsch IE. Early detection of caudal regression syndrome with transvaginal scanning. Obstet Gynecol 1990;75:486-489.

Caudal Regression

112. Stocker JT, Heifetz SA. Sirenomelia. A morphological study of 33 cases and review of the literature. Perspect Pediatr Pathol 1987;10:7-50.

Sirenomelia

113. Stevenson RE, Jones KL, Phelan MC, et al. Vascular steal: the pathogenetic mechanism producing sirenomelia and associated defects of the viscera and soft tissues. Pediatrics 1986;78:451-457.
114. Bloechle M, Bollmann R, Zienert A, et al. [Fetal teratoma: diagnosis and management]. Zentralbl Gynakol 1992;114:175-180.

Sacrococcygeal Teratoma; Presacral Fetal Mass

115. Altman RP, Randolph JG, Lilly JR. Sacrococcygeal teratoma: American Academy of Pediatrics Surgical Section Survey—1973. J Pediatr Surg 1974;9:389-398.
116. Sheth S, Nussbaum AR, Sanders RC, et al. Prenatal diagnosis of sacrococcygeal teratoma: sonographic-pathologic correlation. Radiology 1988;169:131-136.
117. Bond SJ, Harrison MR, Schmidt KG, et al. Death due to high-output cardiac failure in fetal sacrococcygeal teratoma. J Pediatr Surg 1990;25:1287-1291.
118. Langer JC, Harrison MR, Schmidt KG, et al. Fetal hydrops and death from sacrococcygeal teratoma: rationale for fetal surgery. Am J Obstet Gynecol 1989;160:1145-1150.
119. Gross SJ, Benzie RJ, Sermer M, et al. Sacrococcygeal teratoma: prenatal diagnosis and management. Am J Obstet Gynecol 1987;156:393-396.
120. Teal LN, Angtuaco TL, Jimenez JF, Quirk Jr JG. Fetal teratomas: antenatal diagnosis and clinical management. J Clin Ultrasound 1988;16:329-336.
121. Robertson FM, Crombleholme TM, Frantz 3rd ID, et al. Devascularization and staged resection of giant sacrococcygeal teratoma in the premature infant. J Pediatr Surg 1995;30:309-311.

CHAPTER 36

The Fetal Chest

Rola Shaheen and Deborah Levine

Chapter Outline

$\mathcal{F}$amiliarity with the normal development of the fetal chest is important both for recognizing chest anomalies and for understanding the consequences of these anomalies. Accurate prenatal diagnosis of noncardiac thoracic lesions is essential in providing appropriate recommendations for fetal karyotyping and in planning for in utero intervention and mode of delivery. Sonography is important for recognition of thoracic lesions and assessment of their impact on mediastinal structures, because chest lesions can lead to compromised cardiac function and hydrops. Chest abnormalities may be associated with lethal pulmonary hypoplasia, fatal chromosomal abnormalities, and lethal structural anomalies. However, some chest lesions resolve in utero with minimal sequelae. In cases with unclear sonographic diagnosis or planned in utero interventions, fetal magnetic resonance imaging (MRI) is helpful.

DEVELOPMENT OF STRUCTURES IN THE CHEST

Pulmonary Development

In the human lung, there are five distinct stages of development, during which the lung matures and the number of alveoli increases.[1,2] At birth, the lungs are functional but structurally immature; the greatest increase in number of alveoli occurs postnatally. During the first 3 years of life, the alveoli are formed through a septation process that increases the gas exchange surface area. It is important to understand that this lung development process is ongoing, and that **space-occupying lesions,** or extrinsic abnormalities that do not allow for normal lung growth, can lead to improper lung development.

Normal Sonographic Features of the Fetal Chest

The fetal lungs are identified by ultrasound as homogeneously echogenic tissue surrounding the heart, separated by the hypoechoic, dome-shaped diaphragm from the abdominal organs (Fig. 36-1, *A* and *B*). The fetal ribs are highly echogenic, curved bony structures arising near the spine and extending anteriorly to encompass more than half the thoracic circumference. Lung echogenicity varies during gestation, in general increasing in echogenicity as lung development progresses.

Assessment of pulmonary size is important for evaluation of fetuses at risk for pulmonary hypoplasia, particularly in cases of **congenital diaphragmatic hernia (CDH)**, **pleural effusions,** prolonged **oligohydramnios,** and **skeletal deformities.** Methods to assess pulmonary size include measurement of the thoracic circumference[3] (Table 36-1), lung area (defined as internal thoracic area minus cardiac area in diastole on a transverse four-chamber view[4]), and three-dimensional (3-D) lung volumetry with ultrasound or MRI.[5-7]

The fetal lungs, thorax, and heart grow at similar rates, such that the normal cardiothoracic ratio remains

STAGES OF HUMAN LUNG DEVELOPMENT

1. **Embryonic stage.** Extends to about 7 weeks.
2. **Pseudoglandular stage.** Extends from 6 to 16 weeks; the lungs resemble tubuloacinar glands, with epithelial tubes sprouting and branching into the surrounding mesenchyme.
3. **Canalicular stage.** Extends from 16 to 28 weeks; the cuboid epithelium differentiates into type I and type II cells, with production of surfactant and formation of the first, thin, air-blood barriers.
4. **Saccular stage.** Extends from 28 to 36 weeks; the pulmonary parenchyma forms, the surrounding connective tissues thins, and the surfactant system matures.
5. **Alveolar stage.** Extends from the 36th week of gestation to the first 3 years of life.

constant in the second and third trimesters. On a normal four-chamber transverse view of the heart, the heart should occupy approximately one-third to one-half the sonographic diameter of the thorax.

The cardiac position and axis are constant in normal fetuses. The apex of the heart points left and touches the anterior chest wall. The posterior aspect of the right atrium lies to the right of midline.[8]

Familiarity with the normal anatomy and position of the fetal heart is crucial, along with in utero establishment of the right and left sides of the fetus. The reference to cardiac position and **situs** is identified by noting the left atrium lies posteriorly, closest to the spine, and the right ventricle lies anteriorly, close to the chest wall. Any deviation in the position of the heart should prompt a search for cardiac or pulmonary abnormality. Anatomy of the fetal heart, including size and position, can be easily influenced by extracardiac thoracic anomalies.

Normal Diaphragm

Early in embryogenesis, the narrow pleuroperitoneal duct connects the **pleural and peritoneal cavities.** The development of the **diaphragm,** at about 9 weeks, divides the two cavities. The normal diaphragm and diaphragm motion can be visualized as early as 10 weeks of gestation.[9-11] The diaphragm appears as a thin, hypoechoic, arched line separating the chest from intra-abdominal contents (Fig. 36-1, *C, D,* and *F*). It is best recognized as a dome on each side on sagittal and coronal views, with no difference in the height of the diaphragm on either side.[12] The intact left hemidiaphragm is emphasized by the presence of the fluid-filled stomach in the abdomen. On the right side, however, meticulous effort may be required to identify the hypoechoic linear muscular diaphragm between the liver and lung.

Normal Thymus

The fetal thymus can be identified as early as 14 weeks' gestation in the anterior mediastinum. By the third trimester, the thymus is visualized as an ovoid, relatively hypoechoic structure[13,14] (Fig. 36-1, *G* and *I*). The thymus contains spindle-shaped echogenicities that differentiate it from the surrounding lungs.[15] Thymus size varies greatly during gestation. Thymic imaging and measurements are not performed routinely on prenatal scans. However, prenatal identification and measurement of the fetal thymus is important when **DiGeorge syndrome** is suspected. In addition, a large thymus will sometimes be confused with a mediastinal mass. It is therefore important to recognize the normal appearance of the thymus. The normal thymic average transverse measurement is 12 mm at 19 weeks' gestation and 33 mm at 33 weeks.[15] The normal thymic average perimeter is 128 mm at 38 weeks.[13] Acute fetal thymic involution has been reported in association with chorioamnionitis.[16]

PULMONARY HYPOPLASIA AND APLASIA

Pulmonary hypoplasia is defined as a reduction in the number of cells, airways, and alveoli that results in an absolute decrease in the size and weight of the fetal lungs relative to gestational age.[17-19] The earlier the insult to the fetal lungs, the more severe is the degree of pulmonary hypoplasia.[20] Pulmonary hypoplasia is a relatively common process that results in severe postnatal respiratory distress and associated high neonatal mortality,[21] with a high incidence of stillbirths (6.7%).[18] The immaturity of the lungs contributes to the nonviability of fetuses less than 24 weeks.

Pulmonary hypoplasia can be primary or secondary and can be unilateral or bilateral depending on the etiology and time of insult to the lungs. **Primary** pulmonary hypoplasia is very rare and is caused by a primary process in which the lung does not form normally. **Unilateral pulmonary agenesis,** in which no normal lung forms, has an incidence of 1 in 15,000 births and is associated with other congenital anomalies.[22] **Bilateral pulmonary agenesis** is incompatible with postnatal life.

Secondary causes of pulmonary hypoplasia include masses that compress the lungs (e.g., CDH), skeletal malformations that do not allow the lungs to grow (e.g., thanatophoric dysplasia), and severe prolonged oligohydramnios (e.g., bilateral renal agenesis). Other factors that contribute to pulmonary hypoplasia include hormonal influences, pulmonary fluid dynamics, and abnormal fetal breathing movements.[23] The majority of cases of pulmonary hypoplasia are associated with major structural or chromosomal abnormalities (Table 36-2).

Prenatal prediction of pulmonary hypoplasia and the degree of severity are crucial for parental counseling as

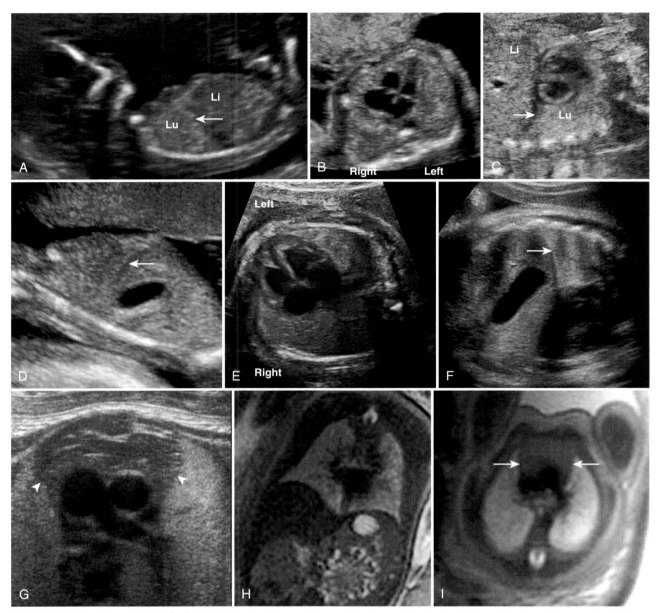

FIGURE 36-1. Normal fetal chest. A, Sagittal view of torso at 13 weeks. Note liver *(Li),* lungs *(Lu),* and diaphragm. **B,** Four-chamber view of the heart surrounded by the homogeneous echogenic lungs at 18 weeks. **C,** Coronal, and **D,** sagittal, views of chest at 18 weeks show the dome-shaped hemidiaphragms *(arrow)* separating the lungs *(Lu)* from intraabdominal organs and the relative hypoechoic appearance of the liver *(Li).* **E** and **F,** Axial and sagittal views of fetal chest at 37 weeks. **G,** Normal appearance of fetal **thymus** *(arrowheads)* at 37 weeks' gestation. **H,** Coronal T2-weighted MR image shows normal lungs and diaphragm at 37 weeks. **I,** Axial T2-weighted MR image of thymus *(arrows)* anterior to heart. The thymus is relatively hypoechoic to the surrounding lungs on ultrasound and relatively low intensity on MRI.

well as for postnatal management planning, especially for neonates requiring intensive respiratory care immediately after birth.[24] Proposed methods for prediction of prenatal pulmonary hypoplasia[25] include estimation of lung volumes by 3-D ultrasound[26,27] or by MRI,[28,29] thoracic circumference[30,31] (Table 36-1), lung-to-head ratio,[9,32] lung-to-body weight ratio,[24] and Doppler studies of pulmonary arteries.[33]

Prognosis and management are variable and depend on the severity and nature of the associated conditions. For example, absence of fetal breathing movements in

the setting of oligohydramnios in pregnancies resulting from **premature rupture of membranes** (PROM) is an accurate predictor for pulmonary hypoplasia.[4] Clinically, the spectrum of outcomes ranges from mild respiratory insufficiency to neonatal death.

In cases of **unilateral** pulmonary hypoplasia or aplasia, there is mediastinal shift to the side of the hypoplastic lung, with no associated mass in the contralateral lung to explain the degree of mediastinal shift[34] (Fig. 36-2). The contralateral lung will often be enlarged and echogenic.[22] Unilateral pulmonary hypoplasia can also be

TABLE 36-1. NORMAL THORACIC CIRCUMFERENCE AND LENGTH CORRELATED WITH MENSTRUAL (GESTATIONAL) AGE*

AGE (WK)	Predictive Percentiles								
	2.5	5	10	25	50	75	90	95	97.5
Thoracic Circumference (CM)									
16	5.9	6.4	7.0	8.0	9.1	10.3	11.3	11.9	12.4
17	6.8	7.3	7.9	8.9	10.1	11.2	12.2	12.8	13.3
18	7.7	8.2	8.8	9.8	11.0	12.1	13.1	13.7	14.2
19	8.6	9.1	9.7	10.7	11.9	13.0	14.0	14.6	15.1
20	9.5	10.0	10.6	11.7	12.9	13.9	15.0	15.5	16.0
21	10.4	11.0	11.6	12.6	13.7	14.8	15.8	16.4	16.9
22	11.3	11.9	12.5	13.5	14.6	15.7	16.7	17.3	17.8
23	12.2	12.8	13.4	14.4	15.5	16.6	17.6	18.2	18.8
24	13.2	13.7	14.3	15.3	16.4	17.5	18.5	19.1	19.7
25	14.1	14.6	15.2	16.2	17.3	18.4	19.4	20.0	20.6
26	15.0	15.5	16.1	17.1	18.2	19.3	20.3	21.0	21.5
27	15.9	16.4	17.0	18.0	19.1	20.2	21.3	21.9	22.4
28	16.8	17.3	17.9	18.9	20.0	21.2	22.2	22.8	23.3
29	17.7	18.2	18.8	19.8	21.0	22.1	23.1	23.7	24.2
30	18.6	19.1	19.7	20.7	21.9	23.0	24.0	24.6	25.1
31	19.5	20.0	20.6	21.6	22.8	23.9	24.9	25.5	26.0
32	20.4	20.9	21.5	22.6	23.7	24.8	25.8	26.4	26.9
33	21.3	21.8	22.5	23.5	24.6	25.7	26.7	27.3	27.8
34	22.2	22.8	23.4	24.4	25.5	26.6	27.6	28.2	28.7
35	23.1	23.7	24.3	25.3	26.4	27.5	28.5	29.1	29.6
36	24.0	24.6	25.2	26.2	27.3	28.4	29.4	30.0	30.6
37	24.9	25.5	26.1	27.1	28.2	29.3	30.3	30.9	31.5
38	25.9	26.4	27.0	28.0	29.1	30.2	31.2	31.9	32.4
39	26.8	27.3	27.9	28.9	30.0	31.1	32.2	32.8	33.3
40	27.7	28.2	28.8	29.8	30.9	32.1	33.1	33.7	34.2
Thoracic Length (cm)									
16	0.9	1.1	1.3	1.6	2.0	2.4	2.8	3.0	3.2
17	1.1	1.3	1.5	1.8	2.2	2.6	3.0	3.2	3.4
18	1.3	1.4	1.7	2.0	2.4	2.8	3.2	3.4	3.6
19	1.4	1.6	1.8	2.2	2.7	3.0	3.4	3.6	3.8
20	1.6	1.8	2.30	2.4	2.8	3.2	3.6	3.8	4.0
21	1.8	2.0	2.2	2.6	3.0	3.4	3.7	4.0	4.1
22	2.0	2.2	2.4	2.8	3.2	3.6	3.9	4.1	4.3
23	2.2	2.4	2.6	3.0	3.4	3.8	4.1	4.3	4.5
24	2.4	2.6	2.8	3.1	3.5	3.9	4.3	4.5	4.7
25	2.6	2.8	3.0	3.3	3.7	4.1	4.5	4.7	4.9
26	2.8	2.9	3.2	3.5	3.9	4.3	4.7	4.9	5.1
27	2.9	3.1	3.3	3.7	4.1	4.5	4.9	5.1	5.3
28	3.1	3.3	3.5	3.9	4.3	4.7	5.0	5.4	5.4
29	3.3	3.5	3.7	4.1	4.5	4.9	5.2	5.5	5.6
30	3.5	3.7	3.9	4.3	4.7	5.1	5.4	5.6	5.8
31	3.7	3.9	4.1	4.5	4.9	5.3	5.6	5.8	6.0
32	3.9	4.1	4.3	4.6	5.0	5.4	5.8	6.0	6.2
33	4.1	4.3	4.5	4.8	5.2	5.6	6.0	6.2	6.4
34	4.2	4.4	4.7	5.0	5.4	5.8	6.2	6.4	6.6
35	4.4	4.6	4.8	5.2	5.6	6.0	6.4	6.6	6.8
36	4.6	4.8	5.0	5.4	5.8	6.2	6.5	6.8	7.0
37	4.8	5.0	5.2	5.6	6.0	6.4	6.7	7.0	7.1
38	5.0	5.2	5.4	5.8	6.2	6.6	6.9	7.1	7.3
39	5.2	5.4	5.6	6.0	6.4	6.8	7.1	7.3	7.5
40	5.4	5.6	5.8	6.1	6.5	6.9	7.3	7.5	7.7

*From Chitkara U, Rosenberg J, Chevanak FA, et al. Prenatal sonographic assessment of thorax: normal values. Am J Obstet Gynecol 1987;156:1069-1074.

produced by space-occupying lesions, such as congenital cystic adenomatoid malformation (CCAM), CDH, or pleural effusion. The extent of pulmonary hypoplasia for a given amount of visualized lung is greater in fetuses with CDH than with CCAM, suggesting that in CDH there is a mechanism other than mass effect that limits pulmonary development.

CONGENITAL PULMONARY MALFORMATION SPECTRUM

An echogenic lesion in the fetal thorax (Table 36-3) or a cystic lesion in the fetal thorax (Table 36-4) can be part of the congenital pulmonary airway malformation

(CPAM) spectrum. This spectrum includes lesions that have been historically called **congenital cystic adenomatoid malformation, bronchopulmonary sequestration,** and **congenital lobar emphysema.** CCAM is a congenital hamartomatous lung lesion,[35] and sequestration is normally developed lung tissue with systemic circulation. However, these lesions often occur together.[36-38] For clarity, we describe these lesions separately, but the reader should be aware that careful histologic inspection will often find regions of CCAM in what appears to be a sequestration, as well as lesions that resemble a CCAM that often have both pulmonic and systemic feeding vessels. Both of these types of lesions can have air trapping postnatally and therefore may have elements of congenital lobar emphysema.

Congenital Cystic Adenomatoid Malformation

Congenital cystic adenomatoid malformation accounts for about 25% of congenital lung masses,[39] with an incidence of 1 in 25,000 live births.[40] It is comprised of pulmonary tissue with abnormal bronchial proliferation that may involve either lung or any lobe. In greater than 95% of cases, CCAM is limited to one lobe or segment, with 2% to 3% of CCAMs occurring bilaterally and with the right and left lungs equally affected.[41]

Cystic adenomatoid malformation results from a pulmonary insult during embryologic development of the

---

TABLE 36-2. CAUSES OF PULMONARY HYPOPLASIA

PRIMARY PULMONARY HYPOPLASIA OR APLASIA	DEVELOPMENTAL ABNORMALITY
Thoracic space-occupying process	Congenital diaphragmatic hernia (CDH)
	Congenital lung masses such as CCAM, sequestration, and bronchogenic cyst
	Mediastinal mass: cardiac masses such as teratomas (rare)
	Large pleural effusions
Oligohydramnios	Bilateral renal agenesis
	Prolonged preterm rupture of membranes
Skeletal and neural malformations	Skeletal dysplasias such as thanatotropic dysplasia or osteogenesis imperfecta
	Chest wall tumors
	Phrenic nerve abnormalities
	Neuromuscular and CNS anomalies
Chromosomal anomalies and syndromes	Trisomies 13, 18, and 21
	Robert syndrome

CCAM, Congenital cystic adenomatoid malformation; *CNS,* central nervous system.

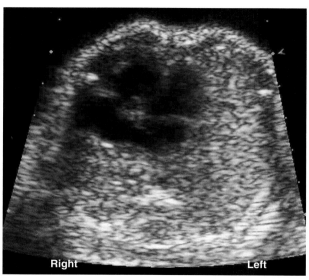

FIGURE 36-2. Pulmonary hypoplasia. Axial sonogram demonstrates mediastinal shift to the right. No lung mass is present. Presumptive diagnosis was pulmonary hypoplasia, confirmed postnatally. *(Courtesy Richard Barth, MD, Stanford University.)*

TABLE 36-3. DIFFERENTIAL DIAGNOSIS OF ECHOGENIC LESION IN FETAL THORAX

ABNORMALITY	LOCATION	DISTINGUISHING FEATURES
Congenital cystic adenomatoid malformation (CCAM)	Unilateral (2%-3% bilateral)	Cystic and solid
Sequestration	Unilateral; left lower lobe most often	Systemic blood supply
Congenital lobar emphysema	Unilateral; upper lobe most often	Similar to microcystic CCAM; enlarged echogenic lung with mediastinal shift
Congenital diaphragmatic hernia (CDH)	Typically unilateral; left sided most often	Peristalsis of bowel in chest
		Stomach above diaphragm
		Absence of part of the diaphragm
Congenital high airway obstruction (CHAOS)	Bilateral	Distended trachea and main central airways
		Symmetrical bilateral enlarged lungs with eversion of hemidiaphragms

TABLE 36-4. DIFFERENTIAL DIAGNOSIS OF CYSTIC LESION IN FETAL THORAX

ABNORMALITY	BILATERAL VS. UNILATERAL	DISTINGUISHING FEATURES
Congenital cystic adenomatoid malformation (CCAM)	Unilateral (2%-3% bilateral)	Associated with echogenic lung mass, typically multiple cysts
Congenital diaphragmatic hernia (CDH)	Typically unilateral	Peristalsis of bowel in chest
Teratoma		Stomach above diaphragm
Neurenteric cyst		Mass does not obey lobar boundaries; may have calcifications.
Bronchogenic cyst		Adjacent to spine
Esophageal duplication		Typically single cyst
Lymphangioma		Adjacent to esophagus
		Crosses anatomic boundaries

bronchial tree before the seventh week of gestation, resulting in failure of bronchial maturation and lack of normal alveoli. Histologically, CCAM is differentiated from other lung masses by the absence of bronchial cartilage and bronchial tubular glands, with overproduction of terminal bronchiolar structures without alveolar differentiation, except in the subpleural areas.[42-44] The resulting cystic lesions result in enlargement of the affected lobe (or segment). If sufficiently large, CCAM will result in mediastinal shift and interfere with normal alveolar development in the adjacent lung. Communication with the tracheobronchial tree usually is retained, with vascular supply and venous drainage to the pulmonary circulation, unless CCAM is associated with sequestration.

Typically, CCAMs are divided into three types. **Type I** is the most common, with variably sized cysts measuring 2 to 10 cm. **Type II** has uniform cysts less than 2 cm in greatest diameter. **Type III** CCAM has small cysts less than 0.5 cm and appears grossly solid.[45]

Sonographic diagnosis is made as early as 16 weeks. CCAM may appear as a solid echogenic lung mass or as a mixed, cystic and solid mass (Fig. 36-3; **Video 36-1**). Color Doppler ultrasound may demonstrate vascular flow to the lesion from a branch of the pulmonary artery. Typically, there is no systemic feeding vessel, although as mentioned, CCAM can occur in concert with sequestration. The lesions with microcysts appear solid and echogenic, whereas the macrocystic CCAM has easily demonstrable cysts. Occasionally, only a single large cyst is visualized.

As with any chest mass, it is important to assess for associated mediastinal shift, polyhydramnios, and hydrops because these factors impact prognosis and management.[46,47] It is the size of the CCAM rather than the size of the cysts that determines whether or not the fetus develops **hydrops.** Large CCAMs result in cardiac compression, leading to altered hemodynamics and hydrops as a result of elevated central venous pressure.[48] Untreated hydrops as a result of CCAM has an anticipated mortality of 100%. Hydrops is therefore an indication for in utero fetal therapy, which generally consists of either draining

the largest cyst with a single stick procedure (Fig. 36-3, *G*) or placing a shunt. Rarely is open fetal surgery indicated. A 2006 meta-analysis showed that shunting of CCAMs improved survival in fetuses with hydrops, versus no effect on survival in fetuses with chest masses without hydrops.[49] The success with open fetal surgery in cases of CCAM ranges between 29% and 62%, but has the limitation of expected preterm delivery.[50] Antenatal aspiration of a macrocystic CCAM is an effective treatment at times[51] but frequently is ineffective because of rapid reaccumulation of the cysts. Steroid therapy may also be beneficial, given the hypothesis that increasing lung maturity improves survival.[52]

Associated anomalies, most often renal, intestinal, and cardiac, are present in up to 26% of cases,[36,45] more frequently when CCAM is bilateral.[41] Chromosomal anomalies in association with CCAM are rare. Thus, if no other structural abnormalities are detected, karyotyping usually is not performed.

Magnetic resonance imaging can be helpful in evaluation and management of CCAM (Fig. 36-3, *H, I*), particularly for fetal surgeons when hydrops and polyhydramnios necessitate surgery.[53] Type I or type II CCAM lesions have very high signal intensity on T2-weighted imaging, almost equal to that of amniotic fluid, and much higher than that of the surrounding unaffected lung tissue. Type III CCAM lesions have moderately high signal intensity and are relatively homogeneous. As the lesions regress, they develop low signal intensity on T2-weighted imaging[54] and may be associated with a small pleural effusion.

If the fetus does not develop hydrops before 26 weeks, the prognosis is generally good.[55,56] Therefore, surveillance of the growth of these lesions is typically performed at frequent intervals (every 1-2 weeks) throughout the second trimester. CCAMs tend to regress in the third trimester. As they regress, they may become isoechoic with normal adjacent lung and thus may become inapparent late in gestation. If originally present, mediastinal shift can resolve. Although regression of CCAM on prenatal ultrasound is common, the lesion does not completely disappear.[55] Up to 40% of neonates with prenatal

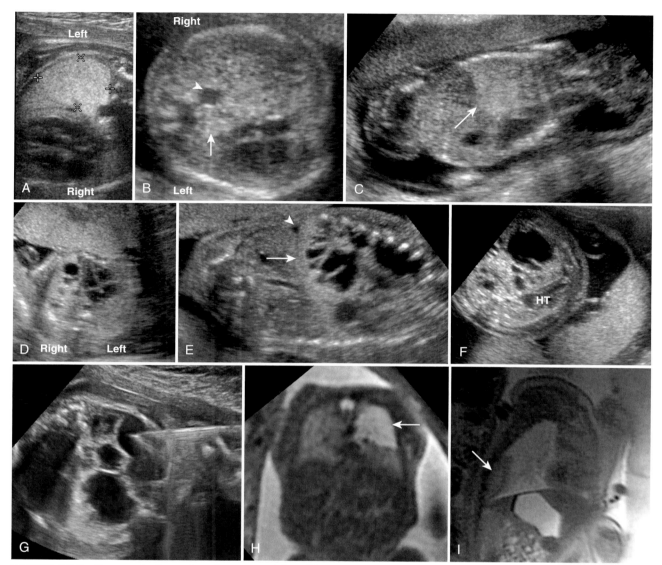

FIGURE 36-3. Congenital cystic adenomatoid malformation (CCAM). A, Axial sonogram at 28 weeks shows a homogeneously echogenic mass *(calipers)* in the mid–left hemithorax with no large cysts or feeding vessels. There is mild mediastinal shift to the right. **B,** Axial sonogram of right-sided CCAM *(arrow)* at 20 weeks with small cysts, the largest of which is 8 mm *(arrowhead)*. There is moderate mediastinal shift to the left. **C,** Sagittal oblique sonogram shows CCAM everting the hemidiaphragm *(arrow)*. **D,** Transverse view of chest with CCAM containing small cysts and mild mediastinal shift. **E** and **F,** Axial and oblique coronal images at 25 weeks in a macrocystic CCAM *(arrow)* with eversion of the hemidiaphragm, trace ascites *(arrowhead)*, and severe mediastinal shift with compression of the heart *(HT)*. **G,** Ultrasound-guided percutaneous drainage of CCAM. A 20-gauge needle was inserted into the largest cyst with relief of cardiac compression. **H,** Coronal T2-weighted MR image shows a well-circumscribed area of T2 hyperintensity *(arrow)* in the left upper lobe. **I,** Oblique coronal T2-weighted MR image shows a well-circumscribed area of low T2 signal, in a fetus with a typical, resolving CCAM.

diagnosis of CCAM are symptomatic at birth and require intervention or respiratory support.[57] Therefore, delivery should be at a site with appropriate neonatal intensive care unit (NICU) services. Because the lesion may be inapparent on chest radiography after birth, postnatal computed tomography (CT) or MRI may be needed to visualize the lesion. Postnatal removal of asymptomatic masses is performed because of potential secondary infection, hemorrhage, and risk of carcinomas arising in CCAM.[58] In addition, CCAM may prevent future normal lung growth if the lung lesion is not resected.[59]

The timing of surgical resection of CCAM remains controversial, but most centers favor elective surgical resection early in life.[60]

Bronchopulmonary Sequestration

Bronchopulmonary sequestration is an anomaly in which nonfunctioning pulmonary tissue is not in normal continuity with the native tracheobronchial tree[61] and has a blood supply from the systemic circulation. Sequestrations account for up to 6% of congenital lung malformations.[62,63] Concomitant anomalies associated with sequestration include CDH, diaphragmatic eventration and paralysis, bronchogenic cyst, ectopic pancreas, vertebral anomalies, and foregut duplication.

There are two main types of sequestration: intralobar and extralobar. A third variant is suggested when communicating bronchopulmonary foregut malformation is present.[64]

Extralobar sequestration represents the vast majority of fetal sequestrations. This lesion is a supernumerary lung bud invested by its own pleura, typically deriving its blood supply from the splanchnic vessels surrounding the foregut, which results in the systemic blood supply.[65] The venous drainage is usually through a single vessel into the azygous, hemiazygos, and/or the vena cava system. In up to 25% of cases, however, the extralobar sequestration is partially drained through pulmonary veins. Extralobar sequestration is typically found in the left posterior costodiaphragmatic sulcus between the lower lobe and the hemidiaphragm.[66] Extralobar sequestrations occur below the diaphragm in suprarenal locations in 10% to 15% of cases (with a differential diagnosis of neuroblastoma and adrenal hemorrhage).[67] Rarely, sequestration may present as a mediastinal or pericardial mass.[68]

Intralobar sequestration comprises abnormal lung tissue with systemic arterial supply within the normal lung, sharing the visceral pleura and draining to pulmonary veins.[66] It occurs more often in the lower lobe than upper lobe and slightly more often on the left.[63]

Sequestration can be detected on prenatal sonogram as early as 16 weeks' gestation.[69] Typically, a sequestration appears as a well-defined, homogeneous, echogenic wedge-shaped pulmonary mass in the lower lobe adjacent to the hemidiaphragm (Fig. 36-4). Classically, these lesions do not have cysts. However, cysts can result from

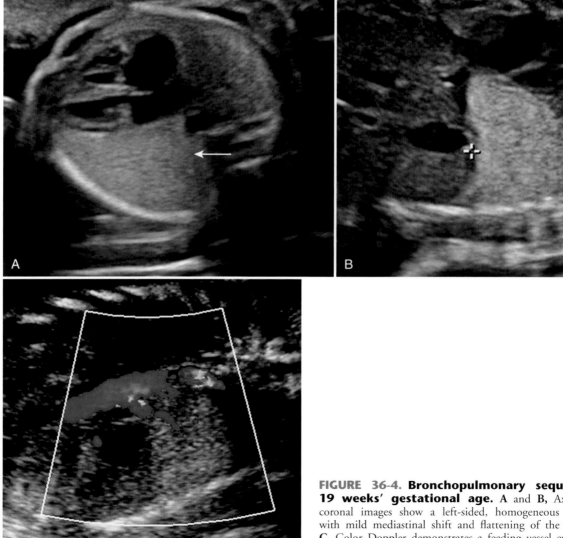

FIGURE 36-4. Bronchopulmonary sequestration at 19 weeks' gestational age. A and **B,** Axial and oblique coronal images show a left-sided, homogeneous echogenic mass with mild mediastinal shift and flattening of the hemidiaphragm. **C,** Color Doppler demonstrates a feeding vessel extending directly from the infradiaphragmatic aorta to the mass, thus proving it is a sequestration.

dilated bronchioles or hybrid lesions of concomitant CCAM. Sequestration can be distinguished from other congenital lung masses by identifying on Doppler interrogation a systemic artery arising from the thoracic or abdominal aorta feeding the mass. Determination of where the vessel arises is important for counseling parents about the approach that will be needed for postnatal surgical removal of the mass.

Small sequestrations with minimal mediastinal shift have a benign clinical course.[38] As with other chest masses, a large sequestration may result in mediastinal shift. However, most prenatally detected sequestrations are of small or medium size. These lesions usually regress in size during gestation.[38,47] Large sequestrations can be complicated by pleural effusions and with hydrops can lead to increased prenatal mortality. For such complicated cases, the pleural effusion can be treated with pleuroamniotic shunting and drainage.[70,71]

Congenital Lobar Emphysema

Congenital lobar emphysema (CLE) is a rare congenital lung malformation manifesting as progressive lobar overinflation of the lung without destruction of alveolar septa. CLE results from maldevelopment of a lobar or segmental bronchus. It occurs in the upper lobes more than lower lobes. On prenatal ultrasound, CLE is similar in appearance to microcystic CCAM, manifesting as an echogenic mass that is relatively large and typically causes mediastinal shift because of its size[72] (Fig. 36-5). As with CCAM, the lesion can regress in utero.[73] Because of the nonspecific appearance, even if it regresses in size, postnatal follow-up is required because air trapping and respiratory distress may necessitate lobar resection early in neonatal life.[74]

CONGENITAL HIGH AIRWAY OBSTRUCTION

Congenital high airway obstruction (CHAOS) is a spectrum of conditions characterized by incomplete or complete obstruction of the high fetal airway.[75,76] Any fetal abnormality that obstructs the larynx or trachea, causing intrinsic atresia or extrinsic compression results in CHAOS. **Laryngeal atresia** is the most frequent cause. Other etiologies include **laryngeal** or **tracheal webs, laryngeal cysts, tracheal atresia, subglottic stenosis** or **atresia,** and **laryngeal** or **tracheal agenesis.**[77] If untreated, CHAOS is almost always lethal.[76]

Although sporadic with unknown incidence, CHAOS can be part of various chromosomal disorders.[78,79] It can also be familial with autosomal dominant inheritance and variable expression.[80] Laryngeal atresia can occur as part of **Fraser syndrome** (tracheal or laryngeal atresia, renal agenesis, microphthalmia, and syndactyly or polydactyly) with autosomal recessive inheritance.[79,81]

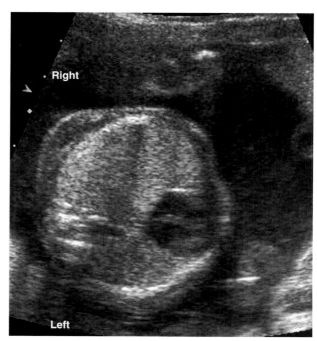

FIGURE 36-5. Congenital lobar emphysema. Axial image of the chest shows an enlarged, diffusely echogenic right lung. Although this appearance would more often be caused by a congenital cystic adenomatoid malformation, the postnatal diagnosis was congenital lobar emphysema. *(Courtesy Richard Barth, MD, Stanford University.)*

Prenatal ultrasound findings can be visualized as early as 16 weeks' gestation.[82] Findings include bilateral symmetrically enlarged echogenic lungs, dilated fluid-filled trachea and central bronchi, and flattened or everted diaphragms[83,84] (Fig. 36-6). The heart usually assumes a more central and anterior position than normal and is often compressed as the size of the lungs increases.[77] Frequently, there are associated findings of ascites and other signs of hydrops. The mechanism of ascites may be from compression of the heart and great vessels by the enlarged lungs.[85] Either polyhydramnios or oligohydramnios may be present.

The lungs are distended and appear homogeneously echogenic because of increased fluid and increased lung growth induced by the upper airway obstruction.[77] The increased number of tissue-fluid interfaces produces the hyperechoic appearance of the lungs. Lung volume can increase up to 15 times the expected size. The hyperplastic lungs are edematous but otherwise histologically normal.[77]

Magnetic resonance imaging can be used to identify the region of obstruction and assist in decisions regarding in utero intervention and intrapartum procedures. Characteristic findings include increased lung volume, diffuse increase in lung intensity on T2-weighted images, and a dilated fluid-filled trachea.[83]

Greater than 50% of fetuses with laryngeal obstruction have associated abnormalities, most often in the

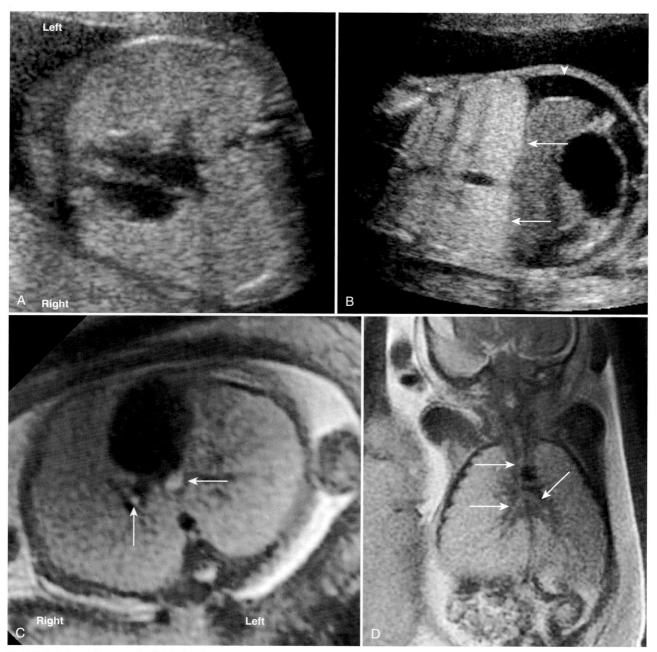

FIGURE 36-6. Congenital high airway obstruction syndrome (CHAOS) at 19 weeks. A and **B,** Axial and coronal views of the chest show diffusely enlarged, echogenic lungs bilaterally with eversion of the hemidiaphragms *(arrows)* and ascites *(arrowhead).* **C** and **D,** Axial and coronal T2-weighted MR images show increased lung volume and fluid-filled airways *(arrows). (Courtesy Katherine Fong, MD, University of Toronto.)*

renal system and central nervous system (CNS). At times, CHAOS can be present in association with a **tracheoesophageal fistula.** This fistula acts as an alternative pathway for the accumulated fluid, leading to a decrease in lung volume, reversal of diaphragmatic eversion, and resolution of ascites and polyhydramnios.[75]

If untreated, laryngeal and tracheal atresia can lead to death either in utero from hydrops or within minutes after birth from respiratory compromise. Neonatal survival is possible if the delivery is performed with the **ex utero intrapartum treatment** (EXIT) procedure.[86,87] The EXIT procedure involves tracheostomy placement below the level of the obstruction while maternal placental circulation is maintained.

BRONCHOGENIC CYST

Bronchogenic cysts are rare anomalies that result from abnormal budding or branching of the tracheobronchial

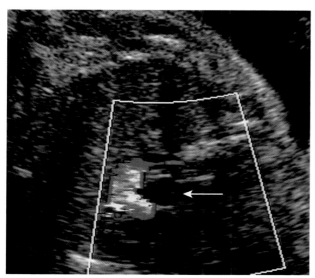

FIGURE 36-7. Bronchogenic cyst at 22 weeks. Color Doppler transverse image shows a cyst *(arrow)* adjacent to vessels without associated solid mass.

tree. They are most often located in the mediastinum in the subcarinal region.[88] However, 15% of bronchogenic cysts occur in the lungs, pleura, and diaphragm. They account for 11% to 18% of mediastinal masses in infants and children.[89,90] The cyst is lined by ciliated mucus-secreting bronchial epithelium and may be mucus filled. Although the mediastinal cysts do not communicate with the bronchopulmonary tree, intrapulmonary cysts usually do.

Bronchogenic cysts range in size from a few millimeters to more than 5 cm. On prenatal ultrasound, they usually appear as anechoic unilocular intrathoracic cysts (Fig. 36-7), at times with layering echogenic material.[91,92] If the cyst does not cause mass effect, it typically will not cause a problem in utero. However, if the cyst compresses the airway, it can lead to airway obstruction at birth.[93] The main differential diagnosis is CCAM. However, CCAM usually has more than one cyst and an associated echogenic mass with mass effect. If a bronchogenic cyst causes obstruction, it may lead to the distal lung accumulating fluid, masquerading as an echogenic lung lesion such as CCAM or sequestration. Fetal MRI can be helpful in cases with unclear diagnosis.[93] Surgical resection for bronchogenic cysts is performed postnatally because of the associated increased risk for hemorrhage, infection, or malignancy.[94]

NEURENTERIC CYST

Neurenteric cysts represent a posterior enteric remnant caused by incomplete separation of the notochord from the foregut during embryogenesis. They typically occur in the posterior mediastinum or in the spinal canal. The

cysts can have a septated or bilobed appearance. Associated spinal abnormalities are typically present.[95-98]

PLEURAL EFFUSION

Fetal pleural effusion is rare, with an incidence of up to 1 in 15,000 pregnancies.[99,100] Males are slightly more affected than females.[101] Any fluid in the pleural space is abnormal. If sufficiently large, pleural effusion may result in mass effect, leading to compression of the heart and hydrops as well as compression of the lungs, resulting in pulmonary hypoplasia.[102]

Primary pleural effusion is most often caused by chylothorax,[103] which results from defective development of the lymphatic system. Any insult to the course of the thoracic duct in the posterior mediastinum in the fetal chest can result in chylous fetal pleural effusion.[104] This can be on either the right or the left side, because the thoracic duct in the posterior mediastinum crosses from right to left at the fifth thoracic level. Primary pleural effusion is suspected when the effusion is unilateral or is much larger on one side than the other, and no other signs of hydrops are present. However, once hydrops develops (cardiac compression from unilateral effusion), this distinction can be difficult.

Primary chylothorax is associated with aneuploidy in 1.8% to 5.8% of cases.[105,106] By definition, chylothorax in neonates is identified when fluid contains more than 1.1 mmol/L triglycerides with oral fat intake, with lymphocyte proportion exceeding 80%.[107] However, the fetus is fasting in utero, and the mean percentage of lymphocytes in the blood of normal fetuses is normally greater than 80%.[108] Therefore, these parameters do not apply in utero.

Secondary pleural effusion occurs in association with aneuploidy, infection, genetic syndromes, and other structural malformations.[105,109] These syndromes typically present with bilateral pleural effusions (particularly in fetuses with hydrops),[104] but occasionally with unilateral effusion.

Pleural effusions appear on prenatal ultrasound as anechoic fluid collections in the pleural space, leading to the appearance of the lung floating in the fluid, surrounded by the chest wall and diaphragm[110] (Fig. 36-8; **Video 36-2**). Small effusions appear as an anechoic thin rim outlining the lungs and the mediastinum. Larger unilateral effusions result in mass effect causing mediastinal shift and flattening or eversion of the diaphragm. If isolated and small, pleural effusions have a benign course. If large with mass effect, untreated fetal pleural effusion has a mortality rate of 22% to 53%.[99,101,104,111,112]

Small pleural effusions do not shift the mediastinum. Pleural effusions associated with hydrops may be unilateral or bilateral, often beginning as unilateral collections that progress bilaterally. If mediastinal shift is visualized in association with a small pleural effusion, a chest mass

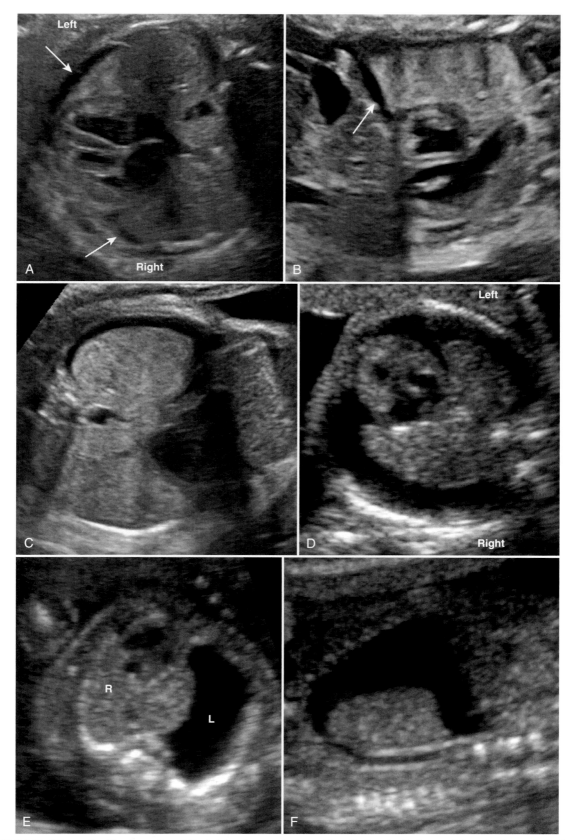

FIGURE 36-8. Pleural effusion. A and **B,** Axial and coronal views of small pleural effusions at 25 weeks *(arrows).* **C,** Axial view of effusion at 28 weeks with mild mediastinal shift. **D,** Axial view shows moderate bilateral effusions outlining the lungs. The effusions are about the same size, so there is no mediastinal shift. **E** and **F,** Axial and oblique sagittal views at 17 weeks show a large left effusion *(L)* with severe mediastinal shift to the right *(R).*

such as a hernia or congenital pulmonary malformation should be sought. Larger effusions will lead to flattening of the hemidiaphragms, and when sufficiently large, mediastinal shift.

Prenatal pleural effusion has a variable natural course ranging from spontaneous resolution to progressive development of hydrops fetalis and polyhydramnios with high risk for perinatal morbidity and mortality.[104] Good prognostic factors include absence of associated abnormalities, unilateral effusion, no associated hydrops, and spontaneous resolution, which may occur in up to 20% (has been associated with 100% survival).[101,104,112] Poor perinatal outcome is associated with pleural effusion in association with hydrops, underlying structural abnormalities, pulmonary hypoplasia, and early gestational age at diagnosis.[101,102]

Pleural effusions are treated by drainage if the effusion is isolated (or asymmetrical) without additional anomalies, typically in fetuses at risk for developing hydrops (i.e., those with severe mediastinal shift or with other signs of hydrops already present).[49] Typically, a pleural effusion is drained with a single stick procedure.[113] If it recurs, placement of a thoracoamniotic shunt is an option.[114] A recent systematic review of prenatal intervention for isolated primary pleural effusion without hydrops suggested that survival rates after prenatal intervention are as high as 60%.[100] Case reports of other treatment options include pleurodesis and intrapleural injection of autologous blood, which have a survival rate of 80%.[115,116] A series of 44 fetuses found thoracoamniotic shunts to have a high survival rate in nonhydropic fetuses of 100%, with survival of 50% in the hydropic group.[4] Risks of prenatal thoracoamniotic shunts include fetal hemorrhage, blockage or migration of the shunt, and placental abruption or preterm labor. In cases of large effusions, drainage immediately before delivery can assist in airway management at birth.

PERICARDIAL EFFUSION

In contrast to pleural effusions that surround the lungs and compress the tissue medially, pericardial effusions are anteromedial fluid collections. Fluid collections of up to 2 mm in thickness are common, and a small amount of pericardial fluid (up to 7 mm, in isolation) can be a normal finding.[117] A large pericardial effusion compresses the lungs against the posterior chest wall (Fig. 36-9). The heart is visualized as "floating" within the anterior thoracic fluid collection.

CONGENITAL DIAPHRAGMATIC HERNIA

Congenital diaphragmatic hernia results from failure of the pleuroperitoneal canal to close at the end of

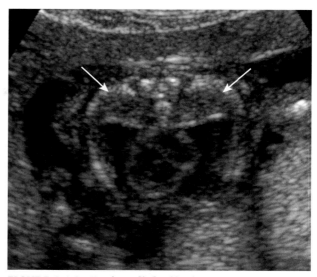

FIGURE 36-9. Pericardial effusion. Note how the lungs *(arrows)* are compressed posteriorly by the effusion surrounding the heart.

organogenesis.[118] A "dual hit" hypothesis suggests that the defect arises in the embryologic period (first hit) and during further gestation, lung development is impaired (second hit).[119] The defect in the diaphragm allows herniation of viscera into the chest. Mass effect from visceral organs in the chest has an adverse impact on the normal development of the fetal cardiac and pulmonary systems. Thus, CDH is associated with substantial morbidity and mortality.[120-123] The incidence of CDH is about 1 in 3000 births.

The majority of hernias are on the left (84%) and occur predominantly through the posterolateral **foramen of Bochdalek.** CDHs occur on the right in 10% to 15% of cases and are bilateral in less than 5%.[124,125] Only a few cases of **Morgagni hernia** (anterior diaphragmatic defect) have been reported prenatally.[126-128] Complete **agenesis of the diaphragm,** herniation of the central tendinous part, **pericardial hernia,** and **eventration of the diaphragm** are rare manifestations.[9]

Left-Sided Hernia

Left-sided CDH is most often diagnosed when the stomach is in the chest near the left atrium, with absence of the normal stomach below the diaphragm (Fig. 36-10; **Videos 36-3** and **36-4**). Small and large bowel as well as the liver, spleen, and kidney can herniate into the thorax. As the abdominal contents herniate into the chest, mediastinal shift occurs with the heart deviating to the right.[9,125,129] In large hernias, mediastinal shift is severe, leading to vascular compromise. Compression of the heart, impaired swallowing, and partial obstruction of the gastrointestinal tract lead to polyhydramnios, which is present in up to 69% of cases, particularly late in gestation (by the third trimester).[121,130,131]

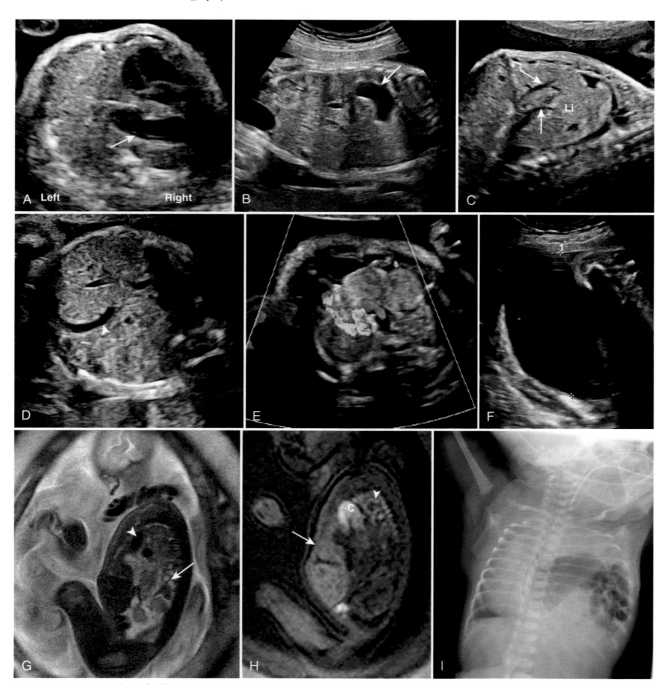

FIGURE 36-10. Left-sided congenital diaphragmatic hernia (CDH). A, Axial view of chest at 28 weeks' gestation shows the stomach *(arrow)* in the chest with mediastinal shift to the right. **B,** Coronal image in a different fetus at 28 weeks shows a slightly distended stomach *(arrow)* in the chest. **C,** Oblique sagittal image shows a large amount of liver *(Li)* in the chest. Note the hepatic vessels *(arrows)*. **D,** Axial view of abdomen shows abnormal course of umbilical vein *(arrowhead)* resulting from the liver herniation into the chest. **E,** Oblique axial view of chest shows kinked hepatic vessels. **F,** Axial view in the right lower quadrant shows the associated polyhydramnios complicating the pregnancy in the same fetus. **G,** Sagittal T2-weighted fetal MR image shows the small bowel *(arrow)* and colon *(arrowhead)* in chest with small pleural effusion. **H,** Sagittal T1-weighted fetal MR image shows liver *(arrow)* in chest. Note bright signal of meconium in colon *(C)* in chest, as well as small bowel loops *(arrowhead)* in chest. **I,** Postnatal radiograph shows the bowel in the left chest, nasogastric tube in the left chest, and a tiny, hypoplastic right lung.

Because left-sided hernias with mediastinal shift compress the left heart, they can lead to underdevelopment of the left heart. Mediastinal shift often makes it difficult to assess for hypoplastic left-sided heart in association with CDH, versus compression caused by mediastinal shift. Because of the high rate of associated cardiac abnormalities, formal fetal echocardiography is indicated in fetuses with CDH.

Prenatal sonographic diagnosis of CDH can be made as early as the first trimester.[124,132] With the increased use of first-trimester nuchal translucency screening, it is expected that early diagnosis of CDH will increase.[124] Overall prenatal detection rate is 59% in European countries. However, detection rate in centers with screening programs is as high as 74%, with an increased detection rate when CDH is associated with other anomalies.[133] Paradoxical movement of abdominal contents during fetal inspiration on real-time sonogram may help to confirm CDH, along with traditional sonographic findings.[121] Fetal MRI is a helpful modality to diagnose or confirm the presence of diaphragmatic defect and to assess involvement of the liver in the hernia.[54,134] MRI also allows lung volumetry to be performed.[9]

At times, a left-sided hernia will be present with the stomach in the abdomen and only small bowel loops in the chest. Real-time ultrasound can demonstrate peristalsis of the bowel in the chest. The abdominal circumference is often small, with a scaphoid shape of the abdomen secondary to displacement of viscera into the chest.[135]

In most left-sided hernias the left lobe of the liver herniates into the chest. The diagnosis of liver in the chest is made by direct visualization of the liver (**Video 36-5**). At times, sonographic detection of intrathoracic liver is difficult because of the liver's isoechoic appearance with the fetal lung. In these cases, examination of the course of the portal and hepatic veins is helpful to demonstrate hepatic vessels extending into the chest.[124] The intra-abdominal hepatic vein takes a curved course, and the left portal vein branches will be seen at or above the diaphragm.[136]

Right-Sided Hernia

In a right-sided hernia, the liver herniates into the chest, and mediastinal shift is to the left (Fig. 36-11; **Video 36-6**). Liver echogenicity can appear similar to the lung, so visualization of gallbladder and hepatic vessels in the thorax are helpful in confirming the diagnosis. Bowel can also herniate, but the stomach is located below the diaphragm. Because of kinking of the intrahepatic inferior vena cava, ascites (with fluid extending into the chest) and hydrops are common. Absence of the hypoechoic muscular diaphragm on the right helps in differentiating CDH from other fetal chest masses.

Other Hernias and Eventration

In **bilateral hernias** the falciform ligament is drawn into the hernia.[137,138] Mediastinal shift is variable, but typically the heart is displaced anteriorly and superiorly. Features of both right and left CDH are present.

Pericardial hernias result from failure of the retrosternal portion of the septum transversum to close the communication between the pericardial and peritoneal cavities.[139] The liver may herniate into the pericardial sac.[127,128,139] Pericardial effusion results from mass effect on the heart and obstruction of venous return or from mechanical irritation of membranes.[1,140] Because the differential diagnosis of a pericardial mass includes pericardial tumors such as teratoma, it is important to recognize the liver as part of the hernial sac contents by identifying the hepatic vessels in the mass.[127]

In **diaphragmatic eventration** the intact diaphragm is displaced cephalad at the weakened muscular portion, without communication between the abdominal and thoracic cavities[141] (Fig. 36-12). Diaphragmatic eventration is associated with lower perinatal mortality compared to CDH and may not require surgical repair.[1] Thus it is crucial to make the distinction between the two diagnoses to provide appropriate counseling. Diaphragmatic eventration can be diagnosed on both ultrasound and fetal MRI.[54]

Associated Anomalies

Congenital diaphragmatic hernia may be an isolated defect or may be associated with other structural, chromosomal, or syndromal anomalies. Associated anomalies are present in 25% to 55% of cases. **Congenital heart disease** is the most common association, with hemodynamically significant heart disease in 11% of cases.[142] Because of the high rate of associated cardiac abnormalities, formal fetal echocardiography is indicated in fetuses with CDH.

Associated CNS anomalies are second in frequency of associated structural abnormalities in CDH fetuses, including **anencephaly, ventriculomegaly,** and **neural tube defects.**[143,144] Chromosomal abnormalities occur in 10% to 20% of antenatally detected CDH, the most common being **trisomy 18.**[9,133,144,145] Chromosomal abnormalities are most common when CDH is present in association with other structural abnormalities. Given the high association with aneuploidy, amniocentesis for fetuses diagnosed at the appropriate gestational age is typically performed. Associated syndromes include **Fryn, Beckwith-Wiedemann, Simpson-Golabi-Behmel, Brachmann–de Lange,** and **Perlman.**[146]

Morbidity and Mortality

It is difficult to give precise figures for mortality of CDH, because survival is improving with better care. However, prenatally detected CDH has a worse prognosis than CDH diagnosed at birth. Mortality varies widely depending on gestational age at diagnosis, side of the hernia (right-sided hernias have poorer survival than left-sided hernias,[9,147] and bilateral hernias have worse prognosis than do unilateral hernias), associated abnormalities, size of hernia, liver position,[74,134] presence of hydrops, degree of mediastinal shift,[32,120,124,131,148-150] polyhydramnios,[131] and size of the residual lung.[32] Table 36-5 provides examples of using imaging findings to predict prognosis (survival predictors).

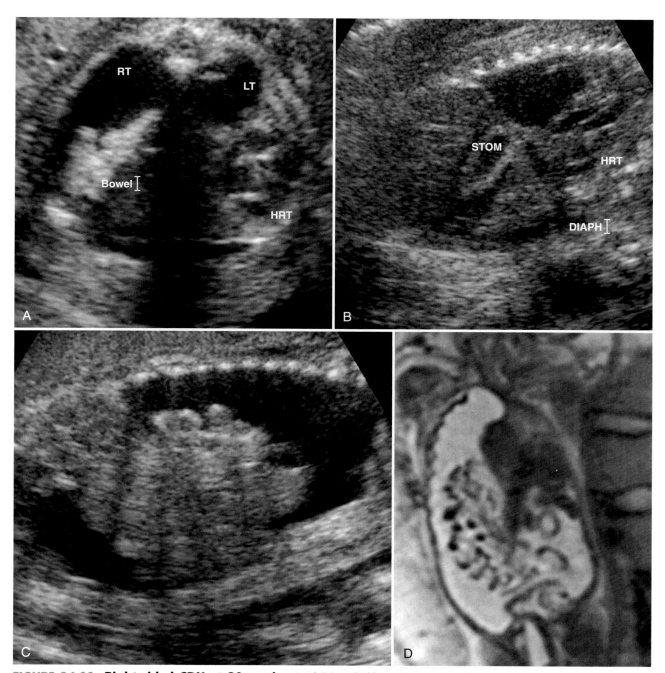

FIGURE 36-11. Right-sided CDH at 30 weeks. Axial **(A)** and oblique **(B, C)** sagittal images show bilateral pleural effusions *(RT, LT)* and bowel loops in the right hemithorax with mediastinal shift with heart *(HRT)* displaced to the left. The left hemidiaphragm *(DIAPH)* is intact, with the stomach *(STOM)* below the diaphragm. **D,** Coronal T2-weighted MR image shows fluid extending from the abdomen into the chest with mediastinal shift to left. Note the lack of a right hemidiaphragm, as well as bowel in the right chest.

Mortality from CHD is high because of termination of pregnancy and in utero demise (secondary to associated abnormalities and hydrops). After birth, CDH has high morbidity and mortality because of pulmonary hypoplasia, pulmonary hypertension, and iatrogenic trauma to the airways from mechanical ventilation. In a 2000 meta-analysis of studies from 1975 to 1998, of 676 prenatally diagnosed fetuses, 142 (21%) were terminated, 36 (5%) died in utero, 333 (49%) died postnatally, and only 165 (24%) survived. More recent studies show improved survival rates. In a 1999-2001 trial, survival of fetuses (without in utero intervention) with lung-to-head ratio of <1.4 and liver in the chest (i.e., fetuses presumed to have poor survival rates) was 77%.[151] Improved overall survival rates in recent years have been attributed to alterations in clinical care for CDH, including minimization of iatrogenic lung injury by gentle ventilation and nutritional support.[124,152-154]

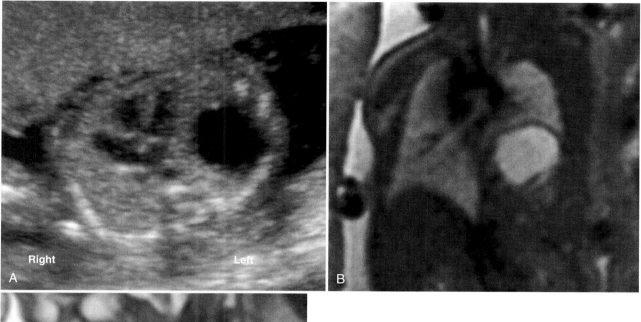

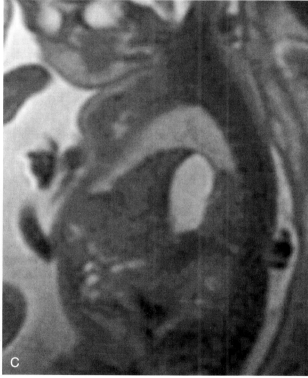

FIGURE 36-12. Eventration of the hemidiaphragm.
A, Transverse view of the thorax demonstrates the stomach in the thorax with mild mediastinal shift. **B** and **C,** Coronal and sagittal T2-weighted MR images show the high position of stomach with intact diaphragm.

Pulmonary hypertension in newborns in association with CDH is thought to be caused by the wall thickening of the small pulmonary arteries. Severity of pulmonary hypoplasia and pulmonary hypertension is related to the volume and timing of herniation of abdominal viscera into the hemithorax.[155]

In Utero Therapy

Options for treatment of CDH focus on lung development. Small hernias with a large amount of visualized lung or hernias diagnosed late in pregnancy can be delivered at a tertiary care center where NICU services are available. In fetuses where pulmonary hypoplasia is a concern, delivery can be done by an EXIT procedure, with testing of the fetus to maintain oxygen saturation before severing the umbilical cord. Fetuses who can maintain oxygen saturation can then be delivered. Those who cannot maintain oxygen saturation can be placed on extracorporeal membrane oxygenation (ECMO) before clamping the cord, to avoid prolonged episodes of hypoxia.

POOR PROGNOSTIC FACTORS IN CONGENITAL DIAPHRAGMATIC HERNIA

Right-sided or bilateral hernia
Early gestational age at diagnosis
Small lung size (measured by lung/head ratio or volumetry)
Associated abnormalities (structural or chromosomal)
Hydrops
Polyhydramnios
Degree of mediastinal shift
Intrauterine growth restriction (IUGR)
Liver in chest

TABLE 36-5. SAMPLE STUDIES OF PREDICTORS OF SURVIVAL IN LEFT-SIDED CDH*

IMAGING FINDING	SIGN/VALUE	OUTCOME (% SURVIVAL)
Liver position[120]	Liver up	43%
	Liver down	93%
Lung-to-head ratio at <25 weeks[32]	<0.6	0%
	0.6-1.35	63%
	>1.35	100%
Fetal lung volume[160] at 22-39 weeks	<5 mL	29%
	>25 mL	100%
Percent predicted lung volume[161]	<15%	40%
	>15%	100%

*Data in this table should be interpreted with caution. Other studies list different rates. Survival rates depend on selection bias of the population, methodology of assessing the imaging findings, and care of neonates at birth.

Fetal surgery can be performed at specialized centers for fetuses least likely to survive with conventional postnatal therapies.[123] Surgery is performed to aid in lung growth and typically is not directed at repair of the diaphragmatic defect, because open fetal surgery is associated with PROM and premature labor. In addition, repair of CDH is associated with intraoperative death caused by kinking of the umbilical vein and ductus venosus as the liver is reduced into the abdomen.[156]

Current in utero therapy is aimed at **fetal endoscopic tracheal occlusion** (FETO), by balloon or clips, which stimulates lung growth.[2] The procedure is performed under combined spinal and epidural anesthesia and fetal analgesia. A 1.2-mm endoscope within a 3.0-mm sheath is introduced into the trachea to place a detachable balloon between the carina and vocal cords.[157] FETO has improved prognosis of severe CDH, with its effect dependent on the preexisting lung size.[9] Other treatment options, such as combining FETO with other modalities (e.g., surfactant, corticosteroids), are being investigated.[158,159]

CONCLUSION

When an abnormality of the fetal thorax is visualized, it is important to have a thorough approach to the fetal evaluation. The echogenicity of the lesion, whether it is cystic or solid, location of the heart, size of normal-appearing lung, evidence of hydrops, and associated abnormalities are important at initial diagnosis. Follow-up to assess interval change in appearance and development of hydrops is important for prognosis. The specific diagnosis is important in determining potential in utero therapy, guiding the appropriate mode of delivery, and explaining to the parents the types of postnatal therapy that may be needed.

References

Development of Structures in the Chest

1. Wayne ER, Campbell JB, Burrington JD, Davis WS. Eventration of the diaphragm. J Pediatr Surg 1974;9:643-651.
2. Wigglesworth JS, Desai R, Hislop AA. Fetal lung growth in congenital laryngeal atresia. Pediatr Pathol 1987;7:515-525.
3. Abu Musa AA, Hata T, Hata K, et al. Ultrasonographic measurement of fetal lung. Gynecol Obstet Invest 1990;30:139-142.
4. Blott M, Greenough A, Nicolaides KH, Campbell S. The ultrasonographic assessment of the fetal thorax and fetal breathing movements in the prediction of pulmonary hypoplasia. Early Hum Dev 1990;21:143-151.
5. Cannie M, Jani J, Meersschaert J, et al. Prenatal prediction of survival in isolated diaphragmatic hernia using observed to expected total fetal lung volume determined by magnetic resonance imaging based on either gestational age or fetal body volume. Ultrasound Obstet Gynecol 2008;32:633-639.
6. Osada H, Iitsuka Y, Masuda K, et al. Application of lung volume measurement by three-dimensional ultrasonography for clinical assessment of fetal lung development. J Ultrasound Med 2002;21:841-847.
7. Osada H, Kaku K, Masuda K, et al. Quantitative and qualitative evaluations of fetal lung with MR imaging. Radiology 2004;231:887-892.
8. Tegnander E, Eik-Nes SH, Linker DT. Incorporating the four-chamber view of the fetal heart into the second-trimester routine fetal examination. Ultrasound Obstet Gynecol 1994;4:24-28.
9. Gucciardo L, Deprest J, Done E, et al. Prediction of outcome in isolated congenital diaphragmatic hernia and its consequences for fetal therapy. Best Pract Res Clin Obstet Gynaecol 2008;22:123-138.
10. Blaas HG, Eik-Nes SH. Sonographic development of the normal foetal thorax and abdomen across gestation. Prenat Diagn 2008;28:568-580.
11. De Vries JI, Visser GH, Prechtl HF. The emergence of fetal behaviour. I. Qualitative aspects. Early Hum Dev 1982;7:301-322.
12. Malas MA, Evcil EH, Desdicioglu K. Size and location of the fetal diaphragm during the fetal period in human fetuses. Surg Radiol Anat 2007;29:155-164.
13. Zalel Y, Gamzu R, Mashiach S, Achiron R. The development of the fetal thymus: an in utero sonographic evaluation. Prenat Diagn 2002;22:114-117.
14. Felker RE, Cartier MS, Emerson DS, Brown DL. Ultrasound of the fetal thymus. J Ultrasound Med 1989;8:669-673.
15. Cho JY, Min JY, Lee YH, et al. Diameter of the normal fetal thymus on ultrasound. Ultrasound Obstet Gynecol 2007;29:634-638.
16. Toti P, De Felice C, Stumpo M, et al. Acute thymic involution in fetuses and neonates with chorioamnionitis. Hum Pathol 2000;31:1121-1128.

Pulmonary Hypoplasia and Aplasia

17. Askenazi SS, Perlman M. Pulmonary hypoplasia: lung weight and radial alveolar count as criteria of diagnosis. Arch Dis Child 1979;54:614-618.

18. Wigglesworth JS, Desai R. Use of DNA estimation for growth assessment in normal and hypoplastic fetal lungs. Arch Dis Child 1981;56:601-605.

19. Lauria MR, Gonik B, Romero R. Pulmonary hypoplasia: pathogenesis, diagnosis, and antenatal prediction. Obstet Gynecol 1995;86:466-475.

20. Rotschild A, Ling EW, Puterman ML, Farquharson D. Neonatal outcome after prolonged preterm rupture of the membranes. Am J Obstet Gynecol 1990;162:46-52.

21. Laudy JA, Wladimiroff JW. The fetal lung. 2. Pulmonary hypoplasia. Ultrasound Obstet Gynecol 2000;16:482-494.

22. Yancey MK, Richards DS. Antenatal sonographic findings associated with unilateral pulmonary agenesis. Obstet Gynecol 1993;81:847-849.

23. Hislop A, Hey E, Reid L. The lungs in congenital bilateral renal agenesis and dysplasia. Arch Dis Child 1979;54:32-38.

24. Ruano R, Martinovic J, Aubry MC, et al. Predicting pulmonary hypoplasia using the sonographic fetal lung volume to body weight ratio: how precise and accurate is it? Ultrasound Obstet Gynecol 2006;28:958-962.

25. Harstad TW, Twickler DM, Leveno KJ, Brown CE. Antepartum prediction of pulmonary hypoplasia: an elusive goal? Am J Perinatol 1993;10:8-11.

26. Jani JC, Cannie M, Peralta CF, et al. Lung volumes in fetuses with congenital diaphragmatic hernia: comparison of 3D US and MR imaging assessments. Radiology 2007;244:575-582.

27. Ruano R, Aubry MC, Barthe B, et al. Three-dimensional sonographic measurement of contralateral lung volume in fetuses with isolated congenital diaphragmatic hernia. J Clin Ultrasound 2008;36:273-278.

28. Cannie M, Neirynck V, De Keyzer F, et al. Prenatal magnetic resonance imaging demonstrates linear growth of the human fetal kidneys during gestation. J Urol 2007;178:1570-1574.

29. Tanigaki S, Miyakoshi K, Tanaka M, et al. Pulmonary hypoplasia: prediction with use of ratio of MR imaging–measured fetal lung volume to ultrasound-estimated fetal body weight. Radiology 2004;232:767-772.

30. Peralta CF, Cavoretto P, Csapo B, et al. Assessment of lung area in normal fetuses at 12-32 weeks. Ultrasound Obstet Gynecol 2005;26:718-724.

31. Fong K, Ohlsson A, Zalev A. Fetal thoracic circumference: a prospective cross-sectional study with real-time ultrasound. Am J Obstet Gynecol 1988;158:1154-1160.

32. Metkus AP, Filly RA, Stringer MD, et al. Sonographic predictors of survival in fetal diaphragmatic hernia. J Pediatr Surg 1996;31:148-151; discussion 151-152.

33. Laudy JA, Gaillard JL, Anker JN, et al. Doppler ultrasound imaging: a new technique to detect lung hypoplasia before birth? Ultrasound Obstet Gynecol 1996;7:189-192.

Congenital Pulmonary Airway Malformation Spectrum

34. Bromley B, Benacerraf BR. Unilateral lung hypoplasia: report of three cases. J Ultrasound Med 1997;16:599-601.

35. Ch'In KY, Tang MY. Congenital adenomatoid malformation of one lobe of a lung with general anasarca. Arch Pathol (Chic) 1949;48:221-229.

36. Stocker JT, Kagan-Hallet K. Extralobar pulmonary sequestration: analysis of 15 cases. Am J Clin Pathol 1979;72:917-925.

37. Bratu I, Flageole H, Chen MF, et al. The multiple facets of pulmonary sequestration. J Pediatr Surg 2001;36:784-790.

38. Lopoo JB, Goldstein RB, Lipshutz GS, et al. Fetal pulmonary sequestration: a favorable congenital lung lesion. Obstet Gynecol 1999;94:567-571.

39. Rosado-de-Christenson ML, Stocker JT. Congenital cystic adenomatoid malformation. Radiographics 1991;11:865-886.

40. Laberge JM, Flageole H, Pugash D, et al. Outcome of the prenatally diagnosed congenital cystic adenomatoid lung malformation: a Canadian experience. Fetal Diagn Ther 2001;16:178-186.

41. Thorpe-Beeston JG, Nicolaides KH. Cystic adenomatoid malformation of the lung: prenatal diagnosis and outcome. Prenat Diagn 1994;14:677-688.

42. Adzick NS, Harrison MR, Glick PL, et al. Fetal cystic adenomatoid malformation: prenatal diagnosis and natural history. J Pediatr Surg 1985;20:483-488.

43. Bunduki V, Ruano R, da Silva MM, et al. Prognostic factors associated with congenital cystic adenomatoid malformation of the lung. Prenat Diagn 2000;20:459-464.

44. Fine C, Adzick NS, Doubilet PM. Decreasing size of a congenital cystic adenomatoid malformation in utero. J Ultrasound Med 1988;7:405-408.

45. Stocker JT, Madewell JE, Drake RM. Congenital cystic adenomatoid malformation of the lung: classification and morphologic spectrum. Hum Pathol 1977;8:155-171.

46. Bromley B, Parad R, Estroff JA, Benacerraf BR. Fetal lung masses: prenatal course and outcome. J Ultrasound Med 1995;14:927-936; quiz p1378.

47. Adzick NS, Harrison MR, Crombleholme TM, et al. Fetal lung lesions: management and outcome. Am J Obstet Gynecol 1998;179:884-889.

48. Mahle WT, Rychik J, Tian ZY, et al. Echocardiographic evaluation of the fetus with congenital cystic adenomatoid malformation. Ultrasound Obstet Gynecol 2000;16:620-624.

49. Knox EM, Kilby MD, Martin WL, Khan KS. In-utero pulmonary drainage in the management of primary hydrothorax and congenital cystic lung lesion: a systematic review. Ultrasound Obstet Gynecol 2006;28:726-734.

50. Harrison MR, Adzick NS, Jennings RW, et al. Antenatal intervention for congenital cystic adenomatoid malformation. Lancet 1990;336:965-967.

51. Crombleholme TM, Coleman B, Hedrick H, et al. Cystic adenomatoid malformation volume ratio predicts outcome in prenatally diagnosed cystic adenomatoid malformation of the lung. J Pediatr Surg 2002;37:331-338.

52. Tsao K, Hawgood S, Vu L, et al. Resolution of hydrops fetalis in congenital cystic adenomatoid malformation after prenatal steroid therapy. J Pediatr Surg 2003;38:508-510.

53. Hubbard AM, States LJ. Fetal magnetic resonance imaging. Top Magn Reson Imaging 2001;12:93-103.

54. Levine D, Barnewolt CE, Mehta TS, et al. Fetal thoracic abnormalities: MR imaging. Radiology 2003;228:379-388.

55. Van Leeuwen K, Teitelbaum DH, Hirschl RB, et al. Prenatal diagnosis of congenital cystic adenomatoid malformation and its postnatal presentation, surgical indications, and natural history. J Pediatr Surg 1999;34:794-798; discussion 798-799.

56. Cavoretto P, Molina F, Poggi S, et al. Prenatal diagnosis and outcome of echogenic fetal lung lesions. Ultrasound Obstet Gynecol 2008;32:769-783.

57. Duncombe GJ, Dickinson JE, Kikiros CS. Prenatal diagnosis and management of congenital cystic adenomatoid malformation of the lung. Am J Obstet Gynecol 2002;187:950-954.

58. Stacher E, Ullmann R, Halbwedl I, et al. Atypical goblet cell hyperplasia in congenital cystic adenomatoid malformation as a possible preneoplasia for pulmonary adenocarcinoma in childhood: a genetic analysis. Hum Pathol 2004;35:565-570.

59. MacSweeney F, Papagiannopoulos K, Goldstraw P, et al. An assessment of the expanded classification of congenital cystic adenomatoid malformations and their relationship to malignant transformation. Am J Surg Pathol 2003;27:1139-1146.

60. Marshall KW, Blane CE, Teitelbaum DH, van Leeuwen K. Congenital cystic adenomatoid malformation: impact of prenatal diagnosis and changing strategies in the treatment of the asymptomatic patient. AJR Am J Roentgenol 2000;175:1551-1554.

61. Rosado de Christensen ML, Frazier AA, Stocker JT, Templeton PA. From the archives of the AFIP. Extralobar sequestration: radiologic-pathologic correlation. Radiographics 1993;13:425-441.

62. Halkic N, Cuenoud PF, Corthesy ME, et al. Pulmonary sequestration: a review of 26 cases. Eur J Cardiothorac Surg 1998;14:127-133.

63. Savic B, Birtel FJ, Tholen W, et al. Lung sequestration: report of seven cases and review of 540 published cases. Thorax 1979;34:96-101.

64. Corbett HJ, Humphrey GM. Pulmonary sequestration. Paediatr Respir Rev 2004;5:59-68.

65. Sade RM, Clouse M, Ellis Jr FH. The spectrum of pulmonary sequestration. Ann Thorac Surg 1974;18:644-658.

66. Frazier AA, Rosado de Christensen ML, Stocker JT, Templeton PA. Intralobar sequestration: radiologic-pathologic correlation. Radiographics 1997;17:725-745.

67. Chan YF, Oldfield R, Vogel S, Ferguson S. Pulmonary sequestration presenting as a prenatally detected suprarenal lesion in a neonate. J Pediatr Surg 2000;35:1367-1369.

68. Levi A, Findler M, Dolfin T, et al. Intrapericardial extralobar pulmonary sequestration in a neonate. Chest 1990;98:1014-1015.

69. Langer B, Donato L, Riethmuller C, et al. Spontaneous regression of fetal pulmonary sequestration. Ultrasound Obstet Gynecol 1995;6:33-39.

70. Yildirim G, Gungorduk K, Aslan H, Ceylan Y. Prenatal diagnosis of an extralobar pulmonary sequestration. Arch Gynecol Obstet 2008;278:181-186.

71. Hayashi S, Sago H, Kitano Y, et al. Fetal pleuroamniotic shunting for bronchopulmonary sequestration with hydrops. Ultrasound Obstet Gynecol 2006;28:963-967.

72. Babu R, Kyle P, Spicer RD. Prenatal sonographic features of congenital lobar emphysema. Fetal Diagn Ther 2001;16:200-202.

73. Quinton AE, Smoleniec JS. Congenital lobar emphysema: the disappearing chest mass—antenatal ultrasound appearance. Ultrasound Obstet Gynecol 2001;17:169-171.

74. Walsh DS, Hubbard AM, Olutoye OO, et al. Assessment of fetal lung volumes and liver herniation with magnetic resonance imaging in congenital diaphragmatic hernia. Am J Obstet Gynecol 2000;183:1067-1069.

Congenital High Airway Obstruction

75. Lim FY, Crombleholme TM, Hedrick HL, et al. Congenital high airway obstruction syndrome: natural history and management. J Pediatr Surg 2003;38:940-945.

76. Hedrick MH, Ferro MM, Filly RA, et al. Congenital high airway obstruction syndrome (CHAOS): a potential for perinatal intervention. J Pediatr Surg 1994;29:271-274.

77. Vidaeff AC, Szmuk P, Mastrobattista JM, et al. More or less CHAOS: case report and literature review suggesting the existence of a distinct subtype of congenital high airway obstruction syndrome. Ultrasound Obstet Gynecol 2007;30:114-117.

78. Kanamori Y, Kitano Y, Hashizume K, et al. A case of laryngeal atresia (congenital high airway obstruction syndrome) with chromosome 5p deletion syndrome rescued by ex utero intrapartum treatment. J Pediatr Surg 2004;39:E25-E28.

79. King SJ, Pilling DW, Walkinshaw S. Fetal echogenic lung lesions: prenatal ultrasound diagnosis and outcome. Pediatr Radiol 1995;25:208-210.

80. Vanhaesebrouck P, De Coen K, Defoort P, et al. Evidence for autosomal dominant inheritance in prenatally diagnosed CHAOS. Eur J Pediatr 2006;165:706-708.

81. Witters I, Moerman P, Fryns JP. Prenatal echographic diagnosis of laryngeal atresia as part of a multiple congenital anomalies (MCA) syndrome. Genet Couns 2000;11:215-219.

82. Morrison PJ, Macphail S, Williams D, et al. Laryngeal atresia or stenosis presenting as second-trimester fetal ascites: diagnosis and pathology in three independent cases. Prenat Diagn 1998;18:963-967.

83. Mong A, Johnson AM, Kramer SS, et al. Congenital high airway obstruction syndrome: MR/US findings, effect on management, and outcome. Pediatr Radiol 2008;38:1171-1179.

84. Langer JE, Coleman BG. Case 2. Diagnosis: congenital high airway obstruction syndrome. Ultrasound Q 2007;23:67-70.

85. Kalache KD, Chaoui R, Tennstedt C, Bollmann R. Prenatal diagnosis of laryngeal atresia in two cases of congenital high airway obstruction syndrome (CHAOS). Prenat Diagn 1997;17:577-581.

86. Crombleholme TM, Sylvester K, Flake AW, Adzick NS. Salvage of a fetus with congenital high airway obstruction syndrome by ex utero intrapartum treatment (EXIT) procedure. Fetal Diagn Ther 2000;15:280-282.

87. Bui TH, Grunewald C, Frenckner B, et al. Successful EXIT (ex utero intrapartum treatment) procedure in a fetus diagnosed prenatally with congenital high-airway obstruction syndrome due to laryngeal atresia. Eur J Pediatr Surg 2000;10:328-333.

Bronchogenic Cyst

88. Rogers LF, Osmer JC. Bronchogenic cyst: a review of 46 cases. Am J Roentgenol Radium Ther Nucl Med 1964;91:273-290.

89. Snyder ME, Luck SR, Hernandez R, et al. Diagnostic dilemmas of mediastinal cysts. J Pediatr Surg 1985;20:810-815.

90. Parikh D, Samuel M. Congenital cystic lung lesions: is surgical resection essential? Pediatr Pulmonol 2005;40:533-537.

91. Albright EB, Crane JP, Shackelford GD. Prenatal diagnosis of a bronchogenic cyst. J Ultrasound Med 1988;7:90-95.

92. Reece EA, Lockwood CJ, Rizzo N, et al. Intrinsic intrathoracic malformations of the fetus: sonographic detection and clinical presentation. Obstet Gynecol 1987;70:627-632.

93. Levine D, Jennings R, Barnewolt C, et al. Progressive fetal bronchial obstruction caused by a bronchogenic cyst diagnosed using prenatal MR imaging. AJR Am J Roentgenol 2001;176:49-52.

94. Eber E. Antenatal diagnosis of congenital thoracic malformations: early surgery, late surgery, or no surgery? Semin Respir Crit Care Med 2007;28:355-366.

Neurenteric Cyst

95. Uludag S, Madazli R, Erdogan E, et al. A case of prenatally diagnosed fetal neurenteric cyst. Ultrasound Obstet Gynecol 2001;18:277-279.

96. Macaulay KE, Winter 3rd TC, Shields LE. Neurenteric cyst shown by prenatal sonography. AJR Am J Roentgenol 1997;169:563-565.

97. Perera GB, Milne M. Neurenteric cyst: antenatal diagnosis by ultrasound. Australas Radiol 1997;41:300-302.

98. Wilkinson CC, Albanese CT, Jennings RW, et al. Fetal neurenteric cyst causing hydrops: case report and review of the literature. Prenat Diagn 1999;19:118-121.

Pleural Effusion

99. Longaker MT, Laberge JM, Dansereau J, et al. Primary fetal hydrothorax: natural history and management. J Pediatr Surg 1989;24:573-576.

100. Deurloo KL, Devlieger R, Lopriore E, et al. Isolated fetal hydrothorax with hydrops: a systematic review of prenatal treatment options. Prenat Diagn 2007;27:893-899.

101. Weber AM, Philipson EH. Fetal pleural effusion: a review and meta-analysis for prognostic indicators. Obstet Gynecol 1992;79:281-286.

102. Castillo RA, Devoe LD, Hadi HA, et al. Nonimmune hydrops fetalis: clinical experience and factors related to a poor outcome. Am J Obstet Gynecol 1986;155:812-816.

103. Lange IR, Manning FA. Antenatal diagnosis of congenital pleural effusions. Am J Obstet Gynecol 1981;140:839-840.

104. Aubard Y, Derouineau I, Aubard V, et al. Primary fetal hydrothorax: a literature review and proposed antenatal clinical strategy. Fetal Diagn Ther 1998;13:325-333.

105. Achiron R, Weissman A, Lipitz S, et al. Fetal pleural effusion: the risk of fetal trisomy. Gynecol Obstet Invest 1995;39:153-156.

106. Nicolaides KH, Rodeck CH, Gosden CM. Rapid karyotyping in non-lethal fetal malformations. Lancet 1986;1:283-287.

107. Buttiker V, Fanconi S, Burger R. Chylothorax in children: guidelines for diagnosis and management. Chest 1999;116:682-687.

108. Poblete A, Roberts A, Trespidi L, et al. Fetal and maternal white cells and B- and T-lymphocyte subpopulations in pregnant women with recent infection. Fetal Diagn Ther 2001;16:378-383.

109. Sherer DM, Abramowicz JS, Sanko SR, Woods Jr JR. Trisomy 21 presented as a transient unilateral pleural effusion at 18 weeks' gestation. Am J Perinatol 1993;10:12-13.

110. Carroll B. Pulmonary hypoplasia and pleural effusions associated with fetal death in utero: ultrasonic findings. AJR Am J Roentgenol 1977;129:749-750.

111. Klam S, Bigras JL, Hudon L. Predicting outcome in primary fetal hydrothorax. Fetal Diagn Ther 2005;20:366-370.

112. Hagay Z, Reece A, Roberts A, Hobbins JC. Isolated fetal pleural effusion: a prenatal management dilemma. Obstet Gynecol 1993;81:147-152.

113. Petres RE, Redwine FO, Cruikshank DP. Congenital bilateral chylothorax: antepartum diagnosis and successful intrauterine surgical management. JAMA 1982;248:1360-1361.

114. Roberts AB, Clarkson PM, Pattison NS, et al. Fetal hydrothorax in the second trimester of pregnancy: successful intra-uterine treatment at 24 weeks gestation. Fetal Ther 1986;1:203-209.

115. Okawa T, Takano Y, Fujimori K, et al. A new fetal therapy for chylothorax: pleurodesis with OK-432. Ultrasound Obstet Gynecol 2001;18:376-377.

116. Tanemura M, Nishikawa N, Kojima K, et al. A case of successful fetal therapy for congenital chylothorax by intrapleural injection of OK-432. Ultrasound Obstet Gynecol 2001;18:371-375.

Pericardial Effusion

117. Di Salvo DN, Brown DL, Doubilet PM, et al. Clinical significance of isolated fetal pericardial effusion. J Ultrasound Med 1994;13:291-293.

Congenital Diaphragmatic Hernia

118. Chinn DH, Filly RA, Callen PW, et al. Congenital diaphragmatic hernia diagnosed prenatally by ultrasound. Radiology 1983;148:119-123.
119. Keijzer R, Liu J, Deimling J, et al. Dual-hit hypothesis explains pulmonary hypoplasia in the nitrofen model of congenital diaphragmatic hernia. Am J Pathol 2000;156:1299-1306.
120. Albanese CT, Lopoo J, Goldstein RB, et al. Fetal liver position and perinatal outcome for congenital diaphragmatic hernia. Prenat Diagn 1998;18:1138-1142.
121. Sista AK, Filly RA. Paradoxical movement of abdominal contents: a real-time sonographic finding indicating a congenital diaphragmatic hernia. J Ultrasound Med 2007;26:1617-1619.
122. Harrison MR, Adzick NS, Estes JM, Howell LJ. A prospective study of the outcome for fetuses with diaphragmatic hernia. JAMA 1994;271:382-384.
123. Conforti AF, Losty PD. Perinatal management of congenital diaphragmatic hernia. Early Hum Dev 2006;82:283-287.
124. Deprest J, Jani J, Van Schoubroeck D, et al. Current consequences of prenatal diagnosis of congenital diaphragmatic hernia. J Pediatr Surg 2006;41:423-430.
125. Deprest JA, Flemmer AW, Gratacos E, Nicolaides K. Antenatal prediction of lung volume and in-utero treatment by fetal endoscopic tracheal occlusion in severe isolated congenital diaphragmatic hernia. Semin Fetal Neonatal Med 2009;14:8-13.
126. Benacerraf BR, Greene MF. Congenital diaphragmatic hernia: ultrasound diagnosis prior to 22 weeks gestation. Radiology 1986;158:809-810.
127. Jain KK, Sen J, Rathee SK, Saini J. Antenatal diagnosis of a Morgagni hernia in the second trimester. J Clin Ultrasound 2008;36:116-118.
128. Robnett-Filly B, Goldstein RB, Sampior D, Hom M. Morgagni hernia: a rare form of congenital diaphragmatic hernia. J Ultrasound Med 2003;22:537-539.
129. Done E, Gucciardo L, van Mieghem T, et al. Prenatal diagnosis, prediction of outcome and in utero therapy of isolated congenital diaphragmatic hernia. Prenat Diagn 2008;28:581-591.
130. Harrison MR, Adzick NS, Nakayama DK, deLorimier AA. Fetal diaphragmatic hernia: fetal but fixable. Semin Perinatol 1985;9:103-112.
131. Adzick NS, Vacanti JP, Lillehei CW, et al. Fetal diaphragmatic hernia: ultrasound diagnosis and clinical outcome in 38 cases. J Pediatr Surg 1989;24:654-657; discussion 657-658.
132. Daskalakis G, Anastasakis E, Souka A, et al. First trimester ultrasound diagnosis of congenital diaphragmatic hernia. J Obstet Gynaecol Res 2007;33:870-872.
133. Garne E, Haeusler M, Barisic I, et al. Congenital diaphragmatic hernia: evaluation of prenatal diagnosis in 20 European regions. Ultrasound Obstet Gynecol 2002;19:329-333.
134. Kitano Y, Nakagawa S, Kuroda T, et al. Liver position in fetal congenital diaphragmatic hernia retains a prognostic value in the era of lung-protective strategy. J Pediatr Surg 2005;40:1827-1832.
135. Teixeira J, Sepulveda W, Hassan J, et al. Abdominal circumference in fetuses with congenital diaphragmatic hernia: correlation with hernia content and pregnancy outcome. J Ultrasound Med 1997;16:407-410.
136. Bootstaylor BS, Filly RA, Harrison MR, Adzick NS. Prenatal sonographic predictors of liver herniation in congenital diaphragmatic hernia. J Ultrasound Med 1995;14:515-520.
137. Bingham JA. Herniation through congenital diaphragmatic defects. Br J Surg 1959;47:1-15.
138. Lanteri R, Santangelo M, Rapisarda C, et al. Bilateral Morgagni-Larrey hernia: a rare cause of intestinal occlusion. Arch Surg 2004;139:1299-1300.
139. Einzig S, Munson DP, Singh S, et al. Intrapericardial herniation of the liver: uncommon cause of massive pericardial effusion in neonates. AJR Am J Roentgenol 1981;137:1075-1077.
140. Iliff PJ, Eyre JA, Westaby S, et al. Neonatal pericardial effusion associated with central eventration of the diaphragm. Arch Dis Child 1983;58:147-149.
141. Jeanty C, Nien JK, Espinoza J, et al. Pleural and pericardial effusion: a potential ultrasonographic marker for the prenatal differential diagnosis between congenital diaphragmatic eventration and congenital diaphragmatic hernia. Ultrasound Obstet Gynecol 2007;29:378-387.
142. Graziano JN. Cardiac anomalies in patients with congenital diaphragmatic hernia and their prognosis: a report from the Congenital Diaphragmatic Hernia Study Group. J Pediatr Surg 2005;40:1045-1049; discussion 1049-1050.
143. Bollmann R, Kalache K, Mau H, et al. Associated malformations and chromosomal defects in congenital diaphragmatic hernia. Fetal Diagn Ther 1995;10:52-59.
144. Sabharwal AJ, Davis CF, Howatson AG. Post-mortem findings in fetal and neonatal congenital diaphragmatic hernia. Eur J Pediatr Surg 2000;10:96-99.
145. Geary MP, Chitty LS, Morrison JJ, et al. Perinatal outcome and prognostic factors in prenatally diagnosed congenital diaphragmatic hernia. Ultrasound Obstet Gynecol 1998;12:107-111.
146. Enns GM, Cox VA, Goldstein RB, et al. Congenital diaphragmatic defects and associated syndromes, malformations, and chromosome anomalies: a retrospective study of 60 patients and literature review. Am J Med Genet 1998;79:215-225.
147. Jani J, Nicolaides KH, Benachi A, et al. Timing of lung size assessment in the prediction of survival in fetuses with diaphragmatic hernia. Ultrasound Obstet Gynecol 2008;31:37-40.
148. Stringer MD, Goldstein RB, Filly RA, et al. Fetal diaphragmatic hernia without visceral herniation. J Pediatr Surg 1995;30:1264-1266.
149. Lipshutz GS, Albanese CT, Feldstein VA, et al. Prospective analysis of lung-to-head ratio predicts survival for patients with prenatally diagnosed congenital diaphragmatic hernia. J Pediatr Surg 1997;32:1634-1636.
150. Harrison MR, Mychaliska GB, Albanese CT, et al. Correction of congenital diaphragmatic hernia in utero IX: fetuses with poor prognosis (liver herniation and low lung-to-head ratio) can be saved by fetoscopic temporary tracheal occlusion. J Pediatr Surg 1998;33:1017-1022; discussion 1022-1023.
151. Harrison MR, Keller RL, Hawgood SB, et al. A randomized trial of fetal endoscopic tracheal occlusion for severe fetal congenital diaphragmatic hernia. N Engl J Med 2003;349:1916-1924.
152. Javid PJ, Jaksic T, Skarsgard ED, Lee S. Survival rate in congenital diaphragmatic hernia: the experience of the Canadian Neonatal Network. J Pediatr Surg 2004;39:657-660.
153. Stege G, Fenton A, Jaffray B. Nihilism in the 1990s: the true mortality of congenital diaphragmatic hernia. Pediatrics 2003;112:532-535.
154. Kitano Y. Prenatal intervention for congenital diaphragmatic hernia. Semin Pediatr Surg 2007;16:101-108.
155. Harrison MR, Adzick NS, Nakayama DK, deLorimier AA. Fetal diaphragmatic hernia: pathophysiology, natural history, and outcome. Clin Obstet Gynecol 1986;29:490-501.
156. Harrison MR, Adzick NS, Flake AW, et al. Correction of congenital diaphragmatic hernia in utero: VI. Hard-earned lessons. J Pediatr Surg 1993;28:1411-1417; discussion 1417-1418.
157. Jani J, Keller RL, Benachi A, et al. Prenatal prediction of survival in isolated left-sided diaphragmatic hernia. Ultrasound Obstet Gynecol 2006;27:18-22.
158. David AL, Weisz B, Gregory L, et al. Ultrasound-guided injection and occlusion of the trachea in fetal sheep. Ultrasound Obstet Gynecol 2006;28:82-88.
159. Davey MG, Danzer E, Schwarz U, et al. Prenatal glucocorticoids and exogenous surfactant therapy improve respiratory function in lambs with severe diaphragmatic hernia following fetal tracheal occlusion. Pediatr Res 2006;60:131-135.
160. Busing KA, Kilian AK, Schaible T, et al. MR lung volume in fetal congenital diaphragmatic hernia: logistic regression analysis—mortality and extracorporeal membrane oxygenation. Radiology 2008;248:233-239.
161. Barnewolt CE, Kunisaki SM, Fauza DO, et al. Percent predicted lung volumes as measured on fetal magnetic resonance imaging: a useful biometric parameter for risk stratification in congenital diaphragmatic hernia. J Pediatr Surg 2007;42:193-197.

CHAPTER 37

The Fetal Heart

Elizabeth R. Stamm and Julia A. Drose

Chapter Outline

Sonographic evaluation of the fetal heart can identify cardiac abnormalities that impact obstetric care in a variety of ways, including mode of delivery, place of delivery, opportunity for termination, intrauterine therapy, and parental reassurance. Congenital heart disease (CHD) is a significant problem, with an incidence of 2 to 6.5 cases per 1000 live births. Greater than 20% of perinatal deaths caused by congenital malformations are the result of a congenital heart defect.[1] In 85% of CHD cases, both environmental and genetic factors are involved (Table 37-1).[2-5] The remaining 15% of cardiac anomalies are associated with a single gene or chromosomal abnormality.[3] The risk of CHD increases to 2% to 3% with an affected sibling and to approximately 10% with two affected siblings or an affected mother.[3,6] The risk to offspring of affected mothers is substantially higher than for those with affected fathers, suggesting that cytoplasmic inheritance may play a role in the genetics of CHD (Tables 37-2 and 37-3). Only 50% of recurrent heart lesions are of the same type as the previously diagnosed defect.[7]

Extracardiac malformations occur in 25%,[8] and chromosomal anomalies occur in 13% of live-born neonates with CHD.[9-11] About 50% of fetuses with nonimmune hydrops and cardiac anomalies have a chromosomal anomaly, and an additional 10% will have extracardiac anomalies.[12] Hydrops in the setting of CHD is predictive of a very poor prognosis.

Although the most common indications for formal **fetal echocardiography** are family history of CHD and fetal arrhythmia, the majority of these fetuses will have normal hearts. The highest incidence of CHD occurs in patients referred for an abnormal four-chamber view on a screening obstetric ultrasound, fetal hydrops, or significant polyhydramnios.[13,14] Literature suggests a ninefold increase in the incidence of CHD in monochorionic, diamniotic twin gestations.[1] Most fetuses with CHD have no known risk factors, which underscores the importance of a meticulous evaluation of the four-chamber heart view and outflow tracts on all routine obstetric ultrasound. When severe structural cardiac anomalies are identified before viability, termination may be offered. Certainly, one of the most important aspects of fetal echocardiography is the psychological relief it affords parents whenever normal cardiac anatomy and function are documented in a fetus at risk.

NORMAL FETAL CARDIAC ANATOMY AND SCANNING TECHNIQUES

The fetal heart is similar to that of the adult, with several anatomic and physiologic differences. The long axis of the fetal heart is perpendicular to the body, such that a transverse section through the fetal thorax demonstrates the four cardiac chambers in a single view. The adult heart, in contrast, is obliquely oriented with its long axis along a line between the left hip and the right shoulder. The four-chamber view is important because 10% to 96% of structural anomalies are detectable on this view.[15-20]

TABLE 37-1. CONGENITAL HEART DISEASE AND ASSOCIATED RISK FACTORS

FACTOR	FREQUENCY	MOST COMMON LESIONS
		Maternal Conditions
Diabetes	3%-5%	TGA, VSD, coarctation
Lupus erythematosus	30%-50%	Heart block
Phenylketonuria	25%-50%	TOF, VSD, ASD, coarctation
Infection		Cardiomyopathy
Rubella	35%	TOF, PS, VSD, ASD, PDA, cardiomegaly
		Drugs
Accutane (retinoic acid)		Truncus, TGA, TOF, DORV, VSD, AO arch interruption, or hypoplasia
Alcohol	25%-30%	VSD, ASD, PDA, DORV, PA, TOF, dextrocardia
Amantadine		Single vent with PA
Amphetamines	5%-10%	VSD, TGA, PDA
Azathioprine		PS
Carbamazepine		ASD, PDA
Chlordiazepoxide		Unspecified CHD
Codeine		Unspecified CHD
Cortisone		VSD, coarctation
Coumadin		Unspecified CHD
Cyclophosphamide		TOF
Cytarabine		TOF
Daunorubicin		TOF
Dextroamphetamine		ASD
Diazepam		Unspecified CHD
Dilantin (hydantoin)		AS, VSD, ASD, coarctation
Lithium	10%	Ebstein anomaly, TA, ASD, dextrocardia, MA
Methotrexate		Dextrocardia
Oral contraceptives		Unspecified CHD
Paramethadione		TOF
Penicillamine		VSD
Primidone		VSD
Progesterone		TOF, truncus, VSD
Quinine		Unspecified CHD
Thalidomide	5%-10%	TOF, VSD, ASD, truncus
Trifluoperazine		TGA
Trimethadione	15%-30%	ASD, VSD, TGA, TOF, HLHS, AS, PS
Valproic acid		TOF, coarctation, HLHS, AS, ASD, VSD, interrupted AO arch, PA without VSD
Warfarin (Coumadin)		Unspecified CHD
		Syndromes
Apert		VSD, coarctation, TOF
Arthrogryposis multiplex congenita		VSD, coarctation, AS, PDA
Atrial myxoma, familial		Myxoma
Beckwith-Wiedemann		Cardiomegaly
C syndrome (Opitz trigonocephaly)		PDA
Carpenter		VSD, PS, TGA, PDA
Cat's eye (22 partial trisomy)	40%	TAPVR, VSD, ASD
CHARGE		VSD, ASD
CHILD		VSD, ASD
Conradi-Hünermann (chondrodysplasia punctata)		VSD, PDA
De Lange	29%	VSD, TOF, DORV, PDA
DiGeorge		VSD, coarctation, truncus
Ellis–van Creveld (chondroectodermal dysplasia)	50%	ASD, single atrium
Fanconi's pancytopenia		ASD, PDA
Goldenhar		TOF, VSD, ASD
Holt-Oram		ASD, VSD
Kartagener		Dextrocardia
Klippel-Feil		VSD, TGA, TAPVR
Laurence-Moon (Bardet-Biedl)		VSD
Leopard		PS
Meckel-Gruber		VSD, ASD, coarctation, PS, PDA
Noonan		PS, VSD, ASD, PDA
Pallister-Hall		Unspecified CHD
Pierre Robin		ASD
Poland		TOF, ASD, PDA, VSD
Refsum		A-V conduction defects
Seckel		VSD, PDA
Smith-Lemli-Opitz		VSD, PDA
Treacher Collins		VSD, ASD, PDA

Continued

TABLE 37-1. CONGENITAL HEART DISEASE AND ASSOCIATED RISK FACTORS—cont'd

FACTOR	FREQUENCY	MOST COMMON LESIONS
Rubinstein-Taybi		ASD, VSD, PDA
Silver		TOF, VSD
Short rib polydactyly (non-Majewski type)		TGA, DOLV, DORV, HRH, AVSD
Thrombocytopenia absent radius (TAR)		ASD, TOF, dextrocardia
VACTERL		Unspecified CHD
Waardenburg		VSD
Weill-Marchesani		PS, VSD
Williams		Supravalvular AS, PS, VSD, ASD
Zellweger		VSD, ASD, PDA
Chromosomal		
Trisomy 13 (Patau)	90%	VSD, ASD, dextroposition, PDA
Trisomy 18 (Edward)	99%	Bicuspid AV, PS, VSD, ASD, PDA
Trisomy 21 (Down)	50%	A-V canal, VSD, ASD, PDA
Triploidy		ASD, VSD
5p− (cri du chat)	30%	Unspecified CHD
9p−		VSD, PS, PDA
Partial trisomy 10q	50%	Unspecified CHD
13q−		Unspecified CHD
T 20p syndromes		VSD, TOF
Turner (45,X)	20%	Bicuspid AV, AS, coarctation, VSD, ASD, AVSD
8 trisomy (mosaic)	50%	VSD, ASD, PDA
9 trisomy (mosaic)	50%	VSD, coarctation, DORV
13q	25%	VSD
+14q	50%	ASD, TOF, PDA
18q	50%	VSD
XXXXY	14%	ASD, ARCA, PDA
Diseases/Conditions		
Crouzon		Coarctation, PDA
Neurofibromatosis		PS, coarctation
Tuberous sclerosis		Rhabdomyoma, angioma
Thalassemia major		Cardiomyopathy

Data also from Lachman RS, Taybi H. *Taybi and Lachman's radiology of syndromes, metabolic disorders, and skeletal dysplasias.* 5th ed. Philadelphia, 2007, Mosby-Elsevier.

AO, Aorta, *ARCA,* anomalous right coronary artery; *AS,* aortic stenosis; ASD, atrial septal defect; *AV,* aortic valve; *A-V,* atrioventricular; *AVSD,* atrioventricular septal defect; *CHD,* congenital heart disease; *DOLV,* double-outlet left ventricle; *DORV,* double-outlet right ventricle; *HLHS,* hypoplastic left heart syndrome; *HRH,* hypoplastic right heart, *MA,* mitral atresia; *PA,* pulmonary atresia; *PDA,* patent ductus arteriosus; *PS,* pulmonary stenosis; *TA,* tricuspid atresia; *TAPVR,* total anomalous pulmonary venous return; *TGA,* transposition of great arteries; *TOF,* tetralogy of Fallot; *truncus,* truncus arteriosus; *VSD,* ventricular septal defect.

TABLE 37-2. RECURRENCE RISKS IN SIBLINGS FOR ANY CONGENITAL HEART DEFECT*

DEFECT	*Suggested Risk (%)*	
	IF 1 SIBLING	IF 2 SIBLINGS
Fibroelastosis	4	12
Ventricular septal defect	3	10
Patent ductus arteriosus	3	10
Atrioventricular septal defect	3	10
Atrial septal defect	2.5	8
Tetralogy of Fallot	2.5	8
Pulmonary stenosis	2	6
Coarctation of aorta	2	6
Aortic stenosis	2	6
Hypoplastic left heart	2	6
Transposition	1.5	5
Tricuspid atresia	1	3
Ebstein anomaly	1	3
Truncus	1	3
Pulmonary atresia	1	3

From Nora JJ. *Medical genetics: principles and practice.* 4th ed. Philadelphia, 1994, Lea & Febiger.

*Combined data published during two decades from European and North American populations.

TABLE 37-3. SUGGESTED OFFSPRING RECURRENCE RISK FOR CONGENITAL HEART DEFECTS GIVEN ONE AFFECTED PARENT

DEFECT	*Affected Parent*	
	FATHER	MOTHER
Aortic stenosis	3	13-18
Atrial septal defect	1.5	4-4.5
Atrioventricular septal defect	1	14
Coarctation of aorta	2	4
Pulmonary stenosis	2	4-6.5
Tetralogy of Fallot	1.5	2.5
Ventricular septal defect	2	6-10

From Nora JJ. *Medical genetics: principles and practice.* 4th ed. Philadelphia, 1994, Lea & Febiger.

COMMON INDICATIONS FOR FETAL ECHOCARDIOGRAPHY

Abnormal heart on screening ultrasound
Hydrops
Polyhydramnios
Fetal arrhythmia
Chromosomal anomalies
Extracardiac anomalies
Family history (CHD, syndromes associated with CHD)
Maternal disease (diabetes, collagen vascular, phenylketonuria)
Teratogen exposure
Increased nuchal translucency on first-trimester screening
Monitoring response to intrauterine therapy
Monitoring fetus at risk for decompensation (persistent tachyarrhythmia, hydrops)

CHD, Congenital heart disease.

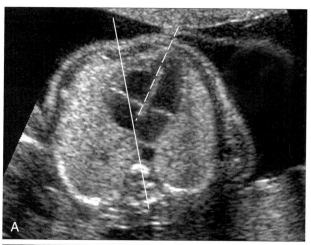

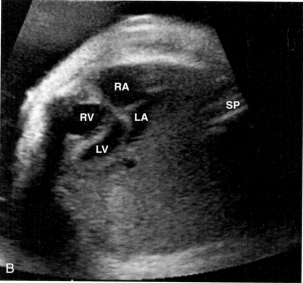

FIGURE 37-1. Heart position. A, Normal position of the heart. The heart is predominantly in the left chest, with only the right atrium in the right chest. There is a normal cardiac axis of *(dashed line)* of 40 degrees from the midline *(solid line).* **B, Dextroposition** of fetal heart caused by a large, congenital cystic adenomatoid malformation. Transverse image through the fetal chest shows the heart displaced to the right, but the apex remaining leftward. *LA,* Left atrium; *LV,* left ventricle; *RA,* right atrium; *RV,* right ventricle; *SP,* spine.

Cardiac axis and position are normally such that the apex of the heart points to the left and the bulk of the heart is in the left chest (Fig. 37-1, *A*). This is **levocardia**. In **mesocardia** the heart is central with the apex pointing anteriorly. In **dextrocardia** the apex is directed rightward, and the heart is primarily in the right chest. This abnormality must be distinguished from **dextroposition** (Fig. 37-1, *B*), in which the heart maintains a normal axis but is displaced to the right by an external process, such as a left chest mass or pleural effusion. **Abnormal cardiac axis** is associated with a 50% mortality and **abnormal cardiac position** with an 81% mortality.[21]

The fetal cardiovascular system contains several unique shunts: the **ductus venosus, foramen ovale,** and **ductus arteriosus** (Fig. 37-2). Antenatally, the placenta rather than the lungs is the fetus' sole source of oxygen. Oxygenated blood leaves the placenta through the umbilical vein and travels through the ductus venosus and inferior vena cava to the fetal right atrium. As a result of laminar flow, much of this blood is shunted across the foramen ovale to the left atrium and then into the left ventricle, aorta, and the fetal brain. Poorly oxygenated blood from the superior vena cava also enters the right atrium but preferentially enters the right ventricle and pulmonary artery because of the unique flow pattern. Most of this blood is shunted through the ductus arteriosus into the descending aorta. Thus, these shunts function so that the majority of output from both ventricles enters the systemic circulation, rather than a substantial portion entering the pulmonary circulation, as in the adult. Normal values for measurements of the fetal heart and great vessels are shown in Figures 37-3 and 37-4.

Fetal echocardiography is best accomplished between 18 and 22 weeks of gestation.[22] Before 18 weeks, resolution is frequently limited by the small size of the fetal heart. After 22 weeks the examination may be compromised by progressive ossification of the fetal skull, spine, and long bones; the relatively smaller amniotic fluid volume; and unaccommodating fetal position. In some cases, first-trimester evaluation of the fetal heart may be accomplished with endovaginal ultrasound as early as 11 to 14 weeks.[23-25]

However, first-trimester fetal echocardiography is limited and should be considered an *adjunct* to second-trimester evaluation, not a replacement.

Scanning the fetal heart requires a systematic approach, beginning with determination of the position of the fetus

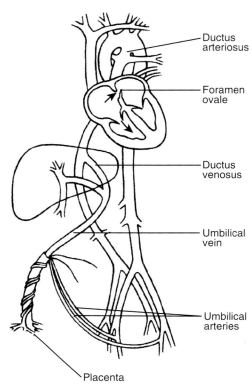

FIGURE 37-2. Diagram of fetal circulation. Blood from the umbilical vein is shunted through the ductus venosus to the right atrium and then across the foramen ovale to the left atrium. Most of the fetal cardiac output is shunted to the descending aorta through the ductus arteriosus.

within the uterus and the heart within the fetal chest. A transverse view through the fetal thorax above the level of the diaphragm demonstrates four cardiac chambers. **Four-chamber views** can be obtained with the angle of insonation parallel to the interventricular septum (**apical** four-chamber view; Fig. 37-5, *A;* **Video 37-1**) or perpendicular to the septum (**subcostal** four-chamber view; Fig. 37-5, *B;* **Video 37-2**). In a four-chamber view the echogenic foraminal flap of the foramen ovale can be observed moving into the left atrium at twice the heart rate. With slight angulation, the superior pulmonary veins may be seen entering the spherical left atrium (Fig. 37-5, *C*). The **atrioventricular valves** are visible in the four-chamber view. The septal leaflet of the tricuspid valve inserts more apically than that of the mitral valve. The left ventricle has a relatively smooth inner wall. The internal surface of the right ventricle is coarse, particularly near the apex, where the moderator band of the trabecula septomarginalis is frequently recognized as a small, bright, echogenic focus. This helps identify the morphologic right ventricle.

From the subcostal four-chamber view, angling the transducer towards the fetus' right shoulder permits evaluation of the continuity of the left ventricle with the ascending aorta (Fig. 37-6). Further angulation in the same direction shows the right ventricle in continuity with the pulmonary artery (Fig. 37-7; **Videos 37-3** and **37-4**). The diameter of the pulmonary artery is

approximately 9% larger than that of the aorta between 14 and 42 weeks. The measured differences in these vessels and with M-mode versus two-dimensional (2-D) imaging are negligible (2%-5%) for both the pulmonary artery and the aorta.[26] Further rightward rotation produces a sagittal view of the fetal thorax and a short-axis view of the ventricles (Fig. 37-8; **Video 37-5**). Angulation toward the left fetal shoulder from this view shows the aorta as a central circle, with the pulmonary artery draping anteriorly and to the left (Fig. 37-9).

The apical four-chamber view may also be used as a starting point when evaluating normal cardiac anatomy. Yagel et al.[27] describe a series of planes arising from the apical four-chamber view, all accomplished by moving the transducer in a cephalad direction. A slight cephalad advancement will show an apical **five-chamber view,** which is useful in accessing continuity of the ascending aorta with the left ventricle (Fig. 37-10). Continued cephalad movement should result in visualization of the bifurcating pulmonary artery and its relationship to the right ventricle. **A three-vessel and trachea view** should be visualized next (Fig. 37-11; **Video 37-6**). This view allows evaluation of the main pulmonary artery–ductus arteriosus confluence, the transverse aortic arch, and the superior vena cava. Comparison of vessel size, confirmation of vessel presence, and direction of blood flow with color Doppler can all be assessed at this level. Additionally, correct location of both great vessels to the left of

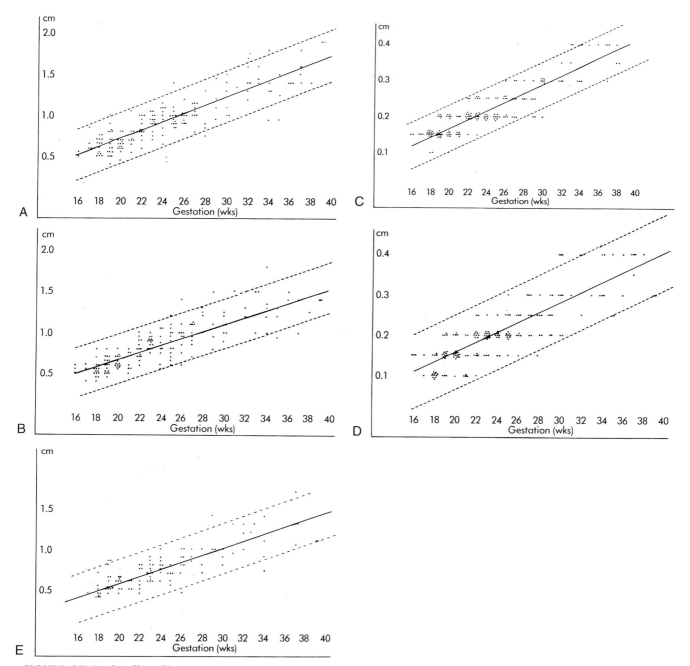

FIGURE 37-3. Cardiac dimensions. A, Left ventricular internal dimension versus gestational age. $y = 0.049x - 0.262$. **B,** Right ventricular internal dimension versus gestational age. $y = 0.045x - 0.228$. **C,** Posterior left ventricular wall thickness versus gestational age. $y = 0.012x - 0.063$. **D,** Septal thickness versus gestational age. $y = 0.012x - 0.088$. **E,** Left atrial internal dimension versus gestational age. $y = 0.040x - 0.214$. In each graph, the 95% confidence limits represent twice the standard error of the mean. *(From Allan LD, Joseph MC, Boyd EG, et al. M-mode echocardiography in the developing human fetus. Br Heart J 1982;47:573-583.)*

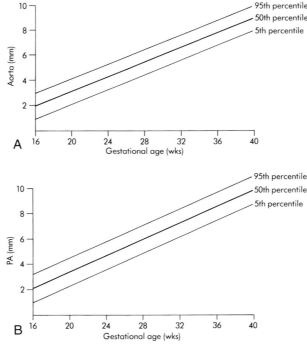

FIGURE 37-4. **Diameter of aortic root and pulmonary artery.** A, Diameter of aortic root versus gestational age. B, Diameter of pulmonary artery *(PA)* versus gestational age. Norms and confidence limits for echocardiographic measurements. *(From Cartier MS, Davidoff A, Warneke LA, et al. The normal diameter of the fetal aorta and pulmonary artery: echocardiographic evaluation in utero. AJR Am J Roentgenol 1987;149:1003-1007.)*

the trachea can be determined.[27] Returning to a sagittal plane of the fetus, directing the transducer from the left shoulder to the right hemithorax, demonstrates the distinctive candy-cane shape of the **aortic arch** (Fig. 37-12; **Videos 37-7** and **37-8**). The three major vessels to the head and neck and the ductus arteriosus may be seen. The aortic arch should not be confused with the **ductal arch** (Fig. 37-13), which is formed by the right ventricular outflow tract, pulmonary artery, and ductus arteriosus. The ductal arch is broader and flatter than the aortic arch. Lastly, sliding the transducer to the right while maintaining a sagittal plane on the fetus should allow visualization of the inferior and superior vena cava entering the right atrium.

M-mode echocardiography provides a 2-D image of motion over time. It is useful in evaluating heart rate, chamber size, wall thickness, and wall motion (Fig. 37-14). Simultaneous M-mode imaging through an atrium and ventricle is helpful in analyzing arrhythmias (Fig. 37-15). Chamber size and function should be evaluated at the level of the atrioventricular valves.[28]

Spectral Doppler ultrasound evaluation of the fetal heart can be used to determine the velocity of flow through the vessels or valves (Fig. 37-16) as well as regurgitant flow into the chambers of the heart (Fig. 37-17). Variation in flow velocity may reflect structural or functional cardiac abnormalities. For example, a stenotic atrioventricular valve will be associated with an abnormal flow pattern through the affected valve. Spectral Doppler

ultrasound is useful in assessing the functional significance of structural abnormalities and arrhythmias.

Color Doppler ultrasound permits a rapid interrogation of flow patterns within the heart and great vessels (Fig. 37-18), allowing functional and structural abnormalities to be more rapidly characterized. For example, valvular stenosis is clearly demonstrated with color Doppler ultrasound, as is reversed flow through insufficient valves or in the great vessels. Color Doppler ultrasound reduces the amount of time required for Doppler ultrasound evaluation of the heart, while improving the accuracy of fetal echocardiography, particularly in the setting of complex cardiac anomalies.[29-32] Subtle lesions such as small ventricular septal defects may be more reliably and easily identified with the use of color flow Doppler ultrasound.

Interest continues to focus on applying three-dimensional (3-D) and four-dimensional (4-D) technologies to fetal echocardiography. These technologies are becoming more readily available on ultrasound equipment, and 2-D fetal echocardiography requires considerable expertise to perform and interpret correctly. The major drawbacks to applying 3-D/4-D technologies to the fetal heart have been long acquisition time and the need for cardiac gating. Recent improvements allow for almost real-time examination. Current 3-D techniques depend on the type of equipment used[33-35] and include spatiotemporal image correlation (STIC), multiplanar

Text continued on p. 1305

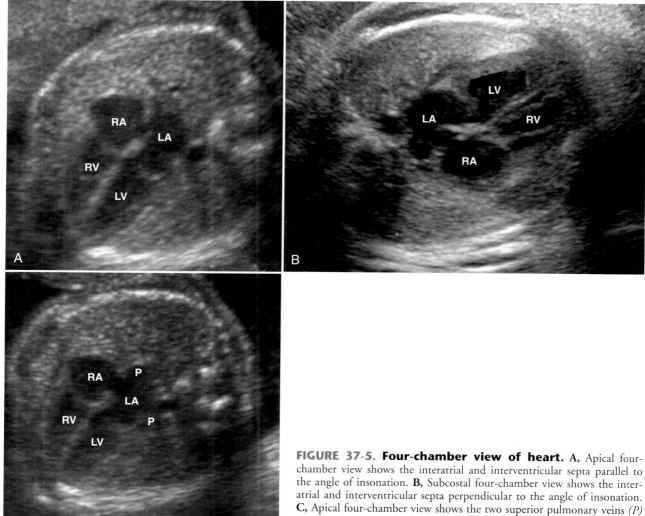

FIGURE 37-5. Four-chamber view of heart. A, Apical four-chamber view shows the interatrial and interventricular septa parallel to the angle of insonation. **B,** Subcostal four-chamber view shows the interatrial and interventricular septa perpendicular to the angle of insonation. **C,** Apical four-chamber view shows the two superior pulmonary veins *(P)* entering the left atrium *(LA); LV,* left ventricle; *RA,* right atrium; *RV,* right ventricle.

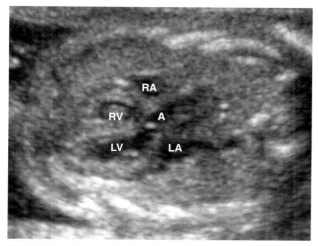

FIGURE 37-6. Continuity of aorta *(A)* with left ventricle *(LV); LA,* left atrium; *RA,* right atrium; *RV,* right ventricle.

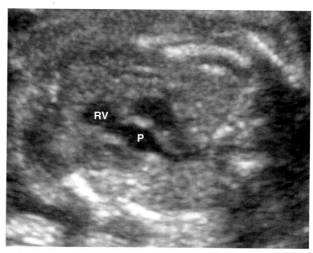

FIGURE 37-7. Continuity of pulmonary artery *(P)* with right ventricle (RV).

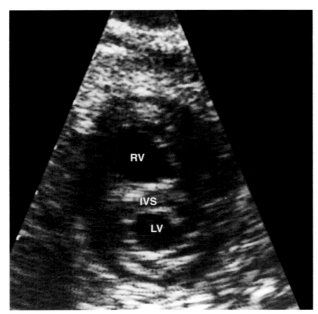

FIGURE 37-8. Short-axis view of ventricles. Anterior right ventricle *(RV)* is normally slightly larger than the left ventricle *(LV); IVS,* interventricular septum.

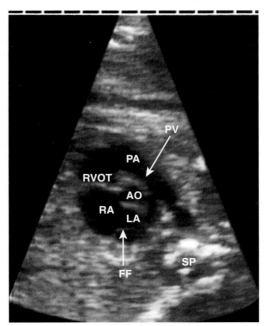

FIGURE 37-9. Short-axis view of great vessels. Aorta *(AO)* in center with pulmonary artery *(PA)* draping anteriorly; *RVOT,* right ventricular outflow tract; *LA,* left atrium; *RA,* right atrium; *PV,* pulmonic valve; *FF,* foraminal flap; *SP,* spine.

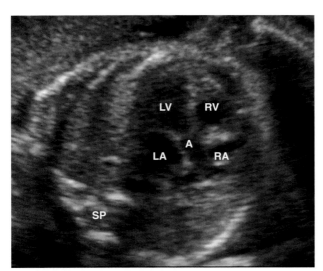

FIGURE 37-10. Apical five-chamber view shows continuity of the aorta *(A)* with the left ventricle *(LV); LA,* left atrium; *RA,* right atrium; *RV,* right ventricle; *SP,* spine.

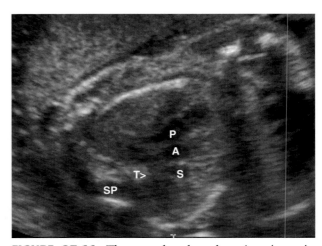

FIGURE 37-11. Three-vessel and trachea view shows the correct orientation of the main pulmonary artery–ductus arteriosus confluence *(P),* the transverse aortic arch *(A),* and the superior vena cava *(S).* This view also shows the two great vessels correctly positioned on the left side of the trachea *(T). SP,* Spine.

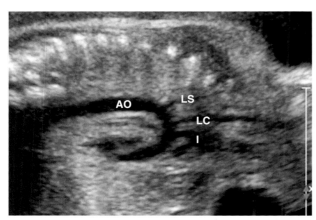

FIGURE 37-12. Normal aortic arch. Sagittal view shows the rounded, "candy cane" appearance of aortic arch and the head and neck vessels arising from it; *LS,* left subclavian artery; *LC,* left carotid artery; *I,* innominate artery; *AO,* descending aorta.

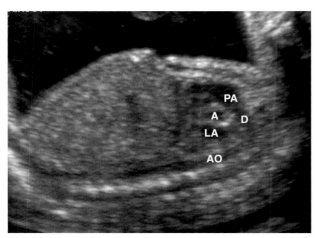

FIGURE 37-13. Normal ductal arch. Sagittal view shows pulmonary artery *(PA)* draping over the aorta *(A)* and joining the ductus arteriosus *(D),* which then joins the descending aorta *(AO); LA,* left atrium.

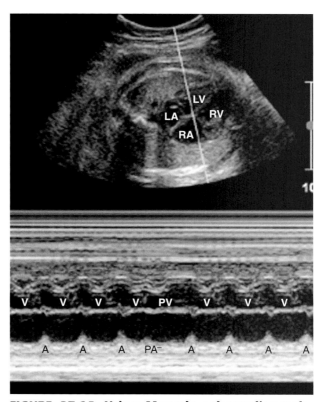

FIGURE 37-15. Using M-mode echocardiography to analyze an arrhythmia: conducted premature atrial contractions. The cursor is placed simultaneously through the left ventricle *(LV)* and right atrium *(RA).* The M-mode tracing shows normal atrial beats *(A)* followed by a premature atrial contraction *(PA).* The ventricles show normal ventricular contraction *(V)* following each atrial beat and a premature beat *(PV)* following the premature atrial contraction. *LA,* Left atrium; *RV,* right ventricle.

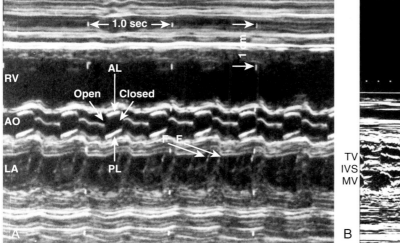

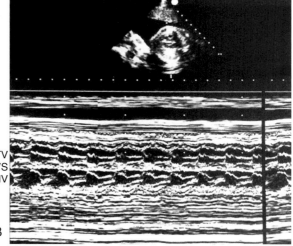

FIGURE 37-14. M-mode echocardiography. A, M-mode tracing through the aortic root shows the aortic valve opening and closing. The foraminal flap can be seen opening into the left atrium *(LA). RV,* Right ventricle; *AL,* anterior leaflet of aortic valve; *PL,* posterior leaflet of aortic valve. **B,** M-mode tracing shows opening and closing of the mitral valve *(MV)* and **tricuspid valve** *(TV); IVS,* interventricular septum.

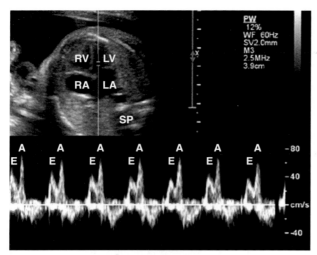

FIGURE 37-16. Spectral Doppler ultrasound used to interrogate a normal mitral valve. Spectral Doppler sample volume is placed distal to the mitral valve in the left ventricle *(LV)*. A normal mitral valve waveform is appreciated above the baseline, showing the normal early diastolic *(E)* and atrial contraction *(A)* wave points. *LA,* Left atrium; *RA,* right atrium; *RV,* right ventricle; *SP,* spine.

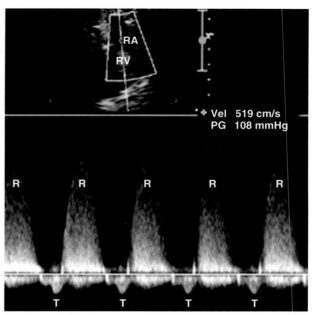

FIGURE 37-17. Tricuspid insufficiency. Spectral Doppler sample volume is placed proximal to the tricuspid valve in the right atrium *(RA)*. The regurgitant flow *(R)* can be seen above the baseline. This implies that the valve has not closed completely during systole, and therefore blood flow is retrograde into the right atrium. *RV,* Right ventricle.

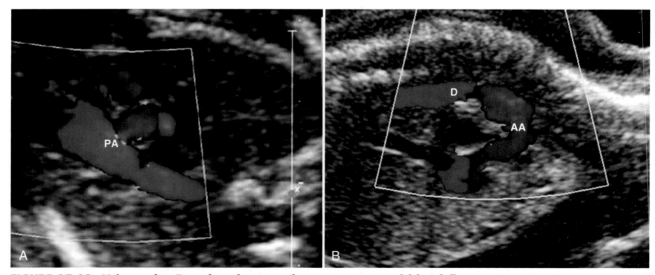

FIGURE 37-18. Using color Doppler ultrasound to access normal blood flow. A, Color Doppler ultrasound shows normal flow through the pulmonary artery *(PA)*. **B,** Color Doppler ultrasound to access normal blood flow through the aortic arch *(AA)* and descending aorta *(D)*. Note that flow is continuous through the descending aorta, but due to angle of 0 degrees in the middle of the image, an artifact gives the appearance of narrowing, and the color of flow changes from red to blue.

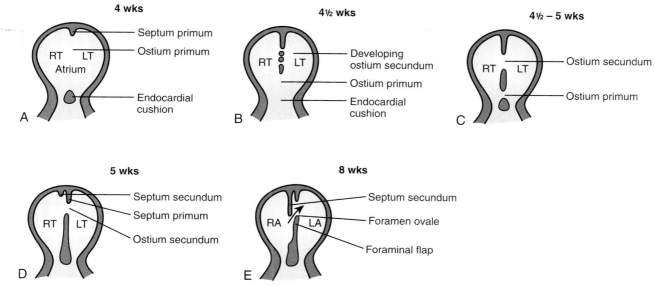

FIGURE 37-19. Development of intra-atrial septum (viewed facing patient). A, At 4 weeks' gestation the septum primum is small. A large ostium primum is present. **B,** At 4.5 weeks, enlargement of the septum primum results in reduction in size of the ostium primum. Perforations in the septum primum develop. **C,** Perforations in the septum primum coalesce to form the ostium secundum. **D,** At 5 weeks the septum primum has fused to the endocardial cushions, and the septum secundum begins to develop to the right of the septum primum. **E,** At 8 weeks the septum secundum has enlarged, now covering the ostium secundum. Blood flows from the right atrium through the valve mechanism (foraminal flap) of the foramen ovale.

reconstruction, tissue Doppler gating, inversion mode, and matrix array real-time 3-D. Because of various limitations associated with all these technologies, 3-D fetal echocardiography should always be used as an adjunct to standard 2-D ultrasound. Limitations include fetal motion artifact, equipment limitations (based on manufacturer), and decreased resolution of rendered images.

STRUCTURAL ANOMALIES

Atrial Septal Defect

An atrial septal defect (ASD) results from an error in the amount of tissue resorbed or deposited in the interatrial septum. It is the fifth most common form of congenital heart disease and is the most common form in adult patients.[36,37] ASDs occur in 1 per 1500 live births[38,39] and comprise 6.7% of CHD in live-born infants.[36] ASDs occur twice as often in females as males.[40,41] ASDs are associated with a variety of cardiac, extracardiac, and chromosomal abnormalities. ASDs can be classified by embryogenesis, size, or relationship to the fossa ovalis.

Embryologically, between the fourth and sixth weeks of gestation, the primitive atrium is divided into right and left halves. The **septum primum,** a crescent-shaped membrane, develops along the cephalad portion of the atrium and grows caudally toward the **endocardial cushions.** The space between these two structures, termed the **ostium primum,** disappears when the septum primum fuses with the endocardial cushion. Before complete fusion, however, multiple small fenestrations

develop in the septum primum, coalescing to form the **ostium secundum.** A second crescent-shaped membrane subsequently develops just to the right of the septum primum. As this membrane grows toward the endocardial cushion, it partially covers the ostium secundum. Its crescent-shaped lower border never entirely fuses with the endocardial cushion, leaving an opening, the **foramen ovale** (Fig. 37-19).

Ostium secundum ASDs make up more than 80% of all ASDs and generally occur in isolation. This ASD is caused by excessive resorption of the septum primum (foraminal flap) or by inadequate growth of the septum secundum (Fig. 37-20, *A*). The **ostium primum ASD** is the second most common type and is located low in the atrial septum, near the atrioventricular (A-V) valves. Although the ostium primum ASD may occur alone, it is more frequently associated with a more complex congenital cardiac anomaly, the **atrioventricular septal defect** (Fig. 37-20, *B*).

The **sinus venosus ASD** is a rare defect that can be divided into two types: (1) sinus venosus ASD of the superior vena cava (SVC), with the defect adjacent to the SVC, and (2) sinus venosus ASD of the inferior vena cava (IVC), with the defect adjacent to the IVC. The first type is often associated with **anomalous pulmonary venous return** (Fig. 37-20, *C*).

The prenatal sonographic diagnosis of ASD is difficult because the normal patent foramen ovale, which allows blood to flow from the right to the left atrium in utero, itself represents an ASD. It can be difficult to distinguish a small, pathologic ASD from the normal patent foramen ovale. The foraminal flap, or septum primum, is clearly

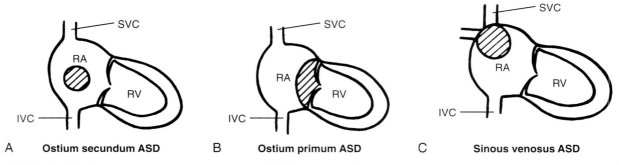

FIGURE 37-20. **Types of atrial septal defect (ASD).** Schema of the atrial septum viewed from the right atrium. **A,** Ostium secundum ASD. **B,** Ostium primum ASD. **C,** Sinus venosus ASD.

visualized on the four-chamber view. It has a "loose pocket" configuration, appearing either circular or linear in shape as it opens into the left atrium[42,43] (Fig. 37-21).

The **septum secundum,** which is thick and relatively stationary, makes up the majority of the atrial septum. The foramen ovale is an opening in the septum secundum. The septum secundum and foramen ovale are well visualized in the four-chamber views. The maximal size of the normal foramen ovale differs by 1 mm or less from the aortic root diameter at all gestational ages.[44] An ostium secundum ASD appears as a larger than expected defect in the central portion of the atrial septum near the foramen ovale. Alternatively, it can appear as a deficient foraminal flap.

If the lowest portion of the atrial septum (just adjacent to the A-V valves) is deficient, an ostium primum defect should be suspected (Fig. 37-22). Color Doppler ultrasound may be helpful in the diagnosis of larger ASDs. However, small ASDs are commonly obscured by the normal flow through the patent foramen ovale.[45,46]

A large, right-to-left shunt is physiologic in utero, and thus an ASD generally does not compromise the fetus hemodynamically. After birth, the shunt may cause right ventricular overload and pulmonary hypertension. Spontaneous closure of an ASD will occur in approximately two thirds of cases.[47] Patients with small ASDs may remain asymptomatic into their fifties.[48]

Ventricular Septal Defect

Isolated ventricular septal defect (VSD) is the most common cardiac anomaly, accounting for 30% of heart defects diagnosed in live-born infants and 9.7% diagnosed in utero.[36,37,49] VSDs are associated with other cardiac anomalies in half the cases.[50] Of the structural cardiac defects, VSDs have the highest recurrence rate and the highest association with teratogen exposure. They are classified according to their position in the interventricular septum (Fig. 37-23) as **membranous** or **muscular** VSD (inlet, trabecular, outlet).[50]

About 80% of VSDs occur in the membranous portion of the septum.[51] However, because most membranous

defects also involve a portion of the muscular septum, they are usually referred to as **perimembranous** defects. The subcostal four-chamber view provides optimal evaluation of the interventricular septum. At sonography, a VSD appears as an area of discontinuity in the interventricular septum. When the defect is small, this diagnosis is problematic, and at least one third of VSDs are missed on the four-chamber view.[15,45,52-56] Color Doppler ultrasound imaging may improve the diagnostic accuracy for VSD. However, most are missed on fetal echocardiography.[45,56,57] Small VSDs not detectable on gray-scale echocardiography may be documented with color Doppler ultrasound[30] (Fig. 37-24). In the setting of an isolated VSD, color Doppler ultrasound imaging typically shows bidirectional interventricular shunting, with a systolic right-to-left shunt and a late diastolic left-to-right shunt.

The prognosis for an infant with an isolated VSD is excellent, and many such defects go undetected. About 40% of VSDs close in the first year of life, and 60% resolve by 5 years of age.[58-60] However, large defects detected in the fetus are associated with an 84% mortality.[61] Concurrent cardiac, extracardiac, and chromosomal anomalies (trisomy 13, 18, 21, and 22) are associated with a worse prognosis.

Ventricular septal defects may be extremely difficult to diagnose in utero, particularly when small in size. Additionally, many small VSDs will close in utero or shortly after birth. A "pseudo" VSD in the membranous portion of the septum may be appreciated when evaluating the interventricular septum from an apical four-chamber view. This occurs when the angle of insonation is parallel to the septum, causing an artifactual dropout of the thin, membranous septum.

Atrioventricular Septal Defect

Atrioventricular septal defect (AVSD) refers to a spectrum of cardiac abnormalities involving various degrees of deficiency of the interatrial and interventricular septa and of the mitral and tricuspid valves. These defects arise when the endocardial cushions fail to fuse properly and were previously called **endocardial cushion defects** or

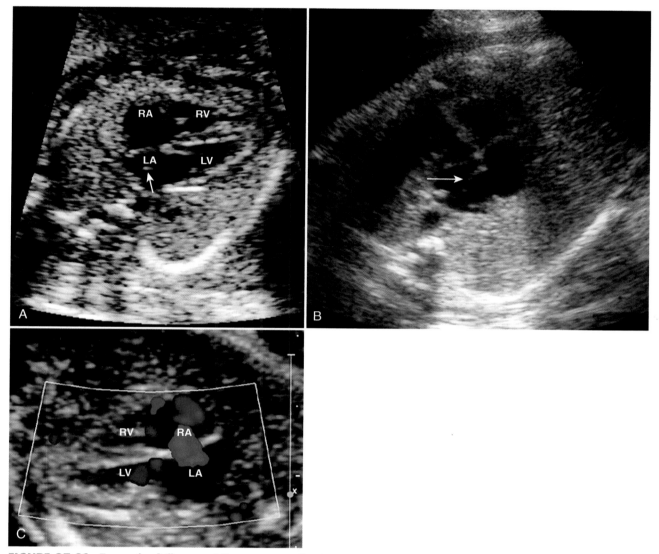

FIGURE 37-21. Foraminal flap and foramen ovale. A, Linear appearance of the foraminal flap *(arrow)* as it enters the left atrium, LA. **B,** Circular appearance of the foraminal flap *(arrow)* entering the left atrium. **C,** Color Doppler ultrasound subcostal four-chamber view shows normal flow through the foramen ovale; *LV,* left ventricle; *RA,* right atrium; *RV,* right ventricle.

A-V canal defects. Almost two thirds of fetuses with AVSD have additional cardiac anomalies.[62-64] About one third are associated with left atrial **isomerism** (both atria anatomically resemble the left), and of these the majority have complete heart block.[61,62] Chromosomal (especially **trisomy 21**) or extracardiac anomalies are associated in 78% of AVSDs.[61]

Embryologically, in the primitive heart, the common atrium and ventricle communicate through the A-V canal. Development of the endocardial cushion results in division of the single, large A-V canal into two separate orifices, separating the atria from the ventricles (Fig. 37-25). The interatrial and interventricular septa develop concurrently, eventually dividing the single atrium and ventricle into right and left portions. When the endocardial cushions fail to fuse properly, normal development

of the mitral and tricuspid valves cannot occur, and an AVSD results (Fig. 37-26).

Atrioventricular septal defects are divided into complete and partial or incomplete forms.[65] In both, the A-V valves are abnormal. In the **complete** type a single, multileaflet valve is present, whereas in the **incomplete** form, two of the leaflets (bridging leaflets) are connected by a narrow strip of tissue, resulting in the appearance of two valve orifices. Complete AVSD has variable amounts of deficient tissue in the atrial and ventricular septa. The incomplete form is associated with an ostium primum ASD. At fetal echocardiography, 97% of AVSDs are complete, although after birth only 69% are complete.[57,61] The fetal incidence of AVSD is four times greater than that in the live-born population, indicating a high incidence of in utero demise.[36,37,66]

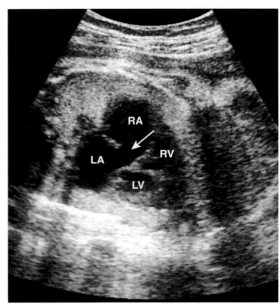

FIGURE 37-22. Four-chamber view shows an **ostium primum atrial septal defect** *(arrow)* in a fetus with an atrioventricular septal defect; *LA,* left atrium; *LV,* left ventricle; *RA,* right atrium; *RV,* right ventricle.

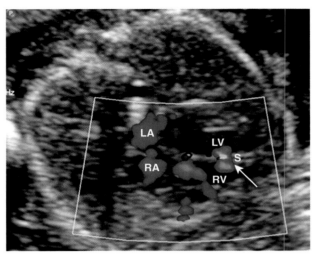

FIGURE 37-24. Muscular ventricular septal defect (VSD). Subcostal four-chamber color Doppler ultrasound view shows a muscular VSD *(arrow)* across the interventricular septum *(S); RA,* right atrium; *RV,* right ventricle; *LA,* left atrium; *LV,* left ventricle.

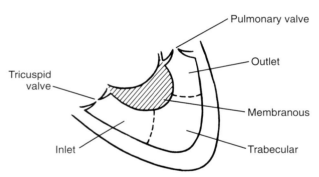

FIGURE 37-23. Interventricular septum viewed from right ventricle. The membranous septum and the three portions of the muscular septum (inlet, outlet, and trabecular) are demonstrated. Ventricular septal defects may occur in any of these locations.

Atrioventricular septal defects are considered **balanced** when the A-V junction is connected to both the right and the left ventricle, such that blood flow is relatively evenly distributed. If this connection exists with primarily one ventricle, such as in the setting of a hypoplastic left ventricle, it is termed an **unbalanced** AVSD.

Sonographically, a defect in the atrial or ventricular septum with an associated single abnormal A-V valve is seen in a four-chamber view (Fig. 37-27). The defect is better visualized in diastole than in systole. The abnormal valve should be suspected when the normal offset of the A-V valves is not visualized. Demonstration of two A-V valve orifices allows for differentiation between complete and incomplete forms of AVSD.[52]

Color Doppler ultrasound demonstrates an open area of flow across the atrioventricular septal defect and the abnormal A-V valve. Color Doppler ultrasound imaging is particularly useful in the detection of valvular insufficiency.[67] **Holosystolic valvular insufficiency** is closely associated with fetal hydrops and a worsening prognosis.[68] Frequently, a left ventricular–to–right atrial jet can be identified across the ostium primum defect before the onset of holosystolic valvular insufficiency.[29] **Cardiac malformations** associated with AVSD include septum secundum ASD, hypoplastic left heart syndrome, valvular pulmonary stenosis, coarctation of the aorta, and tetralogy of Fallot. A recent meta-analysis of published cases of AVSD diagnosed prenatally confirms that chromosomal anomalies are common, occurring in 25% to 58% of affected fetuses.[69] Therefore, karyotyping is indicated. Associated **extracardiac anomalies** are common, including omphalocele, duodenal atresia, tracheoesophageal atresia, facial clefts, cystic hygroma, neural tube defects, and multicystic kidneys.[69]

The fetus with AVSD and associated defects has a poor prognosis. When hydrops is present, few survive the neonatal period.[70] Despite advances in pediatric cardiothoracic surgery, the overall outcome for antenatally diagnosed AVSD remains poor, with most studies reporting 5-year to 15-year survival rates well below 50%.[69]

Ebstein Anomaly

Ebstein anomaly is characterized by inferior displacement of the tricuspid valve, frequently with tethered attachments of the leaflets, tricuspid dysplasia, and right

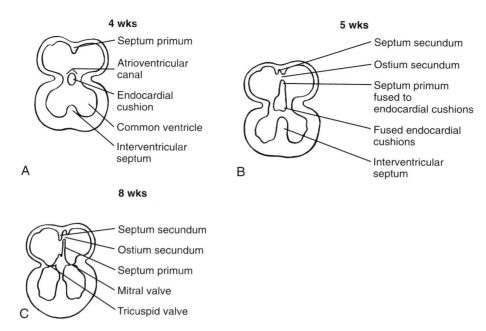

4 wks
- Septum primum
- Atrioventricular canal
- Endocardial cushion
- Common ventricle
- Interventricular septum

A

5 wks
- Septum secundum
- Ostium secundum
- Septum primum fused to endocardial cushions
- Fused endocardial cushions
- Interventricular septum

B

8 wks
- Septum secundum
- Ostium secundum
- Septum primum
- Mitral valve
- Tricuspid valve

C

FIGURE 37-25. Normal development of endocardial cushions. A, In the fourth week the endocardial cushions divide the atrioventricular canal into two orifices. **B,** By the fifth week the communication between the atria, the ostium secundum, is smaller. The ventricular septum has grown, almost obliterating the communication between the ventricles. **C,** At 8 weeks, complete development of the endocardial cushions and atrioventricular valves results in four distinct cardiac chambers.

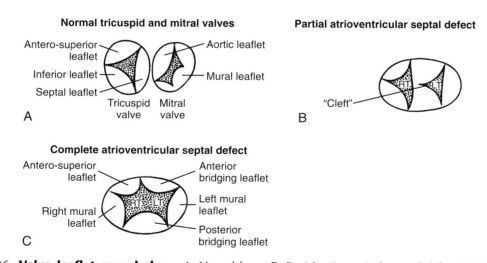

Normal tricuspid and mitral valves
- Antero-superior leaflet
- Inferior leaflet
- Septal leaflet
- Tricuspid valve
- Aortic leaflet
- Mural leaflet
- Mitral valve

A

Partial atrioventricular septal defect
- "Cleft"

B

Complete atrioventricular septal defect
- Antero-superior leaflet
- Right mural leaflet
- Anterior bridging leaflet
- Left mural leaflet
- Posterior bridging leaflet

C

FIGURE 37-26. Valve leaflet morphology. A, Normal heart. **B,** Partial atrioventricular septal defect (AVSD). **C,** Complete AVSD.

ventricular dysplasia[71-75] (Fig. 37-28). Ebstein anomaly makes up approximately 7% of cardiac anomalies in the fetal population and has an incidence of 0.5% to 1% in high-risk populations.[54,76,77] It occurs in approximately 1 per 20,000 live births.[78]

Early data from biased retrospective studies suggested that lithium use during pregnancy was associated with an estimated 500-fold increase in the incidence of Ebstein anomaly in exposed fetuses.[78-83] It is now clear that the increased risk is no more than 28% and may be nonexistent.[84] Ebstein anomaly may be associated with a variety of structural cardiovascular defects, particularly

pulmonary atresia or stenosis,[85] **arrhythmias,** and **chromosomal anomalies.**[73,86-89]

Ebstein anomaly is readily detected in utero.[86,90] The sonographic diagnosis rests on recognition of apical displacement of the tricuspid valve into the right ventricle, an enlarged right atrium containing a portion of the "atrialized" right ventricle, and a reduction in size of the functional right ventricle. Differential diagnosis includes tricuspid valvular dysplasia, Uhl anomaly, and idiopathic right atrial enlargement, but none of these has an inferiorly displaced tricuspid valve, the most reliable sign of Ebstein anomaly. Ebstein anomaly is one of the few

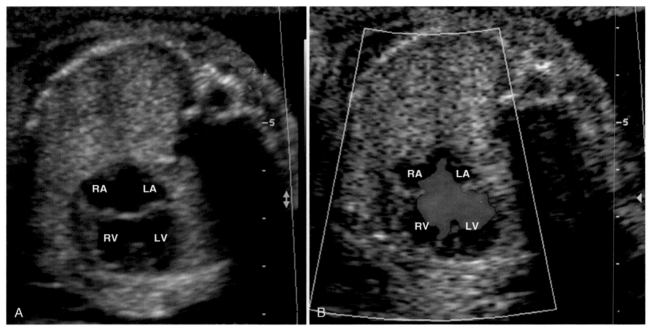

FIGURE 37-27. Atrioventricular septal defect (AVSD). A, Apical four-chamber view shows absent atrial septum, resulting in a single, large atrium (RA-LA). A VSD is seen between the left ventricle *(LV)* and right ventricle *(RV)*. A single, multileaflet atrioventricular valve is also appreciated. **B,** Apical four-chamber color Doppler ultrasound view shows the **atrioventricular septal defect**.

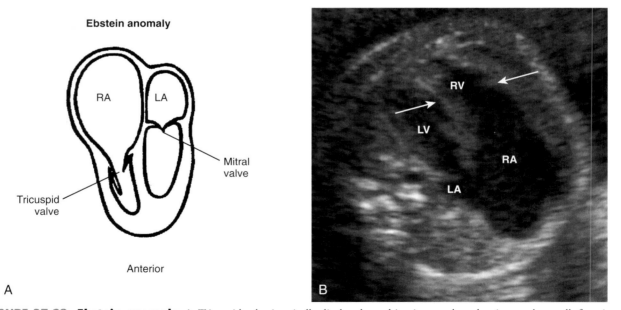

FIGURE 37-28. Ebstein anomaly. A, Tricuspid valve is apically displaced, resulting in an enlarged atrium and a small, functional right ventricle. **B,** Gray-scale image shows tricuspid valve *(arrows)* displaced inferiorly, resulting in an "atrialized" right ventricle *(RV)* and enlarged right atrium *(RA); LV,* left ventricle; *LA,* left atrium.

structural defects that may cause substantial **cardiac dysfunction** in utero, frequently with cardiomegaly, hydrops, and tachyarrhythmias.[73] Examination with spectral and color Doppler ultrasound is helpful in demonstrating **tricuspid valve regurgitation,** which causes further enlargement of the right atrium and ventricle.[91] Tethered distal attachments of the tricuspid valve, marked right atrial enlargement, and left ventricular

compression with narrowing of the pulmonary outflow tract are all associated with a poor prognosis.[73]

Arrhythmias, particularly **supraventricular tachycardias,** are common with Ebstein anomaly and can further compromise the fetus. Overall, the 3-month mortality rate of patients diagnosed in utero is 80%.[73,90] Surgical correction of Ebstein anomaly in young children is associated with a low mortality and an excellent quality of life.[92-94] Because clinical presentation, treatment options, and prognosis are inconsistent, case-by-case management is variable.[95]

Hypoplastic Right Ventricle

Hypoplastic right ventricle generally occurs secondary to **pulmonary atresia** with intact interventricular septum. It has an incidence of 1.1% among stillbirths.[36] **Tricuspid atresia** may be associated with a hypoplastic right ventricle but this is not as common.[96] Pathophysiologically, hypoplasia of the right ventricle develops because of a reduction in blood flow secondary to inflow impedance from tricuspid atresia or outflow impedance from pulmonary arterial atresia. Typical sonographic findings include a small, hypertrophic right ventricle and a small or absent pulmonary artery[96] (Fig. 37-29). Pulsed Doppler ultrasound may be helpful in demonstrating decreased flow through the tricuspid valve or pulmonary artery. Congestive heart failure and hydrops may develop from tricuspid regurgitation. After birth, closure of the ductus arteriosus frequently results in neonatal death. Prognosis improves with preoperative prostaglandin infusion to maintain the patency of the ductus.[97]

Hypoplastic Left Heart Syndrome

In hypoplastic left heart syndrome (HLHS), the left ventricular cavity is pathologically reduced in size. HLHS constitutes approximately 7% to 9% of all congenital cardiac lesions.[98] It has a 2:1 male predominance and a recurrence risk of 0.5%.[98,99] The small left ventricle results from decreased blood flow into or out of the left ventricle. The primary abnormalities include aortic atresia, aortic stenosis, and mitral valve atresia. It is associated with **coarctation of the aorta** in 80% of cases.[100] The primary sonographic feature of HLHS is a small left ventricle (Fig. 37-30). The mitral valve is typically hypoplastic or atretic, as is the aorta.[101] Color Doppler ultrasound is extremely helpful in the setting of HLHS, usually demonstrating the absence of flow through the mitral and aortic valves.[30]

This syndrome has an extremely poor prognosis, with 25% mortality in the first week of life, and untreated infants dying within 6 weeks.[102] Prenatal diagnosis of HLHS is beneficial for preventing ductal shock and keeping affected infants stable in the preoperative stage.[103-105] Monophasic blood flow across the mitral valve, restricted flow through the foramen ovale, and retrograde flow through the aorta are all considered poor prognostic signs in utero. Despite significant advancements in medical-surgical management over the past 20 years, follow-up studies demonstrate that HLHS children often experience major developmental delays[106] and decreased exercise performance, even after heart transplantation.[107]

Univentricular Heart

In univentricular heart, two atria empty into a single ventricle, via two A-V valves or a common A-V valve. Univentricular heart is rare, accounting for approximately 2% of CHD.[37] It results from a failure of the interventricular septum to develop. The single chamber has a left ventricular morphology in 85% of cases.[108] Associated cardiac anomalies are common,[109] with **asplenia** or **polysplenia** occurring in 13%.[110] Sonographically, a single ventricle with absence of the

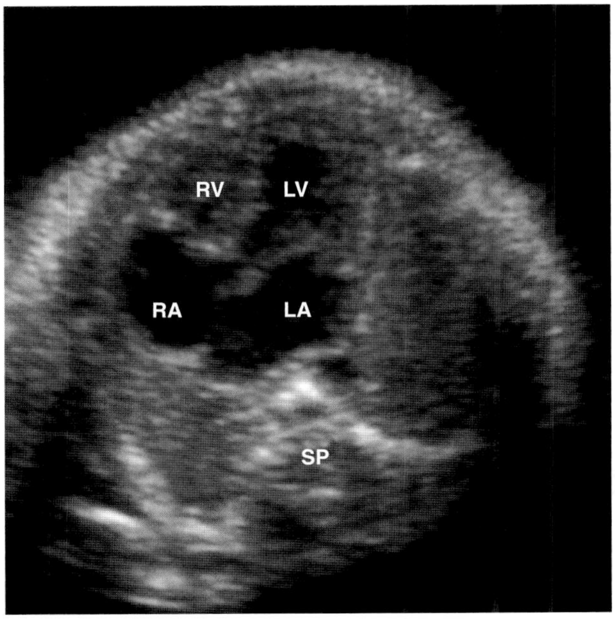

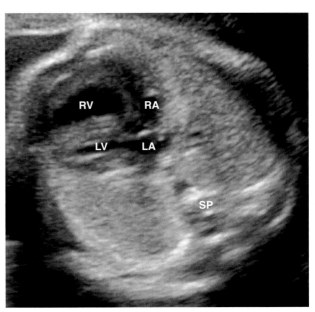

FIGURE 37-29. Hypoplastic right ventricle. Apical four-chamber view shows small, right ventricular chamber *(RV)*; *RA*, right atrium; *LV*, left ventricle; *LA*, left atrium; *SP*, spine.

FIGURE 37-30. Hypoplastic left heart syndrome. The left atrium *(LA)* and left ventricle *(LV)* are small; *RA*, right atrium; *RV*, right ventricle; *SP*, spine.

interventricular septum is seen. Doppler ultrasound examination is helpful in determining if a normal outflow tract is present. A nonfunctioning, rudimentary accessory ventricle may be present in some cases. Differential diagnosis includes a large VSD and hypoplastic right or left ventricle.

Patients with outflow tract stenosis have a poorer prognosis.[111] Death is typically caused by congestive heart failure or arrhythmia.[66] Pulmonary artery banding and shunts yield a 70% 5-year survival rate. Ventricular septation has a postoperative survival rate of approximately 56%.[109,112]

Tetralogy of Fallot

Tetralogy of Fallot consists of (1) VSD, (2) overriding aorta, (3) hypertrophy of the right ventricle, and (4) stenosis of the right ventricular outflow tract (Fig. 37-31; **Video 37-9**). It accounts for 5% to 10% of CHD in live births[36] and is associated with a variety of cardiac and extracardiac abnormalities and chromosomal anomalies.[61] A recent study of 129 fetuses diagnosed in utero with tetralogy of Fallot reported additional cardiac anomalies in 57%, extracardiac anomalies in 50%, and chromosomal anomalies in 49%. The nuchal translucency was above the 95th centile in 47% of fetuses.[113]

Tetralogy of Fallot occurs when the conus septum is located too far anteriorly, thus dividing the conus into a smaller, anterior right ventricular portion and a larger posterior part. Closure of the interventricular septum is incomplete, causing the aorta to override both ventricles.[114] The VSD typically occurs in the perimembranous portion of the septum. Right ventricular hypertrophy rarely occurs in utero, but the overriding aorta is reliably seen.[115,116] Pulmonary atresia or stenosis, or a dilated pulmonary artery secondary to absence of the valve, may be appreciated. The diagnosis of tetralogy of Fallot has

been made before 15 weeks' gestation using transvaginal ultrasound.[24] Color Doppler imaging is helpful in making the diagnosis of tetralogy of Fallot.[117]

The newborn with the classic form of tetralogy of Fallot who has pulmonary stenosis rather than pulmonary atresia is generally asymptomatic at birth but develops cyanosis and a murmur in the first weeks of life. Typical cases of tetralogy of Fallot are repaired at 4 to 6 months of age, with close to 90% survival at 1 year.[118] Patients surviving early surgery (before 5 years old) have a 32-year survival of 90%.[119] The presence of **congestive heart failure** in the fetus or newborn is associated with 17% to 41% mortality.[120,121]

Truncus Arteriosus

Truncus arteriosus accounts for 1.3% of fetal cardiac anomalies and is characterized by a single large vessel arising from the base of the heart. This vessel supplies the coronary arteries and the pulmonary and systemic circulations. Aortic anomalies occur in 20% and noncardiac anomalies in 48% of patients with truncus arteriosus.[122] In almost all cases, a VSD is present. The truncal valve may have two to six cusps and generally overrides the ventricular septum. Four types of truncus arteriosus have been identified by Collett and Edwards,[123] as follows:

- **Type I** has a pulmonary artery that bifurcates into right and left branches after it arises from the ascending portion of the truncal vessel.
- **Type II** has right and left pulmonary arteries arising separately from the posterior truncus.
- **Type III** has pulmonary arteries that arise from the sides of the proximal truncus.
- **Type IV** has systemic collateral vessels from the descending aorta as the source of flow.

The single, large truncal artery with overriding of the ventricular septum and an associated VSD is identified on four-chamber and outflow tract views (Fig. 37-32). This anomaly has been diagnosed before 15 weeks' gestation with transvaginal ultrasound.[24] Color Doppler imaging is particularly helpful in the setting of truncus arteriosus because it facilitates accurate localization of the pulmonary arteries and rapidly detects truncal valvular insufficiency. In the past, prognosis was poor, with an overall mortality of 70%.[122] More recent studies indicate that 10-year to 20-year survival and level of function are excellent for infants undergoing complete repair of truncus arteriosus.[124]

Double-Outlet Right Ventricle

Double-outlet right ventricle (DORV) represents less than 1% of all CHD and occurs when more than 50% of both the aorta and the pulmonary artery arise from the right ventricle.[125,126] DORV is classified into the following three types:

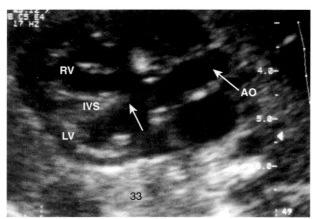

FIGURE 37-31. Tetralogy of Fallot. The aorta *(AO)* overrides both the right ventricle *(RV)* and the left ventricle *(LV)*. A ventricular septal defect *(arrows)* is also appreciated. *IVS,* Interventricular septum.

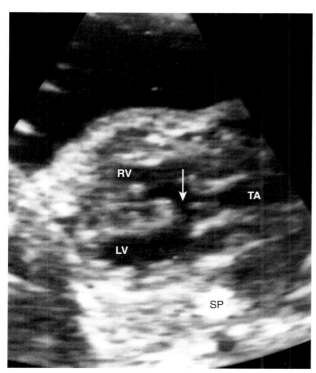

FIGURE 37-32. **Truncus arteriosus.** The single truncal artery *(TA)* overrides both the right ventricle *(RV)* and left ventricle *(LV)*. A ventricular septal defect *(arrow)* is present. No pulmonary artery was seen, helping to differentiate from tetralogy of Fallot. *SP,* Spine.

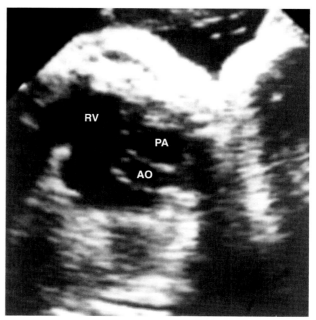

FIGURE 37-33. **Double-outlet right ventricle.** The aorta *(AO)* and pulmonary artery *(PA)* both arise from the right ventricle *(RV)* in a parallel fashion.

- Aorta posterior and to the right of the pulmonary artery.
- Aorta and pulmonary artery parallel, with the aorta to the right (Taussig-Bing type).
- Aorta and pulmonary artery parallel, with the aorta anterior and to the left.

Double-outlet RV is associated with other cardiac defects (particularly VSD), various extracardiac defects, fetal chromosomal anomalies, maternal diabetes, and maternal alcohol consumption.[3,126,127] With surgical intervention, 10-year survival is up to 97%.[125] When extracardiac or chromosomal anomalies are present, prognosis is poor, with 69% mortality when the diagnosis of DORV is made in utero.[127] Sonographically, the aorta and pulmonary artery arise predominantly from the right ventricle (Fig. 37-33). Differential diagnosis includes transposition of the great vessels and tetralogy of Fallot.

Transposition of Great Arteries

Transposition of the great arteries (TGA) is subdivided into two types: (1) complete or **dextrotransposition** (D-TGA) in 80% and (2) congenitally corrected or **levotransposition** (L-TGA) in 20% of fetuses with transposition. In both types, **ventriculoarterial** (V-A) **discordance** is present (aorta arises from right ventricle,

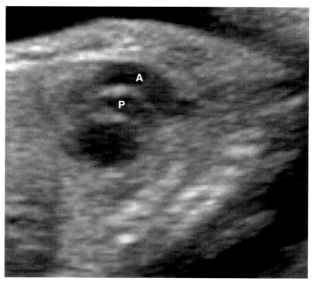

FIGURE 37-34. **Complete transposition of great arteries.** The aorta *(A)* is anterior to the pulmonary artery *(P)*. This abnormal arrangement results in both vessels running parallel to each other in this short-axis view.

and pulmonary artery arises from left ventricle). **Complete transposition** (D-TGA) is defined as A-V concordance (atria and ventricles are correctly paired) with V-A discordance (Fig. 37-34). It comprises 5.5% of heart disease in the fetal population.[37] D-TGA is also classified into two types, depending on the absence (70%) or presence (30%) of a VSD. A variety of cardiac anomalies are associated with D-TGA, including **pulmonic stenosis,** which rarely occurs in the absence of a VSD. In 8% of cases, other organ systems are involved. Chromosomal anomalies are not associated with TGA.

In D-TGA, the aorta arises from the right ventricle, receives systemic blood, and returns it to the systemic circulation. The pulmonary artery arises from the left ventricle, receives pulmonary venous blood, and returns it to the lungs. Generally, the aortic root lies anterior and slightly to the right of the pulmonary outflow tract. With closure of the ductus arteriosus and foramen ovale after birth, this condition is incompatible with life unless an associated shunt allows mixing of the separate right and left circulations.

Sonographic diagnosis depends on demonstrating that the great vessels exit the heart in parallel, rather than crossing in normal fashion. This is optimally seen in a long-axis or short-axis view of the great vessels. A three-vessel view is also useful because only one great vessel (aorta) is usually visualized at this level, in this setting.

Most neonates with D-TGA require immediate treatment. Initially, a temporizing shunt is created before definitive treatment. With surgical intervention, 12-month survival can be expected in 80%.[128]

Corrected transposition (L-TGA) is characterized by A-V discordance with V-A discordance (Fig. 37-35). It comprises 1% of CHD and 20% of cases of fetal TGA.[37] The aorta, which arises from the left sided, morphologic right ventricle, is anterior and to the left of the pulmonary artery. The pulmonary artery arises from the right sided, morphologic left ventricle. VSD and pulmonic stenosis occur in approximately half the cases.[108,129] Malformation and inferior displacement of the morphologic tricuspid valve may be present.

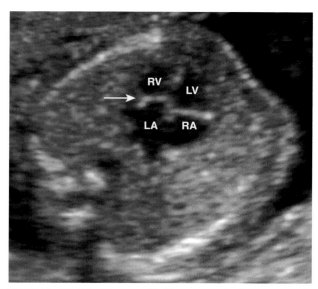

FIGURE 37-35. Congenitally corrected transposition of great arteries. An apical four-chamber view shows the morphologic right ventricle *(RV)* and morphologic left ventricle *(LV)* located on the incorrect sides of the heart. This is evidenced by identifying the atrioventricular valve leaflet insertion *(arrow)* on the left side of the heart in a more apical location than the right-sided atrioventricular valve leaflet insertion.

Pathophysiologically, the flow of blood through the heart to the pulmonic and systemic circulations is normal, even though the morphologic right ventricle is on the left and the morphologic left ventricle is on the right.

The antenatal sonographic diagnosis hinges on demonstrating a parallel arrangement to the great vessels, similar to D-TGA. Differentiating D-TGA from L-TGA entails identification of the morphologic right and left ventricles. The **moderator band** will be seen on the anatomic left side. Additionally, the tricuspid valve will be situated on the anatomic left side, so its more apical septal leaflet should be identified. Associated cardiac defects are common and diverse, including VSD, pulmonary stenosis/atresia, ASD, DORV, tricuspid valve anomalies, dextrocardia, mesocardia, and situs inversus. Fetal A-V block is also common.[130]

In the absence of associated cardiac anomalies, patients with corrected TGA may remain asymptomatic throughout their lives.

Anomalous Pulmonary Venous Return

Anomalous pulmonary venous return can be divided into two subgroups: **total anomalous pulmonary venous return** (TAPVR), in which none of the pulmonary veins drains into the left atrium, and **partial anomalous pulmonary venous return** (PAPVR), in which at least one of the pulmonary veins has an anomalous connection. TAPVR constitutes 2.3% of cases of CHD.[131,132] The four types of anomalous pathways are as follows:

1. The pulmonary veins drain into a vertical vein that empties into the innominate vein and then into the superior vena cava.
2. The pulmonary veins drain into the coronary sinus and then into the right atrium.
3. The pulmonary veins drain directly into the right atrium.
4. The pulmonary vein drains into the portal vein and into the inferior vena cava via the ductus venosus.

Embryologically, TAPVR is thought to result from failure of obliteration of the normal connections between the primitive pulmonary vein and the splanchnic, umbilical, vitelline, and cardinal veins. TAPVR is associated with AVSDs, polysplenia, and asplenia syndromes.

The antenatal sonographic diagnosis of TAPVR is difficult because the anomalous veins are generally extremely small and variable in their course. Often the first sign of APVR is mild right ventricular and pulmonary artery prominence, in which case a careful search for the four normal pulmonary veins should be undertaken. This can be difficult because the two inferior pulmonary veins are usually more difficult to visualize than the two superior veins, even in a normal fetal heart. Color and spectral Doppler ultrasound are helpful in documenting the normal pulmonary venous anatomy

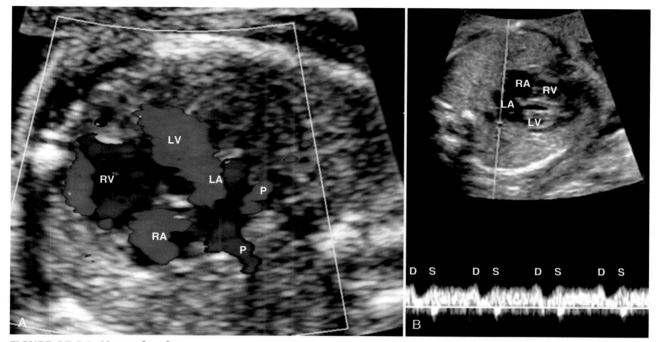

FIGURE 37-36. Normal pulmonary venous anatomy. A, Four-chamber color Doppler ultrasound view shows two superior pulmonary veins *(P)* entering the left atrium *(LA)*. **B,** Subcostal four-chamber view using pulsed Doppler ultrasound shows normal waveform and direction of pulmonary venous flow into the left atrium. *LV,* left ventricle; *RA,* right ventricle; *RV,* right ventricle; *S,* systolic peak; *D,* diastolic peak.

and in detecting and following the anomalous connections (Fig. 37-36). Spectral Doppler imaging is used to evaluate blood flow across the A-V valves or aortic and pulmonic valves. A ratio of right flow/left flow greater than 2:1 is highly suspicious for TAPVR.[133]

The diagnosis of TAPVR is suspected when no pulmonary veins are seen entering the left atrium (Fig. 37-37). A small left atrium resulting from decreased blood return and lack of normal incorporation of the common pulmonary vein into the left atrium is also suggestive of TAPVR. Approximately one third of patients with TAPVR have variable associated cardiac anomalies.[134] **Right atrial isomerism** is common. Associated extracardiac anomalies include gut malrotation and midline liver and stomach.[135,136] TAPVR causes minimal hemodynamic disturbance in utero, although hydrops occasionally results. Left untreated, the majority of infants die before 1 year of age.[134] Although it has also been diagnosed in utero, PAPVR is more difficult and can only be diagnosed when pulmonary veins are seen entering the left atrium as well as the right atrium or an accessory pathway to the right atrium.[137] APVR is associated with a high morbidity and mortality, largely because of the high incidence of additional cardiac anomalies.[135,137]

Coarctation of Aorta

Coarctation is a narrowing of the aortic lumen, usually occurring between the insertion of the ductus arteriosus

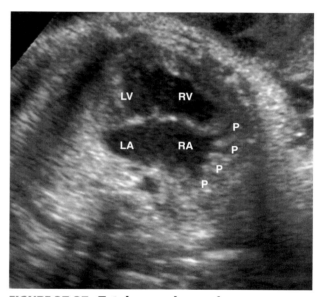

FIGURE 37-37. Total anomalous pulmonary venous return. Apical four-chamber view shows anomalous insertion of all four pulmonary veins *(P)* into the right atrium *(RA); RV,* right ventricle; *LA,* left atrium; *LV,* left ventricle.

and the left subclavian artery. Its severity ranges from a slight narrowing at the distal end of the arch to severe hypoplasia of the entire arch. Coarctation has an incidence of 6% prenatally.[37] Almost 90% of the cases are associated with other cardiac anomalies, including abnormal aortic valve (bicuspid or stenotic), VSD, DORV, and AVSD. Chromosomal abnormalities occur

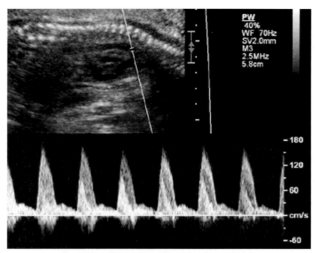

FIGURE 37-38. Coarctation of aorta. Spectral Doppler tracing shows increased velocity through the aortic arch.

in 5%, and almost 5% of coarctations are associated with maternal diabetes.[49,138]

Three embryologic theories have been proposed to explain the origin of coarctation of the aorta: (1) a primary developmental defect with failure of connection of the fourth and sixth aortic arches with the descending aorta;[139] (2) aberrant ductal tissue at the level of the aortic arch;[140,141] and (3) decreased blood flow through the aortic isthmus.[142]

Sonographic detection of coarctation is difficult.[19] Ventricular size discrepancy with a prominent right ventricle and relatively small left ventricle,[45,142] with a right-to-left ventricle diameter ratio greater than 2 standard deviations (SD) above the norm,[143,144] suggests coarctation of the aorta. Likewise, a discrepancy in pulmonary artery–to–ascending aorta diameter that falls greater than 2 SD above the normal ratio of 1.18 to 0.06[144] is suggestive of coarctation.[143] Color Doppler ultrasound is useful in identifying the area of narrowing. Spectral Doppler ultrasound may detect increased flow distal to the narrowed segment (Fig. 37-38). Many coarctations do not become evident until closure of the ductus arteriosus at birth. Additionally, infants with coarctation of the aorta may not develop clinical or echocardiographic signs of coarctation until 6 to 12 weeks after closure of the ductus arteriosus. If coarctation of the aorta is suspected on fetal echocardiogram, the infant should be followed to at least 1 year of age.[145] Although isolated coarctation has a good prognosis, 39% mortality is reported when associated anomalies are present.[146]

Aortic Stenosis

Aortic stenosis is a stricture or obstruction of the ventricular outflow tract occurring in 5.2% of newborns.[36] Aortic stenosis is divided into supravalvular, valvular, and subvalvular types. **Supravalvular** aortic stenosis

occurs above the sinuses of Valsalva and is associated with William's syndrome. **Valvular** aortic stenosis is more frequent in males and associated with a bicuspid aortic valve and chromosomal abnormalities.[147] **Subvalvular** aortic stenosis is associated with inherited disorders, **asymmetrical septal hypertrophy** (ASH), and hypertrophic obstructive cardiomyopathy. Infants of diabetic mothers may have a transient form of left ventricular outflow tract obstruction secondary to ASH.

The supravalvular type of aortic stenosis has not been reported in utero. Thickening of the aortic valve, post-stenotic dilation of the aorta, and ventricular enlargement are clues to valvular aortic stenosis. Thickening of the interventricular septum may be seen in subvalvular aortic stenosis. In all cases, increased velocity through the aortic valve will be identified on pulsed Doppler ultrasound. Early-onset aortic stenosis results in endocardial fibroelastosis and hypoplastic left ventricle.[148]

Aortic stenosis progresses in utero and may not be apparent on early (<16 weeks) fetal echocardiograms. In some cases these defects may not be apparent until after birth.[149] A mortality rate of 23% in the first year of life is reported with aortic stenosis.[150] Prognosis has improved with appropriate surgery, with mortality between 1.9% and 9%.[151,152] In cases of critical aortic stenosis, in utero balloon valvoplasty has been attempted. Technical success has been achieved in many cases, along with reduced sequelae. However, long-term follow-up is not yet available.[153]

Pulmonic Stenosis

Pulmonic stenosis may occur at the valve level or at the infundibulum. It occurs in 7.4% of newborns.[36] Dysplastic and stenotic pulmonic valves are seen in **Noonan syndrome** and with **maternal rubella.** Pulmonic stenosis is associated with TAPVR, ASD, supravalvular aortic stenosis, and tetralogy of Fallot. Pulmonic stenosis can occur in the recipient twin of a pregnancy affected with twin-twin transfusion syndrome. In this setting the recipient's heart becomes hypertrophic secondary to increased preload. This is similar to the ASH present in fetuses of diabetic mothers and results in anatomic obstruction of the outflow tract.[148]

Increased velocity through the pulmonic valve and hypertrophy of the right ventricle suggest pulmonic stenosis. As with aortic stenosis, pulmonic stenosis tends to progress in utero. Pulmonic stenosis has a variable outcome and can be managed with closed transventricular valvotomy or percutaneous balloon valvoplasty.[154,155] In utero pulmonary balloon valvuloplasty has also been attempted but is still in its early phase.[155]

Cardiosplenic Syndrome

Cardiosplenic syndromes are syndromes associated with **asplenia** (right isomerism) and **polysplenia** (left

ASPLENIA AND POLYSPLENIA: ASSOCIATED FINDINGS

ASPLENIA
Bilateral right-sidedness
Right atrial isomerism
Bilateral trilobed lungs
Bilateral right bronchi
Bilateral right pulmonary arteries
Ipsilateral location of both aorta and IVC
Absence of the spleen
Midline horizontal liver
Bilateral superior vena cavae
Severe and complex heart anomalies

POLYSPLENIA
Bilateral left-sidedness
Left atrial isomerism
Interruption of IVC
Azygous continuation of IVC
Multiple spleens
Complete atrioventricular block

IVC, Inferior vena cava.

isomerism; see Fig. 38-5). Both are defects of lateralization in which symmetrical development of normally asymmetrical organs or organ systems occurs.[156] Asplenia **(Ivemark's syndrome)** and polysplenia syndromes are usually considered separate clinical entities. However, they have many characteristics in common, including situs inversus or situs ambiguus of various visceral organs and complex congenital heart defects.[157]

Pathologically, in asplenia or bilateral right-sidedness, left-sided organs are a mirror image of normally right-sided organs. This results in right atrial isomerism, bilateral trilobed lungs, bilateral right bronchi and pulmonary arteries, ipsilateral location of both the aorta and inferior vena cava (either left or right side), absence of the spleen, a midline horizontal liver, and bilateral superior vena cavae.[158] In polysplenia or bilateral left-sidedness, the right lung and bronchial tree morphologically mirror those of the left. In many cases, intrahepatic interruption of the IVC with azygous continuation is present, as are multiple spleens and left atrial isomerism.[159]

Cardiac anomalies associated with these syndromes include TAPVR or PAPVR, ASD, VSD, univentricular heart, TGA, DORV, and pulmonic/aortic stenosis or atresia. Coarctation, hypoplastic left ventricle, mitral stenosis, cor triatriatum, dextrocardia, right atrial hypoplasia, AVSD, truncus arteriosus, and tetralogy of Fallot have also been observed.[159-163] Complete A-V block with an AVSD is associated with polysplenia. **Polysplenia syndrome** is the second most common disease associated with fetal heart block (after L-TGA).[161]

Cardiosplenic syndromes should be considered when CHD occurs with an arrhythmia. If these syndromes are suspected, a careful search is made for the fetal spleen, which has been visualized at 20 weeks' gestation, and for the fetal stomach.[161,164] Other abnormal relationships, such as ipsilateral aorta and IVC (associated with asplenia) or interruption of the IVC with continuation of the azygous vein (associated with polysplenia), may be documented prenatally.

The mortality rate with cardiosplenic syndromes is extremely high. Treatment for polysplenia and asplenia depends largely on the type and number of associated anomalies. Because cardiac malformations associated with polysplenia are often less severe, they are more amenable to surgical correction than lesions associated with asplenia.[164,165] Neonates with asplenia have a higher mortality and postoperative morbidity because of the high frequency of associated complex cardiac malformations. In polysplenia the greatest attrition occurs in the prenatal period and is often related to heart block with resultant hydrops.[163]

Cardiac Tumors

Fetal cardiac tumors are rare, although 10% are malignant.[166,167] Until the infant is 1 year of age, the majority of tumors and cysts of the heart and pericardium are **rhabdomyomas** (58%) and **teratomas** (19%). Cardiac **fibromas** account for approximately 12% of the tumors in this age group. Other, less frequent tumors include **mesothelioma** of the A-V node and cardiac **hemangioma** (~2% each). Although myxomas are the most common heart neoplasm (50% of cardiac tumors over all age groups), they are virtually nonexistent in the neonatal population.[167]

Sonographically, fetal cardiac **rhabdomyomas** appear as solid, echogenic masses. Rhabdomyomas (cardiac hamartomas) can be singular or multiple, typically arising from the interventricular septum[168-174] (Fig. 37-39). Rhabdomyomas may develop in utero after an initially normal fetal echocardiogram.[149] Of patients with cardiac rhabdomyomas, 30% to 78% have **tuberous sclerosis.**[168-170] Other signs of tuberous sclerosis are rarely found in fetal life, with the exception of subependymal tubers in the brain, which can be detected by fetal magnetic resonance imaging (MRI).[168] Unfortunately, the absence of cardiac neoplasms in a fetus at risk for tuberous sclerosis does not exclude this diagnosis.[171]

Several series report the appearance or enlargement of fetal rhabdomyomas on sequential examinations.[171,175-177] This finding underscores the importance of serial fetal echocardiograms in fetuses at risk for rhabdomyomas.

Cardiac tumors may become hemodynamically significant by causing obstruction to the outflow tracts or A-V valves, resulting in congestive heart failure, hydrops, pericardial effusion, and arrhythmias.[168] Prognosis depends on the size, number, and exact location of the

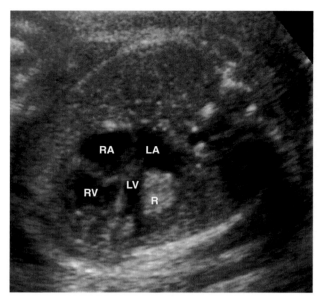

FIGURE 37-39. Rhabdomyoma. Apical four-chamber view shows an echogenic mass in the left ventricle *(LV)*, consistent with a rhabdomyoma *(R)*; *LA,* left atrium; *RA,* right atrium; *RV,* right ventricle.

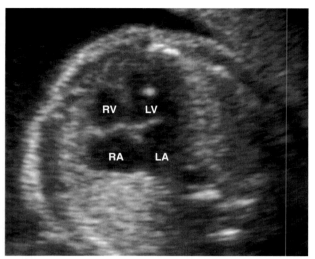

FIGURE 37-40. Echogenic intracardiac focus. Apical four-chamber view of a fetal heart with an echogenic focus in the left ventricle *(LV)*; *LA,* left atrium; *RA,* right atrium; *RV,* right ventricle.

tumor as well as associated arrhythmias and anomalies. A meta-analysis of 138 published cases of fetal cardiac rhabdomyomas found that size greater than 20 mm, presence of arrhythmia, and hydrops were significantly associated with increased morbidity.[175] Infants with cardiac rhabdomyomas have a guarded prognosis. Although spontaneous regression of the tumor has been reported, sudden death may occur.[167] Before reaching their second year, 60% to 75% of infants die.[176]

Teratomas may appear as cystic, complex, or solid masses. These are intrapericardial in origin, with attachment to the aortic root or pulmonary artery, and are virtually always associated with a pericardial effusion. Fetal teratomas are weakly associated with tuberous sclerosis.[171]

Rare cardiac tumors include fibromas and hemangiomas. **Fibromas** are almost always single and typically have central necrosis and calcification.[176] Fibromas are usually located in the ventricular myocardium, making resection problematic. **Hemangiomas** are even rarer and usually associated with the right atrium, often with an intracavitary component or pericardial effusion. Cardiac hemangiomas are heterogeneous with cystic and solid components, often with calcifications.[176]

Echogenic foci within a ventricle should not be mistaken for a cardiac tumor. These are thought to represent areas of mineralization of papillary muscle or chordae tendineae. These usually occur in the left ventricle (93%) but may occur in the right ventricle (5%) or both ventricles (2%) and are generally clinically insignificant[178-180] (Fig. 37-40). As ultrasound equipment resolution advances, echogenic foci are more frequently appreciated, particularly in the apical four-chamber view. Echogenic foci have been associated with chromosomal anomalies such as trisomy 21 and 13. However, more recent literature suggests that in isolation, in an otherwise low-risk pregnancy, an increased risk of aneuploidy does not exist.[180]

Cardiomyopathy

Cardiomyopathy encompasses a diverse group of cardiac disorders with variable etiologies and anatomic and functional characteristics, and all result in an alteration in cardiac function. Cardiomyopathies account for 8% to 11% of fetal cardiovascular disease,[181] but only 1.8% of CHD in live-born infants.[132] Approximately one third of fetuses with cardiomyopathy die in utero, which accounts for the difference in these numbers.[182]

A variety of conditions can cause fetal cardiomyopathy (Fig. 37-41), including viral and bacterial infections, inborn errors of metabolism, endocardial fibroelastosis, familial cardiomyopathy and maternal diabetes. Infectious agents act by damaging the myocardium and producing a myocarditis with resultant cardiomyopathy.[183] In the setting of storage diseases, the myocardium becomes hypertrophic secondary to the accumulation of various products within the myocardial cells. Many cases are idiopathic.[184]

Endocardial fibroelastosis (EF) is a poorly understood process in which diffuse endocardial thickening develops in one or more cardiac chambers. EF is divided into two broad categories, primary and secondary. Primary or isolated endocardial fibroelastosis occurs in the absence of other structural cardiac anomalies. In **primary** EF the affected ventricle may be dilated or constricted.[185] Viral

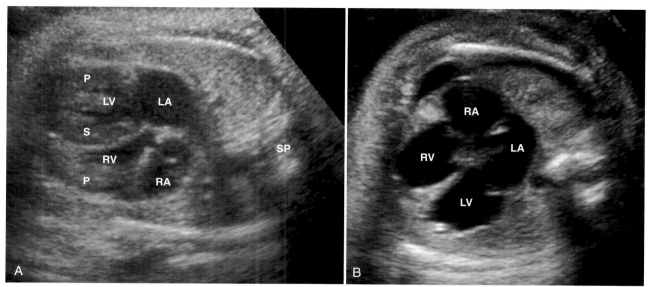

FIGURE 37-41. Cardiomyopathy. A, Concentric hypertrophy of the ventricular heart walls *(P)* and the interventricular septum *(S)* in fetus with **hypertrophic cardiomyopathy. B,** All four cardiac chambers are enlarged, occupying more than half the fetal chest in this fetus with **dilated cardiomyopathy.** A pleural effusion is also seen. *RA,* Right atrium; *RV,* right ventricle; *LA,* left atrium; *LV,* left ventricle; *SP,* spine.

myocarditis is thought to be the cause of primary fetal EF, with **mumps** and **coxsackievirus B** the most common infections.[184,185] **Secondary** EF occurs in the setting of a structural cardiac anomaly and usually results in dilation of the affected chambers. The dilated form occurs with coarctation of the aorta, aortic valvular disease, mitral valvular disease, and other lesions. The constricted form is frequently associated with aortic stenosis or atresia. In both types of EF the mural endocardium is largely replaced by collagen and elastic tissue, giving it a glistening-white appearance grossly[184] and a striking echogenic appearance at echocardiography (Fig. 37-42).

An increased incidence of **asymmetrical septal hypertrophy** or **concentric hypertrophy** has long been recognized in infants of diabetic mothers.[186] The characteristics of these types of cardiomyopathy have been well documented echocardiographically.[186-189] Overall cardiac size in fetuses of diabetic mothers can be increased as a result of the hypertrophy.[190]

Regardless of the etiology, severe cardiomyopathy results in decreased cardiac function and a tendency to congestive heart failure. This may be secondary to obstruction of ventricular emptying in obstructive forms of cardiomyopathy or to pump failure in nonobstructive forms. The sonographic diagnosis of obstructive cardiomyopathy depends on the demonstration of hypertrophy of the ventricular wall or septum. Nonobstructive cardiomyopathy can be diagnosed by demonstrating dilation of one or more cardiac chambers along with poor ventricular contractility. About 37% of live-born infants with cardiomyopathy have associated anomalies.[132] The prognosis for fetal cardiomyopathy is variable, depending on the severity of the cardiac lesion, the

underlying etiology, and associated anomalies. When hydrops accompanies cardiomyopathy, the prognosis is poor.

Ectopia Cordis

Ectopia cordis is a rare malformation in which the heart is located outside the thoracic cavity. It results from failure of fusion of the lateral body fold in the thoracic region. Ectopia cordis is classified by the following four types[191]:

1. **Thoracic** (60%). The heart is displaced from the thoracic cavity through a sternal defect.
2. **Abdominal** (30%). The heart is displaced into the abdomen through a diaphragmatic defect.
3. **Thoracoabdominal** (7%). The heart is displaced from the chest through a defect in the lower sternum, with an associated diaphragmatic or ventral abdominal wall defect (pentalogy of Cantrell).
4. **Cervical** (3%). The heart is displaced into the neck area.

Although most cases are isolated, ectopia cordis may be associated with **pentalogy of Cantrell,** a condition characterized by a sternal cleft, ventral diaphragmatic hernia, omphalocele, intracardiac anomalies, and ectopia cordis.[192] A variety of cardiac and chromosomal anomalies are associated with ectopia cordis. The sonographic diagnosis is generally not difficult and has been made as early as 10 weeks' gestation,[193] although the abdominal and cervical types have not been reported in utero (Fig. 37-43). The prognosis is poor, with most infants dying within a few days of birth.[194]

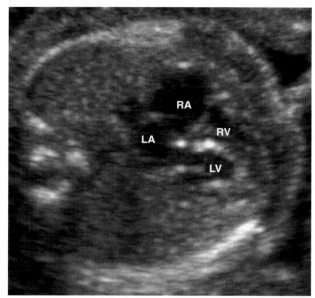

FIGURE 37-42. Endocardial fibroelastosis. Subcostal four-chamber view shows echogenic walls of the left ventricle *(LV); LA,* left atrium; *RA,* right atrium; *RV,* right ventricle.

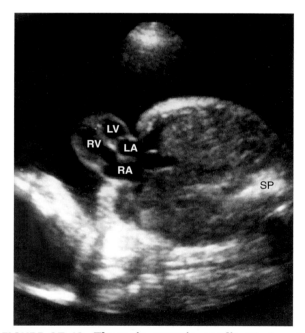

FIGURE 37-43. Thoracic ectopia cordis. The heart is located outside the thorax; *LA,* left atrium; *LV,* left ventricle; *RA,* right ventricle; *RV,* right ventricle.

ARRHYTHMIAS

Premature Atrial and Ventricular Contractions

Premature atrial contractions (PACs) and **premature ventricular contractions** (PVCs) are abnormal atrial or ventricular contractions originating from locations other than the sinus node. PACs account for almost 75% and

PVCs for 8% of fetal arrhythmias.[31,195] PACs are associated with redundancy of the foraminal flap (atrial septal aneurysm), maternal caffeine ingestion, and smoking.[196,197] In 1% to 2% of PACs, a structural cardiac anomaly is present.[28]

Premature atrial contractions may be conducted or nonconducted. In either case, the atrial pacemaker is "reset" so that the next normal atrial beat is also early. PVCs have an early ventricular contraction that is not preceded by an atrial contraction. The atrial pacemaker is not reset, and the next normal beat occurs when expected, as if the rhythm were regular. Thus, PVCs are compensatory, allowing the preexisting rhythm to continue, whereas PACs are generally less than compensatory. PACs and PVCs may be distinguished by M-mode or spectral Doppler sonography (see Fig. 37-15) by placing the M-mode cursor or spectral Doppler sample volume simultaneously through an atrial and ventricular structure. PACs followed by ventricular contraction are described as "conducted," whereas a PAC that is not followed by a ventricular contraction is "blocked." These must be differentiated from A-V block, in which a PAC does not occur. Conducted PACs can be distinguished from PVCs by noting that a PAC precedes the early ventricular beat and that, in the majority of cases, PACs are less than compensatory whereas PVCs are generally compensatory.

Premature contractions are benign arrhythmias in most cases. Most disappear in utero or in the early neonatal period. From 1% to 2% of PACs may evolve into sustained tachyarrhythmia.[198]

Tachycardia

Fetal tachycardia is a heart rate greater than 180 beats per minute. **Supraventricular tachycardias** (SVTs) are more common in the fetus than ventricular tachycardias. SVTs are classified as follows:

- **Paroxysmal supraventricular tachycardia:** atrial rate of 180 to 300 beats/min and a conduction rate of 1:1 (Fig. 37-44).
- **Atrial flutter:** atrial rate of 300 to 400 beats/min, frequently associated with heart block, and a conduction rate of 2:1 to 4:1, yielding a ventricular rate from 60 to 200 beats/min.
- **Atrial fibrillation:** atrial rate of greater than 400 beats/min and an irregular ventricular response at a rate of 120 to 160 beats/ min.

Ventricular tachycardia is defined as a rapid heart rate associated with three or more consecutive premature ventricular systoles. Of cases of SVT, 5% to 10% are associated with CHD.[199]

Fetal cardiac rhythm disturbances are usually first suspected on the basis of auscultatory findings. M-mode and pulsed Doppler echocardiography are useful in identifying and characterizing tachycardias by observing the atrial and ventricular rates. The M-mode tracing is obtained through the heart to allow independent

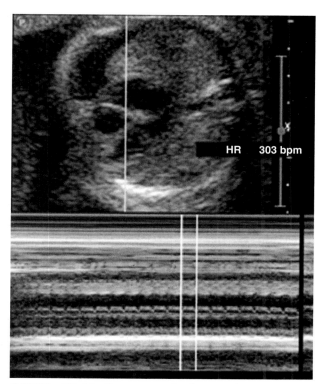

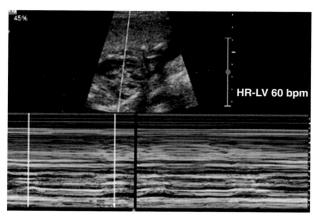

FIGURE 37-45. Fetal bradycardia. M-mode tracing shows ventricular rate of 60 beats/min.

FIGURE 37-44. Supraventricular tachycardia. M-mode tracing through the right atrium and left ventricle, shows a fetal heart rate of 303 beats/min and a 1:1 conduction.

assessment of atrial and ventricular wall motion. Further information is obtained from simultaneous recordings of the atrial and ventricular walls or A-V and semilunar valve motion. Spectral Doppler ultrasound evaluation can demonstrate decreased flow velocities and cardiac output during SVT.[200] Fetal supraventricular tachyarrhythmia can lead to fetal cardiovascular compromise, hydrops, and death.

Most fetal tachycardias have a good prognosis and can be treated in utero with various pharmacologic agents. Careful interrogation of the tricuspid valve with color and spectral Doppler ultrasound imaging is warranted in the setting of fetal tachycardia because tricuspid valvular dysfunction with tricuspid regurgitation can be the first indication of imminent congestive failure and hydrops.[201,202] In the presence of hydrops, immediate and aggressive therapy is warranted.[195,198,203-208] Several antiarrhythmic drugs are available to attempt to cardiovert SVTs in utero. Prognosis in the setting of fetal tachyarrhythmia depends on a number of factors, including type and duration of arrhythmia, presence of structural cardiac anomalies, gestational age, and response to intrauterine therapy.[201]

Bradycardia

Fetal bradycardia is a "prolonged" heart rate of 100 beats/min or less (Fig. 37-45). Approximately 5% of

fetal arrhythmias are classified as bradycardia.[28] Transient bradycardia can be related to an increase in intrauterine pressure, occasionally secondary to the pressure of an ultrasound transducer or fetal compression of the umbilical cord.[209,210] This is often seen during fetal sonograms and is of no clinical consequence, unless the bradyarrhythmia is sustained.

Sinus bradycardia without fetal hypoxia is rare.[210] If less than 80 beats/min, sinus bradycardia may be associated with fetal asphyxia. Heart rates lower than 100 beats/min during the first trimester have an increased risk of fetal demise.[211] When bradycardia is associated with an increased nuchal translucency, risk for CHD is increased, and early transvaginal fetal echocardiogram should be considered. Complex CHD has been detected in the first trimester in this clinical setting.[211] The fetus with sustained bradycardia should have careful follow-up and monitoring for signs of cardiac failure. Persistent bradycardia may warrant early delivery. In utero treatment has had limited success.[212]

Congenital Heart Block

Failure of transmission of impulses from the atrium to the ventricles results in atrioventricular block (AVB). AVB is classified into the following three types:
- **First-degree block:** a prolonged PR interval results in a conduction delay, but without markedly abnormal rate or rhythm. (This has not been diagnosed in utero.)
- **Second-degree block:** with blockage of a single atrial beat (Mobitz type I) or with intermittent conduction abnormalities, such that the ventricular rate is a fraction of the atrial rate (Mobitz type II).
- **Third-degree** or **complete heart block:** the ventricular and atrial rates are entirely dissociated.

In the normal heart, an electrical impulse originates from the sinoatrial (SA) node, travels to the A-V node, and through the Purkinje system to the ventricles. AVB results from immaturity or complete absence of the conducting system or from abnormalities at the level of the A-V node. This rare disorder is associated with **maternal collagen vascular disease (systemic lupus erythematosus).**[213] After one affected child, further pregnancies carry a 30% risk for AVB.[214] Serial fetal echocardiograms are useful in the fetus at risk for congenital complete heart block related to maternal lupus. This monitoring allows early detection and treatment of the immune-mediated fetal myocarditis and congenital complete heart block.[215-217]

In the absence of associated structural abnormalities, the prognosis for a fetus with congenital heart block is good. However, at least 40% of fetuses with complete heart block have structural cardiac abnormalities.[28] When associated cardiac anomalies exist, the prognosis is poor. Fetuses with AVB are at risk for heart failure and should be monitored closely. Overall, the vast majority of fetuses with arrhythmias have a good outcome. The incidence of associated structural cardiac disease is as low as 0.3%, similar to that in the general population, and the incidence of significant arrhythmia is only 1.6%.[217]

References

1. Young ID, Clarke M. Lethal malformations and perinatal mortality: a 10 year review with comparison of ethnic differences. Br Med J Clin Res Ed 1987;295:89-91.
2. Jones KL, Smith DW. Smith's recognizable patterns of human malformation. 6th ed. Philadelphia: Saunders-Elsevier; 2006.
3. Nora JJ. Medical genetics: principles and practice. 4th ed. Philadelphia: Lea & Febiger; 1994.
4. Nyberg DA, Mahony BS, Pretorius D. Diagnostic ultrasound of fetal anomalies : text and atlas. Chicago: Year Book Medical Publishers; 1990.
5. Romero R. Prenatal diagnosis of congenital anomalies. Norwalk, Conn: Appleton & Lange; 1988.
6. Nora JJ, Nora AH. Maternal transmission of congenital heart diseases: new recurrence risk figures and the questions of cytoplasmic inheritance and vulnerability to teratogens. Am J Cardiol 1987;59:459-463.
7. Reed KL. Fetal echocardiography. Semin Ultrasound CT MR 1991;12:2-10.
8. Greenwood RD, Rosenthal A, Parisi L, et al. Extracardiac abnormalities in infants with congenital heart disease. Pediatrics 1975;55:485-492.
9. Berg KA, Boughman JA, Astemborski JA, et al. Implications for prenatal cytogenetic analysis from Baltimore-Washington study of liveborn infants with confirmed congenital heart defects (CHD). Am J Hum Genet 1986;39:A50.
10. Berg KA, Clark EB, Astemborski JA, Boughman JA. Prenatal detection of cardiovascular malformations by echocardiography: an indication for cytogenetic evaluation. Am J Obstet Gynecol 1988;159:477-481.
11. Wladimiroff JW, Stewart PA, Sachs ES, Niermeijer MF. Prenatal diagnosis and management of congenital heart defect: significance of associated fetal anomalies and prenatal chromosome studies. Am J Med Genet 1985;21:285-290.
12. Allan LD. Fetal echocardiography. Clin Obstet Gynecol 1988;31:61-79.
13. Callan NA, Maggio M, Steger S, Kan JS. Fetal echocardiography: indications for referral, prenatal diagnoses, and outcomes. Am J Perinatol 1991;8:390-394.
14. Bromley B, Estroff JA, Sanders SP, et al. Fetal echocardiography: accuracy and limitations in a population at high and low risk for heart defects. Am J Obstet Gynecol 1992;166:1473-1481.

Normal Fetal Cardiac Anatomy and Scanning Techniques

15. Vergani P, Mariani S, Ghidini A, et al. Screening for congenital heart disease with the four-chamber view of the fetal heart. Am J Obstet Gynecol 1992;167:1000-1003.
16. Copel JA, Pilu G, Green J, et al. Fetal echocardiographic screening for congenital heart disease: the importance of the four-chamber view. Am J Obstet Gynecol 1987;157:648-655.
17. Kirk JS, Riggs TW, Comstock CH, et al. The prospective evaluation of fetal cardic anatomy: a comparison of 4 and 5 chamber views in 5967 patients. Am J Obstet Gynecol 1993;168:291.
18. Wyllie J, Wren C, Hunter S. Screening for fetal cardiac malformations. Br Heart J 1994;71:20-27.
19. Sharland GK, Allan LD. Screening for congenital heart disease prenatally: results of a 2½-year study in the South East Thames Region. Br J Obstet Gynaecol 1992;99:220-225.
20. Tegnander E, Eik-Nes SH, Johansen OJ, Linker DT. Prenatal detection of heart defects at the routine fetal examination at 18 weeks in a non-selected population. Ultrasound Obstet Gynecol 1995;5:372-380.
21. Comstock CH. Normal fetal heart axis and position. Obstet Gynecol 1987;70:255-259.
22. AIUM Technical Bulletin. Practice Guidelines for the Performance of Fetal Echocardiography. February 5, 2010.
23. Dolkart LA, Reimers FT. Transvaginal fetal echocardiography in early pregnancy: normative data. Am J Obstet Gynecol 1991;165:688-691.
24. Achiron R, Weissman A, Rotstein Z, et al. Transvaginal echocardiographic examination of the fetal heart between 13 and 15 weeks' gestation in a low-risk population. J Ultrasound Med 1994;13:783-789.
25. Weiner Z, Lorber A, Shalev E. Diagnosis of congenital cardiac defects between 11 and 14 weeks' gestation in high-risk patients. J Ultrasound Med 2002;21:23-29.
26. Cartier MS, Davidoff A, Warneke LA, et al. The normal diameter of the fetal aorta and pulmonary artery: echocardiographic evaluation in utero. AJR Am J Roentgenol 1987;149:1003-1007.
27. Yagel S, Cohen SM, Achiron R. Examination of the fetal heart by five short-axis views: a proposed screening method for comprehensive cardiac evaluation. Ultrasound Obstet Gynecol 2001;17:367-369.
28. Reed KL. Fetal arrhythmias: etiology, diagnosis, pathophysiology, and treatment. Semin Perinatol 1989;13:294-304.
29. Gembruch U, Chatterjee MS, Bald R, et al. Color Doppler flow mapping of fetal heart. J Perinat Med 1991;19:27-32.
30. Chiba Y, Kanzaki T, Kobayashi H, et al. Evaluation of fetal structural heart disease using color flow mapping. Ultrasound Med Biol 1990;16:221-229.
31. Benacerraf BR, Sanders SP. Fetal echocardiography. Radiol Clin North Am 1990;28:131-147.
32. Sharland GK, Chita SK, Allan LD. The use of colour Doppler in fetal echocardiography. Int J Cardiol 1990;28:229-236.
33. Yagel S, Cohen SM, Shapiro I, Valsky DV. 3D and 4D ultrasound in fetal cardiac scanning: a new look at the fetal heart. Ultrasound Obstet Gynecol 2007;29:81-95.
34. Acar P, Dulac Y, Taktak A, Abadir S. Real-time three-dimensional fetal echocardiography using matrix probe. Prenat Diagn 2005;25:370-375.
35. Brekke S, Tegnander E, Torp HG, Eik-Nes SH. Tissue Doppler gated (TDOG) dynamic three-dimensional ultrasound imaging of the fetal heart. Ultrasound Obstet Gynecol 2004;24:192-198.

Structural Anomalies

36. Hoffman JI, Christianson R. Congenital heart disease in a cohort of 19,502 births with long-term follow-up. Am J Cardiol 1978;42:641-647.
37. Allan LD, Crawford DC, Anderson RH, Tynan M. Spectrum of congenital heart disease detected echocardiographically in prenatal life. Br Heart J 1985;54:523-526.
38. Keith JD. Atrial septal defect: ostium secundum, ostium primum, and atrioventricularis communis (common AV canal). In: Keith JD, Rowe RD, Vlad P, editors. Heart disease in infancy and childhood. 3rd ed. New York: Macmillan; 1978. p. 330-404.
39. Samanek M. Children with congenital heart disease: probability of natural survival. Pediatr Cardiol 1992;13:152-158.
40. Fyler DC. Atrial septal defect secundum. In: Fyler DC, editor. Nadas' pediatric cardiology. Philadelphia: Hanley and Belfus; 1992. p. 513-524.

41. Feldt RH, Avasthey P, Yoshimasu F, et al. Incidence of congenital heart disease in children born to residents of Olmsted County, Minnesota, 1950–1969. Mayo Clin Proc 1971;46:794-799.

42. Crelin ES. Anatomy of the newborn: an atlas. Philadelphia: Lea & Febiger; 1969.

43. Kachalia P, Bowie JD, Adams DB, Carroll BA. In utero sonographic appearance of the atrial septum primum and septum secundum. J Ultrasound Med 1991;10:423-426.

44. Wilson AD, Rao PS, Aeschlimann S. Normal fetal foramen flap and transatrial Doppler velocity pattern. J Am Soc Echocardiogr 1990;3:491-494.

45. Benacerraf BR, Pober BR, Sanders SP. Accuracy of fetal echocardiography. Radiology 1987;165:847-849.

46. DeVore GR, Horenstein J, Siassi B, Platt LD. Fetal echocardiography. VII. Doppler color flow mapping: a new technique for the diagnosis of congenital heart disease. Am J Obstet Gynecol 1987;156:1054-1064.

47. Cockerham JT, Martin TC, Gutierrez FR, et al. Spontaneous closure of secundum atrial septal defect in infants and young children. Am J Cardiol 1983;52:1267-1271.

48. Steele PM, Fuster V, Cohen M, et al. Isolated atrial septal defect with pulmonary vascular obstructive disease: long-term follow-up and prediction of outcome after surgical correction. Circulation 1987;76:1037-1042.

49. Ferencz C, Rubin JD, McCarter RJ, et al. Cardiac and noncardiac malformations: observations in a population-based study. Teratology 1987;35:367-378.

50. Goor DA, Lillehei CW. Congenital malformations of the heart: embryology, anatomy, and operative considerations. New York: Grune & Stratton; 1975.

51. Grahm TP, Bender HW, Spach M. Ventricular septal defects. In: Moss AJ, Adams FH, Emmanouilides GC, editors. Heart disease in infancy, childhood, and adolescence. 2nd ed. Baltimore: Williams & Wilkins; 1977.

52. Allan LD, Crawford DC, Anderson RH, Tynan MJ. Echocardiographic and anatomical correlations in fetal congenital heart disease. Br Heart J 1984;52:542-548.

53. Allan LD, Tynan M, Campbell S, Anderson RH. Identification of congenital cardiac malformations by echocardiography in midtrimester fetus. Br Heart J 1981;46:358-362.

54. Parness IA, Yeager SB, Sanders SP, et al. Echocardiographic diagnosis of fetal heart defects in mid trimester. Arch Dis Child 1988;63:1137-1145.

55. Yagel S, Sherer D, Hurwitz A. Significance of ultrasonic prenatal diagnosis of ventricular septal defect. J Clin Ultrasound 1985;13:588-590.

56. Brown DL, Emerson DS, Cartier MS, et al. Congenital cardiac anomalies: prenatal sonographic diagnosis. AJR Am J Roentgenol 1989;153:109-114.

57. Sutherland GR, Smyllie JH, Ogilvie BC, Keeton BR. Colour flow imaging in the diagnosis of multiple ventricular septal defects. Br Heart J 1989;62:43-49.

58. Hoffman JI. Natural history of congenital heart disease: problems in its assessment with special reference to ventricular septal defects. Circulation 1968;37:97-125.

59. Hoffman JI, Rudolph AM. The natural history of isolated ventricular septal defect with special reference to selection of patients for surgery. Adv Pediatr 1970;17:57-79.

60. Hoffman JI, Rudolph AM. The natural history of ventricular septal defects in infancy. Am J Cardiol 1965;16:634-653.

61. Crawford DC, Chita SK, Allan LD. Prenatal detection of congenital heart disease: factors affecting obstetric management and survival. Am J Obstet Gynecol 1988;159:352-356.

62. Machado MV, Crawford DC, Anderson RH, Allan LD. Atrioventricular septal defect in prenatal life. Br Heart J 1988;59:352-355.

63. Carvalho JS, Rigby ML, Shinebourne EA, Anderson RH. Cross-sectional echocardiography for recognition of ventricular topology in atrioventricular septal defect. Br Heart J 1989;61:285-288.

64. Freedom RM, Culham JAG, Moes CAF. Angiography of congenital heart disease. New York: Macmillan; 1984.

65. Becker AE, Anderson RH. Atrioventricular septal defects: what's in a name? J Thorac Cardiovasc Surg 1982;83:461-469.

66. Fontana RS, Edwards JE. Congenital cardiac disease. Philadelphia, 1962, Saunders.

67. Shenker L, Reed KL, Marx GR, et al. Fetal cardiac Doppler flow studies in prenatal diagnosis of heart disease. Am J Obstet Gynecol 1988;158:1267-1273.

68. Gembruch U, Knopfle G, Chatterjee M, et al. Prenatal diagnosis of atrioventricular canal malformations with up-to-date echocardiographic technology: report of 14 cases. Am Heart J 1991;121:1489-1497.

69. Rasiah SV, Ewer AK, Miller P, et al. Outcome following prenatal diagnosis of complete atrioventricular septal defect. Prenat Diagn 2008;28:95-101.

70. Allan LD, Crawford DC, Sheridan R, Chapman MG. Aetiology of non-immune hydrops: the value of echocardiography. Br J Obstet Gynaecol 1986;93:223-225.

71. Genton E, Blount Jr SG. The spectrum of Ebstein's anomaly. Am Heart J 1967;73:395-425.

72. Lev M, Liberthson RR, Joseph RH, et al. The pathologic anatomy of Ebstein's disease. Arch Pathol 1970;90:334-343.

73. Roberson DA, Silverman NH. Ebstein's anomaly: echocardiographic and clinical features in the fetus and neonate. J Am Coll Cardiol 1989;14:1300-1307.

74. Zuberbuhler JR, Becker AE, Anderson RH, Lenox CC. Ebstein's malformation and the embryological development of the tricuspid valve. With a note on the nature of "clefts" in the atrioventricular valves. Pediatr Cardiol 1984;5:289-295.

75. Anderson KR, Zuberbuhler JR, Anderson RH, et al. Morphologic spectrum of Ebstein's anomaly of the heart: a review. Mayo Clin Proc 1979;54:174-180.

76. Stewart PA, Wladimiroff JW, Reuss A, Sachs ES. Fetal echocardiography: a review of six years experience. Fetal Ther 1987;2:222-231.

77. Sharland GK, Chita SK, Allan LD. Tricuspid valve dysplasia or displacement in intrauterine life. J Am Coll Cardiol 1991;17:944-949.

78. Nora JJ, Nora AH, Toews WH. Lithium, Ebstein's anomaly, and other congenital heart defects (letter). Lancet 1974;2:594-595.

79. Nora JJ, Nora AH. The evolution of specific genetic and environmental counseling in congenital heart diseases. Circulation 1978;57:205-213.

80. Schou M, Goldfield MD, Weinstein MR, Villeneuve A. Lithium and pregnancy. I. Report from the Register of Lithium Babies. Br Med J 1973;2:135-136.

81. Weinstein MR, Goldfield M. Cardiovascular malformations with lithium use during pregnancy. Am J Psychiatry 1975;132:529-531.

82. Park JM, Sridaromont S, Ledbetter EO, Terry WM. Ebstein's anomaly of the tricuspid valve associated with prenatal exposure to lithium carbonate. Am J Dis Child 1980;134:703-704.

83. Kallen B, Tandberg A. Lithium and pregnancy. A cohort study on manic-depressive women. Acta Psychiatr Scand 1983;68:134-139.

84. Zalzstein E, Koren G, Einarson T, Freedom RM. A case-control study on the association between first trimester exposure to lithium and Ebstein's anomaly. Am J Cardiol 1990;65:817-818.

85. Anderson RH, Silverman NH, Zuberbuhler JR. Congenitally unguarded tricuspid orifice: its differentiation from Ebstein's malformation in association with pulmonary atresia and intact ventricular septum. Pediatr Cardiol 1990;11:86-90.

86. Oberhoffer R, Cook AC, Lang D, et al. Correlation between echocardiographic and morphological investigations of lesions of the tricuspid valve diagnosed during fetal life. Br Heart J 1992;68:580-585.

87. Handler JB, Berger TJ, Miller RH, et al. Partial atrioventricular canal in association with Ebstein's anomaly: echocardiographic diagnosis and surgical correction. Chest 1981;80:515-517.

88. Fink BW. Congenital heart disease: a deductive approach to its diagnosis. 2nd ed. Chicago: Year Book Medical Publishers; 1985.

89. Copel JA, Cullen M, Green JJ, et al. The frequency of aneuploidy in prenatally diagnosed congenital heart disease: an indication for fetal karyotyping. Am J Obstet Gynecol 1988;158:409-413.

90. Hornberger LK, Sahn DJ, Kleinman CS, et al. Tricuspid valve disease with significant tricuspid insufficiency in the fetus: diagnosis and outcome. J Am Coll Cardiol 1991;17:167-173.

91. Gembruch U, Hansmann M, Redel DA, Bald R. Fetal two-dimensional Doppler echocardiography (colour flow mapping) and its place in prenatal diagnosis. Prenat Diagn 1989;9:535-547.

92. Boston US, Dearani JA, O'Leary PW, et al. Tricuspid valve repair for Ebstein's anomaly in young children: a 30-year experience. Ann Thorac Surg 2006;81:690-695; discussion 695-696.

93. Brown ML, Dearani JA, Danielson GK, et al. The outcomes of operations for 539 patients with Ebstein anomaly. J Thorac Cardiovasc Surg 2008;135:1120-1136, 1136 e1-e7.

94. Palmen M, de Jong PL, Klieverik LM, et al. Long-term follow-up after repair of Ebstein's anomaly. Eur J Cardiothorac Surg 2008;34: 48-54.

95. Paranon S, Acar P. Ebstein's anomaly of the tricuspid valve: from fetus to adult: congenital heart disease. Heart 2008;94:237-243.

96. Grundy H, Burlbaw J, Gowdamarajan R, et al. Antenatal detection of hypoplastic right ventricle with fetal M-mode echocardiography: a report of two cases. J Reprod Med 1987;32:301-304.

97. De Leval M, Bull C, Stark J, et al. Pulmonary atresia and intact ventricular septum: surgical management based on a revised classification. Circulation 1982;66:272-280.

98. Schaffer RM, Corio FJ. Sonographic diagnosis of hypoplastic left heart syndrome in utero. J Diag Med Sonogr 1988;6:319-320.

99. Yagel S, Mandelberg A, Hurwitz A, Jlaser Y. Prenatal diagnosis of hypoplastic left ventricle. Am J Perinatol 1986;3:6-8.

100. Hawkins JA, Doty DB. Aortic atresia: morphologic characteristics affecting survival and operative palliation. J Thorac Cardiovasc Surg 1984;88:620-626.

101. Saied A, Folger Jr GM. Hypoplastic left heart syndrome: clinicopathologic and hemodynamic correlation. Am J Cardiol 1972;29: 190-198.

102. Doty DB. Aortic atresia. J Thorac Cardiovasc Surg 1980;79:462-463.

103. Satomi G, Yasukochi S, Shimizu T, et al. Has fetal echocardiography improved the prognosis of congenital heart disease? Comparison of patients with hypoplastic left heart syndrome with and without prenatal diagnosis. Pediatr Int 1999;41:728-732.

104. Mahle WT, Clancy RR, McGaurn SP, et al. Impact of prenatal diagnosis on survival and early neurologic morbidity in neonates with the hypoplastic left heart syndrome. Pediatrics 2001;107: 1277-1282.

105. Tworetzky W, McElhinney DB, Reddy VM, et al. Improved surgical outcome after fetal diagnosis of hypoplastic left heart syndrome. Circulation 2001;103:1269-1273.

106. Mahle WT, Wernovsky G. Neurodevelopmental outcomes in hypoplastic left heart syndrome. Semin Thorac Cardiovasc Surg Pediatr Card Surg Annu 2004;7:39-47.

107. Jenkins PC, Chinnock RE, Jenkins KJ, et al. Decreased exercise performance with age in children with hypoplastic left heart syndrome. J Pediatr 2008;152:507-512.

108. Becker AE, Anderson RH. Pathology of congenital heart disease. London: Butterworth; 1981.

109. Moodie DS, Ritter DG, Tajik AH, et al. Long-term follow-up after palliative operation for univentricular heart. Am J Cardiol 1984;53: 1648-1651.

110. Moodie DS, Ritter DG, Tajik AJ, O'Fallon WM. Long-term follow-up in the unoperated univentricular heart. Am J Cardiol 1984;53: 1124-1128.

111. Hallermann FJ, Davis GD, Ritter DG, Kincaid OW. Roentgenographic features of common ventricle. Radiology 1966;87:409-423.

112. McKay R, Pacifico AD, Blackstone EH, et al. Septation of the univentricular heart with left anterior subaortic outlet chamber. J Thorac Cardiovasc Surg 1982;84:77-87.

113. Poon LC, Huggon IC, Zidere V, Allan LD. Tetralogy of Fallot in the fetus in the current era. Ultrasound Obstet Gynecol 2007;29: 625-627.

114. Netter F. The Ciba Collection of medical illustrations. V. Heart. New Jersey: CIBA; 1978.

115. Lev M, Rimoldi JA, Rowlatt UF. The quantitative anatomy of cyanotic tetralogy of Fallot. Circulation 1964;30:531-538.

116. DeVore GR, Siassi B, Platt LD. Fetal echocardiography. VIII. Aortic root dilatation: a marker for tetralogy of Fallot. Am J Obstet Gynecol 1988;159:129-136.

117. Anderson CF, McCurdy Jr CM, McNamara MF, Reed KL. Case of the day. 8. Diagnosis: color Doppler aided diagnosis of tetralogy of Fallot. J Ultrasound Med 1994;13:341-342.

118. Gibbs JL, Monro JL, Cunningham D, Rickards A. Survival after surgery or therapeutic catheterisation for congenital heart disease in children in the United Kingdom: analysis of the central cardiac audit database for 2000-2001. BMJ 2004;328:611.

119. Murphy JG, Gersh BJ, Mair DD, et al. Long-term outcome in patients undergoing surgical repair of tetralogy of Fallot. N Engl J Med 1993;329:593-599.

120. Kleinman CS, Donnerstein RL, DeVore GR, et al. Fetal echocardiography for evaluation of in utero congestive heart failure. N Engl J Med 1982;306:568-575.

121. Lakier JB, Stanger P, Heymann MA, et al. Tetralogy of Fallot with absent pulmonary valve: natural history and hemodynamic considerations. Circulation 1974;50:167-175.

122. Fyler DC. Report of the New England Regional Infant Cardiac Program. Pediatrics 1980:375-461.

123. Collett RW, Edwards JE. Persistent truncus arteriosus; a classification according to anatomic types. Surg Clin North Am 1949;29: 1245-1270.

124. Rajasinghe HA, McElhinney DB, Reddy VM, et al. Long-term follow-up of truncus arteriosus repaired in infancy: a twenty-year experience. J Thorac Cardiovasc Surg 1997;113:869-878; discussion 878-879.

125. Kirklin JW, Pacifico AD, Blackstone EH, et al. Current risks and protocols for operations for double-outlet right ventricle: derivation from an 18 year experience. J Thorac Cardiovasc Surg 1986;92: 913-930.

126. Stewart PA, Wladimiroff JW, Becker AE. Early prenatal detection of double outlet right ventricle by echocardiography. Br Heart J 1985;54:340-342.

127. Kim N, Friedberg MK, Silverman NH. Diagnosis and prognosis of fetuses with double outlet right ventricle. Prenat Diagn 2006;26: 740-745.

128. Trusler GA, Castaneda AR, Rosenthal A, et al. Current results of management in transposition of the great arteries, with special emphasis on patients with associated ventricular septal defect. J Am Coll Cardiol 1987;10:1061-1071.

129. Allwork SP, Bentall HH, Becker AE, et al. Congenitally corrected transposition of the great arteries: morphologic study of 32 cases. Am J Cardiol 1976;38:910-923.

130. Rutledge JM, Nihill MR, Fraser CD, et al. Outcome of 121 patients with congenitally corrected transposition of the great arteries. Pediatr Cardiol 2002;23:137-145.

131. DiSessa TG, Emerson DS, Felker RE, et al. Anomalous systemic and pulmonary venous pathways diagnosed in utero by ultrasound. J Ultrasound Med 1990;9:311-317.

132. Ferencz C, Rubin JD, McCarter RJ, et al. Congenital heart disease: prevalence at livebirth. The Baltimore-Washington Infant Study. Am J Epidemiol 1985;121:31-36.

133. Allan LD. Structural cardiac abnormalities. In Allan LD, editor. Manual of fetal echocardiography. Lancaster, UK: MTP Press; 1986. p. 75-79.

134. Carter RE, Capriles M, Noe Y. Total anomalous pulmonary venous drainage: a clinical and anatomical study of 75 children. Br Heart J 1969;31:45-51.

135. Patel CR, Lane JR, Spector ML, et al. Totally anomalous pulmonary venous connection and complex congenital heart disease: prenatal echocardiographic diagnosis and prognosis. J Ultrasound Med 2005;24:1191-1198.

136. Hashmi A, Abu-Sulaiman R, McCrindle BW, et al. Management and outcomes of right atrial isomerism: a 26-year experience. J Am Coll Cardiol 1998;31:1120-1126.

137. Valsangiacomo ER, Hornberger LK, Barrea C, et al. Partial and total anomalous pulmonary venous connection in the fetus: two-dimensional and Doppler echocardiographic findings. Ultrasound Obstet Gynecol 2003;22:257-263.

138. Allan LD, Crawford DC, Tynan M. Evolution of coarctation of the aorta in intrauterine life. Br Heart J 1984;52:471-473.

139. Rosenberg H. Coarctation of the aorta: morphology and pathogenesis considerations. In: Rosenberg HS, Bolande RP, editors. Perspectives in pediatric pathology Vol I. Chicago: Year Book Medical Publishers; 1973.

140. Bruins C. Twelfth Edgar Mannheimer lecture. Competition between aortic isthmus and ductus arteriosus: reciprocal influence of structure and flow. Eur J Cardiol 1978;8:87-97.

141. Hutchins GM. Coarctation of the aorta explained as a branch-point of the ductus arteriosus. Am J Pathol 1971;63:203-214.

142. Benacerraf BR, Saltzman DH, Sanders SP. Sonographic sign suggesting the prenatal diagnosis of coarctation of the aorta. J Ultrasound Med 1989;8:65-69.

143. Hornberger LK, Sahn DJ, Kleinman CS, et al. Antenatal diagnosis of coarctation of the aorta: a multicenter experience. J Am Coll Cardiol 1994;23:417-423.

144. Sahn DJ, Lange LW, Allen HD, et al. Quantitative real-time cross-sectional echocardiography in the developing normal humam fetus and newborn. Circulation 1980;62:588-597.

145. Head CE, Jowett VC, Sharland GK, Simpson JM. Timing of presentation and postnatal outcome of infants suspected of having coarctation of the aorta during fetal life. Heart 2005;91:1070-1074.

146. Hesslein PS, Gutgesell HP, McNamara DG. Prognosis of symptomatic coarctation of the aorta in infancy. Am J Cardiol 1983;51:299-303.

147. Clark CE, Henry WL, Epstein SE. Familial prevalence and genetic transmission of idiopathic hypertrophic subaortic stenosis. N Engl J Med 1973;289:709-714.

148. Barrea C, Alkazaleh F, Ryan G, et al. Prenatal cardiovascular manifestations in the twin-to-twin transfusion syndrome recipients and the impact of therapeutic amnioreduction. Am J Obstet Gynecol 2005;192:892-902.

149. Yagel S, Weissman A, Rotstein Z, et al. Congenital heart defects: natural course and in utero development. Circulation 1997;96:550-555.

150. Campbell M. The natural history of congenital aortic stenosis. Br Heart J 1968;30:514-526.

151. Messina LM, Turley K, Stanger P, et al. Successful aortic valvotomy for severe congenital valvular aortic stenosis in the newborn infant. J Thorac Cardiovasc Surg 1984;88:92-96.

152. Jones M, Barnhart GR, Morrow AG. Late results after operations for left ventricular outflow tract obstruction. Am J Cardiol 1982;50:569-579.

153. Selamet Tierney ES, Wald RM, McElhinney DB, et al. Changes in left heart hemodynamics after technically successful in-utero aortic valvuloplasty. Ultrasound Obstet Gynecol 2007;30:715-720.

154. Merrill WH, Shuman TA, Graham Jr TP, et al. Surgical intervention in neonates with critical pulmonary stenosis. Ann Surg 1987;205:712-718.

155. Marantz PM, Huhta JC, Mullins CE, et al. Results of balloon valvuloplasty in typical and dysplastic pulmonary valve stenosis: Doppler echocardiographic follow-up. J Am Coll Cardiol 1988;12:476-479.

156. Galindo A, Gutierrez-Larraya F, Velasco JM, de la Fuente P. Pulmonary balloon valvuloplasty in a fetus with critical pulmonary stenosis/atresia with intact ventricular septum and heart failure. Fetal Diagn Ther 2006;21:100-104.

157. Niikawa N, Kohsaka S, Mizumoto M, et al. Familial clustering of situs inversus totalis, and asplenia and polysplenia syndromes. Am J Med Genet 1983;16:43-47.

158. Rose V, Izukawa T, Moes CA. Syndromes of asplenia and polysplenia: a review of cardiac and non-cardiac malformations in 60 cases with special reference to diagnosis and prognosis. Br Heart J 1975;37:840-852.

159. Peoples WM, Moller JH, Edwards JE. Polysplenia: a review of 146 cases. Pediatr Cardiol 1983;4:129-137.

160. Zlotogora J, Elian E. Asplenia and polysplenia syndromes with abnormalities of lateralisation in a sibship. J Med Genet 1981;18:301-302.

161. Stewart PA, Becker AE, Wladimiroff JW, Essed CE. Left atrial isomerism associated with asplenia: prenatal echocardiographic detection of complex congenital cardiac malformations. J Am Coll Cardiol 1984;4:1015-1020.

162. Garcia OL, Metha AV, Pickoff AS, et al. Left isomerism and complete atrioventricular block: a report of six cases. Am J Cardiol 1981;48:1103-1107.

163. Berg C, Geipel A, Smrcek J, et al. Prenatal diagnosis of cardiosplenic syndromes: a 10-year experience. Ultrasound Obstet Gynecol 2003;22:451-459.

164. Schmidt W, Yarkoni S, Jeanty P, et al. Sonographic measurements of the fetal spleen: clinical implications. J Ultrasound Med 1985;4:667-672.

165. De Araujo LM, Silverman NH, Filly RA, et al. Prenatal detection of left atrial isomerism by ultrasound. J Ultrasound Med 1987;6:667-670.

166. McAllister Jr HA. Primary tumors of the heart and pericardium. Pathol Annu 1979;14(Pt 2):325-355.

167. Dennis MA, Appareti K, Manco-Johnson ML, et al. The echocardiographic diagnosis of multiple fetal cardiac tumors. J Ultrasound Med 1985;4:327-329.

168. Smythe JF, Dyck JD, Smallhorn JF, Freedom RM. Natural history of cardiac rhabdomyoma in infancy and childhood. Am J Cardiol 1990;66:1247-1249.

169. Simcha A, Wells BG, Tynan MJ, Waterston DJ. Primary cardiac tumours in childhood. Arch Dis Child 1971;46:508-514.

170. Crawford DC, Garrett C, Tynan M, et al. Cardiac rhabdomyomata as a marker for the antenatal detection of tuberous sclerosis. J Med Genet 1983;20:303-304.

171. Groves AM, Fagg NL, Cook AC, Allan LD. Cardiac tumours in intrauterine life. Arch Dis Child 1992;67:1189-1192.

172. Bender BL, Yunis EJ. The pathology of tuberous sclerosis. Pathol Annu 1982;17(Pt 1):339-382.

173. Journel H, Roussey M, Plais MH, et al. Prenatal diagnosis of familial tuberous sclerosis following detection of cardiac rhabdomyoma by ultrasound. Prenat Diagn 1986;6:283-289.

174. DeVore GR, Hakim S, Kleinman CS, Hobbins JC. The in utero diagnosis of an interventricular septal cardiac rhabdomyoma by means of real-time-directed, M-mode echocardiography. Am J Obstet Gynecol 1982;143:967-969.

175. Chao AS, Chao A, Wang TH, et al. Outcome of antenatally diagnosed cardiac rhabdomyoma: case series and a meta-analysis. Ultrasound Obstet Gynecol 2008;31:289-295.

176. Holley DG, Martin GR, Brenner JI, et al. Diagnosis and management of fetal cardiac tumors: a multicenter experience and review of published reports. J Am Coll Cardiol 1995;26:516-520.

177. Gava G, Buoso G, Beltrame GL, et al. Cardiac rhabdomyoma as a marker for the prenatal detection of tuberous sclerosis: case report. Br J Obstet Gynaecol 1990;97:1154-1157.

178. Levy DW, Mintz MC. The left ventricular echogenic focus: a normal finding. AJR Am J Roentgenol 1988;150:85-86.

179. Petrikovsky BM, Challenger M, Wyse LJ. Natural history of echogenic foci within ventricles of the fetal heart. Ultrasound Obstet Gynecol 1995;5:92-94.

180. Arda S, Sayin NC, Varol FG, Sut N. Isolated fetal intracardiac hyperechogenic focus associated with neonatal outcome and triple test results. Arch Gynecol Obstet 2007;276:481-485.

181. Pedra SR, Smallhorn JF, Ryan G, et al. Fetal cardiomyopathies: pathogenic mechanisms, hemodynamic findings, and clinical outcome. Circulation 2002;106:585-591.

182. Yinon Y, Yagel S, Hegesh J, et al. Fetal cardiomyopathy: in utero evaluation and clinical significance. Prenat Diagn 2007;27:23-28.

183. Drose JA, Dennis MA, Thickman D. Infection in utero: ultrasound findings in 19 cases. Radiology 1991;178:369-374.

184. Schryer MJ, Karnauchow PN. Endocardial fibroelastosis; etiologic and pathogenetic considerations in children. Am Heart J 1974;88:557-565.

185. Griffin LD, Kearney D, Ni J, et al. Analysis of formalin-fixed and frozen myocardial autopsy samples for viral genome in childhood myocarditis and dilated cardiomyopathy with endocardial fibroelastosis using polymerase chain reaction (PCR). Cardiovasc Pathol 1995;4:3-11.

186. Sheehan PQ, Rowland TW, Shah BL, et al. Maternal diabetic control and hypertrophic cardiomyopathy in infants of diabetic mothers. Clin Pediatr (Phila) 1986;25:266-271.

187. Lendrum B, Pildes RS, Serratto M, et al. The spectrum of myocardial abnormality in infants of diabetic mothers. Pediatr Cardiol 1979;1:172.

188. Gutgesell HP, Speer ME, Rosenberg HS. Characterization of the cardiomyopathy in infants of diabetic mothers. Circulation 1980;61:441-450.

189. Halliday HL. Hypertrophic cardiomyopathy in infants of poorly controlled diabetic mothers. Arch Dis Child 1981;56:258-263.

190. Veille JC, Hanson R, Sivakoff M, et al. Fetal cardiac size in normal, intrauterine growth retarded, and diabetic pregnancies. Am J Perinatol 1993;10:275-279.

191. Kanagasuntheram R, Verzin JA. Ectopia cordis in man. Thorax 1962;17:159-167.

192. Cantrell JR, Haller JA, Ravitch MM. A syndrome of congenital defects involving the abdominal wall, sternum, diaphragm, pericardium, and heart. Surg Gynecol Obstet 1958;107:602-614.

193. Liang RI, Huang JE, Chang FM. Prenatal diagnosis of ectopia cordis at 10 weeks of gestation using two-dimensional ultrasonography. Ultrasound Obstet Gynecol 2002;10:137-139.

194. Ghidini A, Sirtori M, Romero R, Hobbins JC. Prenatal diagnosis of pentalogy of Cantrell. J Ultrasound Med 1988;7:567-572.

Arrhythmias

195. Lingman G, Lundstrom NR, Marsal K, Ohrlander S. Fetal cardiac arrhythmia: clinical outcome in 113 cases. Acta Obstet Gynecol Scand 1986;65:263-267.
196. Stewart PA, Wladimiroff JW. Fetal atrial arrhythmias associated with redundancy/aneurysm of the foramen ovale. J Clin Ultrasound 1988;16:643-650.
197. Rice MJ, McDonald RW, Reller MD. Fetal atrial septal aneurysm: a cause of fetal atrial arrhythmias. J Am Coll Cardiol 1988;12:1292-1297.
198. Kleinman CS. Prenatal diagnosis and management of intrauterine arrhythmias. Fetal Ther 1986;1:92-95.
199. Shenker L. Fetal cardiac arrhythmias. Obstet Gynecol Surg 1971;34:561.
200. Reed KL, Sahn DJ, Marx GR, et al. Cardiac Doppler flows during fetal arrhythmias: physiologic consequences. Obstet Gynecol 1987;70:1-6.
201. Chao RC, Ho ES, Hsieh KS. Fetal atrial flutter and fibrillation: prenatal echocardiographic detection and management. Am Heart J 1992;124:1095-1098.
202. Silverman NH, Kleinman CS, Rudolph AM, et al. Fetal atrioventricular valve insufficiency associated with nonimmune hydrops: a two-dimensional echocardiographic and pulsed Doppler ultrasound study. Circulation 1985;72:825-832.
203. Cameron A, Nicholson S, Nimrod C, et al. Evaluation of fetal cardiac dysrhythmias with two-dimensional, M-mode, and pulsed Doppler ultrasonography. Am J Obstet Gynecol 1988;158:286-290.
204. Kleinman CS, Copel JA, Weinstein EM, et al. Treatment of fetal supraventricular tachyarrhythmias. J Clin Ultrasound 1985;13:265-273.
205. Kleinman CS, Donnerstein RL, Jaffe CC, et al. Fetal echocardiography: a tool for evaluation of in utero cardiac arrhythmias and monitoring of in utero therapy: analysis of 71 patients. Am J Cardiol 1983;51:237-243.
206. Wiggins Jr JW, Bowes W, Clewell W, et al. Echocardiographic diagnosis and intravenous digoxin management of fetal tachyarrhythmias and congestive heart failure. Am J Dis Child 1986;140:202-204.
207. Komaromy B, Gaal J, Lampe L. Fetal arrhythmia during pregnancy and labour. Br J Obstet Gynaecol 1977;84:492-496.
208. Mendoza GJ, Almeida O, Steinfeld L. Intermittent fetal bradycardia induced by midpregnancy fetal ultrasonographic study. Am J Obstet Gynecol 1989;160:1038-1040.
209. Minagawa Y, Akaiwa A, Hidaka T, et al. Severe fetal supraventricular bradyarrhythmia without fetal hypoxia. Obstet Gynecol 1987;70:454-456.
210. Laboda LA, Estroff JA, Benacerraf BR. First trimester bradycardia: a sign of impending fetal loss. J Ultrasound Med 1989;8:561-563.
211. Sciarrone A, Masturzo B, Botta G, et al. First-trimester fetal heart block and increased nuchal translucency: an indication for early fetal echocardiography. Prenat Diagn 2005;25:1129-1132.
212. Carpenter Jr RJ, Strasburger JF, Garson Jr A, et al. Fetal ventricular pacing for hydrops secondary to complete atrioventricular block. J Am Coll Cardiol 1986;8:1434-1436.
213. McCue CM, Mantakas ME, Tingelstad JB, Ruddy S. Congenital heart block in newborns of mothers with connective tissue disease. Circulation 1977;56:82-90.
214. Crawford D, Chapman M, Allan L. The assessment of persistent bradycardia in prenatal life. Br J Obstet Gynaecol 1985;92:941-944.
215. Friedman DM. Fetal echocardiography in the assessment of lupus pregnancies. Am J Reprod Immunol 1992;28:164-167.
216. Buyon J, Roubey R, Swersky S, et al. Complete congenital heart block: risk of occurrence and therapeutic approach to prevention. J Rheumatol 1988;15:1104-1108.
217. Copel JA, Liang RI, Demasio K, et al. The clinical significance of the irregular fetal heart rhythm. Am J Obstet Gynecol 2000;182:813-817; discussion 817-819.

CHAPTER 38

The Fetal Abdominal Wall and Gastrointestinal Tract

Jodi F. Abbott

Chapter Outline

*I*dentification and confirmation of a normal fetal abdominal wall and gastrointestinal (GI) tract is critical to ascertain the risk of isolated and multiple fetal abnormalities. Anomalies of the fetal abdomen may be the only sonographic evidence of multisystem organ derangement. The National Center for Biotechnical Information (NCBI) with the Online Mendelian Inheritance in Man has recommended new diagnostic categorization (recategorization) of abdominal wall defects. This chapter places these updated diagnostic categories in the context of previous information, sonographic diagnostic criteria, hypothesized etiology, and current management of these abnormalities. Detection of fetal intra-abdominal masses or abnormalities is important because they may be undetected on newborn examinations.

EMBRYOLOGY OF THE DIGESTIVE TUBE

The lumens of both the digestive and the respiratory tubes are lined by the embryonic endoderm, which differentiates distal to the pharynx after formation of the pharyngeal pouches. The digestive tubes are a differentiation of the lateral plate endoderm. The stomach forms as an inferior outpouching below the pharynx. The regional specification of the digestive tube into the esophagus, stomach, and small and large intestines is in response to different mesodermal mesenchymes.[1-3]

The sonic hedgehog gene *(Shh)* has been implicated in this differentiation.[4] As digestive differentiation progresses, the expressivity of *Shh* increases from proximal to distal.[5]

STOMACH

The fetal stomach can be seen as early as 7 weeks and should be noted routinely by 13 to 14 weeks' gestation[6] (Fig. 38-1). The stomach should be in the left upper abdomen. It is important in every fetal survey to confirm situs of the stomach because a midline or right-sided stomach is associated with heterotaxy syndromes. Presence of a right-sided stomach and a right-sided heart is termed **total situs inversus.** A right-sided stomach and a left-sided heart result in **partial situs inversus.** During the 11 to 14-week evaluation of the fetal abdomen, numerous abnormal findings have been reported, including ascites, abdominal cysts, and intestinal obstruction.[7]

Small or Absent Fetal Stomach

Fluid in the stomach should be reliably visualized on first-trimester screening or fetal anatomic survey and all subsequent fetal evaluations. The absence of a visualized stomach on an anatomic survey, although potentially a normal finding, has an increased risk of fetal

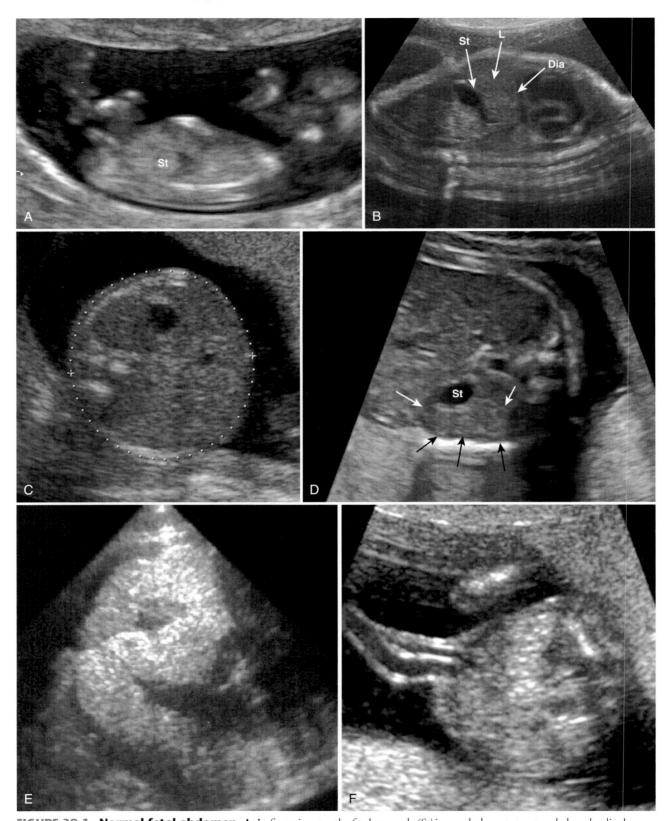

FIGURE 38-1. Normal fetal abdomen. A, In first trimester the fetal stomach *(St)* is an echolucent structure below the diaphragm. Note similar echogenicity of liver, lung, and bowel. **B,** In second trimester in sagittal view, the stomach *(St)* is seen below the diaphragm *(Dia),* and the liver *(L)* extends anteriorly to the abdominal wall. **C,** In second trimester in transverse view with the spine to the left, the stomach is superior, and bowel echogenicity is similar to liver. The liver occupies most of the right abdomen and is relatively homogeneous. **D,** Normal spleen *(arrows)* in the transverse view of second-trimester fetal abdomen. **E,** Normal echogenic appearance of meconium filling the colon in the third trimester. **F,** Normal cord insertion site in midtrimester fetus. *(E from McNamara A, Levine D. Intraabdominal fetal echogenic masses: a practical guide to diagnosis and management. Radiographics 2005;25:633-645.)*

ABSENT STOMACH

Normal stomach that recently emptied
Displaced stomach into chest in hernia
Displaced stomach into abdominal wall defect
Esophageal atresia
Aneuploidy
Anhydramnios
Microgastria

abnormality, including aneuploidy, tracheoesophageal fistula, and oligohydramnios.

When the stomach appears small or absent, it is important to allow sufficient time for it to fill, in case it has recently emptied. Generally, the stomach will fill during a 30-minute examination. Careful attention must be paid to the thorax; the stomach can be herniated into the chest in **congenital diaphragmatic hernia.**

In one retrospective study, an abnormal outcome (structural abnormalities, intrauterine fetal or postnatal death) occurred in 23 (85%) of 27 fetuses with an absent stomach and 27 (52%) of 52 fetuses with a small stomach (combined, 63%). Karyotype was abnormal in eight (38%) of 21 fetuses with an absent stomach and two (4%) of 46 fetuses with a small stomach.[8] Amniotic fluid in cases of absent stomach is typically normal early in the second trimester, but polyhydramnios is common by the third trimester. The finding of a persistently absent stomach on serial ultrasound scans should trigger genetic counseling and consideration of chromosomal testing.

Esophageal Atresia

Developmentally, the trachea and esophagus differentiate inferiorly from the posterior pharynx. Incomplete differentiation of the respiratory and GI tracts can lead to esophageal atresia with or without tracheoesophageal (TE) fistulas. The incidence of TE fistulas, all types, is 2.8 per 10,000 pregnancies.[9,10] Most types of esophageal atresia (90%)[11] are associated with TE fistulas, and therefore the stomach (although often small) will be visualized on ultrasound. Occasionally, fluid in the upper esophagus can be appreciated (Fig. 38-2). For this reason, the term "tracheoesophageal fistula" is usually the working in utero diagnosis when esophageal atresia is suspected, even though this diagnosis cannot be definitively made in utero. The ability of prenatal diagnosis to detect this condition is 42%.[12]

The combination of inability to see a stomach on ultrasound and the presence of polyhydramnios is more suggestive of esophageal atresia than absent stomach alone. The positive predictive value of this combination is still relatively modest, 56% in the largest study.[12] Esophageal atresia is associated with other systemic anomalies, and a detailed evaluation, including echocardiography, should be performed in a fetus with

this suspected diagnosis. It is reported that as many as half of TE fistulas are part of the **VACTERL** sequence,[9] a nonrandom group of coexisting defects: *v*ertebral defects, *a*nal atresia, *c*ardiac anomalies, **tracheoesophageal fistula** with *e*sophageal atresia, *r*enal and radial dysplasia, and *l*imb defects. VACTERL has sporadic inheritance. The corrective surgery for esophageal atresia has a success rate of 90% and is related to the presence of associated anomalies.[11]

Dilated Fetal Stomach

In the second or third trimester a prominent or transiently dilated fetal stomach may be seen on ultrasound. However, diagnosing a dilated fetal stomach requires that the stomach be persistently dilated throughout a 30-minute assessment. Use of a nomogram can aid in identifying true outliers (Table 38-1).[13] The differential diagnosis of a dilated fetal stomach includes normal fetus (Fig. 38-3) and **gastrointestinal atresia** (primarily duodenal atresia). For a dilated stomach when other fetal parameters are normal, follow-up is recommended.

Midline or Right-Sided Stomach

When an apparently malpositioned stomach is noted, the situs must again be carefully determined. Complete situs inversus is uncommon but can be prenatally detected. A **midline stomach** can represent intestinal malrotation[14] (Fig. 38-4). However, **heterotaxy syndrome,** including right isomerism and left isomerism is more common. It is characterized by an abnormal symmetry of the viscera and veins and may be associated with complex cardiac anomalies, intestinal malrotation, and splenic (asplenia or polysplenia; Fig. 38-5), and hepatic abnormalities.[15,16] The incidence of asplenia/polysplenia heterotaxy syndromes is 0.45 per 10,000 pregnancies.[17] Because of the combined cardiovascular and GI abnormalities, infant mortality is high, with 1-year mortality reaching 32% in a Canadian retrospective trial.[18]

LIVER

The fetal liver is clearly visualized in the upper abdomen in the second half of gestation, although earlier in gestation it has an echogenicity similar to renal echoes. In the fetus, the left side of the liver is larger than the right side.[19] The liver increases in size during pregnancy.[20] Hepatic enlargement has been documented in **fetal anemia** caused by isoimmunization,[21] **glycogen storage diseases,** and **fetal infection.**[22]

Hepatic calcifications may be noted in utero (Fig. 38-6). The pathophysiology of the calcifications in otherwise normal fetuses is unknown. These are typically isolated and of no clinical consequence.[23] However, hepatic calcifications have been reported in aneuploid or

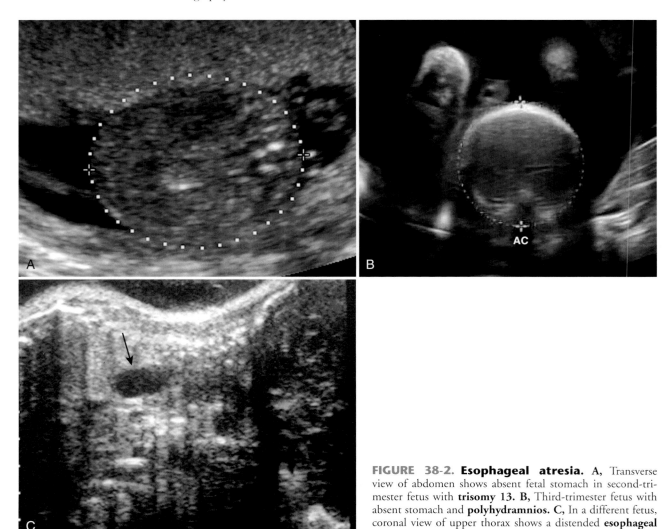

FIGURE 38-2. Esophageal atresia. A, Transverse view of abdomen shows absent fetal stomach in second-trimester fetus with **trisomy 13. B,** Third-trimester fetus with absent stomach and **polyhydramnios. C,** In a different fetus, coronal view of upper thorax shows a distended **esophageal pouch** *(arrow).*

TABLE 38-1. DIAMETER MEASUREMENTS OF FETAL STOMACH*

GESTATIONAL AGE (WK)	N	ANTEROPOSTERIOR (CM)	TRANSVERSE (CM)	LONGITUDINAL (CM)
13-15	15	0.4 ± 0.1	0.6 ± 0.2	0.9 ± 0.3
16-18	29	0.6 ± 0.2	0.8 ± 0.2	1.3 ± 0.4
19-21	17	0.8 ± 0.2	0.9 ± 0.2	1.6 ± 0.5
22-24	11	0.9 ± 0.3	1.8 ± 0.3	1.9 ± 0.6
25-27	14	1.0 ± 0.5	1.9 ± 0.5	2.3 ± 1.0
28-30	17	1.2 ± 0.3	1.6 ± 0.4	2.3 ± 0.5
31-33	18	1.4 ± 0.3	1.6 ± 0.4	2.8 ± 0.2
34-36	15	1.4 ± 0.4	1.6 ± 0.4	2.8 ± 0.9
37-39	16	1.6 ± 0.4	2.0 ± 0.4	3.2 ± 0.9

From Goldstein I, Reece EA, Yakoni S, et al. Growth of the normal stomach in normal pregnancies. Obstet Gynecol 1987;70:641.
*Data are presented as mean ±2 SD.

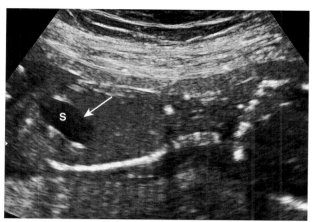

FIGURE 38-3. Dilated fetal stomach in the second trimester. In sagittal view the stomach is visible extending inferiorly into the pelvis. Although this fetus had a persistently dilated stomach during an anatomic survey, it resolved by the next ultrasound, and the fetus had a normal outcome.

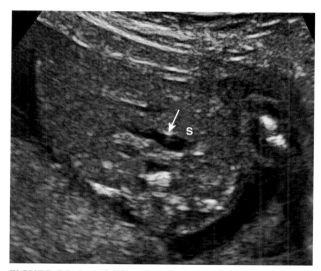

FIGURE 38-4. Midline fetal stomach in fetus with heterotaxy. Transverse view of the abdomen shows a midline stomach *(arrow).* This was the only abnormality seen at time of fetal survey; fetal echocardiogram revealed anomalous pulmonary venous return, and the diagnosis of heterotaxy was confirmed postnatally.

CMV-infected fetuses with additional anomalies.[24] In the largest series of pregnancy outcomes of isolated, prenatally diagnosed calcifications, both trisomy 21 and parvovirus were noted (each 3%).[24] Calcifications associated with vascular insult have also been reported. When hepatic calcifications are visualized, it is important to assess for any associated hepatic mass, for normal flow in the liver, for signs of infection, and for any structural or growth abnormalities. These calcifications in the hepatic parenchyma need to be distinguished from calcifications that line the liver and peritoneal cavity in fetuses with meconium peritonitis.

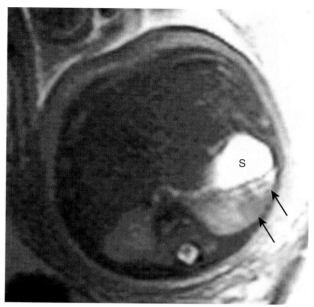

FIGURE 38-5. Polysplenia. Transverse MR image of fetus with complex congenital heart disease (not shown) with multiple splenules *(arrows)* in the left upper quadrant; *S,* stomach.

Hepatic or intra-abdominal masses can also be identified in utero. Solid masses include **hamartoma, adenoma,** and **hepatoblastoma.** Hypoechoic liver masses include **hepatic cyst** (Fig. 38-7, *A*), **hemangioma** (Fig. 38-7, *B*), and **abnormal myelopoiesis** in fetuses with trisomy 21.[25] Color flow Doppler ultrasound is recommended to distinguish vascular lesions. Vascular hepatic lesions have been noted to serve as vascular reservoirs, leading to high-output cardiac failure and fetal hydrops.[26-30] These vascular lesions include **hemangiomas, hemangioendotheliomas,** and **hepatoblastomas** and are associated with fetal hydrops. Therefore, following these fetuses sonographically with middle cerebral artery and ductus venosus Doppler imaging may be helpful because of the ability to predict fetal anemia of other etiologies.[31-42]

BILIARY SYSTEM

The normal fetal gallbladder is an oblong, echolucent structure in the anterior liver (Fig. 38-8), generally located 45 degrees to the right of midline and inferior to the umbilical vein. The gallbladder increases in size with gestational age.[43] In multiple series, visualization of the gallbladder was most common from 20 to 32 weeks.[44,45] Nonvisualization of the gallbladder is associated with **cystic fibrosis, gallbladder atresia,** and **biliary atresia.**[44,46] In a series of 578 fetuses, Hertzberg et al.[44] demonstrated the gallbladder between 12 and 40 weeks in 82.5%, but none of the fetuses with isolated nonvisualization of the gallbladder had any adverse neonatal outcome. Blazer et al.[45] reported on 29,749

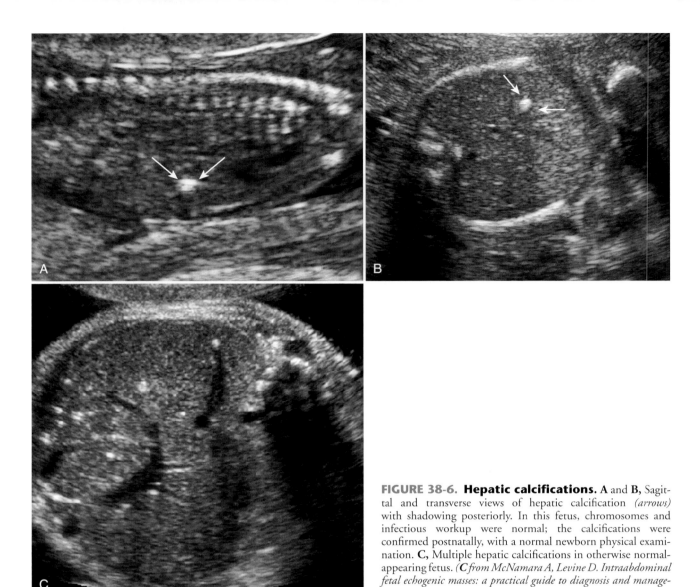

FIGURE 38-6. Hepatic calcifications. A and **B,** Sagittal and transverse views of hepatic calcification *(arrows)* with shadowing posteriorly. In this fetus, chromosomes and infectious workup were normal; the calcifications were confirmed postnatally, with a normal newborn physical examination. **C,** Multiple hepatic calcifications in otherwise normal-appearing fetus. *(C from McNamara A, Levine D. Intraabdominal fetal echogenic masses: a practical guide to diagnosis and management. Radiographics 2005;25:633-645.)*

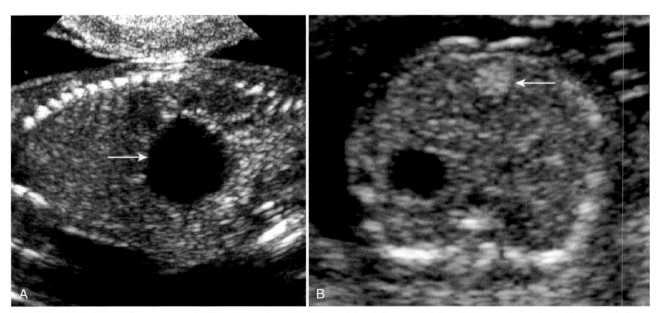

FIGURE 38-7. Hepatic masses. A, Hepatic cyst in sagittal view of the abdomen. **B,** Hepatic hemangioma *(arrow)* in 18-week fetus. *(B from McNamara A, Levine D. Intraabdominal fetal echogenic masses: a practical guide to diagnosis and management. Radiographics 2005;25:633-645.)*

consecutive pregnant women whose fetuses were imaged by both transabdominal and transvaginal sonography at 14 to 16 weeks for gallbladder detection. Maternal scans were repeated in 1 week if the fetal gallbladder was not seen on the initial examination. Of these, only 34 fetuses were identified with nonvisualization of the gallbladder (0.1%); all these women were offered amniocentesis for karyotype and cystic fibrosis screening. In 14 of these fetuses, other anomalies were identified. In the other 20 fetuses, the gallbladder nonvisualization was isolated, and all 20 had a normal karyotype and appeared normal after birth. Therefore, confirmation of a normal gallbladder is not considered a requisite of a detailed fetal anatomic survey.

Echodensities in the fetal gallbladder can be either sludge or gallstones. They are primarily seen in the third trimester.[47-49] **Gallstones** are generally reported to have acoustic shadowing (Fig. 38-9). If there is no shadowing, it is assumed that the echogenic debris represents **sludge,** a precursor of gallstones. In most cases, postnatal resolution occurs, and children are asymptomatic.

Enlarged gallbladder is associated with fetal aneuploidy, but all reported fetuses also had other prenatally visualized anomalies.[50]

Cystic lesions of the biliary tree have been identified in utero. These cysts may be anechoic, may have echogenic debris, or may represent a bilobed gallbladder. **Choledochal cysts** most often represent dilation of the common bile duct[51] (Fig. 38-10). There are numerous case reports of infrahepatic cystic masses representing both choledochal cysts and biliary atresias.[52-54] Although prenatal sonographic appearance is not diagnostic; two case series suggest that infrahepatic cysts with some echogenicity that enlarge in the third trimester are more likely to be choledochal cysts.[52,55]

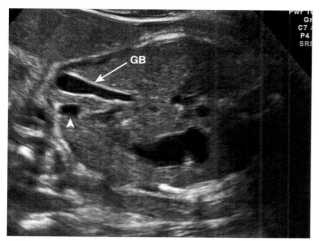

FIGURE 38-8. Normal gallbladder. Transverse view of a third-trimester fetal abdomen shows the gallbladder *(arrow)* as an elongated cystic structure to the right of the umbilical vein *(arrowhead).*

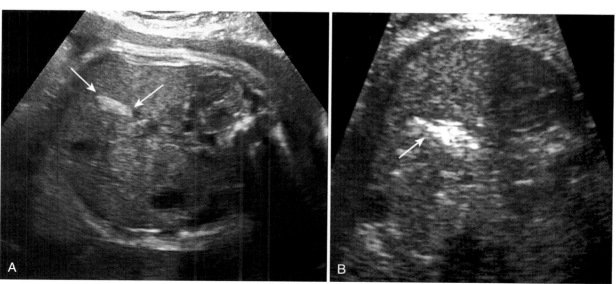

FIGURE 38-9. Gallbladder sludge and stones. A, Transverse third-trimester abdomen shows the lumen of the gallbladder surrounding echogenic material consistent with sludge. This fetus had a normal newborn course. **B,** A fetus with gallstones.

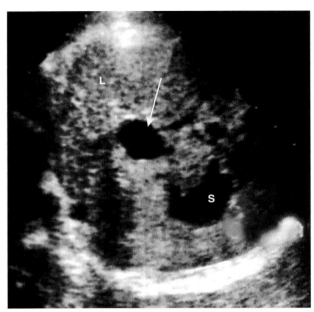

FIGURE 38-10. Choledochal cyst. Transverse view of abdomen shows a cyst *(arrow)* with stomach *(s)* on the left and liver *(L)* on the right.

PANCREAS

Pancreatic abnormalities reported prenatally include **polycystic pancreas**[56] and **annular pancreas.**[57] The diagnoses of annular pancreas were triggered by sonographic assessment for a dilated duodenum. Annular pancreas is associated with as many as 33% of fetuses with prenatally diagnosed duodenal atresias.[58]

SPLEEN

The fetal spleen can be visualized as an echogenic organ in the left upper abdomen, lateral to the spine and the upper renal pole. The relationship to the fetal stomach can vary (Fig. 38-1, *D*). Nomograms are available for splenic size from 18 weeks until term.[59,60] Abnormalities of the fetal spleen (asplenia or polysplenia) are associated with heterotaxy syndromes and warrant a detailed fetal cardiac examination. Splenomegaly in isoimmunized fetuses correlates to the severity of fetal anemia.[61] In addition, splenomegaly in utero has been reported due to viral infection.[62]

SMALL BOWEL AND COLON

In the first trimester and early in the second trimester, the small and large bowel appear somewhat heterogeneous, with echogenicity similar to but increased, compared to liver (see Fig. 38-1). Later in pregnancy, fluid can be seen in small bowel loops. Meconium can be seen in the colon. All GI atresias are thought to represent a failure of recanalization of the bowel lumen, which is a solid tube early in fetal life.

Duodenal Stenosis and Atresia

Dilation of the duodenum resulting from stenosis (obstruction) or atresia is the most common bowel obstruction in the fetus; occurring in 1 or 2 per 10,000 live births.[63-65] Of cases reported up through the 1990s, between 34% and 57% were diagnosed prenatally.[66-69] Other anomalies are usually involved; most notably, 30% to 44% have trisomy 21.[63,67] Familial cases of duodenal atresia have also been reported.[70] Duodenal atresia is also associated with anomalies of the VACTERL spectrum (vertebral abnormalities, anal atresia, cardiac abnormalities, TE fistula, renal agenesis, limb defects).[71,72]

Diagnosis of **duodenal stenosis** is most common in the third trimester. In the early second trimester, false-negative diagnoses as well as false-positives have been reported.[73,74] The infrequent diagnosis in the second trimester may be caused by the relatively small amount of swallowed amniotic fluid by the fetus at this time. In the early second trimester, the fetus normally swallows 2 to 7 mL of fluid, compared to 450 mL at term.[75] Duodenal obstruction may result from preampullary obstruction, a diaphragm or web causing partial or complete obstruction, or complete absence of a duodenal segment.[76-79]

The classic **"double bubble" sign** of a second echolucent mass medial to the stomach (in a transverse view of fetal abdomen) is considered diagnostic of duodenal obstruction. This image represents the dilated duodenum proximal to the atretic area. Because an abdominal fluid collection can have other etiologies, it is important to demonstrate a continuum between the stomach and the cystic mass. A prominent incisura angularis of the stomach may be mistaken for a "double bubble" if these are in different planes, but a careful real-time longitudinal examination of the stomach can eliminate this possibility. Apparent double-bubble sign is also associated with postnatal diagnoses of choledochal cyst and duodenal duplication cyst.[67,80] Second-trimester cases have resolved in pregnancy, with normal outcomes.[73,74] Double-bubble sign has been found the late second or the third trimester in fetuses with echogenic bowel, in both those with trisomy 21 and fetuses with normal karyotypes[81] (Fig. 38-11).

When **duodenal atresia** is suspected based on a "double bubble," the presence of polyhydramnios significantly increases the likelihood of a correct diagnosis. **Polyhydramnios** is frequently present in cases of duodenal atresia by the late second trimester,[66,82,83] but typically is absent in the early second trimester, at the time of routine fetal survey. In a European study of 138 cases of postnatally confirmed duodenal atresia, polyhydramnios was present in only 33%.[58] In this series, the

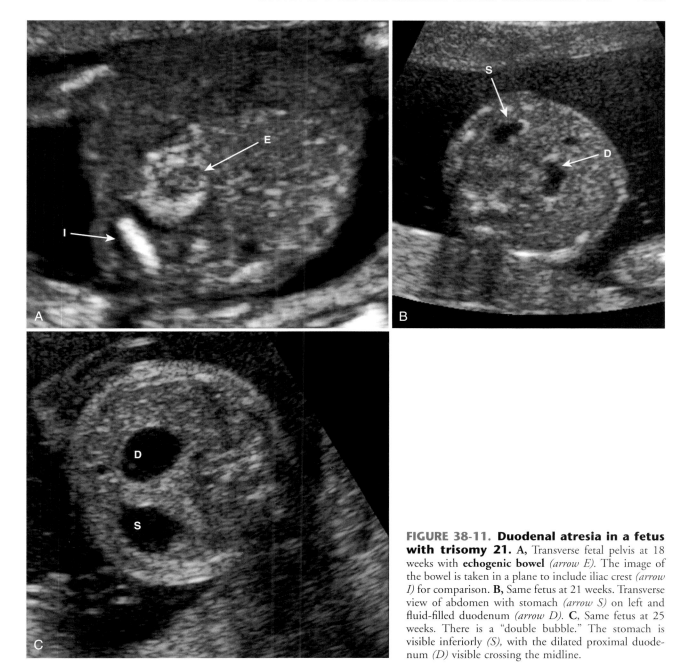

FIGURE 38-11. Duodenal atresia in a fetus with trisomy 21. A, Transverse fetal pelvis at 18 weeks with **echogenic bowel** *(arrow E)*. The image of the bowel is taken in a plane to include iliac crest *(arrow I)* for comparison. **B,** Same fetus at 21 weeks. Transverse view of abdomen with stomach *(arrow S)* on left and fluid-filled duodenum *(arrow D)*. **C,** Same fetus at 25 weeks. There is a "double bubble." The stomach is visible inferiorly *(S)*, with the dilated proximal duodenum *(D)* visible crossing the midline.

pregnancies with polyhydramnios were also more likely to be born preterm. Finding the double-bubble sign should trigger genetic counseling and consideration of amniocentesis because of the association with trisomy 21. Careful renal and cardiac testing should be performed, including fetal echocardiography.

Jejunal and Ileal Atresias

The prevalence of **jejunoileal atresias** (usually reported together) range from .54 to 1.11 cases per 10,000 live births.[84] Jejunal atresias are slightly more common (51%) than ileal.[85] The most common etiology hypothesized for jejunoileal atresias is isolated vascular compromise.[86] In animals, induced vascular compromise leads to isolated bowel atresias.[87] Jejunal atresias have been associated with nonbowel anomalies in up to 42% of cases, with ileal obstructions associated with nonbowel anomalies only in up to 2%.[58,88] Jejunal atresias, however, are more likely to be multiple and less often associated with in utero perforation than ileal atresias, likely because of the lower compliance of the ileum. **"Apple peel" jejunal atresia** is a subtype that involves agenesis of the mesentery, is more often familial,[58,89,90] and is likely of a

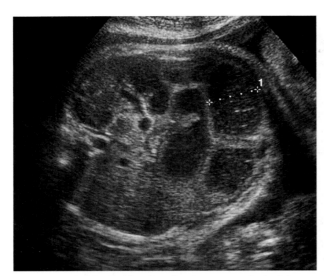

FIGURE 38-12. Ileal atresia. Transverse fetal abdomen with multiple dilated loops of bowel. The bowel lumen is measured in the largest transverse diameter *(calipers)*.

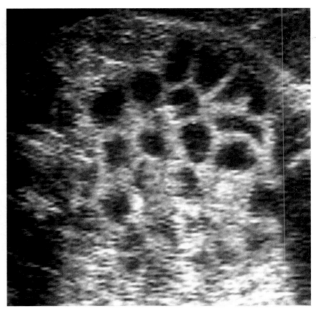

FIGURE 38-13. Hirschsprung disease. Note multiple dilated loops of bowel throughout the abdomen.

different etiology. **Cystic fibrosis** (CF) is a common underlying etiology for ileal obstruction, with or without meconium-increased echogenicity noted prenatally.[81,91] In ileal obstructions without meconium echogenicity, the frequency of CF in newborns is 6% to 8%.[92-94]

Diagnosis of **jejunoileal obstruction** is based on dilated loops of bowel, most frequently without a dilated stomach and sometimes with hyperperistalsis (Fig. 38-12). If peristalsis is not observed, dilated small bowel can be difficult to distinguish from dilated colon. The top normal lumen diameter used to diagnose bowel dilation is 7 mm.[81] The diagnosis of jejunoileal atresia is typically not made until late in the second trimester, when the bowel dilates. Polyhydramnios is less common in lower bowel obstructions than in duodenal atresia, not occurring in any reported ileal atresias,[95] but occurring in one third of jejunal atresias.[95]

Anorectal Atresias

Of the large colon atresias, anorectal atresia is the most common. The incidence is 0.8 to 4 per 10,000 live births.[96] Isolated cases of prenatal diagnosis of midcolon obstruction have also been noted.[97] **Anorectal malformations** have the highest incidence of associated anomalies of any of the GI atresias, 48% to 98%.[96,98,99] The associated abnormalities are chromosomal and genitourinary. Additionally, anal atresia is a part of the VACTERL sequence.[98-100] However, prenatal detection is not as high as for upper bowel obstructions, with anal atresia detected in only 7% to 24% of affected fetuses.[68,93,101]

In prenatally detected cases, there are dilated loops of small bowel or colon in the absence of polyhydramnios.[102,103] In a large series of neonates diagnosed postnatally with VACTERL association, none of the fetuses

with anorectal atresia were detected prenatally.[104] Because of the association of colonic obstruction with non-GI anomalies, a detailed fetal survey, fetal echocardiogram, genetic counseling, and discussion of aneuploidy risk should be included in the management of suspected cases in utero.

Megacystis and Microcolon

In **megacystis-microcolon–intestinal hypoperistalsis syndrome,** there is a distended bladder and at times a dilated small bowel. There is a 4:1 female predominance, which aids in distinguishing the large bladder associated with posterior urethral valves. Magnetic resonance imaging (MRI) can be helpful in identifying the microcolon.[105,106] **Hirschsprung disease** (congenital megacolon) can be detected in utero. In these cases, there are multiple dilated loops of bowel (Fig. 38-13). Hirschsprung disease or congenital aganglionosis of a segment of the colon can cause functional bowel obstruction.

Echogenic Bowel

Hyperechogenicity of the bowel is described when echoes of the bowel are as echogenic as the iliac crest with the ultrasound gain at the lowest gain, where bone looks white in the second trimester of pregnancy (Fig. 38-14; see also Fig. 38-11, *A;* **Video 38-1**). Use of a high-frequency probe (8 MHz) increases the frequency of interpreting fetal bowel as echogenic.[107] A low-frequency (≤5 MHz) probe should be used to confirm this finding.

When strict diagnostic criteria are used, the incidence of echogenic bowel in a general obstetrics population is 0.2% to 0.7%.[93,108] As the echogenicity of normal bowel

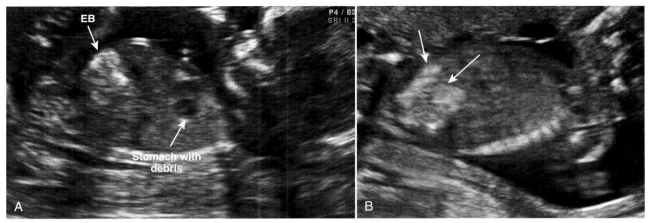

FIGURE 38-14. Echogenic bowel. A, Echogenic bowel *(arrow EB)* in a fetus with previously seen subchorionic hemorrhage. Note small amount of debris in stomach. **B,** Echogenic bowel *(arrows)* in fetus with **cytomegalovirus** infection.

ECHOGENIC BOWEL: COMMON ASSOCIATED RISKS

Aneuploidy
Cystic fibrosis
Swallowed fetal blood
Infection
Gastrointestinal atresias
Intrauterine growth restriction
Fetal demise

increases throughout pregnancy, the finding of echogenic bowel becomes normal in the third trimester. In particular, meconium in the colon can be seen normally as echogenic material in the third trimester.

Echogenic bowel is associated with numerous etiologies. In most cases the lumen of the bowel itself is later found to be normal. However, the in utero diagnosis is associated with fetal and placental abnormalities and an increased risk of poor pregnancy outcome, even when the second-trimester evaluation is otherwise normal. Because of these implications, an experienced sonographer must carefully evaluate the fetus and placenta and offer counseling and follow-up. In most fetuses with echogenic bowel in the second trimester, the bowel findings become normal as the pregnancy progresses. However, this should not eliminate the possibility of an abnormal pregnancy, because many of the associated complications do not occur until the third trimester.

Aneuploidy

The confirmation of hyperechoic bowel on second-trimester ultrasound requires careful evaluation of the fetus because of the association with chromosomal abnormalities. The most common abnormal karyotype is trisomy 21, but trisomies 13 and 18, 45,X, and triploidies have all been reported in fetuses with echogenic bowel.[109-113] In all series, fetuses with chromosomal abnormalities are likely to have other abnormal sonographic findings. The risk of aneuploidy in fetuses with echogenic bowel as an isolated finding is 1.4% to 5%.[109-113] Trisomy 21 is associated with GI dysfunction and dysmotility.[114] Thus, it is hypothesized that the dysmotility is the pathophysiologic cause of the echogenicity in aneuploid fetuses. However, most fetuses with trisomy 21 and echogenic bowel show no GI complication postnatally.[50]

Cystic Fibrosis

Echogenic bowel, meconium cysts, and peritonitis are the sonographic findings visible in the second trimester in fetuses with CF. With confirmed diagnosis of CF, the echogenic appearance of the bowel is caused by the biochemical alterations in the secretory-digestive-absorptive function of the small intestinal mucosa, leading to meconium obstruction in small bowel, primarily meconium ileus.[115] The incidence of CF in fetuses with isolated echogenic bowel varies from 1.3% to 5%.[108,116,117]

Swallowed Fetal Blood

Echogenic bowel has been noted in pregnancies complicated by vaginal bleeding, in those with asymptomatic subchorionic hemorrhage, and with the unexpected finding of new or old blood on amniocentesis performed for chromosomal analysis. In some fetuses with known second-trimester bleeding, the swallowed blood is visible in the fetal stomach on ultrasound, along with the hyperechoic bowel. In these fetuses it was concluded that the increased density of the swallowed blood causes the increased echogenicity. In a case series of pregnancies with isolated echogenic bowel undergoing amniocentesis, even pregnancies without evidence of bleeding and with normal-appearing amniotic fluid had evidence of blood in the fluid on spectrophotometry.[50] In one series, 19% of fetuses with isolated echogenic bowel had sonographic findings of intrauterine bleeding, of which 70% were confirmed to have intra-amniotic bleeding on amniocentesis.[118]

Fetal Viral Infection

Fetal viral infections including **cytomegalovirus** (CMV) and **parvovirus** infection are other associated etiologies of echogenic bowel. The range in incidence of viral infections in fetuses with echogenic bowel is 0.5% to 6.3%.[118-120] The etiology of the echogenic bowel in fetuses with viral infection is not known.

Later Diagnosis of Gastrointestinal Atresias

As previously noted, fetuses with trisomy 21 or CF and those with normal chromosomes and negative for CF have echogenic bowel as a second-trimester finding of a later-diagnosed GI atresia (see Fig. 38-11).

Intrauterine Growth Restriction and Fetal Demise

The risk of both intrauterine growth restriction (IUGR) and fetal demise increases in the second and third trimesters after the second-trimester diagnosis of echogenic bowel. Incidence is 10% for IUGR[116] and 5.8% to 15% for fetal demise.[116,121,122] Subchorionic hematoma is associated with IUGR and fetal demise,[123] and in some pregnancies, echogenic bowel may be the only clinical evidence of abnormal placentation, which could explain some of the poor outcomes in these fetuses.

Summary

Because of the association of echogenic bowel with fetal abnormalities, the following are recommended when echogenic bowel is identified in the second trimester: genetic counseling, consideration of karyotype, evaluation for fetal viral infection, and CF testing. In addition, regardless of whether the patient chooses amniocentesis, serial fetal growth ultrasound and antenatal testing should be done later in pregnancy.

MECONIUM PERITONITIS AND PSEUDOCYST

Meconium peritonitis is a result of in utero small bowel perforation and subsequent extrusion of meconium intraperitoneally. Calcifications can be seen in the peritoneum, outlining bowel or liver (Fig. 38-15). When the extruded meconium becomes walled off in the peritoneum and develops a heterogeneous cystic appearance,

MECONIUM PERITONITIS: NEED FOR POSTNATAL SURGERY (%)
Isolated calcifications: 0%
Calcifications and pseudocyst, ascites, or bowel dilation: 52%
Calcifications and two of pseudocyst, ascites, or bowel dilation: 80%
Calcifications, pseudocyst, ascites, and bowel dilation: 100%
Polyhydramnios and any of above findings: 69%

this is termed a **meconium pseudocyst** (Figs. 38-15, C, and 38-16). Associated ultrasound findings include ascites, polyhydramnios, and dilated bowel.[124,125] Both meconium ileus and meconium peritonitis are associated with CF in 8% to 40% of cases.[124,126] Meconium peritonitis has been classified to predict a postnatal surgical requirement.[127] The risk of need for postnatal surgery increases with the number of findings. Once meconium peritonitis or ileus has been diagnosed, serial fetal sonography in recommended. Because of the association with postnatally diagnosed fetal anomalies, delivery at a center with a neonatal intensive care unit (NICU) and pediatric surgery is suggested.

ENTERIC DUPLICATION CYST

Duplication cysts of the enteric tract are classified by the region of associated bowel, not by the histology of the mucosal lining.[128] The incidence is estimated at 1 per 10,000 infants.[129] Enteric duplication cysts may be associated with any area of the alimentary tract and can present in utero or postnatally as obstructions.[129,130] Associated anomalies occur in 30% of cases, most often gastrointestinal.[130] The majority of duplications are ileal.[130]

Gastric duplication cysts present at ultrasound as cystic or echogenic tubular structures with defined borders. They are classically anechoic and cystic, but at times are filled with echogenic material. The borders typically have double lumens[130] (Fig. 38-17; **Video 38-2**). Depending on the site of presentation, the differential diagnosis includes hepatic or choledochal cysts, bowel atresias, and ovarian cysts. Peristalsis of the cysts has been reported and can differentiate these masses from those of non-GI origin.[131] Postnatally, the standard treatment is surgical, because of the association with delayed obstructions.[129]

ABDOMINAL WALL

Embryology

The embryonic abdominal wall develops from the lateral plate mesoderm and endoderm in later embryonic

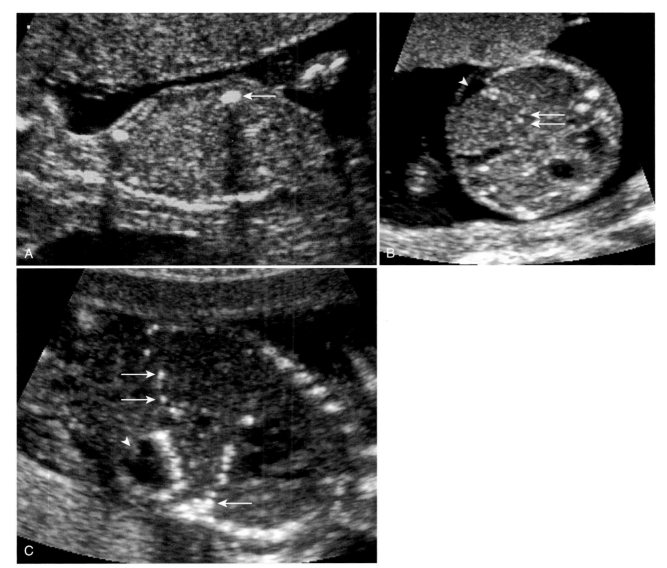

FIGURE 38-15. Meconium peritonitis. A, Sagittal view of fetus with a single calcification *(arrow)* in the abdomen with shadowing. **B,** Transverse view of the abdomen with multiple punctate calcifications *(arrows)* scattered within the fetal abdomen, without shadowing. Note the small amount of ascites *(arrowhead).* **C,** Oblique sagittal view of the torso shows multiple calcifications on the peritoneal surface of the liver in a fetus with a **meconium pseudocyst** *(arrowhead),* with an irregularly calcified wall. *(From McNamara A, Levine D. Intraabdominal fetal echogenic masses: a practical guide to diagnosis and management. Radiographics 2005;25:633-645.)*

development (days 16-26). Each lateral plate splits horizontally into the parietal and visceral mesoderm.[132] The space between these layers becomes the body cavity (**coelom** or celum).[5] The coelom differentiates into the peritoneal, pericardial, and pleural cavities. Normal development of the abdominal wall requires enfolding of the lateral plate around the coelom in several dimensions: caudally, cephalad, and laterally. In the normal enfolding process, the lateral folds come together before the normal gut rotation, leaving a physiologic gut herniation into the coelomic outpouching of the umbilical cord insertion[133] (Fig. 38-18). This herniation is usually visible on ultrasound from 9 to 11 weeks. In several large series of sequentially scanned fetuses, the bowel was no longer evident at the base of the umbilical cord in normal fetuses after 11 weeks.[7] Therefore, if prominent material is seen at the cord insertion site, and it is unclear whether it is caused by an abdominal wall defect or physiologic bowel herniation, a follow-up scan in 1 week will resolve the issue.

Abdominal wall defects include gastroschisis, omphalocele, ectopia cordis, cloacal exstrophy, and amniotic band syndrome (limb–body wall defects). The overall incidence of abdominal wall defects is 6.3 per 10,000 pregnancies.[134] Because of the loss of integrity in the epidermal covering, abdominal wall defects are associated with elevations of maternal serum alpha-fetoprotein (MS-AFP). In the last 3 decades, with both maternal serum screening and fetal anatomic surveys recommended and available in the second trimester, the majority of abdominal wall defects are diagnosed in the second trimester. Centers that practice universal first-trimester screening have documented confirmation of diagnoses before 14 weeks.[6,7] With increased access to early scanning in the United States, earlier diagnosis is expected to become more common.

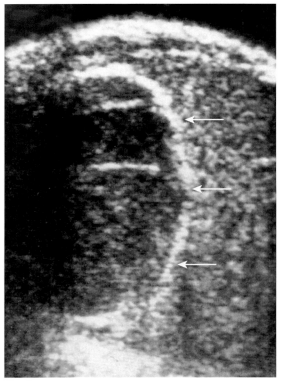

FIGURE 38-16. Meconium pseudocyst. Note cyst with debris with calcified rim *(arrows).*

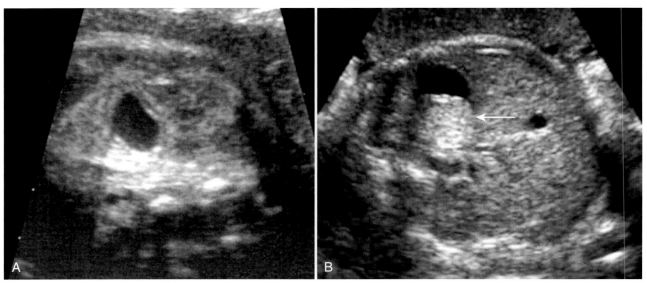

FIGURE 38-17. Enteric duplication cyst. A, Note the characteristic double line around the wall, which distinguishes a gut duplication from other abdominal cysts. **B,** Atypical appearance of gastric duplication cyst with echogenic material *(arrow).* Note how cyst impinges on stomach. (*B from McNamara A, Levine D. Intraabdominal fetal echogenic masses: a practical guide to diagnosis and management. Radiographics 2005;25:633-645.*)

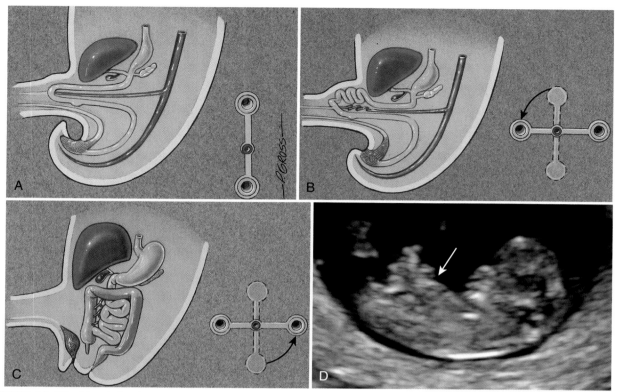

FIGURE 38-18. Physiologic gut herniation. A, Physiologic gut herniation into the coelomic outpouching of the umbilical cord insertion at 9 weeks. **B,** Ninety-degree rotation of the bowel at the axis of the superior mesenteric artery. **C,** At 12 weeks the bowel reverts to its intra-abdominal placement, undergoing an additional 180-degree rotation along the axis of the superior mesenteric artery. **D,** In a fetus at 11 weeks, prominent material is seen at the cord insertion site *(arrow)*. At 12 weeks this fetus was confirmed to have a normal abdominal cord insertion.

Gastroschisis

Gastroschisis is a full-thickness paraumbilical defect of the abdominal wall, most often right sided, although when diagnosed in later pregnancy, the paraumbilical location may be more difficult to demonstrate on prenatal ultrasound. Unlike omphalocele, free-floating loops of bowel in the amniotic fluid are the key finding on ultrasound. In population-based studies in Europe, Australia, and Japan, the incidence of gastroschisis has increased from 0.4 to 1.6 per 10,000 up to 1.4 to 4 per 10,000 live births during the last 25 years.[135-139] There is no gender predilection in the affected fetuses. There is a dramatically increased incidence in teenage mothers, with the largest population-based study showing a tenfold increased incidence in 15- to 19-year-old compared to 20- to 25-year-old women; the incidence in the 15- to 19-year-old age group also increased from 4.0 to 26.5 per 10,000 births.[136]

Particularly in young women, gastroschisis is associated with use of **tobacco, illicit drugs,** and **pseudoephedrine.**[135,136,139-141] Gastroschisis is infrequently associated with **aneuploidy** (0%-1.3%).[139,142-144] The risk of non-GI anomalies is also small, up to 3%.[142,143,145] Increased risk of preterm birth weight (<10%) and a relatively high stillbirth rate (4.5%-12%) have been

reported.[138,142,146] Associated GI abnormalities (atresias, stenosis, perforations, or volvulus) are common (11%-31%).[134,143,145] These anomalies are hypothesized to result from the requisite malrotation or nonrotation in the herniated bowel, often through a relatively small abdominal wall defect. Morbidity and mortality are more common in infants diagnosed postnatally with these complications.[134,145,146]

It is unknown whether one or more etiologies explain the abdominal wall defects in fetuses with gastroschisis. One theory cites isolated vascular compromise of the abdominal wall in the first trimester, which is supported by the increased relative risk in teenage mothers who use vasoactive substances. Other proposed etiologies include failed development of the mesoderm and the lateral mesodermal enfolding.[147] However, these do not account for the paramedian full-thickness defect.

The diagnosis is gastroschisis is relatively straightforward when the defect is limited, and free-floating loops of bowel are identified intra-amniotically. Most often the defect is paraumbilical, right sided (Fig. 38-19; **Video 38-3**), and limited. Less often the defect extends upward or laterally. Extended abdominal wall defects with free-floating bowel or liver are less common. Gastroschisis with inability to identify abdominal wall on prenatal

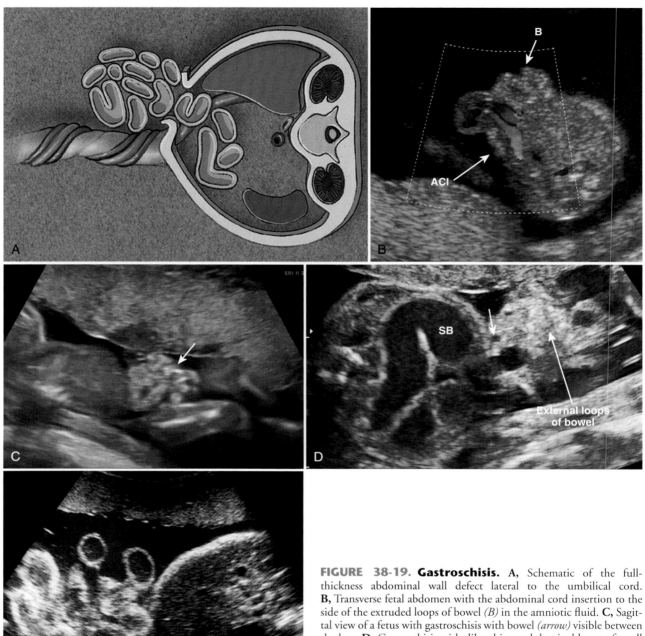

FIGURE 38-19. Gastroschisis. A, Schematic of the full-thickness abdominal wall defect lateral to the umbilical cord. **B,** Transverse fetal abdomen with the abdominal cord insertion to the side of the extruded loops of bowel *(B)* in the amniotic fluid. **C,** Sagittal view of a fetus with gastroschisis with bowel *(arrow)* visible between the legs. **D,** Gastroschisis with dilated intra-abdominal loops of small bowel *(SB)*. This fetus was born with torsion of loops of bowel at the cord insertion site, but they were able to be reduced without requiring bowel resection. **E,** Gastroschisis with dilated loops of bowel floating in the amniotic fluid.

ultrasound has a significantly poorer prognosis than the more common limited defects, with no survivors in one large series. First-trimester diagnosis is possible.[136,148]

Initial management of gastroschisis involves detailed sonographic fetal evaluation and genetic counseling. Although risk of aneuploidy is low, amniocentesis is not unreasonable; given the young age of most mothers, the low risk of aneuploidy is still above age-based risk expectation for this population. Care must be taken to assess if the borders of the defect can be delineated, looking for

the defect extending into the pelvis or up to the sternum. Gastroschisis is associated with IUGR, fetal demise,[149] and evolving GI obstructions or perforations, serial sonography is recommended to continue to evaluate fetal growth and evaluate the bowel. Dilated stomach and dilated loops of bowel, either within the fetal abdomen or within the amniotic cavity, can be identified.

The increased stillbirth rate has led to many series attempting to predict fetuses at risk for in utero demise or poor postnatal outcome and to help optimize timing

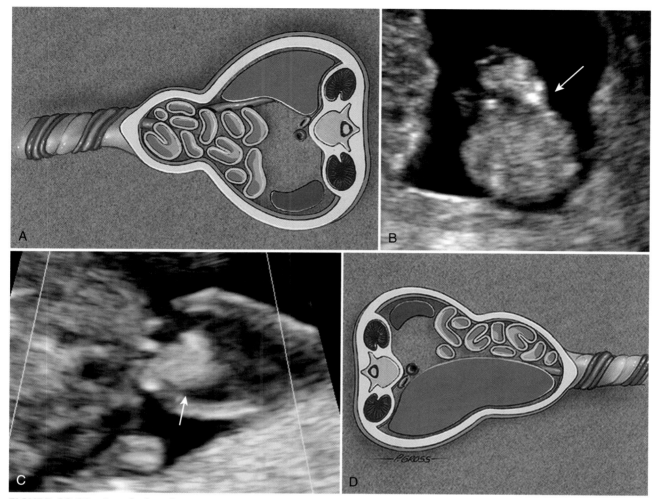

FIGURE 38-20. **Omphalocele. A,** Schematic of membrane covered omphalocele containing only bowel. **B,** Transverse abdomen with loop of bowel herniated into base of umbilical cord *(arrow)* at 13 weeks. **C,** Isolated loop of bowel in omphalocele sac. This is a small, small bowel–only omphalocele. The fetus had a karyotype of trisomy 18. **D,** Schematic of bowel and liver herniated into omphalocele sac.

Continued

of delivery. Some series have reported that a dilated fetal stomach is associated with both increased risk of fetal demise and postnatal morbidity.[146,150,151] Badillo et al.,[152] however, showed that the presence or absence of bowel findings failed to predict in utero or postnatal outcome. Loss of reactivity on fetal heart rate monitoring is a more reliable predictor of poor fetal outcome.[153] Due to concern that prolonged in utero exposure of the bowel to amniotic fluid may worsen outcomes, two trials looked at outcome in fetuses born preterm (average, 35 weeks) versus those delivered at term or for abnormal fetal testing.[154,155] Neither trial showed an improved outcome in preterm fetuses. Based on this information, although sonographic monitoring of the fetus is recommended throughout pregnancy, in addition to antenatal testing, preterm delivery is recommended only in cases of abnormal fetal testing, with or without growth delay.

Omphalocele

Omphalocele is a midline abdominal wall defect into which the abdominal contents are extruded. It is covered by amnion and peritoneum (Fig. 38-20). The incidence of omphalocele varies geographically, from 0.6 per 10,000 births in Japan[139] to 6 per 10,000 births in the British Isles.[143] British rates are also increased compared to European centers in the EUROCAT trials across the same time periods.[142,156] In contrast to gastroschisis, omphalocele is most common in women 35 to 40 years old.[139] Omphaloceles have a higher risk (10%-30%) of chromosome abnormalities than gastroschisis.[139,143] The most common aneuploidies are trisomies 13 and 18, with trisomy 21, 45,X, and triploidy being reported.[157,158] Fetuses with liver herniated into the omphalocele sac have a lower risk of chromosomal abnormality

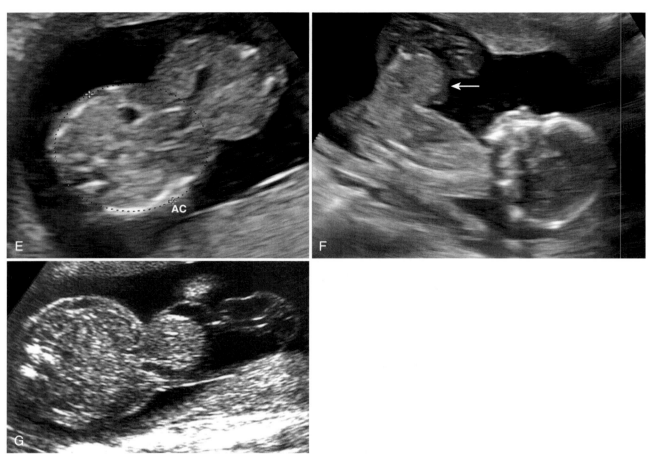

FIGURE 38-20, cont'd. E and **F,** Transverse and sagittal abdominal image of omphalocele with herniated liver and bowel. **G,** Omphalocele. It is difficult to tell if the material in the sac is liver and/or bowel.

than those with small bowel–only omphalocele (Fig. 38-20, *C*).

Omphalocele has a 55% to 58% risk of associated anomalies,[143,159] including midline defects (cardiac, clefting, and spinal/vertebral anomalies), clubfoot, and central nervous system anomalies.[159] Because of the common association with aneuploidies and multisystem anomalies, most published rates of pregnancy termination are high, potentially biasing outcome data. Inherited syndromes associated with omphalocele include autosomal dominant, autosomal recessive, and X-linked recessive.[160] Omphalocele is also part of several syndromes, most notably Beckwith-Weidemann (Fig. 38-21). **Beckwith-Weidemann syndrome** is associated with mutation or deletion of imprinted genes within the chromosome 11p15.5 region. Its hallmarks are omphalocele, macroglossia, and gigantism in the newborn.

The etiology of development of omphalocele is multifactorial when isolated.[161] Other hypotheses include the failure of closure of the lateral mesodermal folds.[162]

Identification of omphalocele in the second trimester is straightforward when close attention is paid to the abdominal cord insertion to ascertain that there is no evidence of bowel herniation into the base of the umbilical cord. In the first trimester, physiologic umbilical herniation can be mistaken for early omphalocele detection. This finding does not persist into the second trimester, so even small herniations into the umbilical cord (Fig. 38-20, *A-C*) are diagnostic of omphalocele in the second trimester. Liver can also be herniated into larger lesions (Fig. 38-20, *D-F*). Liver is never physiologically herniated, and if seen in the late first trimester, this should be considered abnormal. During the evaluation, attempts should be made to assess the boundaries of the abdominal wall lesion for appropriate parental counseling. The finding of fetal omphalocele should trigger a detailed fetal evaluation, including fetal echocardiography, because of the frequency of cardiac defects.[156] Genetic counseling is recommended, with consideration of fetal chromosomal evaluation. Serial fetal sonography should be performed, as well as fetal testing. Parents should be counseled about the risk of stillbirth.[139]

Ectopia Cordis

Ectopia cordis is a midline fetal defect with all or part of the heart extruded out of a sternal defect, with or without a membrane (Fig. 38-22). Whether part of an extended gastroschisis or omphalocele or an isolated finding, the

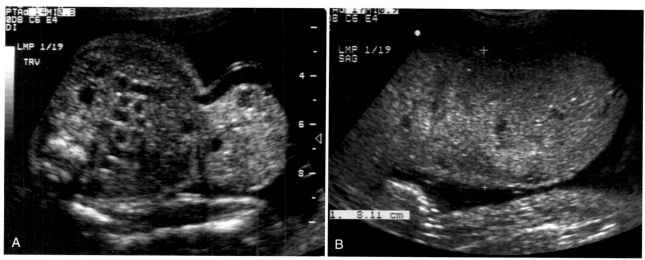

FIGURE 38-21. Beckwith-Weidemann syndrome. A, Transverse view of abdomen demonstrates an **omphalocele** *(calipers)*.
B, View shows an 8-cm-thick placenta, consistent with **placentomegaly.**

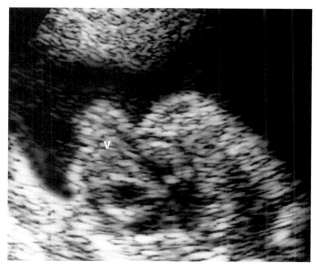

FIGURE 38-22. Ectopia cordis. Transverse color Doppler view of the fetal chest shows that the heart is outside the divergent sternum; *V,* ventricle. *(Courtesy Leo Drolshagen, MD, Fort Smith, Ariz.)*

et al.[167] proposed that these defects result from a developmental field disorder, which is now the accepted working hypothesis. Ectopia cordis therefore may be present independent of or associated with thoracoabdominal syndrome.

Amniotic Band Syndrome and Limb–Body Wall Complex

Amniotic band syndrome can affect any part of the fetus. If a band has disrupted development of the anterior abdominal wall, the defect can appear similar to a gastroschisis (Fig. 38-23). Extended and complex midline defects of the abdominal wall or thorax are generally categorized as **limb–body wall complex** or **body stalk anomaly.**[168] These defects are often one aspect of a fetus with multiple anomalies and are associated with limb or spinal defects, craniofacial defects, exencephaly, or encephaloceles. The incidence is 1.3 per 10,000 pregnancies at 11 to 14 weeks,[169] with spontaneous pregnancy loss leading to decreased incidence later in gestation and at birth. Many suggest that limb–body wall complex encompasses two subtypes of midline defects with entirely different etiologies.[170-175] The first type, phenotypically characterized by craniofacial defects, amnion bands, and adhesions, is caused by **vascular disruption** or **amnion rupture** in very early pregnancy. The second type has no craniofacial defects but rather urogenital anomalies (including cloacal and bladder exstrophies), anal atresia, and abnormalities of the placental attachment site, as well as persistence of the extra-embryonic coelom. This type is thought to be caused by **fetal maldevelopment.**

Sonographic diagnosis is suggested when there is extrusion of abdominal contents into amniotic fluid with the presence of a shortened and two-vessel umbilical

prognosis is poor, although survivors have been reported.[163] Trisomy 18 is associated with this diagnosis.[164,165] **Pentalogy of Cantrell** was first described as a combination of abnormalities, including diaphragmatic and ventral hernias, hypoplastic lung, and cardiac anomalies such as transposition of the great vessels and patent ductus arteriosus.[166] Later, geneticists recommended including fetuses or infants with ectopia cordis and other midline defects within this categorization. With this definition, prenatal diagnosis can only be suspected, and not confirmed in utero. The NCBI Online Mendelian Inheritance in Man (OMIM) registry recommends the term **thoracoabdominal syndrome** for the combinations of these disorders, now including other midline defects such as facial clefting and encephalocele. Martin

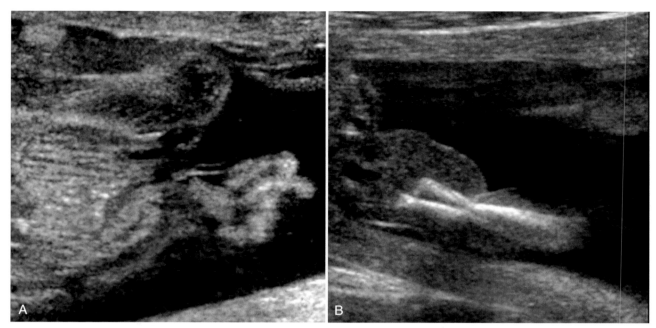

FIGURE 38-23. Amniotic band syndrome. A, Transverse view of abdomen shows anterior abdominal wall defect. **B,** View of lower extremity shows constriction ring caused by amniotic bands. The constellation of findings is consistent with amniotic band syndrome.

cord.[173] Oligohydramnios is common. Distinguishing the subtypes may not be possible because of the difficulty visualizing the fetal face. Fetal MRI may be helpful in illustrating these complex abdominal wall defects.[172,176] Although the subtypes have different developmental etiologies, the prognosis for both types, in the absence of amniotic fluid, is universally fatal.

Bladder Exstrophy

Bladder exstrophy–epispadias complex (BEEC) is defined in OMIM as the combination of infraumbilical abdominal defects, including the pelvis, urinary tract, and external genitalia.[177] Both familial and sporadic cases occur. The etiology is multifactorial; many fetuses have multisystem anomalies, including kyphoscoliosis, renal defects, and clubfoot.[178,179] There is no reported association with aneuploidy.

Sonographic diagnostic criteria include the presence of an infra-abdominal mass and inability to visualize a bladder. There is an inferiorly displaced umbilical cord, usually with a unilateral umbilical artery (Fig. 38-24). Neonatal outcome has low mortality, but repair of these defects is complex, often requiring staged procedures with a mixed outcome, to maintain continence and functional genital tissue.[180,181]

Omphalocele-Exstrophy–Imperforate Anus–Spinal Defects

Omphalocele-exstrophy–imperforate anus–spinal defects (OEIS) complex was formerly known as **cloacal exstro-**

phy (Fig. 38-25). This group of birth defects consists of omphalocele, exstrophy of the cloaca, imperforate anus, and spinal abnormalities. Genital abnormalities are also common.[182] This disorder is sporadic, occurring at a higher rate in monozygous than dizygous twins,[183] suggesting a vascular component.

The OEIS defects probably result from failure of fusion of the abdominal cloaca and exstrophy of the common cloaca that receives ureters, ileum, and a rudimentary hindgut. Additional findings occur in the genital tubercles and pubic rami, with incomplete development of the lower vertebrae. Imperforate anus, cryptorchidism, and epispadias occur in males, with anomalies of the müllerian duct derivatives in females, as well as a wide range of urinary tract anomalies, including renal agenesis.[161]

Criteria for sonographic diagnosis of OEIS are nonvisualization of the bladder associated with a visualized persistent cloaca, presence of an omphalocele, and spinal defects, typically neural tube defects or tethered cord. Single umbilical artery is a common associated finding. Although fetuses also have genital abnormalities, defining these in utero is difficult.[184]

Diagnosis of OEIS has been reported as early as 13 weeks.[95] Tiblad et al.[185] reported 100% diagnostic accuracy in the second trimester, although other series reported diagnostic difficulties differentiating from limb–body wall complex and pentalogy of Cantrell.[182,183,186] Once this diagnosis has been made, genetic counseling is suggested. In patients continuing pregnancy, amniocentesis may be considered to identify gender prior to birth.

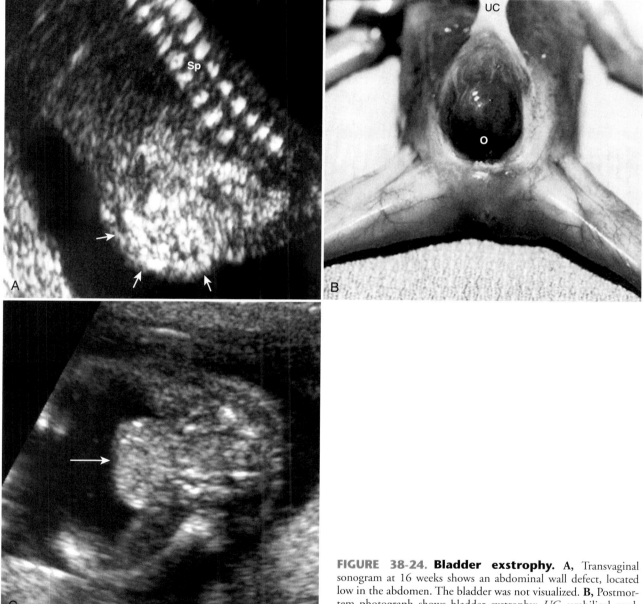

FIGURE 38-24. Bladder exstrophy. A, Transvaginal sonogram at 16 weeks shows an abdominal wall defect, located low in the abdomen. The bladder was not visualized. **B,** Postmortem photograph shows bladder exstrophy; *UC,* umbilical cord. **C,** Bladder exstrophy *(arrow)* in a different fetus.

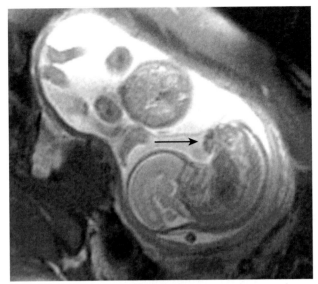

FIGURE 38-25. Omphalocele-exstrophy–imperforate anus–spinal defects (cloacal exstrophy). T2-weighted MR image of twins. The upper twin was normal with normal amniotic fluid. The lower twin had oligohydramnios with a lower anterior abdominal wall defect *(arrow)*.

CONCLUSION

A wide spectrum of abdominal abnormalities can be detected in utero. Appropriate description of these abnormalities is important to assess for associated structural abnormalities. Since many abdominal abnormalities are associated with aneuploidy and syndromes, genetic counseling is important. Follow-up for growth and assessment of interval progression of bowel obstruction in many abnormalities are also important.

Acknowledgments

Many thanks to Aaron and Evan Brown for their valuable technical support.

References

Embryology of the Digestive Tube

1. Fong GH, Rossant J, Gertensetein M, Breitman ML. Role of the Flt-1 receptor tyrosine kinase in regulating the assembly of vascular endothelium. Nature 1995;376:66-70.
2. Fukamachi H, Takayama S. Epithelial-mesenchymal interaction in differentiation of duodenal epithelium of fetal rats in organ culture. Experientia 1980;36:335-336.
3. Gannon M, Wright C. Endodermal patterning and organogenesis. In: Moody SA, editor. Cell lineage and fate determination. San Diego: Academic Press; 1999. p. 583-615.
4. Roberts D, Johnson RL, Burke AC, et al. Sonic hedgehog is an endodermal signal inducing Bmp-4 and Hox genes during induction and regionalization of the chick hindgut. Development 1995;121:3163-3174.
5. Gilbert S. Developmental biology. 6th ed. Sunderland, Mass: Sinauer; 2000.

Stomach

6. Blaas HG, Eik-Nes SH, Kiserud T, et al. Early development of the abdominal wall, stomach and heart from 7 to 12 weeks of gestation: a longitudinal ultrasound study. Ultrasound Obstet Gynecol 1995;6:240-249.
7. Carvalho MHB, Brizot ML, Lopes LM, et al. Detection of fetal structural abnormalities at the 11-14 week ultrasound scan. Prenat Diagn 2002;22:1-4.
8. McKenna KM, Goldstein RB, Stringer MD. Small or absent fetal stomach: prognostic significance. Radiology 1995;197:729-733.
9. Shaw-Smith C. Oesophageal atresia, tracheo-oesophageal fistula, and the VACTERL association: review of genetics and epidemiology J Med Genet 2006;43:545-554.
10. Torfs CP, Curry CJR, Bateson TF. Population-based study of tracheoesophageal fistula and esophageal atresia. Teratology 1995;52:1B-51B.
11. Houben CH, Curry JI. Current status of prenatal diagnosis, operative management and outcome of esophageal atresia/tracheo-esophageal fistula. Prenat Diagn 2008;28:667-675.
12. Stringer MD, McKenna KM, Goldstein RB, et al. Prenatal diagnosis of esophageal atresia. J Pediatr Surg 1995;30:1258-1263.
13. Goldstein I, Reese EA, Yarkoni S, et al. Growth of the fetal stomach in normal pregnancies. Obstet Gynecol 1987;70:645-656.
14. Cassart M. Sonographic prenatal diagnosis of malpositioned stomach as a feature of uncomplicated intestinal malrotation. Pediatr Radiol 2006;36:358-360.
15. Bartram U, Wirbelauer J, Speer CP. Heterotaxy syndrome: asplenia and polysplenia as indicators of visceral malposition and complex congenital heart disease. Biol Neonate 2005;88:278-290.
16. Lin JH, Chang CI, Wang JK, et al. Intrauterine diagnosis of heterotaxy syndrome. Am Heart J 2002;143:1002-1008.
17. Webber SA, Sandor GGS, Patterson MWH, et al. Prognosis in asplenia syndrome: a population-based review. Cardiol Young 1992;2:129-135.
18. Gilljam T, McCrindle BW, Smallhorn JF, et al. Outcomes of left atrial isomerism over a 28-year period at a single institution. J Am Coll Cardiol 2000;36:908-916.

Liver

19. Gross BH, Harter L, Filly R. Disproportionate left hepatic lobe size in the fetus: ultrasonic determination. J Ultrasound Med 1982;1:79-81.
20. Vintzileos AM, Neckles S, Campbell W, Andreoli J. Fetal liver ultrasound measurements during normal pregnancy. Obstet Gynecol 1985;66:477-480.
21. Stiller RJ, Herzlinger R, Siegel SDO, Whetham JCG. Fetal ascites associated with ABO incompatibility: case report and review of the literature. Am J Obstet Gynecol 1996;175:1371-1372.
22. Ceola AF, Angtuaco TL. Ultrasound case of the day. Radiographics 1999;19:1385-1387.
23. Stein B, Bromley B, Michlewitz H, et al. Fetal liver calcifications: sonographic appearance and postnatal outcome. Radiology 1995;197:489-492.
24. Simchen MJ, Toi A, Bona M, et al. Fetal hepatic calcifications: prenatal diagnosis and outcome. Am J Obstet Gynecol 2002;187:1617-1622.
25. Hamada H, Yamada N, Watanabe H, et al. Hypoechoic hepatomegaly associated with transient abnormal myelopoiesis provides clues to trisomy 21 in the third-trimester fetus. Ultrasound Obstet Gynecol 2001;17:442-444.
26. Foucar E, Williamson RA, Yiu-Chiu V, et al. Mesenchymal hamartoma of the liver identified by fetal sonography. AJR Am J Roentgenol 1983;140:970-972.
27. Horgan JG, King DL, Taylor KJW. Sonographic detection of prenatal liver mass. J Clin Gastroenterol 1984;6:277-280.
28. Platt LD, De Vore GR, Benner P, et al. Antenatal diagnosis of a fetal liver mass. J Ultrasound Med 1983;2:521-522.
29. Pott Bartsch EM, Paek BW, Yoshizawa J, et al. Giant fetal hepatic hemangioma: case report and literature review. Fetal Diagn Ther 2003;18:59-64.
30. Morris J, Abbott J, Burrows P, et al. Antenatal diagnosis of fetal hepatic hemangioma treated with maternal corticosteroids. Obstet Gynecol 1999;94:813-815.
31. Dukler D, Oepkes D, Seaward G, et al. Noninvasive tests to predict fetal anemia: a study comparing Doppler and ultrasound parameters. Am J Obstet Gynecol 2003;188:1310-1314.
32. Detti L, Mari G, Akiyama M, et al. Longitudinal assessment of the middle cerebral artery peak systolic velocity in healthy fetuses and

in fetuses at risk for anemia. Am J Obstet Gynecol 2002;187: 937-939.

33. Detti L, Oz U, Guney I, et al. Doppler ultrasound velocimetry for timing the second intrauterine transfusion in fetuses with anemia from red cell alloimmunization. Am J Obstet Gynecol 2001;185: 1048-1051.

34. Mari G. Middle cerebral artery peak systolic velocity for the diagnosis of fetal anemia: the untold story. Ultrasound Obstet Gynecol 2005;25:323-330.

35. Mari G, Deter RL, Carpenter RL, et al. Noninvasive diagnosis by Doppler ultrasonography of fetal anemia due to maternal red-cell alloimmunization. Collaborative Group for Doppler Assessment of the Blood Velocity in Anemic Fetuses. N Engl J Med 2000;342: 9-14.

36. Teixeira J, Duncan K, Letsky E, Fisk NM. Middle cerebral artery peak systolic velocity in the prediction of fetal anemia. Ultrasound Obstet Gynecol 2000;15:205-208.

37. Zimmerman R, Carpenter Jr RJ, Durig P, Mari G. Longitudinal measurement of peak systolic velocity in the fetal middle cerebral artery for monitoring pregnancies complicated by red cell alloimmunisation: a prospective multicentre trial with intention-to-treat. BJOG 2002;109:746-752.

38. Abdel-Fattah SA, Soothill PW, Carroll SG, Kyle PM. Noninvasive diagnosis of anemia in hydrops fetalis with the use of middle cerebral artery Doppler velocity. Am J Obstet Gynecol 2001;185:1411-1415.

39. Deren O, Onderoglu L. The value of middle cerebral artery systolic velocity for initial and subsequent management in fetal anemia. Eur J Obstet Gynecol Reprod Biol 2002;101:26-30.

40. Oepkes D, Seaward PG, Vandenbussche FP, et al. Doppler ultrasonography versus amniocentesis to predict fetal anemia. N Engl J Med 2006;355:156-164.

41. Scheier M, Hernandez-Andrade E, Carmo A, et al. Prediction of fetal anemia in rhesus disease by measurement of fetal middle cerebral artery peak systolic velocity. Ultrasound Obstet Gynecol 2004;23:432-436.

42. Moise KJ. The usefulness of middle cerebral artery Doppler assessment in the treatment of the fetus at risk for anemia. Am J Obstet Gynecol 2008;198:161-164.

Biliary System

43. Goldstein I, Tamir A, Weisman A, et al. Growth of the fetal gallbladder in normal pregnancies. Ultrasound Obstet Gynecol 1994;4: 289-293.

44. Hertzberg BS, Kliewer MA, Maynor C, et al. Nonvisualization of the fetal gallbladder: frequency and prognostic importance. Radiology 1996;199:679-682.

45. Blazer S, Zimmer EZ, Bronshtein M. Nonvisualization of the fetal gallbladder in early pregnancy: comparison with clinical outcome. Radiology 2002;224:379-382.

46. Bronshtein M, Weiner Z, Abramovici H, et al. Prenatal diagnosis of gallbladder anomalies: report of 17 cases. Prenat Diagn 1993;13: 851-861.

47. Brown DL, Teele RL, Doubilet PM, et al. Echogenic material in the fetal gallbladder: sonographic and clinical observations. Radiology 1992;182:73-76.

48. Suma V, Marini A, Bucci N, et al. Fetal gallstones: sonographic and clinical observations. Ultrasound Obstet Gynecol 1998;12: 439-441.

49. Kiserud T, Gjelland K, Bognø H, et al. Echogenic material in the fetal gallbladder and fetal disease. Ultrasound Obstet Gynecol 1997; 10:103-106.

50. Sepulveda W, Hollingsworth J, Bower S, et al. Fetal hyper-echogenic bowel following intra-amniotic bleeding. Obstet Gynecol 1994;83: 947-950.

51. Gallivan EK, Crombleholme TM, D'Alton ME. Early prenatal diagnosis of choledochal cyst. Prenat Diagn 1996;16:934-937.

52. Matsubara H, Oya N, Suzuki Y, et al. Is it possible to differentiate between choledochal cyst and congenital biliary atresia (type I cyst) by antenatal ultrasonography? Fetal Diagn Ther 1997;12:306-308.

53. Redkar R, Davenport M, Howard E. Antenatal diagnosis of congenital anomalies of the biliary tract. J Pediatr Surg 1998;33: 700-704.

54. Schroeder D, Smith L, Prain HC. Antenatal diagnosis of choledochal cyst at 15 weeks gestation etiologic implications and management. J Pediatr Surg 1989;24:936-938.

55. Casaccia G, Bilancioni E, Nahom A, et al. Cystic anomalies of biliary tree in the fetus: Is it possible to make a more specific prenatal diagnosis? J Pediatr Surg 2002;37:1191-1194.

Pancreas

56. Bronstein M, Reichler A, Borochowitz Z, et al. Early prenatal diagnosis of polycystic pancreas with narrow thorax and short limb dwarfism. Am J Med Genet 1994;49:6-9.

57. Pachì A, Maggi E, Giancotti A, et al. Ultrasound diagnosis of fetal annular pancreas. J Perinat Med 1989;17:361-364.

58. Dalla Vecchia L, Grosfeld J, West K, et al. Intestinal atresia and stenosis: a 25-year experience with 277 cases. Arch Surg 1998;133: 490-497.

Spleen

59. Schmidt W, Yarkoni S, Jeanty P, et al. Sonographic measurements of the fetal spleen: clinical implications. J Ultrasound Med 1985;4: 667-672.

60. Hata T, Kuno A, Dai SY, et al. Three-dimensional sonographic volume measurement of the fetal spleen. J Obstet Gynaecol Res 2007;33:600-605.

61. Oepkes DM, Robertjan H, Vandenbussche FP, et al. Ultrasonographic fetal spleen measurements in red blood cell–alloimmunized pregnancies. Am J Obstet Gynecol 1993;169:121-128.

62. Chaoui R, Zodan-Marin R, Wisser J. Marked splenomegaly in fetal cytomegalovirus infection: detection supported by three-dimensional power Doppler ultrasound. Ultrasound Obstet Gynecol 2002;20:299-302.

Small Bowel and Colon

63. Murshed RN, Spitz LG. Intrinsic duodenal obstruction: trends in management and outcome over 45 years (1951-1995) with relevance to prenatal counselling. BJOG 1999;106:1197-1199.

64. Bittencourt DB, Marba SR, Sbragia L. Congenital duodenal obstruction: does prenatal diagnosis improve the outcome? Pediat Surg Int 2004;20:582-585.

65. Fonkalsrud EW, DeLorimier AA, Hays DM. Congenital atresia and stenosis of the duodenum: a review compiled from the members of the surgical section of the American Academy of Pediatrics. Pediatrics 1969;43:79-83.

66. Cohen-Overbeek TE, Niemeijer ND, Hop WC, et al. Isolated or non-isolated duodenal obstruction: perinatal outcome following prenatal or postnatal diagnosis. Ultrasound Obstet Gynecol 2008;32: 784-792.

67. Romero R, Ghidini A, Costigan K, et al. Prenatal diagnosis of duodenal atresia: does it make any difference? Obstet Gynecol 1988; 71:739-741.

68. Stoll CA, Dott BY, Roth D. Evaluation of prenatal diagnosis of congenital gastrointestinal atresias. Eur J Epidemiol 1996;12: 1573-1584.

69. Haeusler M, Stoll A, Barisic C, Clementi I. Prenatal ultrasonographic detection of gastrointestinal obstruction: results from 18 European congenital anomaly registries. The EuroScan Study Group. Prenat Diagn 2002;22:616-623.

70. Poki H, Pitkin J. Double bubble, double trouble. Pediatr Surg Int 2005;21:428-431.

71. Quan L, Smith D. The VATER association: vertebral defects, anal atresia, T-E fistula with esophageal atresia, radial and renal dysplasia: a spectrum of associated defects. J Pediatr 1973;82:104-107.

72. Traubici J. The double bubble sign. Radiology 2001;220:463-464.

73. Zimmer EB. Early diagnosis of duodenal atresia and possible sonographic pitfalls. Prenat Diagn 1996;16:564-566.

74. Petrikovsky B. First-trimester diagnosis of duodenal atresia. Am J Obstet Gynecol 1994;171:569-570.

75. Grand RJ, Watkins JB, Torti FM. Development of the human gastrointestinal tract: a review. Gastroenterology 1976;70:790-810.

76. Calisti A, Oriolo L, Cozzi DA, et al. Prenatal diagnosis of duodenal obstruction selects cases with a higher risk of maternal-foetal complications and demands in utero transfer to a tertiary centre. Fetal Diagn Ther 2008;24:478-482.

77. De Silva NT, Young JA, Wales PW. Understanding neonatal bowel obstruction: building knowledge to advance practice. Neonatal Network 2006;25:303-318.

78. Grosfeld F. Duodenal atresia and stenosis: reassessment of treatment and outcome based on antenatal diagnosis, pathologic variance, and long-term follow-up. World J Surg 1993;17:301-309.

79. Touloukian R. Diagnosis and treatment of jejunoileal atresia. World J Surg 1993;17:1422-1423.

80. Malone FD, Crombleholme TM, Nores JA, et al. Pitfalls of the "double bubble" sign: a case of congenital duodenal duplication. Fetal Diagn Ther 1997;12:298-300.

81. Font GE, Solari M. Prenatal diagnosis of bowel obstruction initially manifested as isolated hyperechoic bowel. J Ultrasound Med 1998; 17:721-723.

82. Kimble RH, Kolbe AJ. Does gut atresia cause polyhydramnios? Pediatr Surg Int 1998;13:115-117.

83. Filkins LR, Flowers JW. Third trimester ultrasound diagnosis of intestinal atresia following clinical evidence of polyhydramnios. Prenat Diagn 1985;5:215-220.

84. Hemming V. Small intestinal atresia in a defined population: occurrence, prenatal diagnosis and survival. Prenat Diagn 2007;27:1205-1211.

85. Sai Prasad TR. Intestinal atresia. Indian J Pediatr 2000;67:671-678.

86. Komuro HA, Hori T, Hirai M, et al. Placental vascular compromise in jejunoileal atresia. J Pediatr Surg 2004;39:1701-1705.

87. Patricolo M, Noia G, Rossi L, et al. An experimental animal model of intestinal obstruction to simulate in utero therapy for jejunoileal atresia. Fetal Diagn Ther 1998;13:298-301.

88. Piper H, Alesbury J, Waterford S, Zurakowski D. Intestinal atresias: factors affecting clinical outcomes. J Pediatr Surg 2008;43:1244-1248.

89. Blyth H. Apple peel syndrome (congenital intestinal atresia): a family study of seven index patients. J Med Genet 1969;6:275-277.

90. Seashore J, Collins F, Markowitz R, Seashore M. Familial apple peel jejunal atresia: surgical, genetic, and radiographic aspects. Pediatrics 1987;80:540-544.

91. Irish MR, Karamanoukian HJ, Borowitz D, et al. Prenatal diagnosis of the fetus with cystic fibrosis and meconium ileus. Pediatr Surg Int 1997;12:434-436.

92. Casaccia G, Trucchi A, Nahom A, et al. The impact of cystic fibrosis on neonatal intestinal obstruction: the need for prenatal/neonatal screening. Pediatr Surg Int 2003;19:75-78.

93. Corteville J, Langer J. Obstetrics: bowel abnormalities in the fetus—correlation of prenatal ultrasonographic findings with outcome. Am J Obstet Gynecol 1996;175:724-729.

94. Chaudry G, Levine D, Oudjhane K. Abdominal manifestations of cystic fibrosis in children. Pediatr Radiol 2006;36:233-240.

95. Wax J, Hamilton T, Cartin A, et al. Congenital jejunal and ileal atresia: natural prenatal sonographic history and association with neonatal outcome. J Ultrasound Med 2006;25:337-342.

96. Cho SM, Fangman TS. One hundred three consecutive patients with anorectal malformations and their associated anomalies. Arch Pediatr Adolesc Med 2001;155:587-591.

97. Anderson NM, Robertson RT. Prenatal diagnosis of colon atresia. Pediatr Radiol 1993;23:63-64.

98. Jenetzky E. Prevalence estimation of anorectal malformations using German diagnosis related groups system. Pediatr Surg Int 2007;23:1161-1165.

99. Rich M, Brock W, Peña A. Spectrum of genitourinary malformations in patients with imperforate anus. Pediatr Surg Int 1988;3:120-123.

100. Martinez-Frias MB, Rodriguez-Pinilla EE. Anal atresia, vertebral, genital, and urinary tract anomalies: a primary polytopic developmental field defect identified through an epidemiological analysis of associations. Am J Med Genet 2000;95:169-173.

101. Brantberg AB, Haugen SE, Isaksen CV, Eik-Nes SH. Imperforate anus: a relatively common anomaly rarely diagnosed prenatally. Ultrasound Obstet Gynecol 2006;28:904-910.

102. Harris RN, Mack LD, Weinberger E. Anorectal atresia: prenatal sonographic diagnosis. AJR Am J Roentgenol 1987;149:395-400.

103. Taipale PR, Hiilesmaa VL. First-trimester diagnosis of imperforate anus. Ultrasound Obstet Gynecol 2005;25:187-188.

104. Tongsong TW, Piyamongkol WC, Sudasana J. Prenatal sonographic diagnosis of VATER association. J Clin Ultrasound 1999;27:378-384.

105. Veyrac C, Couture A, Saguintaah M, Baud C. MRI of fetal GI tract abnormalities. Abdom Imaging 2004;29:411-420.

106. Garel C, Dreux S, Philippe-Chomette P, et al. Contribution of fetal magnetic resonance imaging and amniotic fluid digestive enzyme assays to the evaluation of gastrointestinal tract abnormalities. Ultrasound Obstet Gynecol 2006;28:282-291.

107. Vincoff N, Smith-Bindman R, Goldstein R. Effect of ultrasound transducer frequency on the appearance of the fetal bowel. J Ultrasound Med 1999;18:799-803.

108. Al-Kouatly HB, Chasen ST, Streltzoff J, Chervenak FA. The clinical significance of fetal echogenic bowel. Am J Obstet Gynecol 2001; 185:1035-1038.

109. Scioscia AL, Pretorius DH, Budorick NE, et al. Second-trimester echogenic bowel and chromosomal abnormalities. Am J Obstet Gynecol 1992;167:889-894.

110. Nyberg DA, Resta RG, Mahony BS, et al. Fetal hyperechogenic bowel and Down's syndrome. Ultrasound Obstet Gynecol 1993; 3:330-333.

111. Strocker AS, Carlson DR, Greene N, et al. Fetal echogenic bowel: parameters to be considered in differential diagnosis. Ultrasound Obstet Gynecol 2002;16:519-523.

112. Goetzinger K, Dicke J, Macones G, Odibo A. Evaluating the incidence and likelihood ratios for chromosomal abnormalities in fetuses with common central nervous system malformations. Am J Obstet Gynecol 2008;199:285 e1-285 e6.

113. Leung WC, Waters JJ, Chitty L. Prenatal diagnosis by rapid aneuploidy detection and karyotyping: a prospective study of the role of ultrasound in 1589 second-trimester amniocenteses. Prenat Diagn 2004;24:790-795.

114. Antonarakis SE. The challenge of Down syndrome. Trends Mol Med 2006;12:473-479.

115. Eggermont E. Gastrointestinal manifestations in cystic fibrosis. Eur J Gastroenterol Hepatol 1993;8:731-738.

116. Ghose I, Martinez D, Harrison K, et al. Hyperechogenic fetal bowel: a prospective analysis of sixty consecutive cases. BJOG 2000; 107:426-429.

117. Monaghan K, Feldman G. The risk of cystic fibrosis with prenatally detected echogenic bowel in an ethnically and racially diverse North American population. Prenat Diagn 1999;19:604-609.

118. Yaron YH, Geva ES, Kupferminc M, et al. Evaluation of fetal echogenic bowel in the second trimester. Fetal Diagn Ther 1999; 14:176-180.

119. Simon-Bouy BS, Ferec CV, Malinge M, et al. Hyperechogenic fetal bowel: a large French collaborative study of 682 cases. Am J Med Genet 2003;121A:209-213.

120. Muller F, Dommergues M, Aubry M, et al. Fetus-placenta-newborn. Hyperechogenic fetal bowel: an ultrasonographic marker for adverse fetal and neonatal outcome. Am J Obstet Gynecol 1995;173: 508-513.

121. Sepulveda W, Nicolaidis P, Mai AM, et al. Is isolated second trimester hyperechogenic bowel a predictor of suboptimal fetal growth? Ultrasound Obstet Gynecol 1996;7:104.

122. Al-Kouatly HB, Chasen ST, Karam AK, et al. Factors associated with fetal demise in fetal echogenic bowel. Am J Obstet Gynecol 2001;185:1039-1043.

Meconium Peritonitis and Pseudocyst

123. Ball RA, Schoenborn J, Crane J. The clinical significance of ultrasonographically detected subchorionic hemorrhages. Am J Obstet Gynecol 1996;174:996-1002.

124. Konje J, de Chazal R, MacFadyen U, Taylor DJ. Antenatal diagnosis and management of meconium peritonitis: a case report and review of the literature. Ultrasound Obstet Gynecol 1995;6:66-69.

125. Foster MA, Nyberg DA, Mahony BS, et al. Meconium peritonitis: prenatal sonographic findings and their clinical significance. Radiology 1987;165:661-665.

126. Dirkes K, Crombleholme TM, Craigo SD, et al. The natural history of meconium peritonitis diagnosed in utero. J Pediatr Surg 1995; 60:979-982.

127. Zangheri G, Ciriello E, Urban G, et al. Fetal intra-abdominal calcifications from meconium peritonitis: sonographic predictors of postnatal surgery. Prenat Diagn 2007;7:960-963.

Enteric Duplication Cyst

128. Gross RE. Duplications of the alimentary tract. In: The surgery of infancy and childhood. Philadelphia: Saunders; 1953. p. 221-245.

129. O'Neil J, Rowe M, editors. Duplications of the gastrointestinal tract. St Louis: Mosby; 1995.

130. Richards D, Anderson C. The prenatal sonographic appearance of enteric duplication cysts. Ultrasound Obstet Gynecol 1996;7: 17-20.

131. Spottswood S. Peristalsis in duplication cyst: a new diagnostic sonographic finding. Pediatr Radiol 1994;24:344-345.

Abdominal Wall

132. Duhamel B. Embryology of exomphalus and allied malformations. Arch Dis Child 1963;38:142.

133. Hutchin P. Somatic anomalies of the umbilicus and anterior abdominal wall. Surg Gynecol Obstet 1965;120:1075.

134. Molik KG, West KC, Rescorla C, et al. Gastroschisis: a plea for risk categorization. J Pediatr Surg 2001;36:51-55.

135. Penman DF, Noblett HR, Soothill R. Increase in incidence of gastroschisis in the South West of England in 1995. BJOG 1998; 105:328-331.

136. Nichols CD, Pemberton PJ. Rising incidence of gastroschisis in teenage pregnancies. J Matern Fetal Med 1997;6.

137. Tan KH, Kilby MD, Whittle MJ, et al. Congenital anterior abdominal wall defects in England and Wales 1987-1993: retrospective analysis of OPCS data. BMJ 1996;313:903-906.

138. Reid KD, Doherty DJ. The epidemiologic incidence of congenital gastroschisis in Western Australia. Am J Obstet Gynecol 2003;189: 764-768.

139. Suita T, Yamamoto N, Handa Y, et al. Changing profile of abdominal wall defects in Japan: results of a national survey. J Pediatr Surg 2003;35.

140. Hume RF, Gingas JL, Martin LS, et al. Ultrasound diagnosis of fetal anomalies associated with in utero cocaine exposure: further support for cocaine-induced vascular disruption teratogenesis. Fetal Diagn Ther 1994;9:239-245.

141. Haddow JE, Palomaki GE, Holman MS. Young maternal age and smoking during pregnancy as risk factors for gastroschisis. Teratology 1993;47:225.

142. Barisic I, Clementi M, Häusler R, et al. Evaluation of prenatal ultrasound diagnosis of fetal abdominal wall defects by 19 European registries. Ultrasound Obstetr Gynecol 2001;18:309-316.

143. Rankin J, Dillon E, Wright C. Congenital anterior abdominal wall defects in the north of England, 1986-1996: occurrence and outcome. Prenat Diagn 1999;19:662-668.

144. Mastroiacovo PL, Castilla EA, Martinez-Frias M, et al. Gastroschisis and associated defects: an international study. Am J Med Genet 2003;143:660-670.

145. Snyder C. Outcome analysis for gastroschisis. J Pediatr Surg 1999;34.

146. Santiago-Munoz PM, Barber DD, Megison S, et al. Outcomes of pregnancies with fetal gastroschisis. Obstet Gynecol 2007;110: 663-668.

147. Feldkamp M, Carey JC, Sadler TW. Development of gastroschisis: review of hypotheses, a novel hypothesis, and implications for research. Am J Med Genet 2007;143:639.

148. Economides DB. First trimester ultrasonographic diagnosis of fetal structural abnormalities in a low risk population. BJOG 1998; 105:53-57.

149. Netta D, Wilson R, Visintainer P, et al. Gastroschisis: growth patterns and a proposed prenatal surveillance protocol. Fetal Diagn Ther 2007;22:352-357.

150. Bisulli M, Wood J, Visintine J, et al. Stomach dilatation may be associated with fetal demise in fetuses with isolated gastroschisis. Ultrasound Obstet Gynecol 2008;32:352.

151. Aina-Mumuney A, Blakemore K, Crino K, et al. A dilated fetal stomach predicts a complicated postnatal course in cases of prenatally diagnosed gastroschisis. Am J Obstet Gynecol 2004;190: 1326-1330.

152. Badillo A, Wilson R, Danzer E, et al. Prenatal ultrasonographic gastrointestinal abnormalities in fetuses with gastroschisis do not correlate with postnatal outcomes. J Pediatr Surg 2008;43.

153. Adair C, Frye A, Burrus R, et al. The role of antepartum surveillance in the management of gastroschisis. Int J Gynecol Obstet 1996; 52:141-144.

154. Logghe H, Thornton J, Stringer M. A randomized controlled trial of elective preterm delivery of fetuses with gastroschisis. J Pediatr Surg 2006;40:1726-1731.

155. Puligandla A, Flageole S, Bouchard E, et al. The significance of intrauterine growth restriction is different from prematurity for the outcome of infants with gastroschisis. Pediatr Surg Int 2004;39: 1200-1204.

156. Calzolari EB, Dolk HF, Milan M. Omphalocele and gastroschisis in Europe: a survey of 3 million births 1980-1990. EUROCAT Working Group. Am J Med Genet 1995;58:187-194.

157. Brantberg A, Blaas H, Haugen S, Eik-Nes S. Characteristics and outcome of 90 cases of fetal omphalocele. Ultrasound Obstet Gynecol 2005;26:527.

158. Henrich KH, Reingruber BH, Weber PG. Gastroschisis and omphalocele: treatments and long-term outcomes. Pediatr Surg Int 2008;24.

159. Blazer S, Zimmer E, Gover A, Bronshtein M. Fetal omphalocele detected early in pregnancy: associated anomalies and outcomes. Radiology 2004;232:191-195.

160. DiLiberti JH. Familial omphalocele: analysis of risk factors and case report. Am J Med Genet 1982;13:263-268.

161. Hamosh A, Amberger J, Bocchini C, et al. Omphalocele. In Online Mendelian Inheritance in Man, 2002, National Center for Biotechnical Information.

162. Kurkchubasche AG. The fetus with an abdominal wall defect. Med Health R 2001;84:159-161.

163. Falkensammer C, Altman C, Ge S, et al. Fetal cardiac malposition: incidence and outcome of associated cardiac and extracardiac malformations. Am J Perinatol 2008;25:277-281.

164. Fox JE, Gloster E, Mirchandani R. Trisomy 18 with Cantrell pentalogy in a stillborn infant. Am J Med Genet 1988;31:391-394.

165. Bick DM. Trisomy 18 associated with ectopia cordis and occipital meningocele. Am J Med Genet 1988;30:805-810.

166. Cantrell JR, Haller JA, Ravitch MM. A syndrome of congenital defects involving the abdominal wall, sternum, diaphragm, pericardium and heart. Surg Gynecol Obstet 1958;107:602-614.

167. Martin RAC, Erickson LC, Jones KL. Pentalogy of Cantrell and ectopia cordis, a familial developmental field complex. Am J Med Genet 1992;42:839-841.

168. Moerman P, Vandenberghe K, et al. Constrictive amniotic bands, amniotic adhesions and limb–body wall complex: discrete disruption sequences with pathologic overlap. Am J Med Genet 1992;42: 470-479.

169. Daskalakis G, Sebire J, Jurkovic D, et al. Body stalk anomaly at 10-14 weeks of gestation. Ultrasound Obstet Gynecol 1999;10: 416-418.

170. Deruelle P, Subtil D, Chauvet M, et al. Antenatal diagnosis of limb–body wall complex. J Gynecol Obstet Biol Reprod 2000;29: 395-400.

171. Evans JA, Vitez M, Czeizel A. Congenital abnormalities associated with limb deficiency defects: a population study based on cases from the Hungarian Congenital Malformation Registry (1975-1984). Am J Med Genet 1994;49:52-66.

172. Daltro P, Fricke BL, Kline-Fath BM, et al. Prenatal MRI of congenital abdominal and chest wall defects. AJR Am J Roentgenol 2005;184:1010-1016.

173. Ginsbe NE, Cadkin A, Strom C. Prenatal diagnosis of body stalk anomaly in the first trimester of pregnancy. Ultrasound Obstet Gynecol 1997;10:419-421.

174. Russo R, Angrisani P, Vecchione R. Limb–body wall complex: a critical review and a nosological proposal. Am J Med Genet 1993; 7:893-900.

175. Heyroth-Griffis CA, Weaver DD, Faught PW, et al. On the spectrum of limb–body wall complex, exstrophy of the cloaca, and urorectal septum malformation sequence. Am J Med Genet 2007; 143A:1025-1031.

176. Shinmoto H, Kuribayashi S. MRI of fetal abdominal abnormalities. Abdom Imaging 2003;28:877-886.

177. Gearhart JJ. Exstrophy-epispadias complex and bladder anomalies. In: Walsh PC, Vaughan ED, Wein AJ, editors. Campbell's urology. 7th ed. Philadelphia: Saunders; 1998.

178. Martinez-Frias ML, Bermejo E, Rodriguez-Pinilla E, Frias JL. Exstrophy of the cloaca and exstrophy of the bladder: two different expressions of a primary developmental field defect. Am J Med Genet 1999;99:261-269.

179. Mirk P, Calisti A, Fileni A. Prenatal sonographic diagnosis of bladder extrophy. J Ultrasound Med 1986;5:291-293.

180. Baird AD, Mathews RI, Gearhart JP. The use of combined bladder and epispadias repair in boys with classic bladder exstrophy: outcomes, complications and consequences. J Urol 2005;174 Pt 1: 1421-1424.

181. Borer JG, Gargollo PC, Hendren WH, et al. Early outcome following complete primary repair of bladder exstrophy in the newborn. J Urol 2005;174(Pt 2):1674-1678; discussion 678-679.

182. Keppler-Noreuil K, Gorton S, Foo F, et al. Prenatal ascertainment of OEIS complex/cloacal exstrophy: 15 new cases and literature review. Am J Med Genet 2007;143A:2122-2128.

183. Lam Y, Lee M, Tse H. Echogenic bowel in fetuses with homozygous β-thalassemia-1 in the first and second trimesters. Ultrasound Obstet Gynecol 1999;14:180-182.

184. Pajkrt E, Petersen OB, Chitty LS. Fetal genital anomalies: an aid to diagnosis. Prenat Diagn 2008;28:389-398.

185. Tiblad E, Wilson RD, Carr M, et al. OEIS sequence: a rare congenital anomaly with prenatal evaluation and postnatal outcome in six cases. Prenat Diagn 2008;28:141-147.

186. Kallen K, Castilla EE, Robert E, et al. OEIS complex: a population study. Am J Med Genet 2000;92:62-68.

CHAPTER 39

The Fetal Urogenital Tract

Katherine W. Fong, Julie E. Robertson, and Cynthia V. Maxwell

Chapter Outline

$\mathcal{E}$valuation of the fetal urogenital tract is an integral part of the obstetric ultrasound examination. Sonography depicts normal developmental anatomy and allows detection and characterization of many genitourinary abnormalities. In addition, assessment of the amniotic fluid volume often provides important prognostic information regarding fetal renal function. Accurate and early prenatal diagnosis is important because this may influence obstetric and neonatal management.

Urinary tract anomalies account for 33% of all malformations detected by routine prenatal sonography.[1] A systematic sonographic approach is proposed, which includes a search for associated anomalies and detailed evaluation of renal structure and function.

THE NORMAL URINARY TRACT

Embryology

The **permanent kidney** (metanephros) is the third in a series of excretory organs in the human embryo, forming after the pronephros and mesonephros.[2] In the seventh menstrual week, the metanephros begins to develop from two sources: the metanephric diverticulum (ureteric bud) and the metanephric mass of intermediate mesoderm (Fig. 39-1). The **ureteric bud** is an outgrowth from the mesonephric duct, near its entrance into the cloaca. It elongates and branches in a dichotomous pattern, giving rise to the ureter, renal pelvis, calyces, and collecting tubules. Through interaction with the metanephric mesoderm, the ureteric bud induces the formation of nephrons. In early embryonic life, the kidneys are located in the pelvis, but they "ascend" to their adult position by the 11th menstrual week. At this gestation, the kidneys start to produce urine.

By the ninth menstrual week, the **cloaca** (caudal part of hindgut) is divided by the urorectal septum into the rectum posteriorly and the urogenital sinus anteriorly (Fig. 39-1). The urinary bladder, the female urethra, and most of the male urethra develop from the urogenital sinus and the surrounding splanchnic mesenchyme. Initially, the bladder is continuous with the **allantois,** but this structure soon constricts and becomes a fibrous cord, the **urachus,** which extends from the apex of the bladder to the umbilicus.

Sonographic Appearance

In the **first trimester** the fetal kidneys are best examined by transvaginal sonography. The kidneys are seen as oval, hyperechoic structures in the paravertebral regions, with a small, central sonolucent area caused by fluid in the renal pelvis[3] (Fig. 39-2, *A*). By 12 to 13 weeks of gestation, the kidneys could be visualized in 99% of cases with combined transabdominal and transvaginal sonography.[4] In the **second trimester** the kidneys often appear as isoechoic structures adjacent to the fetal spine on

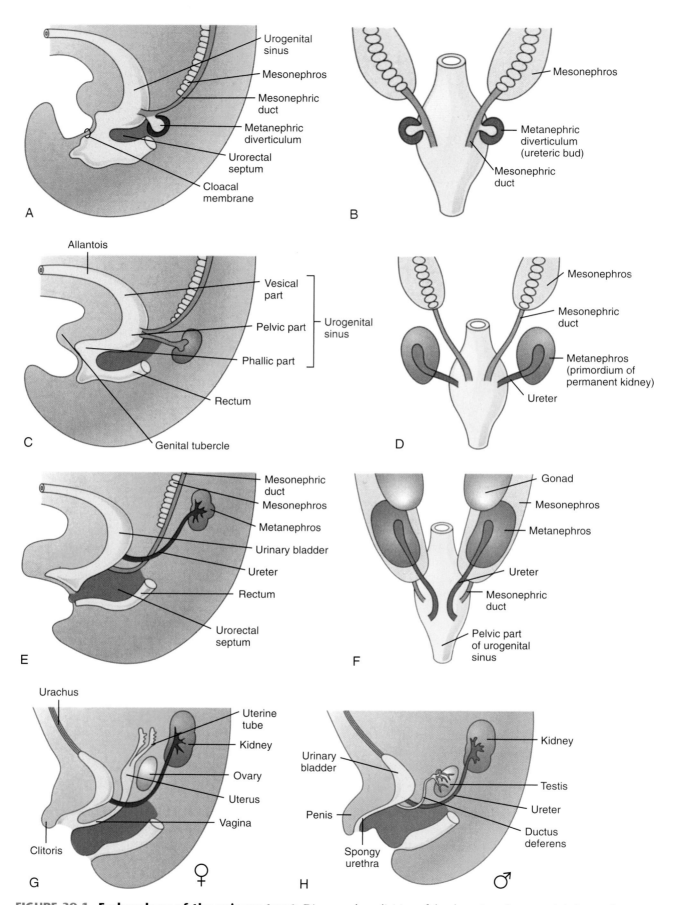

FIGURE 39-1. Embryology of the urinary tract. Diagrams show division of the cloaca into the urogenital sinus and rectum; absorption of the mesonephric ducts; development of the permanent kidneys (metanephroi), urinary bladder, urethra, and urachus; and changes in the location of the ureters. **A,** Lateral view of the caudal half of a 5-week-old embryo. **B, D,** and **F,** Dorsal views. **C, E, G,** and **H,** Lateral views. The stages shown in **G** and **H** are reached by the 12th week. *(From Moore KL, Persaud TVN: The developing human: clinically oriented embryology. 7th ed. Philadelphia, 2003, Saunders.)*

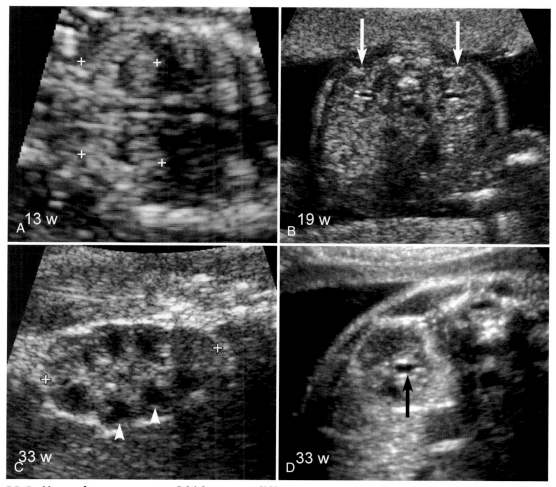

FIGURE 39-2. Normal appearance of kidneys at different gestational ages. A, Transvaginal scan at **13 weeks** of gestation in the coronal plane shows normal kidneys *(calipers)*, which appear hyperechoic, with small central sonolucent areas caused by fluid in the renal pelves. **B,** Transabdominal scan at **19 weeks** in the transverse plane shows the kidneys *(arrows)* as paired isoechoic structures adjacent to the fetal spine. **C** and **D,** Longitudinal and transverse scans at **33 weeks** show the kidney well outlined by perinephric fat, with normal corticomedullary differentiation. The pyramids *(arrowheads)* are hypoechoic. There is a small amount of fluid in the central collecting system *(black arrow)*.

transabdominal sonography (Fig. 39-2, *B*). As the fetus matures, corticomedullary differentiation becomes more obvious, especially in the third trimester (Figs. 39-2, *C* and *D*). The renal pyramids orient in anterior and posterior rows and are hypoechoic relative to the renal cortex. In the **third trimester** the renal cortex is isoechoic or slightly hyperechoic to liver and spleen. With fat deposition in the perinephric region, an echogenic border develops, and the kidney becomes better delineated. Normal fetal lobations are often visible and give the kidneys an undulating contour.

The kidneys grow throughout pregnancy. Table 39-1 provides a **nomogram of renal lengths** at 14 to 42 weeks of gestation.[5] The often-quoted rule of thumb that "renal length in millimeters approximates gestational age in weeks" only applies to a narrow gestational age range of 18 to 21 weeks. There are also published charts of renal anterior-posterior diameter, transverse diameter, and volume.[5] Sometimes, it is difficult to define the exact

renal borders, especially at the upper pole, because of shadowing from ribs or poor distinction from the adrenal gland. Fetal breathing can aid in renal visualization. It is also important to avoid using an oblique section through the kidney for measurement. The **renal/abdominal circumference** ratio remains constant at 0.27 to 0.30 throughout pregnancy.[6]

The calyces are not normally visualized, but some fluid is typically seen in the renal pelvis. The highly characteristic **renal pelvic echo** is often the key to finding the kidneys in the second trimester. Measurements of the renal pelvis are discussed in the section on hydronephrosis. The normal ureter is 1 to 2 mm in diameter and is not normally visible.

By using transvaginal sonography, the **bladder** can be seen as early as 11 weeks of gestation.[3] By 12 to 13 weeks, the bladder is visualized in 98% of cases using both transabdominal and transvaginal sonography.[4] The bladder is thin walled and situated anteriorly in the

TABLE 39-1. RENAL LENGTHS AT 14-42 WEEKS' GESTATION

WEEK	N	Fixed Centiles				
		3rd	10th	50th	90th	97th
14	3	7.5	8.0	9.3	10.8	11.6
15	3	8.8	9.5	11.0	12.8	13.7
16	2	10.2	11.0	12.7	14.8	15.8
17	12	11.6	12.5	14.5	16.8	18.1
18	10	13.1	14.1	16.3	18.9	20.3
19	15	14.6	15.6	18.2	21.1	22.6
20	15	16.1	17.2	20.0	23.2	24.9
21	15	17.5	18.8	21.8	25.4	27.2
22	14	19.0	20.4	23.6	27.4	29.4
23	16	20.4	21.9	25.4	29.5	31.6
24	17	21.8	23.4	27.1	31.5	33.8
25	18	23.1	24.8	28.8	33.4	35.8
26	20	24.4	26.2	30.4	35.3	37.8
27	24	25.6	27.5	31.9	37.1	39.7
28	18	26.8	28.7	33.4	38.7	41.5
29	19	27.9	29.9	34.7	40.3	43.2
30	19	28.9	31.0	36.0	41.8	44.8
31	23	29.9	32.1	37.2	43.2	46.3
32	23	30.8	33.0	38.3	44.5	47.7
33	22	31.6	33.9	39.4	45.7	49.0
34	19	32.4	34.7	40.3	46.8	50.2
35	20	33.1	35.4	41.1	47.8	51.2
36	23	33.7	36.1	41.9	48.7	52.2
37	14	34.2	36.7	42.6	49.4	53.0
38	17	34.7	37.2	43.2	50.1	53.8
39	13	35.1	37.6	43.7	50.7	54.4
40	14	35.4	38.0	44.1	51.2	54.9
41	26	35.7	38.3	44.5	51.6	55.4
42	17	36.0	38.6	44.8	52.0	55.7

From Chitty LS, Altman DG. Charts of fetal size: kidney and renal pelvis measurements. Prenat Diag 2003;23:891-897.

N = Number of fetuses for each week of gestation.

pelvis. The **umbilical** (superior vesical) **arteries** run lateral to the bladder as they course toward the umbilicus (Fig. 39-3). The hourly fetal urine production increases with advancing gestation, from a mean value of 4 to 5 mL/hr at 20 weeks to 52 to 56 mL/hr at 40 weeks.[7,8] Three-dimensional (3-D) ultrasound measurements demonstrate reproducible urine production rates based on bladder volumes, but tend to estimate higher rates in the third trimester compared to the standard two-dimensional (2-D) technique.[9,10] The **maximum bladder volume** increases from a mean value of 1 mL at 20 weeks to 36 mL at 41 weeks.[7] The normal bladder fills and empties (either partially or completely) approximately every 25 minutes (range, 7-43 min). Therefore, changes in bladder volume should be observed during the course of the obstetric sonogram.

Amniotic Fluid Volume

Evaluation of amniotic fluid volume (AFV) provides important information about fetal renal and placental function. Evaluation of AFV is a key component of fetal biophysical assessment. After 16 weeks, fetal urine production becomes the major source of amniotic fluid.[11] Several methods are used to assess AFV. Subjective assessment can be combined with semiquantitative techniques, such as measurement of the **largest single pocket** (free of umbilical cord and fetal small parts) and **amniotic fluid index** (AFI). Intraobserver and interobserver studies have shown that the subjective assessment of AFV by experienced sonographers is reliable.[12] Significant oligohydramnios results in compression of the fetus,

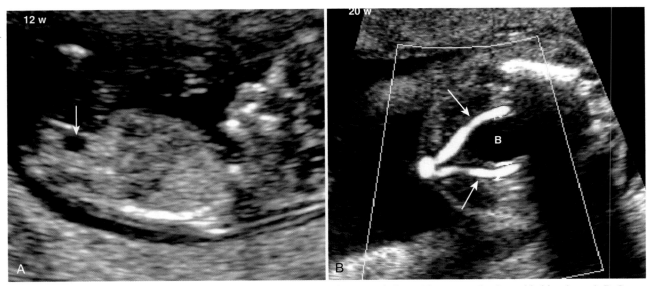

FIGURE 39-3. Normal urinary bladder. A, Sagittal image of a 12-week fetus. Note normal urinary bladder *(arrow)*. **B,** Power Doppler image of the umbilical arteries *(arrows)* at 20 weeks' gestation helps in the identification of any questionable fluid-filled structure in the pelvis as the urinary bladder *(B)*.

AMNIOTIC FLUID ASSESSMENT*

Vertical Depth
<2 cm   Oligohydramnios
2-8 cm   Normal
>8 cm   Polyhydramnios

*Largest single pocket method.

marked crowding of fetal parts, and poor definition of fetal interfaces. The following classification has been proposed for the largest single pocket method: vertical depth of the pocket less than 2 cm indicates moderate to severe oligohydramnios, 2 to 8 cm is normal, and greater than 8 cm indicates polyhydramnios.[13]

The AFI is obtained by measuring the vertical depth (mm) of the largest cord-free amniotic fluid pocket in the four quadrants of the uterus, and the sum of the four measurements is the index.[14,15] AFI varies with gestational age (Table 39-2). **Oligohydramnios** should be defined as more than two standard deviations (2 SD) below the mean for the specific gestational age, although the 5th centile value is recommended for screening. The AFI is a reproducible, objective method for amniotic fluid measurement.[15] It is useful for following AFV on serial examinations, particularly by multiple examiners of varying experience.

However, the semiquantitative methods have several technical and interpretative limitations.[16] If the fetus is active, fetal movement may rapidly change the size of pockets. A large pocket may be replaced by multiple small pockets between extremities. Measuring pockets filled with cord, or pockets with large vertical dimensions but small widths (<1 cm), leads to overestimation. It is recommended that when AFI is less than 10 cm, three measurements should be averaged.[15] The AFI is not a substitute for experience in assessment of AFV. A meta-analysis comparing the use of AFI versus the single deepest vertical pocket method as predictors of poor perinatal outcome failed to show an advantage of one method over the other.[17]

URINARY TRACT ABNORMALITIES

The prevalence of urinary tract malformations varies among studies, likely because of differences in study population and methods of surveillance. In a recent analysis of 709,030 births in 12 European countries, the prevalence of congenital malformations of the urinary tract was 1.6 per 1000 births.[18] The overall prenatal detection rate was high: 82% and 88.5% in two studies.[1,18] However, it varied from 36% to 100% in different centers.[18] Many factors could account for the variation of prenatal detection rates, including the study

TABLE 39-2. AMNIOTIC FLUID INDEX (AFI) VALUES IN NORMAL PREGNANCY

WEEK	AFI (MM)				
	2.5th	5th	50th	95th	97.5th
16	73	79	121	185	201
17	77	83	127	194	211
18	80	87	133	202	220
19	83	90	137	207	225
20	86	93	141	212	230
21	88	95	143	214	233
22	89	97	145	216	235
23	90	98	146	218	237
24	90	98	147	219	238
25	89	97	147	221	240
26	89	97	147	223	242
27	85	95	146	226	245
28	86	94	146	228	249
29	84	92	145	231	254
30	82	90	145	234	258
31	79	88	144	238	263
32	77	86	144	242	269
33	74	83	143	245	274
34	72	81	142	248	278
35	70	79	140	249	279
36	68	77	138	249	279
37	66	75	135	244	275
38	65	73	132	239	269
39	64	72	127	226	255
40	63	71	123	214	240
41	63	70	116	194	216
42	63	69	110	175	192

From Moore TR, Cayle JE. The amniotic fluid index in normal human pregnancy. Am J Obstet Gynecol 1990;162:1168-1173.

PRENATAL DIAGNOSIS OF URINARY TRACT ABNORMALITIES

Assessment of amniotic fluid volume
Localization and characterization of urinary tract abnormalities
Search for associated abnormalities

population (high risk vs. unselected), timing of the ultrasound scan, expertise of the operator, quality of the ultrasound equipment, extent of follow-up, and ascertainment of congenital anomalies. For major urinary tract anomalies, 57% were detected before 24 weeks.[1] Lethal urinary tract anomalies account for 10% of pregnancy terminations.[19]

A systematic approach to the prenatal diagnosis of urinary tract abnormalities includes assessment of amniotic fluid volume, localization and characterization of urinary tract abnormalities, assessment of fetal gender, and search for associated abnormalities.

Normal AFV in the second half of pregnancy implies at least one functioning kidney and a patent urinary conduit to the amniotic cavity. If **oligohydramnios** is present without a history of ruptured membranes, maternal drug intake (e.g., ACE inhibitors,[20] angiotensin II receptor antagonists,[21] COX-2 selective and nonselective inhibitors,[22] nonsteroidal anti-inflammatory drugs,[23] cocaine[24]), or evidence of intrauterine growth restriction (IUGR), urinary tract anomalies must be strongly suspected. In the setting of a urinary tract abnormality, normal AFV indicates a good prognosis. Oligohydramnios in the early second trimester carries a very poor prognosis because of the associated pulmonary hypoplasia. Occasionally and paradoxically, **polyhydramnios** may occur, especially with unilateral obstructive uropathy, with mesoblastic nephroma, or when there are concomitant abnormalities of the central nervous system (CNS) or gastrointestinal (GI) tract.

The following questions are helpful in defining and characterizing the urinary tract abnormality:

- Is the bladder identified and normal in appearance?
- Are kidneys present? Are they normal in position, size, and echogenicity? Are renal cysts identified?
- Is the urinary tract dilated? If so, to what degree, at which level, and what is the cause?
- Is the involvement unilateral or bilateral, symmetrical or asymmetrical?
- What is the fetal gender?

It is important to perform a detailed anatomic scan to search for associated abnormalities, which may indicate the presence of a syndrome or chromosomal abnormality. Renal anomalies may be part of the **VATER association** (vertebral defects, anal atresia, tracheoesophageal fistula, radial defects and renal anomalies). An expansion of this syndrome, **VACTERL,** includes cardiac and non-radial limb defects. When there are additional malformations, the risk for fetal chromosomal abnormalities is substantially increased compared to the maternal age-related risk: 30 times higher for multiple defects versus 3 times higher for isolated renal defect.[25]

In addition, renal ultrasound is recommended for parents (and siblings) of fetuses suspected to have certain renal abnormalities (polycystic kidney disease, renal agenesis or severe dysgenesis), because it may help to diagnose the type of polycystic kidney disease in the fetus, detect asymptomatic renal pathology in parents (and siblings), and counsel parents regarding the recurrence risk.[26,27]

Bilateral Renal Agenesis

Bilateral renal agenesis is a lethal congenital anomaly with an incidence of approximately 1 in 4000 births and a 2.5:1 male preponderance.[28] The ureteric bud fails to develop; nephrons do not form; no urine is produced; and severe oligohydramnios results. Pulmonary hypoplasia is the major cause of neonatal death. Other features of "Potter's sequence" include typical facies (beaked nose, low-set ears, prominent epicanthic folds, hypertelorism), limb deformities, and IUGR.

EVALUATION OF THE FETAL URINARY TRACT

Bladder
Presence
Appearance and size

Kidneys
Presence
Number
Position
Appearance (echogenicity, cysts)
Unilateral or bilateral

Collecting System
Dilation
Level of obstruction
Cause of obstruction
Unilateral or bilateral

Fetal Gender

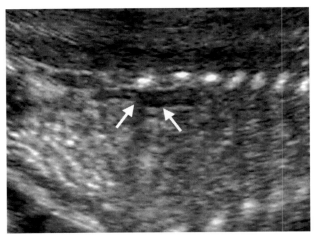

FIGURE 39-4. "Lying down" adrenal sign. Longitudinal scan through the renal fossa shows absence of the kidney and the flattened adrenal gland *(arrows)*. The lying-down adrenal sign is an indication of renal agenesis or ectopia.

The ultrasound findings include severe oligohydramnios and nonvisualization of the kidneys and bladder. Before 16 weeks' gestation, AFV is not dependent on urine production and may be normal despite absent renal function. The absence of fetal kidneys should be the most specific finding, but this may be difficult to document because of poor image quality associated with oligohydramnios. In addition, bowel or adrenal glands in the renal fossae may be mistaken for kidneys.[29] However, recognition of the distinctive, flattened appearance of the adrenal gland on longitudinal sonogram **("lying down" adrenal sign)** helps to confirm that the kidney did not develop in the flank[30] (Fig. 39-4).

Repeated and consistent nonvisualization of the urinary bladder (over 1 hour) is a secondary sign of

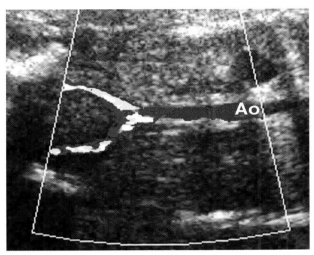

FIGURE 39-5. Absent renal arteries. Color Doppler ultrasound shows no renal artery arising from the aorta *(Ao)* in a fetus with bilateral renal agenesis.

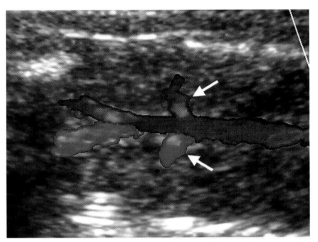

FIGURE 39-6. Normal renal arteries. Color Doppler ultrasound maps out the renal arteries bilaterally *(arrows)* in a 20-week fetus, confirming the presence of kidneys, which are poorly visualized on this image.

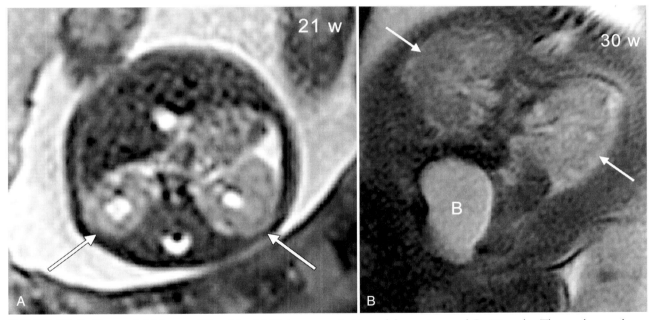

FIGURE 39-7. Normal kidneys. T2-weighted MR images at **A,** 21 weeks' gestation, and **B,** 30 weeks. The renal parenchyma *(arrows)* shows low to intermediate signal intensity. The renal collecting system and bladder *(B)* shows high signal intensity. *(A courtesy Sophia Pantazi, MD, Mount Sinai Hospital, Toronto; B courtesy Susan Blaser, MD, Hospital for Sick Children, Toronto.)*

bilateral renal agenesis. Conversely, identification of a normal bladder excludes this diagnosis. A small urachal diverticulum may mimic the bladder, but its lack of filling and emptying distinguishes it from the bladder. Furosemide challenge is not a useful test because it does not reliably distinguish between fetuses with renal agenesis and those with impaired renal function from other causes (e.g., IUGR).[31]

Other techniques have been proposed to improve visualization of fetal structures: intra-amniotic and intraperitoneal infusion of isotonic saline,[32] transvaginal ultrasound,[33] and color Doppler ultrasound imaging.[34,35]

The transvaginal probe is particularly useful in the second trimester and with breech presentation. Color Doppler imaging can be used to diagnose absent renal arteries, providing further evidence for the diagnosis of bilateral renal agenesis (Fig. 39-5). More importantly, it helps to map out the renal arteries in difficult cases of oligohydramnios, thereby confirming the presence of kidneys and avoiding confusion (Fig. 39-6).

Fetal magnetic resonance imaging (MRI) may help to identify the kidneys when sonographic visualization is limited by anhydramnios (or severe oligohydramnios) and large maternal body habitus[36,37] (Fig. 39-7).

BILATERAL RENAL AGENESIS

SONOGRAPHIC FINDINGS
Severe oligohydramnios
Absent kidneys
"Lying down" adrenal sign
Absent renal arteries on color Doppler imaging
Nonvisualization of bladder (over 1 hour)

TECHNICAL LIMITATIONS
Poor image quality caused by oligohydramnios
Fetal position (breech presentation)

PITFALLS IN INTERPRETATION
Amniotic fluid volume may be normal before 16 weeks' gestation.
Bowel or adrenal glands can be mistaken for kidneys.
Urachal diverticulum may mimic the bladder.
Empty bladder may be caused by impaired renal function from other causes.

However, the image quality of MRI is also affected by patient size and oligohydramnios, although to a lesser degree. Therefore, it may be difficult for MRI to exclude renal agenesis, if the kidneys are not seen before 24 weeks' gestation. Associated anomalies are quite common, including genital, cardiac, skeletal, and GI abnormalities.

In the majority of cases, bilateral renal agenesis is a multifactorial disorder. Parents should be counseled about two risks. First, the recurrence risk of having another child with bilateral renal agenesis is approximately 4%.[26,38] Second, parents and "unaffected" siblings have an increased risk of having silent genitourinary malformations; 9% of first-degree relatives have asymptomatic renal malformations, most often unilateral renal agenesis. Therefore, screening family members with renal ultrasound is recommended.[26]

Unilateral Renal Agenesis

Unilateral renal agenesis is three to four times more common than bilateral renal agenesis, occurring 1 in 1000 births.[2] It may be difficult to diagnose prenatally because AFV is normal and the bladder appears normal. A common pitfall is failure to image the renal fossa in the far field because of acoustic shadowing from the spine, especially in the transverse plane. Meticulous attention to technique is necessary (rotating the transducer, changing the maternal position, or repeated observations). If a kidney is not found in the renal fossa, most are either congenitally absent or ectopic.[39,40] The contralateral kidney may be enlarged because of compensatory hypertrophy.[41] There is a high incidence of contralateral renal abnormalities, the most common being

vesicoureteral reflux (VUR).[42] Unilateral renal agenesis may be associated with genital, cardiac, skeletal and GI abnormalities. Isolated unilateral renal agenesis has a good prognosis. Neonatal urologic workup is necessary, including a voiding cystourethrogram.

The recurrence risk to parents of a baby with isolated unilateral renal agenesis is about 1% if the parents have normal renal ultrasound. However, if one parent has a congenital solitary kidney, the risks to offspring are 7% for congenital solitary kidney and 1% for bilateral renal agenesis.[43]

Renal Ectopia

One or both kidneys may be in an abnormal position. The incidence of renal ectopia varies between 1:500 and 1:1200 births, with pelvic kidney being the most common form.[44] The ectopic kidney may be hypoplastic or dysplastic. When the renal fossa is empty, careful scanning may demonstrate the ectopic kidney adjacent to the bladder or iliac wing. Less frequently, the ectopic kidney is located on the opposite side of the abdomen relative to its ureteral insertion into the bladder, resulting in crossed renal ectopia with or without fusion. In most cases the crossed kidney fuses with the normally located kidney (cross-fused ectopia), and an enlarged bilobed kidney is seen. Renal ectopia is associated with a high incidence of urologic abnormalities, most often VUR. It may be associated with genital, skeletal, and GI abnormalities. Neonatal urologic workup is necessary, including renal ultrasound, technetium-99m succimer (⁹⁹ᵐTc DMSA) scan and a voiding cystourethrogram (in renal ectopia with pelvic dilation and in crossed renal ectopia).[45]

Horseshoe Kidney

Horseshoe kidney is the most common fusion anomaly of the kidney, occurring 1:400 to 1:500 births.[2,44] Prenatal sonographic findings include abnormal longitudinal axis of both kidneys and a bridge of renal tissue connecting the lower poles (Fig. 39-8). Despite its relative frequency, this disorder is seldom diagnosed because the findings are subtle, and surrounding bowel can obscure the fused isthmus. The majority of horseshoe kidneys have an abnormal anterior orientation of the renal pelvis bilaterally. Measurement of the renal pelvic angle on a true axial image of both kidneys is useful for diagnosis, and angles less than 140 degrees are highly suggestive of horseshoe kidney.[46] A horseshoe kidney is frequently associated with other anomalies (e.g., urogenital, cardiac, skeletal, CNS) and chromosomal abnormalities such as Turner syndrome, trisomy 18, and trisomy 9. Isolated horseshoe kidney is a relatively benign disorder that requires postnatal urologic follow-up because of higher prevalence of VUR, renal calculi, urinary tract infections (UTIs), and hydronephrosis.

Renal Cystic Disease

Renal cystic disease consists of a heterogeneous group of hereditary, developmental, and acquired disorders. Because of their diverse etiology, histology, and clinical presentation, a widely accepted classification does not exist. The Potter classification is based on histology and does not take into account recent advances in molecular biology and genetics.[47] A more recent approach is to group the abnormalities based on underlying cell biology, such as **aberrant early development** (with failure of induction between ureteric bud and metanephric mesenchyme) or defects in terminal maturation.[48] The aberrant early development group includes **dysplastic kidneys.** Typical histopathologic changes characterize renal dysplasia, including architectural distortion, metaplasia, and primitive glomeruli and tubules. Cystic changes are not universal but can be found in most forms of renal dysplasia.[49] Defects in terminal maturation are observed in polycystic kidney disease. Initial nephron and collecting duct formation is unremarkable in these kidneys, but cystic dilation of these structures occurs later, causing secondary loss of adjacent normal structures. We find the following classification simple and practical:

1. **Dysplastic cysts,** including the isolated multicystic dysplastic kidney and dysplastic kidney resulting from early severe obstruction.
2. **Hereditary cysts,** including polycystic kidney disease and the inherited syndromes.
3. **Nondysplastic nonhereditary cysts,** such as simple cysts.

Multicystic Dysplastic Kidney

A multicystic dysplastic kidney (MCDK) is the most common form of renal cystic disease in childhood and represents one of the most common abdominal masses in the neonate. The majority of cases are associated with an **atretic ureter** and **pelvoinfundibular atresia.** The kidney is replaced by multiple cysts of varying sizes. Between the cysts is a dense stroma, but usually no normal renal parenchyma. MCDK is almost always nonfunctional, so the prognosis depends entirely on the contralateral kidney. Multicystic renal dysplasia usually affects the whole kidney. However, it can be segmental and can occur in the portion of the duplex kidney supplied by the atretic ureter.

The sonographic findings correlate with the gross pathologic appearance. The malformed kidney is usually enlarged but may be normal or small. There are multiple cysts of varying sizes that do not communicate with each other and are randomly distributed (Fig. 39-9). Large peripheral cysts distort the reniform contour. The renal

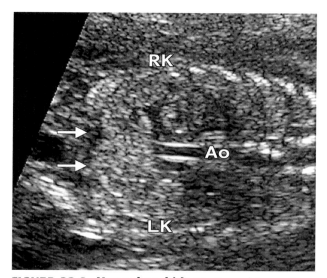

FIGURE 39-8. Horseshoe kidney. Coronal image shows the bridge of renal parenchyma *(arrows)* connecting the lower poles of the kidneys *(RK, LK)*, anterior to the aorta *(Ao)*.

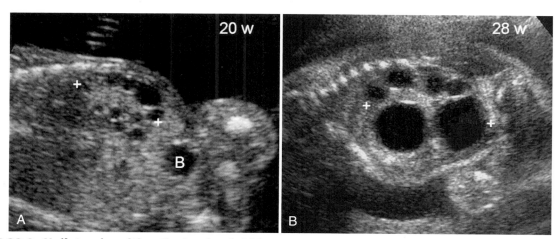

FIGURE 39-9. Unilateral multicystic dysplastic kidney. A, Image of the fetus at 20 weeks' gestation demonstrates multiple small cysts in a slightly enlarged kidney *(calipers); B,* bladder. **B,** Follow-up image at 28 weeks' gestation demonstrates a greatly enlarged kidney *(calipers).* Cysts have increased in size, do not communicate, and are randomly distributed.

pelvis and ureter are usually atretic and not visible. On color Doppler evaluation, the renal artery is either absent or very small. Occasionally, a MCDK with a large central cyst and small peripheral cysts can mimic hydronephrosis from ureteropelvic junction (UPJ) obstruction (see later discussion). In hydronephrosis, however, the dilated calyces are of uniform size and anatomically aligned and communicate with the dilated renal pelvis. The kidney usually maintains the reniform contour, with renal parenchyma present peripherally.

The appearance and size of the MCDK may change markedly over time (Fig. 39-9). On serial examinations, the kidney and its cysts may increase or decrease in size or may initially enlarge and later involute.[50] This variable appearance may result from residual renal function and progressive fibrosis.

Assessment of the contralateral kidney is very important. In utero, multicystic renal dysplasia is bilateral in 19% to 24% of cases[51,52] (Fig. 39-10). In unilateral multicystic renal dysplasia, 13% to 26% is associated with contralateral renal abnormalities, including renal agenesis and UPJ obstruction.[51,53] In fetuses with MCDK, severe oligohydramnios, and nonvisualization of the urinary bladder imply lethal renal disease, either bilateral MCDK or contralateral renal agenesis. Normal AFV is reassuring. If there is contralateral hydronephrosis, follow-up ultrasound is necessary to monitor any progressive dilation or oligohydramnios that may affect obstetric management. Unilateral MCDK, without associated renal or nonrenal abnormalities, is associated with a favorable outcome.[54] Because the incidence of VUR in the contralateral kidney can be up to 23%, prophylactic antibiotic therapy should be initiated soon after birth. A complete urologic workup is necessary, including a voiding cystourethrogram in the first month of life.[52]

The natural history of MCDK is toward spontaneous **involution.** This has been well documented both before and after birth.[50,52] The longer the duration of follow-up, the higher is the likelihood that the dysplastic kidney will disappear completely. The risk of developing hypertension and malignancy in MCDK is low.[55] However, there is still controversy regarding routine prophylactic nephrectomy.[53,56] Increasing evidence shows that the complication rates are similar between children who did and did not undergo neonatal nephrectomy.[56,57] Conservative management (long-term follow-up with serial ultrasound) is favored in most centers.[48,55,56] Most cases of MCDK are sporadic, with a low recurrence risk.

Obstructive Cystic Renal Dysplasia

Experimental work in lambs has shown that urinary obstruction in the first half of gestation produces renal dysplasia.[58,59] Unilateral disease can be caused by ureteropelvic or vesicoureteral junction obstruction. Bilateral disease is caused by severe bladder outlet obstruction, usually urethral atresia or posterior urethral valves. The severity of renal dysplasia is related to the timing and severity of obstruction to urine flow. The size of the kidneys varies from small, normal, to greatly enlarged. In some cases the enlargement is caused partly by the presence of cysts and partly by hydronephrosis. Cysts are usually present in the subcapsular area of the cortex. In a fetus with obstructive uropathy, the sonographic identification of **cortical cysts** is indicative of renal dysplasia (i.e., irreversible renal damage)[60] (Fig. 39-11). Dysplastic kidneys may also demonstrate increased echogenicity relative to the surrounding fetal structures, presumably from abundant fibrous tissue (Fig. 39-12). However,

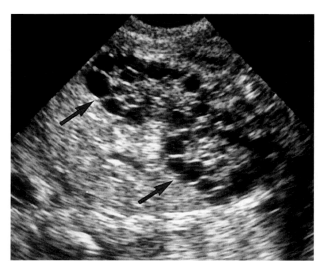

FIGURE 39-10. Bilateral multicystic dysplastic kidneys. Transvaginal image in a 16-week fetus demonstrates numerous small bilateral cysts *(arrows)* and no normal renal parenchyma. Note anhydramnios due to nonfunctioning kidneys.

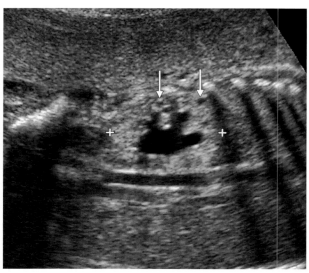

FIGURE 39-11. Obstructive cystic dysplasia. Coronal scan of fetus at 23 weeks with ureteropelvic junction obstruction shows increased echogenicity of the kidney *(calipers)* with small cortical cysts *(arrows),* indicative of irreversible renal damage.

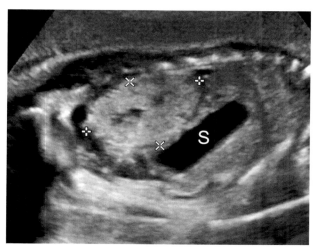

FIGURE 39-12. Echogenic dysplastic kidney. Longitudinal scan of fetus at 32 weeks with urethral obstruction. The kidney *(calipers)* demonstrates increased echogenicity, with no visible cysts. There is loss of corticomedullary differentiation. With severe chronic obstruction, the kidney becomes dysplastic and ceases to function. Note lack of pelvicaliectasis. *S,* Stomach.

increased cortical echogenicity is not a specific finding,[60,61] and a diagnosis of renal dysplasia cannot be made on the basis of increased parenchymal echogenicity alone. Furthermore, it is important to recognize that not all dysplastic kidneys have sonographically visible cysts or increased cortical echogenicity, so one cannot accurately predict the absence of renal dysplasia. Renal function relates directly to the degree of dysplasia, which determines the prognosis of patients surviving the perinatal period.

In general, if the obstruction is early and complete, the renal parenchymal findings will be predominantly macroscopic cysts and will simulate multicystic renal dysplasia. Sonographic distinction between MCDK and obstructive cystic renal dysplasia may be difficult, especially in the absence of hydronephrosis. In obstructive cystic renal dysplasia, recognizable parenchyma surrounds the relatively small cysts, whereas in MCDK, no normal renal parenchyma can be identified between cysts. Obstructive cystic renal dysplasia most often occurs with urethral obstruction. Therefore, sonographic evidence of urethral obstruction is helpful in suggesting the diagnosis. In addition, renal dysplasia from lower urinary tract obstruction frequently involves both kidneys, but bilateral MCDK occurs in only 19% to 24% of cases.[51,52]

Autosomal Recessive (Infantile) Polycystic Kidney Disease

Autosomal recessive polycystic kidney disease (ARPKD) involves both the kidneys and the liver. There is a wide clinical spectrum, which varies from the **perinatal form,** with severe renal disease, minimal hepatic fibrosis, and early death from pulmonary hypoplasia, to the **juvenile form,** with minimal renal disease, marked hepatic fibrosis, and longer survival. Diffuse dilation of the renal collecting tubules produces numerous 1-mm to 2-mm cysts, predominantly in the medulla. Both kidneys are enlarged, but a smooth contour is maintained. The cut surface has a spongelike appearance, with small cysts that tend to be arranged perpendicular to the renal capsule (Fig. 39-13).

Sonography reveals **bilateral reniform enlargement** of the kidneys (Fig. 39-13). There is poor delineation of the intrarenal structures. The numerous tiny cysts are usually smaller than the limit of sonographic resolution, but they create multiple acoustic interfaces, accounting for the characteristic increased renal echogenicity and loss of corticomedullary differentiation.[60,62] Sometimes, a peripheral hypoechoic rim may be seen, surrounding the centrally increased echogenicity. When renal function is abnormal, there is oligohydramnios, and the bladder is small or absent.

Autosomal recessive PKD may be diagnosed by ultrasound in the early second trimester based on the characteristic renal abnormalities, especially if the fetus is at risk.[63] However, because of the variability in expression and gestational age at onset, the kidneys may appear normal initially, only becoming abnormal later.[63,64] Thus, a normal sonogram in a fetus at risk for ARPKD does not exclude this disease, and prenatal diagnosis using sonography can be unreliable, especially in early pregnancy. Usually, but not always, ultrasound shows evidence of recurrent ARPKD by 24 to 26 weeks' gestation.[63,65] Couples who have a child with ARPKD have a 25% risk of having another affected child with each subsequent pregnancy. ARPKD is caused by mutation in the *PKHD1* gene, which has been mapped to **chromosome 6p,** allowing first-trimester genetic diagnosis in at-risk families.[66]

Autosomal Dominant (Adult) Polycystic Kidney Disease

Autosomal dominant polycystic kidney disease (ADPKD) is the most common of the hereditary renal cystic diseases. It is characterized by cyst formation in the kidneys and liver. Cysts may also be present in the pancreas, spleen, and CNS. In the early stage of the disease, only a small percentage of nephrons show cystic dilation. In the established adult disease, the kidneys are enlarged and contain multiple cysts of varying sizes.

Autosomal dominant PKD typically is not recognized in the fetal period because the kidneys typically appear normal. In rare cases, ADPKD can present during the fetal or neonatal period with symmetrically enlarged hyperechogenic kidneys, within which small cysts may be identified[67] (Fig. 39-14). The bladder is usually present, and AFV is often normal. In contrast to ARPKD, where corticomedullary differentiation is absent,[62] increased corticomedullary differentiation has

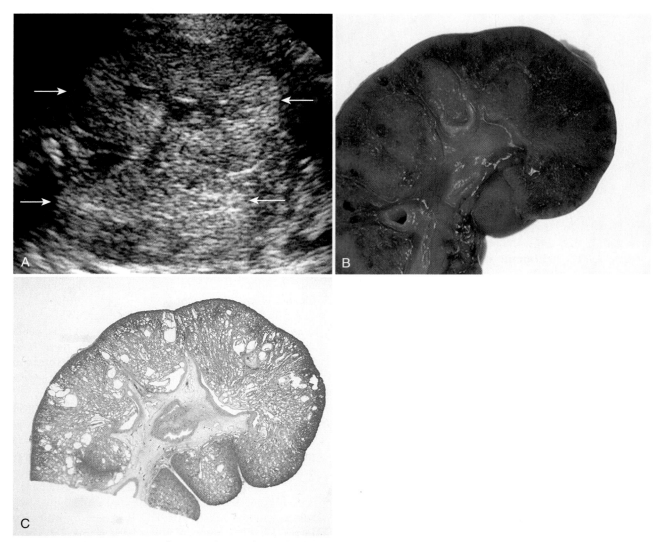

FIGURE 39-13. Autosomal recessive polycystic kidney disease. A, Coronal scan of a 27-week fetus shows enlarged kidneys with increased echogenicity *(arrows)*. Note anhydramnios. **B,** Photograph of cut surface of kidney shows a spongelike appearance. The small cysts are very difficult to see. **C,** Photograph of whole-mount section shows small cysts that tend to be arranged perpendicular to the renal capsule (hematoxylin and eosin stain). (**B** and **C** courtesy Sarah Keating, MD, Department of Pathology and Laboratory Medicine, Mount Sinai Hospital, Toronto.)

been reported in ADPKD (20 of 27 cases).[68] Only a few cases showed absent or decreased corticomedullary differentiation, and one case had normal corticomedullary differentiation. Since the kidneys may appear normal in the second trimester, follow-up scans are necessary in fetuses at risk for ADPKD.

A family history of ADPKD is critical in making the diagnosis of ADPKD in the fetus, because the recurrence risk is 50%. In one review, however, only 38% of the affected parents were aware of their disease before the diagnosis in the affected child.[67] Therefore, ultrasound of the parents' kidneys is necessary (Fig. 39-14, *D*). When there is a positive family history, prenatal diagnosis is possible.[69] ADPKD is caused by mutation in three genes, *PKD1, PKD2,* and *PKD3.* In 90% of cases, the condition is linked to the *PKD1* gene on **chromosome 16p.**

The prognosis for the fetus with ADPKD diagnosed by ultrasound is uncertain because of limited data on prenatal ultrasound findings and postnatal renal evolution.[70] The most useful indicator is the outcome of a previously affected sibling, because there is a high degree of correlation.[69] In the absence of a previously affected pregnancy, counseling may be based on the following data. Of 83 reported cases of ADPKD presenting in utero (excluding termination of pregnancy) or in the first few months of life, 43% died before 1 year.[69] Longitudinal follow-up studies of 24 survivors for a mean of 5 years showed that 67% developed hypertension, three of whom had end-stage renal failure at a mean age of 3 years.[71,72] More recently, a series of 26 consecutive cases demonstrated good prognosis in childhood, with 73% remaining asymptomatic, 19% with hypertension, and

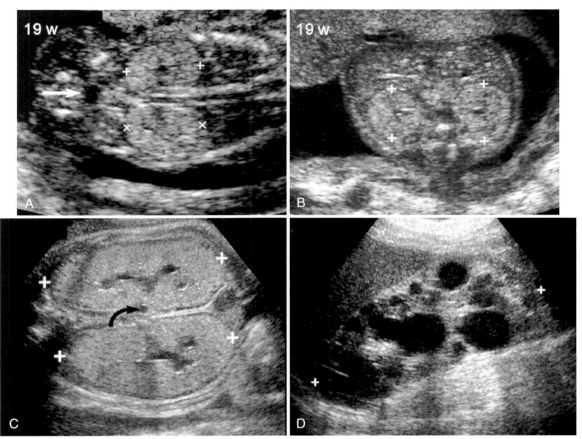

FIGURE 39-14. Autosomal dominant polycystic kidney disease. A and **B,** Coronal and transverse scans of 19-week fetus show slightly enlarged, echogenic kidneys *(cursors).* Note normal amniotic fluid volume and bladder *(arrow).* **C,** Coronal scan at 35 weeks shows greatly enlarged kidneys *(cursors).* They measure 9 cm in length, and multiple small cortical cysts *(curved arrow)* can be seen. **D,** Maternal autosomal dominant polycystic kidney disease. Classic ultrasound appearance of large kidney *(cursors)* with multiple cysts.

of which only two developed chronic renal insufficiency during the 5-year follow-up.[73]

Syndromes Associated with Renal Cystic Disease

A number of rare inherited syndromes and genetic and chromosomal disorders are associated with renal cystic disease.[74] Approximately 30% of fetuses with **trisomy 13** and 10% of fetuses with **trisomy 18** have cystic kidneys.

Meckel-Gruber syndrome is a lethal autosomal recessive disorder that carries a 25% risk of recurrence. It can be detected by sonography at 11 to 14 weeks' gestation, particularly in families with prior affected pregnancies.[75] Sonographic diagnosis requires identification of at least two features of the classic triad: **cystic dysplastic kidneys** (present in almost 100% of cases), **occipital encephalocele** (60%-85%), and **postaxial polydactyly** (55%)[76] (Fig. 39-15). During second-trimester sonography, it can be difficult to detect the encephalocele and polydactyly because of the presence of oligohydramnios. Microcephaly can be a useful clue to the presence of an encephalocele. The kidneys are usually

large and echogenic. Small, discrete cysts may be visible. The diagnosis of Meckel-Gruber syndrome is particularly important for counseling future pregnancies in families not previously known to be at risk.

Recent genetic studies reveal that individuals with renal cystic disease, other than ARPKD and ADPKD, have a high prevalence of *TCF2* gene anomalies, which code for the hepatocyte nuclear factor-1 beta (HNF-1β) transcription factor.[77,78] Individuals with these *TCF2* anomalies may also demonstrate abnormalities of the liver, pancreas, intestine and genital organs.

Hyperechogenic (Bright) Kidneys

Hyperechogenic or "bright" kidneys seen on prenatal ultrasound represent a diagnostic dilemma, particularly in the presence of normal AFV (Fig. 39-16). Fetal kidneys are considered hyperechogenic when they appear more echogenic than expected, compared with the adjacent liver or spleen. There is a wide differential diagnosis,[48,74] and the proposed algorithm is useful for evaluation of hyperechogenic kidneys[79] (Fig. 39-17). A detailed examination of the fetus is necessary to search

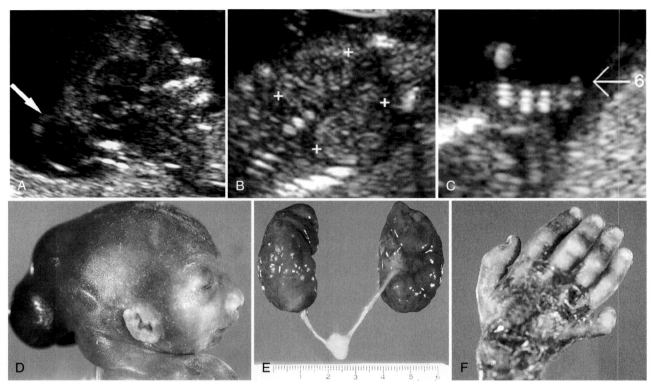

FIGURE 39-15. Meckel-Gruber syndrome. A to C, Ultrasound images of a 12-week fetus show classic features of Meckel-Gruber syndrome: an occipital encephalocele *(thick arrow)*, large echogenic kidneys *(cursors)*, and postaxial polydactyly *(thin arrow)*. **D to F,** Postmortem photographs of the fetus (at 18 weeks' gestation) demonstrate occipital encephalocele, large kidneys, and postaxial polydactyly.

SELECT SYNDROMES ASSOCIATED WITH RENAL CYSTIC DISEASE

Autosomal Dominant
Tuberous sclerosis
Von Hippel–Lindau disease (hemangioblastomas)

Autosomal Recessive
Bardet-Biedl syndrome (blindness, obesity, polydactyly)
Jeune syndrome (asphyxiating thoracic dystrophy)
Meckel-Gruber syndrome (encephalocele and polydactyly)
Short-rib polydactyly syndromes
Zellweger (cerebrohepatorenal) syndrome

X-Linked
Orofaciodigital syndrome type 1

Chromosomal
Trisomy 13
Trisomy 18

---

for associated abnormalities. If there is sonographic evidence of urinary tract obstruction, renal dysplasia is a possibility, especially when the kidneys are small or normal in size and there are peripheral cortical cysts.[61] When other malformations are detected, karyotyping is indicated to exclude aneuploidy (especially **trisomy 13**). If the kidneys and the biometric measurements are above the 95th centile, an overgrowth syndrome (Beckwith-Wiedemann syndrome, Perlman syndrome) should be considered. In both conditions, there is generalized organomegaly. AFV may be normal or increased. In **Beckwith-Wiedemann syndrome** there may be macroglossia and omphalocele. In **Perlman syndrome** there may be micrognathia and depressed nasal bridge.

In recent prospective and retrospective series of prenatally diagnosed, isolated, bilaterally enlarged hyperechogenic kidneys, the most common underlying diagnosis was ARPKD, followed by ADPKD.[80,81] Kidney size and AFI were the best predictors of perinatal outcome.[80] A detailed family history and an ultrasound examination of the parents' kidneys are important. In ADPKD, one parent has the disease, and sonography usually establishes the diagnosis. Normal AFV favors ADPKD. In ARPKD there is usually oligohydramnios, and there may be a previously affected sibling.

Other, less common causes of enlarged hyperechogenic kidneys include **Finnish nephrosis** (an autosomal recessive disorder that may be associated with elevated maternal serum alpha-fetoprotein levels), **renal vein thrombosis** (usually unilateral), **cytomegalovirus** (CMV) infection, **nephrocalcinosis,** and **bilateral renal tumors.** In many cases a definitive diagnosis will require postnatal investigations, including histology. Bilateral

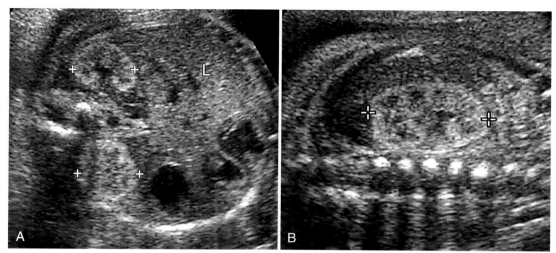

FIGURE 39-16. Hyperechogenic kidneys. A and B, Transverse and longitudinal scans of a 24-week fetus shows increased cortical echogenicity of both kidneys *(calipers),* more than expected when compared with liver *(L)* and increased corticomedullary differentiation. The kidneys are normal in size, and AFV is normal. Ultrasound at 32 weeks (not shown) showed similar findings. Postnatal ultrasound (not shown) on day 8 confirmed normal-sized kidneys with increased cortical echogenicity, and there were several tiny cortical cysts. Subsequent ultrasound scans showed increasing number of cysts. The child, now 3 years old, has normal renal function and blood pressure. Parents have normal kidneys. Genetic testing for ARPKD and *TCF2* was negative. Thus far, there is no definitive diagnosis for the polycystic kidney disease.

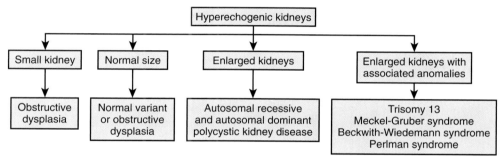

FIGURE 39-17. Algorithm for evaluation of hyperechogenic kidneys. *(Modified from Twining P: Genitourinary malformations. In Nyberg DA, McGahan JP, Pretorius DH, Pilu G, editors:* Diagnostic imaging of fetal anomalies. *Philadelphia, 2003, Lippincott–Williams & Wilkins.)*[7]

hyperechogenic kidneys that are normal in size with preservation of medullary pyramids, and that are associated with normal AFV, have a favorable outcome and may represent a normal variant.[61,82]

Simple Renal Cysts

Simple renal cysts have been reported in the fetus as early as 14 to 16 weeks' gestation.[83] Ultrasound usually shows a small, solitary, unilocular cyst near the periphery of the kidney. It should be differentiated from a cyst arising from structures close to the kidney, such as a duplication or mesenteric cyst. Most simple cysts resolve by 20 to 24 weeks' gestation. However, one study documented a simple renal cyst seen at 14 weeks that developed into a MCDK at 18 weeks.[83] Therefore, if simple cysts are seen in either the first or the second trimester, follow-up scans are indicated.

Renal Neoplasm

Congenital mesoblastic nephroma is the most common renal neoplasm in the fetus and newborn.[84] It is a benign hamartoma composed of mesenchymal tissue (spindle cells), as opposed to the epithelial tissue of Wilms' tumor. **Wilms' tumor** is a malignant lesion that is extremely rare in the fetus. Sonographically, mesoblastic nephroma is indistinguishable from Wilms' tumor. Mesoblastic nephroma is usually seen as a moderately echogenic, solid mass completely replacing the kidney or localized to part of the kidney[85] (Fig. 39-18). The mass may demonstrate increased vascularity and cystic components. **Polyhydramnios** is a frequent association[84] and may lead to preterm labor and preterm birth. Perinatal complications are likely, including acute fetal distress, neonatal hypertension, and hypercalcemia.[84]

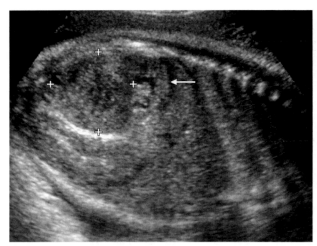

FIGURE 39-18. Congenital mesoblastic nephroma. Longitudinal scan of a 35-week fetus shows a large, heterogeneous solid mass *(calipers)* replacing most of the right kidney, except for the upper pole *(arrow).*

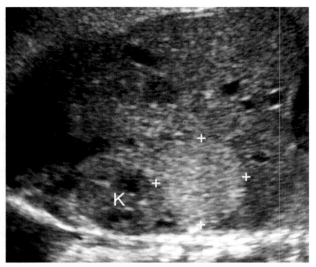

FIGURE 39-20. Adrenal neuroblastoma. Longitudinal scan shows a large solid mass *(cursors)* adjacent to the upper pole of the left kidney *(K). (Courtesy John R Mernagh, MD, McMaster University Medical Center, Hamilton, Ontario.)*

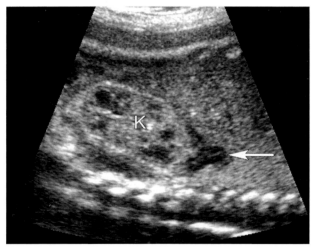

FIGURE 39-19. Normal adrenal gland. Longitudinal scan of a 31-week fetus demonstrates the Y- or V-shaped adrenal gland *(arrow)* at the superior border of the kidney *(K).*

Adrenal Mass

At the end of the first trimester, the normal adrenal glands appear as pyramid-shaped hypoechoic structures at the superior aspect of the hyperechoic kidneys. They are quite prominent, approximately half the size of the kidney. The size of the adrenal gland increases with gestation, but relatively less than the kidney. During the second and third trimesters, corticomedullary differentiation is apparent, with a hyperechoic medulla and a hypoechoic cortex. On longitudinal sonogram, the adrenals are seen as V- or Y-shaped structures superior to the kidneys (Fig. 39-19).

Abnormalities of the adrenal gland include hemorrhage, cyst, hypertrophy, and tumor. The differential diagnosis for fetal suprarenal masses includes adrenal neuroblastoma, adrenal hemorrhage or adrenal cyst, intra-abdominal pulmonary sequestration, enteric duplication cysts, and renal masses, including mesoblastic nephroma, upper-pole cystic dysplasia, or hydronephrosis in a duplex kidney.[86]

Neuroblastoma is the most common abdominal malignancy in neonates, and the adrenal gland is the most common primary site. On prenatal sonography, the retroperitoneal mass can be cystic, solid, or of mixed echogenicity[87,88] (Fig. 39-20). Most reported cases of neuroblastoma have been identified in the third trimester. Metastases (liver, placenta) and hydrops have been reported.[89] Fetal MRI is useful for detailed anatomic characterization of the tumor and extent of disease.[90] There may be maternal symptoms of hypertension, tachycardia, or preeclampsia, which result from elevated catecholamines and correlate with a more advanced stage of disease.[91] Prenatally detected neuroblastomas generally have a favorable outcome, and surgical resection is usually curative.[92] A short period of close observation is recommended for small tumors (<3 cm) and particularly for cystic forms; this strategy may avoid surgery in some neonates whose tumors regress spontaneously.[88]

Adrenal hemorrhage, which is much more common in the neonate, can have a sonographic appearance similar to that of an adrenal or renal neoplasm. Color Doppler ultrasound may be helpful in differentiation.[93] The key to the diagnosis of adrenal hemorrhage is evolution of the lesion over time; serial sonograms demonstrate a change in echogenicity (from solid to cystic) and a decrease in size of the mass.[94,95] Because neuroblastomas may also regress, however, it is important to obtain postnatal follow-up in fetuses with presumed adrenal hemorrhage.

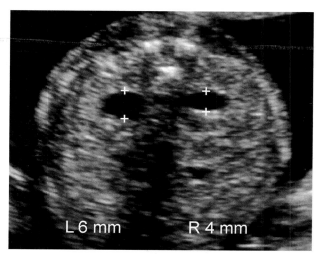

FIGURE 39-21. **Measurement of renal pelvis.** Transverse scan of the abdomen in a 21-week fetus shows prominent renal pelves *(cursors)*. The anteroposterior diameter measures 6 mm on the left side *(L)* and 4 mm on the right side *(R)*.

Upper Urinary Tract Dilation

Dilation of the upper urinary tract accounts for approximately 50% of all prenatally detected renal abnormalities.[96] It may be unilateral or bilateral and is more common in males than females.[97] Several prospective studies in unselected populations have reported a prevalence of 0.7% to 3.9% in the second trimester.[98-100] **Hydronephrosis** refers to abnormal dilation of the renal pelvis and calyces. The term **pyelectasis** implies a milder form of hydronephrosis, with dilation of the renal pelvis only. Dilation of the urinary tract can be obstructive or nonobstructive.

Hydronephrosis

Measurement of the anteroposterior (intra-) **renal pelvic diameter** (RPD) on a transverse scan of the fetal abdomen is the simplest and most common technique used to evaluate and classify renal pelvic dilation (Fig. 39-21). The **Society for Fetal Urology** (SFU) proposed a different classification system based on the degree of renal pelvic dilation (mild, moderate, marked), calyceal dilation, and parenchymal atrophy; with five grades (0-4) of increasing severity[101,102] (Fig. 39-22).

The size of the renal pelvis increases throughout gestation and there are published nomograms for RPD.[5,103] However, controversy surrounds the definition and clinical importance of mild renal pelvic dilation, and different threshold values of RPD have been used for the antenatal diagnosis of hydronephrosis. In general, the cutoff values for RPD vary between 4 mm and 5 mm in the second trimester and between 7 and 10 mm in the third trimester.[97,98,100,104-108] In our study of 328 fetuses, the 95th centile value for RPD was 4.4 mm at 20 weeks, 5.1 mm at 23 weeks, and 6.6 mm at 33 weeks—similar

ULTRASOUND GRADING SYSTEM OF HYDRONEPHROSIS

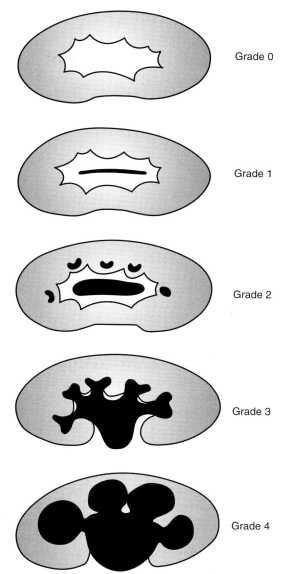

FIGURE 39-22. **Society for Fetal Urology grading system.** This classification is based on the appearance of the renal pelvis, calyces (calices), and renal parenchyma. **Grade 0:** no hydronephrosis; intact central renal complex. **Grade 1:** only dilated renal pelvis; there is some fluid in the renal pelvis. **Grade 2:** dilated renal pelvis and a few calices are visible. **Grade 3:** all the calices are dilated. **Grade 4:** further dilation of renal pelvis and calices, with thin renal parenchyma. *(Modified from Baskin LS: Prenatal hydronephrosis. In Baskin LS, Kogan B, Duckett J, editors: Handbook of pediatric urology. Philadelphia, 1997, Lippincott-Raven.)*

values to the published nomograms.[5,103] We consider the following measurements as abnormal:

- RPD of 5 mm or greater at 18 to 23 weeks
- RPD of 7 mm or greater in the third trimester

Although decreasing the cutoff value to 4 mm in midgestation can increase the sensitivity for the detection of renal pathology, it can lead to a high false-positive rate, perhaps generating unnecessary parental anxiety.[109] On the other hand, it should be recognized that a normal-appearing renal pelvis at midtrimester ultrasound does not exclude obstruction.[110] Factors such as maternal hydration status, maternal pyelectasis, and size of the fetal bladder may affect the RPD measurement.[111-114] Furthermore, RPD can vary greatly over 2 hours of ultrasound observation.[115] These findings suggest caution when considering the implications of renal collecting system dilation based on a single RPD measurement. **Calyceal dilation** is an important finding and is always pathologic, independent of the pelvic size.[100,109]

The detection of **fetal pyelectasis** is important for two reasons: **aneuploidy** and **postnatal uropathy.** The significance of pyelectasis as a marker for aneuploidy is discussed in Chapter 31. Pyelectasis is usually an isolated finding, but a detailed ultrasound examination should be performed to detect other urinary tract pathologic processes and nonrenal anomalies. Renal pelvic dilation may be transient or physiologic, but it may be the first manifestation of a urinary tract abnormality, including **ureteropelvic or vesicoureteral junction obstruction, VUR, duplex kidney,** and **urethral obstruction.** In a meta-analysis of 17 studies (104,572 patients screened), Lee et al.[116] examined antenatal hydronephrosis (1308 subjects) as a predictor of postnatal outcome.[116] Hydronephrosis was classified into mild, moderate, or severe (based on RPD of <7 mm, 7-10 mm, and >10 mm, respectively, if ultrasound was performed in the second trimester; <9 mm, 9-15 mm, and >15 mm if in the third trimester). The risk of any postnatal pathology was 12% for mild, 45% for moderate, and 88% for severe hydronephrosis (Table 39-3). There was a significant increase in the risk of postnatal pathology with increasing degree of hydronephrosis.

A prospective study by Sairam et al.[100] reported on the natural history of hydronephrosis diagnosed in 227 fetuses on midtrimester ultrasound in an unselected population. They demonstrated that 96% of the fetuses with mild hydronephrosis (RPD >4 mm and <7 mm at 18-23 weeks) experienced resolution in either the third trimester or the early neonatal period; none required postnatal surgery. However, approximately one in three fetuses with moderate/severe hydronephrosis (RPD >7 mm or presence of caliectasis at 18-23 weeks) required postnatal surgery. The overall third-trimester resolution rate was 67% and postnatal resolution rate was 21%.[100] Different definition of third-trimester hydronephrosis (RPD >7 mm instead of >10 mm) and preselected study populations weighted by more severe cases of hydronephrosis likely account for the lower third-trimester resolution rates (~30%) in other studies.[109,117] A meta-analysis by Sidhu et al.[118] combined data from seven studies and reported on the findings of serial postnatal renal ultrasonography in children with isolated antenatal hydronephrosis.[118] There was resolution, improvement, or stabilization of hydronephrosis in 98% of patients with SFU grades 1 and 2 and stabilization of hydronephrosis in 51% of those with SFU grades 3 and 4. These results suggest that mild hydronephrosis is a relatively benign condition.

It is important to identify those cases of prenatal pyelectasis most at risk of postnatal renal pathology, using the RPD and the SFU grading system. When a maximum prenatal RPD of 15 mm is used as a threshold, it predicts postnatal obstruction and the need for surgery in 80% of fetuses.[119] In utero progression also increases the likelihood of postnatal uropathy and urologic surgery.[108,120,121] There is a greater likelihood for bilateral renal pelvic

TABLE 39-3. RISK OF POSTNATAL PATHOLOGY BY DEGREE OF ANTENATAL HYDRONEPHROSIS

PATHOLOGY	Degree of Antenatal Hydronephrosis, % (95% CI)			TREND (P)
	MILD	**MODERATE**	**SEVERE**	
Any pathology	11.9 (4.5-28.0)	45.1 (25.3-66.6)	88.3 (53.7-98.0)	<.001
UPJ	4.9 (2.0-11.9)	17.0 (7.6-33.9)	54.3 (21.7-83.6)	<.001
VUR	4.4 (1.5-12.1)	14.0 (7.1-25.9)	8.5 (4.7-15.0)	.10
PUV	0.2 (0.0-1.4)	0.9 (0.2-2.9)	5.3 (1.2-21.0)	<.001
Ureteral obstruction	1.2 (0.2-8.0)	9.8 (6.3-14.9)	5.3 (1.4-18.2)	.025
Other*	1.2 (0.3-4.0)	3.4 (0.5-19.4)	14.9 (3.6-44.9)	.002

Modified from Lee RS, Cendron M, Kinnanmon DD, et al. Antenatal hydronephrosis as a predictor of postnatal outcome: a meta-analysis. Pediatrics 2006;118:586-593.
Hydronephrosis was classified based on anteroposterior diameter of renal pelvis:
    Second trimester: mild <7 mm, moderate 7-10 mm, severe >10 mm.
    Third trimester: mild <9 mm, moderate 9-15 mm, severe >15 mm.
CI, Confidence interval. *UPJ,* ureteropelvic junction obstruction; *VUR,* vesicoureteral reflux; *PUV,* posterior urethral valve.
* Includes prune belly syndrome, VATER syndrome, and unclassified.

dilation to progress (26%) compared with unilateral renal pelvic dilation (3%).[122] Some investigators have found an abnormal RPD in the third trimester to be the best ultrasound criterion to predict postnatal uropathy.[108] Although serial follow-up scans every 3 to 4 weeks are not necessary, a repeat ultrasound in the third trimester may be useful.

The majority of infants identified prenatally as having renal dilation are asymptomatic at birth. Pediatric nephrologists and urologists vary greatly in their management of antenatally diagnosed hydronephrosis, because an evidence-based protocol is lacking.[123] There are no uniformly accepted guidelines regarding antibiotic prophylaxis, postnatal workup, and surgery. However, a postnatal renal ultrasound is the first examination of choice. In the neonate, the relative state of dehydration and physiologic oliguria in the first 24 to 48 hours of life can result in underestimation of the degree of hydronephrosis and a false-negative renal ultrasound.[124] Therefore, ultrasound should not be performed before 72 hours after delivery, unless severe bilateral hydronephrosis or severe hydronephrosis in a solitary kidney may require early intervention. Because a normal ultrasound does not exclude VUR, some authors have recommended routine voiding cystourethrogram regardless of postnatal ultrasound findings.[107,125,126] However, other authors would perform voiding cystourethrogram only when postnatal renal ultrasound is abnormal.[127,128] It has been shown that screening with two successive renal ultrasound examinations performed at day 5 and 1 month has high sensitivity and negative predictive value for prediction of significant uropathy.[129] The indication for renal scintigraphy depends on the particular clinical situation. The preferred isotope scan in the infant is the mercaptoacetyl triglycine (MAG3) renal scan. It provides a dynamic study of the urinary tract, assessment of drainage, and estimation of differential renal function. The static renal scan using dimercaptosuccinic acid (DMSA, succimer) is indicated for detection of focal parenchymal abnormalities. In renal failure and bilateral dilation, it helps to distinguish between two equally affected kidneys or markedly asymmetrical renal function.

In summary, we propose the following management protocol for hydronephrosis detected in the second trimester with regard to repeat antenatal ultrasound, postnatal ultrasound, and antibiotics prophylaxis after delivery. In fetuses with mild renal dilatation (RPD <7 mm), parents are counseled that it is a common finding and may be physiologic or transient, and that the risk of postnatal uropathy is small. The important message is that prediction of outcome after a single scan is difficult, and postnatal renal ultrasound is necessary. Antibiotic prophylaxis is initiated after delivery to prevent UTIs. In addition to postnatal renal ultrasound and antibiotic prophylaxis, a repeat ultrasound in the third trimester is recommended in fetuses with greater degrees of renal pelvic dilation.

The effect of urinary obstruction on subsequent renal development depends on the time of onset and severity of the obstruction. The fetal urinary tract responds differently to chronic obstruction than the adult urinary tract. In adults with chronic urethral obstruction, the pelvicalyceal system is usually greatly dilated; in the fetus there may be a relative lack of pelvicalyceal dilation and possible development of macroscopic renal cysts. Experimental work in lambs has shown that ureteral obstruction originating in the last half of gestation causes simple hydronephrosis and parenchymal atrophy.[58] However, if ureteral obstruction originates during the first half of gestation, **renal dysplasia** and sometimes cyst formation will occur[130] (Fig. 39-23). Therefore, in fetuses with

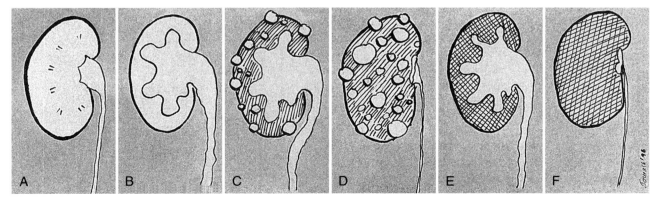

FIGURE 39-23. Urinary tract obstruction produces a varied response from the kidneys. **A,** Normal kidney. **B,** Pelvicaliectasis, with or without parenchymal atrophy. **C,** Renal cystic dysplasia, with parenchymal cysts. **D,** The dysplastic kidney may cease to function (lack of pelvicaliectasis). **E and F,** Alternatively, the kidney may show increased echogenicity, with no visible cysts but with pelvicaliectasis (**E**) or without pelvicaliectasis (**F**). In these cases, dysplasia is probably, but not invariably, present.

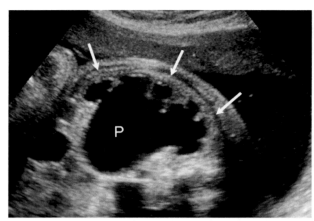

FIGURE 39-24. Ureteropelvic junction obstruction. Longitudinal scan shows moderate caliectasis and extremely dilated renal pelvis *(P)*, with thinning of the cortex *(arrows)*.

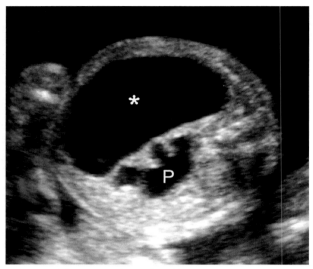

FIGURE 39-25. Perirenal urinoma. Transverse scan of fetal abdomen at 22 weeks' gestation shows a large perirenal urinoma (*) displacing and compressing the kidney, which demonstrates dilated calyces and pelvis *(P)* caused by ureteropelvic junction obstruction.

dilation of the renal pelvis, assessment of renal parenchymal echogenicity, thickness, and cysts are important, because thinned parenchyma, echogenic parenchyma, and cysts suggest more severe and long-standing obstruction with likely loss of renal function on the affected side.

Ureteropelvic Junction Obstruction

Obstruction at the ureteropelvic junction is the most common cause of nonphysiologic neonatal hydronephrosis, with an incidence of 1 in 2000 live births.[131] Most cases of UPJ obstruction are functional (caused by a muscular abnormality) rather than the result of fixed anatomic lesions such as fibrous adhesions, kinks, valves, or aberrant vessels. UPJ obstruction is more common in males and is often unilateral. In 10% to 30% of cases, it is bilateral.

On sonography, a dilated renal pelvis with or without caliectasis is identified. The ureter and the bladder are not dilated. Severe chronic obstruction leads to effacement of the calyces and thinning of the renal cortex (SFU grade 4) (Fig. 39-24). Rarely, the renal pelvis may be extremely dilated, presenting as a large, unilocular cystic mass. Rupture of the collecting system results in the development of a perirenal urinoma (Fig. 39-25; **Video 39-1**). This "pop-off" mechanism may protect the obstructed kidney from further prenatal damage and may diminish the degree of hydronephrosis. The affected kidney should be carefully assessed for renal dysplasia, however, because the probability of a nonfunctional dysplastic ipsilateral kidney is about 80%.[132]

The AFV is usually normal but may be increased paradoxically. When unilateral hydronephrosis is accompanied by oligohydramnios, a search for contralateral renal pathology is warranted (e.g., renal agenesis, multicystic renal dysplasia). UPJ obstruction may be associated with VUR and extrarenal abnormalities, including **anorectal anomalies, congenital heart disease, VATER**

syndrome, and **esophageal atresia.** When the contralateral kidney is normal, the prenatal detection of unilateral UPJ obstruction should not alter obstetric management. In cases of unilateral UPJ obstruction diagnosed before 24 weeks, severe dilation (RPD >15 mm) is predictive of impaired postnatal renal function in the affected kidney.[133] When there is bilateral UPJ obstruction, the prognosis depends on the severity and duration of obstruction and on the AFV. Serial ultrasound evaluations are necessary to assess the AFV, progression of hydronephrosis, and development of renal dysplasia. Early delivery is rarely indicated, except when there is progressive bilateral obstruction with severe oligohydramnios. Prophylactic antibiotic therapy is initiated soon after birth, and neonatal urologic workup is necessary.

Vesicoureteral Junction Obstruction (Primary Nonrefluxing Megaureter)

Vesicoureteral junction obstruction is caused by a structural anomaly of the distal segment of the ureter, with localized dysfunction or obstruction. It is more common in males and is bilateral in up to 25% of cases.[134] Coexisting anomalies of the urinary tract (VUR, UPJ obstruction, multicystic dysplasia) are frequently present. **Megaureters** are classified into three types according to their morphologic appearance. Type I megaureter dilation involves only the distal ureter, with a normal-appearing upper tract. Type II extends to both ureter and pelvis. Type III is associated with severe hydronephrosis and ureteric tortuosity.

On sonography, the affected kidney may demonstrate dilation of the ureter and renal pelvis. A slightly dilated

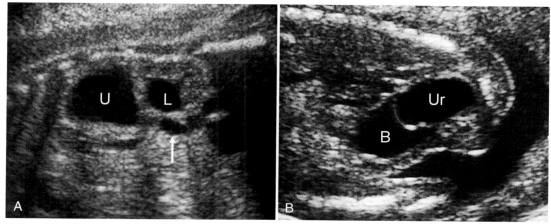

FIGURE 39-26. Duplication anomalies. A, Longitudinal scan shows two separate collecting systems. The hydronephrotic, upper-pole renal pelvis (U) is continuous with the dilated ureter (arrow). The lower-pole collecting system (L) is dilated because of reflux. **B,** Longitudinal scan of the pelvis shows the ureterocele (Ur) separated from the lumen of the bladder (B) by a thin, curvilinear wall of the ureterocele.

ureter may be difficult to recognize or may be mistaken for bowel, although bowel contents are usually more echogenic than urine. Identification of peristalsis in a fluid-filled tubular structure does not confirm bowel because it is often seen with hydroureter as well. To be certain, the serpiginous cystic segments must be traced to the renal pelvis and bladder. In addition, the ureter generally comes into close contact with the spine, but the small bowel does not. The ureteral dilation can be severe, so size alone does not preclude megaureter as a possible diagnosis. On prenatal sonography, nonobstructive causes such as VUR usually cannot be differentiated from primary megaureter or vesicoureteral junction obstruction.

Prophylactic antibiotic therapy is commenced soon after birth. Postnatal investigations are necessary to exclude VUR, duplication anomalies, and bladder outlet obstruction. Most cases of primary megaureter either resolve spontaneously or improve when managed conservatively.[135,136] The presenting hydronephrosis grade (SFU classification) and megaureter type are significant predictors of the spontaneous resolution rate.[135,137] In children with grade IV or V hydronephrosis or a retrovesical ureteral diameter of greater than 1 cm, the condition may persist or resolve slowly and may require surgery.

Duplication Anomalies

Unlike most urinary tract disorders, duplication of the renal collecting system is more common in females. Two ureteral buds arise from the mesonephric duct to grow into the metanephric blastema. The duplex kidney contains two separate pelvicalyceal systems, with either complete or partial duplication of the ureters. When **complete duplication** exists, the upper-pole ureter may end in the bladder (where it often forms an ureterocele) or

---

ectopically, usually into the vagina or urethra. Classically, the upper-pole moiety obstructs, whereas the lower-pole moiety refluxes. Sonographic findings useful for prenatal diagnosis include identification of two separate noncommunicating renal pelves, hydronephrosis in the upper or lower pole, ipsilateral dilated ureter, and ureterocele.[138-140] The most common sonographic appearance is hydronephrosis of the upper-pole moiety, often associated with a dilated ureter and a ureterocele within the bladder[138,139] (Fig. 39-26). If the dilated ureter appears to insert at a level below the bladder base, an ectopic ureter should be considered. The lower-pole moiety may also appear hydronephrotic because of VUR. However, identification of two separate collecting systems, or the nondilated lower pole of a duplex kidney, may be difficult because of its small size and displacement by the dilated upper renal pelvis and ureter.

A careful evaluation of the urinary bladder is necessary to detect the **ureterocele,** which is seen as a thin-walled, cystlike structure within the bladder (Fig. 39-26). The diagnosis is easy when the bladder is partially full but can be overlooked if the bladder is empty or only minimally distended. A full bladder can compress the ureterocele, resulting in nonvisualization. If ureteroceles become sufficiently large, they may also obstruct the contralateral ureteric orifice or cause bladder outlet obstruction. Antibiotic prophylaxis is initiated at birth when upper-pole hydronephrosis is detected antenatally in a duplex kidney.

Vesicoureteral Reflux

Vesicoureteral reflux (VUR) can be **primary** (incompetent valve mechanism at the ureterovesical junction) or **secondary** (due to an obstruction in the urinary tract and high detrusor pressures). The main prenatal sonographic finding is hydronephrosis, which may be unilateral or bilateral. The ureter may be dilated. Intermittent dilation of the collecting system favors VUR. Fluctuation or variation in the RPD (changing by more than 3 mm) during the course of an obstetric sonogram was strongly associated with high-grade VUR (grades IV-V).[141] VUR may be associated with other renal abnormalities, including **UPJ obstruction, duplex kidney, MCDK, and unilateral renal agenesis**.[125]

The reported prevalence of VUR in children with prenatally detected hydronephrosis varies widely because different RPD cutoff values are used for inclusion and different protocols for postnatal investigations (voiding cystourethrogram either in all cases or only after an abnormal postnatal renal ultrasound). A recent systematic review of 18 studies showed a mean prevalence of 15% for postnatal primary VUR after prenatally detected hydronephrosis.[142]

A normal postnatal ultrasound does not exclude VUR. However, if two successive renal ultrasound examinations (at day 5 and at 1 month) were normal (RPD <7 mm), voiding cystourethrography showed abnormalities in only 6.7% of patients.[143] Neonatal reflux is more common in male infants. It is often of low grade, with a high rate of spontaneous resolution by 2 years of age.[144] However, in those children with high-grade VUR, spontaneous resolution is rare. There is a significant correlation between high-grade VUR and findings of either renal dysplasia on ultrasound or renal damage scars on DMSA renal scan.[144,145] Most neonates with VUR are managed conservatively with antibiotic prophylaxis.

Lower Urinary Tract (Urethral) Obstruction

Fetal megacystis has been reported as early as 10 to 14 weeks' gestation when the longitudinal bladder diameter is 7 mm or more[146] (Fig. 39-27). The incidence is 0.3% at 11 to 15 weeks.[147] In the largest case series of 145 fetuses with early megacystis, chromosomal abnormalities were detected in 21%.[148] In the chromosomally normal group, severe megacystis (bladder length >15 mm) was invariably associated with progressive obstructive uropathy.[148] However, if the bladder length was 7 to 15 mm, there was spontaneous resolution of the megacystis by 20 weeks in 90% of cases. Therefore, follow-up ultrasound is necessary to interpret correctly the importance of megacystis detected in the first

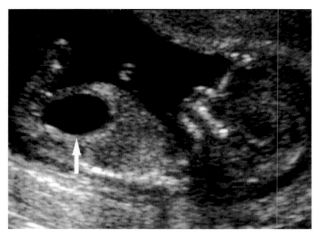

FIGURE 39-27. Megacystis in first trimester. Transabdominal sagittal image of a 12-week fetus shows a distended thick-walled bladder *(arrow)*, measuring 13 mm in length. There is no hydronephrosis.

CAUSES OF FETAL MEGACYSTIS

Posterior urethral valves
Urethral atresia/stricture
Prune belly syndrome
Megalourethra
Cloacal malformation
Megacystis-microcolon–intestinal hypoperistalsis
    syndrome

---

trimester. The role of early vesicocentesis and shunt placement needs further investigation.[149] In fetuses with severe megacystis, survival to the neonatal period was poor even with intervention, and the survivors are at risk of developing renal failure.[147,150]

Posterior urethral valves are the most common cause of lower urinary tract obstruction, followed by **urethral atresia** or stricture. Posterior urethral valves are seen exclusively in males and may cause total, intermittent, or partial obstruction, with variable prognosis. Most cases are sporadic, occurring in 1 in 5000 male births; and the recurrence risk is small.[149] Back pressure causes a persistently dilated urinary bladder, with a dilated proximal urethra **(keyhole sign)** (Fig. 39-28, *A*). There may be thickening of the bladder wall (>2 mm) or a severely distended thin-walled bladder, bilateral tortuous hydroureters, and hydronephrosis (Fig. 39-28, *B*). If the obstruction is severe and of long-standing, progressive renal parenchymal fibrosis and dysplasia develop, resulting in severe oligohydramnios, pulmonary hypoplasia, and compression deformities (Potter's syndrome). There may be spontaneous bladder rupture with urinary ascites or a calyceal rupture with perirenal urinoma[151] (Fig. 39-29). If spontaneous decompression occurs, this

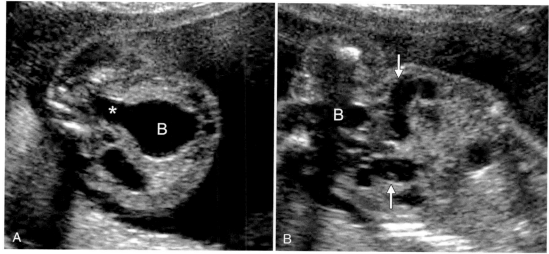

FIGURE 39-28. Posterior urethral valves causing urethral level obstruction. A, Dilated urinary bladder *(B)* and proximal urethra (*) give the appearance of a keyhole, characteristic of urethral obstruction in a 21-week fetus. **B,** Coronal scan shows dilated tortuous ureters *(arrows).*

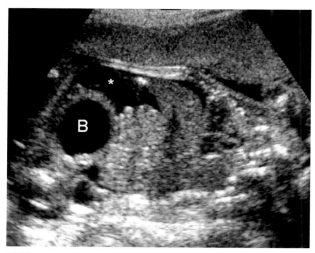

FIGURE 39-29. Urinary ascites. Longitudinal scan of a 22-week fetus shows a thick-walled bladder *(B)* and urinary ascites (*) caused by spontaneous rupture of severe megacystis.

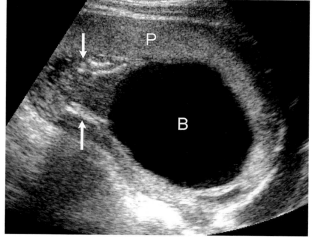

FIGURE 39-30. Urethral atresia. Coronal scan of a 17-week fetus shows a greatly distended bladder *(B)* that occupies the entire abdomen. The thorax *(arrows)* is compressed and bell shaped because of **pulmonary hypoplasia.** There is anhydramnios. *P,* Placenta.

"safety valve" may protect the kidneys from further prenatal damage and may diminish the degree of hydronephrosis.

Urethral atresia causes the most severe form of obstructive uropathy. The sonographic features include a greatly distended bladder and anhydramnios after the first trimester (Fig. 39-30). In the absence of antenatal treatment, urethral atresia is almost always fatal, because of associated renal dysplasia and pulmonary hypoplasia.[152] A small number of survivors have been reported after antenatal intervention.[153]

Prune belly syndrome is characterized by the classic triad of **absent abdominal musculature, undescended testes,** and **urinary tract abnormalities** (megacystis, ureterectasis). Although some authors believe that the

syndrome results from a primary mesodermal defect, others explain the pathogenesis as a urethral obstruction malformation complex (the muscular defect is secondary to distended urinary system).[154] The bladder is typically very large. The prostatic urethra is dilated, and the appearance resembles posterior urethral valves. The ureters tend to be tortuous and dilated. The kidneys may be normal, hydronephrotic, or dysplastic. Other abnormalities may be present, including intestinal malrotation, congenital heart disease, and musculoskeletal deformities. Although not all infants have urethral obstruction at birth, it has been suggested that transient in utero obstruction may initiate the sequence responsible for this syndrome.[155]

PRUNE BELLY SYNDROME

Absent abdominal musculature
Undescended testes
Very large bladder
Dilated prostatic urethra
Ureters tortuous and dilated
Kidneys normal, hydronephrotic, or dysplastic

Megalourethra is characterized by a congenital deficiency of the mesodermal tissues of the phallus, with dilation of the penile urethra and enlargement of the penis (Fig. 39-31). This condition has been classified into two types, fusiform and scaphoid urethra, but it is preferable to consider it as a spectrum rather than two distinct entities. Urinary stasis in the dilated penile urethra results in functional obstruction of the urinary tract. The prenatal sonographic findings include those of

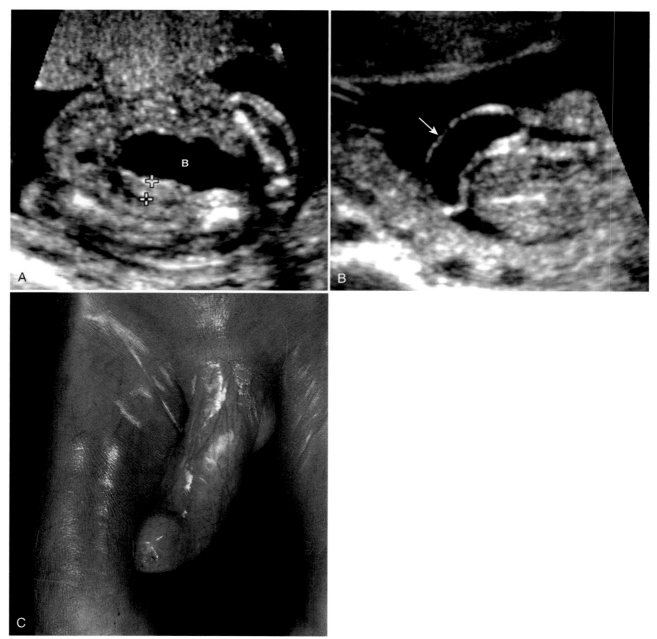

FIGURE 39-31. Megacystis and megalourethra. A, Oblique scan of the fetal pelvis at 21 weeks' gestation shows a dilated urinary bladder *(B)* with thick walls *(calipers)*. **B,** Transverse view of the perineum shows a dilated penile urethra *(arrow)* with deficient mesodermal tissues in the phallus. **C,** Postmortem photograph of the fetus at 23 weeks' gestation shows enlarged penis. The penile urethra was patent (not shown). *(A and B courtesy Ants Toi, MD, Department of Medical Imaging; C courtesy Sarah Keating, MD, Department of Pathology and Laboratory Medicine; Mount Sinai Hospital, Toronto.)*

lower urinary tract obstruction, with dilation and elongation of the penile urethra[156] (Fig. 39-31; **Video 39-2**). Associated malformations of the urinary tract include **urethral atresia, posterior urethral valves, prune belly syndrome,** and **horseshoe kidney.** Abnormalities involving the GI tract, spine, and VACTERL association have been reported. The prognosis depends on the degree of renal dysfunction and the severity of associated anomalies. Survivors are at risk of renal insufficiency, impotence, and infertility.

Megacystis-microcolon–intestinal hypoperistalsis syndrome (MMIHS) is a rare, nonobstructive cause of megacystis, with a 4 : 1 female predominance. The syndrome involves not only a distended bladder but also functional small bowel obstruction and **microcolon.** It is important to differentiate this syndrome from the more common **posterior urethral valves** because it carries a dismal prognosis, and fetal bladder shunting is not indicated. The key features are (1) the amniotic fluid is usually normal or increased; (2) the fetus is usually female; and (3) rarely a dilated small bowel may be present.[157] MRI is a useful adjunct for diagnosis; it can confirm the presence of microcolon when an enlarged bladder is visualized on ultrasound.[158] An abnormal amniotic fluid digestive enzyme profile has shown a sensitivity of 80% and specificity of 89% for detection of MMIHS.[159] No genetic locus for MMIHS has yet been found, although reports of inheritance in families exist.

Cloacal malformation (persistent cloaca) results from failure of the urorectal septum to reach the perineum. It occurs exclusively in phenotypic females, with an incidence of 1 in 50,000 births. The etiology is unknown but is thought to be heterogeneous. Recent studies have suggested that limb–body wall complex, cloacal exstrophy, and urorectal septum malformation sequence may represent a continuous spectrum of abnormalities with a common etiology.[160] The typical patient has a single perineal opening that serves as the outlet for urine, genital secretions, and meconium. Lower urinary tract abnormalities (reflux, ureteral ectopia, duplication of bladder) and genital abnormalities (duplication or atresia of uterus and vagina) are common, as are abnormalities of the bony pelvis and kidneys. Additional complications are related to **urinary tract obstruction, hydrometrocolpos,** and **bowel obstruction.** Prenatal sonographic findings include normal or diminished AFV; a normal, distended, or nonvisualized bladder with a cystic mass containing calcifications (meconium mixed with urine) (Fig. 39-32); ascites; hydronephrosis; ambiguous genitalia; and vertebral anomalies.[161,162]

In Utero Intervention: Vesicoamniotic Shunting

For a carefully selected group of fetuses with severe lower urinary tract obstruction, permanent in utero bladder drainage may be a therapeutic option. The objective of vesicoamniotic shunting is to allow free drainage of urine from the bladder into the amniotic cavity. This relieves back pressure on the urinary tract and should prevent or stabilize renal dysplastic change, correct oligohydramnios, and allow unimpeded lung development. This approach assumes that renal function has not been destroyed by the original insult resulting in the anatomic obstruction. Careful selection of suitable cases is critical, and the goal is often the identification and rigorous evaluation of reliable predictors of postnatal renal function.[147,163-170]

A detailed sonographic evaluation of the fetus is a prerequisite, including a diligent search for associated structural or chromosomal abnormalities. The sonographic appearances and clinical sequelae of severe lower urinary tract obstruction are discussed earlier. A thorough assessment of the urinary tract is necessary to define the probable cause and evaluate prognosis. Intervention is not indicated if the ultrasound suggests either MMIHS

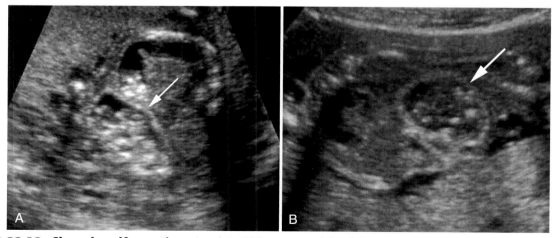

FIGURE 39-32. Cloacal malformation. A and **B,** Oblique views of the abdomen in a fetus with nonvisualized bladder show a complex, fluid-filled structure *(arrow)* in the middle to lower abdomen with calcifications caused by cloacal malformation.

or severe cloacal dysgenesis, because of their dismal prognosis. This procedure is discussed in more detail in Chapter 46.

Fine-needle aspiration under ultrasound guidance (**vesicocentesis**) temporarily relieves the megacystis and allows urine to be analyzed for assessment of renal function and karyotype.[25,164-166] If the urine reaccumulates rapidly (which itself may indicate function) and the other prognostic factors are favorable, placement of a permanent vesicoamniotic shunt may be considered.

ANTENATAL PREDICTORS OF POOR POSTNATAL RENAL FUNCTION

Ultrasound
Severe oligohydramnios, especially if early onset
Increased renal echogenicity
Renal cortical cysts
Slow bladder refilling after vesicocentesis

Fetal Urine
↑Sodium level (Na$^+$)
↑Calcium level (Ca^{2+})
↑β$_2$-Microglobulin level
↑Osmolality

Fetal Blood
↑β$_2$-Microglobulin level

Fetal urinary sodium (Na$^+$), calcium (Ca^{2+}), osmolality, and β$_2$-microglobulin (in combination) appear to be the most predictive of outcome[163-168,170] and form the mainstay of biochemical evaluation (Table 39-4).

Initially, fixed cutoff values were suggested for each variable as predictors of poor prognosis.[59] However, the normal levels of many parameters vary with gestational age and must be interpreted accordingly. Specifically, sodium and β$_2$-microglobulin levels decrease throughout gestation, whereas calcium and creatinine values rise.[163,164,169] In general, more hypotonic fetal urine correlates with a more favorable outcome. Some groups advocate that the last of three sequential urine samplings at 48- to 72-hour intervals is most reflective of true renal function.[163,171,172] A systematic review of 572 pregnancies showed the two most accurate tests of fetal renal function were calcium above 95th centile for gestation and sodium above 95th centile for gestation, with β$_2$-microglobulin being less accurate.[173] It has been suggested that fetal blood levels of β$_2$-microglobulin may better assess glomerular filtration rate than urinary markers, which generally reflect tubular function.[174] Blood sampling for electrolytes and β$_2$-microglobulin may also be useful in cases when no urine can be collected by vesicocentesis.[172] A **urinary function profile,** which combines a number of biochemical and sonographic predictors, appears to be of most clinical value. Only carefully selected fetuses with adequate renal function, despite significant oligohydramnios, are likely to benefit from in utero

TABLE 39-4. PREDICTIVE VALUE OF FETAL URINALYSIS FOR POOR POSTNATAL RENAL FUNCTION

STUDY	THRESHOLD	SENSITIVITY	SPECIFICITY	PPV	NPV
	Sodium				
Muller et al.[169]	>50 mmol/L	0.82	0.64	0.6	
Nicolini et al.[164]	>95th centile** (mmol/L)	0.87	0.8		
Johnson et al.[163]*	>100 mg/dL	1.0	0.79	0.7	1.0
Nicolaides et al.[170]	>95th centile** (mmol/L)			0.9	0.7
	β$_2$-microglobulin				
Muller et al.[166]	>2 mg/L	0.8	0.83	0.8	
Johnson et al.[163]*	>4 mg/L	0.22	1.0	1.0	0.68
	Calcium				
Muller et al.[166]	>0.95 mmol/L	0.53	0.84	0.6	
Nicolini et al.[164]	>95th centile** (mmol/L)	1.0	0.6		
Johnson et al.[163]*	>8 mg/dL	0.88	0.47	0.47	0.88
	Osmolality				
Johnson et al.[163]*	>200 mOsm/L	1.0	0.84	0.77	1.0
	Creatinine				
Nicolaides et al.[170]	>95th centile** (mmol/L)			1.0	0.4
Muller et al.[166]	>200 mmol/L (at 20 weeks, but increases with gestational age)	0.64	0.89	0.85	
	Total protein				
Muller et al.[166]	>0.04 g/L	0.65	0.89	1.0	
Johnson et al.[163]*	>20 mg/dL	0.88	0.71	0.64	0.91

Definitions of "normal" renal function: Muller, serum creatinine ≦50 mmol/L at 1 year of age; Johnson, urine creatinine <1.0 mg/dL at 2 years of age; Nicolaides, serum creatinine <70 mmol/L at 1 to 6 years of age; Nicolini, not stated.
 * Results from third of three sequential samples.
 ** For gestational age.
 PPV, Positive predictive value; *NPV,* negative predictive value.

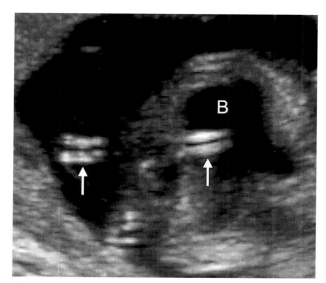

FIGURE 39-33. Vesicoamniotic shunt. Arrows indicate catheter in the decompressed bladder *(B)* and amniotic fluid. Note normal amniotic fluid volume.

intervention; and in our center, only a handful of the fetuses who are referred with lower urinary tract obstruction go on to such treatment.

Our approach is to counsel the parents extensively beforehand, with input from a multidisciplinary team of fetal medicine, pediatrics, urology, nephrology, and social work. Parents are also given the opportunity to speak to others who have faced similar dilemmas. Before any decision is made, we try to ensure that they have an unbiased and complete account of the situation and are fully aware that, despite successful shunt placement, renal failure or pulmonary hypoplasia may still ensue.[174-177]

The technique involves the insertion of a small, plastic, double-coiled Silastic "pigtail" catheter into the bladder under continuous ultrasound guidance. To facilitate insertion, amnioinfusion is always undertaken beforehand. Antibiotic prophylaxis and tocolysis (rectal indomethacin and topical nitroglycerin) are used for 24 hours. We strive to place the shunt anteriorly in the midline, ideally below the umbilical cord insertion[172] (Fig. 39-33). Color Doppler ultrasound is used to help avoid maternal and fetal blood vessels. **Early intervention** is probably necessary for this procedure to be successful in the prevention of pulmonary hypoplasia and preservation of renal function.[149] Usually, **significant oligohydramnios** is a prerequisite for shunting. Occasionally, intervention may be considered in light of documented worsening of renal function on urinalysis or progressively abnormal renal appearance on ultrasound, despite a normal AFV. Rarely, it may be warranted to place the shunt directly into a dilated renal pelvis rather than the bladder. Shunts may become blocked or dislodged and will require replacement in a few cases.

Few studies have looked at long-term outcomes in children treated with prenatal vesicoamniotic shunting. Retrospective series report 22% to 67% survivors among those treated, with renal function preserved in 0% to 50% of survivors.[163,175-177] A systematic review and meta-analysis of 16 observational studies involving 210 fetuses in whom a bladder drainage procedure was attempted concluded that prenatal bladder drainage improved perinatal survival in the most severe cases, but high-quality evidence is lacking.[178] In a recent series of 20 children treated with in utero vesicoamniotic shunts, 10% died from pulmonary hypoplasia.[179] The survivors were followed for a mean age of 5.8 years; 40% of those treated had acceptable renal function, 20% had mild renal insufficiency, and 30% required dialysis and eventual renal transplant. The majority had acceptable bladder function, normal neurologic development, and satisfactory quality of life.

Antenatal management of lower urinary tract obstruction is difficult because the natural history is highly variable and dependent on etiology, severity, duration, and age of onset of the obstruction. Currently, there is a multicenter randomized controlled trial in the United Kingdom to evaluate the safety and effectiveness of in utero vesicoamniotic shunting compared to conservative management (the Pluto trial; www.pluto.bham.ac.uk).

Bladder Exstrophy

This severe anomaly occurs once in 10,000 to 40,000 births, more often in males.[2] Bladder exstrophy is caused by incomplete median closure of the inferior part of the anterior abdominal wall. The defect also involves the anterior wall of the urinary bladder. There is exposure and protrusion of the posterior wall of the bladder. This anomaly is associated with separation of the pubic bones, a low-set umbilicus, and abnormal genitalia. Sonographically, AFV and kidneys are normal, but a fluid-filled bladder is not identified. Instead, the everted bladder

---

NONVISUALIZATION OF FETAL BLADDER: ETIOLOGY

FAILURE OF URINE PRODUCTION
Bilateral renal agenesis
Bilateral multicystic dysplastic kidneys
Bilateral severe renal dysplasia
Bilateral severe ureteropelvic junction obstruction
Bilateral combinations of any of the above
Autosomal recessive polycystic kidney disease
Severe intrauterine growth restriction

FAILURE TO STORE URINE
Bladder exstrophy
Cloacal exstrophy
Bilateral single-system ectopic ureters

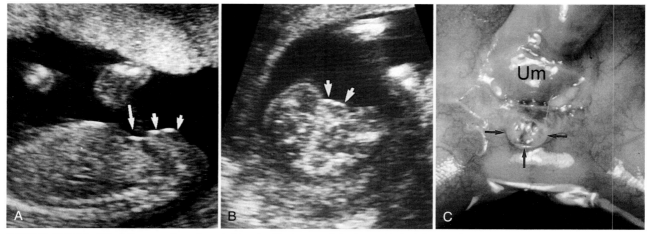

FIGURE 39-34. Bladder exstrophy. A, Longitudinal scan of the lower fetal abdomen shows an irregular mass on the anterior abdominal wall *(small arrows)*, below the umbilical cord insertion *(large arrow)*, which is more caudad than usual. No bladder can be identified. Note normal amniotic fluid volume. **B,** Transverse view of the perineum shows two small excrescences *(small arrows)* that represent the everted bladder with heaped-up mucosa. **C,** Corresponding photograph of the exposed bladder with heaped-up mucosa *(arrows); Um,* umbilical cord. *(Courtesy Ants Toi, MD, Department of Medical Imaging, Mount Sinai Hospital, Toronto.)*

with heaped-up mucosa may be seen as an irregular mass on the anterior abdominal wall, inferior to the umbilicus (Fig. 39-34). Other findings include a low umbilical cord insertion site into the abdomen, widening of the pubic bones, and small penis.[180] Bladder exstrophy is usually a sporadic and isolated defect. Rarely, it has been reported with the **OEIS complex:** omphalocele, exstrophy of bladder, imperforate anus, and spinal defects. Renal anomalies and abnormalities of the lower limbs are often found.[181,182]

THE GENITAL TRACT

Normal Genitalia

Documentation of fetal gender has medical as well as social implications. These include (1) history of X-linked disorders, (2) assignment of dizygosity in twin pregnancies, (3) exclusion of maternal cell contamination during amniocentesis (with mixed cell population on karyotype), (4) need to confirm fetal gender to diagnose certain structural abnormalities (e.g., posterior urethral valves, ovarian cysts), and (5) familial syndromes in which genital abnormalities are common.

In the second trimester the external genitalia can be visualized in 84% to 91% of fetuses, and the fetal gender can be correctly assigned in 93% to 99% of these cases.[183-185] A male fetus is diagnosed when the penis and scrotum are demonstrated, and the female fetus is diagnosed when the labia majora are shown (Fig. 39-35). Inopportune fetal position, oligohydramnios, maternal obesity, and operator inexperience represent the major limitations in fetal gender assessment. Errors may occur when the rounded, apposed labia are mistaken for a

small, empty scrotum or when the umbilical cord is mistaken for the penis.

Fetal gender can also be identified in the first trimester. During embryologic development, the male and female genitalia are identical until the 11th week of gestation, so gender determination is not possible before 11 weeks. In the first trimester the most useful scanning plane is the midsagittal plane, where there is a different orientation of the phallus related to the gender. In males the penis is seen as a cranially or vertically directed phallus; in females the clitoris is represented by a caudally or horizontally directed phallus (Fig. 39-36). Three-dimensional sonography allows the midsagittal plane to be obtained and the genitalia to be visualized more easily.[186] At 12 weeks' gestation, fetal gender can be identified in 87% to 100% of fetuses and is accurately predicted in 86% to 100% of these cases.[187-189]

Testicular descent into the scrotum occurs after 25 weeks' gestation.[190] After 32 weeks, both testes have descended in 97% of the fetuses. Small hydroceles are common in third-trimester male fetuses (15%) and are usually of no clinical importance[191] (Fig. 39-37). However, large hydroceles, especially if they increase in size over time, suggest an open communication between the processus vaginalis and peritoneal cavity. In such cases, postnatal evaluation for inguinal hernia should be performed.[192]

Abnormal Genitalia

An abnormality of the genitalia may be an isolated finding or associated with other major malformations. In a male fetus, abnormal ultrasound findings include **micropenis, penile chordee** (ventral curvature of penis), a shawl or **bifid scrotum, hypospadias,** and

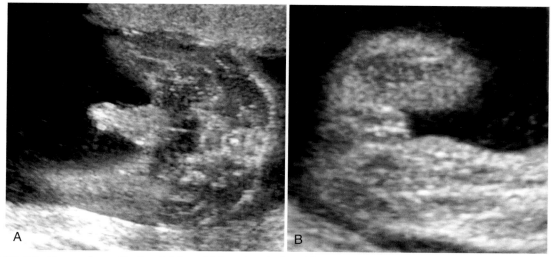

FIGURE 39-35. Normal genitalia. A, Normal 20-week male fetus. Transverse scan of the perineum shows the penis and scrotum. **B,** Normal 21-week female fetus. Transverse scan of the perineum shows the labial folds.

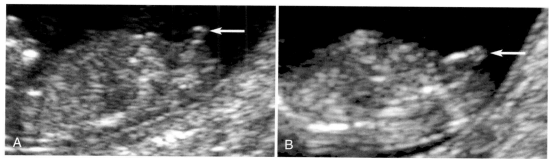

FIGURE 39-36. First-trimester gender identification. A, Sagittal scan of a 12-week male fetus shows the vertical and relatively cranially directed phallus *(arrow)*. **B,** Sagittal scan of a 12-week female fetus shows the horizontal/caudally directed phallus *(arrow)*.

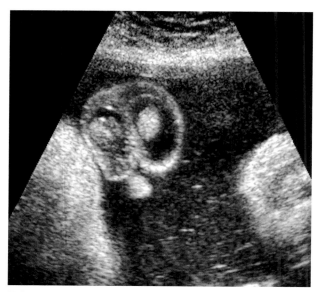

FIGURE 39-37. Hydroceles. Scan of the scrotal sac in a 38-week male fetus demonstrates testes and bilateral hydroceles.

undescended testes (in third trimester).[193-196] In the female, an enlarged clitoris is the most common finding. It can be difficult to define **ambiguous genitalia** accurately (Fig. 39-38). A male fetus with micropenis, bifid scrotum, and undescended testes may not be distinguished from the virilized female who has clitoral enlargement (and labial fusion). If ambiguous genitalia are suspected, a karyotype is obtained to determine the genetic make-up of the fetus. Ambiguous genitalia, syndactyly, and multiple other anomalies would raise the suspicion of **Smith-Lemli-Opitz syndrome,** an autosomal recessive inborn error in cholesterol metabolism. This diagnosis is also suggested by low maternal serum estriol in the second trimester. Elevated 7-dehydrocholesterol in amniotic fluid in the second trimester or at chorionic villus sampling in the first trimester is a reliable marker for prenatal diagnosis of Smith-Lemli-Opitz syndrome.[197]

When ultrasound suggests male genitalia and the fetus is genetically female, **congenital adrenal hyperplasia** is

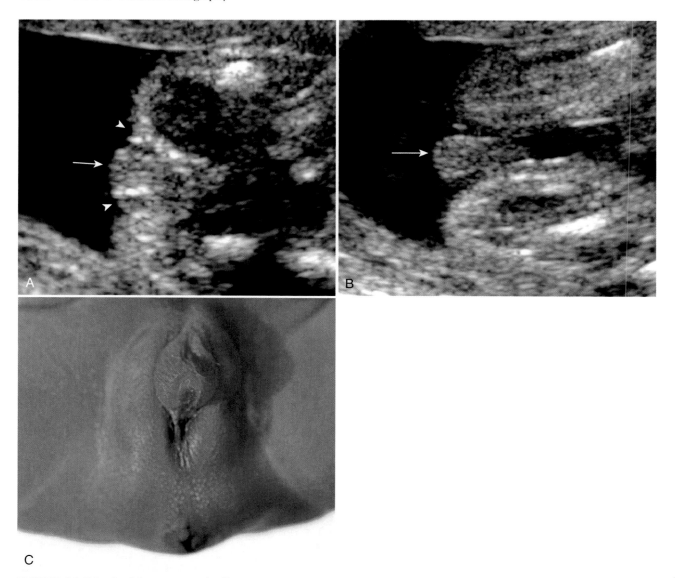

FIGURE 39-38. Ambiguous genitalia. A and **B,** Transverse views of the perineum in a 28-week growth-restricted fetus show ambiguous genitalia: abnormal incurved penis *(arrows)* located between the two labial-like swellings *(arrowheads).* **C,** Postnatal photograph of the newborn (genetically a male) shows micropenis, which is severely incurved with hypospadias, bifid scrotal sac, and cryptorchidism (the latter is normal for a 28-week fetus). *(**C** courtesy Sarah Keating, MD, Department of Pathology and Laboratory Medicine, Mount Sinai Hospital, Toronto.)*

the most common cause. The condition is autosomal recessive, so there may be a previously affected sibling. More than 90% of cases result from mutations of CYP21, leading to 21-hydroxylase deficiency. When a proband exists, early prenatal diagnosis is possible by direct molecular analysis in the first trimester, and fetal adrenal suppression with maternal dexamethasone therapy can reverse or reduce masculinization of the external genitalia.[198] In the absence of a family history, the ultrasound finding of enlarged fetal adrenal glands in addition to genital ambiguity is suggestive of congenital adrenal hyperplasia.[199] Measurement of 17-OHP and Δ4-androstenedione in amniotic fluid can confirm the diagnosis.[200-202]

Prenatal diagnosis of female **pseudohermaphroditism** with bilateral luteoma of pregnancy has been

reported.[203] In a genetic male with female external genitalia, **testicular feminization** is likely. Intersex states may be divided into hormonally and nonhormonally mediated abnormalities. The latter often have associated cloacal anomalies or chromosomal aberrations or may conform to one of numerous multimalformation syndromes. In many cases, an accurate diagnosis and final gender assignment can only be made postnatally.

Hydrometrocolpos

Hydrometrocolpos, enlargement of the obstructed uterus and vagina from retained secretions, results from a number of causes, including vaginal or cervical atresia, imperforate hymen, and vaginal membranes. Sono-

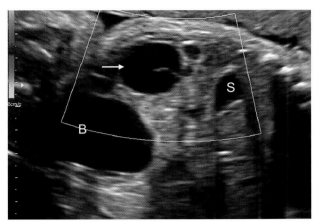

FIGURE 39-39. Ovarian cyst. Coronal scan demonstrates a simple cyst *(arrow)* in the lower abdomen of a 35-week female fetus, separate from the kidneys (not shown), bladder *(B)*, and stomach *(S)*. *(Courtesy of John R Mernagh, MD, McMaster University Medical Center, Hamilton, Ontario.)*

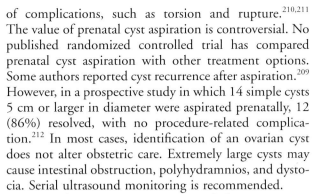

of complications, such as torsion and rupture.[210,211] The value of prenatal cyst aspiration is controversial. No published randomized controlled trial has compared prenatal cyst aspiration with other treatment options. Some authors reported cyst recurrence after aspiration.[209] However, in a prospective study in which 14 simple cysts 5 cm or larger in diameter were aspirated prenatally, 12 (86%) resolved, with no procedure-related complication.[212] In most cases, identification of an ovarian cyst does not alter obstetric care. Extremely large cysts may cause intestinal obstruction, polyhydramnios, and dystocia. Serial ultrasound monitoring is recommended.

Postnatal management options include surgery, percutaneous cyst aspiration, and observation alone. Simple cysts smaller than 5 cm are managed conservatively with serial ultrasound. Complex cysts, simple cysts larger than 5 cm, symptomatic cysts, and cysts that persist or increase in size are indications for surgery.[213,214]

CONCLUSION

The most common antenatally detected fetal anomalies are genitourinary in origin. A thorough sonographic evaluation of renal structure, function, and associated anomalies will improve the accuracy of antenatal diagnosis, thus enabling optimal obstetric and neonatal management.

graphically, an ovoid mass, either cystic or complex, is seen posterior to the bladder. This should be differentiated from the rectosigmoid colon (either normally filled with meconium or obstructed), which is seen as a tubular structure. The enlarged uterus may compress the urinary tract and cause hydronephrosis or hydroureter. Hydrometrocolpos may be associated with a spectrum of malformations, and therefore a detailed sonographic examination should be performed. MRI may be useful as an adjunct to ultrasound when pelvic anatomy is not well identified or to aid in diagnosis of cloacal malformation or other associated GI abnormalities.[204-206]

Ovarian Cysts

The vast majority of fetal ovarian cysts are benign functional cysts.[207] They probably result from excessive stimulation of the fetal ovary by placental and maternal hormones. They are usually detected in the second half of pregnancy. The main criteria for diagnosis are the presence of a cystic mass, usually located on one side of the pelvis or lower abdomen; normal urinary and GI tracts; and female gender. The diagnosis is always presumptive because other lesions, such as **enteric duplication cysts, mesenteric cysts, meconium pseudocysts,** or **urachal cysts,** cannot be ruled out with certainty. Most ovarian cysts are small and anechoic (Fig. 39-39). When complicated by torsion or hemorrhage, ovarian cysts may appear complex or even solid (**Video 39-3**). A fluid-debris level, a retracting clot, or internal septa may be demonstrated.[208] The wall may be echogenic from dystrophic calcification.

The outcome depends on the cyst size and sonographic patterns. The natural course for most ovarian cysts (>50%) is spontaneous resolution, either prenatally or postnatally (within 6 months of birth).[207,209,210] With simple cysts larger than 5 cm, there is an increased risk

References

1. Grandjean H, Larroque D, Levi S. The performance of routine ultrasonographic screening of pregnancies in the Eurofetus Study. Am J Obstet Gynecol 1999;181:446-454.

The Normal Urinary Tract
2. Moore KL, Persaud TVN, editors. The developing human: clinically oriented embryology. 7th ed. Philadelphia: Saunders; 2003.
3. Bronshtein M, Yoffe N, Brandes JM, Blumenfeld Z. First- and early second-trimester diagnosis of fetal urinary tract anomalies using transvaginal sonography. Prenat Diagn 1990;10:653-666.
4. Braithwaite JM, Armstrong MA, Economides DL. Assessment of fetal anatomy at 12 to 13 weeks of gestation by transabdominal and transvaginal sonography. Br J Obstet Gynaecol 1996;103:82-85.
5. Chitty LS, Altman DG. Charts of fetal size: kidney and renal pelvis measurements. Prenat Diagn 2003;23:891-897.
6. Grannum P, Bracken M, Silverman R, Hobbins JC. Assessment of fetal kidney size in normal gestation by comparison of ratio of kidney circumference to abdominal circumference. Am J Obstet Gynecol 1980;136:249-254.
7. Rabinowitz R, Peters MT, Vyas S, et al. Measurement of fetal urine production in normal pregnancy by real-time ultrasonography. Am J Obstet Gynecol 1989;161:1264-1266.
8. Fagerquist M, Fagerquist U, Oden A, Blomberg SG. Fetal urine production and accuracy when estimating fetal urinary bladder volume [see comment]. Ultrasound Obstet Gynecol 2001;17: 132-139.
9. Touboul C, Boulvain M, Picone O, et al. Normal fetal urine production rate estimated with 3-dimensional ultrasonography using the rotational technique (virtual organ computer-aided analysis). Am J Obstet Gynecol 2008;199:57 e1-57 e5.
10. Lee SM, Park SK, Shim SS, et al. Measurement of fetal urine production by three-dimensional ultrasonography in normal pregnancy. Ultrasound Obstet Gynecol 2007;30:281-286.
11. Abramovich D. The volume of amniotic fluid and its regulating factors. In: Fairweather D, Eskers T, editors. Amniotic fluid research

and clinical application. 2nd ed. Amsterdam: Excerpta Medica; 1978. p. 31-49.

12. Goldstein RB, Filly RA. Sonographic estimation of amniotic fluid volume: subjective assessment versus pocket measurements. J Ultrasound Med 1988;7:363-369.

13. Chamberlain PF, Manning FA, Morrison I, et al. Ultrasound evaluation of amniotic fluid. Vol I. The relationship of marginal and decreased amniotic fluid volumes to perinatal outcome. Am J Obstet Gynecol 1984;150:245-249.

14. Phelan JP, Ahn MO, Smith CV, et al. Amniotic fluid index measurements during pregnancy. J Reprod Med 1987;32:601-604.

15. Moore TR, Cayle JE. The amniotic fluid index in normal human pregnancy. Am J Obstet Gynecol 1990;162:1168-1173.

16. Hashimoto BE, Kramer DJ, Brennan L. Amniotic fluid volume: fluid dynamics and measurement technique. Semin Ultrasound CT MR 1993;14:40-55.

17. Nabhan AF, Abdelmoula YA, Nabhan AF, Abdelmoula YA. Amniotic fluid index versus single deepest vertical pocket as a screening test for preventing adverse pregnancy outcome. Cochrane Database Syst Rev 2008:CD006593.

Urinary Tract Abnormalities

18. Wiesel A, Queisser-Luft A, Clementi M, et al. Prenatal detection of congenital renal malformations by fetal ultrasonographic examination: an analysis of 709,030 births in 12 European countries. Eur J Med Genet 2005;48:131-144.

19. Thomas DF. Prenatally detected uropathy: epidemiological considerations. Br J Urol 1998;81(Suppl 2):8-12.

20. Murki S, Kumar P, Dutta S, et al. Fatal neonatal renal failure due to maternal enalapril ingestion. J Matern Fetal Neonatal Med 2005;17:235-237.

21. Saji H, Yamanaka M, Hagiwara A, Ijiri R. Losartan and fetal toxic effects [see comment]. Lancet 2001;357:363.

22. Locatelli A, Vergani P, Bellini P, et al. Can a cyclo-oxygenase type-2 selective tocolytic agent avoid the fetal side effects of indomethacin? BJOG 2001;108:325-326.

23. Kaplan BS, Restaino I, Raval DS, et al. Renal failure in the neonate associated with in utero exposure to non-steroidal anti-inflammatory agents [see comment]. Pediatr Nephrol 1994;8:700-704.

24. Mitra SC. Effect of cocaine on fetal kidney and bladder function. J Matern Fetal Med 1999;8:262-269.

25. Nicolaides KH, Cheng HH, Abbas A, et al. Fetal renal defects: associated malformations and chromosomal defects. Fetal Diagn Ther 1992;7:1-11.

26. Roodhooft AM, Birnholz JC, Holmes LB. Familial nature of congenital absence and severe dysgenesis of both kidneys. N Engl J Med 1984;310:1341-1345.

27. Deshpande C, Hennekam RCM. Genetic syndromes and prenatally detected renal anomalies. Semin Fetal Neonatal Med 2008;13:171-180.

28. Potter EL. Bilateral absence of ureters and kidneys: a report of 50 cases. Obstet Gynecol 1965;25:3-12.

29. Bronshtein M, Amit A, Achiron R, et al. The early prenatal sonographic diagnosis of renal agenesis: techniques and possible pitfalls. Prenat Diagn 1994;14:291-297.

30. Hoffman CK, Filly RA, Callen PW. The "lying down" adrenal sign: a sonographic indicator of renal agenesis or ectopia in fetuses and neonates. J Ultrasound Med 1992;11:533-536.

31. Raghavendra BN, Young BK, Greco MA, et al. Use of furosemide in pregnancies complicated by oligohydramnios. Radiology 1987;165:455-458.

32. Haeusler MC, Ryan G, Robson SC, et al. The use of saline solution as a contrast medium in suspected diaphragmatic hernia and renal agenesis. Am J Obstet Gynecol 1993;168:1486-1492.

33. Benacerraf BR. Examination of the second-trimester fetus with severe oligohydramnios using transvaginal scanning. Obstet Gynecol 1990;75:491-493.

34. DeVore GR. The value of color Doppler sonography in the diagnosis of renal agenesis. J Ultrasound Med 1995;14:443-449.

35. Sepulveda W, Stagiannis KD, Flack NJ, Fisk NM. Accuracy of prenatal diagnosis of renal agenesis with color flow imaging in severe second-trimester oligohydramnios. Am J Obstet Gynecol 1995;173:1788-1792.

36. Martín C, Darnell A, Durán C, et al. Magnetic resonance imaging of the intrauterine fetal genitourinary tract: normal anatomy and pathology. Abdom Imaging 2004;29:286-302.

37. Dialani V, Mehta T, Levine D. MR imaging of the fetal abdomen and pelvis. In: Levine D, editor. Atlas of fetal MRI. Boca Raton, Fla: Taylor & Francis; 2005. p. 113-129.

38. Carter CO, Evans K, Pescia G. A family study of renal agenesis. J Med Genet 1979;16:176-188.

39. Chow JS, Benson CB, Lebowitz RL. The clinical significance of an empty renal fossa on prenatal sonography. J Ultrasound Med 2005;24:1049-1054.

40. Yuksel A, Batukan C. Sonographic findings of fetuses with an empty renal fossa and normal amniotic fluid volume. Fetal Diagn Ther 2004;19:525-532.

41. Hill LM, Nowak A, Hartle R, Tush B. Fetal compensatory renal hypertrophy with a unilateral functioning kidney. Ultrasound Obstet Gynecol 2000;15:191-193.

42. Cascio S, Paran S, Puri P. Associated urological anomalies in children with unilateral renal agenesis. J Urol 1999;162:1081-1083.

43. McPherson E, McPherson E. Renal anomalies in families of individuals with congenital solitary kidney. Genet Med 2007;9:298-302.

44. Dunnick NR, Sandler CM, Newhouse JH, Amis Jr ES, editors. Textbook of uroradiology. 4th ed. Philadelphia: Lippincott–Williams & Wilkins; 2008.

45. Arena F, Arena S, Paolata A, et al. Is a complete urological evaluation necessary in all newborns with asymptomatic renal ectopia? Int J Urol 2007;14:491-495.

46. Cho JY, Lee YH, Toi A, Macdonald B. Prenatal diagnosis of horseshoe kidney by measurement of the renal pelvic angle. Ultrasound Obstet Gynecol 2005;25:554-558.

47. Osathanondh V, Potter EL. Pathogenesis of polycystic kidneys: historical survey. Arch Pathol 1964;77:459-465.

48. Winyard P, Chitty L. Dysplastic and polycystic kidneys: diagnosis, associations and management. Prenat Diagn 2001;21:924-935.

49. Matsell DG. Renal dysplasia: new approaches to an old problem. Am J Kidney Dis 1998;32:535-543.

50. Dungan JS, Fernandez MT, Abbitt PL, et al. Multicystic dysplastic kidney: natural history of prenatally detected cases. Prenat Diagn 1990;10:175-182.

51. Kleiner B, Filly RA, Mack L, Callen PW. Multicystic dysplastic kidney: observations of contralateral disease in the fetal population. Radiology 1986;161:27-29.

52. Lazebnik N, Bellinger MF, Ferguson Jr JE, et al. Insights into the pathogenesis and natural history of fetuses with multicystic dysplastic kidney disease. Prenat Diagn 1999;19:418-423.

53. Van Eijk L, Cohen-Overbeek TE, den Hollander NS, et al. Unilateral multicystic dysplastic kidney: a combined pre- and postnatal assessment. Ultrasound Obstet Gynecol 2002;19:180-183.

54. Eckoldt F, Woderich R, Smith RD, et al. Antenatal diagnostic aspects of unilateral multicystic kidney dysplasia: sensitivity, specificity, predictive values, differential diagnoses, associated malformations and consequences [see comment]. Fetal Diagn Ther 2004;19:163-169.

55. Gordon AC, Thomas DF, Arthur RJ, Irving HC. Multicystic dysplastic kidney: is nephrectomy still appropriate? J Urol 1988;140:1231-1234.

56. Rudnik-Schoneborn S, John U, Deget F, et al. Clinical features of unilateral multicystic renal dysplasia in children. Eur J Pediatr 1998;157:666-672.

57. Eckoldt F, Woderich R, Wolke S, et al. Follow-up of unilateral multicystic kidney dysplasia after prenatal diagnosis. J Matern Fetal Neonatal Med 2003;14:177-186.

58. Beck AD. The effect of intra-uterine urinary obstruction upon the development of the fetal kidney. J Urol 1971;105:784-789.

59. Harrison MR, Filly RA. The fetus with obstructive uropathy: pathophysiology, natural history, selection and treatment. In: Harrison MR, Golbus MS, Filly RA, editors. The unborn patient: prenatal diagnosis and treatment. 2nd ed. Philadelphia: Saunders; 1991. p. 328-393.

60. Mahony BS, Filly RA, Callen PW, et al. Fetal renal dysplasia: sonographic evaluation. Radiology 1984;152:143-146.

61. Estroff JA, Mandell J, Benacerraf BR. Increased renal parenchymal echogenicity in the fetus: importance and clinical outcome. Radiology 1991;181:135-139.

62. Avni FE, Garel L, Cassart M, et al. Perinatal assessment of hereditary cystic renal diseases: the contribution of sonography. Pediatr Radiol 2006;36:405-414; erratum 36:731.

63. Reuss A, Wladimiroff JW, Stewart PA, Niermeijer MF. Prenatal diagnosis by ultrasound in pregnancies at risk for autosomal recessive polycystic kidney disease. Ultrasound Med Biol 1990;16:355-359.

64. Romero R, Cullen M, Jeanty P, et al. The diagnosis of congenital renal anomalies with ultrasound. II. Infantile polycystic kidney disease. Am J Obstet Gynecol 1984;150:259-262.

65. Barth RA, Guillot AP, Capeless EL, Clemmons JJ. Prenatal diagnosis of autosomal recessive polycystic kidney disease: variable outcome within one family. Am J Obstet Gynecol 1992;166:560-561.

66. Zerres K, Mucher G, Becker J, et al. Prenatal diagnosis of autosomal recessive polycystic kidney disease (ARPKD): molecular genetics, clinical experience, and fetal morphology. Am J Med Genet 1998; 76:137-144.

67. Pretorius DH, Lee ME, Manco-Johnson ML, et al. Diagnosis of autosomal dominant polycystic kidney disease in utero and in the young infant. J Ultrasound Med 1987;6:249-255.

68. Brun M, Maugey-Laulom B, Eurin D, et al. Prenatal sonographic patterns in autosomal dominant polycystic kidney disease: a multicenter study. Ultrasound Obstet Gynecol 2004;24:55-61.

69. MacDermot KD, Saggar-Malik AK, Economides DL, Jeffery S. Prenatal diagnosis of autosomal dominant polycystic kidney disease (PKD1) presenting in utero and prognosis for very early onset disease. J Med Genet 1998;35:13-16.

70. Sinibaldi D, Malena S, Mingarelli R, Rizzoni G. Prenatal ultrasonographic findings of dominant polycystic kidney disease and postnatal renal evolution. Am J Med Genet 1996;65:337-341.

71. Fick GM, Johnson AM, Strain JD, et al. Characteristics of very early onset autosomal dominant polycystic kidney disease. J Am Soc Nephrol 1993;3:1863-1870.

72. Zerres K, Rudnik-Schoneborn S, Deget F. Childhood onset autosomal dominant polycystic kidney disease in sibs: clinical picture and recurrence risk. German Working Group on Paediatric Nephrology (Arbeitsgemeinschaft fur Padiatrische Nephrologie). J Med Genet 1993;30:583-588.

73. Boyer O, Gagnadoux MF, Guest G, et al. Prognosis of autosomal dominant polycystic kidney disease diagnosed in utero or at birth. Pediatr Nephrol 2007;22:380-388.

74. Wellesley D, Howe DT. Fetal renal anomalies and genetic syndromes. Prenat Diagn 2001;21:992-1003.

75. Sepulveda W, Sebire NJ, Souka A, et al. Diagnosis of the Meckel-Gruber syndrome at eleven to fourteen weeks' gestation. Am J Obstet Gynecol 1997;176:316-319.

76. Nyberg DA, Hallesy D, Mahony BS, et al. Meckel-Gruber syndrome: importance of prenatal diagnosis. J Ultrasound Med 1990;9:691-696.

77. Ulinski T, Lescure S, Beaufils S, et al. Renal phenotypes related to hepatocyte nuclear factor-1beta (TCF2) mutations in a pediatric cohort. J Am Soc Nephrol 2006;17:497-503.

78. Decramer S, Parant O, Beaufils S, et al. Anomalies of the TCF2 gene are the main cause of fetal bilateral hyperechogenic kidneys. J Am Soc Nephrol 2007;18:923-933.

79. Twining P. Genitourinary malformations. In: Nyberg DA, McGahn JP, Pretorius DH, Pilu G, editors. Diagnostic imaging of fetal anomalies. Philadelphia: Lippincott–Williams & Wilkins; 2003.

80. Tsatsaris V, Gagnadoux MF, Aubry MC, et al. Prenatal diagnosis of bilateral isolated fetal hyperechogenic kidneys. Is it possible to predict long term outcome? BJOG 2002;109:1388-1393.

81. Chaumoitre K, Brun M, Cassart M, et al. Differential diagnosis of fetal hyperechogenic cystic kidneys unrelated to renal tract anomalies: a multicenter study. Ultrasound Obstet Gynecol 2006;28:911-917.

82. Carr MC, Benacerraf BR, Estroff JA, Mandell J. Prenatally diagnosed bilateral hyperechoic kidneys with normal amniotic fluid: postnatal outcome. J Urol 1995;153:142-144.

83. Blazer S, Zimmer EZ, Blumenfeld Z, et al. Natural history of fetal simple renal cysts detected in early pregnancy. J Urol 1999;162: 812-814.

84. Leclair MD, El-Ghoneimi A, Audry G, et al. The outcome of prenatally diagnosed renal tumors. J Urol 2005;173:186-189.

85. Chen WY, Lin CN, Chao CS, et al. Prenatal diagnosis of congenital mesoblastic nephroma in mid-second trimester by sonography and magnetic resonance imaging. Prenat Diagn 2003;23:927-931.

86. Rubenstein SC, Benacerraf BR, Retik AB, Mandell J. Fetal suprarenal masses: sonographic appearance and differential diagnosis. Ultrasound Obstet Gynecol 1995;5:164-167.

87. Heling KS, Chaoui R, Hartung J, et al. Prenatal diagnosis of congenital neuroblastoma: analysis of 4 cases and review of the literature. Fetal Diagn Ther 1999;14:47-52.

88. Sauvat F, Sarnacki S, Brisse H, et al. Outcome of suprarenal localized masses diagnosed during the perinatal period: a retrospective multicenter study. Cancer 2002;94:2474-2480.

89. Toma P, Lucigrai G, Marzoli A, Lituania M. Prenatal diagnosis of metastatic adrenal neuroblastoma with sonography and MR imaging. AJR Am J Roentgenol 1994;162:1183-1184.

90. Blackman SC, Evenson AR, Voss SD, et al. Prenatal diagnosis and subsequent treatment of an intermediate-risk paraspinal neuroblastoma: case report and review of the literature. Fetal Diagn Ther 2008;24:119-125.

91. Jennings RW, LaQuaglia MP, Leong K, et al. Fetal neuroblastoma: prenatal diagnosis and natural history. J Pediatr Surg 1993; 28:1168-1174.

92. Ho PT, Estroff JA, Kozakewich H, et al. Prenatal detection of neuroblastoma: a ten-year experience from the Dana-Farber Cancer Institute and Children's Hospital [see comment]. Pediatrics 1993; 92:358-364.

93. Schwarzler P, Bernard JP, Senat MV, Ville Y. Prenatal diagnosis of fetal adrenal masses: differentiation between hemorrhage and solid tumor by color Doppler sonography. Ultrasound Obstet Gynecol 1999;13:351-355.

94. Rahman S, Ohlsson A, Fong KW, Glanc P. Fetal adrenal hemorrhage in a diamniotic, dichorionic twin: case report and review of controversies in diagnosis and management. J Ultrasound Med 1997;16:297-300.

95. Schrauder MG, Hammersen G, Siemer J, et al. Fetal adrenal haemorrhage: two-dimensional and three-dimensional imaging. Fetal Diagn Ther 2008;23:72-75.

96. Reddy PP, Mandell J. Prenatal diagnosis: therapeutic implications. Urol Clin North Am 1998;25:171-180.

97. Chudleigh T. Mild pyelectasis. Prenat Diagn 2001;21:936-941.

98. Thompson MO, Thilaganathan B. Effect of routine screening for Down's syndrome on the significance of isolated fetal hydronephrosis. Br J Obstet Gynaecol 1998;105:860-864.

99. Chudleigh PM, Chitty LS, Pembrey M, Campbell S. The association of aneuploidy and mild fetal pyelectasis in an unselected population: the results of a multicenter study. Ultrasound Obstet Gynecol 2001;17:197-202.

100. Sairam S, Al-Habib A, Sasson S, Thilaganathan B. Natural history of fetal hydronephrosis diagnosed on mid-trimester ultrasound. Ultrasound Obstet Gynecol 2001;17:191-196.

101. Fernbach SK, Maizels M, Conway JJ. Ultrasound grading of hydronephrosis: introduction to the system used by the Society for Fetal Urology. Pediatr Radiol 1993;23:478-480.

102. Baskin LS. Prenatal hydronephrosis. In: Baskin LS, Kogan B., Duckett J, editors. Handbook of pediatric urology. Philadelphia: Lippincott-Raven; 1997. p. 15.

103. Odibo AO, Marchiano D, Quinones JN, et al. Mild pyelectasis: evaluating the relationship between gestational age and renal pelvic anterior-posterior diameter. Prenat Diagn 2003;23:824-827.

104. Livera LN, Brookfield DS, Egginton JA, Hawnaur JM. Antenatal ultrasonography to detect fetal renal abnormalities: a prospective screening programme. BMJ 1989;298:1421-1423.

105. Benacerraf BR, Mandell J, Estroff JA, et al. Fetal pyelectasis: a possible association with Down syndrome. Obstet Gynecol 1990;76: 58-60.

106. Corteville JE, Dicke JM, Crane JP. Fetal pyelectasis and Down syndrome: is genetic amniocentesis warranted? Obstet Gynecol 1992;79:770-772.

107. Anderson NG, Abbott GD, Mogridge N, et al. Vesicoureteric reflux in the newborn: relationship to fetal renal pelvic diameter. Pediatr Nephrol 1997;11:610-616.

108. Ismaili K, Hall M, Donner C, et al. Results of systematic screening for minor degrees of fetal renal pelvis dilatation in an unselected population. Am J Obstet Gynecol 2003;188:242-246.

109. Corteville JE, Gray DL, Crane JP. Congenital hydronephrosis: correlation of fetal ultrasonographic findings with infant outcome [see comment]. Am J Obstet Gynecol 1991;165:384-388.

110. Anderson N, Clautice-Engle T, Allan R, et al. Detection of obstructive uropathy in the fetus: predictive value of sonographic measurements of renal pelvic diameter at various gestational ages. AJR Am J Roentgenol 1995;164:719-723.

111. Babcook CJ, Silvera M, Drake C, Levine D. Effect of maternal hydration on mild fetal pyelectasis. J Ultrasound Med 1998;17:539-544.

112. Graif M, Kessler A, Hart S, et al. Renal pyelectasis in pregnancy: correlative evaluation of fetal and maternal collecting systems. Am J Obstet Gynecol 1992;167:1304-1306.

113. Petrikovsky BM, Cuomo MI, Schneider EP, et al. Isolated fetal hydronephrosis: beware the effect of bladder filling. Prenat Diagn 1995;15:827-829.

114. Damen-Elias HAM, Stigter RH, De Jong TPVM, Visser GHA. Variability in dilatation of the fetal renal pelvis during a bladder filling cycle. Ultrasound Obstet Gynecol 2004;24:750-755.

115. Persutte WH, Hussey M, Chyu J, Hobbins JC. Striking findings concerning the variability in the measurement of the fetal renal collecting system. Ultrasound Obstet Gynecol 2000;15:186-190.

116. Lee RS, Cendron M, Kinnamon DD, et al. Antenatal hydronephrosis as a predictor of postnatal outcome: a meta-analysis. Pediatrics 2006;118:586-593.

117. Adra AM, Mejides AA, Dennaoui MS, Beydoun SN. Fetal pyelectasis: is it always "physiologic"? Am J Obstet Gynecol 1995;173:1263-1266.

118. Sidhu G, Beyene J, Rosenblum ND. Outcome of isolated antenatal hydronephrosis: a systematic review and meta-analysis. Pediatr Nephrol 2006;21:218-224.

119. Coplen DE, Austin PF, Yan Y, et al. The magnitude of fetal renal pelvic dilatation can identify obstructive postnatal hydronephrosis, and direct postnatal evaluation and management [see comment]. J Urol 2006;176:724-727; discussion 727.

120. Wickstrom E, Maizels M, Sabbagha RE, et al. Isolated fetal pyelectasis: assessment of risk for postnatal uropathy and Down syndrome. Ultrasound Obstet Gynecol 1996;8:236-240.

121. Ek S, Lidefeldt KJ, Varricio L. Fetal hydronephrosis; prevalence, natural history and postnatal consequences in an unselected population. Acta Obstet Gynecol Scand 2007;86:1463-1466.

122. Bobrowski RA, Levin RB, Lauria MR, et al. In utero progression of isolated renal pelvis dilation. Am J Perinatol 1997;14:423-426.

123. Ismaili K, Avni FE, Piepsz A, et al. Current management of infants with fetal renal pelvis dilation: a survey by French-speaking pediatric nephrologists and urologists. Pediatr Nephrol 2004;19:966-971.

124. Laing FC, Burke VD, Wing VW, et al. Postpartum evaluation of fetal hydronephrosis: optimal timing for follow-up sonography. Radiology 1984;152:423-424.

125. Zerin JM, Ritchey ML, Chang ACH. Incidental vesicoureteral reflux in neonates with antenatally detected hydronephrosis and other renal abnormalities. Radiology 1993;187:157-160.

126. Clautice-Engle T, Anderson NG, et al. Diagnosis of obstructive hydronephrosis in infants: comparison sonograms performed 6 days and 6 weeks after birth. AJR Am J Roentgenol 1995;164:963-967.

127. De Bruyn R, Gordon I. Postnatal investigation of fetal renal disease. Prenat Diagn 2001;21:984-991.

128. Lidefelt KJ, Ek S, Mihocsa L, et al. Is screening for vesicoureteral reflux mandatory in infants with antenatal renal pelvis dilatation? Acta Paediatr 2006;95:1653-1656.

129. Ismaili K, Avni FE, Wissing KM, Hall M. Long-term clinical outcome of infants with mild and moderate fetal pyelectasis: validation of neonatal ultrasound as a screening tool to detect significant nephrouropathies. J Pediatr 2004;144:759-765.

130. Glazer GM, Filly RA, Callen PW. The varied sonographic appearance of the urinary tract in the fetus and newborn with urethral obstruction. Radiology 1982;144:563-568.

131. Pates JA, Dashe JS. Prenatal diagnosis and management of hydronephrosis. Early Hum Dev 2006;82:3-8.

132. Gorincour G, Rypens F, Toiviainen-Salo S, et al. Fetal urinoma: two new cases and a review of the literature. Ultrasound Obstet Gynecol 2006;28:848-852.

133. Barker AP, Cave MM, Thomas DF, et al. Fetal pelvi-ureteric junction obstruction: predictors of outcome. Br J Urol 1995;76:649-652.

134. Liu HY, Dhillon HK, Yeung CK, et al. Clinical outcome and management of prenatally diagnosed primary megaureters. J Urol 1994;152:614-617.

135. McLellan DL, Retik AB, Bauer SB, et al. Rate and predictors of spontaneous resolution of prenatally diagnosed primary nonrefluxing megaureter. J Urol 2002;168:2177-2180.

136. Shukla AR, Cooper J, Patel RP, et al. Prenatally detected primary megaureter: a role for extended follow-up. J Urol 2005;173:1353-1356.

137. Calisti A, Oriolo L, Perrotta ML, et al. The fate of prenatally diagnosed primary nonrefluxing megaureter: do we have reliable predictors for spontaneous resolution? Urology 2008;72:309-312.

138. Abuhamad AZ, Horton Jr CE, Horton SH, Evans AT. Renal duplication anomalies in the fetus: clues for prenatal diagnosis. Ultrasound Obstet Gynecol 1996;7:174-177.

139. Vergani P, Ceruti P, Locatelli A, et al. Accuracy of prenatal ultrasonographic diagnosis of duplex renal system. J Ultrasound Med 1999;18:463-467.

140. Whitten SM, McHoney M, Wilcox DT, et al. Accuracy of antenatal fetal ultrasound in the diagnosis of duplex kidneys. Ultrasound Obstet Gynecol 2003;21:342-346.

141. Anderson NG, Allan RB, Abbott GD, et al. Fluctuating fetal or neonatal renal pelvis: marker of high-grade vesicoureteral reflux. Pediatr Nephrol 2004;19:749-753.

142. Van Eerde AM, Meutgeert MH, De Jong TPVM, Giltay JC. Vesicoureteral reflux in children with prenatally detected hydronephrosis: a systematic review. Ultrasound Obstet Gynecol 2007;29:463-469.

143. Ismaili K, Avni FE, Hall M. Results of systematic voiding cystourethrography in infants with antenatally diagnosed renal pelvis dilation. J Pediatr 2002;141:21-24.

144. Ismaili K, Hall M, Piepsz A, et al. Primary vesicoureteral reflux detected in neonates with a history of fetal renal pelvis dilatation: a prospective clinical and imaging study. J Pediatr 2006;148:222-227.

145. Penido Silva JM, Oliveira EA, Diniz JS, et al. Clinical course of prenatally detected primary vesicoureteral reflux. Pediatr Nephrol 2006;21:86-91.

146. Sebire NJ, von Kaisenberg C, Rubio C, et al. Fetal megacystis at 10-14 weeks of gestation. Ultrasound Obstet Gynecol 1996;8:387-390.

147. Favre R, Kohler M, Gasser B, et al. Early fetal megacystis between 11 and 15 weeks of gestation. Ultrasound Obstet Gynecol 1999;14:402-406.

148. Liao AW, Sebire NJ, Geerts L, et al. Megacystis at 10-14 weeks of gestation: chromosomal defects and outcome according to bladder length. Ultrasound Obstet Gynecol 2003;21:338-341.

149. Carroll SG, Soothill PW, Tizard J, Kyle PM. Vesicocentesis at 10-14 weeks of gestation for treatment of fetal megacystis. Ultrasound Obstet Gynecol 2001;18:366-370.

150. Jouannic JM, Hyett JA, Pandya PP, et al. Perinatal outcome in fetuses with megacystis in the first half of pregnancy. Prenat Diagn 2003;23:340-344.

151. Perks AE, MacNeily AE, Blair GK. Posterior urethral valves. J Pediatr Surg 2002;37:1105-1107.

152. Yerkes EB, Cain MP, Padilla LM. In utero perinephric urinoma and urinary ascites with posterior urethral valves: a paradoxical pop-off valve? J Urol 2001;166:2387-2388.

153. Bierkens AF, Feitz WF, Nijhuis JG, de Wildt MJ, et al. Early urethral obstruction sequence: a lethal entity? Fetal Diagn Ther 1996;11:137-145.

154. Cilento Jr BG, Benacerraf BR, Mandell J. Prenatal diagnosis of cloacal malformation. Urology 1994;43:386-388.

155. Greskovich 3rd FJ, Nyberg Jr LM. The prune belly syndrome: a review of its etiology, defects, treatment and prognosis. J Urol 1988;140:707-712.

156. Sepulveda W, Elorza C, Gutierrez J, et al. Congenital megalourethra: outcome after prenatal diagnosis in a series of 4 cases. J Ultrasound Med 2005;24:1303-1308.

157. Fitzsimons RB, Keohane C, Galvin J. Prune belly syndrome with ultrasound demonstration of reduction of megacystis in utero. Br J Radiol 1985;58:374-376.

158. Garel C, Dreux S, Philippe-Chomette P, et al. Contribution of fetal magnetic resonance imaging and amniotic fluid digestive enzyme assays to the evaluation of gastrointestinal tract abnormalities. Ultrasound Obstet Gynecol 2006;28:282-291.

159. Muller F, Dreux S, Vaast P, et al. Prenatal diagnosis of megacystis-microcolon-intestinal hypoperistalsis syndrome: contribution of amniotic fluid digestive enzyme assay and fetal urinalysis. Prenat Diagn 2005;25:203-209.

160. Heyroth-Griffis CA, Weaver DD, Faught P, Bellus GA, Torres-Martinez W. On the spectrum of limb-body wall complex, exstrophy

of the cloaca, and urorectal septum malformation sequence. Am J Med Genet A 2007;143A:1025-1031.

161. Gonzalez R, De Filippo R, Jednak R, Barthold JS. Urethral atresia: long-term outcome in 6 children who survived the neonatal period. J Urol 2001;165:2241-2244.

162. Jaramillo D, Lebowitz RL, Hendren WH. The cloacal malformation: radiologic findings and imaging recommendations. Radiology 1990;177:441-448.

163. Johnson MP, Corsi P, Bradfield W, et al. Sequential urinalysis improves evaluation of fetal renal function in obstructive uropathy. Am J Obstet Gynecol 1995;173:59-65.

164. Nicolini U, Fisk NM, Rodeck CH, Beacham J. Fetal urine biochemistry: an index of renal maturation and dysfunction. Br J Obstet Gynaecol 1992;99:46-50.

165. Lipitz S, Ryan G, Samuell C, et al. Fetal urine analysis for the assessment of renal function in obstructive uropathy. Am J Obstet Gynecol 1993;168:174-179.

166. Muller F, Dommergues M, Mandelbrot L, et al. Fetal urinary biochemistry predicts postnatal renal function in children with bilateral obstructive uropathies. Obstet Gynecol 1993;82:813-820.

167. Crombleholme TM, Harrison MR, Golbus MS, et al. Fetal intervention in obstructive uropathy: prognostic indicators and efficacy of intervention. Am J Obstet Gynecol 1990;162:1239-1244.

168. Qureshi F, Jacques SM, Seifman B, et al. In utero fetal urine analysis and renal histology correlate with the outcome in fetal obstructive uropathies. Fetal Diagn Ther 1996;11:306-312.

169. Muller F, Dommergues M, Bussieres L, et al. Development of human renal function: reference intervals for 10 biochemical markers in fetal urine. Clin Chem 1996;42:1855-1860.

170. Nicolaides KH, Cheng HH, Snijders RJ, Moniz CF. Fetal urine biochemistry in the assessment of obstructive uropathy. Am J Obstet Gynecol 1992;166:932-937.

171. Berry SM, Lecolier B, Smith RS, et al. Predictive value of fetal serum beta 2-microglobulin for neonatal renal function. Lancet 1995;345:1277-1278.

172. Nicolini U, Spelzini F. Invasive assessment of fetal renal abnormalities: urinalysis, fetal blood sampling and biopsy. Prenat Diagn 2001;21:964-969.

173. Morris RK, Quinlan-Jones E, Kilby MD, Khan KS. Systematic review of accuracy of fetal urine analysis to predict poor postnatal renal function in cases of congenital urinary tract obstruction. Prenat Diagn 2007;27:900-911.

174. Holmes N, Harrison MR, Baskin LS. Fetal surgery for posterior urethral valves: long-term postnatal outcomes. Pediatrics 2001;108:E7.

175. Makino Y, Kobayashi H, Kyono K, et al. Clinical results of fetal obstructive uropathy treated by vesicoamniotic shunting. Urology 2000;55:118-122.

176. McLorie G, Farhat W, Khoury A, et al. Outcome analysis of vesicoamniotic shunting in a comprehensive population. J Urol 2001;166:1036-1040.

177. Freedman AL, Johnson MP, Smith CA, et al. Long-term outcome in children after antenatal intervention for obstructive uropathies. Lancet 1999;354:374-377.

178. Clark TJ, Martin WL, Divakaran TG, et al. Prenatal bladder drainage in the management of fetal lower urinary tract obstruction: a systematic review and meta-analysis. Obstet Gynecol 2003;102:367-382.

179. Biard JM, Johnson MP, Carr MC, et al. Long-term outcomes in children treated by prenatal vesicoamniotic shunting for lower urinary tract obstruction. Obstet Gynecol 2005;106:503-508.

180. Gearhart JP, Ben-Chaim J, Jeffs RD, Sanders RC. Criteria for the prenatal diagnosis of classic bladder exstrophy. Obstet Gynecol 1995;85:961-964.

181. Ben-Neriah Z, Withers S, Thomas M, et al. OEIS complex: prenatal ultrasound and autopsy findings. Ultrasound Obstet Gynecol 2007;29:170-177.

182. Tiblad E, Wilson RD, Carr M, et al. OEIS sequence: a rare congenital anomaly with prenatal evaluation and postnatal outcome in six cases. Prenat Diagn 2008;28:141-147.

The Genital Tract

183. Reece EA, Winn HN, Wan M, et al. Can ultrasonography replace amniocentesis in fetal gender determination during the early second trimester? Am J Obstet Gynecol 1987;156:579-581.

184. Harrington K, Armstrong V, Freeman J, et al. Fetal sexing by ultrasound in the second trimester: maternal preference and professional ability [see comment]. Ultrasound Obstet Gynecol 1996;8:318-321.

185. Meagher S, Davison G. Early second-trimester determination of fetal gender by ultrasound [see comment]. Ultrasound Obstet Gynecol 1996;8:322-324.

186. Lev-Toaff AS, Ozhan S, Pretorius D, et al. Three-dimensional multiplanar ultrasound for fetal gender assignment: value of the mid-sagittal plane. Ultrasound Obstet Gynecol 2000;16:345-350.

187. Whitlow BJ, Lazanakis MS, Economides DL. The sonographic identification of fetal gender from 11 to 14 weeks of gestation [see comment]. Ultrasound Obstet Gynecol 1999;13:301-304.

188. Efrat Z, Akinfenwa OO, Nicolaides KH. First-trimester determination of fetal gender by ultrasound [see comment]. Ultrasound Obstet Gynecol 1999;13:305-307.

189. Mazza V, Falcinelli C, Paganelli S, et al. Sonographic early fetal gender assignment: a longitudinal study in pregnancies after in vitro fertilization. Ultrasound Obstet Gynecol 2001;17:513-516.

190. Achiron R, Pinhas-Hamiel O, Zalel Y, et al. Development of fetal male gender: prenatal sonographic measurement of the scrotum and evaluation of testicular descent [see comment]. Ultrasound Obstet Gynecol 1998;11:242-245.

191. Pretorius DH, Halsted MJ, Abels W, et al. Hydroceles identified prenatally: common physiologic phenomenon? J Ultrasound Med 1998;17:49-52.

192. Meizner I, Levy A, Katz M, et al. Prenatal ultrasonographic diagnosis of fetal scrotal inguinal hernia. Am J Obstet Gynecol 1992;166:907-909.

193. Mandell J, Bromley B, Peters CA, Benacerraf BR. Prenatal sonographic detection of genital malformations. J Urol 1995;153:1994-1996.

194. Shapiro E. The sonographic appearance of normal and abnormal fetal genitalia. J Urol 1999;162:530-533.

195. Cheikhelard A, Luton D, Philippe-Chomette P, et al. How accurate is the prenatal diagnosis of abnormal genitalia? J Urol 2000;164:984-987.

196. Meizner I. The "tulip sign": a sonographic clue for in-utero diagnosis of severe hypospadias. Ultrasound Obstet Gynecol 2002;19:317.

197. McGaughran JM, Clayton PT, Mills KA, et al. Prenatal diagnosis of Smith-Lemli-Opitz syndrome. Am J Med Genet 1995;56:269-271.

198. Shapiro E, Santiago JV, Crane JP. Prenatal fetal adrenal suppression following in utero diagnosis of congenital adrenal hyperplasia. J Urol 1989;142:663-666; discussion 667-668.

199. Saada J, Grebille AG, Aubry MC, et al. Sonography in prenatal diagnosis of congenital adrenal hyperplasia. Prenat Diagn 2004;24:627-630.

200. Carlson AD, Obeid JS, Kanellopoulou N, et al. Congenital adrenal hyperplasia: update on prenatal diagnosis and treatment. J Steroid Biochem Mol Biol 1999;69:19-29.

201. New MI. An update of congenital adrenal hyperplasia. Ann NY Acad Sci 2004;1038:14-43.

202. Pajkrt E, Petersen OB, Chitty LS. Fetal genital anomalies: an aid to diagnosis. Prenat Diagn 2008;28:389-398.

203. Mazza V, Di Monte I, Ceccarelli PL, et al. Prenatal diagnosis of female pseudohermaphroditism associated with bilateral luteoma of pregnancy: case report. Hum Reprod 2002;17:821-824.

204. Picone O, Laperelle J, Sonigo P, et al. Fetal magnetic resonance imaging in the antenatal diagnosis and management of hydrocolpos. Ultrasound Obstet Gynecol 2007;30:105-109.

205. Hayashi S, Sago H, Kashima K, et al. Prenatal diagnosis of fetal hydrometrocolpos secondary to a cloacal anomaly by magnetic resonance imaging. Ultrasound Obstet Gynecol 2005;26:577-579.

206. Dhombres F, Jouannic JM, Brodaty G, et al. Contribution of prenatal imaging to the anatomical assessment of fetal hydrocolpos. Ultrasound Obstet Gynecol 2007;30:101-104.

207. Garel L, Filiatrault D, Brandt M, et al. Antenatal diagnosis of ovarian cysts: natural history and therapeutic implications. Pediatr Radiol 1991;21:182-184.

208. Nussbaum AR, Sanders RC, Hartman DS, et al. Neonatal ovarian cysts: sonographic-pathologic correlation. Radiology 1988;168:817-821.

209. Heling KS, Chaoui R, Kirchmair F, et al. Fetal ovarian cysts: prenatal diagnosis, management and postnatal outcome. Ultrasound Obstet Gynecol 2002;20:47-50.

210. Meizner I, Levy A, Katz M, et al. Fetal ovarian cysts: prenatal ultrasonographic detection and postnatal evaluation and treatment. Am J Obstetr Gynecol 1991;164:874-878.

211. Giorlandino C. Antenatal ultrasonographic diagnosis and management of fetal ovarian cysts. Int J Gynecol Obstet 1994;44:27-31.

212. Bagolan P, Giorlandino C, Nahom A, et al. The management of fetal ovarian cysts. J Pediatr Surg 2002;37:25-30.

213. Bryant AE, Laufer MR. Fetal ovarian cysts: incidence, diagnosis and management. J Reprod Med 2004;49:329-337.

214. Monnery-Noche ME, Auber F, Jouannic JM, et al. Fetal and neonatal ovarian cysts: is surgery indicated? Prenat Diagn 2008;28:15-20.

CHAPTER 40

The Fetal Musculoskeletal System

Phyllis Glanc, David Chitayat, and Sheila Unger

Chapter Outline

$\mathcal{C}$ongenital bone disorders are a heterogeneous group of disorders primarily affecting the growth and development of the musculoskeletal system. There are three major categories. The skeletal dysplasias are developmental disorders of chondro-osseous tissue caused by single-gene disorders with prenatal and postnatal manifestations. the dysostoses are single-gene disorders resulting in malformations of individual bones caused by transient abnormalities of signaling factors. Disruptions are morphologic defects of an organ or larger region resulting from extrinsic breakdown or interference with an originally normal developmental process.[1] The prevalence of skeletal dysplasias, also called osteochondrodysplasias, diagnosed prenatally or during the neonatal period, excluding limb amputations, is 2.4 to 4.5 per 10,000 births. More than 400 subtypes have been reported[2-5] (Table 40-1).

The number of recognized genetic disorders with a substantial skeletal component is increasing, and the distinction among dysplasias, metabolic bone disorders, dysostoses, and malformation syndromes is constantly evolving. Despite increased knowledge about the genetic etiology of many of these conditions and the improved ability to diagnose and categorize these disorders correctly, the clinical and imaging features remain a fundamental tool for diagnosing and directing the molecular

investigation.[2,6] Although many fetal skeletal dysplasias can be accurately identified by prenatal ultrasound, this remains a challenging task because of the low incidence, phenotypic variability and wide range of appearances.[7] The majority of cases have no family history of a similar condition. Nonetheless, the majority of **lethal skeletal dysplasias,** including **thanatophoric dysplasia, achondrogenesis,** and **osteogenesis imperfecta** type II, can be diagnosed solely on the basis of prenatal ultrasound.[8] Tretter et al.[9] determined that 26 of 27 lethal skeletal dysplasias were identified correctly by prenatal ultrasound; however, only 13 of 27 (48%) received an accurate specific antenatal diagnosis.[9] Eight of 14 (57%) underwent a substantial change in genetic counseling when cytogenetic, molecular (including microarray), pathologic, and radiologic findings were added. Thus, although the ultrasound diagnosis of a lethal skeletal dysplasia is highly accurate (85%-95%), a correct specific diagnosis is obtained in only 40% to 55% of cases.[7-9]

Nonetheless, the highly accurate prenatal determination of the lethality of a given skeletal dysplasia is crucial in helping couples with decision making. Typically, a combination of ultrasound, radiologic, genetic, pathologic, and cytogenetic investigation is required to classify a specific congenital musculoskeletal disorder. A prenatal

TABLE 40-1. BIRTH PREVALENCE OF SKELETAL DYSPLASIAS

SKELETAL DYSPLASIA	PREVALENCE PER 100,000 BIRTHS
Lethal Dysplasias	
Thanatophoric dysplasia	2.4 to 6.9
Achondrogenesis	0.9 to 2.3
Osteogenesis imperfecta type IIA	1.8
Hypophosphatasia congenita	1.0
Variable-Prognosis Dysplasias	
Rhizomelic chondrodysplasia punctata	0.5 to 0.9
Campomelic dysplasia	1.0 to 1.5
Asphyxiating thoracic dystrophy	0.8 to 1.4
Ellis–van Creveld syndrome	0.7
Osteogenesis imperfecta (other types)	1.8
Nonlethal Dysplasias	
Heterozygous achondroplasia	3.3 to 3.8
Overall	24.4 to 75.0

diagnosis of a musculoskeletal anomaly will provide an opportunity for genetic counseling, pregnancy termination, or tertiary-level care when appropriate. A multidisciplinary approach involving the medical imaging team, obstetrician, medical geneticist, and perinatologist is important in optimizing the accuracy of prognosis and recurrence risk. This information is crucial to the family and to medical personnel involved in planning clinical management for both current and future pregnancies. This chapter uses a "key features" approach to the sonographic diagnosis of the common skeletal dysplasias to aid in the classification and differential diagnosis.

NORMAL FETAL SKELETON

Development

The high level of intrinsic contrast of the fetal extremities places them among the earliest structures that can be evaluated by ultrasound. By the end of the embryonic period, the differentiation of bones, joints, and musculature is similar to that of an adult and is associated with increased fetal movements.[10,11] Transvaginal ultrasound can demonstrate the limb buds by 7 weeks' gestation, and the foot and hand plates are visible by 8 weeks.[12] Osteogenesis begins in the clavicle and mandible by 8 weeks as well. By 11 to 12 weeks, the **primary ossification centers** of the long bones (e.g., scapula, ileum), as well as the limb articulations and phalanges, can be identified. The ischium, metacarpals, and metatarsals ossify during the fourth month of gestation. The pubis, calcaneus, and talus ossify during the fifth and sixth months. Ossification of the other tarsal and carpal bones occurs postnatally.[13] The direction of growth in the long bones is from proximal to distal, and the lower extremities lag slightly behind the upper extremities.[11]

Of the **secondary ossification centers** in the long bones, only the distal femoral epiphysis, the proximal tibial epiphysis, and occasionally the proximal humeral epiphysis ossify prenatally (Fig. 40-1). The unossified epiphysis appears hypoechoic, with a variably, mildly echogenic center. Ossification begins centrally. The distal femoral epiphysis can ossify as early as 29 weeks' menstrual age and as late as 34 weeks. When it measures greater than 7 mm, the menstrual age is generally later than 37 weeks.[14,15] The proximal tibial epiphysis begins to ossify by 35 menstrual weeks.[15] In uncomplicated pregnancies the combination of a distal femoral epiphysis of 3 mm or greater and the presence of a proximal tibial epiphysis is considered a reliable marker of pulmonary maturity.[16] **Intrauterine growth restriction** (IUGR) may delay ossification of the distal femoral epiphysis and proximal tibial epiphysis. The earliest secondary epiphysis to ossify is the **calcaneus,** at approximately 20 weeks' gestation, thus marking the earliest point that assessment of delayed ossification of the secondary epiphyseal centers can be attempted.

The fascia within the muscle is highly echogenic compared with the relatively hypoechoic cartilage. The fetal musculature is slightly more echogenic than the relatively hypoechoic cartilage. The fetal joint spaces, in particular the knee, appear echogenic because of the combination of synovium, fat, and microvasculature.[11] The normal development and ultimate function of the fetal musculoskeletal system depend on **fetal movements,** which start by the second half of the first trimester. In the absence of normal fetal motion, the bones and muscles will be underdeveloped, the chest will be narrow, and joint contractures and postural deformities may also occur.

Extremity Measurements

It is a standard practice to assess **femur length** (FL) as part of the evaluation of fetal size and morphology. Although measurement of all the long bones is not required in a routine obstetric ultrasound, an overall evaluation of the fetal skeleton should be performed to ensure the presence and bilateral symmetry of the tubular bones. Available charts provide guidance for correlating the length of the extremities with the gestational age (Table 40-2).

The longest femur measurement, excluding both proximal and distal epiphyses, is usually chosen. The inclusion of the **distal femur point,** or the specular reflection of the lateral aspect of the distal femoral epiphysis cartilage, is the most common reason for overestimating FL[17] (Fig. 40-2, A). An oblique FL measurement will result in undermeasurement. The lateral border of the femur in the near field of the transducer appears straight, whereas the medial border of the femur in the far field has a curved appearance[18] (Fig. 40-2, B).

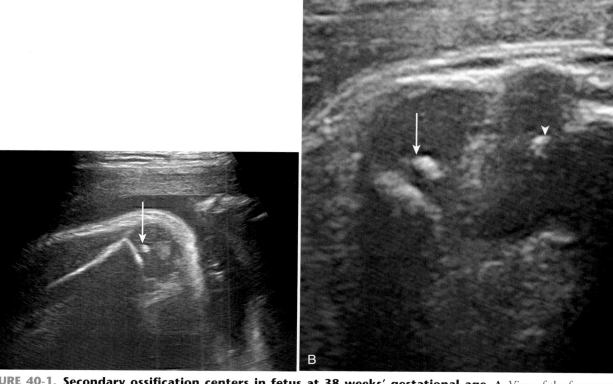

FIGURE 40-1. Secondary ossification centers in fetus at 38 weeks' gestational age. A, View of the femur and distal femoral ossification center *(arrow)*. **B,** View of distal femur and proximal tibia with distal femoral ossification center *(arrow)* and proximal tibial ossification center *(arrowhead)*.

TABLE 40-2. NORMAL EXTREMITY LONG-BONE LENGTHS AND BIPARIETAL DIAMETERS AT DIFFERENT MENSTRUAL AGES*

MENSTRUAL AGE	BIPARIETAL DIAMETER	Bone					
		FEMUR	TIBIA	FIBULA	HUMERUS	RADIUS	ULNA
13	2.3 (0.3)	1.1 (0.2)	0.9 (0.2)	0.8 (0.2)	1.0 (0.2)	0.6 (0.2)	0.8 (0.3)
14	2.7 (0.3)	1.3 (0.2)	1.0 (0.2)	0.9 (0.3)	1.2 (0.2)	0.8 (0.2)	1.0 (0.2)
15	3.0 (0.1)	1.5 (0.2)	1.3 (0.2)	1.2 (0.2)	1.4 (0.2)	1.1 (0.1)	1.2 (0.1)
16	3.3 (0.2)	1.9 (0.3)	1.6 (0.3)	1.5 (0.3)	1.7 (0.2)	1.4 (0.3)	1.6 (0.3)
17	3.7 (0.3)	2.2 (0.3)	1.8 (0.3)	1.7 (0.2)	2.0 (0.4)	1.5 (0.3)	1.7 (0.3)
18	4.2 (0.5)	2.5 (0.3)	2.2 (0.3)	2.1 (0.3)	2.3 (0.3)	1.9 (0.2)	2.2 (0.3)
19	4.4 (0.4)	2.8 (0.3)	2.5 (0.3)	2.3 (0.3)	2.6 (0.3)	2.1 (0.3)	2.4 (0.3)
20	4.7 (0.4)	3.1 (0.3)	2.7 (0.2)	2.6 (0.2)	2.9 (0.3)	2.4 (0.2)	2.7 (0.4)
21	5.0 (0.5)	3.5 (0.4)	3.0 (0.4)	2.9 (0.4)	3.2 (0.4)	2.7 (0.4)	3.0 (0.4)
22	5.5 (0.5)	3.6 (0.3)	3.2 (0.3)	3.1 (0.3)	3.3 (0.3)	2.8 (0.5)	3.1 (0.4)
23	5.8 (0.5)	4.0 (0.4)	3.6 (0.2)	3.4 (0.2)	3.7 (0.3)	3.1 (0.4)	3.5 (0.2)
24	6.1 (0.5)	4.2 (0.3)	3.7 (0.3)	3.6 (0.3)	3.8 (0.4)	3.3 (0.4)	3.6 (0.4)
25	6.4 (0.5)	4.6 (0.3)	4.0 (0.3)	3.9 (0.4)	4.2 (0.4)	3.5 (0.3)	3.9 (0.4)
26	6.8 (0.5)	4.8 (0.4)	4.2 (0.3)	4.0 (0.3)	4.3 (0.3)	3.6 (0.4)	4.0 (0.3)
27	7.0 (0.3)	4.9 (0.3)	4.4 (0.3)	4.2 (0.3)	4.5 (0.2)	3.7 (0.3)	4.1 (0.2)
28	7.3 (0.5)	5.3 (0.5)	4.5 (0.4)	4.4 (0.3)	4.7 (0.4)	3.9 (0.4)	4.4 (0.5)
29	7.6 (0.5)	5.3 (0.5)	4.6 (0.3)	4.5 (0.3)	4.8 (0.4)	4.0 (0.5)	4.5 (0.4)
30	7.7 (0.6)	5.6 (0.3)	4.8 (0.5)	4.7 (0.3)	5.0 (0.5)	4.1 (0.6)	4.7 (0.3)
31	8.2 (0.7)	6.0 (0.6)	5.1 (0.3)	4.9 (0.5)	5.3 (0.4)	4.2 (0.3)	4.9 (0.4)
32	8.5 (0.6)	6.1 (0.6)	5.2 (0.4)	5.1 (0.4)	5.4 (0.4)	4.4 (0.6)	5.0 (0.6)
33	8.6 (0.4)	6.4 (0.5)	5.4 (0.5)	5.3 (0.3)	5.6 (0.5)	4.5 (0.5)	5.2 (0.3)
34	8.9 (0.5)	6.6 (0.6)	5.7 (0.5)	5.5 (0.4)	5.8 (0.5)	4.7 (0.5)	5.4 (0.5)
35	8.9 (0.7)	6.7 (0.6)	5.8 (0.4)	5.6 (0.4)	5.9 (0.6)	4.8 (0.6)	5.4 (0.4)
36	9.1 (0.7)	7.0 (0.7)	6.0 (0.6)	5.6 (0.5)	6.0 (0.6)	4.9 (0.5)	5.5 (0.3)
37	9.3 (0.9)	7.2 (0.4)	6.1 (0.4)	6.0 (0.4)	6.1 (0.4)	5.1 (0.3)	5.6 (0.4)
38	9.5 (0.6)	7.4 (0.6)	6.2 (0.3)	6.0 (0.4)	6.4 (0.3)	5.1 (0.5)	5.8 (0.6)
39	9.5 (0.6)	7.6 (0.8)	6.4 (0.7)	6.1 (0.6)	6.5 (0.6)	5.3 (0.5)	6.0 (0.6)
40	9.9 (0.8)	7.7 (0.4)	6.5 (0.3)	6.2 (0.1)	6.6 (0.4)	5.3 (0.3)	6.0 (0.5)
41	9.7 (0.6)	7.7 (0.4)	6.6 (0.4)	6.3 (0.5)	6.6 (0.4)	5.6 (0.4)	6.3 (0.5)
42	10.0 (0.5)	7.8 (0.7)	6.8 (0.5)	6.7 (0.7)	6.8 (0.7)	5.7 (0.5)	6.5 (0.5)

From Merz E, Kim-Kern MS, Pehl S: Ultrasonic mensuration of fetal limb bones in the second and third trimesters. J Clin Ultrasound 1987;5:175-183.
*Mean values (cm); value of 2 SD in parentheses.

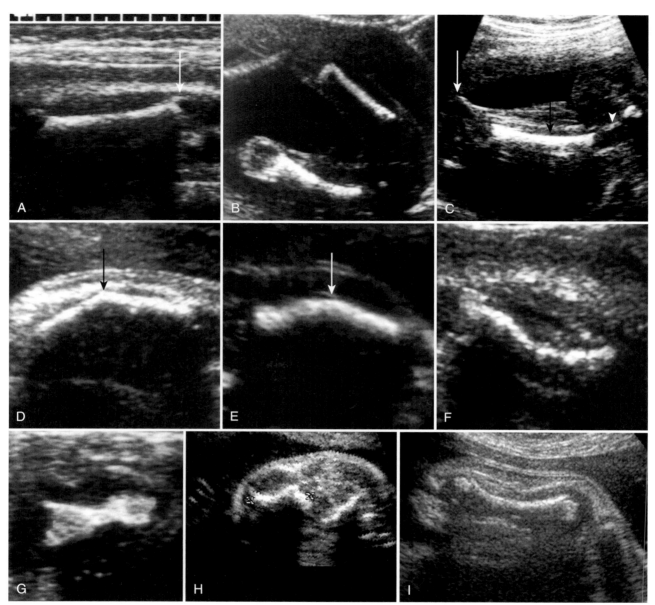

FIGURE 40-2. Normal femur and spectrum of abnormal appearances. A, Normal femur: measure the longest length, excluding the proximal and distal epiphysis and the specular reflection of the lateral aspect of the distal femoral epiphysis *(arrow)*. **B,** Normal femur in the near field, with straight lateral border versus the curved medial border in the far field of the transducer. **C,** Isolated hypoplastic left femur *(arrowhead)*, with normal tibia *(black arrow)* and foot *(white arrow)*. **D,** Osteogenesis imperfecta type I. Isolated femoral fracture with acute angulation *(arrow)*. **E,** Campomelic dysplasia. Mild shortening and a gently curved ventral femoral bowing *(arrow)*. **F,** Osteogenesis imperfecta type IIA. Bowed femur with multiple discontinuities representing fractures. **G,** Hypophosphatasia congenita. Severe micromelia (relatively broad metaphysis, short diaphysis). **H,** Thanatophoric dysplasia. Curved, "telephone receiver" femur. **I,** Chondrodysplasia punctata. Third-trimester appearance of a stippled epiphysis. *(C courtesy Ants Toi, MD; D and E courtesy Shia Salem, MD; University of Toronto.)*

In the **lower extremity** the lateral bone is the fibula and the medial bone is the tibia. The tibia and fibula end at the same level distally. In the **upper extremity,** pronation may cause the radius and ulna to cross, so it can be difficult to distinguish the ulna from the radius using lateral and medial positions. The ulna is distinguished from the radius by its longer proximal extent and its relationship to the fifth digit distally. The radius

and ulna end at the same level distally. Demonstration of this relationship will effectively exclude the majority of radial ray defects.

The **clavicles** grow in a linear fashion, approximately 1 mm per week, and the gestational age in weeks is approximately the length of the clavicle in millimeters from 14 weeks to term. By 40 weeks' gestation, the clavicles measure approximately 40 mm.[19]

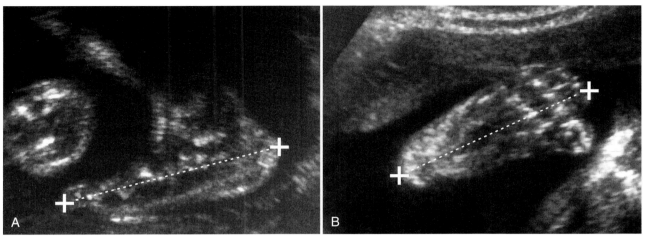

FIGURE 40-3. Foot length measurement. From the skin edge overlying the calcaneus to the distal end of the longest toe. **A,** Sagittal measurement; note the normal squared appearance of the heel. **B,** Plantar measurement.

Foot length is measured from the skin edge overlying the calcaneus to the distal end of the longest toe (the first or second toe) on either the plantar or the sagittal view[20-22] (Fig. 40-3). The ossified femur length is almost equivalent to the foot length, resulting in a normal **femur/foot length ratio** of approximately 1.0. This ratio remains relatively constant from the 14th week of gestation onward. If the fetus is constitutionally small or there is symmetrical IUGR, the ratio is generally 0.9 or greater. In most skeletal **dysplasias** characterized by short limbs, the ratio is generally less than 0.9 because of the relative sparing of the hands and feet. The greater the deviation from the lower limits of the norm, the greater is the severity.

SONOGRAPHIC EVALUATION OF FETUS WITH SKELETAL DYSPLASIA

A prenatal evaluation of a skeletal dysplasia is indicated if there is a positive family history or an abnormal length or appearance of the bones at ultrasound.

ASSESSMENT OF SKELETAL DYSPLASIAS: KEY FEATURES

Family history
Serial measurements
Degree of limb shortening
Pattern of limb shortening
Presence of bowing, fractures, and angulations
Spine
Thoracic measurements
Hands and feet
Calvarium and facial features

Positive Family History

A positive family history of a sibling or parents affected by a skeletal dysplasia or consanguineous parents should prompt an intensive ultrasound investigation with a focus on targeted abnormalities and serial measurements. A history of consanguinity is important because many of the skeletal dysplasias have an autosomal recessive mode of inheritance. **Heterozygous achondroplasia,** the most common nonlethal skeletal dysplasia, has an autosomal dominant pattern of inheritance. Family history may not be helpful because 80% of cases are caused by a new dominant mutation.

Abnormal Bone Length or Appearance

The fetal femur is often the only long bone routinely measured at the second-trimester ultrasound evaluation. An abnormal FL is traditionally defined as below −2 standard deviations (SD) for gestational age.[23,24] Using this cutoff, 2.5% of all fetuses would be classified as having short limbs. This exceeds the expected frequency of skeletal dysplasias, and thus additional investigations are needed to identify the fetus with a skeletal dysplasia.

When one or all of the long bones measure less than −2 SD for gestational age, a follow-up ultrasound should be done in 3 to 4 weeks to evaluate the interval growth. If the interval femur growth is normal, there is a high likelihood that the fetus does not have skeletal dysplasia. However, further deviation from the mean by at least 1 SD should suggest the presence of a skeletal dysplasia or severe IUGR. When FL measures below −4 SD for gestational age, there is a high likelihood of a skeletal dysplasia. Kurtz et al.[23] have shown that the number of millimeters below the −2 SD line is a simple screening tool to evaluate femoral shortening with the following guidelines:

- If FL is 1 to 4 mm below the −2 SD point, further serial measurements are required to determine if a skeletal dysplasia is present.
- If FL is greater than 5 mm below the −2 SD point, there is a high likelihood of a skeletal dysplasia.

The most common etiology of a so-called **short femur** is either inaccurate dating or a normal variant in a constitutionally small fetus, which may be associated with a parental or family history of less-than-average stature. In about 13% of cases, a remeasurement will bring the FL into a normal range, likely representing a false-positive diagnosis rather than a growth-spurt.[25] Isolated, symmetrical short femurs identified at the second midtrimester ultrasound evaluation are helpful in identifying a group of fetuses at increased risk for low birth weight, small for gestational age, or severe IUGR.[25-27] Typically, these fetuses will also have small abdominal circumference measurements.

Occasionally, severe IUGR may present with greatly shortened long bones.[28] Associated findings of normal or decreased skin fold measurements, oligohydramnios, abnormal placental morphology, and abnormal Doppler waveforms suggest the diagnosis of IUGR,[29] whereas redundant, thickened skin folds and polyhydramnios typically accompany short-limb dysplasias.

Nonlethal skeletal dysplasias such as **heterozygous achondroplasia** are generally not evident before 20 weeks' gestation. The findings of short long bones before 20 weeks indicate a more serious and usually fatal skeletal dysplasia. As a rule, the earlier the detection of limb shortening, the worse is the prognosis. Virtually all cases diagnosed in first trimester are considered severe skeletal dysplasias, with the greater majority representing lethal conditions.[30] First-trimester skeletal biometry tables are available.[31] Although mild, isolated shortening of the femur indicates increased risk for **trisomy 21** by 1.5-fold, other factors are more important for assessing this risk.[32]

The **pattern of limb shortening** should be assessed to determine which long-bone segments are most severely affected[8,33] (Fig. 40-4). Rather than millimeters, we find it useful to standardize measurements to "weeks of size" to determine disproportion. There are four main patterns of shortening of the long bones: **rhizomelia,** shortening of the proximal segment (femur and humerus); **mesomelia,** shortening of the middle segment (radius, ulna, tibia, and fibula); **acromelia,** shortening of the distal segment (hands and feet); and **micromelia,** shortening of the entire limb (mild, mild/bowed, or severe).

PATTERNS OF LIMB SHORTENING

Rhizomelia: shortening of proximal segment (femur, humerus).
Mesomelia: shortening of middle segment (radius, ulna/tibia, fibula).
Acromelia: shortening of distal segment (hands, feet).
Micromelia: shortening of entire limb (mild, mild/bowed, severe).

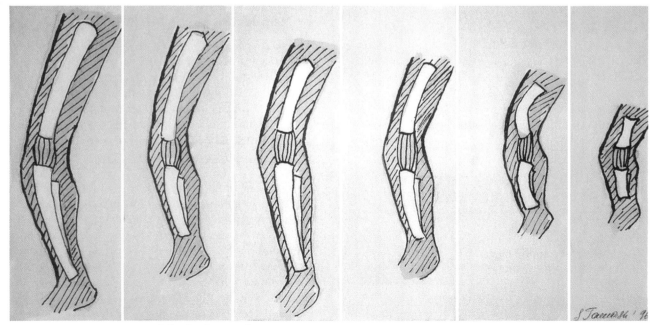

FIGURE 40-4. Patterns of limb shortening. *Left to right,* Normal, mesomelia, rhizomelia, mild micromelia, mild and curved micromelia, and severe micromelia. *(Drawing courtesy J. Tomash, MD, University of Toronto.)*

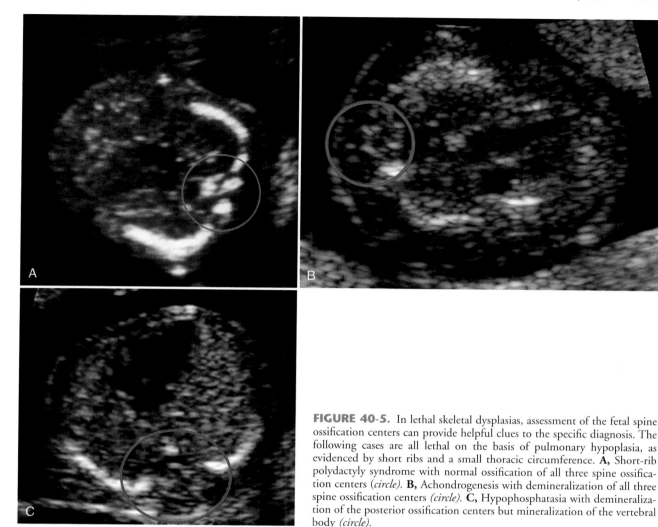

FIGURE 40-5. In lethal skeletal dysplasias, assessment of the fetal spine ossification centers can provide helpful clues to the specific diagnosis. The following cases are all lethal on the basis of pulmonary hypoplasia, as evidenced by short ribs and a small thoracic circumference. **A,** Short-rib polydactyly syndrome with normal ossification of all three spine ossification centers *(circle)*. **B,** Achondrogenesis with demineralization of all three spine ossification centers *(circle)*. **C,** Hypophosphatasia with demineralization of the posterior ossification centers but mineralization of the vertebral body *(circle)*.

The shape, contour, and density of the bones should be assessed for the presence of bowing, angulations, fractures, or thickening. **Bowing** is a nonspecific finding, typically caused by underlying osseous fragility. Although more than 40 distinct disorders can be associated with bowed, bent, or angulated femurs, the majority (63%) belong to three disorders: **campomelic dysplasia** (24.4%), **thanatophoric dysplasia** (23.9%) and **osteogenesis imperfecta** (OI) (18.1%).[34] Patients with OI types I and IV can present with apparent in utero bowing and shortening without frank fractures of the long bones (see Fig. 40-2, *D*). Anterior bowing of the tibia, femur, and humerus may suggest the diagnosis of campomelic dysplasia; associated findings such as **hypoplastic scapulae** and **cervical kyphosis** are typically present. Bone **fractures** may appear as angulations or interruptions in the bone contour or as thick, wrinkled contours corresponding to repetitive cycles of fracture and callus formation (Fig. 40-2, *F*). **Decreased or absent acoustic shadowing** is a marker for decreased mineralization of the long bones. When evident, this is helpful, but in its absence the bone mineralization may still be abnormal.

The **spine** is assessed for **segmentation anomalies, kyphoscoliosis, platyspondyly** (flattened vertebral bodies), **demineralization, myelodysplasia,** and **caudal regression syndromes.** Although platyspondyly is the most common spine abnormality, it is a challenging prenatal diagnosis.[35] Demineralization of the spine can result in the appearance of ghost vertebrae or nonvisualization of one or all of the three ossification centers (Fig. 40-5). A progressively narrowed lumbar interpedicular distance is associated with achondroplasia; a widened interpedicular distance is associated with myelodysplasia.

The most important prognostic determinant of the lethality of a given skeletal dysplasia is the presence of **pulmonary hypoplasia.** Ultrasound is 85% to 95% accurate in the diagnosis of a lethal skeletal dysplasia on the basis of pulmonary hypoplasia.[7,8] The **thoracic circumference** is measured at the level of the four-chamber heart and compared to nomograms (see Table 36-1). A thoracic/abdominal circumference ratio of less than 0.8 is considered abnormal. The **thoracic length** (from the neck to the diaphragm) is also measured, and the ribs are assessed to determine if they are short. At the level of the

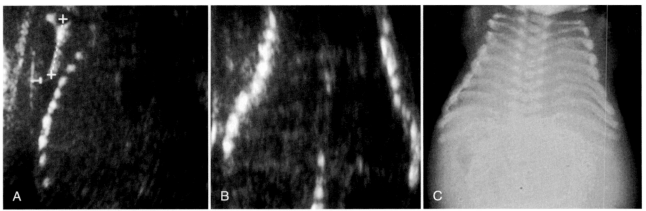

FIGURE 40-6. Triplet B affected with campomelic dysplasia and pulmonary hypoplasia. Coronal ultrasound images of the thorax in triplet pregnancy at 27 weeks' gestation. **A,** Normal triplet A shows normal convex contour of the thorax. Calipers measure the scapula. **B,** Triplet B shows a bell-shaped thorax. **C,** Radiograph of triplet B confirms a bell-shaped thorax consistent with pulmonary hypoplasia.

four-chamber cardiac view, the ribs should normally encircle at least 70% to 80% of the thoracic circumference.[36] The ribs remain in a relatively horizontal plane, as does the cardiac axis, facilitating this evaluation. In a sagittal view, a markedly narrowed anteroposterior (AP) diameter of the thorax is associated with pulmonary hypoplasia. In the coronal view, a concave or bell-shaped contour is associated with pulmonary hypoplasia (Fig. 40-6).

The **hands and feet** are examined for deformities such as **clubfoot** or **clubhand.** A **hitchhiker thumb,** or abducted thumb, is associated with **diastrophic dwarfism.** Fixed postural deformities may suggest the diagnosis of **arthrogryposis multiplex congenita. Polydactyly** is associated with **short-rib polydactyly syndromes, Ellis–van Creveld syndrome, asphyxiating thoracic dystrophy** and some chromosomal abnormalities.

The fetal **cranium** is assessed for the presence of **macrocranium, frontal bossing, cloverleaf skull deformity,** underlying brain abnormalities, and facial abnormalities, such as **saddle nose, hypertelorism,** and **cleft lip and palate.** An abnormal cranial contour may indicate **craniosynostosis** or premature fusion of the sutures. The most reliable sonographic sign of demineralization is increased compressibility of the calvarium. This finding is typically present in **osteogenesis imperfecta type II, achondrogenesis,** and **hypophosphatasia.** The falx may appear abnormally bright or echogenic compared to the demineralized calvarium.

The **ribs** are assessed to ensure an adequate length, thus minimizing the risk of pulmonary hypoplasia, and are examined for abnormal number or appearance.[37] The finding of an abnormal number of fetal ribs is an isolated finding of no clinical importance in the majority of cases,[37] associated with minor anomalies in a smaller group (29%) and only occasionally associated with severe malformations. Associated syndromes include **Poland syndrome, VACTERL** association (vertebral abnormalities, anal atresia, cardiac abnormalities, tracheoesopha-

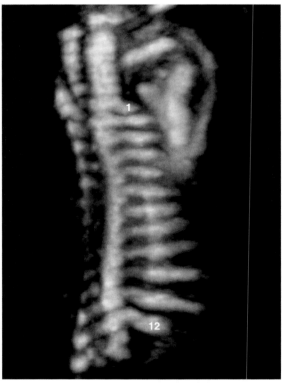

FIGURE 40-7. Normal ribs: 3-D ultrasound.

geal fistula, renal agenesis and dysplasia, limb defects), **cleidocranial dysplasia, campomelic dysplasia,** and chromosome abnormalities. Three-dimensional ultrasound volume images aid in accurately counting the number of ribs (Fig. 40-7).

Ultimately, a detailed examination of each bone may be required to determine the fetal condition. Specific dysmorphic features of bones (e.g., clavicular or scapular hypoplasia; aplasia of fibula, tibia, or radius; platyspondyly) can be helpful to further define a specific skeletal dysplasia. A detailed evaluation of the cardiovascular, genitourinary, gastrointestinal (GI), and central nervous system (CNS) should be done concurrently with the musculoskeletal evaluation.

Dizygotic **twin pregnancies** are at similar risk for skeletal abnormalities as singleton pregnancies, and the frequency is increased two to three times in monozygotic twins. Both monozygotic and dizygotic twins can be discordant for genetic and nongenetic skeletal abnormalities. Twin pregnancies are generally discordant; overall, about 15% of twins are concordant for the same anomaly.[38,39]

Three-Dimensional Ultrasound

Surface-rendering capabilities are proving especially useful in elucidating potentially subtle fetal features, such as low-set ears, facial dysmorphism, clubfoot, cleft lip/palate, or polydactyly. High-contrast structures such as the fetal skeleton are especially amenable to data manipulation. Early studies suggest that 3-D ultrasound may enhance diagnostic capability, especially for cranial, facial, skeletal, and body surface malformations[40-42] (Fig. 40-8).

Additional Imaging

The role of **prenatal radiography** is limited. Typically, two films might be performed: an anteroposterior (AP) view, placing the fetus over the hollow of the pelvis, and an angulated view, with the fetus projected down, away from the sacrum. The appearance of short limbs of normal shape and the presence of growth recovery lines

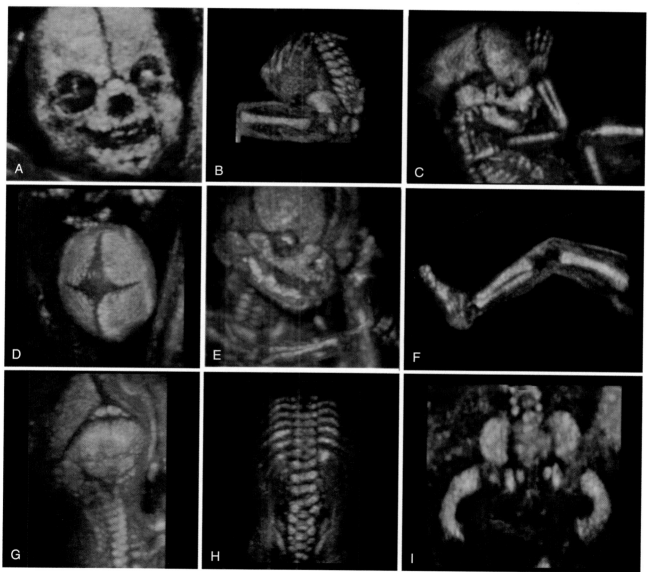

FIGURE 40-8. Collage of 3-D images. A, Normal skull at 22 weeks, frontal aspect. **B,** Femur and iliac bone at 22 weeks. **C,** Upper extremity at 22 weeks. **D,** Normal skull at 22 weeks, superior aspect. **E,** Face and skull at 22 weeks. **F,** Normal lower limb at 22 weeks, profile. **G,** Wormian bones, posterior fontanelle. **H,** Hemivertebrae at 23 weeks. **I,** Osteogenesis imperfecta; note abnormally shortened, curved, and thickened femurs. *(Courtesy Dr. Bernard Benoit.)*

can be useful in distinguishing severe IUGR from a skeletal dysplasia.[29] In contrast, **postnatal radiography** plays an extremely important role in defining the characteristic radiologic features found in many skeletal anomalies. Low-dose 3-D **computed tomography** (CT) scan may have a better diagnostic yield than 2-D ultrasound and may provide a valuable complementary diagnostic tool in the appropriate clinical situation[43,44] (Fig. 40-9). Postmortem 3-D CT scan may provide a "virtual autopsy," particularly for patients who declined autopsy. **Magnetic resonance imaging** (MRI) plays a relatively limited role in fetal skeletal dysplasias. MRI plays an important role in cases with inconclusive ultrasound findings and for cases in which MRI is expected to provide important additional information that may change management.[45]

When the diagnosis remains unknown, the involvement of specialists in skeletal dysplasias may be helpful in determining the diagnosis. It is crucial to obtain postnatal radiographs, fetal DNA, and fibroblast culture to try and delineate the diagnosis, the gene, and gene mutation. This may help in preimplantation or with prenatal diagnosis in future pregnancies.

LETHAL SKELETAL DYSPLASIAS

The lethal skeletal dysplasias are characterized by severe **micromelia** and small thoracic circumference with **pulmonary hypoplasia.**[46] The most important determinant of lethality is the presence and degree of pulmonary hypoplasia. In a prospective series by Krakow et al.,[7] lethality was accurately predicted in 96.8% of cases. This extremely high accuracy of the designation of a lethal skeletal dysplasia is important for the management of the current pregnancy and delivery.

IS THERE A LETHAL SKELETAL DYSPLASIA?

CHARACTERISTIC FEATURES
Severe micromelia
Pulmonary hypoplasia

DISTINGUISHING FEATURES
Abnormal mineralization
Fractures
Presence or absence of macrocranium
Thoracic length

In many fetal skeletal dysplasias, the skin and subcutaneous layers continue to grow at a rate proportionately greater than the long bones, resulting in **relatively thickened skin folds**, on occasion mistaken for hydrops fetalis. **Polyhydramnios** is common and may be related to a variable combination of the following: esophageal compression by the small chest; GI abnormalities; micrognathia or hypotonia.

The three most common lethal skeletal dysplasias are thanatophoric dysplasia; achondrogenesis, and osteogenesis imperfecta type II, overall accounting for 40% to 60% of all lethal skeletal dysplasias.[4,7,47] We use a "key features" approach in assessing degree of micromelia, mineralization, presence of macrocranium, and evaluation of thoracic length and circumference to improve specificity and ease of diagnosis in lethal skeletal dysplasias (Table 40-3).

Thanatophoric Dysplasia

Thanatophoric dysplasia is the most common lethal skeletal dysplasia, with a prevalence of 0.24 to 0.69 per

---

SONOGRAPHIC ASSESSMENT OF BONES

Long Bones
Degree of limb shortening
Pattern of limb shortening
Degree of mineralization
Presence of fractures, bowing, or angulation
Abnormal shape or contour
Limb reduction anomalies
Hypoplastic or aplastic bones

Spine
Degree and pattern of demineralization
Platyspondyly
Segmentation or curvature anomalies
Caudal regression syndrome
Myelodysplasia

Thorax
Thoracic length and circumference
Hypoplastic ribs
Bell-shaped thorax of pulmonary hypoplasia
Convex contour in cross section

Hands and Feet
Postural deformities
Abnormal number of digits
Syndactyly

Calvarium
Macrocranium
Frontal bossing
Craniosynostosis
Compressibility/abnormal degree of mineralization

Facial Features
Cleft lip and palate
Hypertelorism and hypotelorism
Midface hypoplasia/flat nasal bridge

TABLE 40-3. SEVERE MICROMELIA WITH DECREASED THORACIC CIRCUMFERENCE

	MINERALIZATION	FRACTURES	MACROCRANIA	SHORT TRUNK
Thanatophoric dysplasia*†	Normal	No	Yes	No
Achondrogenesis	Patchy demineralization	Occasional	Yes	Yes
Osteogenesis imperfecta type II	Generalized demineralization	Innumerable	No	Yes
Hypophosphatasia congenita	Patchy or generalized demineralization	No	No	No

*Homozygous achondroplasia is similar to thanatophoric dysplasia but distinguishable because both parents are affected with the heterozygous form of achondroplasia.
†Short-rib polydactyly dysplasias are similar to thanatophoric dysplasia, but no macrocrania or polydactyly is present.

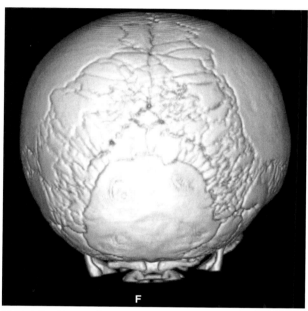

FIGURE 40-9. Three-dimensional CT reconstruction of calvarium in osteogenesis imperfecta type 1. Multiple wormian bones are present in this 3-D surface-rendered CT reconstruction in a 4-week-old neonate.

10,000 births. The key features are severe micromelia with rhizomelic predominance and **macrocrania** (disproportionately large head) in association with decreased thoracic circumference but a normal trunk length. Mineralization is normal, with no fractures present. Typically, the extremities are so foreshortened that they protrude at right angles to the body. The skin folds are thickened and redundant secondary to a relatively greater rate of growth of the skin and subcutaneous layers than the bones. Clinical presentation is usually caused by large-for-date measurements secondary to polyhydramnios (Figs. 40-10 and 40-11; **Video 40-1**).

Langer et al.[48] distinguished two types of thanatophoric dysplasia. The more common **type 1** (TD1), usually caused by the R248C and Y373C mutations in the fibroblast growth factor receptor 3 (FGFR3) gene, displays the typical "telephone receiver" shape of the extremities[49,50] (see Fig. 40-2, *H*). This bowed or curved appearance is secondary to the broadened metaphyses at the ends of the severely shortened tubular bones. TD1 is associated with frontal bossing and a flattened nasal

bridge with midface hypoplasia. Occasionally, craniosynostosis results in a mild variant of cloverleaf skull deformity. Platyspondyly is present. In **type 2** (TD2), usually caused by the K650E mutation in the FGFR3 gene, the femurs are typically straight with flared metaphyses. The most specific feature is the **cloverleaf skull,** a trilobed appearance of the skull in the coronal plane that results from premature craniosynostosis of the lambdoid and coronal sutures (Fig. 40-12). Other conditions that may be associated with this unusual skull deformity are homozygous achondroplasia, campomelic dysplasia, and trisomy 13. Both TD1 and TD2 are autosomal dominant conditions, with all cases caused by new mutations in the FGFR3 gene, which gene also causes hypochondroplasia, achondroplasia, severe achondroplasia with developmental delay, and acanthosis nigricans, as well as craniosynostosis.[50,51]

Thanatophoric dysplasia has many phenotypic similarities to **homozygous achondroplasia.** Both conditions may appear identical from ultrasound and radiographic perspectives. They can be distinguished by the positive family history,[46] in which both parents are affected with the heterozygous form of achondroplasia (Fig. 40-13). Another condition presenting with bowed tubular bones is **campomelic dysplasia,** which is distinguished from thanatophoric dysplasia by a moderate and bowed form of micromelia, typically affecting the tibias with characteristic associated anomalies.

Platyspondyly, or flattened vertebral bodies, is one of the most characteristic features on AP radiographs of a thanatophoric dwarf (see Fig. 40-10, *A*). There is a U or H configuration of the vertebral bodies and a relatively increased height of the disc spaces. Platyspondyly appears on ultrasound as a **wafer-thin vertebral body** with a relatively larger, hypoechoic disc space on either side of the vertebral body (Fig. 40-14). The ratio of vertebral body height to vertebral interspace (disc and body) in thanatophoric dysplasia is lower than in normal cases. Platyspondyly may also occur in cases of achondrogenesis and OI type II.[29,46]

Associated CNS findings may include holoprosencephaly, agenesis of the corpus callosum, polymicrogyria, heterotopia, and ventriculomegaly. Other anomalies may include horseshoe kidneys, hydronephrosis, congenital heart disease (atrial septal defect and tricuspid insufficiency), radioulnar synostosis, and imperforate anus.[52]

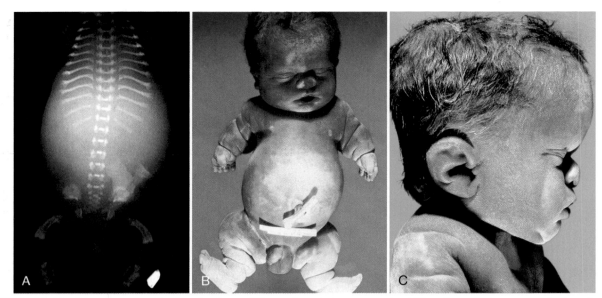

FIGURE 40-10. Thanatophoric dysplasia at 33 weeks. A, Anteroposterior (AP) radiograph shows normal mineralization, short curved extremity bones, severe platyspondyly with U-shaped vertebral bodies, and narrow thorax with short ribs. **B,** AP specimen photograph shows severe micromelia with relative sparing of the feet, telescoping of the redundant skin folds, and small, bell-shaped thorax. **C,** Profile specimen photograph shows macrocranium, frontal bossing, and flattened nasal bridge.

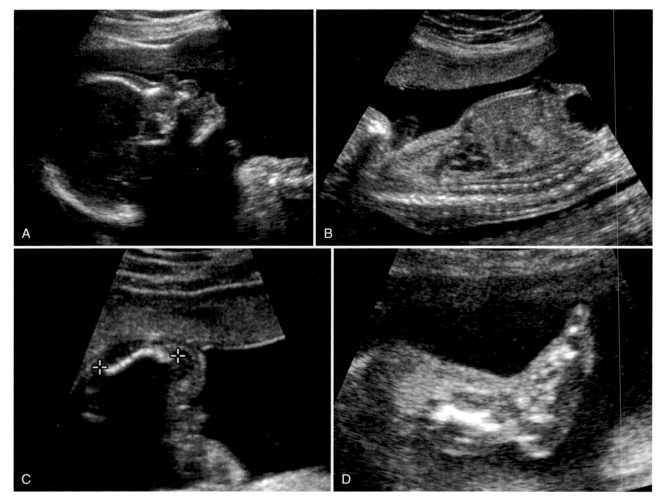

FIGURE 40-11. Thanatophoric dysplasia at 22 weeks. A, Profile; midface hypoplasia with flat nasal bridge. **B,** Sagittal sonogram shows disproportionately narrow thorax and relatively protuberant abdomen, signifying lethal condition on the basis of pulmonary hypoplasia. **C,** Short curved femur. **D,** Sparing of foot length versus extreme shortening of tibia. *(Courtesy Fetal Assessment Unit, University Health Network.)*

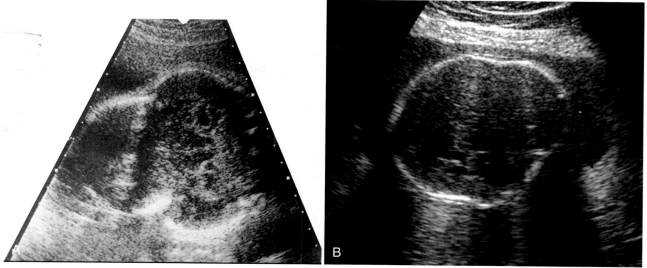

FIGURE 40-12. Cloverleaf deformity of thanatophoric dysplasia. A, Severe variant. **B,** Mild variant. *(Courtesy Greg Ryan, MD, University of Toronto.)*

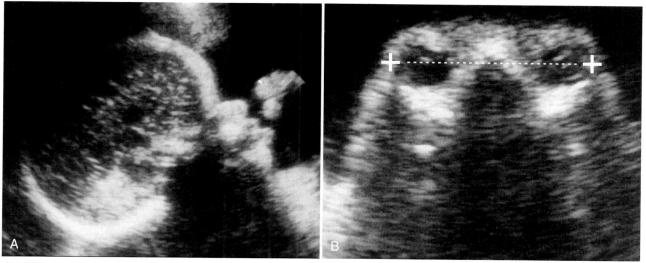

FIGURE 40-13. Homozygous achondroplasia at 34 weeks. A, Lateral profile is similar to thanatophoric dysplasia with macrocranium, frontal bossing, and flat nasal bridge. **B,** Axial image through the orbits (calipers denote outer orbital diameter) and nasal bones confirms a flat nasal bridge.

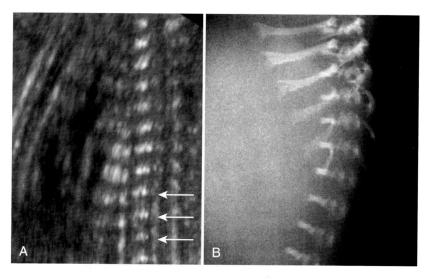

FIGURE 40-14. Thanatophoric dysplasia at 33 weeks. A, Platyspondyly appears on ultrasound as a wafer-thin vertebral body *(arrows)* with relatively larger hypoechoic intervertebral disc space on either side of the vertebral body. **B,** Correlative lateral spine radiograph. Note the short ribs with wide-cupped metaphyseal ends.

Achondrogenesis

Achondrogenesis is the second most common lethal skeletal dysplasia, with a prevalence of 0.09 to 0.23 per 10,000 births. It is a phenotypically and genetically diverse group of chondrodysplasias characterized by severe micromelia, macrocranium, decreased thoracic circumference and trunk length, and decreased mineralization.[52,53] The pattern of demineralization is most marked in the vertebral bodies, ischium, and pubic bones, leading to a greatly shortened trunk length, decreased thoracic circumference, and occasional fractures.[54] Classically, because of predominant demineralization of the vertebral body, only the two echogenic posterior elements or neural arches appear in a transverse image of the spine. This is in contrast to **hypophosphatasia congenita,** in which the predominant spine demineralization involves the posterior elements, with only patchy involvement of the vertebral bodies. Polyhydramnios and thick, redundant skin folds are a common accompaniment of achondrogenesis.[55]

Type 1 achondrogenesis accounts for about 20% of cases and is divided into A and B subtypes (ACH1A and ACH1B).[6,53] ACH1A includes rib fractures, which are not present in ACH1B. Both are autosomal recessive in inheritance and thus have a 25% recurrence risk, but the genetic defect in ACH1A remains unknown. ACH1B is caused by mutations in the diastrophic dysplasia sulfate transporter gene. Both ACH1A and ACH1B have a severe form of **micromelia,** evidenced by short, cuboid bones and metaphyseal scalloping with bone spurs at the periphery. There is partial or complete lack of ossification of the calvarium, vertebral bodies, and sacral and pubic bones. Because of the extremely limited skeletal frame, the subcutaneous tissues can appear grotesquely redundant, with multiple telescoped skin folds that may be mistaken prenatally for hydrops fetalis.

Type 2 (ACH2), or the Langer-Saldino form, accounts for 80% of achondrogenesis cases. It is caused by new dominant mutations in the *COL2A1* gene that encodes type II collagen and has a very small recurrence risk. It is characterized by normal calvarial ossification and by absent ossification in the vertebral column and sacral and pubic bones (Fig. 40-15). ACH2 has the most complete lack of ossification of the vertebral column of all the skeletal dysplasias. The Langer-Saldino form demonstrates relatively longer tubular bones and body length in association with increased survival. **Hypochondrogenesis** is phenotypically similar but less severe with better ossification of the spine, pelvis, and long bones. Another condition to differentiate is **Kniest dysplasia,** characterized by vertebral coronal clefts and metaphyseal expansion (most prominent in the proximal femurs).[1]

These two key features of achondrogenesis—abnormal mineralization and shortened trunk length—distinguishes it from thanatophoric dysplasia, which has normal mineralization and a normal trunk length. Both display macrocrania and severe micromelia.

Osteogenesis Imperfecta

Osteogenesis imperfecta is a clinically and genetically heterogeneous group of collagen disorders characterized by brittle bones resulting in fractures. The incidence is

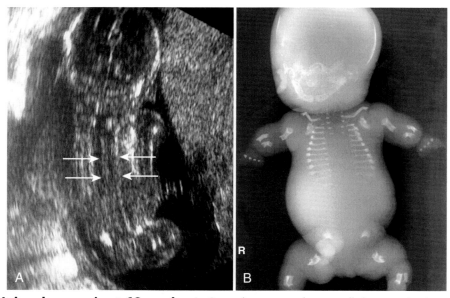

FIGURE 40-15. Achondrogenesis at 18 weeks. A, Coronal sonogram shows small thorax, redundant subcutaneous tissues, absent spine ossification *(arrows),* and decreased calvarial ossification. **B,** Postmortem radiograph demonstrates macrocranium, decreased calvarial ossification, virtually absent spine ossification (only some posterior elements are ossified in the cervical region). There is severe micromelia with strikingly short wide bones with metaphyseal spurs. The ribs are short and horizontal with splayed ends. *(Courtesy Shia Salem, MD, University of Toronto.)*

TABLE 40-4. CLASSIFICATION OF OSTEOGENESIS IMPERFECTA BY TYPE

TYPE	CLINICAL FEATURES	PRENATAL FINDINGS	PROGNOSIS	INHERITANCE	MOLECULAR ABNORMALITIES
I	Normal stature, little or no deformity, blue sclera, hearing loss in 50% of cases Type IA: normal teeth Type IB: opalescent teeth	Occasionally, short and bowed long bones and fractures	Fair	Autosomal dominant	Non-sense or frameshift mutations in COL1A1 gene
II	Lethal; hypomineralization of the skull, beaded ribs, compressed femurs, marked long-bone deformity, blue sclera, triangular face, platyspondyly	Severe micromelia Rib and long-bone fractures Hypomineralization of skull	Lethal	Autosomal dominant (new mutations) Parental gonadal mosaicism responsible for recurrence	Glycine missense mutation in COL1A1 or COL1A2 genes
III	Usually with long-bone fractures; moderate deformity at birth but progressively deforming bones; triangular face, blue sclera, opalescent teeth, hearing loss, short stature	Occasionally, short and bowed long bones and fractures	Wheelchair bound, nonambulatory	Autosomal dominant Parental gonadal mosaicism responsible for recurrence Autosomal recessive (rare)	Glycine missense mutation in COL1A1 or COL1A2 genes
IV	Mild to moderate bone deformity and variable short stature; opalescent teeth in type IVB; hearing loss occurs in some families; white sclera	Occasionally, short and bowed long bones and fractures	Fair	Autosomal dominant Parental gonadal mosaicism responsible for recurrence	Glycine missense mutation in COL1A1 or COL1A2 genes

Modified from Sillence DO, Senn A, Danks DM. Genetic heterogeneity in osteogenesis imperfecta. J Med Genet 1979;16:101-116.

1:60,000 births. Until recently there were four types of OI, all with an autosomal dominant mode of inheritance and associated with mutations in the COL1A1 or COL1A2 genes. In the past several years a few more conditions that can be categorized phenotypically into one of the four categories identified by Sillence et al.,[56,57] but of a different etiologies and some with autosomal recessive modes of inheritance, have been detected (Table 40-4). Nonclassical types of OI, phenotypically indistinguishable from type IV and etiologically noncollagenous, have been identified. Type V also has a triad of callus formation, dense metaphyseal bands, and ossification of the interosseous membranes of the forearm and has an autosomal dominant mode of inheritance. Type VI is of an unknown inheritance and is diagnosed on the basis of a unique histological feature of "fish scale" appearance of bone and elevated alkaline phosphatase. Three autosomal recessive conditions caused by a defect in collagen prolyl 3-hydroxylation complex have also been identified. OI types VII and VIII have manifestations similar to OI types II and III. Those with type VII also have a small head circumference, exophthalmus, and white or light gray sclera. Type VIII is typically more common in people of West African origin. Type VII is caused by a mutation in the gene CRTAP (cartilage-associated protein), and type VIII is caused by a mutation in the P3H1/LEPRE1 gene. OI type IX has recently been delineated as an autosomal recessive condition with clinical manifestations similar to types IV or III and is associated with white sclera and a mutation in the peptidyl-prolyl isomerase B gene (PPIB), which results in a lack of cyclophilin B (CyPB).[58]

Prenatal diagnosis is possible based on DNA from chorionic villus sampling (CVS)[56] or amniotic fluid cells from amniocentesis. A modification of the Sillence classification, based on skeletal radiographic findings, is still used most often to distinguish the subtypes of OI.[57,59] The Sillence classification has become less clinically useful as the molecular abnormalities associated with OI are elucidated. According to genetics subclassification, the key features are the specific molecular abnormality, inheritance pattern, and clinical features, such as blue sclerae and opalescent teeth, and the prognosis.[59]

Osteogenesis imperfecta type II is the classic neonatal lethal form and usually results from a new, dominant null mutation in the COL1A1 gene.[59] The empiric recurrence risk is 6%, most of which are caused by parental germline and somatic mosaicism but can also be the results of one of the autosomal recessive forms of OI, identified previously as type II. Multiple repetitive in utero fractures occur secondary to defective collagen formation, which results in osseous fragility. Prevalence of OI type II is 0.18 per 10,000 births. Most cases are sporadic and can be detected on prenatal ultrasound. The key features are severe micromelia, decreased thoracic circumference and trunk length, decreased mineralization, and multiple bone fractures. The cranial vault remains normal in size (Fig. 40-16).

The generalized demineralization results in innumerable fractures (Fig. 40-17). The tubular bones exhibit a classic "accordion" or wrinkled contour caused by multiple in utero fractures with repetitive callus formation. Angulation and bowing are common in association with severe micromelia (see Fig. 40-2, F). On ultrasound, the

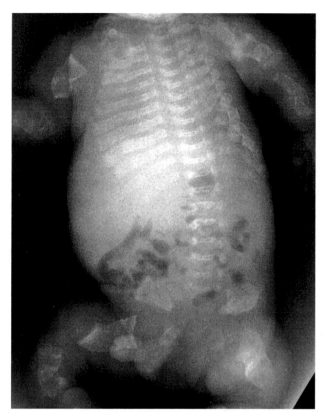

FIGURE 40-16. Osteogenesis imperfecta type IIA at 32 weeks. Postmortem radiograph shows severe micromelia; thickened bones with wavy contours caused by innumerable fractures and exuberant callus formation; shortened ribs with multiple fractures; and platyspondyly.

bones may appear thickened because demineralized bone reflects sound waves less than a normally ossified bone. Acoustic shadowing may be present, absent, or diminished and thus is an unreliable sign. Multiple rib fractures cause the lateral chest contour to be concave rather than convex. The concavity is often most evident at the lateral thorax, and it is speculated that the elbows "bash" in the fragile rib cage. The ribs are hypoplastic, thus appearing shortened. The ribs may have a continuous, beaded, or wavy appearance secondary to repetitive fractures and callus formation. Platyspondyly secondary to multiple compression fractures may be present. Demineralization of the cranial vault can be observed by looking for a **localized deformation of the cranial vault** under gentle transducer pressure (Fig. 40-18) and the **bright falx sign,** in which the falx appears brighter or more echogenic than the demineralized cranial vault, with unusual clarity of detail in the near field. Large fontanelles and wormian bones may be noted (Fig. 40-18). The cranial vault is normal in size. Micrognathia is commonly present (Fig. 40-19).

The three criteria or a specific diagnosis of OI type II are (1) FL greater than 3 SD below the mean, (2) demineralization of the calvarium, and (3) multiple fractures within a single bone.[59] A normal ultrasound examination

after 17 weeks excludes this diagnosis. The diagnosis may be made as early as 13 to 15 weeks' gestational age.

Osteogenesis types I, III, and IV are further described in the section on nonlethal skeletal dysplasias.

Hypophosphatasia

Hypophosphatasia congenita, the lethal neonatal form of hypophosphatasia, is an autosomal recessive skeletal dysplasia caused by a deficiency of tissue-nonspecific alkaline phosphatase mapped to 1p36.1-p34.[60] Frequency of hypophosphatasia congenita is approximately 1 in 100,000 births. The key features are **severe micromelia, decreased thoracic circumference** with normal trunk length, and **decreased mineralization** with occasional fractures. Cranial vault size remains normal.

The demineralized long bones may be bowed with occasional angulations caused by fractures. The bones appear thin and delicate and may appear entirely absent. The cranial vault fails to mineralize and may be compressible under locally applied transducer pressure. In contrast to OI, the demineralization in hypophosphatasia congenita can vary from a patchy distribution to a diffuse form with severe involvement of the spine and calvarium. The ribs are short, resulting in a decreased thoracic circumference, but the trunk length is normal. There is no macrocrania; polyhydramnios is a common finding.

The main differential diagnosis is OI type II. Both hypophosphatasia and OI display a severe form of micromelia, demineralization, decreased thoracic circumference, and a normal-sized cranial vault that is compressible due to demineralization. In OI type II, the greater degree of osseous fragility results in innumerable fractures and a thickened, wavy appearance of the bones, in contrast to the thin, delicate appearance of the bones in hypophosphatasia congenita. The normal trunk length and cranial vault size can aid in distinguishing hypophosphatasia from achondrogenesis. Typically, in hypophosphatasia congenita, the posterior elements are poorly ossified, whereas in achondrogenesis, the vertebral bodies are maximally affected by demineralization with relative sparing of the posterior elements[61] (Fig. 40-20). The cartilage is normally formed in hypophosphatasia; thus the fetus has a more normal gross appearance, despite severe bony abnormalities helping to distinguish it from the other lethal skeletal dysplasias.

Campomelic Dysplasia

Campomelic dysplasia, or **bent-limb dysplasia,** is a rare autosomal-dominant condition that usually results from a new dominant mutation in the *SOX9* gene (sex-determining protein homeobox 9 mapped to 17q24.3). The incidence is 0.5 to 1.0 per 100,000 births. Most cases are lethal because of respiratory insufficiency from laryngotracheomalacia in combination with a mildly narrowed thorax.

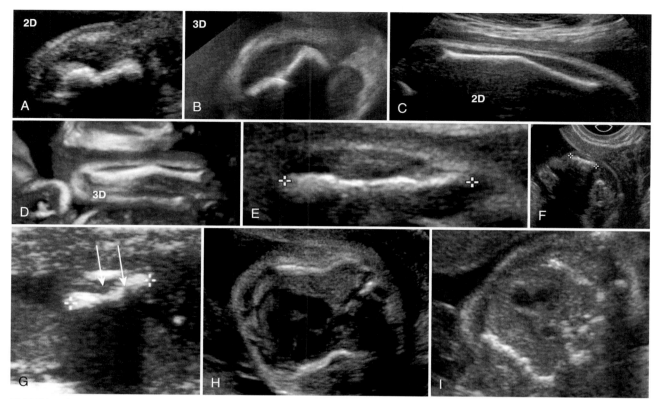

FIGURE 40-17. Osteogenesis imperfecta (OI): spectrum of appearances of fractures. A, Type IIA. Two-dimensional ultrasound image of extremely shortened femur with at least two bone deformities, consistent with fractures. Note redundant overlying soft tissues. **B,** Correlative 3-D ultrasound image demonstrates a midshaft fracture with callus formation. **C, Type I.** Nonlethal variant of OI with a mildly angulated femur of normal length. **D,** Correlative 3-D ultrasound image demonstrates the angulated healed fracture. **E, Type III.** Multiple fractures in the mildly to moderately shortened femur are evidenced by multiple discontinuities in the cortex. The demineralized shaft permits visualization of the thickened cortex. **F, Type II.** Extremely short and thickened femur resulting from repetitive callus formation. Acoustic shadowing is still present in this demineralized fragile bone, and thus its presence is not a reliable sign of normal mineralization. **G, Type II.** At least two discontinuities are present in the shortened tibia *(arrows),* consistent with fractures. Note acoustic shadowing present despite generalized demineralization. **H, Type II.** Cross section of the thorax demonstrates a typical concavity noted at the lateral aspect of the thorax. This may be caused by repetitive in utero fractures as the elbows "hit" the fragile rib cage. **I, Type II.** Cross section of the thorax demonstrates normal-length ribs with multiple fractures within each rib, resulting in a wavy contour.

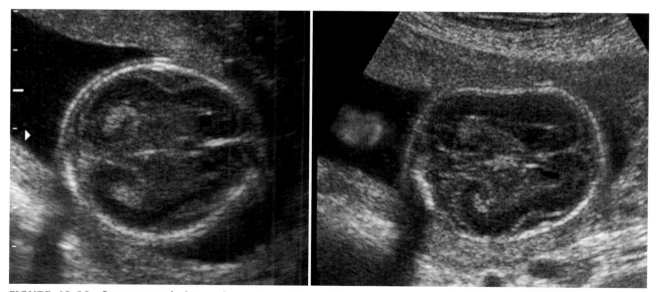

FIGURE 40-18. Osteogenesis imperfecta type IIA at 17 weeks. A, Rounded head contour. **B,** Gentle transducer compression on the demineralized calvarium results in flattening of the cranial contour. Note widened fontanelles and sutures, as well as ease of visualization of intracranial contents in the near field (which would usually have artifacts caused by shadowing from the ossified skull).

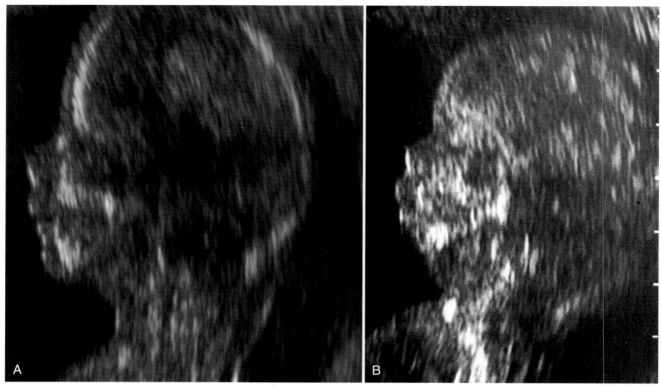

FIGURE 40-19. Facial profile: normal versus osteogenesis imperfecta. A, Normal profile of a 14-week fetus. **B,** Facial profile of a 14-week fetus affected by OI. Note the absent calvarial and nasal ossification and micrognathia.

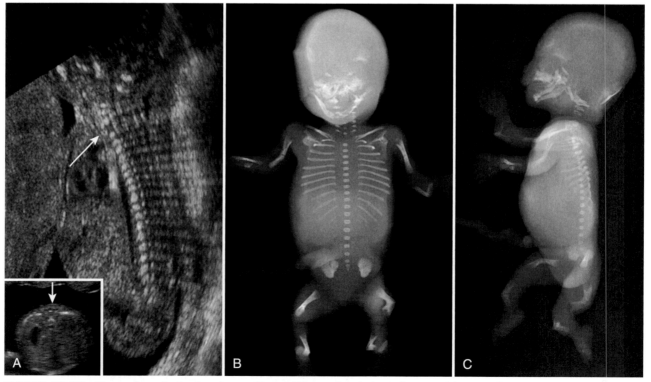

FIGURE 40-20. Hypophosphatasia congenita at 18 weeks. A, Sagittal image of the spine demonstrates absent ossification of posterior elements of the vertebrae. Patchy form of spine demineralization with absent ossification of a cervical vertebral body *(arrow)*. Note narrow anteroposterior (AP) diameter of thorax. *Inset,* Cross-sectional image of the upper abdomen with absent ossification of posterior elements of the spine *(arrow)* and vertebral body maintaining ossification. **B,** AP radiograph confirms absent mineralization of a cervical vertebral body, with absent ossification of posterior elements of the vertebrae. Additional findings include hypoplastic ribs, occasional fractures, micromelia, and decreased cranial vault mineralization. **C,** Lateral radiograph confirms absent mineralization of posterior elements of the spine.

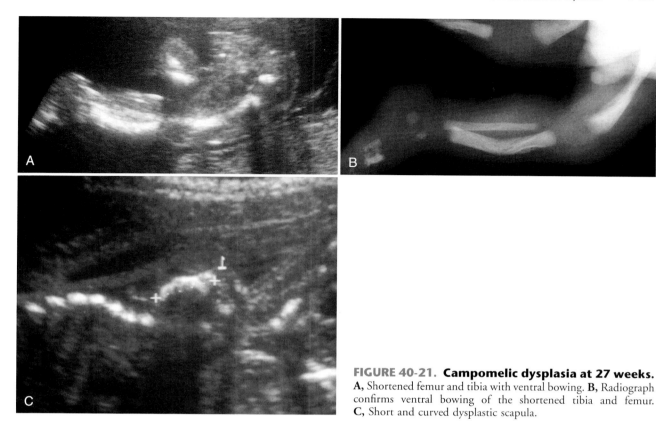

FIGURE 40-21. Campomelic dysplasia at 27 weeks. **A,** Shortened femur and tibia with ventral bowing. **B,** Radiograph confirms ventral bowing of the shortened tibia and femur. **C,** Short and curved dysplastic scapula.

The characteristic skeletal features of campomelic dysplasia are a short and ventrally bowed tibia and femur, a hypoplastic or absent fibula, talipes equinovarus (clubfoot), and hypoplastic scapulae (Fig. 40-21). Bowing may also occur in the upper extremities. Additional skeletal features may include scoliosis; hypoplastic, hypoplastic, or poorly ossified cervicothoracic vertebrae; dislocated hips; 11 rib pairs; and facial abnormalities, including micrognathia and cleft palate (Pierre Robin sequence). Approximately 33% of fetuses have congenital heart disease (CHD) and brain (e.g., ventriculomegaly) and renal (e.g., pyelectasis) abnormalities.

Sex reversal is found in about 75% of the affected 46,XY cases, with a gradation of defects ranging from ambiguous genitalia to normal female genitalia phenotype. The gene responsible for campomelic dysplasia is expressed in the fetal brain, the testes, and the perichondrium and chondrocytes of the long bones and ribs.[62]

Short-Rib Polydactyly Syndromes

Short-rib polydactyly dysplasias are a heterogeneous group of rare and lethal skeletal dysplasias with an autosomal recessive mode of inheritance. All forms are characterized by severe micromelia and decreased thoracic circumference. The cranial vault measurements and bone mineralization are normal. Polydactyly, cardiac, and genitourinary abnormalities are found in most cases.

Thanatophoric dysplasia is distinguished by the absence of polydactyly and the presence of the typical facial features, macrocrania, and platyspondyly. **Ellis–van Creveld syndrome** (Fig. 40-22) and **asphyxiating thoracic dystrophy** have similar features, but the shortening of the limbs and the narrowing of the thorax are less severe.

The short-rib polydactyly syndromes are subdivided into four groups: type I—Saldino-Noonan; type II—Majewski; type III—Verma-Naumoff; and type IV—Beemer-Langer (which can occur without polydactyly).[60,63] Radiographic and clinical features can distinguish them. The genetic basis remains unknown, and thus prenatal diagnosis relies on ultrasound findings.

Fibrochondrogenesis is a rare, lethal, autosomal recessive rhizomelic chondrodysplasia. The typical features include narrow chest (short ribs with cupping), short long bones with irregular metaphyses with peripheral spurs, and extra-articular calcifications giving the appearance of stippling, platyspondyly with decreased ossification (particularly cervical vertebrae), and vertebral midline clefts. Other features include flat facies and cleft palate.[64,65]

Other Dysplasias

Other lethal skeletal dysplasias include **atelosteogenesis, boomerang dysplasia, de la Chapelle dysplasia,** and **Schneckenbecken dysplasia.** These are rare and difficult to diagnose, specifically on ultrasound.

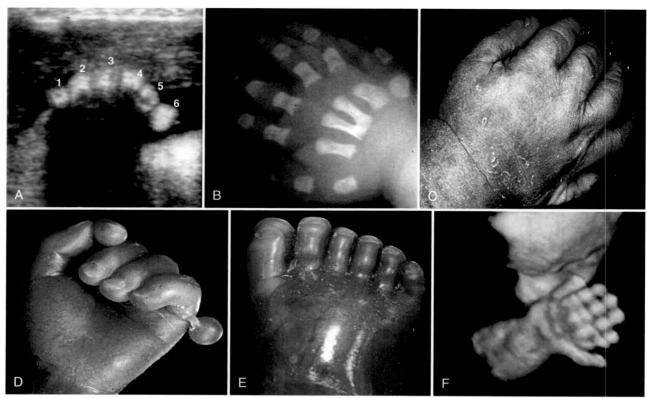

FIGURE 40-22. Collage of polydactyly. A, Ellis–van Creveld syndrome. Postaxial polydactyly on cross section through six digits. **B,** Corresponding radiograph shows postaxial polydactyly. Note hypoplastic distal phalanges and fusion of the third and fourth metacarpals. **C,** Corresponding pathology specimen. **D,** Polydactyly may present as a soft tissue nubbin with no bony elements. **E,** Ellis–van Creveld with toe polydactyly. **F,** 3-D ultrasound image shows isolated familial polydactyly.

NONLETHAL OR VARIABLE-PROGNOSIS SKELETAL DYSPLASIAS

The nonlethal or variable prognosis skeletal dysplasias form a larger group typically presenting with milder and later onset of skeletal abnormalities. Select nonlethal or variable-prognosis skeletal dysplasias with characteristic ultrasound findings are described in Tables 40-5, 40-6, and 40-7.

Heterozygous Achondroplasia

Heterozygous achondroplasia is the most common nonlethal skeletal dysplasia.[4] About 80% of cases are the result of a spontaneous dominant mutation associated with advanced paternal age, and the remainder is inherited from parental heterozygous achondroplasia. The incidence is approximately 1 in 26,000 births. Previously considered a diagnosis of the third trimester, recent studies have shown that a second-trimester diagnosis is possible.[66,67]

The key features are mild to moderate forms of rhizomelic limb shortening (more prominent in upper limbs), macrocranium, frontal bossing, depressed nasal bridge, midface hypoplasia, and brachydactyly, with a trident configuration of the hand. The biparietal diameter (BPD) typically is above the 97th centile at term. The interpedicular distances progressively narrow from the upper to the lower lumbar spine. There is a progressive discrepancy between FL and BPD during the third trimester, with FL falling below the first percentile compared to BPD[67] (Fig. 40-23). This may occur as early as 21 weeks or as late as 27 weeks' gestational age.

It is important to recognize that the pattern of BPD greater than expected with FL less than expected for gestational age, in combination with average abdominal circumference measurements, suggests heterozygous achondroplasia. A reliance on the mean of the three values may result in an average value for gestational age, thus masking the BPD/FL discrepancy. Patel and Filly[66] report that fetuses with heterozygous achondroplasia have FL that exceeds 34 mm at 26 weeks' BPD age, whereas those with homozygous achondroplasia do not. In cases where both parents are heterozygous achondroplasia, fetal ultrasound can differentiate among normal, heterozygous, and homozygous achondroplasia. Fetuses with FL below the third percentile compared with the BPD at 17 weeks' BPD age, with progressive shortening over the following 6 weeks, have homozygous achondroplasia, whereas those with decreasing FL between 17 and 23 weeks' BPD age have heterozygous achondroplasia.[66]

TABLE 40-5. RHIZOMELIC DYSPLASIA: KEY FEATURES

DYSPLASIA	PROGNOSIS	DEGREE OF LIMB SHORTENING	KEY SONOGRAPHIC FEATURES
Heterozygous achondroplasia	Nonlethal	Mild	Progressive discrepancy in femur length and biparietal diameter
Chondrodysplasia punctata, rhizomelic form	Lethal	Moderate-severe	Stippled epiphysis in third trimester
Diastrophic dysplasia	Variably lethal	Mild-moderate	Hitchhiker thumb, postural deformities, dislocations, joint contractures, clubfoot

TABLE 40-6. MICROMELIC DYSPLASIA, MILD: KEY FEATURES

DYSPLASIA	PROGNOSIS	KEY SONOGRAPHIC FEATURES
Asphyxiating thoracic dystrophy	May be lethal	Long narrow thorax, renal anomalies (cystic dysplasia), polydactyly (14%)
Ellis–van Creveld syndrome	May be lethal	Long narrow thorax, congenital heart disease (50% atrial septal defect), polydactyly (100%)

TABLE 40-7. MICROMELIC DYSPLASIA, MILD AND BOWED: KEY FEATURES

DYSPLASIA	PROGNOSIS	KEY SONOGRAPHIC FEATURES
Osteogenesis imperfecta type III	Nonlethal, progressively deforming	Lower extremities demonstrate greater degree of shortening and fractures/bowing
Campomelic dysplasia	Variably lethal	Ventral-bowing femur and tibia, hypoplastic or absent fibula, hypoplastic scapulas

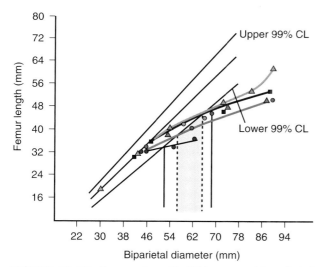

FIGURE 40-23. Femur length (FL) versus biparietal diameter (BPD). Seven cases of recurrent **heterozygous achondroplasia.** The FL falls below the 99% confidence limit (CL) by the time the BPD corresponds to 27 weeks' gestational age (~69 mm). *(From Kurtz AB, Filly RA, Wapner RJ, et al. In utero analysis of heterozygous achondroplasia: variable time of onset as detected by femur length measurements. J Ultrasound Med 1986;5:137-140.)*

The identification of the gene responsible for achondroplasia, FGFR3, mapped to the short arm of chromosome 4, has allowed the early prenatal diagnosis by DNA analysis by CVS when the parents are heterozygous for achondroplasia.[51]

Diastrophic Dysplasia

Diastrophic dysplasia is an autosomal recessive disorder with variable expression and a predominantly rhizomelic form of micromelia. The term *diastrophic* implies "twisted," which reflects the multiple postural deformities, dislocations, joint contractures, and kyphoscoliosis present.[1] The most characteristic feature is the "hitchhiker thumb," caused by a lateral positioning of the thumb in association with a hypoplastic first metacarpal (Fig. 40-24). The first toe may have similar positioning. There is a severe talipes equinovarus (clubfoot), which may be refractory to surgical treatment. Other features include micrognathia, cleft palate (50%), and laryngotracheomalacia. The life span may be normal if the progressive kyphoscoliosis does not compromise cardiopulmonary function. The diastrophic dysplasia gene was mapped to the long arm of chromosome 5 and found to encode a novel sulfate transporter. Mutations in the same gene were reported in ACH1B and atelosteogenesis type II.[68,69]

Asphyxiating Thoracic Dysplasia

Asphyxiating thoracic dysplasia, or **Jeune syndrome,** is an autosomal recessive disorder with variable expressivity. The incidence is 1 in 70,000 to 130,000 births. The perinatal mortality is high as a result of pulmonary hypoplasia. Those who survive may develop renal and hepatic fibrosis[1,68] (see Table 40-7). Key features are a mild to

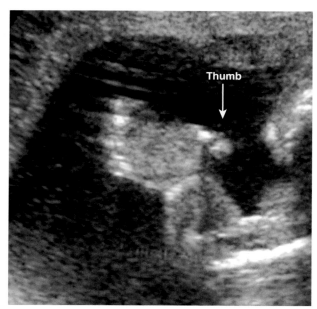

FIGURE 40-24. Diastrophic dysplasia with "hitch-hiker thumb." *(Courtesy Fetal Assessment Unit, University Health Network.)*

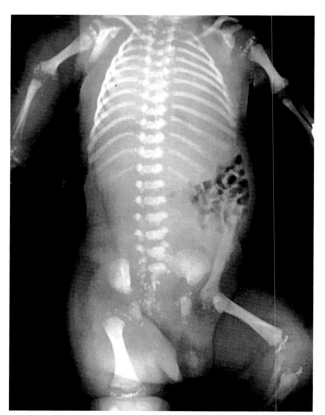

FIGURE 40-25. Chondrodysplasia punctata, rhizomelic form. Radiograph demonstrates stippled calcification within the epiphyseal and paravertebral cartilages. Humeri are very short, the femurs are relatively short.

moderate form of micromelia (60%) with rhizomelic predominance, a long narrow thorax with short horizontal ribs, inverted "handlebar" appearance of the clavicles, renal dysplasia and cysts, and postaxial polydactyly in 14%.

Ellis–van Creveld Syndrome

Ellis–van Creveld syndrome, or **chondroectodermal dysplasia,** is an autosomal-recessive disorder with an incidence of 1 per 150,000 births. The condition has a high prevalence among inbred populations, such as the Amish and the Arabs of the Gaza strip.[60] It is generally a nonlethal disorder, but death can result from pulmonary hypoplasia.[33,60] Key features include mild to moderate form of micromelia with a mesomelic predominance, short horizontal ribs, postaxial or ulnar polydactyly[1] (see Fig. 40-22) that is almost 100% in the hands and 25% in the feet,[52] and CHD (50%), most often atrial septal defect. Additional findings include a progressive distalward shortening of the extremities with hypoplastic distal phalanges. Fusion of the metacarpals and phalanges is common. The presence of polydactyly, CHD, and the absence of renal cysts help to distinguish this condition from asphyxiating thoracic dystrophy.

Chondrodysplasia Punctata

Chondrodysplasia punctata, or **stippled epiphyses**, is a heterogeneous group of disorders with many small calcifications (**ossification centers**) in the cartilage, in the ends of bones, and around the spine. Known associated conditions include single-gene disorders such as rhizo-

melic chondrodysplasia punctata, Conradi-Hünermann syndrome, and Zellweger syndrome (cerebrohepatorenal syndrome); chromosomal abnormalities such as trisomy 21 and 18; maternal autoimmune diseases; and teratogen exposure (e.g., warfarin, alcohol).[70,71]

Rhizomelic chondrodysplasia punctata is an autosomal-recessive condition caused by a peroxisomal disorder that appears as severe, symmetrical, predominantly rhizomelic limb shortening.[60,72] The incidence is approximately 1 in 110,000 births, and it is generally lethal before the second year of life. The humeri tend to be relatively shorter than the femurs and have metaphyseal cupping. The enlarged epiphyses with characteristic stippling may occasionally be identified on ultrasound in the third trimester (Fig. 40-25; see also Fig. 40-2, *I*). Other abnormalities include dysmorphic facial features, joint contractures, coronal clefting of the vertebral bodies, brain abnormalities, and severe mental retardation.

Conradi-Hünermann syndrome, or the **nonrhizomelic** form of chondrodysplasia punctata (**CDPX2),** is an X-linked dominant condition with extreme phenotypic variations, rendering the antenatal diagnosis difficult in the absence of known family history. The widely variable phenotypic presentation may be related to random X inactivation.[73,74] CDPX2 is uncommon, with X-linked dominant inheritance and possible lethality in the hemizygous male (Xp11).[73] The characteristic skeletal abnormalities are asymmetrical shortening of the extremities with punctate calcifications primarily affecting the ends of long bones, the carpal and tarsal regions, paravertebral region, and pelvic bones. Stature is usually reduced; kyphoscoliosis with shortening of the long bones (particularly femur and humerus) and dysmorphic facial features are common.[71]

Dyssegmental Dysplasia

Dyssegmental dysplasia is a rare autosomal recessive skeletal dysplasia characterized by gross vertebral disorganization. The findings typically include micromelia, short narrow thorax, joint rigidity, **anisospondyly** (gross irregularity of the size and shape of the vertebral bodies) which may include malsegmentation, clefting or "oversize" bodies, kyphoscoliosis, and multiple ossification centers (Fig. 40-26). The gross spine disorganization may be recognized as early as the first trimester. The more severe form is referred to as **Silverman-Handmaker** and the milder form as **Rolland-Desbuquois,** although some think that dyssegmental dysplasia may represent a spectrum of findings caused by different mutations in the perlecan gene.[75]

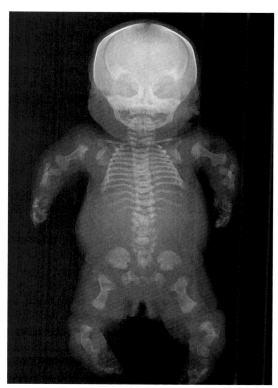

FIGURE 40-26. Dyssegmental dysplasia in stillborn fetus. AP radiograph demonstrates **anisospondyly,** characterized by the varying size and shape of vertebral bodies. The "oversize" large vertebral bodies are characteristic. Note the shortened, wide, and angulated tubular long bones with a characteristic dumbbell configuration. Small thorax with short ribs is associated with pulmonary hypoplasia.

Osteogenesis Imperfecta Types I, III, IV—Nonlethal Types

Osteogenesis imperfecta type I is a mild, "tarda" variant inherited in an autosomal dominant manner as a result of mutation in the *COL1A1* (on chromosome 17) or *COL1A2* (on chromosome 7) and possibly in other collagen genes. OI **type I** is a generalized connective tissue disorder characterized by bone fragility and blue sclerae. The bones are of normal length, and only 5% present at birth with fractures. Most fractures occur from childhood to puberty. There is progressive hearing loss in approximately 50% of type I cases. **Type III** has a heterogeneous mode of inheritance. This is a nonlethal, progressively deforming variety of OI that often spares the humeri, vertebrae, and pelvis. Rib involvement is variable. The blue sclerae will normalize, and there is no associated hearing impairment. **Type IV** is an autosomal dominant form of OI. It is the mildest form, involving isolated fractures. The sclerae are blue at birth but normalize over time. There is no associated hearing impairment.

LIMB REDUCTION DEFECTS AND ASSOCIATED CONDITIONS

This heterogeneous group of disorders is associated with a spectrum of limb defects caused by chromosomal abnormalities, single-gene disorders, and maternal exposures and diseases, causing a variety of limb defects. There are three major categories of limb reduction defects. A **malformation** is a defect resulting from an abnormal developmental process. A **deformation** is an abnormality of form, shape, or position caused by mechanical forces. A **disruption** is a defect caused by the extrinsic breakdown or interference with an originally normal developmental process. The defect can consist of the absence of an entire limb (**amelia**), of part of a limb (**phocomelia**), or of digits (**oligodactyly**), or it can involve an increased number of digits (**polydactyly**).[76] It can also affect only the **radial ray** or **ulnar ray,** with or without involvement of the corresponding fingers (Table 40-8).

The overall incidence of congenital limb reduction deformities is estimated at 0.40 per 10,000 births. An isolated amputation may be caused by amniotic band sequence, teratogen exposure, or a vascular accident. Overall limb abnormalities are detected prenatally in approximately 45% of cases diagnosed postnatally.[77]

Proximal Focal Femoral Deficiency

Proximal focal femoral deficiency is a rare, sporadic condition, and 35% of those affected are infants of diabetic mothers[52] (see Fig. 40-2, *C*). There is an asymmetrical degree of absence of the **subtrochanteric femur,** which

TABLE 40-8. NOMENCLATURE OF LIMB ANOMALIES

ANOMALY	DESCRIPTION
Limb Reduction Anomalies	
Amelia	Absent limb
Adactyly	Absent digits
Acheiria	Absent hand
Apodia	Absent foot
Hemimelia	Absent extremity distal to knee or elbow
Phocomelia	Absent middle segment of limb
Ectrodactyly	Split hand
Ulnar or radial hemimelia	Absent ulnar and ulnar digits paraxial or radius and thumb
Hand and Foot Anomalies	
Clinodactyly	Incurvature of a digit
Camptodactyly	Flexion of a digit
Syndactyly	Fusion of digits
Polydactyly	Extra digits
Oligodactyly	Decreased number of digits

may extend to the femoral head and acetabulum.[60] The femoral hypoplasia is often associated with ipsilateral fibular hemimelia, which may result in a bowed appearance of the tibia, similar to that of campomelic dysplasia; however, proximal focal femoral deficiency is generally unilateral. Hypoplasia or aplasia of other long bones, vertebral anomalies, microcephaly, and facial dysmorphism can also occur. If the defect is unilateral, it may represent the **femur-fibula-ulnar complex,** which is nonfamilial, versus the **femur-tibia-radius complex,** which has a strong genetic association.[78] When associated with the unusual facies syndrome, the femoral hypoplasia is usually bilateral.

Caudal Regression Syndrome and Sirenomelia

Caudal regression syndrome consists of partial to complete **sacral agenesis** and abnormalities of the lumbar spine, pelvis, and lower limbs.[79-81] The majority of cases are associated with maternal diabetes, but familial cases have been reported. **Sirenomelia** is characterized by an absent sacrum, fusion of the lower extremities, anorectal atresia, and renal dysgenesis or agenesis (Fig. 40-27). Severe oligohydramnios and single umbilical artery are typically present. Prevalence is approximately 1:60,000 births.

Amniotic Band Sequence

Amniotic band sequence is suspected to be secondary to first-trimester rupture of the amnion, resulting in **amniotic bands** that extend from the chorionic surface of the amnion to the fetal tissue.[82,83] The incidence is approximately 1:1200 live births but is much higher in

spontaneous abortions. Depending on the timing and orientation of the bands, the resultant disruption of fetal organs includes **amputations** of limbs or digits (Figs. 40-28 and 40-29), bizarre facial or cranial clefting, and thoracoabdominal schisis. The distribution is asymmetrical. Constriction ring defects are the most common finding. Fibrous bands of tissue with a constricting ring and distal elephantiasis or protrusion of uncovered bone distally are pathognomonic for this anomaly (Fig. 40-30). Antenatally, an aberrant band attached to the fetus, with characteristic deformities and restriction of motion, permits the diagnosis. An amniotic sheet is a **synechia,** or scar in the uterus, and is distinguished from an amniotic band by a thickened base and a free edge.[84] Synechiae are not associated with amniotic band sequence.

The **limb–body wall complex** is a sporadic disorder that occurs in approximately 1:4000 live births with a similar, but more severe and lethal, complex of fetal malformations.[85] Additional findings include evisceration of internal organs, myelomeningocele, marked scoliosis, and short straight umbilical cord.

Limb Reduction Defects

The prenatal detection rate of isolated limb reduction defect is estimated at 14.6%, compared to 49.1% when associated anomalies were detected.[86] **Terminal transverse limb defects** are associated with amniotic bands only in some cases, and thus other etiologies (e.g., vascular disruption, fetal hypoxemia, errors in embryologic development) are suspected in other cases.

Radial Ray Defects

Radial ray defects are associated with a wide variety of syndromes. The diagnosis is based on the absence of a visualized distal radius at the same level as the ulna, in association with a radial deviation or clubhand (Fig. 40-31). There may be bowing or hypoplasia of the ulna and a hypoplastic or absent thumb. Ulnar ray defects are rare.

Fanconi pancytopenia (syndrome) is an autosomal recessive blood dyscrasia in which 50% of cases have an associated unilateral or bilateral **aplastic or hypoplastic thumb and radius.** Identification of the thumb hypoplasia or aplasia in association with a radial ray defect suggests this diagnosis, initiating discussion of prenatal diagnosis and potential cesarean section to avoid excessive bleeding (Fig. 40-32). Prenatal diagnosis is based on increased chromosome breakage and sister chromatid exchange in cultured amniotic fluid cells, both before and after exposure to diepoxybutane.[87]

Aase syndrome is an autosomal recessive blood dyscrasia characterized by hypoplastic anemia, a hypoplastic distal radius with radial clubhand, and a **triphalangeal thumb.** Associated cardiac defects (ventricular septal defect, coarctation of aorta) may be present.

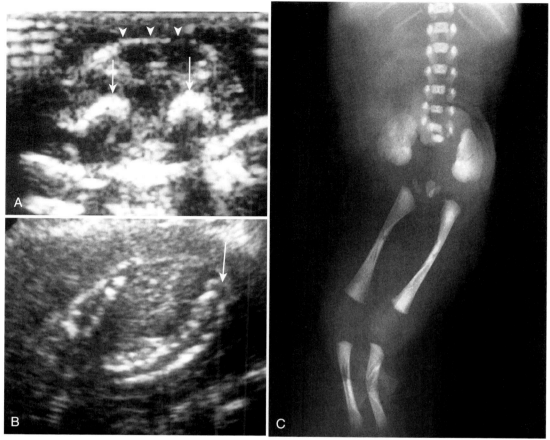

FIGURE 40-27. Sirenomelia. A, Cross section of lower extremities. Femurs *(arrows)* are closer than expected because of fusion of the overlying soft tissues with a continuous layer of overlying skin *(arrowheads)*. **B,** Sacral agenesis with abrupt termination of the lower spine *(arrow)*. **C,** Single, fused lower extremity and sacral agenesis.

Triphalangeal thumb may also be found in Holt-Oram syndrome, Diamond-Blackfan syndrome, chromosomal abnormalities, and fetal hydantoin exposure.

Thrombocytopenia–absent radius syndrome (TAR) is an autosomal recessive blood dyscrasia characterized by hypomegakaryocytic thrombocytopenia and bilateral absence of the radii.[88] The thumb is always present. The humerus and lower extremities are variably involved. One third of such patients have CHD, typically tetralogy of Fallot or septal defects. Fetuses are at risk of intracranial hemorrhage, so delivery by cesarean section is recommended (Fig. 40-33).

Holt-Oram syndrome is an autosomal dominant disorder consisting of a congenital heart defect (atrial or ventricular septal defect) in combination with a variety of upper limb anomalies. The limbs are asymmetrically affected, with the left limb usually showing more effects than the right. The lower extremities are not involved.

Roberts' syndrome, or pseudothalidomide syndrome, is an autosomal recessive disorder characterized by tetraphocomelia and bilateral cleft lip/palate. The limb reductions are most prominent in the upper extremities.

Other conditions associated with radial ray abnormalities include trisomies 18 and 13, the VACTERL association, acrorenal syndrome, Cornelia de Lange syndrome, Goldenhar syndrome, Nager acrofacial dysostosis, and Klippel-Feil syndrome.

Arthrogryposis Multiplex Congenita

Arthrogryposis multiplex congenita is a heterogeneous group of disorders with **multiple joint contractures** of prenatal onset[89] (Fig. 40-34). Normal fetal motion by approximately 7 to 8 weeks onward is required for development of the musculoskeletal system. Some cases result from extrinsic causes, such as oligohydramnios, twinning, or uterine masses, and most of these have a good prognosis. Intrinsic causes include neuromuscular disorders (most cases) and skeletal and connective tissue disorders. Typically, the severity of the deformity increases distally, with maximal deformity in the hands and feet. This may result in the "Buddha position" of the fetus, with arms and legs crossed and ending in clubhand or clubfoot (Fig. 40-34, *D*). The **fetal akinesia sequence** refers to the combination of multiple joint contractures in association with IUGR, underdevelopment of the bones, pulmonary hypoplasia, typical craniofacial abnormalities, and a short umbilical cord.

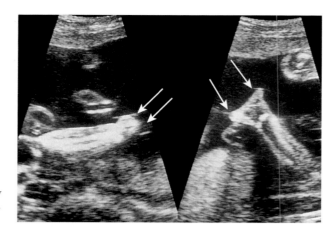

FIGURE 40-28. Amputation of the hand. Upper extremity ends abruptly distal to the wrist, in the midcarpal region *(arrows)*. *(Courtesy Ants Toi, MD, University of Toronto.)*

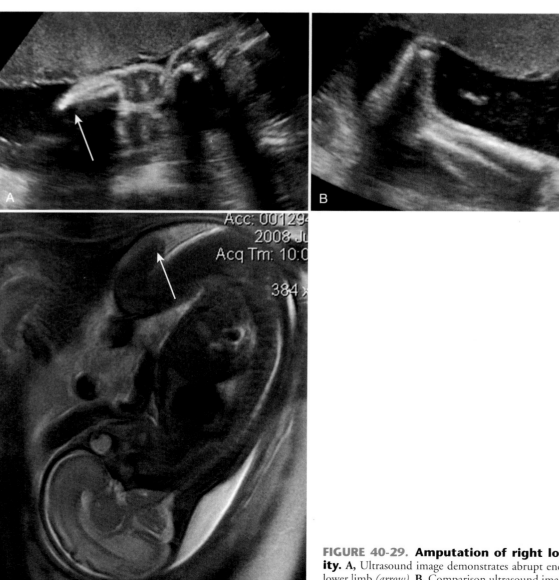

FIGURE 40-29. Amputation of right lower extremity. A, Ultrasound image demonstrates abrupt ending of the right lower limb *(arrow)*. **B,** Comparison ultrasound image shows normal left lower limb. **C,** T2-weighted MR image confirms amputation of the right lower limb *(arrow)*.

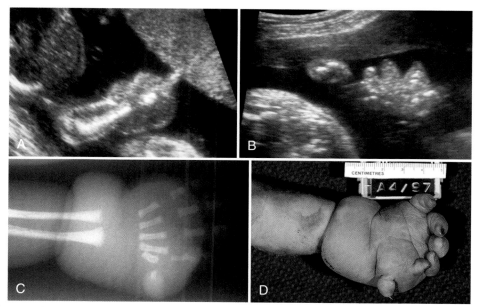

FIGURE 40-30. Amniotic band sequence. Constriction rings with distal elephantiasis. **A,** Ultrasound lateral image of the distal forearm and hand demonstrates the two constriction rings with elephantiasis. **B,** Ultrasound of the digits demonstrates the distal tapering of the digits. **C,** Radiograph demonstrates the two constriction rings in the distal forearm and hand. **D,** Correlative specimen photograph.

Limb pterygium, or webbing of the skin across a joint, can involve a single or several joints[90] and etiologically is a heterogeneous disorder. Popliteal pterygium is the most common dominantly inherited pterygium syndrome.

Asymmetrical **limb enlargement** may be caused by hemihypertrophy, cutaneous hemangioma or lymphangioma, elephantiasis secondary to a constricting band, arteriovenous malformations, neurofibromatosis, or Beckwith-Wiedemann syndrome. **Hereditary lymphedema type 1,** or Nonne-Milroy lymphedema, is a rare autosomal dominant condition secondary to deficient lymphatic drainage, typically affecting the lower extremities. The subcutaneous tissues of the affected extremity appear diffusely thickened. Associated ascites and pleural effusions may be seen. There is variable expressivity and age of onset[91] (Fig. 40-35). Extremity enlargement may also be related to thickened subcutaneous tissues, as in hydrops or large-for-gestational-age infants.

Kyphoscoliosis may be a manifestation of an isolated vertebral defect or may be associated with myelomeningocele or with complex syndromes, such as VACTERL, limb–body wall complex, neurofibromatosis, arthrogryposis, diastrophic dysplasia, and other skeletal dysplasias.

HAND AND FOOT DEFORMITIES

A complete digit evaluation can be performed by 12 to 13 weeks' gestation.[92] The fetus typically maintains open hands with digit extension in the first half of gestation,

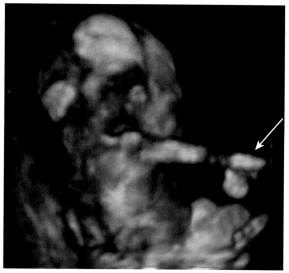

FIGURE 40-31. Radial ray anomaly diagnosed at 13 weeks' gestation. Three-dimensional (3-D) ultrasound surface display demonstrates the hypoplastic radius and ulna in association with talipomanus (clubhand) *(arrow).*

whereas in the second half the fetus may maintain hand closure for relatively prolonged periods, up to 30 minutes, limiting detailed evaluation. The incidence of finger abnormalities is approximately 1:1000 fetuses, of which 60% will have either an associated malformation sequence or karyotypic malformation. The optimal time for evaluation of the hands and feet is during the second trimester.[12,93-95]

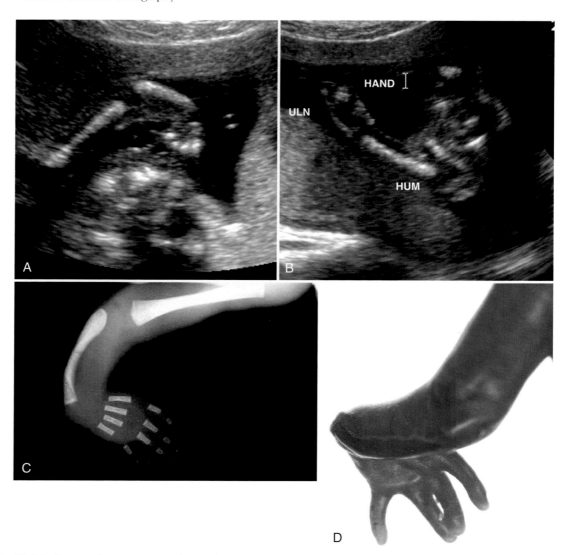

FIGURE 40-32. Fanconi pancytopenia. Radial ray aplasia with talipomanus and bilateral absence of thumbs. **A,** Radial deviation left hand, or clubhand, secondary to radial ray aplasia and ulnar hypoplasia. Note absent thumb. **B,** More extreme example of radial deviation hand or clubhand secondary to radial ray aplasia and ulnar hypoplasia. **C,** Correlative radiograph (of **A**) of left arm. Note absent thumb. **D,** Correlative specimen photograph of **A**. Note absent thumb. *(Courtesy Shia Salem, MD, University of Toronto.)*

Transient findings represent a potential pitfall in the analysis of the distal extremities. During the second half of gestation, the fetus may appear to have **pseudosyndactyly** by maintaining clenched fists for prolonged periods or the appearance of "sandal foot." The diagnosis of an isolated clubfoot can be risky because the fetus can hold the foot in a position to suggest the diagnosis in the absence of a structural defect. An apparent clubfoot may be secondary to positioning against the maternal uterine wall or in the setting of oligohydramnios, which subsequently resolves with a change in fetal position or amniotic fluid volume.

Aneuploidy is associated with an increased risk of hand and foot anomalies, including persistent clenched hand, overlapping digits, clinodactyly, polydactyly, syndactyly, simian creases, talipes equinovarus, rocker-bottom foot, and sandal toes (Fig. 40-36).

Persistent clenched hand with overlapping of digits occurs in more than 50% of trisomy 18 fetuses and is generally bilateral. This characteristic hand appearance is highly suggestive of trisomy 18 but can also occur in other conditions, such as fetal akinesia syndrome and triploidy.

Clinodactyly is the permanent incurvature of a finger. Clinodactyly, caused by asymmetric hypoplasia of the middle phalanx (medial shorter than lateral aspect), most often involves the fifth finger and is associated with trisomies 13, 15, 18, and 21 (Fig. 40-36, *G*). Clinodactyly

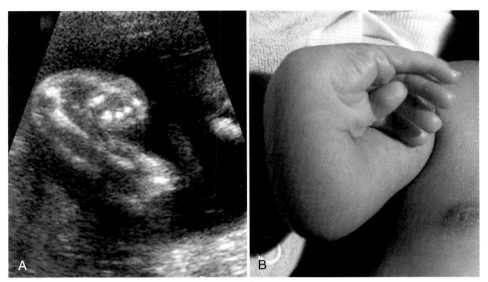

FIGURE 40-33. Thrombocytopenia: absent radius syndrome. A, Absent radius in association with hypoplastic ulna results in talipomanus. Note that thumb is present. **B,** Correlative specimen photograph.

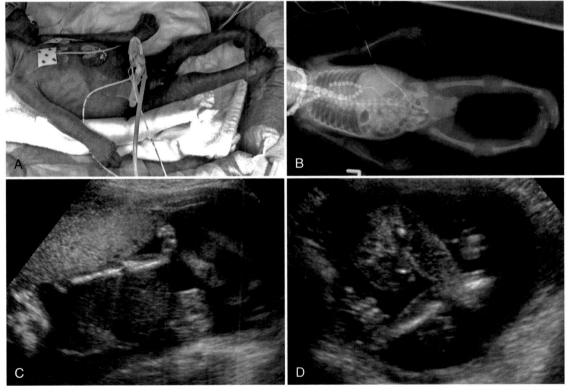

FIGURE 40-34. Arthrogryposis multiplex congenita. Decreased muscle bulk is replaced by a mixture of fat and adipose tissue, resulting in multiple congenital joint contractures, including fixed internal rotation of shoulders, hyperextension of elbows, flexion of wrists, and talipes equinovarus (clubfoot). Note that severity of deformity increases distally. The knees and hips at birth were demonstrated to be nonrigid contractures amenable to conservative postural therapy. **A,** Photograph demonstrates fixed contractures of the elbows, wrists, digits, and ankles. **B,** Radiograph demonstrates similar contractures. **C,** Ultrasound of upper extremity demonstrates fixed extension of the elbow and fixed flexion of the wrist and digits with talipomanus. **D,** "Buddha position" with flexed hips, knees, and ankles and clubfoot distally.

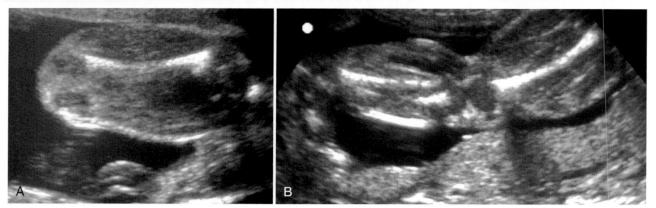

FIGURE 40-35. **Hereditary lymphedema at 21 weeks. A,** Femur surrounded by marked thickening of the subcutaneous tissues. **B,** Lower extremity with marked thickening of subcutaneous tissues.

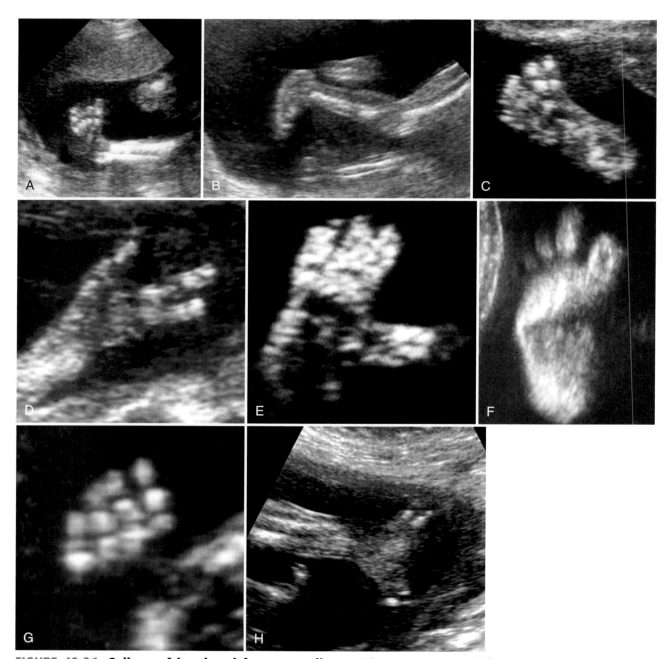

FIGURE 40-36. **Collage of hand and foot anomalies. A, Talipes equinovarus** (clubfoot). Inverted plantar flexion with medial deviation of the foot results in visualization of the long axis of the foot (metatarsals) and lower leg in the same plane. Note the rounded angle between the foot and lower leg. **B, Rocker-bottom foot.** Convex sole contour and rounded soft tissue protrusion posterior to the calf soft tissues. **C, Toe polydactyly,** six digits. **D, Oligodactyly,** three digits. **E, Syndactyly.** Soft tissue fusion of the first and second digits. **F, Sandal toes** in a 37-week fetus with Nager syndrome demonstrates an exaggerated gap between the first and second toes and a plantar skin furrow. **G, Clinodactyly.** Hypoplastic middle phalanx of fifth digit. **H, Ectrodactyly,** or split hand/foot deformity. *(C and E courtesy Ants Toi, MD; D and H courtesy Shia Salem, MD; University of Toronto.)*

occurs in 60% of fetuses with trisomy 21; however, up to 18% of normal fetuses may have a mild degree of clinodactyly.[93] **Camptodactyly** is the permanent flexion of a finger caused by flexion contracture of an interphalangeal joint.

Polydactyly is the presence of extra digits on the foot or hand. Most cases are isolated findings, but extra digits can be associated with syndromes and chromosomal abnormalities. Polydactyly may be diagnosed toward the end of the first trimester. The extra digit may consist of a small, soft tissue projection or a complete digit. **Postaxial polydactyly** (ulnar or fibular) is more common and is found in conditions such as Ellis–van Creveld syndrome, asphyxiating thoracic dystrophy, short-rib polydactyly syndrome, and trisomy 13. **Preaxial** (radial or tibial) **polydactyly** is found in familial conditions, such as Fanconi syndrome, Holt-Oram syndrome, acrocephalosyndactyly, and conditions associated with triphalangeal thumb.[60] Central polydactyly can also occur. Polydactyly may be hereditary and familial. Because this form is associated with a good prognosis, it is important to review the pertinent family history.

Syndactyly refers to soft tissue and/or osseous fusion of digits (Fig. 40-36, E). Syndactyly of the third and fourth fingers in association with IUGR in the second trimester suggests the diagnosis of **triploidy**.

An abducted, low-set thumb, or **hitchhiker thumb** (see Fig. 40-24), is associated with **diastrophic dwarfism**. An adducted thumb may be associated with aqueductal stenosis.

Ectrodactyly, or the split hand/foot "lobster claw" deformity, is a deficiency of the central digits resulting in a cleft. It can occur as an isolated abnormality or in association with other findings, such as cleft lip/palate, as in ectrodactyly–ectodermal dysplasia clefting syndrome, Cornelia de Lange syndrome, and limb-mammary syndrome[96] (Fig. 40-36, H). Many isolated cases are the result of a new dominant mutation or are inherited from parents with minimal manifestations. Thus, a careful examination of the parents is needed before counseling low recurrence risk.[96,97]

Talipomanus, or **clubhand**, can be radial or ulnar. Radial clubhand is more common and is generally associated with the syndromes or karyotype abnormalities previously described with radial ray variants. Trisomies 18 and 21, long arm deletion of chromosome 13, and ring formation of chromosome 4 can be associated with radial clubhand. Other conditions associated with talipomanus include the VACTERL association, Goldenhar syndrome, and Klippel-Feil syndrome. Another abnormality includes a sporadic group of syndromes associated with craniofacial abnormalities, most often cleft lip and palate. Ulnar clubhand, associated with ulnar ray defects, is uncommon and may be an isolated finding.

Talipes equinovarus, or **clubfoot**, occurs in 0.1% to 0.2% of the population. The recurrence risk after the birth of one child with isolated clubfoot is 2% to 3%, and if one of the parents is affected, the recurrence risk is 3% to 4%. The diagnosis is based on the recognition of an inverted and plantar-flexed foot in which the metatarsal long axis is in the same plane as the tibia and fibula, in association with a rounded angle of junction between the foot and the lower leg (Figs. 40-37 and 40-38; **Video 40-2**). The majority are isolated malformations; however,

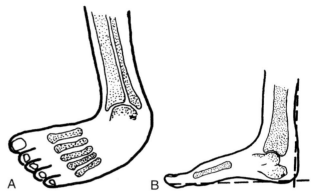

FIGURE 40-37. Sonographic in utero diagnosis of clubfoot. A, Clubfoot. Inverted, plantar-flexed, and medially deviated foot results in visualization of the long axis of the foot and tibia/fibula in the same plane. Note the rounded angle of junction between the lower leg and foot. **B, Normal foot.** Note the normal relationship of tibia and fibula to the metatarsals and the normal squared angle of the lower leg to the foot. *(From Jeanty P, Romero R, d'Altoan M, et al: In utero sonographic detection of hand and foot deformities. J Ultrasound Med 1985;4:595-601.)*

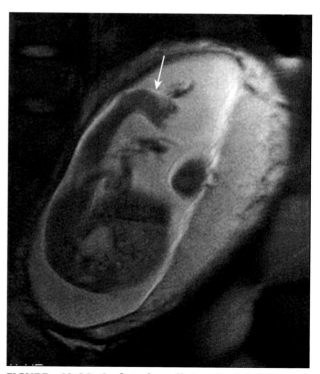

FIGURE 40-38. Isolated unilateral clubfoot. T2-weighted MR image demonstrates a clubfoot.

MRI and fetal karyotyping should be considered when clubfoot is found in association with other structural abnormalities.[98-104] Early amniocentesis is associated with an increased risk of clubfoot. Hindfoot equinus (plantar flexion), hindfoot varus (inward rotation), forefoot adduction, and variable forefoot cavus (plantar flexion) can also occur.

Congenital talipes equinovarus represents a spectrum ranging from "postural" talipes or nonrigid deformity requiring little active management, to a severe, rigid deformity requiring extensive surgery. The foot is fixed in adduction, supination, and varus position, thus appearing to be turned inward. Tillett et al.[99] found that up to 26% of cases of clubfoot required no active postnatal management, presumably in the postural group. It is difficult to determine if this group is positional or a false-positive diagnosis. False-positive results are most often found in the group with an isolated diagnosis of talipes equinovarus made in late pregnancy, although they can occur at the 18- to 22-week evaluation, at a reported rate of 2.3%.[105] The normal foot may achieve extreme dorsiflexion or plantar flexion, and caution is advised when making the initial diagnosis of isolated clubfoot in the third trimester.[101,103] In the setting of isolated clubfoot (unilateral or bilateral) the risk of requiring surgery is approximately 40%.[105]

Rocker-bottom foot is the result of a vertical position of the talus and equinus or vertical position of the calcaneus secondary to a short Achilles tendon (Fig. 40-36, B). The tarsal bones are dislocated dorsally, so there is a convex plantar surface with posterior bulging of the calcaneus. It carries a high risk for fetal chromosomal abnormalities such as trisomies 18 and 13 when associated with other abnormalities, as well as for other syndromes such as fetal akinesia sequence.

Brachydactyly is the abnormal shortening of the digits. There is relative sparing of foot length in many skeletal dysplasias, but the hands may be affected. Achondroplasia has a characteristic configuration with the digits ending at the same level and unable to approximate the second, third, or fourth digits, leading to the appearance of the "trident hand" (Fig. 40-39).

Sandal toes, or an exaggerated gap between the first and second digits, is often visualized in the normal fetus but has a higher prevalence in trisomy 21 fetuses[12] (Fig. 40-36, F). An elevated first digit/toe may cause a false or transient abnormality that mimics sandal toes.

SKELETAL FINDINGS ASSOCIATED WITH ANEUPLOIDY

When an abnormality in the musculoskeletal system is detected during routine ultrasound examination, a systematic search is performed to detect other defects that may lead to the diagnosis of a specific genetic or chromosomal defect.[106,107] During the second trimester, an expected/measured FL ratio below 0.9, based on BPD, should prompt a detailed examination to assess for other possible features of aneuploidy. However, in the third trimester, a mildly shortened femur is generally associated with asymmetrical IUGR or a constitutional small fetus rather than with aneuploidy. A femur/foot ratio greater than 0.9 suggests IUGR rather than a bone dysplasia, whereas a femur/foot ratio of less than 0.9 suggests a skeletal dysplasia.[12,108] In general, chromosomal anomalies are associated with a symmetrical form of IUGR versus asymmetrical IUGR often associated with uteroplacental insufficiency. Triploidy is an exception, occurring with an asymmetrical form of IUGR.

Trisomy 21 (Down syndrome) is the most common chromosome abnormality in newborns, with an incidence of 1:600 to 1:800. About 95% of such cases result from an additional chromosome 21; 3% result from translocation; and 2% are mosaic. Most cases are sporadic; about 33% are born to mothers older than 35. Characteristic skeletal findings include mild shortening of the femur and humerus, clinodactyly of the fifth finger, sandal gap toes, flat nasal bridge, frontal bossing, and brachycephaly.

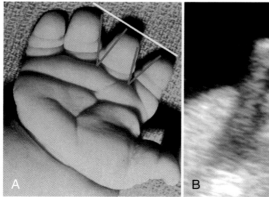
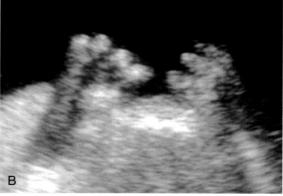

FIGURE 40-39. Achondroplasia and the "trident hand" configuration. A, Homozygous achondroplasia with trident configuration with the digits ending at the same level *(yellow line),* with inability to approximate the second, third, and fourth digits *(pink lines).* **B,** Homozygous achondroplasia with ultrasound appearance of severe brachydactyly with trident configuration.

TRISOMY 21: MUSCULOSKELETAL FEATURES

Mild shortening of femur and humerus
Clinodactyly of fifth finger
Sandal toes
Flat nasal bridge
Frontal bossing
Brachycephaly

Trisomy 18 (Edwards syndrome) is sporadically inherited, with an incidence of 1:5000 live births. The classic appearance is a persistently clenched hand with overlapping of the second and third digits and the fourth and fifth digits, often in association with clinodactyly of the fifth digit. The findings are usually bilateral and occur in more than 50% of trisomy 18 cases. Other musculoskeletal findings include radial ray aplasia variants in 10% to 50%, syndactyly of the second and third toes, simian creases, clubfoot or rocker-bottom foot, incomplete clavicle ossification, and vertebral and rib anomalies. The prognosis is poor; 90% of neonates succumb in the first year of life, and all survivors have profound mental retardation.

TRISOMY 18: MUSCULOSKELETAL FEATURES

Persistent clenched hand with overlapping digits
Radial ray aplasia variants
Syndactyly
Talipes equinovarus (clubfoot)
Rocker-bottom foot
Vertebral and rib anomalies

Trisomy 13 (Patau syndrome) is sporadically inherited with an incidence of 1:10,000 live births. The musculoskeletal anomalies include postaxial polydactyly of hands and feet, possible clenched hand (with or without overlapping digits), clinodactyly, and possibly associated hypoplastic ribs and pelvic bones.

TRISOMY 13: MUSCULOSKELETAL FEATURES

Polydactyly
Persistent clenched hand with or without
   overlapping digits
Clinodactyly
Hypoplastic ribs and pelvic bones
Microcephaly
Hypotelorism
Facial clefts

Triploidy (69,XXX, 69,XXY, or 69,XXY) occurs in 18% of all early miscarriages, but the incidence is only 1:2500 births. In 60% of cases, triploidy results from dispermy, and in 40%, from diploid sperm or diploid egg. The combination of early severe asymmetrical IUGR, oligohydramnios, and an enlarged hydropic placenta suggests this diagnosis. A partial molar pregnancy may be present. Associated musculoskeletal findings include syndactyly of the third and fourth fingers, simian crease, talipes equinovarus, and hitchhiker toe deformity. Other findings may include micrognathia, ventriculomegaly, myelomeningocele, and cardiac abnormalities.

Acknowledgments

Special thanks to Drs. Katherine Fong, Shia Salem, Ants Toi, and Greg Ryan and all the staff at Medical Imaging and Maternal Fetal Medicine Department at the Mount Sinai Hospital, Women's College Hospital, and Sunnybrook Health Science Center in Toronto who have provided many wonderful images and generously shared their knowledge and work.

References

1. Spranger JW, Brill PW, Poznanski AK. Bone dysplasias: an atlas of genetic disorders of skeletal development. 2nd ed. New York: Oxford University Press; 2002.
2. Superti-Furga A, Unger S, Superti-Furga A, Unger S. Nosology and classification of genetic skeletal disorders: 2006 revision [see comment]. Am J Med Genet 2007;143A:1-18.
3. Lachman RS, Rappaport V. Fetal imaging in the skeletal dysplasias. Clin Perinatol 1990;17:703-722.
4. Camera G, Mastroiacovo P. Birth prevalence of skeletal dysplasias in the Italian Multicentric Monitoring System for Birth Defects. Prog Clin Biol Res 1982;104:441-449.
5. Rimoin DL, Cohn D, Krakow D, et al. The skeletal dysplasias: clinical-molecular correlations. Ann NY Acad Sci 2007;1117:302-309.
6. Superti-Furga A, Hastbacka J, Wilcox WR, et al. Achondrogenesis type IB is caused by mutations in the diastrophic dysplasia sulphate transporter gene. Nat Genet 1996;12:100-102.
7. Krakow D, Alanay Y, Rimoin LP, et al. Evaluation of prenatal-onset osteochondrodysplasias by ultrasonography: a retrospective and prospective analysis. Am J Med Genet 2008;146A:1917-1924.
8. Pretorius DH, Rumack CM, Manco-Johnson ML, et al. Specific skeletal dysplasias in utero: sonographic diagnosis. Radiology 1986;159:237-242.
9. Tretter AE, Saunders RC, Meyers CM, et al. Antenatal diagnosis of lethal skeletal dysplasias. Am J Med Genet 1998;75:518-522.

Normal Fetal Skeleton
10. Merz E, Kim-Kern MS, Pehl S. Ultrasonic mensuration of fetal limb bones in the second and third trimesters. J Clin Ultrasound 1987;15:175-183.
11. Mahony BS, Filly RA. High-resolution sonographic assessment of the fetal extremities. J Ultrasound Med 1984;3:489-498.
12. Bromley B, Benacerraf B. Abnormalities of the hands and feet in the fetus: sonographic findings. AJR Am J Roentgenol 1995;165:1239-1243.
13. Greulich WW, Pyle SI. Radiographic atlas of skeletal development of the hand and wrist. 2nd ed. Stanford, Calif: Stanford University Press; 1959.
14. Mahony BS, Callen PW, Filly RA. The distal femoral epiphyseal ossification center in the assessment of third-trimester menstrual age: sonographic identification and measurement. Radiology 1985;155:201-204.

15. Chinn DH, Bolding DB, Callen PW, et al. Ultrasonographic identification of fetal lower extremity epiphyseal ossification centers. Radiology 1983;147:815-818.
16. Goldstein I, Lockwood CJ, Reece EA, Hobbins JC. Sonographic assessment of the distal femoral and proximal tibial ossification centers in the prediction of pulmonic maturity in normal women and women with diabetes. Am J Obstet Gynecol 1988;159:72-76.
17. Goldstein RB, Filly RA, Simpson G. Pitfalls in femur length measurements. J Ultrasound Med 1987;6:203-207.
18. Abrams SL, Filly RA. Curvature of the fetal femur: a normal sonographic finding. Radiology 1985;156:490.
19. Yarkoni S, Schmidt W, Jeanty P, et al. Clavicular measurement: a new biometric parameter for fetal evaluation. J Ultrasound Med 1985;4:467-470.
20. Campbell J, Henderson A, Campbell S. The fetal femur/foot length ratio: a new parameter to assess dysplastic limb reduction. Obstet Gynecol 1988;72:181-184.
21. Platt LD, Medearis AL, DeVore GR, et al. Fetal foot length: relationship to menstrual age and fetal measurements in the second trimester. Obstet Gynecol 1988;71:526-531.
22. Chitkara U, Rosenberg J, Chervenak FA, et al. Prenatal sonographic assessment of the fetal thorax: normal values. Am J Obstet Gynecol 1987;156:1069-1074.

Sonographic Evaluation of Fetus with Skeletal Dysplasia
23. Kurtz AB, Needleman L, Wapner RJ, et al. Usefulness of a short femur in the in utero detection of skeletal dysplasias. Radiology 1990;177:197-200.
24. Goncalves L, Jeanty P. Fetal biometry of skeletal dysplasias: a multicentric study. J Ultrasound Med 1994;13:767-775.
25. Papageorghiou AT, Fratelli N, Leslie K, et al. Outcome of fetuses with antenatally diagnosed short femur [see comment]. Ultrasound Obstet Gynecol 2008;31:507-511.
26. Nelson TR, Ji EK, Lee JH, et al. Stereoscopic evaluation of fetal bony structures. J Ultrasound Med 2008;27:15-24.
27. Weisz B, David AL, Chitty L, et al. Association of isolated short femur in the mid-trimester fetus with perinatal outcome [see comment]. Ultrasound Obstet Gynecol 2008;31:512-516.
28. Zalel Y, Lehavi O, Schiff E, et al. Shortened fetal long bones: a possible in utero manifestation of placental function. Prenat Diagn 2002;22:553-557.
29. Pattarelli P, Pretorius DH, Edwards DK. Intrauterine growth retardation mimicking skeletal dysplasia on antenatal sonography. J Ultrasound Med 1990;9:737-739.
30. Ngo C, Viot G, Aubry MC, et al. First-trimester ultrasound diagnosis of skeletal dysplasia associated with increased nuchal translucency thickness. Ultrasound Obstet Gynecol 2007;30:221-226.
31. De Biasio P, Prefumo F, Lantieri PB, Venturini PL. Reference values for fetal limb biometry at 10-14 weeks of gestation. Ultrasound Obstet Gynecol 2002;19:588-591.
32. Nyberg DA, Souter VL, El-Bastawissi A, et al. Isolated sonographic markers for detection of fetal Down syndrome in the second trimester of pregnancy. J Ultrasound Med 2001;20:1053-1063.
33. Spirt BA, Oliphant M, Gottlieb RH, Gordon LP. Prenatal sonographic evaluation of short-limbed dwarfism: an algorithmic approach. Radiographics 1990;10:217-236.
34. Alanay Y, Krakow D, Rimoin DL, Lachman RS. Angulated femurs and the skeletal dysplasias: experience of the International Skeletal Dysplasia Registry (1988-2006). Am J Med Genet 2007;143A:1159-1168.
35. Rouse GA, Filly RA, Toomey F, Grube GL. Short-limb skeletal dysplasias: evaluation of the fetal spine with sonography and radiography. Radiology 1990;174:177-180.
36. Dugoff L, Coffin CT, Hobbins JC. Sonographic measurement of the fetal rib cage perimeter to thoracic circumference ratio: application to prenatal diagnosis of skeletal dysplasias. Ultrasound Obstet Gynecol 1997;10:269-271.
37. Gindes L, Benoit B, Pretorius DH, et al. Abnormal number of fetal ribs on three-dimensional ultrasonography: associated anomalies and outcomes in 75 fetuses. J Ultrasound Med 2008;27:1263-1271.
38. Quarello E, Roume J, Molho M, et al. Twins discordant for fetal skeletal abnormalities: a natural confrontation between the two siblings. Prenat Diagn 2008;28:21-27.
39. Rustico MA, Baietti MG, Coviello D, et al. Managing twins discordant for fetal anomaly. Prenat Diagn 2005;25:766-771.

40. Xu HX, Zhang QP, Lu MD, Xiao XT. Comparison of two-dimensional and three-dimensional sonography in evaluating fetal malformations. J Clin Ultrasound 2002;30:515-525.
41. Benoit B, Hafner T, Kurjak A, et al. Three-dimensional sonoembryology. J Perinat Med 2002;30:63-73.
42. Benacerraf BR. Three-dimensional fetal sonography: use and misuse. J Ultrasound Med 2002;21:1063-1067.
43. Cassart M, Massez A, Cos T, et al. Contribution of three-dimensional computed tomography in the assessment of fetal skeletal dysplasia. Ultrasound Obstet Gynecol 2007;29:537-543.
44. Ruano R, Molho M, Roume J, Ville Y. Prenatal diagnosis of fetal skeletal dysplasias by combining two-dimensional and three-dimensional ultrasound and intrauterine three-dimensional helical computer tomography. Ultrasound Obstet Gynecol 2004;24:134-140.
45. Nagayama M, Watanabe Y, Okumura A, et al. Fast MR imaging in obstetrics. Radiographics 2002;22:563-580; discussion 580-582.

Lethal Skeletal Dysplasias
46. Lemyre E, Azouz EM, Teebi AS, et al. Bone dysplasia series. Achondroplasia, hypochondroplasia and thanatophoric dysplasia: review and update. Can Assoc Radiol J 1999;50:185-197.
47. Kallen B, Knudsen LB, Mutchinick O, et al. Monitoring dominant germ cell mutations using skeletal dysplasias registered in malformation registries: an international feasibility study. Int J Epidemiol 1993;22:107-115.
48. Langer Jr LO, Yang SS, Hall JG, et al. Thanatophoric dysplasia and cloverleaf skull. Am J Med Genet Suppl 1987;3:167-179.
49. Chen CP, Chern SR, Shih JC, et al. Prenatal diagnosis and genetic analysis of type I and type II thanatophoric dysplasia. Prenat Diagn 2001;21:89-95.
50. Vajo Z, Francomano CA, Wilkin DJ. The molecular and genetic basis of fibroblast growth factor receptor 3 disorders: the achondroplasia family of skeletal dysplasias, Muenke craniosynostosis, and Crouzon syndrome with acanthosis nigricans. Endocr Rev 2000;21:23-39.
51. Tavormina PL, Shiang R, Thompson LM, et al. Thanatophoric dysplasia (types I and II) caused by distinct mutations in fibroblast growth factor receptor 3. Nat Genet 1995;9:321-328.
52. Taybi H, Lachman RS. Radiology of syndromes, metabolic disorders, and skeletal dysplasias. 3rd ed. Chicago: Year Book Medical Publishers; 1990.
53. Hall CM. International nosology and classification of constitutional disorders of bone (2001). Am J Med Genet 2002;113:65-77.
54. DiMaio MS, Barth R, Koprivnikar KE, et al. First-trimester prenatal diagnosis of osteogenesis imperfecta type II by DNA analysis and sonography. Prenat Diagn 1993;13:589-596.
55. Latini G, De Felice C, Parrini S, et al. Polyhydramnios: a predictor of severe growth impairment in achondroplasia. J Pediatr 2002;141:274-276.
56. Sillence DO, Senn A, Danks DM. Genetic heterogeneity in osteogenesis imperfecta. J Med Genet 1979;16:101-116.
57. Sillence DO, Barlow KK, Garber AP, et al. Osteogenesis imperfecta type II delineation of the phenotype with reference to genetic heterogeneity. Am J Med Genet 1984;17:407-423.
58. Barnes AM, Carter EM, Cabral WA, et al: Lack of cyclophilin B in osteogenesis imperfecta with normal collagen folding. N Engl J Med 2010;362(6):521-528.
59. Munoz C, Filly RA, Golbus MS. Osteogenesis imperfecta type II: prenatal sonographic diagnosis. Radiology 1990;174:181-185.
60. Meizner I, Bar-Ziv J. In utero diagnosis of skeletal disorders: an atlas of prenatal sonographic and postnatal radiologic correlation. Boca Raton, Fla: CRC Press; 1993.
61. Bowerman RA. Anomalies of the fetal skeleton: sonographic findings. AJR Am J Roentgenol 1995;164:973-979.
62. Kwok C, Weller PA, Guioli S, et al. Mutations in SOX9, the gene responsible for campomelic dysplasia and autosomal sex reversal. Am J Hum Genet 1995;57:1028-1036.
63. Wu MH, Kuo PL, Lin SJ. Prenatal diagnosis of recurrence of short rib–polydactyly syndrome. Am J Med Genet 1995;55:279-284.
64. Whitley CB, Langer Jr LO, Ophoven J, et al. Fibrochondrogenesis: lethal, autosomal recessive chondrodysplasia with distinctive cartilage histopathology. Am J Med Genet 1984;19:265-275.

65. Kulkarni ML, Matadh PS, Praveen Prabhu SP, Kulkarni PM. Fibrochondrogenesis. Indian J Pediatr 2005;72:355-357.

Nonlethal or Variable-Prognosis Skeletal Dysplasias

66. Patel MD, Filly RA. Homozygous achondroplasia: ultrasound distinction between homozygous, heterozygous, and unaffected fetuses in the second trimester. Radiology 1995;196:541-545.
67. Kurtz AB, Filly RA, Wapner RJ, et al. In utero analysis of heterozygous achondroplasia: variable time of onset as detected by femur length measurements. J Ultrasound Med 1986;5:137-140.
68. Hastbacka J, Superti-Furga A, Wilcox WR, et al. Atelosteogenesis type II is caused by mutations in the diastrophic dysplasia sulfate-transporter gene (DTDST): evidence for a phenotypic series involving three chondrodysplasias. Am J Hum Genet 1996;58:255-262.
69. Kaitila I, Ammala P, Karjalainen O, et al. Early prenatal detection of diastrophic dysplasia. Prenat Diagn 1983;3:237-244.
70. Chitayat D, Keating S, Zand DJ, et al. Chondrodysplasia punctata associated with maternal autoimmune diseases: expanding the spectrum from systemic lupus erythematosus (SLE) to mixed connective tissue disease (MCTD) and scleroderma report of eight cases. Am J Med Genet A 2008;146A:3038-3053.
71. Patel MS, Callahan JW, Zhang S, et al. Early-infantile galactosialidosis: prenatal presentation and postnatal follow-up. Am J Med Genet 1999;85:38-47.
72. Duff P, Harlass FE, Milligan DA. Prenatal diagnosis of chondrodysplasia punctata by sonography. Obstet Gynecol 1990;76:497-500.
73. Umranikar S, Glanc P, Unger S, et al. X-linked dominant chondrodysplasia punctata: prenatal diagnosis and autopsy findings. Prenat Diagn 2006;26:1235-1240.
74. Pryde PG, Bawle E, Brandt F, et al. Prenatal diagnosis of nonrhizomelic chondrodysplasia punctata (Conradi-Hunermann syndrome). Am J Med Genet 1993;47:426-431.
75. Winship WS, Beighton P. Dyssegmental dysplasia in a South African neonate. Clin Dysmorphol 2008;17:95-98.

Limb Reduction Defects and Associated Conditions

76. Koifman A, Nevo O, Toi A, Chitayat D. Diagnostic approach to prenatally diagnosed limb abnormalities. Ultrasound Clin 2008;3:595-608.
77. Holder-Espinasse M, Devisme L, Thomas D, et al. Pre- and postnatal diagnosis of limb anomalies: a series of 107 cases. Am J Med Genet 2004;124A:417-422.
78. Sen Gupta DK, Gupta SK. Familial bilateral proximal femoral focal deficiency: report of a kindred. J Bone Joint Surg Am 1984;66:1470-1472.
79. Sonek JD, Gabbe SG, Landon MB, et al. Antenatal diagnosis of sacral agenesis syndrome in a pregnancy complicated by diabetes mellitus. Am J Obstet Gynecol 1990;162:806-808.
80. Twickler D, Budorick N, Pretorius D, et al. Caudal regression versus sirenomelia: sonographic clues. J Ultrasound Med 1993;12:323-330.
81. Valenzano M, Paoletti R, Rossi A, et al. Sirenomelia: pathological features, antenatal ultrasonographic clues, and a review of current embryogenic theories. Hum Reprod Update 1999;5:82-86.
82. Mahony BS, Filly RA, Callen PW, Golbus MS. The amniotic band syndrome: antenatal sonographic diagnosis and potential pitfalls. Am J Obstet Gynecol 1985;152:63-68.
83. Patten RM, Van Allen M, Mack LA, et al. Limb-body wall complex: in utero sonographic diagnosis of a complicated fetal malformation. AJR Am J Roentgenol 1986;146:1019-1024.
84. Randel SB, Filly RA, Callen PW, et al. Amniotic sheets. Radiology 1988;166:633-636.
85. Van Allen MI, Curry C, Gallagher L. Limb-body wall complex. I. Pathogenesis. Am J Med Genet 1987;28:529-548.
86. Stoll C, Wiesel A, Queisser-Luft A, et al. Evaluation of the prenatal diagnosis of limb reduction deficiencies. EUROSCAN Study Group. Prenat Diagn 2000;20:811-818.
87. Auerbach AD. Fanconi anemia. Dermatol Clin 1995;13:41-49.
88. Hall JG. Thrombocytopenia and absent radius (TAR) syndrome. J Med Genet 1987;24:79-83.
89. Ohlsson A, Fong KW, Rose TH, Moore DC. Prenatal sonographic diagnosis of Pena-Shokeir syndrome type I, or fetal akinesia deformation sequence. Am J Med Genet 1988;29:59-65.
90. Hall JG, Reed SD, Rosenbaum KN, et al. Limb pterygium syndromes: a review and report of eleven patients. Am J Med Genet 1982;12:377-409.
91. Souka AP, Krampl E, Geerts L, Nicolaides KH. Congenital lymphedema presenting with increased nuchal translucency at 13 weeks of gestation. Prenat Diagn 2002;22:91-92.

Hand and Foot Deformities

92. Bronshtein M, Stahl S, Zimmer EZ. Transvaginal sonographic diagnosis of fetal finger abnormalities in early gestation. J Ultrasound Med 1995;14:591-595.
93. Benacerraf BR, Osathanondh R, Frigoletto FD. Sonographic demonstration of hypoplasia of the middle phalanx of the fifth digit: a finding associated with Down syndrome. Am J Obstet Gynecol 1988;159:181-183.
94. Hegge FN, Prescott GH, Watson PT. Utility of a screening examination of the fetal extremities during obstetrical sonography. J Ultrasound Med 1986;5:639-645.
95. Jeanty P, Romero R, d'Alton M, et al. In utero sonographic detection of hand and foot deformities. J Ultrasound Med 1985;4:595-601.
96. Anneren G, Andersson T, Lindgren PG, Kjartansson S. Ectrodactyly–ectodermal dysplasia–clefting syndrome (EEC): the clinical variation and prenatal diagnosis. Clin Genet 1991;40:257-262.
97. Ianakiev P, Kilpatrick MW, Toudjarska I, et al. Split-hand/split-foot malformation is caused by mutations in the p63 gene on 3q27. Am J Hum Genet 2000;67:59-66.
98. Chesney D. Clinical outcome of congenital talipes equinovarus diagnosed antenatally by ultrasound. J Bone Joint Surg 2001;83B:462-463.
99. Tillett RL, Fisk NM, Murphy K, Hunt DM. Clinical outcome of congenital talipes equinovarus diagnosed antenatally by ultrasound. J Bone Joint Surg 2000;82B:876-880.
100. Keret D, Bollini G, Dungl P, et al. The fibula in congenital pseudoarthrosis of the tibia: the EPOS multicenter study. European Paediatric Orthopaedic Society. J Pediatr Orthop 2000;9B:69-74.
101. Treadwell MC, Stanitski CL, King M. Prenatal sonographic diagnosis of clubfoot: implications for patient counseling. J Pediatr Orthop 1999;19:8-10.
102. Bakalis S, Sairam S, Homfray T, et al. Outcome of antenatally diagnosed talipes equinovarus in an unselected obstetric population. Ultrasound Obstet Gynecol 2002;20:226-229.
103. Maffulli N. Prenatal ultrasonographic diagnosis of talipes equinovarus: does it give the full picture? Ultrasound Obstet Gynecol 2002;20:217-218.
104. Farrell SA, Summers AM, Dallaire L, et al. Club foot, an adverse outcome of early amniocentesis: disruption or deformation? Canadian Early and Mid-Trimester Amniocentesis Trial (CEMAT). J Med Genet 1999;36:843-846.
105. Canto MJ, Cano S, Palau J, Ojeda F. Prenatal diagnosis of clubfoot in low-risk population: associated anomalies and long-term outcome. Prenat Diagn 2008;28:343-346.

Skeletal Findings Associated with Aneuploidy

106. Avni EF, Rypens F, Zappa M, et al. Antenatal diagnosis of short-limb dwarfism: sonographic approach. Pediatr Radiol 1996;26:171-178.
107. Snijders RJM, Nicolaides KH. Ultrasound markers for fetal chromosomal defects. New York: Parthenon; 1996.
108. Benacerraf BR, Frigoletto Jr FD, Greene MF. Abnormal facial features and extremities in human trisomy syndromes: prenatal ultrasound appearance. Radiology 1986;159:243-246.

Fetal Hydrops

Deborah Levine

Chapter Outline

*H*ydrops fetalis is an end-stage process for a number of different diseases. It is defined as an abnormal accumulation of interstitial fluid in at least two body cavities (pleural, peritoneal, or pericardial) or one body cavity in association with anasarca (generalized massive edema). Placentomegaly and polyhydramnios are common findings in cases of hydrops but are not needed for the diagnosis.

Hydrops is the late stage of many processes that lead to redistribution of body fluids among the intravascular and interstitial compartments. This imbalance of fluid can have many etiologies (see Table 41-1). There are at least 80 different known causes of fetal hydrops.[1] Many of the causes and associations with hydrops overlap. The basic etiology of hydrops is an imbalance of interstitial fluid, which may be caused by myocardial failure, high-output cardiac failure, decreased colloid oncotic plasma pressure (anemia), increased capillary permeability, and/or obstruction of venous and lymphatic flow.

Hydrops can be **immune** or **nonimmune** in origin. Immune hydrops is defined by a circulating antibody against red blood cells (RBCs) in the mother, whereas in nonimmune hydrops no such antibody is found. Before the widespread introduction of rhesus (Rh) anti-D immune globulin in the 1970s, most cases of hydrops were immune,[2,3] whereas currently, most are nonimmune.[4,5] This chapter reviews the findings of fluid in different body cavities and the etiologies, diagnosis, and treatment of hydrops. The mortality of fetal hydrops generally remains higher than 70%. However, fetal medical and interventional techniques allow for reversal of hydrops (in nonaneuploid cases) and improved survival.[6] Although hydrops is a relatively common indication for tertiary-level fetal evaluation, because of the many causes, each specific etiology is relatively rare.

SONOGRAPHIC FEATURES

It is important to understand the sonographic appearance of fluid in the different interstitial compartments of the fetus. These fluid collections can occur in isolation, as in isolated **ascites** or isolated **pleural** or **pericardial** effusion. When one collection is seen, it is important to assess for a second collection to make the diagnosis of hydrops; the fluid collection must be in at least two body cavities to qualify as hydrops. Other findings in hydrops can include **subcutaneous edema, polyhydramnios,** and **placentomegaly.**

Ascites

Fetal ascites is diagnosed when fluid is seen between **bowel loops,** along the abdominal flanks, around the

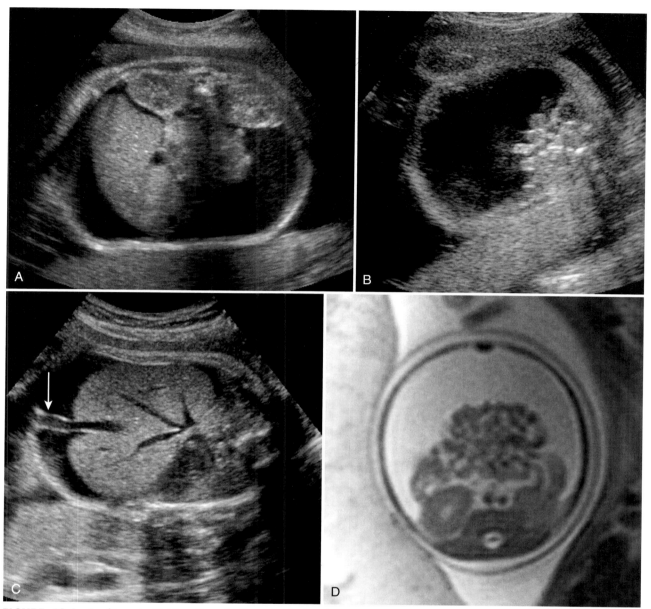

FIGURE 41-1. Ascites. A, Fluid outlines the liver. **B,** Fluid outlines the bowel, compressing it posteriorly. **C,** Ascites outlines the umbilical vein *(arrow)*. **D,** T2-weighted MR image shows the high-signal-intensity fluid in the fetal abdomen.

liver, and outlining the umbilical vessels (Fig. 41-1). In normal fetuses, a small hypoechoic band (<2 mm in thickness) extending along the anterior and lateral fetal abdomen may be present. This "pseudoascites" represents normal abdominal wall muscles or abdominal wall fat, and should not be mistaken for an abnormal fluid collection[7] (Fig. 41-2). The distinction between the pseudoascites appearance and true ascites can be made when the transducer angle is changed and the appearance resolves. Pseudoascites does not surround the liver, but rather stops at the insertion of the ribs. Note that true ascites will extend around bowel loops (Fig. 41-3; **Video 41-1**), whereas pseudoascites is always a subcutaneous finding.

Isolated ascites can be an early sign of hydrops. If truly isolated, it can be caused by an obstructive urinary etiology or gastrointestinal (GI) obstruction. Isolated fetal ascites has a more favorable prognosis than hydrops but requires follow-up to ensure that hydrops does not ensue.

Small collections of ascitic fluid may outline abdominal viscera, including bowel loops or bladder, and may cause an apparent increase in their echogenicity. Larger accumulations outline the liver and spleen (Fig. 41-1, *A* and *B*). The umbilical vessels will be seen as parallel echogenic lines traversing the fluid space (Fig. 41-1, *D*). Bowel loops may be free floating or, when meconium peritonitis is present, may appear as a matted, echogenic posterior mass. In male fetuses, ascitic fluid may track

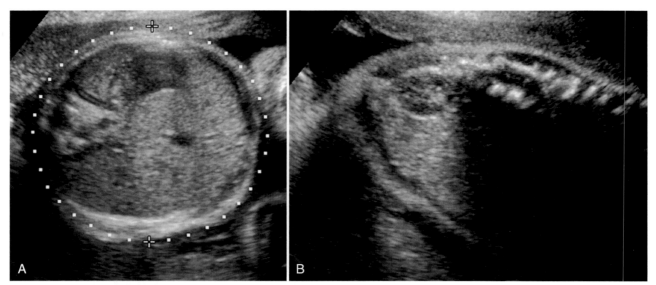

FIGURE 41-2. Pseudoascites. A, Transverse, and **B,** parasagittal, ultrasound views show hypoechoic abdominal musculature and fat mimicking ascites. Note that this appearance will change with transducer angle, and the hypoechoic material will always be visualized in the subcutaneous regions, not surrounding bowel.

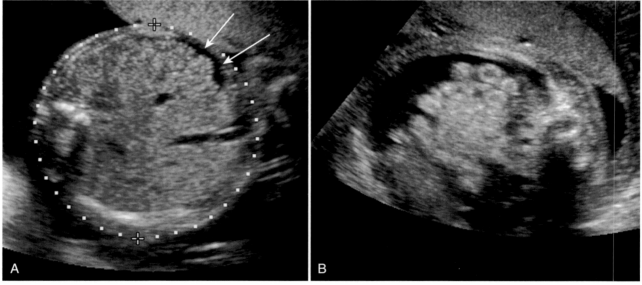

FIGURE 41-3. Ascites. A, Small amount of ascites *(arrows).* **B,** Moderate amount of ascites. Note how the ascites surrounds loops of bowel. The bowel can appear echogenic because of through-transmission from the fluid.

through the patent processus vaginalis into the scrotum, leading to **hydroceles** (Fig. 41-4). Chronic chest compression from massive ascites may result in pulmonary hypoplasia (Fig. 41-5).

Pleural Effusions

Pleural effusions typically occur later in hydrops than does ascites (Fig. 41-6). If isolated and small, pleural effusions tend to have a benign course (Fig. 41-6, *A;* **Video 41-2**). Small effusions are seen as a thin, echolucent rim surrounding lung tissue and may also outline

mediastinal structures. Small pleural effusions do not shift the mediastinum. Pleural effusions associated with hydrops may be **unilateral** or **bilateral**, often beginning as unilateral collections that progress bilaterally (Fig. 41-6, *D*). If mediastinal shift is visualized in association with a small pleural effusion, a chest mass such as a hernia or congenital pulmonary malformation should be sought (Fig. 41-7). Larger effusions will lead to flattening of the hemidiaphragms and, when sufficiently large, mediastinal shift. A large, unilateral effusion suggests a local cause, such as **chylothorax.** Although chylothorax begins as a unilateral effusion, it can progress to cause

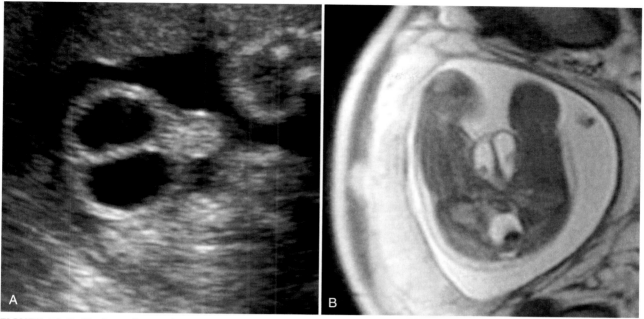

FIGURE 41-4. Hydrocele. A, Ultrasound, and **B,** MRI, appearances of male fetus with hydrops with fluid extending into the scrotum.

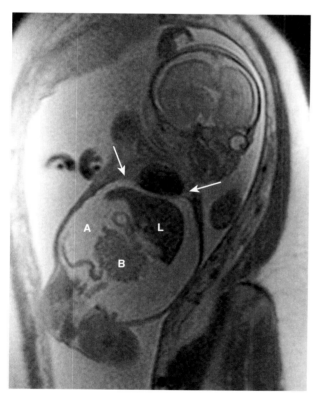

FIGURE 41-5. Massive ascites leading to lung compression. Coronal T2-weighted MR image shows massive ascites *(A)* surrounding the liver *(L)* and bowel *(B)*. Note the compression of the fetal lungs *(arrows).*

mediastinal shift, obstructing venous return and leading to hydrops. In large, bilateral pleural effusions the lungs appear as free-floating "bat wings" beside the heart (Fig. 41-6, *D*). When chronic, large effusions can lead to pulmonary hypoplasia. As pleural effusions enlarge,

compression or kinking of mediastinal vascular structures causes upper body edema and functional esophageal obstruction, leading to secondary polyhydramnios.

Chylothorax is the most common cause of pleural effusion leading to respiratory distress in the newborn. This is an important diagnosis to suggest when associated with hydrops because drainage can be curative. Drainage of the effusion can lead to reversal of hydrops and can prevent pulmonary hypoplasia. Drainage immediately before delivery can assist in peripartum care. When drained, the fluid has a large number of lymphocytes in clear, yellow fluid. The fluid will not be "milky" until after the infant feeds.

Pericardial Effusions

In contrast to pleural effusions that surround the lungs and compress the tissue medially, pericardial effusions are anteromedial fluid collections. Fluid collections of up to 2 mm in thickness are common, and a small amount of pericardial fluid (up to 7 mm, in isolation) can be a normal finding[8] (Fig. 41-8; **Video 41-3**). A large pericardial effusion compresses the lungs against the posterior chest wall (Fig. 41-9). The heart is visualized as "floating" within the anterior thoracic fluid collection.

Subcutaneous Edema

Subcutaneous edema may be localized or generalized, depending on the etiology. A thickness of 5 mm has been suggested as the cutoff value.[9] Edema is most easily seen over the fetal scalp or face, where thickening of skin overlying bone is visualized (Fig. 41-10, *A*). It is important to realize that the **biparietal diameter** and **head**

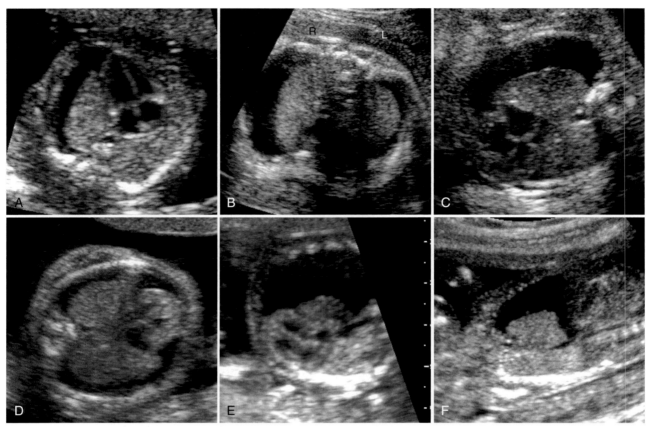

FIGURE 41-6. Fetal pleural effusions. A, Unilateral small right pleural effusions. **B,** Moderate right *(R)* and small left *(L)* effusions. **C,** Moderate right effusion. Note moderate mediastinal shift to the left. **D,** Bilateral moderate effusions. Note how the partially compressed lungs appear as free-floating "bat wings." **E,** Axial, and **F,** oblique, coronal views of large right pleural effusion. Note the severe mediastinal shift in **E.**

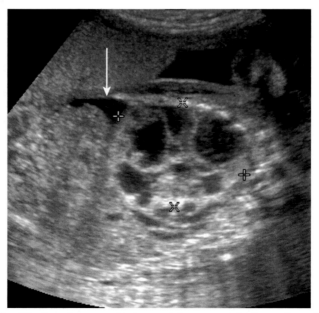

FIGURE 41-7. Small pleural effusion in association with congenital cystic adenomatoid malformation. Note the large cystic mass *(calipers)* and small pleural effusion *(arrow).*

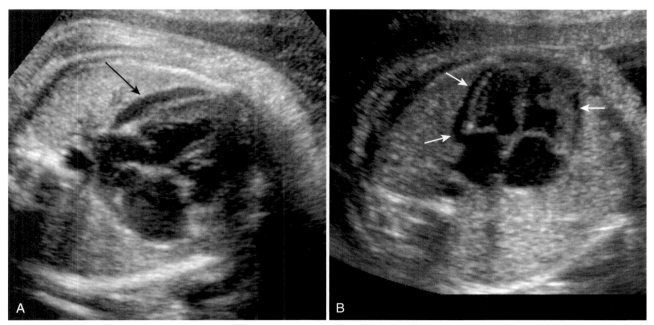

FIGURE 41-8. Normal finding of small amount of pericardial fluid. A and **B,** Note the small rim of anechoic fluid *(arrows)* in two different fetuses.

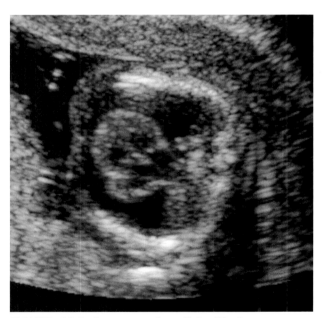

FIGURE 41-9. Large pericardial effusion. Lungs are compressed posteriorly.

circumference measurements are taken around the skull bone, excluding the skin. Subcutaneous edema may also be seen over the limbs and abdominal wall. Care should be taken not to mistake prominent fat in a macrosomic fetus to anasarca in a hydropic fetus. Subcutaneous edema will increase the abdominal circumference measurement, beyond that which is expected for gestational age (Fig. 41-10, *B*). It is important when measuring the fetus to include the entirety of the skin in the abdominal circumference measurement, because this

affects the weight calculation of the fetus. Thus, when performing biometric assessment of the hydropic fetus, the abdominal circumference measurement is included in the weight calculation, but it should be excluded from the gestational age assessment so that the thickened skin does not falsely elevate fetal age. When generalized subcutaneous edema is present, the appearances may be referred to as anasarca (Fig. 41-11, **Video 41-4**). Note that on fetal magnetic resonance imaging (MRI), body wall edema will appear of high signal intensity on T2-weighted images, similar to surrounding fluid (Fig. 41-12).

Placentomegaly

Placental edema is a variable and usually late sign in hydrops (Fig. 41-13). The sonographic texture of the placenta may be altered, and its appearance may be described as **thickened**, **echogenic, spongy,** or **ground glass.** Placental dimensions, especially thickness, are increased above the normal of 5 cm in the third trimester.[9-11] When placental edema is secondary to an hydropic process in the fetus, the entire placenta is usually affected. This finding may be used to exclude the very rare primary placental causes of hydrops (e.g., chorioangioma).

Polyhydramnios

The assessment of amniotic fluid is described in Chapter 46. Polyhydramnios occurs frequently in conjunction with hydrops (Fig. 41-14; see Video 41-1). This increases the risk of prematurity, which adds to the morbidity associated with hydrops.

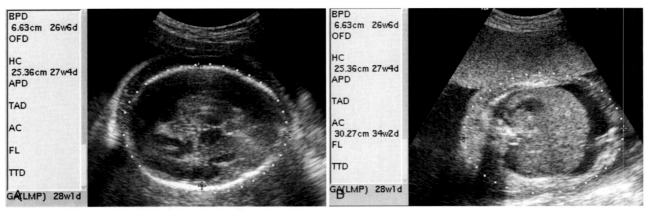

FIGURE 41-10. Scalp and body wall edema are measured differently. A, Fetal scalp edema. Head measurements *(cursors)* are obtained around the bone, not the skin; *BPD,* biparietal diameter; *HC,* head circumference. **B, Abdominal wall thickening.** Abdominal wall measurements are obtained around the abdomen, including the skin thickening; *AC,* abdominal circumference. Note that gestational age is 27 weeks by HC, but 34 weeks if only AC is used.

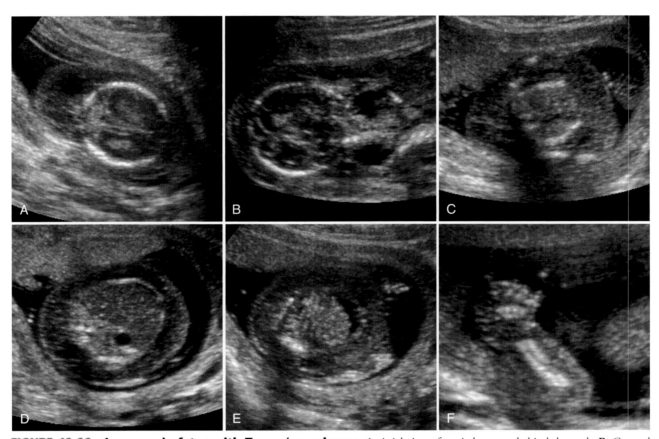

FIGURE 41-11. Anasarca in fetus with Turner's syndrome. A, Axial view of cystic hygroma behind the neck. **B,** Coronal view of diffuse scalp edema and cystic hygroma. **C,** Axial view of thoracic wall edema. **D** and **E,** Axial views of abdomen show body wall edema and ascites. **F,** Arm with anasarca as well.

ETIOLOGY

Before the availability of $Rh_0(D)$ immune globulin (RhoGAM), immune hydrops represented greater than 80% of all cases of hydrops. Now, **nonimmune hydrops** represents 90% of cases. The **distribution, timing,** and **size** of fluid collections and edema as detected by ultrasound may provide a clue to the etiology of hydrops. For example, in **immune hydrops,** ascites appears first, with subcutaneous edema appearing only with more advanced anemia. Intrathoracic collections generally do not occur or occur late in the process.

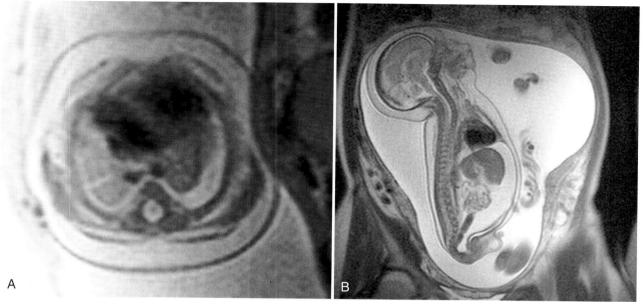

FIGURE 41-12. Fetal body wall edema on MRI. A and **B,** Axial and sagittal T2-weighted MR images show how edema appears as high signal in the skin.

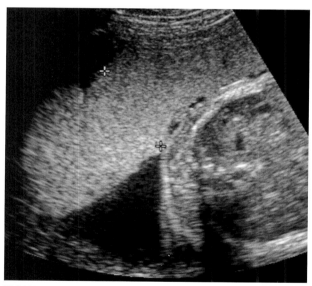

FIGURE 41-13. Placental edema. Placental thickness is normally about 1 mm of thickness per week gestational age, and it should not exceed 5 cm in the third trimester.

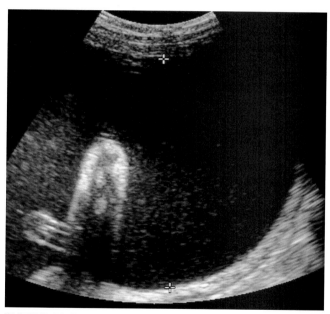

FIGURE 41-14. Polyhydramnios. A 12-cm pocket of fluid *(cursors)* in pregnancy with hydrops.

Generally, pleural and pericardial effusions appear earlier and more prominently with thoracic pathologies, whereas ascites appears earlier and predominates with anemia and primary abdominal pathologies. Massive ascites with associated bowel hyperechogenicity is typical of either **parvovirus** infection (when the ascites is very tense) or a bowel perforation that may be secondary to **meconium peritonitis** (Fig. 41-15). Localized fluid collections may progress to hydrops because of pressure or metabolic effects, and thus the pattern of hydrops may evolve over time.

IMMUNE HYDROPS

Immune hydrops, or **erythroblastosis fetalis,** occurs when a sensitized mother develops antibodies to fetal RBCs that lead to hemolysis. Circulating maternal immunoglobulin G (IgG) antibodies cross the placenta and attack antigen-positive fetal RBCs. The majority of cases still occur in the presence of Rh(D) antibodies. Atypical antibodies such as Kell, Rh(C), and Rh(E) develop in 1% to 2% of individuals after blood

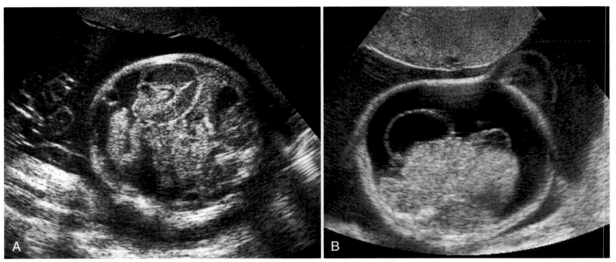

FIGURE 41-15. Meconium peritonitis. A, Matted and dilated echogenic bowel with ascites, typical of meconium peritonitis. **B,** Tense ascites in meconium peritonitis.

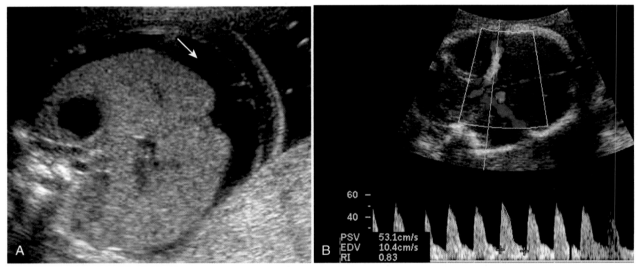

FIGURE 41-16. Immune hydrops. A, Ascites *(arrow).* **B,** Middle cerebral artery measuring peak systolic velocity *(PSV); EDV,* end diastolic velocity; *RI,* resistive index.

transfusion and cause 2% of hemolytic disease of the fetus. The result is anemia, extramedullary erythropoiesis, hepatosplenomegaly, hypoalbuminemia, and congestive heart failure (CHF). Hydrops develops when the **fetal hemoglobin** (HbF) **deficit** exceeds 7 g/dL,[12] probably because of reduced oncotic pressure secondary to hypoalbuminemia, combined with high-output cardiac failure (Fig. 41-16). Eventually, the fetus develops both metabolic and lactic acidosis,[13,14] and once this decompensation occurs, progression of hydrops is rapid, leading to fetal demise within 24 to 48 hours.

Causes of maternal sensitivity include fetal maternal hemorrhage and transplacental hemorrhage. In women with incompatible blood types with respect to the fetus (Rh alloimmunization, other RBC antigen), antibodies can be made. This typically occurs after delivery of the first pregnancy and therefore will affect the second pregnancy. Other times of blood sharing include abortion (spontaneous or therapeutic), amniocentesis, placental abruption, incompatible blood transfusions, and transplacental hemorrhage. An additional blood incompatibility issue is fetal alloimmune thrombocytopenia.

To avoid maternal sensitization, 300 mg of RhoGAM is given at 28 weeks' gestation in sensitized individuals. This protects against 30 mL of fetal blood. If a greater degree of fetomaternal hemorrhage is suspected, a Kleihauer-Betke test can be done to quantify fetal blood in maternal circulation to determine the necessary dose. As a prophylactic measure, RhoGAM is given to Rh-negative women within 48 hours after invasive fetal procedures such as amniocentesis and chorionic villus sampling.

Management of the Fetus

Immune hydrops is an indication for urgent **fetal blood sampling** and transfusion. This technique is performed by **percutaneous ultrasound-guided blood sampling** (PUBS)[15] (see Chapter 46). In a study of 80 fetuses with hydrops secondary to anemia, when hydrops was mild before treatment (only a thin rim of ascites, with or without pericardial effusion), hydrops was reversed in 88%; when hydrops was severe before treatment, hydrops reversed in only 65%. This stresses the importance of early treatment in cases of suspected anemia. After reversal of hydrops, survival rate was 98%.[16] The incremental loss rate after this procedure is about 1.4%.[17]

Noninvasive Assessment of Alloimmunization

Fetuses are screened for risk of alloimmunization by determining the Rh status of the parents. If the pregnant woman is Rh negative, the father is screened. If the father of the baby is also Rh negative, no further screening is needed. If the mother is Rh negative and the father is Rh positive, maternal antibody titers are monitored. If they rise above 1:8, further testing is warranted. In the past, this was done with amniocentesis assessing for optical density (OD_{50}) of amniotic fluid (hemolysis increases OD of amniotic fluid), and serial PUBS was performed as indicated to determine **hematocrit** (Hct). Currently, Hct is indirectly inferred from **middle cerebral artery** (MCA) Doppler studies, in which **peak systolic velocity** (PSV) is elevated in cases of anemia (**Video 41-5;** see Chapter 43).

In response to severe anemia, the **fetal circulation becomes hyperdynamic** with increased blood flow velocities, which are thought to result from increased cardiac output and decreased viscosity of fetal blood. In addition, blood flow in the MCA may be increased further because the brain circulation is known to respond quickly to hypoxemia.[18] Although flow velocities in all fetal vessels will be increased, the MCA is particularly suitable for assessment because of its easy visualization with color Doppler imaging as it courses directly above the greater wing of the sphenoid bone, carrying more than 80% of cerebral blood flow. The MCA has a high-impedance circulation with continuous forward flow. The method for MCA Doppler includes finding the circle of Willis, measuring a pulsed Doppler waveform of the proximal MCA at the base of the brain, and obtaining a PSV measurement with the angle of insonation close to 0 degrees (Fig. 41-16, *B*). Intraobserver and interobserver variability is low.

In hypoxia, there is central redistribution of blood flow with increased blood flow to the brain. This leads to elevated PSV in cases of anemia. PSV is compared to normed measures with respect to gestational age. Using these thresholds, Zimmerman et al.[19] found that overall sensitivity to detect moderate to severe anemia at less than 35 weeks (hemoglobin <0.65 multiples of median) was 88%. Specificity was 87%; positive predictive value (PPV) was 53%, and negative predictive value (NPV) was 98%.

It should be recognized that immune hydrops, even untreated, is not uniformly lethal, and that transfusion is not uniformly lifesaving. If fetuses with anemia and hydrops are untreated, 34% of hydrops cases resolve spontaneously, and 30% of fetuses die in utero. However, if anemia is treated with intrauterine infusions, 53% of hydrops cases resolve and 17.5% of fetuses die in utero.

When performing PUBS, it is important to check that the mean corpuscular volume (MCV) is greater than 100 μm^3 to prove that it is fetal blood being tested. The hematocrit is checked to determine the amount of transfusion needed (Hct <30% is 2.5th centile >20 weeks). To limit the amount of fluid being transfused into the relatively small circulatory capacity of the fetus, packed RBCs (type O negative; Hct >90%) are given. The goal is to transfuse to Hct of 40 mL/dL. Successful treatment of anemia with intravascular blood transfusion has been reported as early as 13 weeks' gestation.[20]

A variable sign of anemia in the fetus is that of **hepatosplenomegaly.** The fetal liver and spleen increase in size because of their increased production of RBCs. However, the fetus may be able to compensate for the breakdown of RBCs and, in such cases, may have a large liver and spleen, but would not necessarily be severely anemic. Conversely, more rapid breakdown of RBCs may prevent the fetus from adapting to hemolysis. Therefore, anemia may develop without hepatosplenomegaly.[21,22]

NONIMMUNE HYDROPS

Nonimmune hydrops occurs in 1:1500 to 1:4000 pregnancies. It is a common pathologic finding in first- and second-trimester spontaneous abortions. The etiology varies geographically and with gestational age. In North America and Europe, most cases are cardiovascular (20%-40%), infective (5%-10%), or chromosomal (16%; usually Turner's syndrome; trisomy 13, 18, and 21; triploidy) in origin.[23,24] In Southeast Asia, however, homozygous **α-thalassemia** is a common cause;[25] in this region, carrier status for α-thalassemia occurs in 5% to 15% of the population. Nonimmune hydrops in homozygous α-thalassemia accounts for 25% of perinatal deaths in Southeast Asia.

Pathophysiology

Nonimmune hydrops represents the terminal stage for many conditions and is frequently multifactorial (Table 41-1). Pathophysiology of hydrops may involve increased hydrostatic pressure, high-output cardiac failure, decreased plasma oncotic pressure, increased capillary permeability, obstruction of lymph flow, or a

TABLE 41-1. NONIMMUNE HYDROPS: COMMON CAUSES AND ASSOCIATIONS

	EXAMPLES	SUBCATEGORY EXAMPLES
Cardiovascular	Structural heart disease	Hypoplastic left or right heart syndrome Atrioventricular canal Atrioventricular septal defect Transposition of great vessels Tetralogy of Fallot Ebstein anomaly
	Myocarditis/cardiomyopathy	
	Valvular disease	
	Myocardial or pericardial tumors	Tuberous sclerosis (e.g., rhabdomyoma)
	Premature closure of foramen ovale or ductus arteriosus	
	Twin-twin transfusion syndrome	
	Arrhythmia	Tachyarrhythmia Bradyarrhythmia (including heart block)
	High-output cardiac failure	Tumors such as maternal chorioangioma or fetal sacrococcygeal teratoma Vein of Galen malformation Acardiac twin (donor)
	Generalized arterial calcification	
	Myocardial infarction	Anomalous left coronary artery
Lymphatics	Abnormal lymphatic drainage	
Neck	Cystic hygroma	
	Congenital high airway obstruction	
Chest	Chylothorax/hydrothorax	
	Congenital cystic adenomatoid malformation	
	Congenital diaphragmatic hernia	
	Pulmonary sequestration	
	Bronchogenic cyst	
	Congenital lymphedema	
Gastrointestinal	Hepatic cirrhosis/fibrosis	
	Hepatitis	
	Tumor	
	Portal vein thrombosis	
	Bowel atresia	
	Volvulus	Malrotation with midgut volvulus
	Meconium peritonitis	
Urinary tract	Finnish nephrosis	
	Urinary tract obstruction	
	Prune belly syndrome	
	Cloacal malformation	
	Renal vein thrombosis	
Chromosomal	45,XO (Turner's syndrome)	
	Trisomy 21	
	Trisomy 18	
	Trisomy 13	
	Other aneuploidies	
Hematologic	α-Thalassemia (homozygous)	
	Parvovirus	
	G6PD deficiency	
	Twin-twin transfusion (donor)	
	Congenital leukemia	
	Hemochromatosis	
	Inferior vena cava thrombosis	
Infection	Cytomegalovirus	
	Parvovirus	
	Toxoplasmosis	
	Syphilis	
	Coxsackievirus	
	Adenovirus	
	Herpes simplex virus	
	Varicella	
Monochorionic twins	Twin-twin transfusion syndrome (donor or recipient)	
	Acardiac twin (donor)	

TABLE 41-1. NONIMMUNE HYDROPS: COMMON CAUSES AND ASSOCIATIONS—cont'd

	EXAMPLES	SUBCATEGORY EXAMPLES
Genetic	Metabolic disorders	Gaucher disease
		GM1 gangliosidosis
		Sialidosis
		Niemann-Pick disease types A and C
		Mucopolysaccharidosis
		Carnitine deficiency
		Pyruvate kinase deficiency
		Glucose phosphate isomerase deficiency
Skeletal dysplasias	Achondroplasia	
	Achondrogenesis	
	Osteogenesis imperfecta	
	Osteochondrodystrophy	
	Osteochondrodysplasia	
	Hypophosphatasia	
	Thanatophoric dysplasia	
	Asphyxiating thoracic dystrophy	
	Short-rib polydactyly syndrome	
Fetal hypokinesis	Arthrogryposis	
	Congenital myotonic dystrophy	
	Neu-Laxova syndrome	
	Pena-Shokeir syndrome	
Other syndromes	Noonan syndrome	
	Cornelia de Lange syndrome	
	Orofaciodigital syndrome	
	Idiopathic recurrent hydrops	
Tumors	Wilms' tumor	
	Sacrococcygeal teratoma	
	Nephroblastoma	
	Neuroblastoma	
	Teratoma	
	Tuberous sclerosis	
	Arteriovenous malformation	
Maternal	Severe diabetes mellitus	
	Severe anemia	
	Severe hypoproteinemia	
	Indomethacin use (premature closure of ductus arteriosus)	
Placental/cord	Placental or umbilical vein thrombosis	
	Cord torsion, knot, or tumor	
	Umbilical artery aneurysm	
	Angiomyxoma of umbilical cord	
	Hemorrhagic endovasculitis of placenta	
	Chorioangioma	

combination of these factors (Fig. 41-17). Fluid collections result from redistribution of fetal body fluids among the intravascular, intracellular, and interstitial compartments, secondary to an imbalance in capillary ultrafiltration and interstitial fluid return.[26] Hypoxia and circulatory failure may result in capillary damage that leads to plasma protein and fluid loss from the intravascular compartment.

Several factors predispose to edema in the fetus versus after birth. Both total body and extracellular fluid compartments are proportionately greater in the fetus, particularly at earlier gestational ages. Colloid osmotic pressure is lower because of lower albumin concentrations. High compliance of the interstitial space facilitates the accumulation of large volumes of fluid. Many causes of fetal hydrops, especially those with a cardiac component, result from an increase in systemic venous pressure, to which the fetus is particularly sensitive. In the fetus,

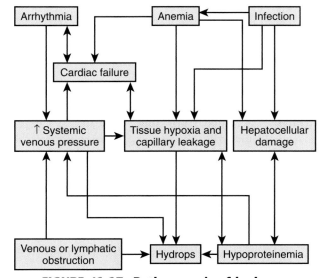

FIGURE 41-17. Pathogenesis of hydrops.

there is a net movement of fluid from the intravascular to the extravascular space. Fivefold larger volumes of fluid are removed by the lymphatics in fetal models than in adult animal models. Thus, small elevations in systemic venous pressure (2-3 mm Hg) in the fetus can substantially reduce lymphatic flow and can drive large amounts of fluid into the extracellular space. This process is further enhanced by the relatively greater permeability of fetal capillaries to protein. The fetus is therefore particularly susceptible to small elevations in venous pressure from a number of causes, all of which can result in hydrops.[12,13,24]

Causes and Associations

Nonimmune hydrops is most commonly of a **fetal** etiology, but also may be caused by maternal or placental factors (Table 41-1). **Maternal** causes (such as poorly controlled diabetes mellitus) are rare and should be differentiated from maternal complications, which are secondary to fetal hydrops (termed **mirror syndrome** because edema develops in the mother of an hydropic fetus, "mirroring" the condition in the fetus).[27,28] Maternal thyrotoxicosis can cause fetal hyperthyroidism and fetal hydrops, with potential for resolution of hydrops after treatment with antithyroid drugs.[29] **Placental** causes, such as **chorioangioma** and other vascular shunts, are relatively rare and are usually associated with high-output failure states and, in some cases, fetal anemia.[30,31] Fetal metabolic causes are rare but important, because diagnosis can lead to appropriate neonatal treatment and appropriate counseling of the patients regarding recurrence risks.

A classification scheme for fetal causes is shown in Table 41-1 and has some overlap in the groupings, some of which may represent associations rather than causations.

Cardiovascular Abnormalities

Cardiovascular abnormalities are the etiology of hydrops in up to 40% of cases.[25,32] Hydrops is a rare complication of *isolated* cardiac abnormality because the fetus has a parallel flow circulation. In chromosomal abnormalities, however, other factors with or without cardiac abnormality lead to hydrops.
Structural Cardiac Anomalies. In hydrops, cardiac structural abnormalities may be causative or may be found as associations[33] (Fig. 41-18). Right-sided lesions, whether obstructive, such as **pulmonary or tricuspid atresia,** or structural lesions that result in right atrial volume or pressure overload, such as **mitral regurgitation,** can result in congestive heart failure and hydrops.[34,35] Left-sided obstructive lesions, such as **aortic stenosis, mitral stenosis,** and **coarctation of the aorta,** can result in a hypoplastic left heart, causing increased blood flow through the fetal right ventricle, which may result in

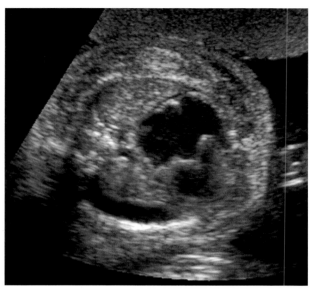

FIGURE 41-18. Hydrops secondary to structural cardiac abnormality. Note the enlarged abnormal heart, pleural effusions, and skin thickening.

hydrops.[36] The presence of hydrops with congenital structural heart disease carries a poor prognosis, with survival as low as 17% for those with tricuspid disease and hydrops.[37] Some fetuses with structural cardiac anomalies also have rhythm disturbances, which contribute to the poor prognosis. In one series of 301 fetuses with atrioventricular (A-V) septal defects, the presence of fetal hydrops, together with **bradycardia** from sinus node dysfunction or **complete heart block,** was associated with a poor outcome.[38]
Cardiac Tumors. Cardiac tumors are a rare cause of fetal hydrops.[39-44] Hydrops may be caused by several mechanisms, depending on the tumor location, size, and number. Cardiac lesions may cause obstruction to blood flow and alteration of A-V valve function and may lead to arrhythmia, cardiac tamponade, pericardial effusion, and hydrops.[41-43]

Rhabdomyomas are the most common fetal cardiac tumor and are seen in association with tuberous sclerosis in more than 80% of cases.[44] Rhabdomyomas are also the most common cardiac tumors to cause hydrops. Usually, these tumors are multiple, well circumscribed, hyperechoic, and homogeneous and mainly involve the ventricular myocardium[42] (Fig. 41-19). Rhabdomyomas tend to grow during the second half of pregnancy,[45] so most are diagnosed during the second and third trimesters. The location, size, and number of lesions correspond to risk for hydrops. Rhabdomyomas may cause hydrops as a result of impaired diastolic filling, altered A-V valve function, or outflow obstruction.

Intrapericardial teratomas are rare, usually appearing as cystic and solid masses outside the cardiac cavities, arising from the pericardium. Teratomas may be larger than the heart, and rapid growth of the tumor within the small, confined space can result in pericardial effusion and hydrops as a result of cardiac compression[46,47] (Fig. 41-20). Drainage of pericardial fluid associated with an intrapericardial teratoma has been reported, with resolution of associated hydrops.[48,49] Frequently, more than one drainage procedure is necessary.[50] At times, a shunt is placed if fluid rapidly reaccumulates after

drainage.[51] Drainage of pericardial effusion secondary to intrapericardial teratoma usually results in a live birth after 32 weeks' gestational age.

Arrhythmias. Arrhythmias associated with hydrops are most often **tachyarrhythmias** (≧200 beats/min) and less frequently bradyarrhythmias. The diagnosis is important because treatment can reverse the hydrops. It is important to avoid premature delivery; treatment of a hydropic preterm fetus is difficult. Fetal tachyarrhythmias are most often **supraventricular tachycardia** (SVT, which includes **atrial fibrillation/flutter**)[52] (Fig. 41-21). The prognosis for a fetus with an isolated arrhythmia is favorable, with a 95% likelihood of survival.[53] However, when hydrops is present (41% in this series) with an otherwise isolated arrhythmia, the survival decreases to 73%.[52] When studying neonates with fetal SVT, most cases are the result of reentry circuits.[54] If the SVT is of limited duration, there are typically no fetal consequences. However, with sustained SVT, hydrops may develop. The presence of hydrops in these cases is associated with more difficult prenatal antiarrhythmic control of the tachycardia and higher mortality. Prenatal control of the tachycardia was achieved in 83% of treated nonhydropic fetuses, compared with 66% of the treated hydropic fetuses.[52]

Tachyarrhythmia treatment is almost always given transplacentally; the pregnant woman is given the drug, which crosses the placenta and enters the fetal circulation. Rarely is direct fetal administration required.[25] Maternal digoxin is the mainstay of treatment,[55-57] and

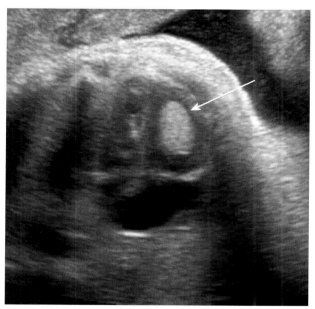

FIGURE 41-19. Cardiac rhabdomyoma. Note the echogenic lesion *(arrow)* adjacent to the myocardium.

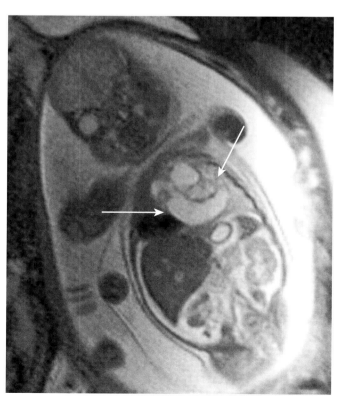

FIGURE 41-20. Mediastinal teratoma. T2-weighted MR image shows heterogeneous mediastinal mass *(arrows)* and ascites in the abdomen.

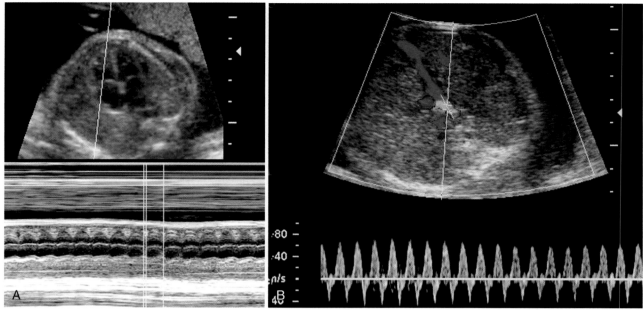

FIGURE 41-21. Supraventricular tachycardia (SVT). A, Atrial rate of 250 beats/min. **B,** Color Doppler ultrasound shows ductus venosus waveform with SVT.

doses causing some maternal toxicity symptoms may be required. Digoxin alone is less likely to be successful in hydropic fetuses, with a response rate of 20%.[52] Numerous other antiarrhythmics, including sotalol, verapamil, flecainide, amiodarone, and adenosine, have also been used.[58-61] Clinical and biochemical fetal hypothyroidism has been associated with the use of amiodarone.[52,57] Treatment for SVT has been described as early as 13 weeks' gestational age.[62] In rare cases of SVT and hydrops, preterm delivery (if at sufficient gestational age) may be the best option, allowing for direct treatment of the tachyarrhythmia. Again, however, treatment of a hydropic preterm infant is difficult, and therefore preterm delivery is usually not indicated.

Heart Block. Congenital heart block (CHB) is a rare cardiac conduction defect, occurring in 1:15,000 to 1:20,000 live births. In fetuses with CHB, hydrops results from a combination of low cardiac output, a structural lesion, and a slow heart rate. The increased venous pressure in association with low colloid oncotic pressure leads to edema. Because approximately one third of fetuses with CHB have associated structural heart defects, a detailed fetal echocardiographic assessment is always warranted. In isolated heart block, maternal rheumatologic disease is common. Maternal serologic testing for anti-Ro/La antibodies is warranted because transplacental passage of maternal anti-Ro and anti-La autoantibodies is seen in 95% of cases of fetal CHB.[63] These antibodies cross the placenta from as early as 16 weeks' gestational age and initiate inflammatory damage to the fetal conduction system and myocardium.[64,65] Hydrops develops with ventricular rates less than 60 beats/min (about 40% of cases with isolated heart block)[66,67] and has a mortality rate of 25%[68] to

100%.[66] Treatment can be given with steroids and plasmapheresis.[69-73]

When structural abnormalities accompany heart block, hydropic fetuses have a combined fetal and neonatal mortality of 83% to 100%.[63,67] Jaeggi et al.[63] reported 29 cases of prenatally diagnosed isolated congenital A-V block; six fetuses presented with hydrops: two died antenatally, and four died in the neonatal period.[63] In these cases, corticosteroid use during pregnancy did not reverse hydrops or reduce the severity of A-V block. In addition to hydrops, other poor prognostic factors include **endocardial fibroelastosis** with ventricular dysfunction and coexistent structural heart disease.[66] Although 95% of mothers tested positive for anti-Ro/La antibodies, fewer than 5% of these pregnant patients had signs and symptoms of connective tissue disease at diagnosis of fetal A-V block.[63]

Decreased Myocardial Function. Fetal cardiomyopathy causes hydrops in 56% of cases.[74] **Cardiomyopathies** can be classified as primary or secondary or by an echocardiographic evaluation as **dilated** or **hypertrophic. Primary** fetal cardiomyopathies may have intrinsic causes (e.g., single-gene disorders, mitochondrial disorders, chromosomal abnormalities, α-thalassemia) or extrinsic causes such as infection, maternal disease (autoantibodies or insulin-dependent diabetes) and twin-twin transfusion syndrome. **Secondary** fetal cardiomyopathies may be associated with structural or functional cardiac disorders and high-output states.[74]

Neck Abnormalities

Neck masses, such as **teratomas** and **lymphangiomas,** may cause fetal hydrops from compression or high-out-

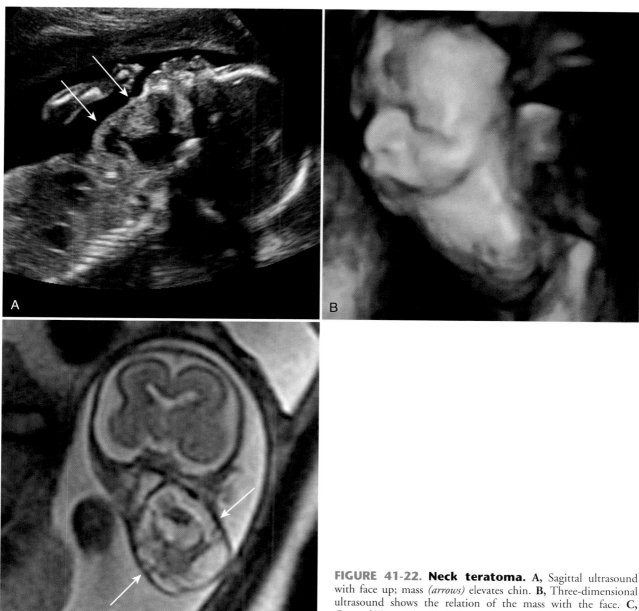

FIGURE 41-22. Neck teratoma. A, Sagittal ultrasound with face up; mass *(arrows)* elevates chin. **B,** Three-dimensional ultrasound shows the relation of the mass with the face. **C,** Coronal T2-weighted MR image shows cervical mass outside fetal calvarium, with normal-appearing brain.

put cardiac failure (Fig. 41-22). A **cystic hygroma** (fluid in posterior neck) may indicate a chromosomal (e.g., Turner's) or other abnormality. Of 42 fetuses with first-trimester cystic hygroma, 14 developed hydrops later in pregnancy. Each of these had a **nuchal translucency** measurement of 3 mm or more at diagnosis of cystic hygroma.[75] For fetuses presenting with hydrops in the first trimester, all have increased nuchal translucency.[76]

Thoracic Anomalies

Hydrops can result from obstruction of venous or lymphatic return due to maldevelopment, compression, kinking, or cardiac tamponade. **Mediastinal masses** (see Fig. 41-20), **pleural effusions,** and **diaphragmatic hernias** (Fig. 41-23) may cause nonimmune hydrops by similar mechanisms.[77]

The incidence of **fetal hydrothorax** is estimated at 1:15,000 pregnancies. Isolated hydrothorax is most often caused by **congenital chylothorax,** a primary lymphatic abnormality. Accumulation of fluid in the pleural space may lead to pulmonary hypoplasia, compression of the heart, and obstruction of venous return, with subsequent development of hydrops and compression of the esophagus leading to polyhydramnios. Untreated, the perinatal mortality is 22% to 53%.[78-82] Associated malformations (~25% of cases) and aneuploidy (~7%) worsen the outcome.[81-84]

In the absence of hydrops, fetuses with isolated hydrothorax have such a good prognosis that invasive prenatal

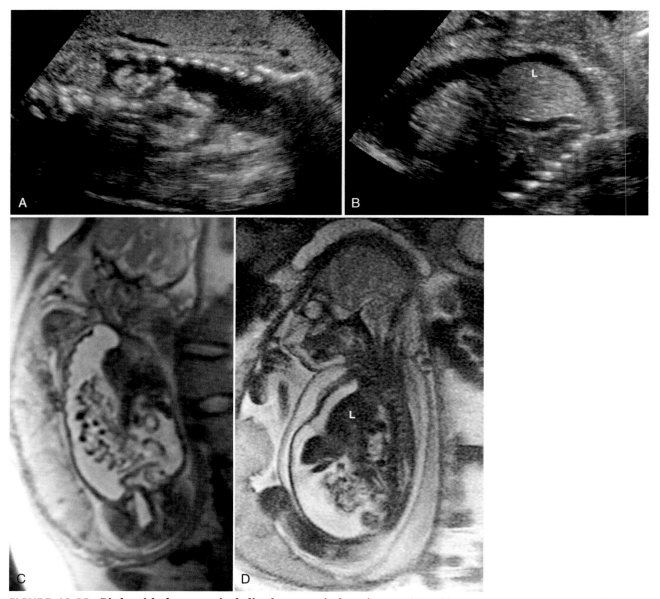

FIGURE 41-23. Right-sided congenital diaphragmatic hernia. A and **B,** Oblique coronal ultrasound views of the torso show fluid, bowel loops, and liver *(L)* extending from the abdomen into the chest. **C** and **D,** Coronal and sagittal T2-weighted MR images show similar findings.

treatment is not indicated.[79,85] However, when hydrops develops, the outcome without intervention is very poor. In a large review, perinatal mortality in the hydropic group was 69% despite prenatal interventions in a number of cases.[81]

An echogenic lung mass is usually a **congenital cystic adenomatoid malformation** (CCAM), a **bronchopulmonary sequestration** (BPS), an airway plug, or rarely, **congenital high airway obstruction syndrome** (CHAOS). Most cases of CCAM/BPS spectrum, regardless of their size, regress spontaneously at least partially during the third trimester, and only a minority become hydropic. Focal lung masses can lead to ipsilateral pleural

effusion (Fig. 41-24; see also Fig. 41-7), mediastinal shift, and ultimately, hydrops. However, the hydrops may not be caused only by the mediastinal shift, but also by high-output cardiac failure because of shunting that may occur in an anomalous systemic artery and venous drainage through pulmonary or systemic veins.[86]

In a report of 67 cases of lung masses, only 7% developed hydrops.[87] Of 134 fetuses with CCAM referred to the two fetal surgical centers in the United States, 101 were followed expectantly, and all 25 hydropic fetuses died, whereas all 76 nonhydropic fetuses survived,[88] suggesting that fetal surgery might be considered for hydropic cases. In the absence of hydrops, and provided

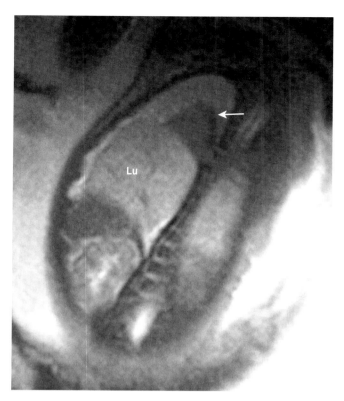

FIGURE 41-24. Resolving sequestration with ipsilateral pleural effusion. T2-weighted MR image shows a low-signal-intensity lung mass *(arrow)* caused by a resolving sequestration. Note the higher signal intensity of the normal lower lung *(Lu)* and surrounding pleural effusion.

there are no other anomalies, survival in these cases is virtually 100%.[89,90]

When a fetus with CCAM develops hydrops, the prognosis is poor, and antenatal intervention is often advisable. Intervention may be in the form of decompression by cyst aspiration or shunt, or open fetal surgery. A 2006 meta-analysis showed that shunting of CCAMs improved survival in fetuses with hydrops, as opposed to no effect on survival in fetuses with chest masses without hydrops.[91] Antenatal predictors of progression to hydrops include a combination of microcystic and macrocystic components and a large volume ratio of the mass to the normal lung (>1.6).[92] For fetuses with no dominant cyst and CCAM volume ratio less than 1.6, 97% did not progress to hydrops, whereas in the group with volume ratio greater than 1.6, 75% progressed to hydrops.[92] The success with open fetal surgery in cases of CCAM is variable, 29% to 62%. Antenatal aspiration of a macrocystic CCAM at times may be an effective treatment,[92] but frequently it is ineffective because of rapid reaccumulation of the cysts. In cases with rapid reaccumulation of fluid, thoracoamniotic shunting may be a better approach.[93] Maternal administration of steroids also may be helpful.[94]

Although nonimmune hydrops fetalis rarely occurs in BPS cases, it is associated with a high rate of perinatal mortality and severe respiratory insufficiency in the neonate.[95,96] However, neonates with BPS and hydrops can survive.[97] Different strategies of in utero treatment have been proposed, such as thoracoamniotic shunting

of pleural effusion,[98-101] thoracentesis and intravascular furosemide and digoxin,[102] alcohol ablation of the vascular pedicle with placement of a shunt,[103] ablation of the abnormal systemic artery from the aorta,[104,105] and open fetal surgery.[95]

In CHAOS the mechanism of hydrops is secondary to cardiac and great vessel compression by the enlarged fetal lungs.[106]

Pleural Drainage. Thoracic causes of hydrops, such as chylothorax and CCAM, have been successfully treated by thoracoamniotic chest shunt insertion in utero.[82,83,93,107] The main rationale for invasive therapy in these cases is to prevent pulmonary hypoplasia and prevent or reverse hydrops and polyhydramnios. Cases must be carefully selected because smaller effusions can resolve spontaneously, whereas others proceed to develop hydrops, polyhydramnios, and premature labor and/or intrauterine death.[82] Aneuploidy is present in about 6% of cases of chylothorax and should be excluded.[108] Isolated large effusions may be drained initially using a fine needle and the fluid sent for lymphocyte count,[109] rapid karyotyping, protein, inclusion bodies, and infection studies. This maneuver also evaluates the ability of the lungs to reexpand and may occasionally be therapeutic. Effusions that recollect rapidly can have multiple drainage procedures or may have shunt placement.[79,110] With treatment, survival is greater than 60%.[111] For large effusions occurring late in pregnancy, therapeutic drainage immediately before delivery facilitates neonatal resuscitation.[112]

Gastrointestinal Anomalies

Anomalies of the GI tract typically cause isolated ascites, rather than hydrops. If there is local obstruction of lymphatic and venous drainage, as from GI obstruction, volvulus, or omphalocele, hydrops may result in rare cases. Abdominal masses presumably act by compression of venous return, although hypoproteinemia or A-V shunting can also play a role.

Meconium peritonitis is associated with fetal **cystic fibrosis** in 70% of cases. Bowel rupture results in a sterile chemical peritonitis, often with ascites[113] (Fig. 41-25; see also Fig. 41-14). The ascites may be clear or particulate on ultrasound, and its appearance may change over time. The bowel will usually have a bunched or matted appearance, and areas of calcification may be visible. If this diagnosis is suspected, the parents should be offered carrier testing for the common cystic fibrosis mutations, approximately 85% of which are now routinely detectable.

Urinary Tract Anomalies

Urinary tract anomalies are rare causes of hydrops. Congenital nephrosis can lead to severe proteinuria and

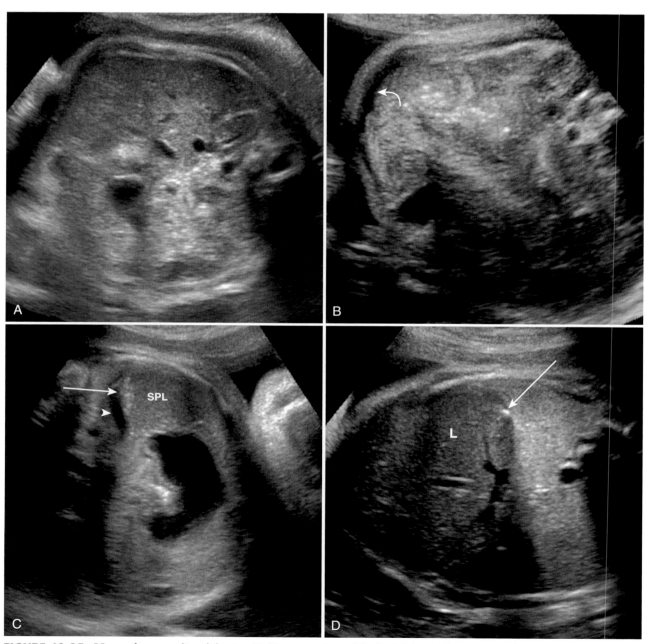

FIGURE 41-25. Meconium peritonitis. A to D, Transverse views of the fetal abdomen demonstrate echogenic bowel and punctate echogenicities *(arrows)* around the spleen *(SPL)* and liver. Note associated ascites *(curved arrow* in **B)** and pleural effusion *(arrowhead* in **C).**

hypoalbuminemia as the etiology of hydrops.[114] Bladder rupture can lead to urinary ascites but rarely hydrops (Fig. 41-26).

Lymphatic Dysplasia

Congenital lymphatic dysplasia may be the source of many cases of hydrops that do not have an obvious cause. Bellini et al.[115] found that six newborns presenting at birth with hydrops of unidentified cause all had lymphatic dysplasia.

Twins

Twins have an increased incidence of hydrops secondary to a higher incidence of congenital anomalies and

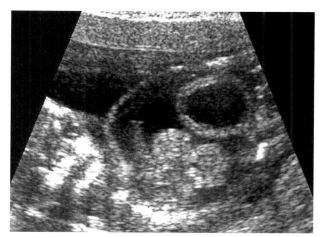

FIGURE 41-26. Lower urinary tract obstruction. Urinary ascites in obstructive uropathy with bladder rupture. Note the thickened bladder wall.

secondary to **twin-twin transfusion syndrome** (TTTS) and acardiac twinning. TTTS accounts for up to 9% of cases of nonimmune hydrops[116,117] and occurs in approximately 15% of **monochorionic twins,** representing the most common major complication for this group. It is responsible for 15% to 20% of perinatal deaths in twins overall.[118] TTTS is caused by a net transfer of blood from a donor fetus to the recipient fetus through unbalanced, unidirectional A-V placental anastomoses. This tends to result from deep unidirectional A-V channels with a paucity of superficial bidirectional channels.[119] It leads to an imbalance in amniotic fluid (polyhydramnios/oligohydramnios sequence) caused by polyuria in the recipient, who is hypervolemic, and has a persistently full bladder. As TTTS worsens, the **recipient** develops cardiomegaly with decreased cardiac function, ultimately leading to hydrops. The **donor** has a persistently empty bladder and is often "stuck" against the uterine wall as a result of severe oligohydramnios (Fig. 41-27). The donor can also be growth restricted secondary to placental insufficiency, with increased resistance in the umbilical arterial Doppler waveforms. The Quintero classification of TTTS is as follows[120]:

I   Donor twin bladder still visible.
II   Donor bladder no longer visible, but no critically abnormal Doppler studies.
III Critically abnormal Doppler studies (absent or reverse end diastolic velocity in umbilical artery, reverse flow in ductus venosus, or pulsatile flow in umbilical vein).
IV   Hydrops.
V   Death of either twin.

Mechanism of Hydrops. Hydrops may develop in either twin in cases of TTTS.[120] The **recipient twin** experiences an elevation in cardiac output and blood pressure due to shunting of blood through the A-V

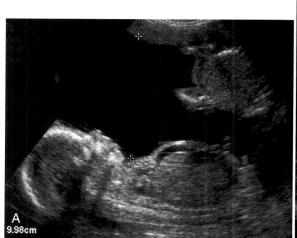
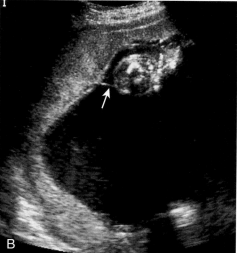

FIGURE 41-27. Twin-twin transfusion syndrome (TTTS) at 20 weeks' gestation. A, Polyhydramnios and hydropic recipient twin. **B,** Note membrane *(arrow)* closely adjacent to the stuck twin.

anastomoses. Initially, the increase in right ventricular (RV) workload is compensated for by ventricular hypertrophy, with minimal hemodynamic dysfunction. With ongoing volume and pressure overload, the RV stretches and the tricuspid regurgitation begins, probably associated with increase in RV end-diastolic pressure, reflected in the end-diastolic pressure of the right atrium. Atrial contractions against an elevated pressure produce retrograde flow during atrial systole in the ductus venosus, hepatic veins, and inferior vena cava. Eventually, metabolic acidosis and congestive heart failure develop.[121]

Conservative management of early-onset severe TTTS is associated with a survival rate of less than 10%.[122] Mortality is caused by extreme prematurity, in association with growth restriction in the donor and cardiac failure and hydrops in the recipient. Current series suggest improved survival and decreased neurologic sequelae if severe TTTS before 26 weeks is treated with endoscopic selective laser ablation of the placental vascular anastomoses.[123,124] Serial therapeutic amnioreduction has also been shown to improve perinatal outcome.[125] Recent studies show that laser treatment has better results than amnioreduction.

In acardiac twins (**twin reversed arterial perfusion [TRAP] sequence**) a monochorionic pair has a pump twin and an acardiac twin. The **pump twin** perfuses the acardiac twin and develops high-output cardiac failure. The **acardiac twin** has anasarca but not true hydrops. Treatment involves interruption of the blood flow to the acardiac twin, typically by radiofrequency ablation,[126-128] laser ablation,[129] or cord ligation.[130]

Chromosomal Anomalies

The incidence of aneuploidy is higher in hydrops cases presenting before 24 weeks than those later in pregnancy. Before 24 weeks, the incidence of aneuploidy in cases of hydrops ranges from 33% to 78%.[131-133] **Turner's syndrome** is classically associated with a cystic hygroma in the first and early second trimesters (Fig. 41-28; see also Fig. 41-14). Many of these disorders result in early spontaneous abortion. **Trisomies 21, 18, and 13** and **triploidy** have been associated with nonimmune hydrops, although it is often unclear why hydrops develops. There are a few reports of transient abnormal myelopoiesis with trisomy 21 as a cause of hepatomegaly and nonimmune hydrops.[134,135] In these cases, PUBS demonstrates fetal anemia and hypoalbuminemia. A hydropic fetus with multiple structural anomalies, prominent cystic hygromas, or increased nuchal translucency likely has a chromosomal abnormality. The physiologic basis for increased nuchal translucency is incompletely understood, but it may be caused by delayed lymphatic development or related to cardiovascular malformations,[136] especially in cases with aneuploidy.[137] After 24 weeks the incidence of aneuploidy in hydrops is as low as 2%.[132]

Tumors

Arteriovenous malformations and arteriovenous shunting in large tumors with a high proportion of solid tissue lead to hydrops by causing high-output cardiac failure and leading to **Kasabach-Merritt sequence** (consumptive coagulopathy). Selected fetuses with tumors, such as large **sacrococcygeal teratoma** associated with hydrops, have undergone in utero procedures, including cyst aspiration and open fetal surgical resection. However, these procedures are complicated by preterm delivery and other obstetric complications.[138]

Anemia

Fetal anemia is caused by decreased RBC production, increased hemolysis, or hemorrhage. If the process is gradual, the fetus mounts a compensatory erythropoietic response, and nonimmune hydrops develops only when the anemia exceeds its ability to keep pace, which is typically when the hemoglobin concentration deficit is 7 g/dL or greater.[13] Hydrops results from a combination of high-output cardiac failure and hypoxic capillary damage, causing protein leakage, as well as infiltration of the liver by erythropoietic tissue, leading to portal hypertension.[13]

Decreased Red Blood Cell Production. Homozygotes with **α-thalassemia** cannot manufacture HbF in utero or hemoglobin A (HbA) after birth.[139] Instead, Hb Bart is formed in utero, which has such a high affinity for oxygen that tissue hypoxia results, leading to capillary damage, protein leakage, cardiac failure, and hydrops. Other causes of decreased RBC production in utero include generalized marrow aplasia, as found in parvovirus infection[20,26] or fetal leukemia.[135]

Hemolysis. Glucose-6-phosphate dehydrogenase (G6PD) deficiency has been reported as a rare cause of nonimmune hydrops resulting from increased hemolysis.[140] Hemolysis may also contribute to anemia caused by in utero infection.

Hemorrhage. Blood loss may occur either into another fetus in TTTS, into the fetus itself (e.g., intracranial), into a tumor (e.g., sacrococcygeal teratoma), or transplacentally.

Infection

Intrauterine infections account for up to 16% of cases of nonimmune hydrops.[116] An autopsy series of fetuses with in utero demise and nonimmune hydrops showed that 33% had infection.[32] Hydrops may result from effects on the bone marrow (**parvovirus, cytomegalovirus** [CMV], **toxoplasmosis**), myocardium (**adenovirus, coxsackievirus, CMV,** leading to CHF), vascular endothelium (hypoxic capillary damage causing protein leakage), or overwhelming sepsis with hepatitis and decreased protein production (**syphilis**).[141-146] In addition to hydrops, signs

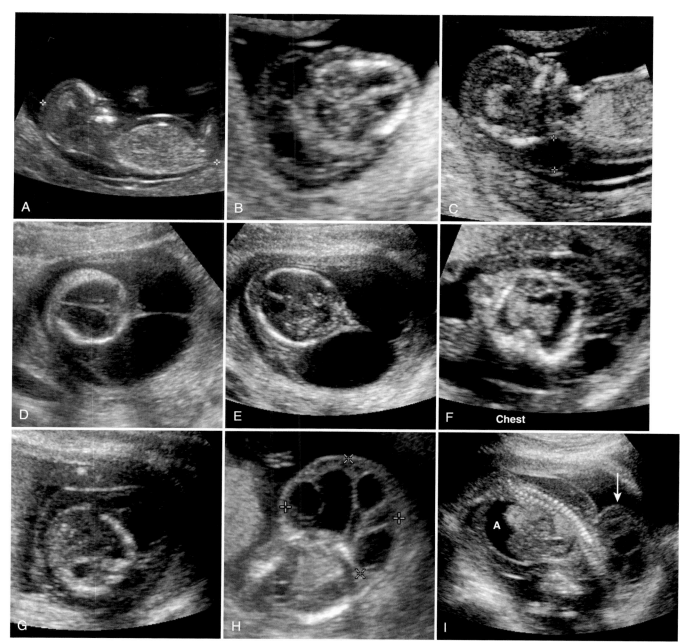

FIGURE 41-28. Turner's syndrome in first and second trimesters. A, Fetus at 12 weeks with diffuse skin thickening and lymphangiectasia. **B** and **C,** Fetus at 13 weeks with nuchal thickening and diffuse body wall edema. **D** to **G,** Fetus at 18 weeks with cystic hygroma and pleural effusion and diffuse body wall edema. **H** and **I,** Fetus at 19 weeks with cystic hygroma *(arrows)* and ascites *(A)*.

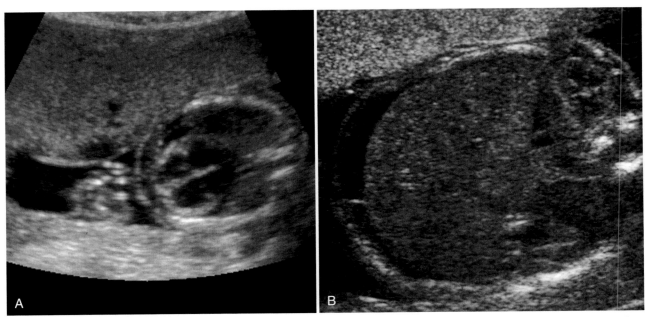

FIGURE 41-29. Hydrops in fetus with parvovirus infection and anemia at 19 weeks. A, Transverse view of the fetal thorax shows a slightly enlarged heart with echogenic myocardium and small pericardial effusion. **B,** Transverse view of abdomen shows ascites. Middle cerebral artery Doppler studies (not shown) showed peak systolic velocity of 55 cm/sec, indicating severe anemia.

of infection include calcifications in the pericardium or brain, as well as ventriculomegaly.

Human Parvovirus B19. Human parvovirus B19 is responsible for up to 27% of cases of nonimmune hydrops.[147] Myocarditis and fetal anemia secondary to bone marrow aplasia are thought to be the mechanisms of hydrops (Fig. 41-29). The marrow is particularly sensitive to parvovirus infection from 16 to 24 weeks' gestation.[141] The impact on RBC aplasia is further pronounced by the shortened life span of RBCs (45-70 days).[148]

Fetal infection occurs in up to 10% of pregnancies with maternal infection. This leads to an excess fetal loss rate of 9% of fetuses infected between 9 and 20 weeks' gestation.[149] In the first trimester, fetal infection can cause miscarriage, whereas in the second trimester, the fetus is at risk for hydrops. In contrast to most other congenital infections, adverse long-term sequelae are rarely associated with parvovirus.[144] Although hydrops associated with parvovirus B19 can spontaneously resolve without transfusion,[150-153] most cases benefit from intrauterine transfusion. Parvovirus infection is suspected when maternal blood shows positive immunoglobulin M (IgM, indicating a recent infection) and high or increasing IgG. Cordocentesis will show aplastic anemia with few reticulocytes, although at times the hydrops is caused by myocarditis.[150] Fetal parvovirus infection is diagnosed by polymerase chain reaction (PCR) testing of amniotic fluid or fetal blood.[154] PCR results can be available within a few hours.

When maternal parvovirus infection is discovered, serial monitoring of the pregnancy is indicated, with weekly sonograms for 8 to 12 weeks after maternal infection. Sonograms are performed to assess for signs of hydrops and include Doppler analysis to assess for elevated MCA velocity, as an indication of fetal anemia.

Toxoplasmosis. Congenital infection with *Toxoplasma gondii* may cause anemia, intracerebral or intrahepatic calcifications, ventriculomegaly, and chorioretinitis, and can present with hydrops, particularly ascites.[155-157] Most pregnant women with congenital toxoplasmosis are asymptomatic or only mildly symptomatic during pregnancy. The rate of fetal infection varies according to the gestational age at the time of vertical transmission, ranging from 26% to 40%.[155] Prenatal diagnosis of toxoplasmosis can be difficult and depends on the demonstration of maternal seroconversion and/or the parasite in amniotic fluid by PCR or isolation techniques.[155] Diagnosis is important because infected mothers are treated with spiramycin throughout pregnancy; if fetal infection was demonstrated, pyrimethamine and sulfadoxine or sulfadiazine are added to the regimen.[155]

Other Infections. Congenital **CMV** infection is responsible for 1% to 2% of cases of nonimmune hydrops and can occur even with recurrent maternal infection.[158] Fetal treatment can be attempted with umbilical vein injection of ganciclovir[159] or intraperitoneal injection of hyperimmunoglobulin.[160] **Rubella, syphilis,** and **varicella** are less common causes of nonimmune hydrops.[161,162] Diagnosis is important; in cases of syphilis, since if the fetus is in the third trimester and the lungs are mature, delivery and treatment with penicillin can lead to resolution of the hydrops. Rare infectious causes of nonimmune hydrops include **herpes simplex virus,**[163,164] **adenovirus,**[165] and acute maternal **hepatitis B** infection.[166]

Genetic Disorders

Multiple nonchromosomal genetic conditions can cause nonimmune hydrops[167] (see Table 41-1). The mechanisms are poorly understood and are multifactorial. In storage diseases, the most likely mechanism is hepatic infiltration resulting in hypoproteinemia or vascular obstruction.

Metabolic Disorders

Inborn errors of metabolism are rare, and these are a rare cause of hydrops. However, diagnosis is important because early treatment of some disorders can lead to improved outcome. Diagnosis is also important for genetic counseling regarding recurrence risk. Lysosomal disorders associated with hydrops fetalis include GM1 gangliosidosis, galactosialidosis, infantile free–sialic acid storage disease, mucopolysaccharidosis types IV and VII, mucolipidosis types I and II, Gaucher disease type II, Farber disease, Niemann-Pick disease, Wolman disease, and multiple sulfatase deficiency.[168] Hydrops fetalis has been associated with deficiencies of G6PD[140] or pyruvate kinase,[169,170] Pearson syndrome[171] and other mitochondrial disorders,[171,172] congenital defects of N-glycosylation,[173] glycogen storage disease type IV,[174] and neonatal hemochromatosis.[175]

Skeletal Disorders

Skeletal dysplasia is a rare cause of hydrops.[167] Examples include achondroplasia, achondrogenesis, osteogenesis imperfecta, hypophosphatasia, and arthrogryposis.

Endocrine Disorders

Fetal endocrine disorders are rare causes of nonimmune hydrops. Fetal hypothyroidism and hyperthyroidism can cause hydrops.[171,176] Hydrops can develop from maternal antibodies crossing the placenta, even if the pregnant patient has already been treated for Graves' disease.[177]

Drugs

In utero exposure to **indomethacin** can result in ductus arteriosus constriction and rarely, hydrops. Because of this, ultrasound evaluation of the ductus arteriosus should be performed within 48 hours of starting indomethacin therapy.[178]

Idiopathic Disorders

The number of idiopathic cases of nonimmune hydrops (for which we still cannot identify a cause) is about 10%[25,116] and will continue to decrease as our investigative abilities improve.

DIAGNOSTIC APPROACH TO HYDROPS

Systematic prenatal evaluation can establish a cause for nonimmune hydrops in up to 90% of cases.[116] This is important not only for the management of the current pregnancy, but also for future genetic counseling.[32]

History

A detailed history may provide the first clues to the etiology and may suggest appropriate investigations. For example, a maternal history of systemic lupus erythematosus or diabetes may be relevant, and homozygous α-thalassemia is particularly prevalent in patients of Southeast Asian origin. Blood type can supply a clue to isoimmunization. Maternal diseases with anemia or infection are important. Previous pregnancy losses may be related to one of the inborn errors of metabolism or chromosome rearrangements, and the family history or presence of consanguinity may suggest other genetic conditions. Parvovirus infection is more likely to occur in teachers or day-care workers.[179] Medication use can at times establish a cause.

Complete Obstetric Ultrasound

A comprehensive sonographic evaluation should be the initial step. However, no sonographic cause is found in 15% to 30% of cases. **Polyhydramnios** is a common association. A common indication for ultrasound is the clinical suspicion of being large for gestational dates. Collections of fluid in the pleural, peritoneal, and pericardial spaces are diagnostic, and their relative distribution and the timing of their development may give a clue to the etiology.[180] Ultrasound markers of aneuploidy suggest a chromosomal cause. The degree of polyhydramnios should be assessed because this may pose an imminent threat of premature rupture of the membranes or preterm labor, and the cervix should be imaged to ensure there is no funneling or shortening.

A systematic detailed survey of fetal anatomy should be performed, searching for other clues to the etiology of the hydrops. The fetal bladder should be visualized to exclude urinary ascites caused by bladder rupture. Bone length, curvature, density, and presence or absence of fractures should be evaluated to exclude skeletal dysplasias. Stigmata of congenital infection should be assessed, such as microcephaly or calcifications within the fetal brain or liver. A dedicated fetal echocardiographic structural and functional assessment is warranted to evaluate fetal heart structure, rhythm, and function in hydrops.

Amniocentesis for fetal karyotype (if at an appropriate gestational age), antigen tests by PCR, and culture for syphilis, CMV, and toxoplasmosis are often indicated. MCA Doppler should be performed, with PUBS when the Doppler indicates anemia.

Maternal Investigations

Maternal blood type, indirect Coombs' test (antiglobulin titer), and presence or absence of RBC antibodies should be checked to exclude immune hydrops. Other baseline tests include a complete blood count (CBC) and indices, Kleihauer-Betke, infection screen (TORCH, parvovirus IgM/IgG), and glucose.

Fetal Investigations

Fetal karyotype can be determined from amniotic fluid, chorionic villus sampling (CVS), fetal blood, or fluid aspirated from one of the fetal body cavities. The most appropriate choice depends on gestational age, accessibility, and urgency of results. A rapid karyotype can be obtained successfully from most collections of fetal body fluid.[181] **Fluorescent in situ hybridization** (FISH) can be used to identify common **aneuploidies** (trisomies 13, 18, and 21; monosomy X or Turner's) as well as other specific deletions and chromosome rearrangements. This technique can provide a result from amniotic fluid in 24 to 48 hours.[182] In practice, the confirmation or exclusion of the most common aneuploidies is often adequate to guide pregnancy management. Amniotic fluid is preferable for both viral culture and PCR for toxoplasmosis[156] and CMV, and it can be used to assess fetal lung maturity at later gestations. CVS is an alternative at any gestation for obtaining a rapid karyotype or DNA testing.

Fetal Blood Sampling. Fetal blood sampling is a key investigation in many cases when the chromosomes do not provide a diagnosis. Basic fetal blood work should include a direct Coombs' test, CBC and indices, karyotype, protein, albumin, and viral-specific IgM. Other tests are done selectively,[183,184] and samples can be stored for subsequent evaluation. With this approach, one can elucidate the etiology of hydrops in most cases. The risk of **fetal loss** from this procedure is 0.8%[185] to 2.8%,[186] although in the sick fetus with nonimmune hydrops, higher loss rates occur.[187] If it is anticipated that the fetus may require transfusion (e.g., parvovirus infection with elevated MCA Doppler velocity), it is prudent to have crossmatched blood and platelets ready to avoid the risks with a second procedure.

Cavity Aspiration. The clinician can usually advance the needle easily into the fetal chest, abdomen, or amniotic fluid at the time of fetal blood sampling or amniocentesis (Fig. 41-30). This can be both diagnostic (e.g., lymphocyte count in chylothorax or for rapid karyotype) and occasionally therapeutic. Simultaneous sampling does not increase the overall procedure risk.

Postnatal Investigations

After birth, the **placenta** should be sent for pathology, and a **skeletal survey** may be helpful. A geneticist may see the neonate to provide additional input. In cases of demise, detailed **autopsy** and placental examination, correlated with antenatal findings, is the best way to determine the etiology of nonimmune hydrops.[188,189] Further investigations may be prompted by additional physical findings at autopsy.[190] If a metabolic condition is suspected as the cause of hydrops, inclusion bodies can be sought on microscopy. In some series the cause of hydrops was identified in only 40% to 50% of patients without autopsy,[132] versus 80% to 90% after postmortem examination.[5,188]

FETAL WELFARE ASSESSMENT IN NONIMMUNE HYDROPS

Noninvasive ultrasound techniques for fetal welfare assessment in pregnancies complicated by nonimmune hydrops include biophysical assessment, pulsed Doppler velocimetry of umbilical and regional fetal vessels, and functional cardiac assessment. Fetal Doppler evaluation may give some indication of anemia, cardiac failure, and well-being.[22] Umbilical vein and intrahepatic vein pulsations, or ductus venosus a-wave reversal, represent cardiac diastolic dysfunction and have been correlated with poor perinatal outcomes.[191]

OBSTETRIC PROGNOSIS

The overall **mortality** in nonimmune hydrops is approximately 70%,[25] with mortality in cases of structural abnormalities not amenable to therapy as high as 100%. In a series of 100 cases of nonimmune hydrops, 74 were thought to have a nontreatable cause, and none of these resulted in a live birth; of 26 with a treatable cause, 18 resulted in a live birth and were alive at 1 year of age.[25] Gestational age at diagnosis of hydrops has been used to predict outcome. A 10-year review of 82 cases presenting after 20 weeks[132] reported an overall mortality of 87%, and those diagnosed after 24 weeks were more likely to be idiopathic or related to cardiothoracic abnormalities. Spontaneous resolution of hydrops has been reported in fetuses with normal chromosomes diagnosed before 24 weeks.

Although the overall prognosis for fetal hydrops has improved in recent years, most series are small with a mixture of causes and thus are difficult to compare. Some improvement in outcome over earlier reports is attributable to the growing number of cases that are amenable to in utero therapy. Unfortunately, many cases still represent a terminal process. Earlier identification and referral, thorough evaluation, and fetal therapy in appropriate cases are the cornerstone to further

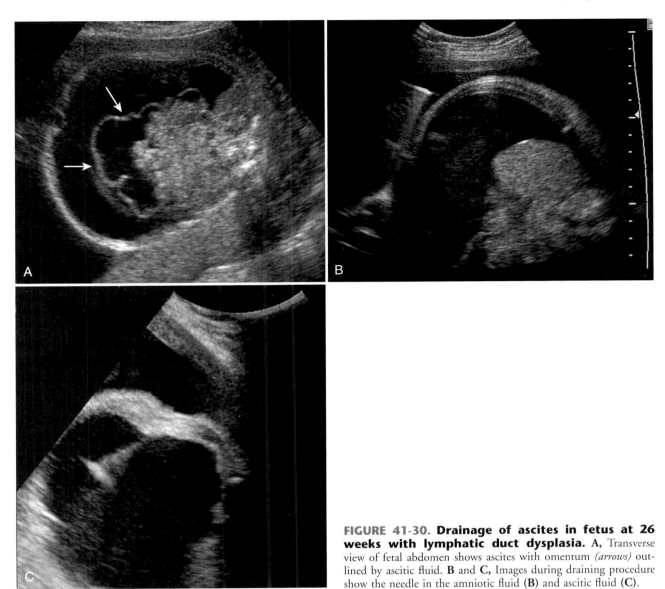

FIGURE 41-30. Drainage of ascites in fetus at 26 weeks with lymphatic duct dysplasia. A, Transverse view of fetal abdomen shows ascites with omentum *(arrows)* outlined by ascitic fluid. **B** and **C,** Images during draining procedure show the needle in the amniotic fluid **(B)** and ascitic fluid **(C).**

improvements in prognosis. Obtaining the best diagnosis is helpful in counseling about recurrence risks.

Maternal Complications (Mirror Syndrome)

Maternal complications may occur in association with fetal hydrops. Hypoproteinemia, edema, weight gain, hypertension, oliguria, and **preeclampsia** may develop.[192] This association has been termed **mirror syndrome** because edema in the pregnant patient mirrors that of the hydropic fetus.[27,193,194] The syndrome has been described in conjunction with hydrops of various etiologies.[192,195,196] Perinatal mortality and morbidity are high. Maternal outcome can be improved by delivery of the fetus and placenta or by fetal intervention to treat the etiology of the hydrops.[194,197-199] If hydrops

cannot be cured, delivery may limit the risk of maternal complications.[28,199]

Espinoza et al.[200] recently suggested the high plasma concentrations of soluble vascular endothelial growth factor receptor 1 (sVEGFR-1) is implicated in the pathophysiology of mirror syndrome. Hypoxia of the villous trophoblast in cases of villous edema leads to increased production and release of sVEGFR-1 and other antiangiogenic factors into the maternal circulation. Excessive concentrations of these products may be responsible for maternal edema in mirror syndrome.

Delivery

Mode and location of delivery are based on obstetric factors, taking into account the underlying prognosis.[201] Uterine overdistention in severe polyhydramnios carries the risks of **placental abruption** and **cord prolapse** after membrane rupture and **postpartum hemorrhage** from uterine atony. Prematurity secondary to polyhydramnios is a major contributing factor to the poor outcome of some neonates. **Therapeutic amniocentesis** before induction of labor may be considered in cases with massive polyhydramnios to decrease the risk of malpresentation or cord prolapse. **Indomethacin** has also been used to decrease the amniotic fluid volume.[202] This drug should be used with caution after 32 weeks' gestation because of the potential for ductal constriction.

Predelivery Aspiration Procedures

Fetal fluid collections may be drained under ultrasound guidance just before delivery to assist with **neonatal resuscitation.** This is particularly relevant if large fetal pleural effusions are present.[112] Massive ascites may also be drained to prevent abdominal dystocia (when vaginal birth is planned) and aid in fetal breathing when ascites has caused elevation of the diaphragms.

Postnatal Outcome

Because of the high incidence of in utero demise, the etiology of hydrops in utero is different from that with a live neonate. In a review of 30 cases of hydrops diagnosed between 10 and 14 weeks of pregnancy, all pregnancies with nonimmune hydrops resulted in abortion, intrauterine fetal death, or pregnancy termination.[133] A 2007 national database review of live-born neonates with hydrops found heart problems (13.7%), abnormalities in heart rate (10.4%), TTTS (9%), congenital anomalies (8.7%), chromosomal abnormalities (7.5%), congenital viral infections (6.7%), isoimmunization (4.5%), and congenital chylothorax (3.2%).[203] Mortality rates were highest among neonates with congenital anomalies (57.7%) and lowest among those with congenital chylothorax (5.9%), and a cause could not be determined in 26%. Factors associated independently with death were younger gestational age, low 5-minute Apgar score, and high levels of support needed the first day after birth.[203] This study reported a 36% death rate before discharge or transfer to another hospital. The severity of hydrops and birth gestational age of the infant are the key determinants for survival. This is important because delivering a fetus early to treat worsening hydrops may not improve survival.

Data are limited regarding long-term outcome of children surviving after hydrops. In one series, 13 of 19 (68%) children surviving beyond 1 year of age were normal; two had mild developmental delay at 1 year of age; one 8-year-old child was mentally retarded; and three (16%) had severe psychomotor impairment with marked growth failure.[204] Haverkamp et al.[205] found that 86% of patients had normal psychomotor development, 86% showed normal neurologic status, 7% had minor neurologic dysfunction, and 4% had spastic cerebral paresis.

CONCLUSION

Hydrops represents a terminal stage for many conditions, the vast majority of which are fetal in origin. The onset of hydrops signifies fetal decompensation. Immune causes can be successfully treated in utero, as can an increasing number of nonimmune causes. Whereas in the past nonimmune hydrops carried virtually 100% mortality, this is no longer the case. A team approach using obstetric imagers, maternal fetal medicine specialists, neonatologists, and geneticists can help to decide which cases are suitable for therapeutic intervention. A comprehensive approach must be taken to the investigation of hydrops, both for the management of the index case and for future counseling. Cornerstones of this investigation are detailed ultrasound, including echocardiography, fetal karyotyping and other diagnostic interventions as appropriate, and pathologic examination of the fetus and placenta.

References

1. Machin GA. Hydrops revisited: literature review of 1,414 cases published in the 1980s. Am J Med Genet 1989;34:366-390.
2. Freda VJ, Gorman JG, Pollack W, et al. Prevention of Rh isoimmunization: progress report of the clinical trial in mothers. JAMA 1967;199:390-394.
3. Macafee CA, Fortune DW, Beischer NA. Non-immunological hydrops fetalis. J Obstet Gynaecol 1970;77:226-237.
4. Andersen HM, Drew JH, Beischer NA, et al. Non-immune hydrops fetalis: changing contribution to perinatal mortality. Br J Obstet Gynaecol 1983;90:636-639.
5. Santolaya J, Alley D, Jaffe R, Warsof SL. Antenatal classification of hydrops fetalis. Obstet Gynecol 1992;79:256-259.
6. Ayida GA, Soothill PW, Rodeck CH. Survival in non-immune hydrops fetalis without malformation or chromosomal abnormalities after invasive treatment. Fetal Diagn Ther 1995;10:101-105.
7. Hashimoto BE, Filly RA, Callen PW. Fetal pseudoascites: further anatomic observations. J Ultrasound Med 1986;5:151-152.

Sonographic Features

8. Di Salvo DN, Brown DL, Doubilet PM, et al. Clinical significance of isolated fetal pericardial effusion. J Ultrasound Med 1994;13:291-293.
9. Bukowski R, Saade GR. Hydrops fetalis. Clin Perinatol 2000;27:1007-1031.
10. Nicolaides KH, Fontanarosa M, Gabbe SG, Rodeck CH. Failure of ultrasonographic parameters to predict the severity of fetal anemia in rhesus isoimmunization. Am J Obstet Gynecol 1988;158:920-926.
11. Fleischer AC, Killam AP, Boehm FH, et al. Hydrops fetalis: sonographic evaluation and clinical implications. Radiology 1981;141:163-168.
12. Nicolaides KH, Warenski JC, Rodeck CH. The relationship of fetal plasma protein concentration and hemoglobin level to the development of hydrops in rhesus isoimmunization. Am J Obstet Gynecol 1985;152:341-344.

Immune Hydrops

13. Nicolaides KH. Studies on fetal physiology and pathophysiology in rhesus disease. Semin Perinatol 1989;13:328-337.
14. Soothill PW, Nicolaides KH, Rodeck CH. Effect of anaemia on fetal acid-base status. Br J Obstet Gynaecol 1987;94:880-883.

15. Daffos F, Capella-Pavlovsky M, Forestier F. Fetal blood sampling during pregnancy with use of a needle guided by ultrasound: a study of 606 consecutive cases. Am J Obstet Gynecol 1985;153:655-660.

16. Van Kamp IL, Klumper FJ, Bakkum RS, et al. The severity of immune fetal hydrops is predictive of fetal outcome after intrauterine treatment. Am J Obstet Gynecol 2001;185:668-673.

17. Tongsong T, Wanapirak C, Kunavikatikul C, et al. Fetal loss rate associated with cordocentesis at midgestation. Am J Obstet Gynecol 2001;184:719-723.

18. Mari G, Deter RL, Carpenter RL, et al. Noninvasive diagnosis by Doppler ultrasonography of fetal anemia due to maternal red-cell alloimmunization. Collaborative Group for Doppler Assessment of the Blood Velocity in Anemic Fetuses. N Engl J Med 2000;342: 9-14.

19. Zimmerman R, Carpenter Jr RJ, et al. Longitudinal measurement of peak systolic velocity in the fetal middle cerebral artery for monitoring pregnancies complicated by red cell alloimmunisation: a prospective multicentre trial with intention-to-treat. BJOG 2002; 109:746-752.

20. Kempe A, Rosing B, Berg C, et al. First-trimester treatment of fetal anemia secondary to parvovirus B19 infection. Ultrasound Obstet Gynecol 2007;29:226-228.

21. Oepkes D, Brand R, Vandenbussche FP, et al. The use of ultrasonography and Doppler in the prediction of fetal haemolytic anaemia: a multivariate analysis. Br J Obstet Gynaecol 1994;101: 680-684.

22. Dukler D, Oepkes D, Seaward G, et al. Noninvasive tests to predict fetal anemia: a study comparing Doppler and ultrasound parameters. Am J Obstet Gynecol 2003;188:1310-1314.

Nonimmune Hydrops

23. Sohan K, Carroll SG, De La Fuente S, et al. Analysis of outcome in hydrops fetalis in relation to gestational age at diagnosis, cause and treatment. Acta Obstet Gynecol Scand 2001;80:726-730.

24. Allan LD, Crawford DC, Sheridan R, Chapman MG. Aetiology of non-immune hydrops: the value of echocardiography. Br J Obstet Gynaecol 1986;93:223-225.

25. Anandakumar C, Biswas A, Wong YC, et al. Management of non-immune hydrops: 8 years' experience. Ultrasound Obstet Gynecol 1996;8:196-200.

26. Apkon M. Pathophysiology of hydrops fetalis. Semin Perinatol 1995;19:437-446.

27. Van Selm M, Kanhai HH, Gravenhorst JB. Maternal hydrops syndrome: a review. Obstet Gynecol Surv 1991;46:785-788.

28. Carbillon L, Oury JF, Guerin JM, et al. Clinical biological features of Ballantyne syndrome and the role of placental hydrops. Obstet Gynecol Surv 1997;52:310-314.

29. Treadwell MC, Sherer DM, Sacks AJ, et al. Successful treatment of recurrent non-immune hydrops secondary to fetal hyperthyroidism. Obstet Gynecol 1996;87:838-840.

30. Makino Y, Horiuchi S, Sonoda M, et al. A case of large placental chorioangioma with non-immunological hydrops fetalis. J Perinat Med 1999;27:128-131.

31. Haak MC, Oosterhof H, Mouw RJ, et al. Pathophysiology and treatment of fetal anemia due to placental chorioangioma. Ultrasound Obstet Gynecol 1999;14:68-70.

32. Rodriguez MM, Chaves F, Romaguera RL, et al. Value of autopsy in nonimmune hydrops fetalis: series of 51 stillborn fetuses. Pediatr Dev Pathol 2002;5:365-374.

33. Knilans TK. Cardiac abnormalities associated with hydrops fetalis. Semin Perinatol 1995;19:483-492.

34. Poeschmann RP, Verheijen RH, van Dongen PW. Differential diagnosis and causes of nonimmunological hydrops fetalis: a review. Obstet Gynecol Surv 1991;46:223-231.

35. Groves AM, Fagg NL, Cook AC, Allan LD. Cardiac tumours in intrauterine life. Arch Dis Child 1992;67:1189-1192.

36. Schmider A, Henrich W, Dahnert I, Dudenhausen JW. Prenatal therapy of non-immunologic hydrops fetalis caused by severe aortic stenosis. Ultrasound Obstet Gynecol 2000;16:275-278.

37. Hornberger LK, Sahn DJ, Kleinman CS, et al. Tricuspid valve disease with significant tricuspid insufficiency in the fetus: diagnosis and outcome. J Am Coll Cardiol 1991;17:167-173.

38. Huggon IC, Cook AC, Smeeton NC, et al. Atrioventricular septal defects diagnosed in fetal life: associated cardiac and extra-cardiac abnormalities and outcome. J Am Coll Cardiol 2000;36: 593-601.

39. Guereta LG, Burgueros M, Elorza MD, et al. Cardiac rhabdomyoma presenting as fetal hydrops. Pediatr Cardiol 1986;7:171-174.

40. Rheuban KS, McDaniel NL, Feldman PS, et al. Intrapericardial teratoma causing nonimmune hydrops fetalis and pericardial tamponade: a case report. Pediatr Cardiol 1991;12:54-56.

41. Tollens T, Casselman F, Devlieger H, et al. Fetal cardiac tamponade due to an intrapericardial teratoma. Ann Thorac Surg 1998;66: 559-560.

42. Geipel A, Krapp M, Germer U, et al. Perinatal diagnosis of cardiac tumors. Ultrasound Obstet Gynecol 2001;17:17-21.

43. Scurry J, Watkins A, Acton C, Drew J. Tachyarrhythmia, cardiac rhabdomyomata and fetal hydrops in a premature infant with tuberous sclerosis. J Paediatr Child Health 1992;28:260-262.

44. Bader RS, Chitayat D, Kelly E, et al. Fetal rhabdomyoma: prenatal diagnosis, clinical outcome, and incidence of associated tuberous sclerosis complex. J Pediatr 2003;143:620-624.

45. Paladini D, Palmieri S, Russo MG, Pacileo G. Cardiac multiple rhabdomyomatosis: prenatal diagnosis and natural history. Ultrasound Obstet Gynecol 1996;7:84-85.

46. Perez-Aytes A, Sanchis N, Barbal A, et al. Non-immunological hydrops fetalis and intrapericardial teratoma: case report and review. Prenat Diagn 1995;15:859-863.

47. Catanzarite V, Mehalek K, Maida C, Mendoza A. Early sonographic diagnosis of intrapericardial teratoma. Ultrasound Obstet Gynecol 1994;4:505-507.

48. Czernik C, Stiller B, Hubler M, et al. Hydrops fetalis caused by a large intrapericardial teratoma. Ultrasound Obstet Gynecol 2006; 28:973-976.

49. Benatar A, Vaughan J, Nicolini U, et al. Prenatal pericardiocentesis: its role in the management of intrapericardial teratoma. Obstet Gynecol 1992;79:856-859.

50. Paw PT, Jamieson SW. Surgical management of intrapericardial teratoma diagnosed in utero. Ann Thorac Surg 1997;64:552-554.

51. Bader R, Hornberger LK, Nijmeh LJ, et al. Fetal pericardial teratoma: presentation of two cases and review of literature. Am J Perinatol 2006;23:53-58.

52. Simpson JM, Sharland GK. Fetal tachycardias: management and outcome of 127 consecutive cases. Heart 1998;79:576-581.

53. Eronen M. Outcome of fetuses with heart disease diagnosed in utero. Arch Dis Child Fetal Neonatal Ed 1997;77:F41-F46.

54. Naheed ZJ, Strasburger JF, Deal BJ, et al. Fetal tachycardia: mechanisms and predictors of hydrops fetalis. J Am Coll Cardiol 1996;27:1736-1740.

55. Hidaka N, Tsukimori K, Hojo S, et al. Transplacental digitalization for nonimmune hydrops fetalis caused by isolated noncompaction of the ventricular myocardium. J Ultrasound Med 2007;26:519-524.

56. Bitar FF, Byrum CJ, Kveselis DA, et al. In utero management of hydrops fetalis caused by critical aortic stenosis. Am J Perinatol 1997;14:389-391.

57. Cuneo BF, Strasburger JF. Management strategy for fetal tachycardia. Obstet Gynecol 2000;96:575-581.

58. Knirsch W, Kretschmar O, Vogel M, et al. Successful treatment of atrial flutter with amiodarone in a premature neonate: case report and literature review. Adv Neonatal Care 2007;7:113-121.

59. Pradhan M, Manisha M, Singh R, Kapoor A. Amiodarone in treatment of fetal supraventricular tachycardia: a case report and review of literature. Fetal Diagn Ther 2006;21:72-76.

60. Krapp M, Baschat AA, Gembruch U, et al. Flecainide in the intrauterine treatment of fetal supraventricular tachycardia. Ultrasound Obstet Gynecol 2002;19:158-164.

61. Allan LD, Chita SK, Sharland GK, et al. Flecainide in the treatment of fetal tachycardias. Br Heart J 1991;65:46-48.

62. Porat S, Anteby EY, Hamani Y, Yagel S. Fetal supraventricular tachycardia diagnosed and treated at 13 weeks of gestation: a case report. Ultrasound Obstet Gynecol 2003;21:302-305.

63. Jaeggi ET, Hamilton RM, Silverman ED, et al. Outcome of children with fetal, neonatal or childhood diagnosis of isolated congenital atrioventricular block: a single institution's experience of 30 years. J Am Coll Cardiol 2002;39:130-137.

64. McCue CM, Mantakas ME, Tingelstad JB, Ruddy S. Congenital heart block in newborns of mothers with connective tissue disease. Circulation 1977;56:882-890.

65. Litsey SE, Noonan JA, O'Connor WN, et al. Maternal connective tissue disease and congenital heart block: demonstration of

immunoglobulin in cardiac tissue. N Engl J Med 1985;312: 98-100.

66. Schmidt KG, Ulmer HE, Silverman NH, et al. Perinatal outcome of fetal complete atrioventricular block: a multicenter experience. J Am Coll Cardiol 1991;17:1360-1366.

67. Groves AM, Allan LD, Rosenthal E. Outcome of isolated congenital complete heart block diagnosed in utero. Heart 1996;75:190-194.

68. Eronen M, Siren MK, Ekblad H, et al. Short- and long-term outcome of children with congenital complete heart block diagnosed in utero or as a newborn. Pediatrics 2000;106:86-91.

69. Carpenter RJ Jr, Strasburger JF, Garson Jr A, et al. Fetal ventricular pacing for hydrops secondary to complete atrioventricular block. J Am Coll Cardiol 1986;8:1434-1436.

70. Buyon JP, Hiebert R, Copel J, et al. Autoimmune-associated congenital heart block: demographics, mortality, morbidity and recurrence rates obtained from a national neonatal lupus registry. J Am Coll Cardiol 1998;31:1658-1666.

71. Martin TC, Arias F, Olander DS, et al. Successful management of congenital atrioventricular block associated with hydrops fetalis. J Pediatr 1988;112:984-986.

72. Bierman FZ, Baxi L, Jaffe I, Driscoll J. Fetal hydrops and congenital complete heart block: response to maternal steroid therapy. J Pediatr 1988;112:646-648.

73. Barclay CS, French MA, Ross LD, Sokol RJ. Successful pregnancy following steroid therapy and plasma exchange in a woman with anti-Ro (SS-A) antibodies: case report. Br J Obstet Gynaecol 1987;94:369-371.

74. Pedra SR, Smallhorn JF, Ryan G, et al. Fetal cardiomyopathies: pathogenic mechanisms, hemodynamic findings, and clinical outcome. Circulation 2002;106:585-591.

75. Kharrat R, Yamamoto M, Roume J, et al. Karyotype and outcome of fetuses diagnosed with cystic hygroma in the first trimester in relation to nuchal translucency thickness. Prenat Diagn 2006;26:369-372.

76. Jauniaux E. Diagnosis and management of early non-immune hydrops fetalis. Prenat Diagn 1997;17:1261-1268.

77. Giacoia GP. Right-sided diaphragmatic hernia associated with superior vena cava syndrome. Am J Perinatol 1994;11:129-131.

78. Estroff JA, Parad RB, Frigoletto FD, Benacerraf BR. The natural history of isolated fetal hydrothorax. Ultrasound Obst Gynecol 1992;3:162-165.

79. Hagay Z, Reece A, Roberts A, Hobbins JC. Isolated fetal pleural effusion: a prenatal management dilemma. Obstet Gynecol 1993;81:147-152.

80. Longaker MT, Laberge JM, Dansereau J, et al. Primary fetal hydrothorax: natural history and management. J Pediatr Surg 1989;24:573-576.

81. Weber AM, Philipson EH. Fetal pleural effusion: a review and meta-analysis for prognostic indicators. Obstet Gynecol 1992;79:281-286.

82. Aubard Y, Derouineau I, Aubard V, et al. Primary fetal hydrothorax: a literature review and proposed antenatal clinical strategy. Fetal Diagn Ther 1998;13:325-333.

83. Nicolaides KH, Azar GB. Thoraco-amniotic shunting. Fetal Diagn Ther 1990;5:153-164.

84. Mussat P, Dommergues M, Parat S, et al. Congenital chylothorax with hydrops: postnatal care and outcome following antenatal diagnosis. Acta Paediatr 1995;84:749-755.

85. Klam S, Bigras JL, Hudon L. Predicting outcome in primary fetal hydrothorax. Fetal Diagn Ther 2005;20:366-370.

86. Morin L, Crombleholme TM, D'Alton ME. Prenatal diagnosis and management of fetal thoracic lesions. Semin Perinatol 1994;18:228-253.

87. Davenport M, Warne SA, Cacciaguerra S, et al. Current outcome of antenatally diagnosed cystic lung disease. J Pediatr Surg 2004;39:549-556.

88. Adzick NS, Harrison MR, Crombleholme TM, et al. Fetal lung lesions: management and outcome. Am J Obstet Gynecol 1998;179:884-889.

89. Barret J, Chitayat D, Sermer M, et al. The prognostic factors in the prenatal diagnosis of the echogenic fetal lung. Prenat Diagn 1995;15:849-853.

90. Adzick NS, Flake AW, Crombleholme TM. Management of congenital lung lesions. Semin Pediatr Surg 2003;12:10-16.

91. Knox EM, Kilby MD, Martin WL, Khan KS. In-utero pulmonary drainage in the management of primary hydrothorax and congenital cystic lung lesion: a systematic review. Ultrasound Obstet Gynecol 2006;28:726-734.

92. Crombleholme TM, Coleman B, Hedrick H, et al. Cystic adenomatoid malformation volume ratio predicts outcome in prenatally diagnosed cystic adenomatoid malformation of the lung. J Pediatr Surg 2002;37:331-338.

93. Ryo E, Okai T, Namba S, et al. Successful thoracoamniotic shunting using a double-flower catheter in a case of fetal cystic adenomatoid malformation associated with hydrops and polyhydramnios. Ultrasound Obstet Gynecol 1997;10:293-296.

94. Peranteau WH, Wilson RD, Liechty KW, et al. Effect of maternal betamethasone administration on prenatal congenital cystic adenomatoid malformation growth and fetal survival. Fetal Diagn Ther 2007;22:365-371.

95. Adzick NS. Management of fetal lung lesions. Clin Perinatol 2003;30:481-492.

96. Dolkart LA, Reimers FT, Helmuth WV, et al. Antenatal diagnosis of pulmonary sequestration: a review. Obstet Gynecol Surv 1992;47:515-520.

97. Da Silva OP, Ramanan R, Romano W, et al. Nonimmune hydrops fetalis, pulmonary sequestration, and favorable neonatal outcome. Obstet Gynecol 1996;88:681-683.

98. Slotnick RN, McGahan J, Milio L, et al. Antenatal diagnosis and treatment of fetal bronchopulmonary sequestration. Fetal Diagn Ther 1990;5:33-39.

99. Salomon LJ, Audibert F, Dommergues M, et al. Fetal thoracoamniotic shunting as the only treatment for pulmonary sequestration with hydrops: favorable long-term outcome without postnatal surgery. Ultrasound Obstet Gynecol 2003;21:299-301.

100. Becmeur F, Horta-Geraud P, Donato L, Sauvage P. Pulmonary sequestrations: prenatal ultrasound diagnosis, treatment, and outcome. J Pediatr Surg 1998;33:492-496.

101. Chan V, Greenough A, Nicolaides KN. Antenatal and postnatal treatment of pleural effusion and extra-lobar pulmonary sequestration. J Perinat Med 1996;24:335-338.

102. Anandakumar C, Biswas A, Chua TM, et al. Direct intrauterine fetal therapy in a case of bronchopulmonary sequestration associated with non-immune hydrops fetalis. Ultrasound Obstet Gynecol 1999;13:263-265.

103. Nicolini U, Cerri V, Groli C, et al. A new approach to prenatal treatment of extralobar pulmonary sequestration. Prenat Diagn 2000;20:758-760.

104. Ruano R, Marques da Silva M, Maksoud JG, Zugaib M. Percutaneous intrauterine laser ablation of the abnormal vessel in pulmonary sequestration with hydrops at 29 weeks' gestation. J Ultrasound Med 2007;26:1235-1241.

105. Oepkes D, Devlieger R, Lopriore E, Klumper FJ. Successful ultrasound-guided laser treatment of fetal hydrops caused by pulmonary sequestration. Ultrasound Obstet Gynecol 2007;29:457-459.

106. Kalache KD, Chaoui R, Tennstedt C, Bollmann R. Prenatal diagnosis of laryngeal atresia in two cases of congenital high airway obstruction syndrome (CHAOS). Prenat Diagn 1997;17:577-581.

107. Morrow RJ, MacPhail S, Johnson JA, et al. Midtrimester thoracoamniotic shunting for the treatment of fetal hydrops. Fetal Diagn Ther 1995;10:92-94.

108. Achiron R, Weissman A, Lipitz S, et al. Fetal pleural effusion: the risk of fetal trisomy. Gynecol Obstet Invest 1995;39:153-156.

109. Eddleman KA, Levine AB, Chitkara U, Berkowitz RL. Reliability of pleural fluid lymphocyte counts in the antenatal diagnosis of congenital chylothorax. Obstet Gynecol 1991;78:530-532.

110. Rodeck CH, Fisk NM, Fraser DI, Nicolini U. Long-term in utero drainage of fetal hydrothorax. N Engl J Med 1988;319:1135-1138.

111. Deurloo KL, Devlieger R, Lopriore E, et al. Isolated fetal hydrothorax with hydrops: a systematic review of prenatal treatment options. Prenat Diagn 2007;27:893-899.

112. Cardwell MS. Aspiration of fetal pleural effusions or ascites may improve neonatal resuscitation. South Med J 1996;89:177-178.

113. Mayock DE, Hickok DE, Guthrie RD. Cystic meconium peritonitis associated with hydrops fetalis. Am J Obstet Gynecol 1982;142:704-705.

114. Mark K, Reis A, Zenker M. Prenatal findings in four consecutive pregnancies with fetal Pierson syndrome, a newly defined congenital nephrosis syndrome. Prenat Diagn 2006;26:262-266.

115. Bellini C, Hennekam RC, Boccardo F, et al. Nonimmune idiopathic hydrops fetalis and congenital lymphatic dysplasia. Am J Med Genet A 2006;140:678-684.

116. Lallemand AV, Doco-Fenzy M, Gaillard DA. Investigation of nonimmune hydrops fetalis: multidisciplinary studies are necessary for diagnosis—review of 94 cases. Pediatr Dev Pathol 1999;2:432-439.

117. Holzgreve W, Curry CJ, Golbus MS, et al. Investigation of nonimmune hydrops fetalis. Am J Obstet Gynecol 1984;150:805-812.

118. Cincotta RB, Fisk NM. Current thoughts on twin-twin transfusion syndrome. Clin Obstet Gynecol 1997;40:290-302.

119. Bajoria R, Wigglesworth J, Fisk NM. Angioarchitecture of monochorionic placentas in relation to the twin-twin transfusion syndrome. Am J Obstet Gynecol 1995;172:856-863.

120. Quintero RA, Morales WJ, Allen MH, et al. Staging of twin-twin transfusion syndrome. J Perinatol 1999;19:550-555.

121. Huhta JC. Right ventricular function in the human fetus. J Perinat Med 2001;29:381-389.

122. Berghella V, Kaufmann M. Natural history of twin-twin transfusion syndrome. J Reprod Med 2001;46:480-484.

123. Senat MV, Deprest J, Boulvain M, et al. Endoscopic laser surgery versus serial amnioreduction for severe twin-to-twin transfusion syndrome. N Engl J Med 2004;351:136-144.

124. Quintero RA, Dickinson JE, Morales WJ, et al. Stage-based treatment of twin-twin transfusion syndrome. Am J Obstet Gynecol 2003;188:1333-1340.

125. Mari G, Detti L, Oz U, Abuhamad AZ. Long-term outcome in twin-twin transfusion syndrome treated with serial aggressive amnioreduction. Am J Obstet Gynecol 2000;183:211-217.

126. Hirose M, Murata A, Kita N, et al. Successful intrauterine treatment with radiofrequency ablation in a case of acardiac twin pregnancy complicated with a hydropic pump twin. Ultrasound Obstet Gynecol 2004;23:509-512.

127. Tsao K, Feldstein VA, Albanese CT, et al. Selective reduction of acardiac twin by radiofrequency ablation. Am J Obstet Gynecol 2002;187:635-640.

128. Rodeck C, Deans A, Jauniaux E. Thermocoagulation for the early treatment of pregnancy with an acardiac twin. N Engl J Med 1998;339:1293-1295.

129. Ville Y, Hyett JA, Vandenbussche FP, Nicolaides KH. Endoscopic laser coagulation of umbilical cord vessels in twin reversed arterial perfusion sequence. Ultrasound Obstet Gynecol 1994;4:396-398.

130. Quintero RA, Reich H, Puder KS, et al. Brief report: umbilical-cord ligation of an acardiac twin by fetoscopy at 19 weeks of gestation. N Engl J Med 1994;330:469-471.

131. Iskaros J, Jauniaux E, Rodeck C. Outcome of nonimmune hydrops fetalis diagnosed during the first half of pregnancy. Obstet Gynecol 1997;90:321-325.

132. McCoy MC, Katz VL, Gould N, Kuller JA. Non-immune hydrops after 20 weeks' gestation: review of 10 years' experience with suggestions for management. Obstet Gynecol 1995;85:578-582.

133. Has R. Non-immune hydrops fetalis in the first trimester: a review of 30 cases. Clin Exp Obstet Gynecol 2001;28:187-190.

134. Hojo S, Tsukimori K, Kitade S, et al. Prenatal sonographic findings and hematological abnormalities in fetuses with transient abnormal myelopoiesis with Down syndrome. Prenat Diagn 2007;27:507-511.

135. Zerres K, Schwanitz G, Niesen M, et al. Prenatal diagnosis of acute non-lymphoblastic leukaemia in Down syndrome. Lancet 1990;335:117.

136. Hyett JA, Perdu M, Sharland GK, et al. Increased nuchal translucency at 10-14 weeks of gestation as a marker for major cardiac defects. Ultrasound Obstet Gynecol 1997;10:242-246.

137. Jenderny J, Schmidt W, Hecher K, et al. Increased nuchal translucency, hydrops fetalis or hygroma colli: a new test strategy for early fetal aneuploidy detection. Fetal Diagn Ther 2001;16:211-214.

138. Hedrick HL, Flake AW, Crombleholme TM, et al. Sacrococcygeal teratoma: prenatal assessment, fetal intervention, and outcome. J Pediatr Surg 2004;39:430-438; discussion 438.

139. Dame C, Albers N, Hasan C, et al. Homozygous alpha-thalassaemia and hypospadias: common aetiology or incidental association? Long-term survival of Hb Bart's hydrops syndrome leads to new aspects for counselling of alpha-thalassaemic traits. Eur J Pediatr 1999;158:217-220.

140. Perkins RP. Hydrops fetalis and stillbirth in a male glucose-6-phosphate dehydrogenase-deficient fetus possibly due to maternal ingestion of sulfisoxazole: a case report. Am J Obstet Gynecol 1971;111:379-381.

141. Barron SD, Pass RF. Infectious causes of hydrops fetalis. Semin Perinatol 1995;19:493-501.

142. Porter HJ, Quantrill AM, Fleming KA. B19 parvovirus infection of myocardial cells. Lancet 1988;1:535-536.

143. Naides SJ, Weiner CP. Antenatal diagnosis and palliative treatment of non-immune hydrops fetalis secondary to fetal parvovirus B19 infection. Prenat Diagn 1989;9:105-114.

144. Morey AL, Keeling JW, Porter HJ, Fleming KA. Clinical and histopathological features of parvovirus B19 infection in the human fetus. Br J Obstet Gynaecol 1992;99:566-574.

145. Oyer CE, Ongcapin EH, Ni J, et al. Fatal intrauterine adenoviral endomyocarditis with aortic and pulmonary valve stenosis: diagnosis by polymerase chain reaction. Hum Pathol 2000;31:1433-1435.

146. Bates Jr HR. Coxsackie virus B3 calcific pancarditis and hydrops fetalis. Am J Obstet Gynecol 1970;106:629-630.

147. Von Kaisenberg CS, Jonat W. Fetal parvovirus B19 infection. Ultrasound Obstet Gynecol 2001;18:280-288.

148. Gray ES, Davidson RJ, Anand A. Human parvovirus and fetal anaemia. Lancet 1987;1:1144.

149. Miller E, Fairley CK, Cohen BJ, Seng C. Immediate and long-term outcome of human parvovirus B19 infection in pregnancy. Br J Obstet Gynaecol 1998;105:174-178.

150. Bhal PS, Davies NJ, Westmoreland D, Jones A. Spontaneous resolution of non-immune hydrops fetalis secondary to transplacental parvovirus B19 infection. Ultrasound Obstet Gynecol 1996;7:55-57.

151. Pryde PG, Nugent CE, Pridjian G, et al. Spontaneous resolution of nonimmune hydrops fetalis secondary to human parvovirus B19 infection. Obstet Gynecol 1992;79:859-861.

152. Humphrey W, Magoon M, O'Shaughnessy R. Severe nonimmune hydrops secondary to parvovirus B-19 infection: spontaneous reversal in utero and survival of a term infant. Obstet Gynecol 1991;78:900-902.

153. Cossart YE, Field AM, Cant B, Widdows D. Parvovirus-like particles in human sera. Lancet 1975;1:72-73.

154. Kovacs BW, Carlson DE, Shahbahrami B, Platt LD. Prenatal diagnosis of human parvovirus B19 in nonimmune hydrops fetalis by polymerase chain reaction. Am J Obstet Gynecol 1992;167:461-466.

155. Daffos F, Forestier F, Capella-Pavlovsky M, et al. Prenatal management of 746 pregnancies at risk for congenital toxoplasmosis. N Engl J Med 1988;318:271-275.

156. Friedman S, Ford-Jones LE, Toi A, et al. Congenital toxoplasmosis: prenatal diagnosis, treatment and postnatal outcome. Prenat Diagn 1999;19:330-333.

157. Zornes SL, Anderson PG, Lott RL. Congenital toxoplasmosis in an infant with hydrops fetalis. South Med J 1988;81:391-393.

158. Inoue T, Matsumura N, Fukuoka M, et al. Severe congenital cytomegalovirus infection with fetal hydrops in a cytomegalovirus-seropositive healthy woman. Eur J Obstet Gynecol Reprod Biol 2001;95:184-186.

159. Revello MG, Gerna G. Diagnosis and management of human cytomegalovirus infection in the mother, fetus, and newborn infant. Clin Microbiol Rev 2002;15:680-715.

160. Negishi H, Yamada H, Hirayama E, et al. Intraperitoneal administration of cytomegalovirus hyperimmunoglobulin to the cytomegalovirus-infected fetus. J Perinatol 1998;18:466-469.

161. Barton JR, Thorpe Jr EM, Shaver DC, et al. Nonimmune hydrops fetalis associated with maternal infection with syphilis. Am J Obstet Gynecol 1992;167:56-58.

162. Harger JH, Ernest JM, Thurnau GR, et al. Frequency of congenital varicella syndrome in a prospective cohort of 347 pregnant women. Obstet Gynecol 2002;100:260-265.

163. Anderson MS, Abzug MJ. Hydrops fetalis: an unusual presentation of intrauterine herpes simplex virus infection. Pediatr Infect Dis J 1999;18:837-839.

164. Ashshi AM, Cooper RJ, Klapper PE, et al. Detection of human herpes virus 6 DNA in fetal hydrops. Lancet 2000;355:1519-1520.

165. Ranucci-Weiss D, Uerpairojkit B, Bowles N, et al. Intrauterine adenoviral infection associated with fetal non-immune hydrops. Prenat Diagn 1998;18:182-185.

166. Schroter B, Chaoui R, Meisel H, Bollmann R. [Maternal hepatitis B infection as the cause of nonimmunologic hydrops fetalis]. Z Geburtshilfe Neonatol 1999;203:36-38.

167. Jauniaux E, van Maldergem L, De Munter C, et al. Nonimmune hydrops fetalis associated with genetic abnormalities. Obstet Gynecol 1990;75:568-572.

168. Wraith JE. Lysosomal disorders. Semin Neonatol 2002;7:75-83.
169. Ravindranath Y, Paglia DE, Warrier I, et al. Glucose phosphate isomerase deficiency as a cause of hydrops fetalis. N Engl J Med 1987;316:258-261.
170. Gilsanz F, Vega MA, Gomez-Castillo E, et al. Fetal anaemia due to pyruvate kinase deficiency. Arch Dis Child 1993;69:523-524.
171. Rotig A, Cormier V, Blanche S, et al. Pearson's marrow-pancreas syndrome: a multisystem mitochondrial disorder in infancy. J Clin Invest 1990;86:1601-1608.
172. Fayon M, Lamireau T, Bioulac-Sage P, et al. Fatal neonatal liver failure and mitochondrial cytopathy: an observation with antenatal ascites. Gastroenterology 1992;103:1332-1335.
173. De Koning TJ, Toet M, Dorland L, et al. Recurrent nonimmune hydrops fetalis associated with carbohydrate-deficient glycoprotein syndrome. J Inherit Metab Dis 1998;21:681-682.
174. Alegria A, Martins E, Dias M, et al. Glycogen storage disease type IV presenting as hydrops fetalis. J Inherit Metab Dis 1999;22:330-332.
175. Knisely AS, Mieli-Vergani G, Whitington PF. Neonatal hemochromatosis. Gastroenterol Clin North Am 2003;32:877-889, vi-vii.
176. Kessel I, Makhoul IR, Sujov P. Congenital hypothyroidism and nonimmune hydrops fetalis: associated? Pediatrics 1999;103:E9.
177. Stulberg RA, Davies GA. Maternal thyrotoxicosis and fetal nonimmune hydrops. Obstet Gynecol 2000;95:1036.
178. Pratt L, Digiosia J, Swenson JN, et al. Reversible fetal hydrops associated with indomethacin use. Obstet Gynecol 1997;90:676-678.

Diagnostic Approach to Hydrops

179. Adler SP, Manganello AM, Koch WC, et al. Risk of human parvovirus B19 infections among school and hospital employees during endemic periods. J Infect Dis 1993;168:361-368.
180. Saltzman DH, Frigoletto FD, Harlow BL, et al. Sonographic evaluation of hydrops fetalis. Obstet Gynecol 1989;74:106-111.
181. Teoh TG, Ryan G, Johnson J, Winsor EJ. The role of fetal karyotyping from unconventional sources. Am J Obstet Gynecol 1996;175:873-877.
182. Cheong Leung W, Chitayat D, Seaward G, et al. Role of amniotic fluid interphase fluorescence in situ hybridization (FISH) analysis in patient management. Prenat Diagn 2001;21:327-332.
183. Soma H, Yamada K, Osawa H, et al. Identification of Gaucher cells in the chorionic villi associated with recurrent hydrops fetalis. Placenta 2000;21:412-416.
184. Galjaard H. Fetal diagnosis of inborn errors of metabolism. Baillieres Clin Obstet Gynaecol 1987;1:547-567.
185. Weiner CP, Wenstrom KD, Sipes SL, Williamson RA. Risk factors for cordocentesis and fetal intravascular transfusion. Am J Obstet Gynecol 1991;165:1020-1025.
186. Ghidini A, Sepulveda W, Lockwood CJ, Romero R. Complications of fetal blood sampling. Am J Obstet Gynecol 1993;168:1339-1344.
187. Acar A, Balci O, Gezginc K, et al. Evaluation of the results of cordocentesis. Taiwan J Obstet Gynecol 2007;46:405-409.
188. Ruiz Villaespesa A, Suarez Mier MP, Lopez Ferrer P, et al. Nonimmunologic hydrops fetalis: an etiopathogenetic approach through the postmortem study of 59 patients. Am J Med Genet 1990;35:274-279.
189. Knisely AS. The pathologist and the hydropic placenta, fetus, or infant. Semin Perinatol 1995;19:525-531.
190. Steiner RD. Hydrops fetalis: role of the geneticist. Semin Perinatol 1995;19:516-524.

Fetal Welfare Assessment in Nonimmune Hydrops

191. Gudmundsson S, Huhta JC, Wood DC, et al. Venous Doppler ultrasonography in the fetus with nonimmune hydrops. Am J Obstet Gynecol 1991;164:33-37.

Obstetric Outcome

192. Kaiser IH. Ballantyne and triple edema. Am J Obstet Gynecol 1971;110:115-120.
193. Kumar B, Nazaretian SP, Ryan AJ, Simpson I. Mirror syndrome: a rare entity. Pathology 2007;39:373-375.
194. Vidaeff AC, Pschirrer ER, Mastrobattista JM, et al. Mirror syndrome: a case report. J Reprod Med 2002;47:770-774.
195. Ordorica SA, Marks F, Frieden FJ, et al. Aneurysm of the vein of Galen: a new cause for Ballantyne syndrome. Am J Obstet Gynecol 1990;162:1166-1167.
196. Dorman SL, Cardwell MS. Ballantyne syndrome caused by a large placental chorioangioma. Am J Obstet Gynecol 1995;173:1632-1633.
197. Livingston JC, Malik KM, Crombleholme TM, et al. Mirror syndrome: a novel approach to therapy with fetal peritoneal-amniotic shunt. Obstet Gynecol 2007;110:540-543.
198. Duthie SJ, Walkinshaw SA. Parvovirus associated fetal hydrops: reversal of pregnancy induced proteinuric hypertension by in utero fetal transfusion. Br J Obstet Gynaecol 1995;102:1011-1013.
199. Heyborne KD, Chism DM. Reversal of Ballantyne syndrome by selective second-trimester fetal termination. A case report. J Reprod Med 2000;45:360-362.
200. Espinoza J, Romero R, Nien JK, et al. A role of the anti-angiogenic factor sVEGFR-1 in the "mirror syndrome" (Ballantyne's syndrome). J Matern Fetal Neonatal Med 2006;19:607-613.
201. McCurdy Jr CM, Seeds JW. Route of delivery of infants with congenital anomalies. Clin Perinatol 1993;20:81-106.
202. Kirshon B, Mari G, Moise Jr KJ. Indomethacin therapy in the treatment of symptomatic polyhydramnios. Obstet Gynecol 1990;75:202-205.
203. Abrams ME, Meredith KS, Kinnard P, Clark RH. Hydrops fetalis: a retrospective review of cases reported to a large national database and identification of risk factors associated with death. Pediatrics 2007;120:84-89.
204. Nakayama H, Kukita J, Hikino S, et al. Long-term outcome of 51 liveborn neonates with non-immune hydrops fetalis. Acta Paediatr 1999;88:24-28.
205. Haverkamp F, Noeker M, Gerresheim G, Fahnenstich H. Good prognosis for psychomotor development in survivors with nonimmune hydrops fetalis. BJOG 2000;107:282-284.

CHAPTER 42

Fetal Measurements: Normal and Abnormal Fetal Growth

Carol B. Benson and Peter M. Doubilet

Chapter Outline

Sonographic measurements of the fetus provide information about fetal age and growth. These data are used to assign gestational age, estimate fetal weight, and diagnose growth disturbances. As discussed in other chapters, fetal measurements are also used in the diagnosis of a number of fetal anomalies, such as skeletal dysplasias[1] and microcephaly.[2] Each of these abnormalities can be diagnosed or suspected on the basis of measurements that deviate from the "normal for dates."

It is important to begin by defining the various terms used in the evaluation of the age of a pregnancy. The true measure of age is the number of days since conception, termed **conceptional age.** Historically, pregnancies were dated by the number of days since the first day of the last menstrual period (LMP), termed **menstrual age.** In women with regular 28-day cycles, menstrual age is 2 weeks more than conceptional age, because conception occurs approximately 2 weeks after the LMP in such women. Currently, the term most often used to date pregnancies is **gestational age,** defined as follows:

$$\text{Gestational age (menstrual age)} = \text{Conceptional age} + 2 \text{ weeks}$$

In women with 28-day cycles, gestational age and menstrual age are equal. In women with longer cycles, gestational age is less than menstrual age; the opposite holds in women with shorter cycles.

Accurate knowledge of gestational age is important for a number of reasons. The timing of chorionic villus sampling and screening tests in the first trimester, genetic amniocentesis in the second trimester, and elective induction or cesarean delivery in the third trimester are all based on the gestational age. The differentiation between term and preterm labor and the characterization of a fetus as "postdates" depend on gestational age. Knowledge of the gestational age can be critical in distinguishing normal from pathologic fetal development. Midgut herniation, for example, is normal up to 11 to 12 weeks of gestation,[3] but signifies omphalocele thereafter. The normal size of a variety of fetal body parts depends on gestational age, as do levels of maternal serum alpha-fetoprotein,[4] human chorionic gonadotropin,[5] and estriol.[6] When a fetal anomaly is detected prenatally, the maternal choices and obstetric management are significantly influenced by gestational age. In fact, virtually all important clinical decisions in obstetrics are influenced by gestational age.

Estimation of the fetal weight, on its own and in relation to the gestational age, can influence obstetric management decisions concerning the timing and route of delivery. Early delivery may benefit a fetus that is small for dates. Such a fetus may be inadequately supplied by its placenta with oxygen and nutrients and therefore may do better in the care of a neonatologist than in utero. When the fetus is large, cesarean section may be the preferred route of delivery, particularly in pregnancies complicated by maternal diabetes. In view of these considerations, fetal measurements should be a component of every complete obstetric sonogram.[7]

GESTATIONAL AGE DETERMINATION

Clinical dating of a pregnancy is usually based on the patient's recollection of the first day of her LMP and on physical examination of uterine size. Unfortunately, both these methods are subject to imprecision, leading to inaccuracies in gestational age assignment. Dating by LMP (menstrual age) may be inaccurate because of variability in length of menstrual cycles (early or late ovulation occurs in 20% of population), faulty memory, recent exposure to oral contraceptives, or bleeding during early pregnancy.[8] Determining gestational age from the palpated dimension of the uterus may be affected by uterine fibroids, multiple pregnancy, and maternal body habitus.

Clinical dating is accurate only if one of two conditions apply: (1) the patient is a good historian with regular menstrual cycles, and the uterine size correlates closely with LMP; and (2) information is available specifying the time of conception, such as a basal body temperature chart or in vitro fertilization. When the pregnancy cannot be dated accurately by clinical evaluation, sonography is accepted as the most useful and accurate tool for estimating gestational age.

First Trimester

Sonographic milestones of early pregnancy and measurement of the embryo once it can be visualized by transvaginal ultrasound allow highly accurate dating from 5 weeks' gestation until the end of the first trimester.

The earliest sign of an intrauterine pregnancy is identification of a **gestational sac** in the uterine cavity. This appears as a round or oval fluid collection surrounded by one and sometimes two echogenic rings formed by the proliferating chorionic villi and the deeper layer of the decidua vera (Fig. 42-1). It is first seen at approximately 5 weeks' gestation.[9-11]

From 5 to 6 weeks' gestation, two methods are used to assign gestational age by ultrasound: (1) measurement of **mean sac diameter** (MSD) or (2) sonographic identification of gestational sac contents. The MSD, the average internal diameter of the gestational sac, is calculated as the mean of the anteroposterior (AP) diameter, the transverse diameter, and the longitudinal diameter. It increases from 2 mm at 5 weeks to 10 mm at 6 weeks,[12] a growth pattern that can be used to assign gestational age during this period (Table 42-1).

The second method, based on the sonographic findings within the gestational sac, is best done by transvaginal sonography and relies on the observation that, on average, the gestational sac is first identifiable at 5.0 weeks, the **yolk sac** at 5.5 weeks (Fig. 42-2), and the embryo and **embryonic heartbeat** at 6.0 weeks[13] (Fig. 42-3). From 6.3 weeks onward, ultrasound will visualize an embryo 5 mm or greater in length, by which time a heartbeat should always be seen if the embryo is alive. The timing of these milestones is subject to some variability, but they usually are seen within 0.5 week of the stated gestational ages. Gestational age can be assigned based on these milestones (Table 42-2).

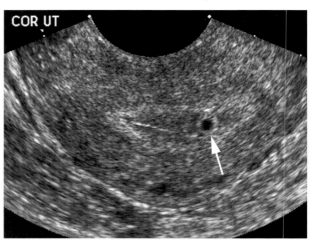

FIGURE 42-1. Gestational sac. At 5.0 weeks' gestation, gestational sac *(arrow)* appears as a small, intrauterine fluid collection with an echogenic rim; *COR UT,* coronal uterus. Note how this is eccentrically located within the endometrium.

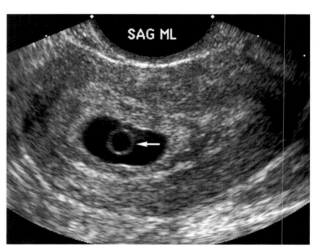

FIGURE 42-2. Yolk sac. Gestational sac contains yolk sac *(arrow)* on transvaginal sonogram at 5.5 weeks' gestation; *SAG ML,* sagittal midline. No embryo is seen.

TABLE 42-1. GESTATIONAL DATING BY MEAN SAC DIAMETER (MSD) IN THE EARLY FIRST TRIMESTER

MSD (mm)	GESTATIONAL AGE (weeks)*
2	5.0
3	5.1
4	5.2
5	5.4
6	5.5
7	5.6
8	5.7
9	5.9
10	6.0

*Values from Daya S, Wood S, Ward S, et al. Early pregnancy assessment with transvaginal ultrasound scanning. CMAJ 1991;144:441-446.
  95% confidence interval = ±0.5 week.

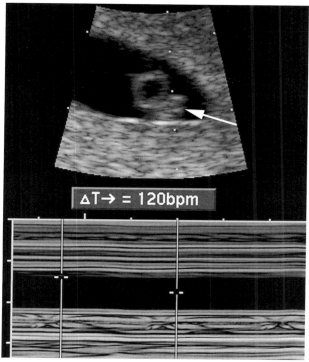

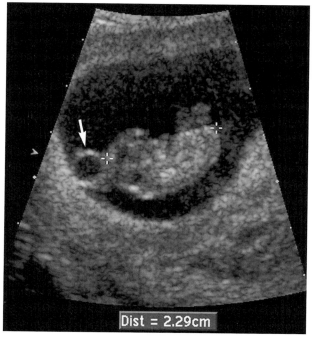

FIGURE 42-4. Crown-rump length (CRL) measurement. Cursors delineate the length of the fetus from the top of its head to the bottom of its torso. The yolk sac (arrow) should not be included in the fetal CRL measurements.

FIGURE 42-3. Embryonic heartbeat. Transvaginal sonogram and M-mode at 6 weeks demonstrate cardiac activity (calipers) originating from tiny embryo (arrow) adjacent to the yolk sac.

TABLE 42-2. GESTATIONAL DATING BY ULTRASOUND IN THE FIRST TRIMESTER

SONOGRAPHIC FINDING	GESTATIONAL AGE (weeks)
Gestational sac, no yolk sac, embryo, or heartbeat	5
Gestational sac with yolk sac, no embryo or heartbeat	5.5
Gestational sac with heartbeat and embryo <5 mm in length	6
Embryo/fetus ≧5 mm in length	Age based on crown-rump length (see Table 42-3)

From 6 weeks until the end of the first trimester, gestational age correlates closely with the **crown-rump length** (CRL) of the embryo or fetus.[14,15] The term **embryo** is used up to 8 to 10 weeks' gestation, and the term **fetus** applies thereafter.[16] The CRL is the length of the embryo or fetus from the top of its head to the bottom of its torso. It is measured as the longest dimension of the embryo, excluding the yolk sac and extremities (Fig. 42-4). The CRL can be used to assign gestational age accurately up to 11 weeks because minimal biologic variability occurs during this time (Table 42-3). After 12 to 13 weeks' gestation, the CRL of the longer, more

developed fetus becomes less reliable. At this later stage, the CRL is affected by the fetal position, measuring shorter in a fetus whose spine is flexed and longer in a fetus whose spine is extended.

The accuracy of gestational age determination by ultrasound, as measured by the width of the 95% confidence range, is approximately ±0.5 week throughout the first trimester.[14,15] The sonographic estimation of gestational age will be within 0.5 week of the actual age in 95% of cases.

Second and Third Trimesters

Many sonographic parameters have been proposed for estimating gestational age in the second and third trimesters. These include several fetal measurements: **biparietal diameter** (BPD),[17,18] **head circumference** (HC),[19] **abdominal circumference** (AC),[20] **femur length** (FL),[18,21-23] **length of other long bones,**[22] and **binocular distance,**[24] as well as combinations of two or more fetal measurements: the **corrected-BPD**[25] and **composite age formulas.**[20,26] Measurements of structurally abnormal fetal body parts should not be used in the assignment of gestational age.

Fetal Head Measurements

Three measurements or parameters involve the fetal head: BPD, corrected-BPD, and HC. All three measurements are taken from transaxial sonograms of the fetal

TABLE 42-3. GESTATIONAL AGE ESTIMATION* BY CROWN-RUMP LENGTH (CRL)

CRL (mm)	GESTATIONAL AGE (weeks)	CRL (mm)	GESTATIONAL AGE (weeks)
5	6.0	45	11.1
6	6.2	46	11.2
7	6.4	47	11.3
8	6.6	48	11.4
9	6.8	49	11.4
10	7.0	50	11.5
11	7.2	51	11.6
12	7.4	52	11.7
13	7.5	53	11.8
14	7.7	54	11.8
15	7.8	55	11.9
16	8.0	56	12.0
17	8.1	57	12.1
18	8.3	58	12.2
19	8.4	59	12.2
20	8.5	60	12.3
21	8.7	61	12.4
22	8.8	62	12.4
23	8.9	63	12.5
24	9.0	64	12.6
25	9.1	65	12.7
26	9.3	66	12.7
27	9.4	67	12.8
28	9.5	68	12.9
29	9.6	69	12.9
30	9.7	70	13.0
31	9.8	71	13.1
32	9.9	72	13.2
33	10.0	73	13.2
34	10.1	74	13.3
35	10.2	75	13.4
36	10.3	76	13.4
37	10.4	77	13.5
38	10.5	78	13.5
39	10.6	79	13.6
40	10.7	80	13.7
41	10.8		
42	10.8		
43	10.9		
44	11.0		

*Values derived from formula in Robinson HP, Fleming JE. A critical evaluation of sonar "crown-rump length" measurements. Br J Obstet Gynaecol 1975;82:702-710.

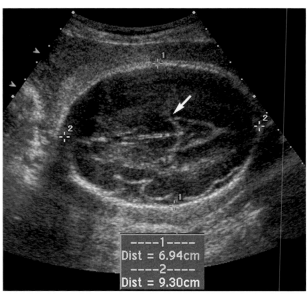

FIGURE 42-5. Biparietal diameter (BPD) and occipitofrontal diameter (OFD) measurements. Transaxial sonogram of the fetal head at the level of the paired thalami *(arrow),* with BPD *(calipers 1)* and OFD *(calipers 2).* Note how the calipers for the BPD are placed from the outer aspect of the skull to the inner aspect of the skull.

head at the level of the paired thalami and cavum septi pellucidi[27] (Fig. 42-5). The BPD is measured from the outer edge of the cranium nearest the transducer to the inner edge of the cranium farthest from the transducer (Fig. 42-5). The **occipitofrontal diameter** (OFD) is obtained from the same transaxial image as the BPD and is measured from midskull to midskull along the long axis of the fetal head (Fig. 42-5). This latter measurement is used in conjunction with the BPD to calculate the corrected-BPD using the following formula[25]:

$$\text{Corrected-BPD} = \sqrt{(\text{BPD} \times \text{OFD})/1.265}$$

The rationale for the corrected-BPD is that it represents the BPD of the standard-shaped head (one with an

OFD/BPD ratio of 1.265) of the same cross-sectional area.[25] The same tables or formulas used to determine gestational age from the BPD are used to determine gestational age from the corrected-BPD (Table 42-4).

The HC is the length of the outer perimeter of the cranium, made on the same transaxial image of the fetal head. It can be measured by using an electronic ellipse available on most ultrasound scanners[28] (Fig. 42-6 and Table 42-5). Alternatively, it can be calculated from the outer-edge-to-outer-edge analogs of the BPD and OFD:

$$\text{HC} = 1.57 \times [(\text{Outer-to-outer BPD}) + (\text{Outer-to-outer OFD})]$$

Although the BPD is simpler to measure than the corrected-BPD or HC, it has the disadvantage of being the only one of the three measurements that disregards head shape. This means that two heads of equal widths but different lengths will have the same BPD, but the longer head will have a greater corrected-BPD and HC than the shorter head (Fig. 42-7). The fetus with the longer head will therefore be assigned a greater gestational age based on the corrected-BPD or HC; however, both fetuses will be assigned the same gestational age if the BPD is used as the basis for age assignment.

Femur Length

The length of the diaphysis of the fetal femur is often used for gestational age prediction.[18,21,22] Careful measurement of the ossified diaphysis of the femur is necessary to obtain an accurate estimate of gestational age by

TABLE 42-4. GESTATIONAL AGE ESTIMATION* BY BIPARIETAL DIAMETER (BPD)

BPD OR BPDc (mm)	GESTATIONAL AGE (weeks)	BPD OR BPDc (mm)	GESTATIONAL AGE (weeks)
20	13.2	60	24.2
21	13.4	61	24.5
22	13.6	62	24.9
23	13.8	63	25.3
24	14.0	64	25.7
25	14.3	65	26.1
26	14.5	66	26.5
27	14.7	67	26.9
28	14.9	68	27.3
29	15.1	69	27.7
30	15.4	70	28.1
31	15.6	71	28.5
32	15.8	72	29.0
33	16.1	73	29.4
34	16.3	74	29.9
35	16.6	75	30.3
36	16.8	76	30.8
37	17.1	77	31.2
38	17.3	78	31.7
39	17.6	79	32.2
40	17.9	80	32.7
41	18.1	81	33.2
42	18.4	82	33.7
43	18.7	83	34.2
44	19.0	84	34.7
45	19.3	85	35.2
46	19.6	86	35.8
47	19.9	87	36.3
48	20.2	88	36.9
49	20.5	89	37.4
50	20.8	90	38.0
51	21.1	91	38.6
52	21.4	92	39.2
53	21.7	93	39.8
54	22.1	94	40.4
55	22.4	95	41.0
56	22.8	96	41.6
57	23.1	≥97	42.0
58	23.5		
59	23.8		

*Values from Doubilet PM, Benson CB. Improved prediction of gestational age in the late third trimester. J Ultrasound Med 1993;12:647-653.
  BPDc, Corrected-BPD.

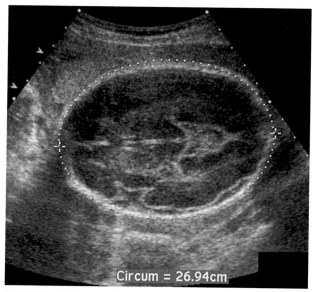

FIGURE 42-6. Head circumference (HC) measurement. HC measurement (*calipers* and *tracing dots*) on transaxial sonogram of the fetal head at the same level as for the biparietal diameter measurement. Note how the HC measurement is obtained from around the bone.

TABLE 42-5. GESTATIONAL AGE ESTIMATION* BY HEAD CIRCUMFERENCE (HC)

HC (mm)	GESTATIONAL AGE (weeks)	HC (mm)	GESTATIONAL AGE (weeks)
80	13.4	225	24.5
85	13.7	230	25.0
90	14.0	235	25.5
95	14.3	240	26.1
100	14.7	245	26.6
105	15.0	250	27.1
110	15.3	255	27.7
115	15.6	260	28.3
120	16.0	265	28.9
125	16.3	270	29.4
130	16.6	275	30.0
135	17.0	280	30.7
140	17.3	285	31.3
145	17.7	290	31.9
150	18.1	295	32.6
155	18.4	300	33.3
160	18.8	305	33.9
165	19.2	310	34.6
170	19.6	315	35.3
175	20.0	320	36.1
180	20.4	325	36.8
185	20.8	330	37.6
190	21.3	335	38.3
195	21.7	340	39.1
200	22.2	345	39.9
205	22.6	350	40.7
210	23.1	355	41.6
215	23.6	360	42.4
220	24.0		

*Values derived from formula in Law RG, MacRae KD. Head circumference as an index of fetal age. J Ultrasound Med 1982;1:281-288.

FL (Fig. 42-8 and Table 42-6). The transducer must be aligned to the long axis of the diaphysis; this can be ensured by demonstrating that both the femoral head or greater trochanter and the femoral condyle are simultaneously in the plane of section. The cursors should be positioned at the junction of the bone with the cartilage, and the thin, bright reflection of the cartilaginous epiphysis should not be included in the measurement.[29]

Abdominal Circumference

The fetal AC is the length of the outer perimeter of the fetal abdomen, measured on transverse scan at the level

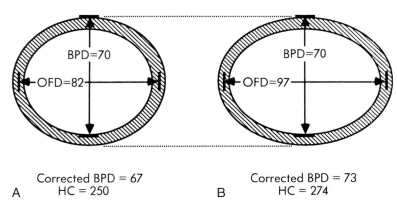

FIGURE 42-7. Effect of head shape on corrected-BPD and HC. Heads **A** and **B** have equal biparietal diameters *(BPD),* but **A** has a smaller occipitofrontal diameter *(OFD)* than **B.** Therefore the corrected-BPD and head circumference *(HC)* are smaller for **A** than **B.** Based on BPD, fetuses **A** and **B** would be assigned the same gestational age. Based on corrected-BPD or HC, however, fetus **A** would be assigned a lower gestational age than fetus **B.**

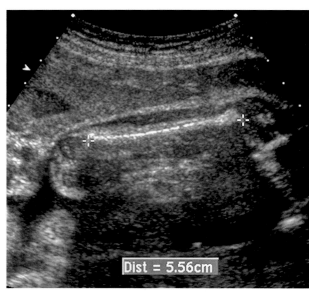

FIGURE 42-8. Femur length (FL) measurement. Electronic calipers measure the ossified diaphysis of the femur. Note how the bone is imaged close to parallel to the transducer, and the femur closest to the maternal abdominal wall is measured.

of the stomach and intrahepatic portion of the umbilical vein (Fig. 42-9). Alternatively, the AC may be calculated with equivalent results from two orthogonal **abdominal diameters** (AD_1, AD_2), one anteroposterior and the other transverse, measured on the same image, as follows[28,30]:

$$AC = 1.57 \times (AD_1 + AD_2)$$

Composite Formulas and Accuracy

Gestational age can be estimated from measurements of the head, abdomen, or femur by means of tables or formulas that present the mean value of each measurement for a given gestational age (see Tables 42-4 to 42-6). Composite age formulas that combine several fetal measurements can also be used to predict gestational age.[21,26]

TABLE 42-6. GESTATIONAL AGE ESTIMATION* BY FEMUR LENGTH (FL)

FL (mm)	GESTATIONAL AGE (weeks)	FL (mm)	GESTATIONAL AGE (weeks)
10	13.7	45	24.5
11	13.9	46	24.9
12	14.2	47	25.3
13	14.4	48	25.7
14	14.6	49	26.2
15	14.9	50	26.6
16	15.1	51	27.0
17	15.4	52	27.5
18	15.6	53	28.0
19	15.9	54	28.4
20	16.2	55	28.9
21	16.4	56	29.4
22	16.7	57	29.9
23	17.0	58	30.4
24	17.3	59	30.9
25	17.6	60	31.4
26	17.9	61	31.9
27	18.2	62	32.5
28	18.5	63	33.0
29	18.8	64	33.6
30	19.1	65	34.1
31	19.4	66	34.7
32	19.7	67	35.3
33	20.1	68	35.9
34	20.4	69	36.5
35	20.7	70	37.1
36	21.1	71	37.7
37	21.4	72	38.3
38	21.8	73	39.0
39	22.2	74	39.6
40	22.5	75	40.3
41	22.9	76	40.9
42	23.3	77	41.6
43	23.7	≥78	42.0
44	24.1		

*Values from Doubilet PM, Benson CB. Improved prediction of gestational age in the late third trimester. J Ultrasound Med 1993;12:647-653.

The accuracy of gestational age determination ranges from 1.2 weeks for the HC and corrected-BPD between 14 and 20 weeks, to 3.5 weeks in the late third trimester for the FL. As pregnancy progresses, each parameter becomes less accurate.[18,31,32] The two fetal

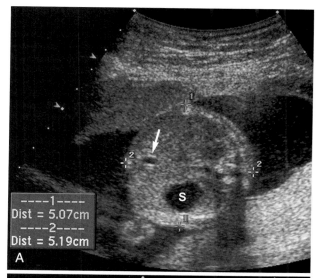

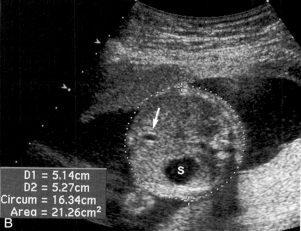

FIGURE 42-9. Abdominal diameter and circumference measurements. A and B, Axial views of the fetal abdomen at the level of the stomach *(S)* and intrahepatic portion of the umbilical vein *(arrow)*. On **A** the transverse *(calipers 1)* and anteroposterior *(calipers 2)* diameters have been measured with electronic calipers. On **B** the circumference of the abdomen has been traced electronically *(calipers and tracing dots)*.

head measurements that take head shape into account, corrected-BPD and HC, are equivalent in accuracy and more accurate than the BPD throughout gestation. In the second trimester, corrected-BPD and HC are the best predictors of gestational age. In the third trimester, these two head measurements, the FL, and the composite age formulas all predict gestational age with comparable accuracy.[18,32,33]

Composite age formulas use two or more measurements in conjunction to estimate gestational age. A potential disadvantage of using such formulas is that an abnormal measurement or anomaly might be obscured. For example, in a fetus with a skeletal dysplasia manifested by shortened long bones and a normal head size, the gestational age based on the composite formula will be an underestimation, falling between that predicted by the corrected-BPD and that predicted by the short FL. As a result, the FL might not appear to be abnormally small when compared to this improperly calculated gestational age.

Assignment of Gestational Age

The recommended approach to gestational age assignment at the time of the first sonogram is presented in Table 42-7. In the second and third trimesters, the choice depends on which measurements are available, because two or more parameters may be equivalent in accuracy. In some cases, especially when the initial scan occurs late in pregnancy, the clinician must decide whether to use clinical or sonographic criteria to determine the gestational age. As a general rule, we recommend using ultrasound criteria up to 24 weeks of gestation and the LMP (if clearly recalled) thereafter.[34]

Because fetal measurements become progressively less accurate predictors of gestational age as pregnancy progresses,[34-36] the age assigned at the time of the first scan

TABLE 42-7. APPROACH TO GESTATIONAL AGE (GA) ASSIGNMENT BY ULTRASOUND ON INITIAL SCAN

STAGE OF PREGNANCY	BASIS FOR GA	TABLES	ACCURACY (weeks)*
	First Trimester		
Early (5-6 weeks)	Sonographic milestones	42-1	±0.5
Mid- to late (6-13 weeks)	CRL	42-2	±0.5
	Second Trimester		
If OFD measurable	BPDc or HC	42-3, 42-4	±1.2 (14-20 wk)
			±1.9 (20-26 wk)
If OFD not measurable	BPD or FL	42-3, 42-5	±1.4 (14-20 wk)
			±2.1-2.5 (20-26 wk)
	Third Trimester		
If OFD measurable	BPDc, HC, or FL	42-3, 42-4, 42-5	±±3.1-3.4 (26-32 wk)
			±±3.5-3.8 (32-42 wk)
If OFD not measurable	FL	42-5	±±3.1 (26-32 wk)
			±±3.5 (36-42 wk)

*Two standard deviations (2 SD), or 95% confidence interval (CI).
  CRL, Crown-rump length; *OFD*, occipitofrontal diameter; *BPD*, biparietal diameter; *BPDc*, corrected-BPD; *HC*, head circumference; *FL*, femur length.

should not be changed thereafter. The age at any time later in pregnancy should be based on the **initial sonographic study,** calculated by taking the gestational age assigned at the time of the first scan and adding the number of weeks that have elapsed since that scan. On subsequent examinations, standard fetal measurements (BPD, OFD, AC, and FL) should be obtained and should be compared to the normal standards for the gestational age, based on the initial sonogram, to determine whether the fetus is appropriate in size.

WEIGHT ESTIMATION AND ASSESSMENT

Estimation of Fetal Weight

Before the availability of ultrasound, manual examination of the maternal abdomen was the only approach that could be used to estimate fetal size. The physical examination, however, provides only a general approximation of fetal weight because the palpated dimensions of the uterus are affected by several factors other than fetal size, including amniotic fluid volume, placental bulk, presence of fibroids, and maternal obesity.

Sonographic measurements of fetal body parts provide a direct way of assessing fetal size. Numerous formulas have been published for estimating fetal weight from one or more of these fetal body measurements: head (BPD or HC), abdomen (AD or AC), and femur (FL).[37-46] Other measurements, such as thigh circumference, have been used as well.[46] Formulas that estimate fetal

weight using three-dimensional (3-D) sonography[47-49] and 3-D magnetic resonance imaging (MRI) have also been published.[50,51]

The accuracy of a weight prediction formula is determined by assessing how well the formula works in a group of fetuses scanned close to delivery. An important measure of a formula's performance is its 95% confidence range. If the 95% confidence range is ±18%, for example, the estimated weight will fall within 18% of the actual weight in 95% of cases, and the error will be greater than 18% in only 5% of cases. The narrower the confidence range, the more reliable is the formula.

Many published studies provide information that allows one to estimate this measure of a formula's accuracy[52,53] (Table 42-8). The following points are noteworthy:

- The accuracy of weight prediction formulas improves as the number of measured body parts increases up to three, achieving greatest accuracy when measurements of the head, abdomen, and femur are used. There is no apparent improvement by adding the thigh circumference as a fourth measurement,[54] and no proven benefit from using 3-D sonography or MRI.
- Even when based on measurements of the head, abdomen, and femur, sonographic weight prediction has a rather wide 95% confidence range of at least ±15%. Based on the abdomen and either the head or femur, the range is at least ±16%-18%. Precision is considerably worse when only the abdomen is used.

TABLE 42-8. ACCURACY OF FETAL WEIGHT PREDICTION FORMULAS

BODY PART(S) INCLUDED IN FORMULA	FORMULA*	95% CONFIDENCE RANGE (%)†
Abdomen	Campbell and Wilkin[37]	±17.1-23.8[43,52]
	Higginbottom et al.[38]	±23.8[43]
	Hadlock et al.[43]	±22.2[43]
	Vintzileos et al.[46]	±22.8[46]
Head and abdomen	Warsof et al.[39]	±17.4-21.2[39,43,57]
	Shepard et al.[40]	±18.2-18.3[40,52]
	Thurneau et al.[41]	±19.8[43]
	Jordaan[42]	±25.8[43]
	Hadlock et al.[43]	±18.2[43]
	Hadlock et al.[44]	±18.2[44]
	Birnholz[45]	±17.7[53]‡
	Vintzileos et al.[46]	±21.2[46]
Abdomen and femur	Hadlock et al.[43]	±16.4[43]
	Hadlock et al.[44]	±16.0[44]
Head, abdomen, and femur	Hadlock et al.[43]	±15.0-15.4[43]
	Hadlock et al.[44]	±14.8-15.0[44]
	Vintzileos et al.[46]	±17.6[46]
Head, abdomen, femur, and thigh	Vintzileos et al.[46]	±15.6-17.8[46]

*Study in which formula was developed.
†Computed as two standard deviations (2 SD) of the relative error, as reported in the study(ies) referenced, unless otherwise indicated.
‡Based on the fraction of cases in which the estimated weight falls within 10% of the actual weight.

- A number of factors have been studied to determine their effect on accuracy of weight prediction. Accuracy appears to be worse in fetuses that weigh under 1000 grams than in larger fetuses.[53] Over the rest of the birth weight range, however, accuracy is fairly constant.[43,44,52,55] Weight prediction is less accurate in diabetic than in nondiabetic mothers. In diabetic mothers, formulas that use measurements of the head, abdomen, and femur have a 95% confidence range of ±24%,[56] wider than the range of ±15% in the general population.[43,44] The presence of oligohydramnios or polyhydramnios has no impact on accuracy.[41,53,57] Scan quality may have an effect on accuracy. Studies have shown a trend toward greater accuracy in scans that were rated "good" compared with those rated "poor" based on ability to visualize anatomic landmarks.[53,58]

Recommended Approach

An attempt should be made to image all three key fetal anatomic regions—head, abdomen, and femur—at the appropriate anatomic levels (Table 42-9). If measurements of all three structures can be obtained, Formula 1 in Table 42-9 should be used to estimate fetal weight. This formula should be used with the corrected-BPD when the OFD is available, and with the BPD itself if not. An alternative approach, equally accurate but more cumbersome, would be to use Formula 1 when the OFD is unavailable, and a formula based on HC, AC, and FL when the OFD is available. If the abdomen and only the head or the femur can be appropriately imaged, Formula 2 or 3 should be used. If the abdomen cannot be measured, or both the head and femur cannot be measured, then a weight estimate should not be calculated. Using the approach outlined in Table 42-9, an accuracy of ±15%-18% can be achieved for weight estimation.

Weight Assessment in Relation to Gestational Age

When an ultrasound is performed in the third trimester, best estimates of gestational age and fetal weight should be established. The gestational age may be based on a prior ultrasound, clinical dating criteria, or current measurements; fetal weight is always calculated from current measurements. The two values should be cross-assessed to determine whether the fetus is appropriate in size for dates. This can be accomplished by using a table that provides norms of values for fetal weight as a function of gestational age (Table 42-10), several of which appear in the literature.[59-64]

As an example, suppose that an obstetric sonogram reveals the best estimated gestational age is **34 weeks.** According to Table 42-10, a weight of 2146 grams (g)

TABLE 42-9. APPROACH TO FETAL WEIGHT ESTIMATION

BODY PARTS IMAGED	FORMULA USED FOR WEIGHT ESTIMATE
Head, Abdomen, and Femur	
OFD measurable	Formula 1, using corrected-BPD in place of BPD
OFD not measurable	Formula 1
Head and Abdomen	
OFD measurable	Formula 2, using corrected-BPD in place of BPD
OFD not measurable	Formula 2
Abdomen and Femur	
—	Formula 3

Formula 1*

$$Log_{10}(EFW>) = 1.4787 - 0.003343 \ AC \times FL + 0.001837 \ BPD_2 + 0.0458 \ AC + 0.158 \ FL$$

Formula 2*

$$Log_{10}(EFW>) = 1.1134 + 0.05845 \ AC - 0.000604 \ AC^2 - 0.007365 \ BPD^2 + 0.00595 \ BPD \times AC + 0.1694 \ BPD$$

Formula 3*

$$Log_{10}(EFW) = 1.3598 + 0.051 \ AC + 0.1844 \ FL - 0.0037 \ AC \times FL$$

*Formulas from Hadlock FP, Harrist RB, Sharman RS, et al. Estimation of fetal weight with the use of head, body, and femur measurements: a prospective study. Am J Obstet Gynecol 1985;151:333-337.

EFW, Estimated fetal weight, in grams (g); *BPD,* biparietal diameter (cm); *AC,* abdominal circumference (cm); *FL,* femur length (cm); *OFD,* occipitofrontal diameter (cm).

TABLE 42-10. FETAL WEIGHT PERCENTILES IN THE THIRD TRIMESTER

GESTATIONAL AGE (weeks)	Weight Percentiles (Grams)		
	10th	**50th**	**90th**
25	490	660	889
26	568	760	1016
27	660	875	1160
28	765	1005	1322
29	884	1153	1504
30	1020	1319	1706
31	1171	1502	1928
32	1338	1702	2167
33	1519	1918	2421
34	1714	2146	2687
35	1919	2383	2959
36	2129	2622	3230
37	2340	2859	3493
38	2544	3083	3736
39	2735	3288	3952
40	2904	3462	4127
41	3042	3597	4254
42	3142	3685	4322
43	3195	3717	4324

From Doubilet PM, Benson CB, Nadel AS, Ringer SA. Improved birth weight table for neonates developed from gestations dated by early ultrasonography. J Ultrasound Med 1997;16:241-249.

corresponds to the 50th percentile, and weights of 1714 g and 2687 g correspond to the 10th and 90th percentiles, respectively. A weight between the 10th and 90th percentiles is generally considered to be "appropriate for gestational age." When the estimated weight falls outside this range, the diagnosis of a small-for-gestational-age or large-for-gestational-age fetus is suggested.

When fetal weight is estimated on a third-trimester sonogram and a weight percentile is determined, correct interpretation of that percentile should take into account how weight percentile tables are derived. Such tables are, of necessity, derived from birth weights of neonates, versus estimated weights of fetuses, because only neonatal weights are known. For example, the mean and standard deviation of weight at 27 weeks' gestation is determined from data on birth weights of babies born at 27 weeks' gestation. It is important to note that several studies have shown that small fetuses have an increased likelihood of early delivery, so neonates born at 27 weeks' gestation are, on average, smaller than fetuses remaining in utero at that gestational age.[65-67] It follows that more than 50% of 27-week fetuses will have an estimated weight above the 50th percentile, and fewer than 10% will fall below the 10th percentile.

The weight gain between two ultrasound examinations can be estimated as the difference between the two estimated weights. Adequacy of weight gain can be assessed by comparing this difference to established normal fetal growth rate as a function of gestational age. Brenner's data indicate that median fetal weight gain per week increases progressively until 36 weeks of gestation, reaching a maximum rate of 220 grams per week.[59,60] After 36 weeks, the rate of weight gain steadily decreases in the normal fetus. The longer the time between scans, the more accurate is the sonographic estimate of interval weight gain. When two scans are performed within 1 week of each other, weight gain cannot be determined reliably, so there is little or no value in computing an estimated weight at the time of the second scan.

When several examinations have been performed, fetal growth can be depicted graphically by means of a trend plot, or growth curve. One form of growth curve plots the **estimated fetal weight versus gestational age,** with the curve for the fetus being examined superimposed on lines depicting the 1st, 10th, 50th, 90th, and 99th percentiles (Fig. 42-10, *A*). An alternative mode of display plots the **estimated weight percentile versus gestational age** (Fig. 42-10, *B*). In this latter format, the graph for a normally growing fetus will be a horizontal line, indicating maintenance of a particular weight percentile throughout gestation. A downsloping line indicates a subnormal growth rate, and an upsloping line indicates accelerated growth.

Calculation of weight percentiles and plotting of growth curves is most easily accomplished by computer, using an obstetric ultrasound software package that performs these tasks.[68-70] Alternatively, similar results can be

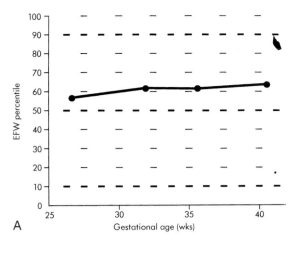

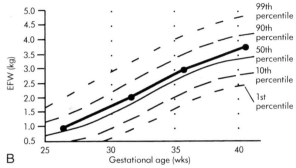

FIGURE 42-10. Fetal growth curves. A, Estimated fetal weight plotted against gestational age, superimposed on 1st, 10th, 50th, 90th, and 99th percentile curves. The fetus depicted here has a normal growth pattern, with estimated fetal weights between the 50th and 90th percentile over four sonograms. **B,** Estimated fetal weight *(EFW)* percentile against gestational age.

achieved by means of a calculator and manual plotting of data.

FETAL GROWTH ABNORMALITIES

The Large Fetus

The **large-for-gestational-age** (LGA) neonate (or fetus) is defined as one whose weight is above the 90th percentile for gestational age.[59,71-73] **Macrosomia,** a related entity, is most often defined on the basis of a weight above 4000 g; other weight cutoffs (4100 g, 4500 g) are sometimes used.[62,64-66] These growth disturbances occur with different frequencies and are associated with different morbidities and mortalities in diabetic mothers than in the general population. Therefore these two patient populations are considered separately.

General Population

About 10% of all infants have birth weights above the 90th percentile for gestational age and are considered

LGA infants. Of all newborns, 8% to 10% have birth weights over 4000 g and thus are classified as "macrosomic," and 2% weigh over 4500 g.[72,74-76] Risk factors for LGA and macrosomia include maternal obesity, diabetes, history of a previous LGA infant, prolonged pregnancy (>40 weeks), excess pregnancy weight gain, multiparity, and advanced maternal age.[71,72,74,77-79]

Large fetuses have an increased incidence of perinatal morbidity and mortality, in large part because of obstetric complications. Shoulder dystocia, fractures, and facial and brachial plexus palsies occur more frequently as a result of traumatic delivery.[77,80,81] The incidence of perinatal asphyxia, meconium aspiration, neonatal hypoglycemia, and other metabolic complications is significantly increased in these pregnancies.[71,74,77]

The most straightforward approach to diagnosing LGA and macrosomia is to use the estimated fetal weight computed from sonographic measurements. An estimated weight above the 90th percentile for gestational age suggests LGA, and a weight estimate above 4000 g suggests macrosomia. Although weight estimation is less accurate in large than in average-sized fetuses,[52,82-84] this approach has been demonstrated to be moderately good for diagnosing LGA and macrosomia. It has a **positive predictive value** (PPV) of up to 51% for LGA and 67% for macrosomia. Other proposed sonographic parameters have lower sensitivity or lower PPV than the estimated fetal weight[52,71,82,85-90] (Table 42-11).

Diabetic Mothers

Fetuses of insulin-dependent and gestational diabetic mothers are exposed to high levels of glucose throughout pregnancy and, as a result, produce excess insulin. This leads to overgrowth of the fetal trunk and abdominal organs, while the head and brain grow at a normal rate.[72,74] Therefore, these fetuses tend to have different body proportions than fetuses of nondiabetic mothers. Sonographic measurements of fetuses of diabetic mothers demonstrate accelerated growth of the fetal thorax and abdomen beginning between 28 and 32 weeks' gestation.[72,73,91]

An LGA weight occurs in 25% to 42% and macrosomia in 10% to 50% of infants of diabetic mothers (IDMs).[72,73,92] As many as 12% of IDMs weigh more than 4500 g at birth. Perinatal complications are more frequent in macrosomic fetuses of diabetic mothers than in those of nondiabetic mothers.[76,80,81,93,94] Shoulder dystocia, for example, occurs in 31% of macrosomic fetuses of diabetic mothers and only 3% to 10% of macrosomic fetuses of nondiabetic mothers.[77,80]

Many sonographic parameters, involving a variety of measurements, formulas, and ratios, have been proposed for diagnosing LGA and macrosomia in the fetus of the diabetic mother[85,95-97] (Table 42-12). As a group, these have higher sensitivities and PPVs than sonographic criteria in the general population, in part because of the higher prevalence of large fetuses in diabetic mothers.

As in the general population, the most straightforward approach to diagnosing LGA and macrosomia in the fetuses of diabetic mothers is by means of the sonographically estimated fetal weight.[56,85,95,98,99] A fetus whose estimated weight falls above the 90th percentile for gestational age has a 74% likelihood of being LGA, versus 19% if the estimated weight lies below the 90th percentile.[95] A weight estimate above 4000 g is associated with a 77% chance of macrosomia, and one above 4500 g with an 86% chance. The chance of macrosomia

---

TABLE 42-11. SONOGRAPHIC CRITERIA FOR LARGE-FOR-GESTATIONAL AGE (LGA) AND MACROSOMIA IN THE GENERAL POPULATION: PERFORMANCE CHARACTERISTICS

	(%)		Predictive Values (%)*	
	SENSITIVITY	**SPECIFICITY**	**POSITIVE**	**NEGATIVE**
Criteria to Predict LGA*				
Elevated AD-BPD[86]	46	79	19	93
Low FL/AC[71,86]	24-75	44-93	13-26	92-94
Elevated AFV[87,88]	12-17	92-98	19-35	91
Elevated ponderal index[71,86]	13-15	85-98	13-36	91-94
High EFW[71,88]	20-74	93-96	6-51	88-94
Elevated growth score[71]	14	91	10	90
Elevated AFV, high EFW[88]	11	99	54	99
Criteria to Predict Macrosomia				
Elevated FL[89]	24	96	52	88
Elevated AC[89]	53	94	63	89
High EFW[53,84,89]	11-65	89-96	38-67	83-91
Elevated BPD[89]	29	98	71	92

From Doubilet PM, Benson CB. Fetal growth disturbances. Semin Roentgenol 1990;25:309-316.
*Predictive values for criteria for LGA computed using Bayes' theorem,[112] assuming an LGA prevalence rate of 10%.
AD, Abdominal diameter; *BPD*, biparietal diameter; *FL/AC*, femur length/abdominal circumference ratio; *AFV*, amniotic fluid volume; *EFW*, estimated fetal weight; *FL*, femur length; *AC*, abdominal circumference.

TABLE 42-12. SONOGRAPHIC CRITERIA FOR LARGE-FOR-GESTATIONAL AGE (LGA) AND MACROSOMIA IN DIABETIC MOTHERS: PERFORMANCE CHARACTERISTICS

	(%)		Predictive Values (%)	
	SENSITIVITY	SPECIFICITY	POSITIVE	NEGATIVE
Criteria to Predict LGA*				
Elevated HC[95]	50	80	64	70
Elevated AC/BPD[96]	83	60	71	75
High EFW[95]	78	78	74	81
Elevated BPD[95]	13	86	75	57
Elevated AC[73,93,95]	71-88	81-85	56-78	81-96
Elevated AC growth[73]	84	85	79	89
Low FL/AC[73,96]	58-79	75-80	68-83	75-76
Elevated AC, high EFW[95]	72	71	89	89
Criteria to Predict Macrosomia				
Elevated AC[93]	84	78	41	96
Low FL/AC[97]	48-64	60-74	36-42	80-83
Elevated TD-BPD[92]	87	72	61	92
High EFW[56]	48	95	77	84

From Doublet PM, Benson CB. Fetal growth disturbances. Semin Roentgenol 1990;25:309-16.

*Predicted values for criteria for LGA computed using Bayes' theorem,[112] assuming an LGA prevalence rate of 10%.

HC, Head circumference; *AC/BPD*, abdominal circumference/biparietal diameter ratio; *EFW*, estimated fetal weight; *FL/AC*, femur length/abdominal circumference ratio; *TD*, thoracic diameter.

is only 16% when the weight estimate is less than 4000 g.[56] It follows that if vaginal delivery is believed to be contraindicated for the macrosomic fetuses of diabetic mothers, the estimated fetal weight should be considered when selecting the route of delivery.

Intrauterine Growth Restriction

Intrauterine growth restriction (IUGR) is a fetal growth disorder most often defined on the basis of a weight below the 10th percentile for gestational age.[100-104] This disorder is sometimes termed **small for gestational age** (SGA); however, it should be recognized that some authors use the term SGA to describe fetuses measuring less than the 10th percentile that are constitutionally small, and differentiate these from fetuses with abnormal growth restriction.

Most cases of growth restriction are caused by placental insufficiency, either primary or secondary to a maternal etiology such as hypertension, collagen vascular disease, poor nutrition, or substance abuse. IUGR may also result from a chromosomal anomaly (e.g., trisomy 18) or intrauterine infection (e.g., cytomegalovirus).[101,104-106]

In many cases, the specific cause of IUGR cannot be determined prenatally. As a group, regardless of the etiology, growth-restricted fetuses have a poor prognosis, with increased perinatal morbidity and mortality. Their mortality rate is four to eight times that of non-IUGR fetuses.[105,106] One half of surviving growth-restricted infants have serious short-term or long-term morbidity, including meconium aspiration, pneumonia, and metabolic disorders.[104,105,107,108]

Intrauterine growth restriction has been categorized as symmetrical or asymmetrical. Fetuses with **symmetrical** IUGR are proportionately reduced in size, whereas in **asymmetrical** IUGR the fetal abdomen is disproportionately small in relation to the head and limbs. There is considerable overlap between these two groups, however, so this categorization is probably not useful clinically.[109]

Numerous sonographic parameters, using both conventional and Doppler ultrasound, have been proposed for antenatal diagnosis of IUGR.[110,111] To be clinically useful for diagnosis, a criterion must detect a substantial fraction of cases of growth restriction (i.e., its sensitivity must be high), and a positive result must be associated with a high likelihood of IUGR (i.e., its PPV must be high). Similarly, to be valuable for excluding IUGR, a criterion must have high specificity and high **negative predictive value** (NPV).[112]

The performance characteristics of conventional sonographic criteria for IUGR are presented in Table 42-13, listed in order of increasing PPV.[110] The best criterion is the HC/AC ratio, with a PPV of 62%. Even when based on this criterion, IUGR cannot be diagnosed with confidence because more than one third (38%) of fetuses with an abnormal HC/AC ratio will not be growth restricted. Other parameters have even lower PPV, with seven of the nine parameters listed having PPV under 50%.

Doppler became readily available for clinical use in the mid-1980s. Early studies evaluated the use of Doppler to diagnose IUGR. In particular, Doppler was used to assess blood flow in the fetoplacental or uteroplacental circulations, both of which are essential for fetal

FETAL AND PLACENTAL RISK FACTORS ASSOCIATED WITH FETAL GROWTH RESTRICTION

FETAL FACTORS
Chromosomal Abnormalities
Trisomy 13, 18, 21
Monosomy (45,XO)
Deletions
Uniparental disomy
Confined placental mosaicism

Congenital Malformations
Absence of fetal pancreas
Anencephaly
Diaphragmatic hernia
Omphalocele
Gastroschisis
Renal agenesis/dysplasia
Multiple malformations

Multiple Gestations
Monochorionic twins
One fetus with malformations
Twin-to-twin transfusion
Discordant twins
Triplets

PLACENTAL FACTORS
Abnormal trophoblastic invasion
Multiple placental infarctions (chronic abruption)
Umbilical-placental vascular anomalies
Abnormal cord insertion (velamentous cord insertion)
Placenta previa
Circumvallate placenta
Chorioangiomata

From Lin CC, Santolaya-Forgas J. Current concepts of fetal growth restriction. Obstet Gynecol 1998;92:1044-1055.

MATERNAL RISK FACTORS ASSOCIATED WITH FETAL GROWTH RESTRICTION

Genetic/Constitutional
Nutrition/Starvation
Inflammatory bowel disease
Ileojejunal bypass
Chronic pancreatitis
Low prepregnancy weight
Poor pregnancy weight gain, second and third trimesters

Hypoxic
Severe lung disease
Cyanotic heart disease
Sickle cell anemia

Vascular
Chronic hypertension
Preeclampsia
Collagen vascular disease
Type 1 diabetes mellitus

Renal
Glomerulonephritis
Lipoid nephritis
Arteriolar nephrosclerosis
Renal transplantation

Antiphospholipid Antibodies
Environment and Drugs
High altitude
Emotional stress
Physical stress
Cigarette smoking
Alcohol abuse
Substance abuse (heroin, cocaine)
Therapeutic drugs
Antimetabolites
Anticonvulsants
Anticoagulants

Poor Obstetric History
Previous stillbirths
Recurrent aborters
Previous birth of growth-restricted fetus
Previous preterm births

From Lin CC, Santolaya-Forgas J. Current concepts of fetal growth restriction. Obstet Gynecol 1998;92:1044-1055.

nourishment and oxygenation, to determine if Doppler criteria were useful for predicting fetal growth restriction. These criteria, however, were found to be poor predictors of IUGR.[111,113,114]

More recent studies of Doppler ultrasound, however, have shown that it can play a useful role in determining the prognosis of fetuses with IUGR.[115-119] In growth-restricted fetuses, **reversed diastolic flow** in the umbilical artery carries a very poor prognosis, an elevated risk of fetal demise. They often die if not delivered soon. An **absent diastolic flow** or an **elevated systolic/diastolic ratio** is associated with poor prognosis, including increased likelihood of fetal distress in labor, admission to the intensive care unit, and perinatal mortality.[116-118,120-125]

Although no single criterion permits confident diagnosis of IUGR, the following three key parameters can be used in combination to establish the diagnosis with greater certainty[126]:

- Estimated fetal weight
- Amniotic fluid volume
- Maternal blood pressure status (normal vs. hypertensive)

Other proposed parameters for diagnosing IUGR can be safely ignored because they add no significant information.[127,128]

The three key parameters can be combined into an **IUGR score** or a table that permits the confident diagnosis or exclusion of growth restriction in most cases[126,127]

TABLE 42-13. CONVENTIONAL SONOGRAPHIC CRITERIA FOR INTRAUTERINE GROWTH RESTRICTION (IUGR): PERFORMANCE CHARACTERISTICS

CRITERION†	(%)		Predictive Values (%)*	
	SENSITIVITY	SPECIFICITY	POSITIVE (PPV)	NEGATIVE (NPV)
Advanced placental grade	62	64	16	94
Elevated FL/AC	34-49	78-83	18-20	92-93
Low TIUV	57-80	72-76	21-24	92-97
Small BPD	24-88	62-94	21-44	92-98
Small BPD and advanced placental grade	59	86	32	95
Slow rate of BPD growth	75	84	35	97
Low EFW	89	88	45	99
Decreased AFV	24	98	55	92
Elevated HC/AC	82	94	62	98

From Benson CB, Doubilet PM, Saltzman DH. Intrauterine growth retardation: predictive value of ultrasound criteria for antenatal diagnosis. Radiology 1986;160:415-417.
*Computed using Bayes' theorem,[112] assuming an IUGR prevalence rate of 10%.
†A range of values is given for a criterion when different studies apply that criterion in two or more ways.
FL/AC, Femur length/abdominal circumference ratio; *TIUV*, total intrauterine volume; *BPD*, biparietal diameter; *EFW*, estimated fetal weight; *AFV*, amniotic fluid volume; *HC/AC*, head circumference/abdominal circumference ratio.

TABLE 42-14. CRITICAL VALUES* FOR ESTIMATED FETAL WEIGHT (IN GRAMS) FOR DIAGNOSING OR EXCLUDING INTRAUTERINE GROWTH RESTRICTION

GA WK	Status of Maternal Blood Pressure and Amniotic Fluid Volume					
	NL BP NL/POLY	NL BP M-M OLIGO	NL BP SEV OLIGO	HTN NL/POLY	HTN M-M OLIGO	HTN SEV OLIGO
26	516-660	646-826	743-950	610-780	763-976	878-1123
27	597-761	745-949	855-1090	704-898	878-1119	1009-1285
28	693-877	859-1087	982-1244	813-1030	1008-1276	1153-1460
29	803-1008	988-1239	1124-1410	937-1176	1152-1446	1312-1646
30	931-1155	1132-1405	1281-1589	1078-1337	1311-1627	1483-1840
31	1075-1317	1293-1584	1452-1779	1234-1512	1484-1819	1667-2042
32	1235-1493	1468-1774	1635-1976	1405-1698	1670-2018	1860-2248
33	1411-1682	1656-1973	1830-2180	1590-1895	1865-2223	2061-2456
34	1600-1880	1853-2177	2031-2386	1785-2098	2067-2429	2266-2662
35	1798-2083	2055-2382	2236-2590	1987-2302	2272-2633	2471-2863
36	1997-2285	2257-2583	2437-2789	2189-2504	2474-2830	2671-3056
37	2192-2479	2452-2774	2631-2976	2383-2696	2666-3016	2861-3236
38	2371-2658	2631-2949	2807-3147	2563-2872	2843-3186	3034-3400
39	2526-2812	2785-3101	2961-3296	2717-3025	2996-3335	3185-3545
40	2645-2933	2906-3223	3083-3419	2838-3147	3118-3458	3307-3668
41	2717-3013	2985-3310	3166-3511	2915-3232	3202-3551	3396-3766
42	2736-3045	3016-3356	3205-3567	2942-3274	3243-3609	3447-3836

From Benson CB, Belville JS, Lentini JF, et al. Intrauterine growth retardation: diagnosis based on multiple parameters: a prospective study. Radiology 1990;177:499-502.
*For each pair, estimated weight less than the lower value allows confident diagnosis of intrauterine growth restriction (IUGR; positive predictive value, 74%). Estimated weight greater than the upper value virtually excludes IUGR (negative predictive value, 97%). Estimated weight between the two values is indeterminate for IUGR (likelihood of IUGR, 13%).
GA, Gestational age; *Nl BP*, normal blood pressure; *Htn*, hypertension; *Nl*, normal fluid; *Poly*, polyhydramnios; *M-M*, mild to moderate; *Oligo*, oligohydramnios; *Sev*, severe.

(Table 42-14). For any gestational age, amniotic fluid volume (subjectively assessed), and maternal blood pressure status, the table presents two values. When a fetus has an estimated weight below the smaller value, IUGR can be diagnosed with confidence. If the estimated weight is above the larger value, growth restriction can be excluded with near certainty. An estimated weight between the two values is indeterminate for IUGR.

When accurate dating by an ultrasound performed before 20 weeks' gestation is available, a simpler rule applies, using only the lower value in the appropriate column. IUGR can be diagnosed if the estimated fetal weight falls below this value and can be excluded if the weight estimate falls above this same value.

To illustrate the use of this table in the diagnosis of IUGR, consider a case in which the gestational age is 34 weeks (based on a 24-week ultrasound), there is moderate oligohydramnios, and the mother is normotensive. On the basis of Table 42-14, if the estimated fetal weight is below 1853 g, IUGR can be diagnosed with confidence, and if it is above 2177 g, growth restriction can be ruled out. A weight estimate between these two values is indeterminate for IUGR. If the age of 34 weeks had been based on a 12-week ultrasound, IUGR could be diagnosed if the estimated weight was below 1853 g and excluded if the weight estimate was above 1853 g. Table 42-14 provides a rational and reliable means for prenatal diagnosis of IUGR. When growth restriction is diagnosed, further evaluation using Doppler velocimetry can help to determine the prognosis.[129]

Once IUGR has been diagnosed, an attempt should be made to determine its etiology, through evaluation of both the mother and the fetus. Maternal assessment should include physical examination and blood tests, directed toward diagnosis of **hypertension, renal disease,** and other maternal conditions that can cause IUGR. Fetal assessment begins with a careful sonographic examination, looking especially for findings suggestive of a **chromosomal** or **viral** etiology (e.g., holoprosencephaly, clenched hands, rocker-bottom feet, intracranial calcifications). If such a finding is present, amniocentesis or umbilical blood sampling can confirm the diagnosis of a chromosomal abnormality. A viral etiology of IUGR may also be diagnosed by these procedures, in some cases.[128]

Growth-restricted fetuses, other than those with a lethal condition such as **trisomy 13 or 18**, should be carefully monitored for the remainder of the pregnancy. The monitoring is usually performed at weekly or semiweekly intervals. Sonographic features to be followed include **amniotic fluid volume, biophysical profile score, estimated fetal weight percentile,** and **umbilical artery Doppler assessment** (see Chapter 43). A worsening trend in one or more of these features should prompt consideration of early delivery.

References

1. Filly RA, Golbus MS, Carey JC, Hall JG. Short-limbed dwarfism: ultrasonographic diagnosis by mensuration of fetal femoral length. Radiology 1981;138:653-656.
2. Chervenak FA, Rosenberg J, Brightman RC, et al. A prospective study of the accuracy of ultrasound in predicting fetal microcephaly. Obstet Gynecol 1987;69:908-910.
3. Bowerman RA. Sonography of fetal midgut herniation: normal size criteria and correlation with crown-rump length. J Ultrasound Med 1993;12:251-254.
4. Wald NJ, Cuckle HS, Densem JW, et al. Maternal serum screening for Down's syndrome in early pregnancy. BMJ 1988;297:883-887.
5. Osathanondh R, Canick JA, Abell KB, et al. Second trimester screening for trisomy 21. Lancet 1989;2:52.
6. Canick JA, Knight GJ, Palomaki GE, et al. Low second trimester maternal serum unconjugated oestriol in pregnancies with Down's syndrome. Br J Obstet Gynaecol 1988;95:330-333.
7. American Institute of Ultrasound in Medicine. Guidelines for performance of the antepartum obstetrical ultrasound examination. 1994.

Gestational Age Determination

8. Campbell S, Warsof SL, Little D, Cooper DJ. Routine ultrasound screening for the prediction of gestational age. Obstet Gynecol 1985; 65:613-620.
9. Bradley WG, Fiske CE, Filly RA. The double sac sign of early intrauterine pregnancy: use in exclusion of ectopic pregnancy. Radiology 1982;143:223-226.
10. Fossum GT, Davajan V, Kletzky OA. Early detection of pregnancy with transvaginal ultrasound. Fertil Steril 1988;49:788-791.
11. Bree RL, Edwards M, Bohm-Velez M, et al. Transvaginal sonography in the evaluation of normal early pregnancy: correlation with HCG level. AJR Am J Roentgenol 1989;153:75-79.
12. Daya S, Woods S, Ward S, et al. Early pregnancy assessment with transvaginal ultrasound scanning. CMAJ 1991;144:441-446.
13. Jain KA, Hamper UM, Sanders RC. Comparison of transvaginal and transabdominal sonography in the detection of early pregnancy and its complications. AJR Am J Roentgenol 1988;151:1139-1143.
14. Robinson HP, Fleming JE. A critical evaluation of sonar "crown-rump length" measurements. Br J Obstet Gynaecol 1975;82:702-710.
15. MacGregor SN, Tamura RK, Sabbagha RE, et al. Underestimation of gestational age by conventional crown-rump length dating curves. Obstet Gynecol 1987;70:344-348.
16. Moore KL, Persaud TVN. The developing human: clinically oriented embryology. 5th ed. Philadelphia: Saunders; 1993.
17. Kurtz AB, Wapner RJ, Kurtz RJ, et al. Analysis of biparietal diameter as an accurate indicator of gestational age. J Clin Ultrasound 1980; 8:319-326.
18. Doubilet PM, Benson CB. Improved prediction of gestational age in the late third trimester. J Ultrasound Med 1993;12:647-653.
19. Law RG, MacRae KD. Head circumference as an index of fetal age. J Ultrasound Med 1982;1:281-288.
20. Hadlock FP, Deter RL, Harrist RB, Park SK. Fetal abdominal circumference as a predictor of menstrual age. AJR Am J Roentgenol 1982;139:367-370.
21. Hadlock FP, Deter RL, Harrist RB, Park SK. Estimating fetal age: computer-assisted analysis of multiple fetal growth parameters. Radiology 1984;152:497-501.
22. Jeanty P, Rodesch F, Delbeke D, Dumont JE. Estimation of gestational age from measurements of fetal long bones. J Ultrasound Med 1984;3:75-79.
23. Honarvar M, Allahyari M, Dehbashi S. Assessment of gestational age based on ultrasonic femur length after the first trimester: a simple mathematical correlation between gestational age (GA) and femur length (FL). Int J Gynaecol Obstet 2000;70:335-340.
24. Jeanty P, Cantraine F, Cousaert E, et al. The binocular distance: a new way to estimate fetal age. J Ultrasound Med 1984;3:241-243.
25. Doubilet PM, Greenes RA. Improved prediction of gestational age from fetal head measurements. AJR Am J Roentgenol 1984;142: 797-800.
26. Hadlock FP, Deter RL, Harrist RB, Park SK. Computer assisted analysis of fetal age in the third trimester using multiple fetal growth parameters. J Clin Ultrasound 1983;11:313-316.
27. Hadlock FP, Deter RL, Harrist RB, Park SK. Fetal biparietal diameter: rational choice of plane of section for sonographic measurement. AJR Am J Roentgenol 1982;138:871-874.
28. Hadlock FP, Kent WR, Loyd JL, et al. An evaluation of two methods for measuring fetal head and body circumferences. J Ultrasound Med 1982;1:359-360.
29. Goldstein RB, Filly RA, Simpson G. Pitfalls in femur length measurements. J Ultrasound Med 1987;6:203-207.
30. Smulian JC, Ranzini AC, Ananth CV, et al. Comparison of three sonographic circumference measurement techniques to predict birth weight. Obstet Gynecol 1999;93:692-696.
31. Guihard-Costa AM, Droulle P, Thiebaugeorges O, Hascoet JM. A longitudinal study of fetal growth variability. Biol Neonate 2000; 78:8-12.
32. Benson CB, Doubilet PM. Fetal measurements for predicting gestational age in the second and third trimesters: a reappraisal with a more reliable gold standard. Radiology 1988;169(P):210.
33. Johnsen SL, Rasmussen S, Sollien R, Kiserud T. Fetal age assessment based on femur length at 10-25 weeks of gestation, and reference ranges for femur length to head circumference ratios. Acta Obstet Gynecol Scand 2005;84:725-733.
34. Verburg BO, Steegers EA, De Ridder M, et al. New charts for ultrasound dating of pregnancy and assessment of fetal growth: longitudinal data from a population-based cohort study. Ultrasound Obstet Gynecol 2008;31:388-396.
35. Caughey AB, Nicholson JM, Washington AE. First- vs second-trimester ultrasound: the effect on pregnancy dating and perinatal

outcomes. Am J Obstet Gynecol 2008;198:703 e1-e5; discussion e5-e6.

36. Kalish RB, Thaler HT, Chasen ST, et al. First- and second-trimester ultrasound assessment of gestational age. Am J Obstet Gynecol 2004;191:975-978.

Weight Estimation and Assessment

37. Campbell S, Wilkin D. Ultrasonic measurement of fetal abdomen circumference in the estimation of fetal weight. Br J Obstet Gynaecol 1975;82:689-697.

38. Higginbottom J, Slater J, Porter G, Whitfield CR. Estimation of fetal weight from ultrasonic measurement of trunk circumference. Br J Obstet Gynaecol 1975;82:698-701.

39. Warsof SL, Gohari P, Berkowitz RL, Hobbins JC. The estimation of fetal weight by computer-assisted analysis. Am J Obstet Gynecol 1977;128:881-892.

40. Shepard MJ, Richards VA, Berkowitz RL, et al. An evaluation of two equations for predicting fetal weight by ultrasound. Am J Obstet Gynecol 1982;142:47-54.

41. Thurneau GR, Tamura RK, Sabbagha R, et al. A simple estimated fetal weight equation based on real-time ultrasound measurements of fetuses less than thirty-four weeks' gestation. Am J Obstet Gynecol 1983;145:557-561.

42. Jordaan HV. Estimation of fetal weight by ultrasound. J Clin Ultrasound 1983;11:59-66.

43. Hadlock FP, Harrist RB, Carpenter RJ, et al. Sonographic estimation of fetal weight: the value of femur length in addition to head and abdomen measurements. Radiology 1984;150:535-540.

44. Hadlock FP, Harrist RB, Sharman RS, et al. Estimation of fetal weight with the use of head, body, and femur measurements: a prospective study. Am J Obstet Gynecol 1985;151:333-337.

45. Birnholz JC. An algorithmic approach to accurate ultrasonic fetal weight estimation. Invest Radiol 1986;21:571-576.

46. Vintzileos AM, Campbell WA, Rodis JF, et al. Fetal weight estimation formulas with head, abdominal, femur, and thigh circumference measurements. Am J Obstet Gynecol 1987;157:410-414.

47. Lee W, Deter RL, Ebersole JD, et al. Birth weight prediction by three-dimensional ultrasonography: fractional limb volume. J Ultrasound Med 2001;20:1283-1292.

48. Song TB, Moore TR, Lee JI, et al. Fetal weight prediction by thigh volume measurement with three-dimensional ultrasonography. Obstet Gynecol 2000;96:157-161.

49. Schild RL, Fimmers R, Hansmann M. Fetal weight estimation by three-dimensional ultrasound. Ultrasound Obstet Gynecol 2000;16:445-452.

50. Uotila J, Dastidar P, Heinonen T, et al. Magnetic resonance imaging compared to ultrasonography in fetal weight and volume estimation in diabetic and normal pregnancy. Acta Obstet Gynecol Scand 2000;79:255-259.

51. Hatab MR, Zaretsky MV, Alexander JM, Twickler DM. Comparison of fetal biometric values with sonographic and 3D reconstruction MRI in term gestations. AJR Am J Roentgenol 2008;191:340-345.

52. Benacerraf BR, Gelman R, Frigoletto Jr FD. Sonographically estimated fetal weights: accuracy and limitation. Am J Obstet Gynecol 1988;159:1118-1121.

53. Townsend RR, Filly RA, Callen PW, Laros RK. Factors affecting prenatal sonographic estimation of weight in extremely low birth-weight infants. J Ultrasound Med 1988;7:183-187.

54. Scioscia M, Scioscia F, Vimercati A, et al. Estimation of fetal weight by measurement of fetal thigh soft-tissue thickness in the late third trimester. Ultrasound Obstet Gynecol 2008;31:314-320.

55. Hill LM, Breckle R, Wolfgram KR, O'Brien PC. Evaluation of three methods for estimating fetal weight. J Clin Ultrasound 1986;14:171-178.

56. Benson CB, Doubilet PM, Saltzman DH. Sonographic determination of fetal weights in diabetic pregnancies. Am J Obstet Gynecol 1987;156:441-444.

57. Chauhan SP, Scardo JA, Hendrix NW, et al. Accuracy of sonographically estimated fetal weight with and without oligohydramnios: a case-control study. J Reprod Med 1999;44:969-973.

58. Pineau JC, Grange G, Kapitaniak B, et al. Estimation of fetal weight: accuracy of regression models versus accuracy of ultrasound data. Fetal Diagn Ther 2008;24:140-145.

59. Doubilet PM, Benson CB, Nadel AS, Ringer SA. Improved birth weight table for neonates developed from gestations dated by early ultrasonography. J Ultrasound Med 1997;16:241-249.

60. Brenner WE, Edelman DA, Hendricks CH. A standard of fetal growth for the United States of America. Am J Obstet Gynecol 1976;126:555-564.

61. Lubchenco LO, Hansman C, Dressler M, Boyd E. Intrauterine growth as estimated from liveborn birth-weight data at 24 to 42 weeks of gestation. Pediatrics 1963;32:793-800.

62. Gruenwald P. Growth of the human fetus. I. Normal growth and its variation. Am J Obstet Gynecol 1966;94:1112-1119.

63. Thomson AM, Billewicz WZ, Hytten FE. The assessment of fetal growth. J Obstet Gynaecol 1968;75:903-916.

64. Hutchins CJ. Delivery of the growth-retarded infant. Obstet Gynecol 1980;56:683-686.

65. Doubilet PM, Benson CB, Wilkins-Haug L, Ringer S. Fetuses subsequently born premature are smaller than gestational age-matched fetuses not born premature. J Ultrasound Med 2003;22:359-363.

66. Lysikiewicz A, Bracero LA, Tejani N. Sonographically estimated fetal weight percentile as a predictor of preterm delivery. J Matern Fetal Med 2001;10:44-47.

67. Mercer BM, Merlino AA, Milluzzi CJ, Moore JJ. Small fetal size before 20 weeks' gestation: associations with maternal tobacco use, early preterm birth, and low birthweight. Am J Obstet Gynecol 2008;198:673 e1-e7; discussion e7-e8.

68. Greenes RA. OBUS: a microcomputer system for measurement, calculation, reporting, and retrieval of obstetric ultrasound examinations. Radiology 1982;144:879-883.

69. Jeanty P. A simple reporting system for obstetrical ultrasonography. J Ultrasound Med 1985;4:591-593.

70. Ott WJ. The design and implementation of a computer-based ultrasound data system. J Ultrasound Med 1986;5:25-32.

Fetal Growth Abnormalities

71. Ott WJ. The diagnosis of altered fetal growth. Obstet Gynecol Clin North Am 1988;15:237-263.

72. Mintz MC, Landon MB. Sonographic diagnosis of fetal growth disorders. Clin Obstet Gynecol 1988;31:44-52.

73. Landon MB, Mintz MC, Gabbe SG. Sonographic evaluation of fetal abdominal growth: predictor of the large-for-gestational-age infant in pregnancies complicated by diabetes mellitus. Am J Obstet Gynecol 1989;160:115-121.

74. Boyd ME, Usher RH, McLean FH. Fetal macrosomia: prediction, risks, proposed management. Obstet Gynecol 1983;61:715-722.

75. Modanlou HD, Dorchester WL, Thorosian A, Freeman RK. Macrosomia: maternal, fetal, and neonatal implications. Obstet Gynecol 1980;55:420-424.

76. Deter RL, Hadlock FP. Use of ultrasound in the detection of macrosomia: a review. J Clin Ultrasound 1985;13:519-524.

77. Golditch IM, Kirkman K. The large fetus: management and outcome. Obstet Gynecol 1978;52:26-30.

78. Rodriguez MH. Ultrasound evaluation of the postdate pregnancy. Clin Obstet Gynecol 1989;32:257-261.

79. Arias F. Predictability of complications associated with prolongation of pregnancy. Obstet Gynecol 1987;70:101-106.

80. Acker DB, Sachs BP, Friedman EA. Risk factors for shoulder dystocia. Obstet Gynecol 1985;66:762-768.

81. Gross SJ, Shime J, Farine D. Shoulder dystocia: predictors and outcome—a five-year review. Am J Obstet Gynecol 1987;156:334-336.

82. Miller Jr JM, Korndorffer 3rd FA, Gabert HA. Fetal weight estimates in late pregnancy with emphasis on macrosomia. J Clin Ultrasound 1986;14:437-442.

83. Sabbagha RE, Minogue J, Tamura RK, Hungerford SA. Estimation of birth weight by use of ultrasonographic formulas targeted to large-, appropriate-, and small-for-gestational-age fetuses. Am J Obstet Gynecol 1989;160:854-860; discussion 860-862.

84. Miller Jr JM, Kissling GA, Brown HL, Gabert HA. Estimated fetal weight: applicability to small- and large-for-gestational-age fetus. J Clin Ultrasound 1988;16:95-97.

85. Doubilet PM, Benson CB. Fetal growth disturbances. Semin Roentgenol 1990;25:309-316.

86. Miller Jr JM, Korndorffer Jr FA, Kissling GE, et al. Recognition of the overgrown fetus: in utero ponderal indices. Am J Perinatol 1987;4:86-89.

87. Chamberlain PF, Manning FA, Morrison I, et al. Ultrasound evaluation of amniotic fluid volume. II. The relationship of increased amniotic fluid volume to perinatal outcome. Am J Obstet Gynecol 1984;150:250-254.

88. Benson CB, Doubilet PM. Amniotic fluid volume in the large-for-gestational-age fetus. Radiology 1989;173(P):248.
89. Miller Jr JM, Brown HL, Khawli OF, et al. Ultrasonographic identification of the macrosomic fetus. Am J Obstet Gynecol 1988;159:1110-1114.
90. Chauhan SP, West DJ, Scardo JA, et al. Antepartum detection of macrosomic fetus: clinical versus sonographic, including soft-tissue measurements. Obstet Gynecol 2000;95:639-642.
91. Basel D, Lederer R, Diamant YZ. Longitudinal ultrasonic biometry of various parameters in fetuses with abnormal growth rate. Acta Obstet Gynecol Scand 1987;66:143-149.
92. Elliott JP, Garite TJ, Freeman RK, et al. Ultrasonic prediction of fetal macrosomia in diabetic patients. Obstet Gynecol 1982;60:159-162.
93. Bochner CJ, Medearis AL, Williams 3rd J, et al. Early third-trimester ultrasound screening in gestational diabetes to determine the risk of macrosomia and labor dystocia at term. Am J Obstet Gynecol 1987;157:703-708.
94. Sandmire HF, O'Halloin TJ. Shoulder dystocia: its incidence and associated risk factors. Int J Gynaecol Obstet 1988;26:65-73.
95. Tamura RK, Sabbagha RE, Depp R, et al. Diabetic macrosomia: accuracy of third trimester ultrasound. Obstet Gynecol 1986;67:828-832.
96. Bracero LA, Baxi LV, Rey HR, Yeh MN. Use of ultrasound in antenatal diagnosis of large-for-gestational age infants in diabetic gravid patients. Am J Obstet Gynecol 1985;152:43-47.
97. Benson CB, Doubilet PM, Saltzman DH, et al. Femur length/abdominal circumference ratio: poor predictor of macrosomic fetuses in diabetic mothers. J Ultrasound Med 1986;5:141-144.
98. Combs CA, Rosenn B, Miodovnik M, Siddiqi TA. Sonographic EFW and macrosomia: is there an optimum formula to predict diabetic fetal macrosomia? J Matern Fetal Med 2000;9:55-61.
99. Colman A, Maharaj D, Hutton J, Tuohy J. Reliability of ultrasound estimation of fetal weight in term singleton pregnancies. NZ Med J 2006;119:U2146.
100. Lugo G, Cassady G. Intrauterine growth retardation: clinicopathologic findings in 233 consecutive infants. Am J Obstet Gynecol 1971;109:615-622.
101. Galbraith RS, Karchmar EJ, Piercy WN, Low JA. The clinical prediction of intrauterine growth retardation. Am J Obstet Gynecol 1979;133:281-286.
102. Divon MY, Chamberlain PF, Sipos L, et al. Identification of the small for gestational age fetus with the use of gestational age-independent indices of fetal growth. Am J Obstet Gynecol 1986;155:1197-1201.
103. Sabbagha RE. Intrauterine growth retardation avenues of future research in diagnosis and management by ultrasound. Semin Perinatol 1984;8:31-36.
104. Reed K, Droegmueller W. Intrauterine growth retardation. In: Centrullo CL, Sbarra AJ, editors. The problem-oriented medical record. New York: Plenum; 1984. p. 174-194.
105. Lockwood CJ, Weiner S. Assessment of fetal growth. Clin Perinatol 1986;13:3-35.
106. Lin CC, Santolaya-Forgas J. Current concepts of fetal growth restriction. Part I. Causes, classification, and pathophysiology. Obstet Gynecol 1998;92:1044-1055.
107. Seeds JW. Impaired fetal growth: definition and clinical diagnosis. Obstet Gynecol 1984;64:303-310.
108. Dobson PC, Abell DA, Beischer NA. Mortality and morbidity of fetal growth retardation. Aust NZ J Obstet Gynaecol 1981;21:69-72.
109. Benson CB, Doubilet PM. Head-sparing in fetuses with intrauterine growth retardation: does it really occur? Radiology 1986;161(P):75.
110. Benson CB, Doubilet PM, Saltzman DH. Intrauterine growth retardation: predictive value of ultrasound criteria for antenatal diagnosis. Radiology 1986;160:415-417.
111. Benson CB, Doubilet PM. Doppler criteria for intrauterine growth retardation: predictive values. J Ultrasound Med 1988;7:655-659.
112. Weinstein MC, Fineberg HV, Elstein AS, et al. Clinical decision analysis. Philadelphia: Saunders; 1980.
113. Ott WJ. Diagnosis of intrauterine growth restriction: comparison of ultrasound parameters. Am J Perinatol 2002;19:133-137.
114. Bahado-Singh RO, Kovanci E, Jeffres A, et al. The Doppler cerebroplacental ratio and perinatal outcome in intrauterine growth restriction. Am J Obstet Gynecol 1999;180:750-756.
115. McCowan LM, Erskine LA, Ritchie K. Umbilical artery Doppler blood flow studies in the preterm, small for gestational age fetus. Am J Obstet Gynecol 1987;156:655-659.
116. Reuwer PJ, Sijmons EA, Rietman GW, et al. Intrauterine growth retardation: prediction of perinatal distress by Doppler ultrasound. Lancet 1987;2:415-418.
117. Rochelson BL, Schulman H, Fleischer A, et al. The clinical significance of Doppler umbilical artery velocimetry in the small for gestational age fetus. Am J Obstet Gynecol 1987;156:1223-1226.
118. Berkowitz GS, Mehalek KE, Chitkara U, et al. Doppler umbilical velocimetry in the prediction of adverse outcome in pregnancies at risk for intrauterine growth retardation. Obstet Gynecol 1988;71:742-746.
119. Westergaard HB, Langhoff-Roos J, Lingman G, et al. A critical appraisal of the use of umbilical artery Doppler ultrasound in high-risk pregnancies: use of meta-analyses in evidence-based obstetrics. Ultrasound Obstet Gynecol 2001;17:466-476.
120. Illyes M, Gati I. Reverse flow in the human fetal descending aorta as a sign of severe fetal asphyxia preceding intrauterine death. J Clin Ultrasound 1988;16:403-407.
121. Brar HS, Platt LD. Reverse end-diastolic flow velocity on umbilical artery velocimetry in high-risk pregnancies: an ominous finding with adverse pregnancy outcome. Am J Obstet Gynecol 1988;159:559-561.
122. Woo JS, Liang ST, Lo RL. Significance of an absent or reversed end diastolic flow in Doppler umbilical artery waveforms. J Ultrasound Med 1987;6:291-297.
123. Trudinger BJ, Giles WB, Cook CM. Flow velocity waveforms in the maternal uteroplacental and fetal umbilical placental circulations. Am J Obstet Gynecol 1985;152:155-163.
124. Baschat AA, Gembruch U, Reiss I, et al. Relationship between arterial and venous Doppler and perinatal outcome in fetal growth restriction. Ultrasound Obstet Gynecol 2000;16:407-413.
125. Fong KW, Ohlsson A, Hannah ME, et al. Prediction of perinatal outcome in fetuses suspected to have intrauterine growth restriction: Doppler ultrasound study of fetal cerebral, renal, and umbilical arteries. Radiology 1999;213:681-689.
126. Benson CB, Boswell SB, Brown DL, et al. Improved prediction of intrauterine growth retardation with use of multiple parameters. Radiology 1988;168:7-12.
127. Benson CB, Belville JS, Lentini JF, et al. Intrauterine growth retardation: diagnosis based on multiple parameters: a prospective study. Radiology 1990;177:499-502.
128. Doubilet PM, Benson CB. Sonographic evaluation of intrauterine growth retardation. AJR Am J Roentgenol 1995;164:709-717.
129. Hecher K, Bilardo CM, Stigter RH, et al. Monitoring of fetuses with intrauterine growth restriction: a longitudinal study. Ultrasound Obstet Gynecol 2001;18:564-570.

CHAPTER 43

Fetal Surveillance: Doppler Assessment of Pregnancy and Biophysical Profile

Maryam Rivaz, Norman L. Meyer, Rebecca A. Uhlmann, and Giancarlo Mari

Chapter Outline

*F*etal surveillance by ultrasound is performed by a combination of assessment of growth (Chapter 42), Doppler ultrasound waveform analysis, and biophysical profile.

Studies have shown that Doppler ultrasound, introduced in obstetrics in 1977, represents an important screening and diagnostic tool in modern obstetrics.[1,2] FitzGerald and Drumm[3] first reported that the **umbilical artery** (UA) **waveforms** are abnormal in fetuses with **intrauterine growth restriction** (IUGR), and that **reversed flow of the UA** is associated with poor prognosis. Their breakthrough concept of studying waveforms resulted in several important clinical applications. For example, the American College of Obstetrics and Gynecology (ACOG) has endorsed the use of UA Doppler ultrasound in high-risk pregnancies.[4] Doppler ultrasound assessment of the UA has become a standard of care for fetuses with IUGR, which helps to decrease the perinatal mortality in high-risk pregnancies.[1] Doppler ultrasound of the **middle cerebral artery** has become the standard care for the diagnosis of fetal anemia, thus avoiding unnecessary invasive procedures.[5-8]

Information obtained with Doppler ultrasound helps manage pregnancies complicated by IUGR, fetal anemia, and multiple gestations. In addition, Doppler sonography is useful in the assessment of medication effects on maternal and fetal circulation.

FETAL CIRCULATION

The fetal blood circulation consists of parallel blood flow pathways and two shunts (Fig. 43-1). The oxygen (O_2)–rich and nutrient-enriched blood goes from the placenta to the umbilical vein, and once it reaches the liver, some blood flows through it, turns right, and joins the transverse portion of the left portal vein. Some blood bypasses the liver via the ductus venosus and enters the right atrium via the **inferior vena cava** (IVC).

A subdiaphragmatic venous vestibulum is formed by the confluence of the three hepatic veins, the ductus venosus, and the IVC just below the level of the right atrium. The **right atrium** receives venous return from the upper part of the body through the **superior vena cava** (SVC) and from the myocardium via the **coronary sinus.** The largest amount of the blood from the right atrium flows through the **foramen ovale** into the **left atrium** and through the mitral valve into the left ventricle. From there, blood empties into the aorta, passes through the aortic arch over the bifurcation in the right and left pulmonary artery, and enters the descending part of the aorta.

In contrast, carbon dioxide (CO_2)–rich, nutrient-poor blood flows from the SVC into the right atrium, is partially mixed with the O_2-rich blood from the placenta, and enters the right ventricle via the tricuspid valve. A small portion of the blood passes through the pulmonary circulation via the pulmonary trunk and the pulmonary arteries and reaches the left atrium through the pulmonary veins, followed by entrance into the systemic circulation system. Because of the high pulmonary arterial pressure in the lungs, however, a substantially larger part flows through the **ductus arteriosus** and goes into the descending aorta and directly into the systemic circulation.

The blood streams to the right atrium carry blood with different concentrations of nutrients and oxygen,

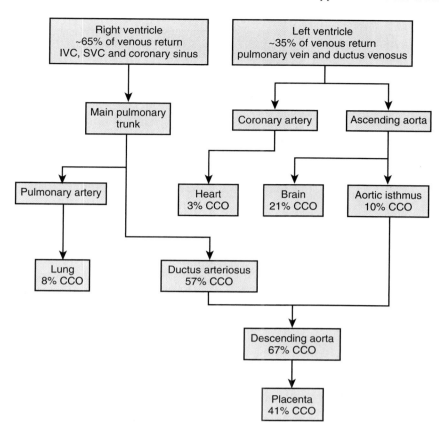

FIGURE 43-1. Diagram of fetal heart. Percentages of combined ventricular output ejected by each ventricle in the circulation of the fetal lamb. Well-oxygenated left ventricular blood supplies the brain and heart while right ventricular blood with lower oxygen content is predominantly distributed to the placenta. The largest proportion of the combined cardiac output (*CCO*) is distributed to the placenta for oxygenation.

so appropriate channeling is necessary to ensure that sufficient nutrient and oxygen is delivered to the vital organs. This is accomplished by several unique features of the ductus venosus foramen ovale, aortic isthmus, and origin of the UA that result in different velocities and directions in venous bloodstreams. The **umbilical vein** transports nutrient-rich blood from the placenta, and a large part of it is channeled through the bed of capillaries in the liver.

A functional sphincter regulates the flow of blood through the **ductus venosus** (DV). The DV develops at approximately 7 weeks' gestation and shows relatively little increase in size, in contrast to the other precordial veins, which grow proportionally with the embryo.[9] After the first trimester, diameter of the DV measures approximately one-third the umbilical vein diameter. As a result, blood from the umbilical vein accelerates on entering the DV.[10] This accelerated blood flow enters the IVC with the left hepatic venous return, and the combined flow is directed through the foramen ovale into the left atrium. By comparison, the venous returns from the right and middle hepatic veins and IVC have slower blood flow velocities and are directed toward the right atrium. There is relatively little mixing of the venous returns from the DV/left hepatic vein and the right and middle hepatic veins/IVC because of the differences in velocity and direction of the incoming bloodstreams. As a result, **O₂-rich blood** reaches the left ventricle through

the foramen ovale, whereas **O₂-poor blood** enters the right ventricle through the tricuspid valve.

Blood from the left ventricular output is circulated through the brachiocephalic vessels to the brain and upper body and through the coronary vessels to the myocardium. Right ventricular output largely bypasses the lungs and reaches the aorta through the ductus arteriosus. The blood from both ventricles is mixed and eventually reaches the placenta through the umbilical arteries.[11]

In the human fetus, 60% to 70% of umbilical venous blood is circulated to the liver and the remainder to the heart. With chronic hypoxemia, this proportion may be adjusted so that a larger proportion of umbilical venous blood can bypass the liver to reach the heart.[12]

INTRAUTERINE GROWTH RESTRICTION

The fetus with IUGR is a fetus that does not reach its potential growth. However, most of the studies that report on IUGR have not differentiated between "constitutionally" small and "pathologically" small fetuses. Additionally, studies on the pathogenesis of IUGR have been limited by the concept that IUGR fetuses represent a homogeneous group. This has created some confusion about the mechanisms of IUGR. We use the term **small**

for gestational age (SGA) for those small fetuses with no maternal pathology and with normal UA and middle cerebral artery (MCA) Doppler ultrasound results. In contrast, growth-restricted fetuses are small fetuses with a recognizable maternal pathology or an abnormal UA or MCA Doppler ultrasound. In many IUGR fetuses, there is an underlying maternal pathology, such as **chronic hypertension** or **advanced-stage diabetes mellitus,** as the basis of **placental insufficiency.** In other fetuses with IUGR, placental insufficiency has no identifiable cause, but there is an abnormal fetal Doppler ultrasound, defined as "idiopathic" IUGR.[13,14]

The concept that placental insufficiency is "the" cause of IUGR is a source of confusion. Placental insufficiency is not the "cause" of the problem, but rather is the *consequence* of a poorly understood disease process.[14,15] Placental insufficiency is a "symptom" with many potential underlying causes. With IUGR, we often view the problem from the wrong direction—as a consequence of placental insufficiency—and we therefore believe that we should treat the placental insufficiency. In reality, we should find and treat the specific *cause* of placental insufficiency.

Optimal management, however, would be the prevention of IUGR entirely. Growth-restricted fetuses undergo a different series of cardiovascular changes that in patients with preeclampsia, or other maternal pathology, and fetuses with idiopathic IUGR. In idiopathic IUGR, Doppler ultrasound changes can be predicted on almost a day-by-day basis. If no sudden adverse event occurs, such as a placental abruption, these fetuses can be followed until fetal cardiac failure occurs. This is not the case in patients with **preeclampsia,** in whom Doppler ultrasound changes of IUGR are unpredictable.[16] The importance of this concept is that in cases of idiopathic IUGR, delivery has the potential of being timed. It is important to emphasize that not all IUGR fetuses are the same, and that they must be categorized into appropriate groups according to severity and etiology.[14-24]

Doppler ultrasound plays a fundamental role in the diagnosis of IUGR and also has the potential to play an important role in timing the delivery of some growth-restricted fetuses. Doppler sonography of the UA and MCA, in combination with biometry, provides the best tool to identify small fetuses at risk for an adverse outcome.[25,26] In addition, Doppler ultrasound studies of the fetal cardiovascular system allow assessment of the blood flow redistribution observed in IUGR.[26] This process is mainly characterized by an **increased UA** and a **decreased MCA pulsatility index,** which suggests increased vascular resistance of the UA and cerebral vasodilation.

Doppler Waveform Analysis

Doppler ultrasound waveforms reflect blood velocity. However, Doppler waveforms also may provide

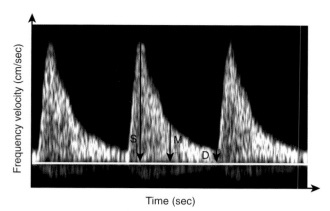

FIGURE 43-2. Typical Doppler waveform of a fetal artery. The beginning of the waveform coincides with the beginning of the cardiac systole; *S,* peak systolic velocity (PSV); *D,* end diastolic velocity (EDV); *M,* mean velocity (MV). Velocity is shown on the Y axis. Note that the velocity is the true velocity if the angle between the ultrasound beam and the blood flow is close to 0 degrees.

information on various aspects of blood flow in circulation, including the presence and direction of flow, velocity profile, volume of flow, and impedance to flow. These waveforms have been used extensively for assessing downstream circulatory impedance. The essential condition for the assessment of true velocity depends on the angle between the ultrasound beam and the direction of the blood flow, which needs to be as close as possible to 0 degrees (Fig. 43-2). As the incident angle increases, blood velocity is progressively underestimated; therefore the following angle-independent indices are used:

1. **Systolic-to-diastolic** (S/D) **ratio** = Peak systolic velocity/End diastolic velocity (PSV/EDV)
2. **Resistive index** (RI) = (PSV − EDV)/PSV
3. **Pulsatility index** (PI) = (PSV − EDV)/Mean velocity

Blood flow velocity of the fetal vascular system can be either pulsatile or continuous. The arteries always have a pulsatile pattern, whereas the veins have either a pulsatile or a continuous pattern (Fig. 43-3). The S/D ratio and RI are easy to calculate. The PI is more complex because it requires the calculation of the **mean velocity** (MV), but modern Doppler ultrasound equipment provides those values in real time. In practice, for the UA, the MCA, and the uterine arteries, no one index is superior to the others, and any of the indices may be used.

These three indices provide information on **vascular impedance,** which is not the same as vascular resistance. In fact, impedance has a more extensive meaning than resistance, because it depends on vascular resistance, preload, heart rate, and cardiac contractility. The term **vascular resistance,** however, has been extensively used in the literature and is commonly accepted. By calculating one of these indices and therefore estimating the vascular resistance, we can obtain information on the amount of blood flow. For example, if we assess the PI

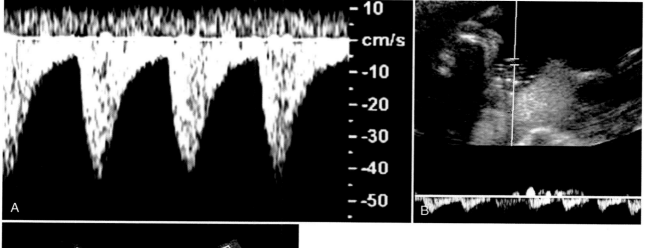

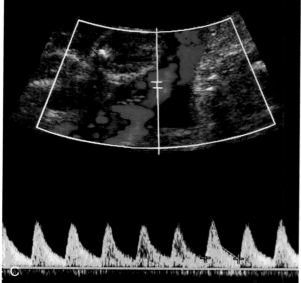

FIGURE 43-3. Umbilical artery and umbilical vein. A, The umbilical vein has a constant velocity, whereas the umbilical artery (UA) is pulsatile because it reflects the systole and diastole of the cardiac cycle. In this case, the umbilical vein blood flow was toward the transducer, and therefore the waveform is represented above the baseline. The UA blood flow was directed away from the transducer, and therefore arterial flow is represented below the baseline. **B,** "Chasing" the cord in gray scale will lead to inadvertently large angles of insonation and the erroneous impression of reduced or even absent end diastolic flow. Magnification of a cord segment followed by use of color flow Doppler ultrasound, detecting blood flow velocity in the vertical plane, allows the pulsed Doppler gate to be placed in each artery with a minimal angle of insonation. **C,** Normal arterial waveform in the same patient as **B.** (*A from Mari G, Detti L. Doppler ultrasound: application to fetal medicine. In Fleischer AC, Manning FA, Jeanty P, Romero R, editors.* Sonography in obstetrics and gynecology: principles and practice. *New York, 2001, McGraw-Hill, pp 247-283.*)

(or the RI or S/D ratio) at the level of the MCA in fetuses **appropriate for gestational age** (AGA) and in growth-restricted fetuses at the same gestational age, the IUGR fetuses will have a lower PI value at the MCA than the AGA fetuses. Our interpretation is that in IUGR fetuses, there is a lower vascular resistance at the MCA than in AGA fetuses. This suggests an increased blood flow to the brain. However, we do not know the true value of the vascular resistance or the true amount of cerebral blood flow.

Uterine Artery

In the first half of pregnancy, trophoblasts invade the uterine vessels and result in dilated spiral arteries, which increase the uterine perfusion 10-fold to 12-fold. These arteries provide nutrient supply and gas exchange for the fetus. Each uterine artery should be sampled soon after the crossing of the iliac vessels (Fig. 43-4).

The uterine arterial blood flow in nonpregnant women is 50 mL per minute and increases to over 700 mL/min

in the third trimester of pregnancy. Thus the diastolic component of the uterine artery Doppler waveform is transformed during normal pregnancy from one of low peak flow velocity and an early diastolic notch, to one of high flow velocity and an early diastolic notch by 18 to 22 weeks.[27] The uterine artery waveform by the mid–second trimester is therefore characterized by high end diastolic velocities (EDVs) with continuous forward blood flow throughout diastole. With advancing gestation, the degree of end diastolic flow typically increases. Indices used to quantify these waveforms include PI, RI, and notching of one or both uterine arteries.

However, failure of normal endovascular trophoblastic invasion of the spiral arteries results in increased uterine artery vascular resistance and decreased perfusion of the placenta.[28,29] If the end diastolic flow does not increase throughout pregnancy, or if a small notch is detected at the beginning of diastole, the fetus is at high risk for developing IUGR.[30] Diastolic blood flow may be absent or even reversed with extreme degrees of placental dysfunction. Such findings are ominous and may precede

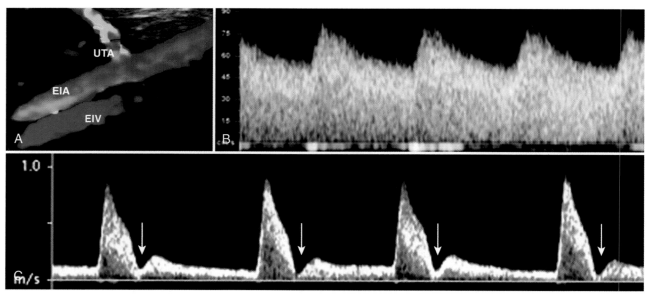

FIGURE 43-4. Uterine artery as it crosses iliac vessels. A, When it appears to originate from the external iliac artery, this is an artifact. The uterine artery *(UTA)* is sampled on color Doppler ultrasound soon after it crosses the iliac vessels. *EIA,* External iliac artery; *EIV,* external iliac vein. **B,** Normal UTA waveform with high diastolic flow. **C,** Abnormal UTA waveform with obvious early diastolic notch. *(From Mari G. Doppler ultrasonography in obstetrics: from the diagnosis of fetal anemia to the treatment of intrauterine growth-restricted fetuses. Am J Obstet Gynecol 2009;200:613 e1-e9.)*

fetal death or signal a high risk of abnormal fetal neurologic outcome.[31] The PI of each uterine artery should be obtained independently, using a PI value of 1.41 to differentiate between normal and abnormal values. Doppler ultrasound studies of the uterine artery in early pregnancy have been evaluated as a screening tool for pregnancies destined to develop preeclampsia or IUGR.[31]

A recent literature review reported that abnormal uterine artery waveforms are a better predictor of preeclampsia than of IUGR when performed after 16 weeks' gestation.[32] However, different indices best predicted preeclampsia or IUGR based on the a priori risk. Thus, an abnormal PI and uterine artery notching in the second trimester best predicted preeclampsia, whereas the best predictor of IUGR in high-risk patients was an increased RI.[33] The following issues, however, remain unclear:

1. When the assessment of uterine arteries should be carried out: at 16, 20, or 24 weeks of gestation.
2. Whether assessment of the maternal uterine arteries notching is useful.
3. If the PI or RI is the most useful parameter.
4. Whether the addition of the PI or RI of both maternal uterine arteries is necessary.

Future studies will have to clarify when to assess the uterine arteries, what cutoff value to use for the uterine artery Doppler RI and PI, and whether biochemical markers need to be added to the Doppler ultrasound assessment for better predictive information.

It is also important to minimize subjective interpretation of the waveforms, especially characterization if a notch is present, which can depend on the speed of recording the Doppler ultrasound tracing. The indications for the assessment of the uterine artery Doppler ultrasound are (1) previous history of preeclampsia, (2) previous child with IUGR, (3) unexplained high maternal serum alpha-fetoprotein levels, and (4) high human chorionic gonadotropin levels. If the PI values of both uterine arteries are normal, the patient can be informed that she most likely will not develop preeclampsia or have an IUGR fetus. This is because of the high negative predictive value (>99%) of the test. If one of the uterine arteries is abnormal, patients are followed with more frequent clinic visits and ultrasounds for growth because the positive predictive value in populations at risk ranges from 50% to 75%.

Umbilical Artery

Placental blood is assessed by studying the umbilical artery. UA waveforms are slightly different at the fetal abdominal wall and at the placental insertion,[34] with indices higher at the wall than the insertion (Fig. 43-5). However, the difference is minimal, so it is not important to obtain the waveforms always at the same level. In practice, the UA is best examined in a segment of **free-floating umbilical cord.** Waveforms are optimized by selecting the vessel to be interrogated, zooming in on the region, and placing the Doppler ultrasound gate in a segment of cord flowing at close to 0 degrees to the transducer. If there is reversed flow, the UA is reexamined close to the placental insertion, because this segment of the UA is the last part to develop reversed flow[16] (Fig. 43-6). UA waveforms change with advancing gestation.[3,35] **End diastolic flow** is often absent in the first trimester,[11] and the diastolic component increases with advancing gestation because of a decreased placental vascular resistance.[25,36,37] Absent end diastolic flow in the umbilical artery is an abnormal finding by the mid–second trimester. UA waveforms should be obtained during periods of fetal apnea because **fetal breathing** affects the waveforms (Fig. 43-7). Similarly, a fetal cardiac arrhythmia, particularly periods of bradycardia, can also lead to abnormal Doppler ultrasound indices.

In pathologic conditions such as IUGR, the UA waveforms change, with a decreased diastolic component, and the angle-independent indices become abnormal, with values above their reference ranges.[38-42] These changes reflect an increased placental vascular resistance.[25] As the placental insufficiency worsens, the **diastolic velocity decreases,** then becomes absent, and later is reversed. Some fetuses have a decreased diastolic velocity that remains constant with advancing gestation and never becomes absent or reversed, which may be caused by a milder form of placental insufficiency. Trudinger et al.[25] demonstrated that the number of placental arteries per high-power field is decreased in cases of abnormal UA Doppler ultrasound.[25] Only in pregnancies with suspected IUGR or hypertensive disease of pregnancy does the use of UA Doppler ultrasound reduce the number of perinatal deaths and unnecessary obstetric interventions.[43]

Middle Cerebral Artery

Anteriorly, the **circle of Willis** is composed of the anterior cerebral arteries (branches of internal carotid artery [ICA] connected by anterior communicating artery); posteriorly, it consists of the two posterior cerebral arteries (branches of basilar artery connected on either side to ICA), which supply the cerebral hemispheres on each side. These arteries have different waveforms,[44] so it is important to know which artery is being interrogated.

The middle cerebral artery is the vessel of choice to assess the fetal cerebral circulation because it is easy to identify, is highly reproducible, and provides information on the brain-sparing effect.[26] In addition, the MCA can be studied easily with an angle of 0 degrees between the ultrasound beam and the direction of blood flow (Fig. 43-8), providing information on the true velocity of the blood flow.[26] The MCA should be sampled soon after its origin from the ICA.[17] Technique is important for obtaining accurate results. In the absence of fetal breathing and movements, the examination takes approximately 5 to 10 minutes with the patient.

Reference values for the **middle cerebral artery pulsatility index** (MCA PI) change throughout gestation (Table 43-1 and Fig. 43-9). The lower PI values early and late in gestation may be caused by the increased metabolic requirements of the brain during these periods.[45] Several conditions are associated with an

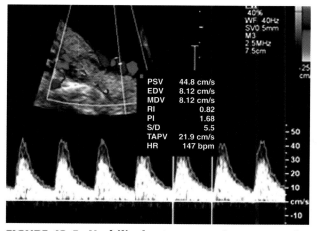

FIGURE 43-5. Umbilical artery waveform near placental insertion.

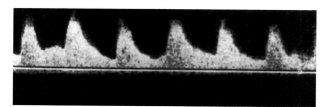

FIGURE 43-7. Umbilical artery waveforms. UA Doppler ultrasound waveforms during fetal breathing are different from each other. *(From Mari G, Detti L. Doppler ultrasound: application to fetal medicine. In Fleischer AC, Manning FA, Jeanty P, Romero R, editors. Sonography in obstetrics and gynecology: principles and practice. New York, 2001, McGraw-Hill, pp 247-283.)*

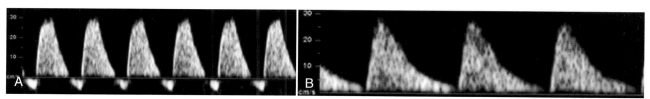

FIGURE 43-6. Umbilical artery (UA) in intrauterine growth restriction (IUGR). A, Reversal of diastolic flow. UA Doppler waveforms obtained in fetus with severe IUGR, 23 days before fetal demise at 26 weeks' gestation. The umbilical cord was sampled in a free-floating segment. **B,** Absent, but not reversed, UA diastolic flow on Doppler ultrasound waveforms sampled at the placental insertion. *(From Mari G. Doppler ultrasonography in obstetrics: from the diagnosis of fetal anemia to the treatment of intrauterine growth-restricted fetuses. Am J Obstet Gynecol 2009;200:613 e1-e9.)*

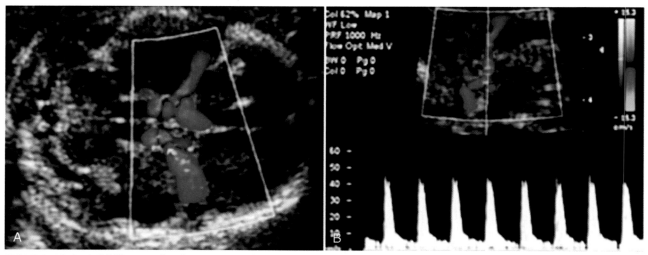

FIGURE 43-8. Middle cerebral artery (MCA) on color Doppler ultrasound. A, Circle of Willis. **B,** Spectral Doppler tracing. Note how Doppler gate is on the MCA just after the origin from the internal carotid artery. Note that the MCA is studied with an angle close to 0 degrees; therefore the velocity is close to the real velocity of the blood flow. *(From Mari G, Abuhamad AZ, Cosmi E, et al. Middle cerebral artery peak systolic velocity: technique and variability. J Ultrasound Med 2005;24:425-430.)*

MEASUREMENT OF MIDDLE CEREBRAL ARTERY (MCA) PEAK SYSTOLIC VELOCITY (PSV)

1. Obtain an axial section of the head at the level of the sphenoid bones.
2. Use color Doppler ultrasound to identify circle of Willis with MCA at angle close to 0 degrees.
3. Enlarge image of MCA.
4. Interrogate MCA soon after its origin from the ICA at angle close to 0 degrees using a 1- to 2-mm sample volume.
5. Measure PSV.
6. Repeat the collection of MCA Doppler ultrasound three to five times.
7. Repeated waveforms should be similar.

TABLE 43-1. MIDDLE CEREBRAL ARTERY PULSATILITY INDEX (MCA PI)*

	Normal Values		
GA (week)	**LOWER LIMIT†**	**PREDICTED VALUE**	**UPPER LIMIT‡**
15	0.99	1.57	2.14
16	1.08	1.71	2.33
17	1.16	1.83	2.51
18	1.23	1.95	2.67
19	1.30	2.05	2.81
20	1.35	2.14	2.93
21	1.40	2.22	3.04
22	1.44	2.29	3.13
23	1.48	2.34	3.20
24	1.51	2.38	3.26
25	1.52	2.41	3.30
26	1.54	2.43	3.32
27	1.54	2.44	3.33
28	1.54	2.43	3.32
29	1.52	2.41	3.30
30	1.50	2.38	3.26
31	1.48	2.34	3.20
32	1.44	2.28	3.12
33	1.40	2.21	3.03
34	1.35	2.13	2.92
35	1.29	2.04	2.79
36	1.22	1.94	2.65
37	1.15	1.82	2.49
38	1.07	1.69	2.32
39	0.98	1.56	2.13
40	0.89	1.40	1.92
41	0.78	1.24	1.70
42	0.67	1.06	1.45

From Mari G, Deter RL. Middle cerebral artery flow velocity waveforms in normal and small-for-gestational-age fetuses. Am J Obstet Gynecol 1992;166:1262-1270.
*PI $= -1.9763 + (0.32737 \, GA^1) + (-0.00611 \, GA^2)$.
†Predicted value $-$ ($2 \times 0.184 \times$ Predicted value).
‡Predicted value $+$ ($2 \times 0.184 \times$ Predicted value).
GA, Gestational age.

increase or decrease of the MCA PI when compared to normal values.

Animal and human experiments have shown that IUGR is associated with increased blood flow to the fetal brain.[46,47] This increase in blood flow during diastole can be demonstrated by Doppler ultrasound of the MCA.[26] This effect is termed the **brain-sparing effect** and is demonstrated by a **lower value of the MCA PI** (Fig. 43-10). It is important to emphasize that the MCA PI changes with increasing gestational age. In IUGR fetuses with a PI below the normal range, there is a greater incidence of adverse perinatal outcome.[26] The brain-sparing effect may be transient, as reported during prolonged hypoxemia in animal experiments,[48] and it may be lost in the overstressed human fetus[49] (Fig. 43-11).

The MCA PI is below the normal range when oxygen tension (P_{O_2}) is reduced.[50] Maximum reduction in PI is

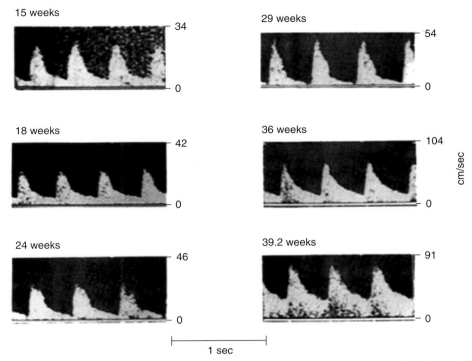

15 weeks

18 weeks

24 weeks

29 weeks

36 weeks

39.2 weeks

cm/sec

1 sec

FIGURE 43-9. Middle cerebral artery. MCA Doppler ultrasound at various gestational ages shows how diastolic flow increases as gestation advances. *(From Mari G, Deter RL. Middle cerebral artery flow velocity waveforms in normal and small-for-gestational-age fetuses. Am J Obstet Gynecol 1992;166:1262-1270.)*

FACTORS ASSOCIATED WITH LOW AND HIGH MIDDLE CEREBRAL ARTERY PULSATILITY INDEX (MCA PI) VALUES

LOW MCA PI
Brain growth spurt
Postuterine contractions
High fetal heart rate
Severe anemia
Post-transfusion
Therapeutic amniocentesis
Ductal constriction and tricuspid insufficiency
Hypoxemia and acidemia

HIGH MCA PI
Uterine contractions
Low fetal heart rate
Oligohydramnios
Fetal head compression
Sustained hypoxemia with acidemia
Hydranencephaly
Indomethacin administration

Modified from Mari G, Detti L. Doppler ultrasound: application to fetal medicine. In Fleischer AC, Manning FA, Jeanty P, Romero R, editors. *Sonography in obstetrics and gynecology: principles and practice.* New York, 2001, McGraw-Hill, pp 247-283.

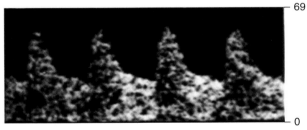

FIGURE 43-10. Middle cerebral artery. MCA Doppler ultrasound in IUGR at 24 weeks' gestation shows how the brain-sparing effect has resulted in relatively high diastolic flow (compare to 24 weeks in Fig. 43-9). The MCA pulsatility index (PI) is abnormal at 24 weeks. *(From Mari G, Detti L. Doppler ultrasound: application to fetal medicine. In Fleischer AC, Manning FA, Jeanty P, Romero R, editors. Sonography in obstetrics and gynecology: principles and practice. New York, 2001, McGraw-Hill, pp 247-283.)*

reached when the fetal Po_2 is 2 to 4 standard deviations (SD) below normal for gestational age. When the O_2 deficit is greater, the PI tends to rise, which presumably reflects the development of brain edema. In growth-restricted fetuses the disappearance of the brain-sparing effect or presence of reversed MCA flow is a critical event for the fetus and precedes fetal death.[49,51-53] Reversed

25 weeks   Umbilical artery   27 weeks

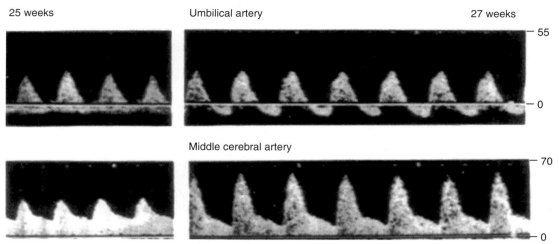

Middle cerebral artery

FIGURE 43-11. Umbilical artery (UA) and middle cerebral artery (MCA) waveforms in severe IUGR. At 25 weeks' gestation, there was absent end diastolic flow of the UA, pulsation of the umbilical vein, and the brain-sparing effect, as shown by high diastolic flow of the MCA. At 27 weeks, there was reverse diastolic flow of the UA, and the brain-sparing effect was not present. The fetus died 24 hours after this study. *(From Mari G, Wasserstrum N. Flow velocity waveforms of the fetal circulation preceding fetal death in a case of lupus anticoagulant. Am J Obstet Gynecol 1991;164:776-778.)*

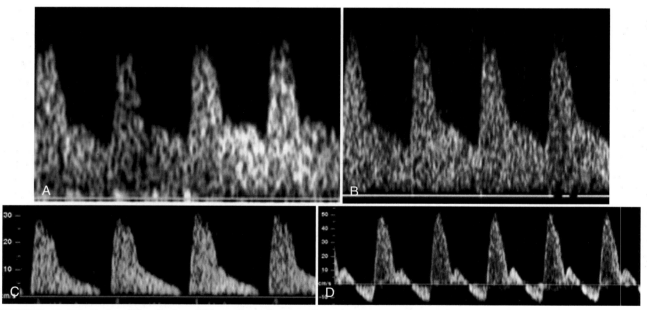

FIGURE 43-12. Pulsatility index (PI) and peak systolic velocity (PSV) in IUGR. A, PI is abnormal, but PSV is normal. **B,** Both PI and PSV are abnormal. These findings indicate a more severe IUGR condition than in cases with normal PSV. **C,** Middle cerebral artery (MCA) waveforms with absent end diastolic flow. **D,** Reversed flow in MCA. *(A and B from Mari G, Hanif F. Intrauterine growth restriction: how to manage and when to deliver. Clin Obstet Gynecol 2007;50:497-509. C and D from Mari G. Doppler ultrasonography in obstetrics: from the diagnosis of fetal anemia to the treatment of intrauterine growth-restricted fetuses. Am J Obstet Gynecol 2009;200: 613 e1-e9.)*

flow of the MCA velocity waveforms can be observed with head compression in normal pregnancies.

The **middle cerebral artery peak systolic velocity (MCA PSV) is increased in IUGR fetuses** (Fig. 43-12). This increase predicts perinatal mortality more accurately than does the MCA PI.[22] This finding can be explained because initially the MCA PI is abnormal in most IUGR fetuses but subsequently increases and trends toward normalization before delivery or fetal

death. Conversely, the MCA PSV progressively increases with advancing gestation in all fetuses and tends to decrease slightly just before fetal biophysical deterioration or fetal demise. Despite this decrease, however, the MCA PSV value remains above the upper limit of normal until a few hours before delivery or fetal demise.

Although the MCA PSV is increased in anemic fetuses, those with IUGR are not anemic, raising the question, what is the mechanism of increased MCA PSV

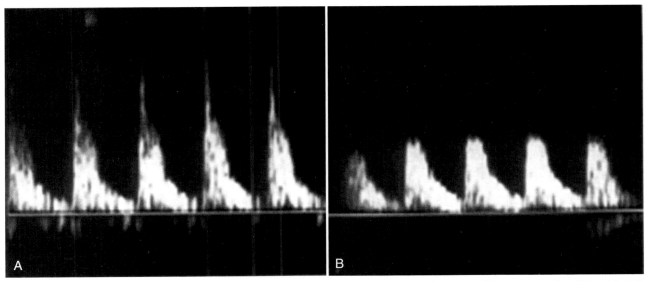

FIGURE 43-13. **Descending aorta. A,** At the level of the diaphragm. **B,** Distal to the origin of the renal arteries. *(From Mari G, Detti L. Doppler ultrasound: application to fetal medicine. In Fleischer AC, Manning FA, Jeanty P, Romero R, editors.* Sonography in obstetrics and gynecology: principles and practice. *New York, 2001, McGraw-Hill, pp 247-283.)*

in anemic and nonanemic fetuses? Hanif et al.[54] showed that the mechanisms determining increased MCA PSV values are different in anemic AGA fetuses compared with nonanemic IUGR fetuses.[54] In anemic fetuses the high MCA PSV is related to a decreased fetal hemoglobin that can decrease blood viscosity; therefore cardiac output increases. In IUGR fetuses, however, the MCA PSV increase is significantly related to hypoxemia and hypercapnia and thus to brain autoregulation.[17,54]

Other Arteries

Many other arteries have been examined in AGA fetuses and those with IUGR, increasing our understanding of fetal physiology and pathophysiology in these conditions. In our experience, however, the study of these vessels as currently performed adds no new information to the study of the UA and MCA in the management of IUGR fetuses.

Descending Aorta. Waveforms from the fetal descending aorta are usually recorded at the level of the diaphragm. Waveforms distal to the origin of the renal arteries are different[55,56] (Fig. 43-13). The PI of the fetal descending aorta is 1.96 ± 0.30 (SD) at the diaphragm and 1.68 ± 0.28 after the origin of the renal arteries.[56] The pulsatility index is the preferred measurement in the descending aorta because end diastolic flow may be absent in normal fetuses. Waveforms in the descending aorta represent the summation of flow to the kidneys, bowel, placenta, and lower extremities. The PI of the fetal descending aorta remains relatively constant throughout gestation because placental and renal resistance decreases while lower extremity vascular resistance increases with advancing gestation.[57] In severe IUGR fetuses, there is reversed flow in the descending aorta.

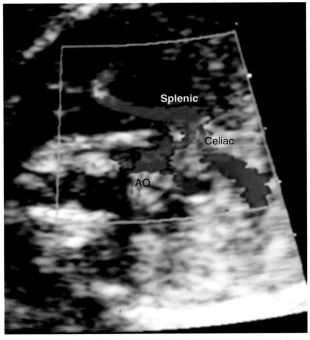

FIGURE 43-14. **Celiac trunk.** Transverse section of the fetal abdomen at the level of the descending aorta, celiac trunk, splenic artery, and hepatic artery. *(From Abuhamad AZ, Mari G, Bogdan D, Evans AT 3rd. Doppler flow velocimetry of the splenic artery in the human fetus: is it a marker of chronic hypoxia? Am J Obstet Gynecol 1995;172:820-825.)*

Splenic Artery. The celiac trunk arises from the aorta between the crura of the diaphragm at the level of the 12th thoracic vertebra (Fig. 43-14). The celiac trunk has three main branches: the splenic, common hepatic, and left gastric arteries. Abuhamad et al.[58] found that IUGR fetuses have a lower splenic artery PI value. This suggests that in cases of chronic hypoxia, there is increased blood flow to the spleen because of increased erythropoiesis.[59,60]

Superior Mesenteric Artery. Superior mesenteric artery fetal waveforms are shown in Fig. 43-15. PI values increase over time.[61] This may reflect increased bowel resistance because of increased bowel length with advancing gestation. However, assessment of these waveforms has not been found to be useful in evaluating IUGR fetuses.[62]

Adrenal Artery. In IUGR fetuses, there is a lower adrenal artery PI, suggesting an adrenal "stress response," as reported in animal studies[63] (Fig. 43-16).

Renal Artery. The renal artery can be studied in a coronal section of the descending aorta and after its origin from the descending aorta in the kidneys (Fig. 43-17). Doppler ultrasound waveforms of the renal artery and vein are displayed on either side of the baseline. The PI must be used to assess the renal artery because EDV is often absent in the second trimester and early third trimester.[64,65] In fetuses with severe IUGR, the renal artery PI is above the reference range.

Femoral, Internal Iliac, and External Iliac Arteries. Femoral artery waveforms are obtained soon after the vessel origin (Fig. 43-18). The normal appearance of the femoral artery waveforms changes during gestation. There is no difference between the femoral artery PI and the external iliac artery PI.[57] The internal iliac artery is the intra-abdominal continuation of the umbilical artery and therefore reflects the UA waveforms.

Superior Cerebellar Artery. The superior cerebellar artery arises from the basilar artery before it divides into the two posterior cerebral arteries. The PI of the superior cerebellar artery is similar to that of the MCA. Uerpairojkit et al.[66] found that the PI of the superior cerebellar artery is lower than normal in IUGR fetuses, whereas it is in the normal range in SGA fetuses.

Fetal Venous System

Most studies on fetal venous blood flow have been performed on the blood flow from the placenta, which returns to the heart through the umbilical vein. Normal flow in the free-floating umbilical vein is monophasic (see Fig. 43-3). Fetuses with pulsation in the umbilical vein in the second and third trimesters have a higher morbidity and mortality, even in the setting of normal UA blood flow. For the umbilical vein, we use a qualitative assessment: continuous versus pulsatile blood flow[67,68] (Fig. 43-19).

Flow from the **umbilical vein** enters the fetal abdomen and at the portal sinus enters the ductus venosus (Fig. 43-20) and inferior vena cava. Approximately 50% of the blood flow from the umbilical vein goes to the liver and 50% to the DV.[69,70] The umbilical vein has a continuous flow that becomes pulsatile at the portal sinus[71,72] (Fig. 43-21). The IVC, before its entrance into the right atrium, has a triphasic pulsatile pattern.[73,74] The first forward wave begins to increase with atrial relaxation, reaches a peak during ventricular systole, and then falls to a nadir at the end of ventricular systole. The second

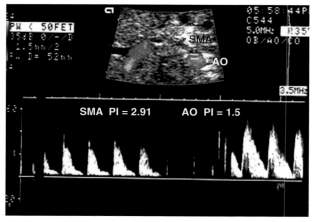

FIGURE 43-15. Superior mesenteric artery (SMA) and descending aorta (AO). The sample volume was initially placed on the SMA and then moved to the AO; *PI*, pulsatility index. *(From Mari G, Detti L. Doppler ultrasound: application to fetal medicine. In Fleischer AC, Manning FA, Jeanty P, Romero R, editors. Sonography in obstetrics and gynecology: principles and practice. New York, 2001, McGraw-Hill, pp 247-283.)*

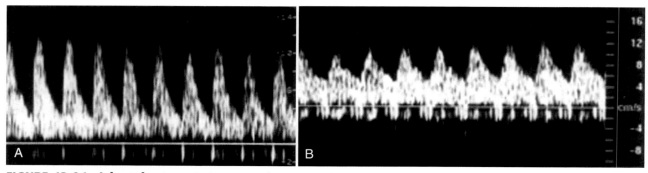

FIGURE 43-16. Adrenal artery. A, Appropriate-for-gestational-age (AGA) fetus. **B,** Fetus with IUGR. *(From Mari G, Uerpairojkit B, Abuhamad AZ, Copel JA. Adrenal artery velocity waveforms in the appropriate and small-for-gestational-age fetus. Ultrasound Obstet Gynecol 1996;8:82-86.)*

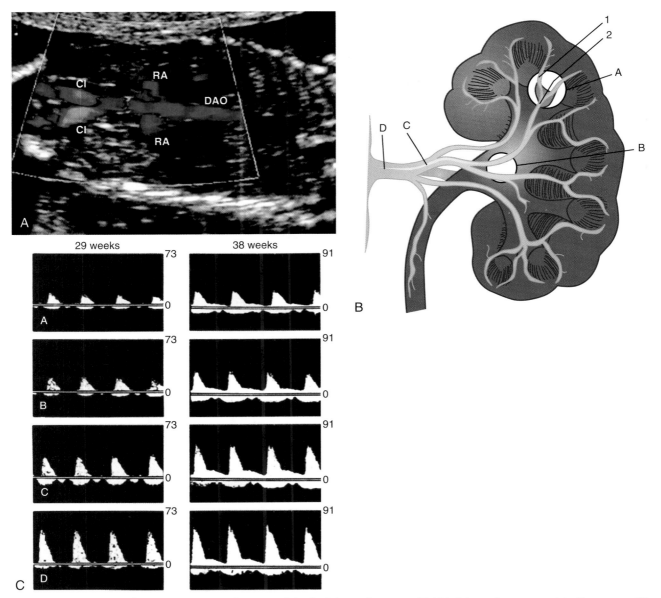

FIGURE 43-17. Renal artery. A, Coronal section of the fetal descending aorta *(DAO); RA,* renal artery at origin from aorta; *CI,* common iliac artery. **B,** Diagram shows where the waveforms in C were obtained. **C,** Waveforms of the renal artery obtained at different levels. *(From Mari G, Detti L. Doppler ultrasound: application to fetal medicine. In Fleischer AC, Manning FA, Jeanty P, Romero R, editors. Sonography in obstetrics and gynecology: principles and practice. New York, 2001, McGraw-Hill, pp 247-283.)*

forward wave occurs during early diastole, and the third wave, characterized by reversed flow, is present in late diastole with atrial contraction. In healthy fetuses, a significant decrease of the reversed flow during atrial contraction is present with advancing gestation.[74] These changes are related to improved ventricular compliance and to the reduction of right ventricular afterload caused by the fall in placental resistance as gestation advances. In IUGR fetuses the IVC is characterized by an increase in reversed flow during atrial contraction.[74] This increase is attributed to abnormal ventricular filling characteristics, an abnormal ventricular chamber, or wall compliance (Fig. 43-22).

The ductus venosus transports oxygenated blood from the umbilical vein to the left atrium and ventricle, then to the myocardium and brain. The DV waveform has a biphasic pattern characterized by two peaks: the "S", or peak systolic velocity (PSV), which corresponds to the highest velocity of the blood in systole and is followed by a period of decreased velocity called isovolumetric relaxation (IRV); and the "D", which corresponds to the rapid filling of the ventricles that is followed by a nadir, the "A wave," which corresponds to atrial contraction.[75] Hemodynamically, these phases reflect the rapid chronologic change in pressure gradients between the umbilical vein and the right atrium. In AGA fetuses, there is

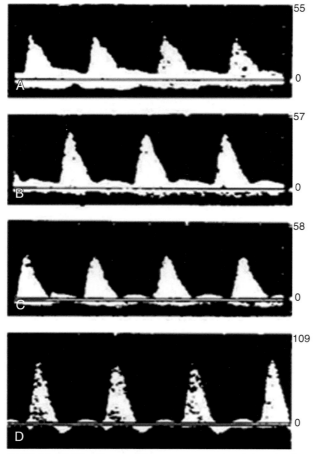

FIGURE 43-18. Femoral artery. A, Forward diastolic flow in femoral artery at 18 weeks' gestation. Presence of a notch at **B,** 24 weeks, and **C,** 30 weeks. **D,** Reversed flow at 39 weeks. *(From Mari G. Arterial blood flow velocity waveforms of the pelvis and lower extremities in normal and growth-retarded fetuses. Am J Obstet Gynecol 1991;165:143-151.)*

forward flow at the DV, and the PI for veins ([S − D]/A) decreases with advancing gestation. In the first trimester, reversed blood flow may be caused by the immaturity of the sphincter of the DV, which also may explain the umbilical vein pulsatile pattern seen in the first trimester.[76] A common error is sampling the left hepatic vein rather than the DV. The left hepatic vein waveform is similar to that of the IVC and has reversed flow in AGA fetuses.

In growth-restricted fetuses, the PI increases in the DV, and in the most severe cases, there is A wave of reversed flow. The presence of DV reversed flow can be explained in light of the transitional phase recently described by Picconi et al.[77] Based on this study, when the DV is longitudinally assessed in IUGR fetuses, the progression follows three steps: (1) normal waveforms, (2) a period with normal and abnormal waveforms, and (3) persistent abnormal waveforms. Picconi et al.[78] also recently developed the S-wave/isovolumetric A-wave (SIA) index for the analysis of the DV waveforms (Fig. 43-23), which allows a much more accurate prediction of fetal outcome compared to A-wave reversed flow alone[78] (Fig. 43-24).

Fetal Cardiac System

Atrioventricular Valves. Atrioventricular (A-V) valve (mitral and tricuspid) velocities may be obtained from a four-chamber view by placing the sample volume just distal to the valve leaflets. Two peaks usually are present in the A-V valve signal; the first peak reflects passive ventricular filling in **early diastole** (E), and the second peak reflects the atrial contraction in **late diastole** (A). Early in gestation, A is much higher than E[79,80] (see Fig. 37-25), indicating that the atrial contraction is

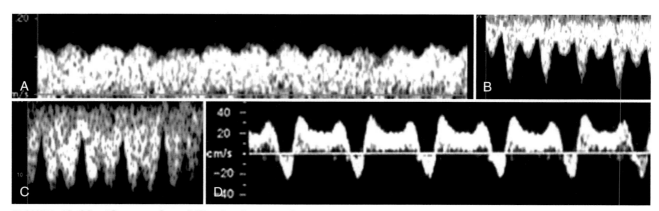

FIGURE 43-19. Abnormal umbilical vein waveforms. A, Single pulsation. **B,** Double pulsation. Waveforms obtained close to the origin of the ductus venosus 48 hours before fetal demise. **C,** Double pulsation; same case as **B.** Waveforms obtained between the origin of the ductus venosus and the umbilicus. **D,** Reversed flow. Fetus died within 24 hours of this finding. *(From Mari G, Hanif F, Kruger M. Sequence of cardiovascular changes in IUGR in pregnancies with and without preeclampsia. Prenat Diagn 2008;28:377-383.)*

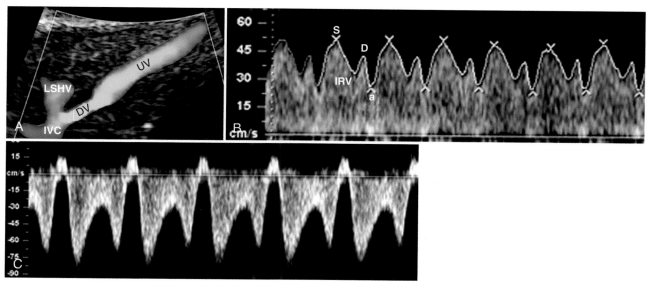

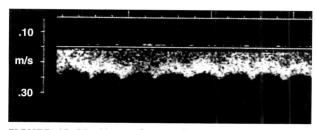

FIGURE 43-20. Ductus venosus. A, Sagittal section of fetal torso. The ductus venosus *(DV)* is brighter than the other vascular areas because of the high blood velocity at this point. When the DV is not clearly visualized, this brighter appearance helps to distinguish the DV from the surrounding vessels. *UV,* Umbilical vein; *IVC,* inferior vena cava; *LHV,* left hepatic vein. **B,** Normal DV waveforms: *S,* peak systolic velocity; *D,* first phase of diastole corresponding to the passive rapid filling of the ventricles; *IRV,* isovolumetric relaxation; *a,* second phase of diastole with atrial contraction. **C,** DV waveforms obtained at 24 weeks' gestation. Note that there is reversal of flow. *(From Mari G. Doppler ultrasonography in obstetrics: from the diagnosis of fetal anemia to the treatment of intrauterine growth-restricted fetuses. Am J Obstet Gynecol 2009;200:613 e1-e9.)*

FIGURE 43-21. Normal portal sinus with pulsatile flow. *(From Mari G, Detti L. Doppler ultrasound: application to fetal medicine. In Fleischer AC, Manning FA, Jeanty P, Romero R, editors.* Sonography in obstetrics and gynecology: principles and practice. *New York, 2001, McGraw-Hill, pp 247-283.)*

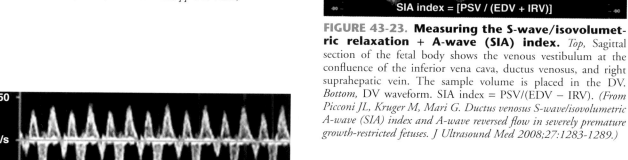

SIA index = [PSV / (EDV + IRV)]

FIGURE 43-23. Measuring the S-wave/isovolumetric relaxation + A-wave (SIA) index. *Top,* Sagittal section of the fetal body shows the venous vestibulum at the confluence of the inferior vena cava, ductus venosus, and right suprahepatic vein. The sample volume is placed in the DV. *Bottom,* DV waveform. SIA index = PSV/(EDV − IRV). *(From Picconi JL, Kruger M, Mari G. Ductus venosus S-wave/isovolumetric A-wave (SIA) index and A-wave reversed flow in severely premature growth-restricted fetuses. J Ultrasound Med 2008;27:1283-1289.)*

FIGURE 43-22. Abnormal inferior vena cava waveform. These values were obtained 48 hours before intrauterine fetal demise. Note the double-reversed flow. *(From Mari G, Hanif F, Kruger M. Sequence of cardiovascular changes in IUGR in pregnancies with and without preeclampsia. Prenat Diagn 2008;28: 377-383.)*

important in the fetus. With advancing gestation, early diastole E increases and reaches late diastole A, suggesting that the atrial systole becomes less important with maturation of the ventricular myocardium.[79,81-84] At birth and after birth, E becomes higher than A, suggesting a less important role for atrial contraction. The index used most to quantify these waveforms is the **early-diastole-to-late-diastole** (E/A) **ratio.** When the A-V

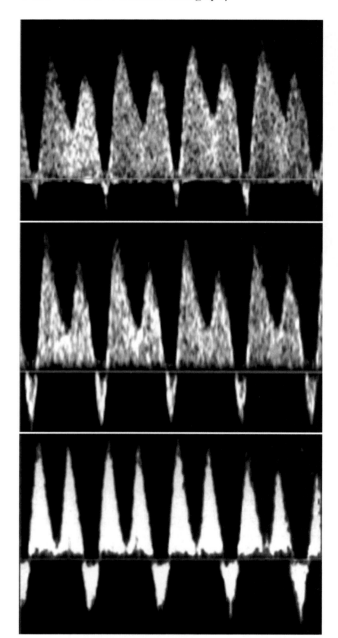

FIGURE 43-24. Ductus venosus waveforms in IUGR. At 16 days *(top)*, 4 days *(middle)*, and 24 hours *(bottom)* before intrauterine death at 23 weeks' gestation. The patient declined intervention because of a fetal weight less than 500 grams and a gestational age of 23 weeks. Note the reversed flow in the A wave that becomes more pronounced closer to the time of fetal demise. *(From Picconi JL, Kruger M, Mari G. Ductus venosus S-wave/iso-volumetric A-wave (SIA) index and A-wave reversed flow in severely premature growth-restricted fetuses. J Ultrasound Med 2008;27: 1283-1239.)*

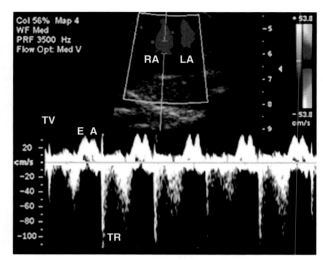

FIGURE 43-25. Tricuspid regurgitation. Tricuspid valve *(TV)* antegrade flow (above baseline) and tricuspid regurgitation *(TR;* below baseline); *RA,* right atrium; *LA,* left atrium; *E,* E wave; *A,* A wave. *(From Mari G, Hanif F, Kruger M. Sequence of cardiovascular changes in IUGR in pregnancies with and without preeclampsia. Prenat Diagn 2008;28:377-383.)*

valve velocity waveforms are studied at a low incident angle, the blood velocity obtained is close to the true velocity. The increase of the E/A ratio with advancing gestation is a sign of progressive improvement in myocardial compliance. Importantly, with advancing gestation, the peak velocity of the late diastolic A wave does not change, whereas the peak velocity of the early diastolic E wave increases.

In growth-restricted fetuses, the E/A ratio is higher than that of normal fetuses controlled for gestational age. These changes are attributed to changes in preload without impairment in fetal myocardial diastolic function. In the most severe cases, there is tricuspid and mitral regurgitation[85] (Fig. 43-25).

Aortic and Pulmonary Valves. Aortic valve (AoV) and pulmonary valve (PuV) velocities are studied at the levels of their respective outflow tracts. The peak velocity of both valves increases with advancing gestation.[86] In IUGR fetuses the AoV and PuV decrease, which may be secondary to increased placental resistance.

Measurement of Fetal Cardiac Output. Many investigators have attempted volumetric studies at the level of the fetal heart,[86-91] based on the formula $Q = TVI \times HR \times A$, where Q is the absolute flow per minute, TVI is the **time velocity integral,** HR is fetal heart rate, and A is the area of the valve.

The velocity of blood passing through a valve is not constant, but rather changes with the cardiac cycle; therefore the TVI, integral to the velocity waveforms over the entire cardiac cycle, is considered to be a measure of the length of the column of blood. The main problem in the calculation of absolute flow per minute *(Q)* is the measurement of the valve area. We can assume that the blood flow at the level of the valvular area is close to laminar, and that the Doppler spectrum reflects all velocities inside the valve. Newer spectral analyzers in many ultrasound machines can provide true intensity-weighted mean flow measurements that take spectral broadening into account. In addition, we can obtain Doppler ultrasound waveforms with an angle close to 0 degrees (<20 degrees) between the ultrasound beam and the blood flow. However, small errors in the calculation of the area ($\frac{1}{2}$ D^2) may substantially affect the measurement. For example, a 0.5-mm error in the measurement of a 4-mm valve will produce a 25% variation in the flow calculation.

Animal studies have demonstrated that the calculation of the blood flow may be reliable.[92] The study of the human fetus, however, is different from the "ideal" situation of animal research. An alternative approach may be used to measure the cardiac output indirectly if the valve diameter (D) remains constant. For example, if measurements are taken in a short interval, valvular area does not change, and an intervention that changes flow will be detected from changes in the TVI, HR, or both. For example, the product of the TVI and HR was measured at the AoV and PuV before and after two doses of nifedipine. No difference was noted in the two sets of measurements. Although the true value of the cardiac output could not be evaluated because the valve diameter was not measured, these results suggest that there were no changes in cardiac output after nifedipine. Subsequently, the effect of fetal transfusion on cardiac output was determined by using the same formula.[93,94] More recently, Gonzalez et al.[95] used the same formula to assess the effect of nitroglycerine on the fetal cardiac output.

In fetuses with IUGR, blood flow is presumably redistributed from the right to the left ventricle, with increased blood flow to the brain. Under these conditions, Doppler ultrasound reportedly may show this redistribution by calculating the amount of blood flow through the two ventricles.

Management: Staging and Classification

Growth-restricted fetuses have been categorized into three stages of severity using nonstress testing and UA Doppler ultrasound velocimetry. Pardi et al.[24] showed that if the nonstress test (NST) and UA Doppler studies were normal (group I fetuses), there was no fetal acidosis or hypoxemia. In contrast, group II fetuses, with a normal NST but an abnormal UA Doppler study (PI >2 SD below mean), showed a 5% rate of hypoxia/acidemia. Group III fetuses, with abnormal NST and UA Doppler studies, showed a 60% rate of hypoxia/acidemia. Although this study is informative, greater clinical utility may be achieved through fetal Doppler ultrasound in additional vessels.

We recently proposed staging guidelines for IUGR fetuses based on fetal biometry, Doppler ultrasound cardiovascular changes, amniotic fluid, and clinical parameters.[23] The Doppler waveforms used for staging are shown in Figs. 43-26, 43-27, and 43-28. Stage I IUGR fetuses are considered mild IUGR, and such patients are usually managed as outpatients, whereas stage II and III patients need to be admitted to the hospital when the

fetuses are considered viable. Stage II patients are admitted for observation, whereas stage III patients are at high risk for fetal demise.

The major advantage for selecting the parameters included in this staging system is the ability to track clearly the progression of abnormal parameters that start at the UA and MCA and later progressively extend to the other parameters, up to fetal demise if the fetus remains undelivered.[16,85] Another advantage is the simplicity of the system. Only four fetal vessels and one cardiac valve need to be investigated with Doppler ultrasound. Furthermore, it is not necessary to determine the parameters reported in a certain stage if the parameters of the previous stage are normal. For example, if the UA PI and the MCA PI are normal, determining these parameters for the next stage is unnecessary.

Stage III fetuses have a lower birth weight than both stage II and stage I fetuses at similar gestational ages. Moreover, stage II and III IUGR fetuses are delivered earlier than fetuses of stage I. In a study from our laboratory, no deaths occurred in stage I fetuses.[23] At the other extreme, the mortality for stage III fetuses was high (50% if there was DV reversed flow; 85% when DV reversed flow was present with one of the other parameters that characterize stage III), whereas the mortality in stage II IUGR fetuses was intermediate between the other two stages. Fetuses could survive for days or weeks when DV reversed flow was present.

DOPPLER ULTRASOUND STAGING GUIDELINES FOR INTRAUTERINE GROWTH RESTRICTION (IUGR)

STAGE I
Abnormal umbilical artery pulsatility index (UA PI)
Abnormal middle cerebral artery pulsatility index (MCA PI)

STAGE II
Umbilical artery absent/reversed flow (UA ARF)
Elevated middle cerebral artery peak systolic velocity (MCA PSV)
Abnormal ductus venosus pulsatility index (DV PI)*
Umbilical vein pulsation

STAGE III
Ductus venosus reversed flow
Umbilical vein reversed flow
Tricuspid valve (TV) E/A ratio >1

Tricuspid Valve Regurgitation (TR)

Modified from Mari G, Hanif F, Drennan K, Kruger M. Staging of intrauterine growth-restricted fetuses. J Ultrasound Med 2007;26:1469-1477.
  E/A, Early diastole/late diastole (velocities).
  *Absent ductus venosus is included in stage II.

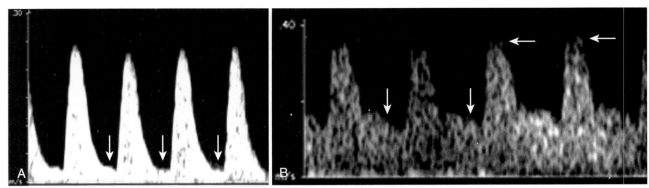

FIGURE 43-26. Stage I IUGR: abnormal waveforms. A, Abnormal umbilical artery (UA) Doppler sonogram. *Arrows,* Low diastole, indicating a high placental resistance. **B,** Abnormal middle cerebral artery (MCA) Doppler sonogram at 27 weeks. *Vertical arrows,* Diastole (increased, indicating "brain-sparing effect"); *horizontal arrows,* peak systolic velocity (PSV, appears normal). An abnormal pulsatility index (PI) of either the UA or MCA characterizes stage I. *(From Mari G, Hanif F, Drennan K, Kruger M. Staging of intrauterine growth-restricted fetuses. J Ultrasound Med 2007;26:1469-1477.)*

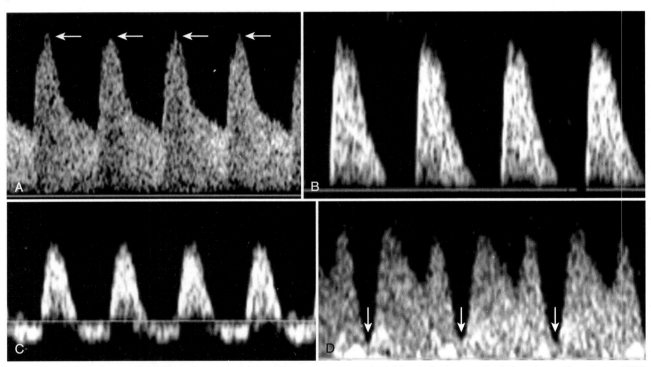

FIGURE 43-27. Stage II IUGR: abnormal waveforms. A, Elevated middle cerebral artery (MCA) peak systolic velocity (PSV; *arrows*) at 27 weeks is abnormal (76 cm/sec). **B,** Umbilical artery absent diastolic flow. **C,** Umbilical artery reversed flow. **D,** Abnormal ductus venosus Doppler sonogram with low "a" wave. Arrows point to "a" wave recorded at atrial contraction; when "a" wave is low, pulsatility index (PI) is abnormal. *(From Mari G, Hanif F, Drennan K, Kruger M. Staging of intrauterine growth-restricted fetuses. J Ultrasound Med 2007;26:1469-1477.)*

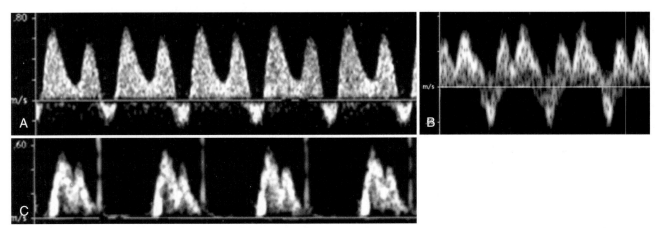

FIGURE 43-28. Stage III IUGR: abnormal waveforms. The presence of one of these findings characterizes stage III intrauterine growth restriction: **A,** Ductus venosus reversed flow. **B,** Umbilical vein reversed flow. **C,** Abnormal tricuspid valve waveform (E/A <1). *(From Mari G, Hanif F, Drennan K, Kruger M. Staging of intrauterine growth-restricted fetuses. J Ultrasound Med 2007;26:1469-1477.)*

Based on the information obtained from our staging system, we have proposed the following steps to classify IUGR fetuses:

1. In the presence of a fetus with an estimated weight below the 10th percentile, determine the stage using Doppler ultrasound examinations and amount of amniotic fluid.
2. Maternal or fetal pathology/anomalies should be identified, if any.
3. The gestational age should be reported.

RED CELL ALLOIMMUNIZATION

Maternal Rh alloimmunization occurs when a pregnant woman develops an immunologic response to a paternally derived red blood cell antigen (D) foreign to the mother and inherited by the fetus. The antibodies cross the placenta, bind to antigens present on the fetal erythrocytes, and cause hemolysis. Hemolysis of the erythrocytes causes anemia in the fetus and, if severe, can result in edema, hydrops, and fetal death. Hemolytic disease of the fetus/neonate can also be caused by other antigens of the Rh blood group system and by the "irregular antigens" of the non-Rhesus blood group system; therefore the term "red cell alloimmunization" is more often used. Red cell alloimmunization remains the most common cause of fetal anemia. In the United States, more than 30,000 fetuses are at risk for anemia each year because of red cell alloimmunization from Rh, Kell, Kidd, Duffy, or other antigens. In 1956, amniocentesis was performed in a pregnancy at risk for anemia to assess the fetal bilirubin through a spectrophotometric analysis of amniotic fluid, which changes optical density at 450 nm (ΔOD_{450}) in fetuses shown to have hemolytic disease. These changes can predict the severity of hemolytic disease. From 1963 on, investigators have used different techniques for fetal blood transfusion, from intrauterine transfusion and intravascular transfusion to umbilical blood sampling under fetoscopy guidance, to the current method of fetal blood sampling under ultrasound guidance.

PREDICTION OF FETAL HEMATOCRIT

Starting in 1987, the effects of **intravascular transfusion** (IVT) on the circulation of the anemic fetus were evaluated by looking at the PI of eight fetal vessels that were studied before, within 2 hours, and the day after IVT.[96-98] A significant decrease in the PI of all the vessels was noted soon after transfusion, with a return to baseline the day after IVT. In all the fetal anemia cases, the MCA waveforms after transfusion had a lower PSV value than before transfusion.[99,100] In 1990, Mari et al.[101] suggested that MCA-PSV was a better parameter than PI in the diagnosis of fetal anemia. In 1993, they reported that in anemic fetuses the MCA PSV had a sensitivity of 100% and a false-positive rate of approximately 50% in detecting anemia secondary to red cell alloimmunization,[102] which they confirmed in 1995 with a prospective study.[103] After applying the MCA PSV in practice and looking at the correlation between it and **fetal hemoglobin** (Hb), Mari et al.[104] noticed that MCA PSV does not diagnose all cases of fetal anemia, because in mildly anemic cases, the velocity does not necessarily change. However, the correlation between Hb and MCA PSV values becomes more accurate as the severity of anemia increases.[104] Additionally, when anemia becomes very severe (Hb 1-3 g/dL), the velocity does not increase further.

A multicenter study determined that 70% of invasive procedures (e.g., amniocentesis and cordocentesis) used to assess a fetus at risk for anemia because of maternal red cell alloimmunization are unnecessary because the fetuses were either nonanemic or only slightly anemic.[6] Using MCA PSV as the criterion for intervention would have avoided those procedures.[17] Normal Hb values are 0.84 multiples of the median (MoM) or greater for gestational age. Fetal anemia is divided into **mild** (Hb <0.84 MoM), **moderate** (Hb <0.65 MoM), and **severe** (Hb <0.55 MoM) (Table 43-2).

In 1997, it was reported that the trend of the MCA-PSV was at least as effective as ΔOD_{450} to predict fetal anemia.[99] However, MCA PSV assessment was less expensive and less invasive than amniocentesis. In 2003, Pereira et al.[105] confirmed the accuracy of the MCA-PSV in a

TABLE 43-2. REFERENCE RANGES FOR FETAL HEMOGLOBIN CONCENTRATION IN NORMAL AND ANEMIC FETUSES*

	Multiples of the Median				
GA†	**1.16**	**1.00 (median)**	**0.84**	**0.65**	**0.55**
18	12.3	10.6	8.9	6.9	5.8
20	12.9	11.1	9.3	7.2	6.1
22	13.4	11.6	9.7	7.5	6.4
24	13.9	12.0	10.1	7.8	6.6
26	14.3	12.3	10.3	8.0	6.8
28	14.6	12.6	10.6	8.2	6.9
30	14.8	12.8	10.8	8.3	7.1
32	15.2	13.1	10.9	8.5	7.2
34	15.4	13.3	11.2	8.6	7.3
36	15.6	13.5	11.3	8.7	7.4
38	15.8	13.6	11.4	8.9	7.5
40	16.0	13.8	11.6	9.0	7.6

From Mari G, Deter RL, Carpenter RL, et al. Noninvasive diagnosis by Doppler ultrasonography of fetal anemia due to maternal red-cell alloimmunization. Collaborative Group for Doppler Assessment of the Blood Velocity in Anemic Fetuses. N Engl J Med 2000;342:9-14. Courtesy Massachusetts Medical Society.

*In grams per deciliter (g/dL). The hemoglobin values at 0.65 and 0.55 multiples of the median (MoM) are the cutoff points for mild anemia and moderate anemia, respectively. The values at 1.16 and 0.84 MoM correspond to the 95th and 5th percentiles, respectively (normal range).

†Gestational age (week of gestation).

retrospective study. A multicenter prospective study later determined that the MCA PSV is actually more reliable than the ΔOD_{450} in the diagnosis of fetal anemia,[7] which has led ACOG to report that the MCA PSV is an excellent tool for the diagnosis of fetal anemia in the hands of trained personnel.[5] Retrospective studies suggest that the MCA PSV can be used for timing subsequent transfusions, but a randomized trial is needed to confirm this.

The technique for obtaining MCA Doppler ultrasound is described earlier in regard to IUGR. In the context of screening for anemia, it is crucial that use of MCA Doppler ultrasound be for anemia, before a high PSV is interpreted as being indication of a low hematocrit. Indiscriminate use of the MCA PSV without a clear indication may cause more harm than good. It is neither wise nor good medical care to screen every patient with the MCA PSV and assume that the fetus is anemic if the value is elevated. This may create unnecessary anxiety and iatrogenic investigation. For example, if fetal-maternal hemorrhage is suspected because of absent fetal movements and a sinusoidal HR tracing, an elevated MCA PSV may strengthen the suspicion. On the other hand, an elevated MCA PSV, in the presence of a reassuring HR tracing and no risk for anemia, does not indicate pathology; rather, it may represent a false-positive case. Therefore, no intervention is indicated when an elevated MCA PSV value is found in the absence of risk for fetal anemia.

The blood velocity is increased in any vessel of the severely anemic fetus, as suggested by van Dongen et al.[106] Again, the advantage of studying the MCA is that it is easy to obtain an angle of 0 degrees between the ultrasound beam and the direction of blood flow. Tricuspid regurgitation precedes the development of ascites and hydrops, and the use of this parameter can help in decreasing false-negative cases.

The lowest intraobserver and interobserver variability is obtained when the MCA proximal to the transducer is sampled soon after its origin from the ICA without the use of an angle corrector and by using a 1 to 2–mm sample volume.[17] A PSV greater than 1.50 MoM in fetuses at risk for anemia has a sensitivity for detecting anemia of 100% (confidence interval, 86%-100%) in red cell alloimmunization cases, as well as in other cases of anemia.[6,8,107] The false-positive rate is 12%, but this percentage may decrease when serial MCA values are obtained.[19]

In fetuses at risk for anemia because of red cell alloimmunization, we use the regression lines reported in Figure 43-29. We initially perform three examinations, 1 week apart, then obtain the regression line of the three points. If the curve is to the right side of the dotted line (nonanemic fetuses), we perform the next MCA Doppler ultrasound in 2 to 4 weeks. For example, if a patient with an anti-D titer of 1:256 is seen at 17 weeks' gestation and her previous pregnancies have not been complicated by fetal anemia, and if the regression line of her first three

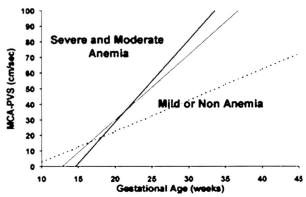

FIGURE 43-29. Fetal anemia. Middle cerebral artery peak systolic velocity (MCA PSV) regression lines for the diagnosis of fetal anemia. Average regression line for nonanemic fetuses (*dotted line, y = −17.28 + 1.99x*); mildly anemic fetuses (*thin line, y = −53.54 + 4.17x*), and severely anemic fetuses (*thick line, y = −76.82 + 5.26x*). (*From Detti L, Mari G, Akiyama M, et al. Longitudinal assessment of the middle cerebral artery peak systolic velocity in healthy fetuses and in fetuses at risk for anemia. Am J Obstet Gynecol 2002;187:937-939.*)

exams is to the right side of the dotted line, we perform the next examination in 4 weeks. However, if the values are between the dotted line (nonanemic fetuses) and one of the continuous lines (mildly or severely anemic fetuses), the next examination is performed in 2 weeks. Finally, if the regression line is to the left of one of the continuous lines (mildly or severely anemic fetuses), and the MCA PSV is below 1.50 MoM, we perform an examination every 2 to 3 days. After 34 weeks, if we use the 1.50 MoM as the cutoff point, we find that the number of false-positive cases increases; therefore we look at serial MCA values rather than a single value. We deliver our patients at risk for fetal anemia at 38 to 39 weeks' gestation.

The MCA PSV can be used to diagnose fetal anemia from causes other than red cell alloimmunization. Cosmi et al.[107] and Delle Chiaie et al.[108] reported that this parameter is useful in cases of fetal anemia secondary to parvovirus infection. Senat et al.[109] reported that the MCA PSV helps to diagnose anemia secondary to **twin-twin transfusion syndrome** (TTTS; see later discussion), and others report that it diagnoses anemia secondary to fetomaternal hemorrhage[110,111] and fetal hydrops.[112,113] In cases with parvovirus infection, we perform an ultrasound every week for 10 weeks after the exposure. We look for signs of anemia and evaluate the MCA PSV. If the value of the velocity becomes higher than 1.5 MoM, ultrasound is repeated twice a week, looking for tricuspid regurgitation and ascites. Often, we do not intervene in cases of parvovirus infection based solely on the MCA PSV because the fetus would not necessarily become hydropic and the anemia might resolve spontaneously without intervention.

Fetomaternal hemorrhage usually occurs in the third trimester. When it is diagnosed, we perform a cesarean delivery. The MCA PSV is elevated in cases of feto-maternal hemorrhage, but we use other signs that might suggest hemorrhage (e.g., absence of fetal movements, sinusoidal pattern in HR tracing) before assessing the MCA PSV. In nonimmune hydrops, if the MCA PSV is below the cutoff point of 1.5 MoM, we do not perform cordocentesis.

MULTIPLE GESTATIONS

The S/D ratio of the umbilical artery in twin pregnancies where both twins are AGA are similar to singleton pregnancy results in the third trimester. Gaziano et al.[114] reported that twins with abnormal UA waveforms tended to be born 3 to 4 weeks earlier and exhibited more stillbirths and structural malformations and greater morbidity than fetuses without abnormal Doppler results. Use of UA Doppler ultrasound in the clinical management of twins leads to a decrease in perinatal mortality and a reduction in the number of infants requiring admission to the neonatal intensive care unit.[115]

Umbilical Artery Doppler Ultrasound in Discordant Twins

Discordant growth in twin gestations can result from placental crowding, TTTS, a poor placental implantation site, placental insufficiency, or chromosomal anomalies. Thus, discordant growth is associated with a substantial increase in perinatal morbidity and mortality. The diagnosis of discordant twins is made primarily with ultrasound. Comparing intertwin differences in sonographically derived fetal weight, biparietal diameter, abdominal circumference, femur length, and UA S/D ratio, Divon et al.[116] reported that the best predictor for the diagnosis of discordant twins was either a difference in S/D ratio greater than 15% or a different estimated fetal weight greater than 15%. They correctly identified 14 of the 18 discordant twins. Degani et al.[117] reported that changes in the Doppler of the ICA and UA preceded sonographic diagnosis of SGA fetuses by a mean interval of 3.7 weeks and demonstrated better sensitivity and specificity. Hecher et al.[118] reported that abnormal UA velocimetry can be observed in small twins more often when they are monochorionic rather than dichorionic.

We assess the fetal growth in twin gestations every 4 weeks. We also assess the UA in twin gestations because in cases of an abnormal UA Doppler ultrasound, we intensify fetal surveillance.

Doppler Ultrasound in Twin-Twin Transfusion Syndrome

One of the most serious complications of **monochorionic** (MC) multiple gestations is TTTS. Cardiovascular changes in response to an unequal sharing of intravascular volume between twins, resulting from anastomosis of intertwined placental blood vessels, complicates 10% to 15% of MC pregnancies and often results in fetal/neonatal mortality. Fetuses who survive are at risk for severe cardiac, neurologic, and developmental disorders. Several fetal vessels have been studied in pregnancies complicated by TTTS.[119] Doppler ultrasound measurement of the UA in either twin is an excellent prognostic parameter to assess patients with TTTS. TTTS patients with absent end diastolic flow have a worse prognosis than patients with forward end diastolic flow. Staging of TTTS is discussed in Chapter 32. Doppler ultrasound measurements are used to assess for stage III; abnormal results include absent of reversed end diastolic flow in the UA or revised flow in the DV or pulsatile flow in the umbilical vein[120] (Fig. 43-30).

Interventions for TTTS include expectant management, amnioreduction, septostomy, selective feticide, and fetoscopic laser ablation of vascular anastomoses. When the twins undergo amnioreduction or laser therapy,[121,122] the MCA PSV allows the diagnosis of fetal anemia and indicates the need for transfusions in the recipient after laser therapy.[109] The preliminary data of Senat et al.[109] appear promising for MCA PSV in the management of MC twins after the death of the co-twin. If pregnancy is evaluated within 2 to 3 days of fetal death, signs of fetal anemia may be evident, with elevated MCA PSV. Documentation of normal MCA Doppler ultrasound and normal fetal activity within days of an MC co-twin death is reassuring. Recently, Robyr et al.[123] reported that in TTTS, fetofetal hemorrhage from recipient to donor occurs in 10% of cases with double survivors as a result of incomplete laser coagulation of anastomoses. Therefore, this parameter should be used as a follow-up for cases of TTTS after laser therapy.

INDOMETHACIN AND DUCTUS ARTERIOSUS

Indomethacin, a prostaglandin synthetase inhibitor, has been used in the management of preterm labor and polyhydramnios. Additional use of indomethacin has been limited, mainly because of concerns about its constrictive effect on the fetal ductus arteriosus. In utero closure of the ductus arteriosus causes increased pulmonary blood flow and can result in neonatal pulmonary hypertension, shunting of blood through the foramen ovale, and ultimately, persistent fetal circulation after birth.

Indomethacin causes constriction of the fetal ductus arteriosus and tricuspid insufficiency.[44,124] This effect is readily reversible and can be monitored using ultrasound (Fig. 43-31). In our experience, 50% of the fetuses exposed to indomethacin show no effect on the ductus arteriosus, although these fetuses still have increased

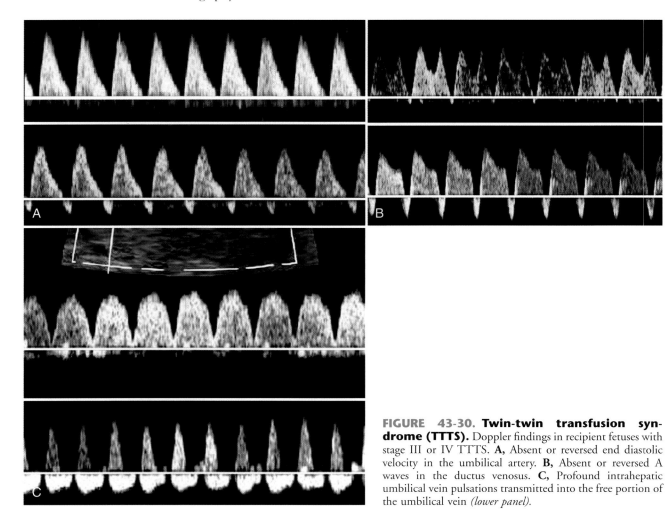

FIGURE 43-30. Twin-twin transfusion syndrome (TTTS). Doppler findings in recipient fetuses with stage III or IV TTTS. **A,** Absent or reversed end diastolic velocity in the umbilical artery. **B,** Absent or reversed A waves in the ductus venosus. **C,** Profound intrahepatic umbilical vein pulsations transmitted into the free portion of the umbilical vein *(lower panel).*

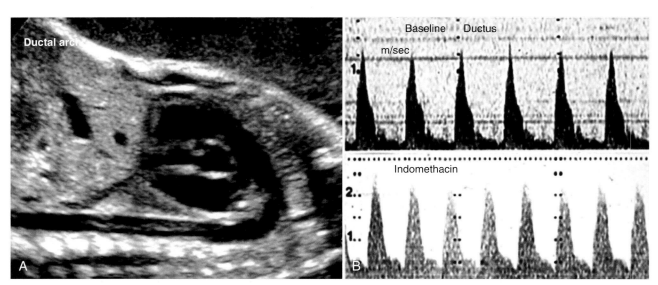

FIGURE 43-31. Ductus arteriosus and indomethacin. A, Image of fetus shows right ventricular outflow tract, ductus arteriosus, and descending aorta. **B,** Ductus arteriosus waveforms of the fetus before *(top)* and after *(bottom)* administration of indomethacin. (**B** *from Mari G, Detti L. Doppler ultrasound: application to fetal medicine. In Fleischer AC, Manning FA, Jeanty P, Romero R, editors. Sonography in obstetrics and gynecology: principles and practice. New York, 2001, McGraw-Hill, pp 247-283.)*

pulmonary arterial vascular impedence.[125] We propose the following classification to define ductal constriction:

- **Mild** constriction (20% of patients treated with indomethacin). The peak systolic velocity of the ductus arteriosus is increased with respect to the baseline value. The end diastolic velocity remains constant.
- **Moderate** constriction (20% of patients treated with indomethacin). The PSV and EDV of the ductus arteriosus increase above baseline values. There is absence of tricuspid insufficiency.
- **Severe** constriction (10% of patients treated with indomethacin). In our experience, after indomethacin therapy, there is at first an increase of the ductus arteriosus PSV, which is followed by an increase of the EDV. Of note, when the EDV is greater than 100 to 120 cm/sec, tricuspid insufficiency is often present.

In our experience with more than 100 fetuses treated with indomethacin, discontinuation of the drug is followed by a return to normal of the Doppler ultrasound ductal parameters within the next 36 hours. Only 50% of the fetuses developing ductal constriction may be explained by different sensitivities to indomethacin. In addition, gestational age plays an important role; for example, we have never seen severe ductal constriction before 22 weeks' gestation. The interaction between ductal constriction and the other neonatal complications of fetal indomethacin exposure requires further investigation.

DOPPLER ULTRASOUND IN FETAL MORPHOLOGIC ABNORMALITIES

Color, pulsed, and power Doppler ultrasound can be used to refine the diagnosis of a variety of fetal structural abnormalities. For example, in the fetal brain, Doppler ultrasound is used to assess **vein of Galen malformations.** In the fetal body, vascularity of tumors such as **sacrococcygeal teratomas** are assessed to evaluate for the vascularity of the lesion and presence of arteriovenous shunting. In the chest, if a **sequestration** is of potential concern, Doppler ultrasound is used to assess for feeding vessel from the aorta. When a **congenital diaphragmatic hernia** is visualized, Doppler ultrasound assessment of the course of the hepatic vasculature is helpful in assessing for intrathoracic position of the liver. Color Doppler ultrasound is helpful in assessing for a two- or three-vessel umbilical cord. Assessment of the umbilical arteries adjacent to the bladder aids in identification of the bladder when this organ is difficult to visualize.

BIOPHYSICAL PROFILE SCORING

The **biophysical profile** (BPP) and fetal heart rate monitoring **nonstress test** (NST) are the most common tests used in the United States to assess fetal well-being in women with high-risk factors for stillbirth. The BPP was developed by Manning et al.[126] in 1980 and incorporates fetal tone, movements, breathing, amniotic fluid, and an NST. A normal BPP is associated with decreased fetal deaths within 1 week.[127]

The fetal BPP is noninvasive and easily applied, can be objectively evaluated, uses universally available equipment, and is highly accurate for predicting the presence of significant fetal hypoxemia or acidemia, which is the most common cause of fetal death or morbidity.[128] A compromised fetus typically exhibits loss of HR accelerations, decreased body movement and breathing, hypotonia, and less acutely, decreased amniotic fluid volume. Sonographic detection of signs of fetal compromise can allow appropriate intervention that ideally will prevent adverse fetal sequelae.

The BPP consists of an NST combined with four variables evaluated by real-time ultrasonography.[129] Thus the BPP comprises five components. Each of the five components is assigned a score of either 2 (normal or present) or 0 (abnormal, absent, or insufficient). For example, monotonous picket-fence breathing or gasping should not be considered normal breathing movements, and seizures should not be counted as normal fetal limb movements.[130-132] A variable may be assigned a normal score as soon as it is observed. Because most fetuses are normal and will demonstrate these biophysical activities, the usual time to complete a normal fetal BPP is less than 5 minutes.[133] The acute variables are subject to fetal sleep-wake cycles, so continuous observation for at least 30 minutes must occur before the variable can be defined as "absent" (abnormal).

COMPONENTS OF BIOPHYSICAL PROFILE (BPP)

1. Nonstress test (NST). Fetal heart rate (HR) accelerations in response to fetal movements, which, if all four ultrasound components are normal, may be omitted without compromising the validity of the test results.[128]
2. Fetal breathing movements. One or more episodes of rhythmic fetal breathing movements of 30 seconds or more within 30 minutes **(Video 43-1)**.
3. Fetal movement. Three or more discrete body or limb movements within 30 minutes **(Video 43-2)**.
4. Fetal tone. One or more episodes of extension of a fetal extremity with return to flexion, or opening or closing of a hand **(Video 43-3)**.
5. Determination of amniotic fluid volume. A single vertical pocket of amniotic fluid exceeding 2 cm is considered evidence of adequate amniotic fluid.[134,147]

INTERPRETATION OF BPP SCORES

- 10/10 or 8/10 (normal fluid): risk of fetal asphyxia within 1 week if no intervention is 1/1000.
- 8/10 (abnormal fluid): risk of fetal asphyxia within 1 week if no intervention is 89/1000.
- 6/10 (normal fluid): equivocal test, possible fetal asphyxia; repeat test within 24 hours or deliver.
- 6/10 (abnormal fluid): risk of fetal asphyxia within 1 week if no intervention is 89/1000.
- 0/10 to 4/10: risk of fetal asphyxia within 1 week if no intervention is 91-600/1000.

Evaluation of the **amniotic fluid** is based on an ultrasound-based objective measurement of the largest visible pocket(s) and is recorded as the vertical diameter relative to the transducer. The selected largest pocket must have a transverse diameter of at least 1 cm. This method does not measure the actual amniotic fluid; rather, it evaluates the distribution of amniotic fluid within the uterine cavity. A highly significant, inverse exponential relationship exists between the largest pocket measurement and perinatal mortality and morbidity. For example, one study comparing the corrected perinatal mortality in association with normal versus decreased qualitative amniotic fluid volume found rates of 1.97 and 109.4 per 1000, respectively.[134] Alternatively, the **amniotic fluid index** (AFI) can be used to assess the adequacy of the amniotic fluid.[135] The **single deepest pocket** technique is preferred to the AFI because of its higher specificity; use of the single deepest pocket decreases the likelihood of intervention for low amniotic fluid volume without adversely affecting outcomes.[136] Both methods have low sensitivity for predicting or preventing adverse outcomes.

All the ultrasound-monitored variables for the BPP can be observed as early as the first trimester. However, characteristics of fetal behavior (breathing, tone, movement, as well as other fetal activities) change with advancing gestational age.[137,138] The ACOG recommends testing in the following situations[126]:

- Women with high-risk factors for significant fetal acidemia.
- Testing may be initiated as early as 26 weeks' gestation when clinical conditions suggest early fetal compromise is likely. Initiating testing at 32 to 34 weeks is appropriate for most pregnancies at increased risk for stillbirth.
- A reassuring test (e.g., BPP of 8-10/10) should be repeated periodically (weekly or twice weekly) until delivery when the high-risk condition persists.
- Any significant deterioration in the clinical status (e.g., worsening preeclampsia, decreased fetal activity) requires fetal reevaluation, regardless of the time elapsed since the last test.
- Severe oligohydramnios (no vertical pocket >2 cm or AFI ≤5 cm) requires either delivery or close maternal and fetal surveillance.
- Normal antepartum testing does not preclude the need for intrapartum fetal monitoring.

Induction of labor may be attempted with abnormal antepartum testing as long as the fetal heart rate and contractions are monitored continuously and are reassuring. Cesarean delivery is indicated if there are repetitive late decelerations. The minimum gestational age for testing should reflect the lower limit that intervention with delivery would be considered. The age has gradually decreased and is now 24 to 25 weeks in most centers. Although typically used for antepartum fetal assessment, BPP can also be performed in the intrapartum period; however, its clinical utility intrapartum is not clear.[139,140]

The BPP has maximum clinical efficacy when interpreted in the context of fetal age and maternal and obstetric factors. A **normal score** predicts no fetal compromise and allows for conservative management in a gravida with discrete high-risk factors, such as diabetes mellitus or hypertension. This affords the fetus the advantage of continued intrauterine maturation, reducing the risk of complications from prematurity. In contrast, an **abnormal score** in a similarly high-risk patient allows for weighing of relative fetal-neonatal risks and selection of delivery at a time when the balance shifts to greater fetal risk.

A change in maternal condition will also affect application of the fetal BPP. The decision to intervene in a patient with deteriorating hypertension, for example, may depend less on the score and more on maternal risk. Similarly, the presence of a favorable cervix for induction may override the fetal BPP results in the mature or postdate fetus.

Modified Profile

The modified BPP combines the NST, as a short-term indicator of **fetal acid-base status**, with the AFI, which is the sum of measurements of the deepest cord-free amniotic fluid pocket in each of the abdominal quadrants, as an indicator of long-term **placental function.**[141] The modified BPP was developed to simplify the examination and reduce the time necessary to complete testing by focusing on those components of the profile that are most predictive of outcomes. The assessment of amniotic fluid volume and an NST appear to be as reliable a predictor of long-term fetal well-being as the full BPP.[142]

In the second- or third-trimester fetus, amniotic fluid reflects fetal urine production. Placental dysfunction may result in diminished fetal renal perfusion, leading to **oligohydramnios.**[143] Amniotic fluid volume assessment can therefore be used to evaluate long-term uteroplacental function. An AFI greater than 5 cm generally represents an adequate volume of amniotic fluid.[144] Thus, the modified BPP is considered **normal** if the NST is reactive and the AFI is more than 5 cm, but **abnormal** if the NST is nonreactive or the AFI is 5 cm or less. A normal modified BPP will occur in 90% of pregnancies tested; thus, proceeding with a full biophysical evaluation is necessary in only a minority of patients.[145] An NST should always be performed if any ultrasound monitored variable is abnormal. However, a BPP of 8/10 by any combination of variables, with or without the NST, is as accurate as a score of 10/10 for the prediction of fetal well-being, as long as no points are deducted for amniotic fluid volume.

Growth-Restricted Fetuses

The addition of Doppler ultrasound studies for the assessment of growth-restricted fetuses is believed to provide a better approach for the treatment of IUGR, but few studies have indicated a relationship between Doppler changes and the BPP in which changes are noted before development of an abnormal BPP score.[13,139] In IUGR fetuses with an abnormal UA Doppler ultrasound result, the BPP is initiated as early as 26 to 28 weeks and is performed twice a week.[126] Despite these guidelines, most obstetricians perform BPPs daily and repeat the NST twice or three times daily.

The BPP has been proposed as the antenatal testing modality of choice in the treatment of IUGR fetuses, even compared with Doppler ultrasound results alone or Doppler results in combination with BPP.[146] The BPP in fetuses with severe IUGR can change rapidly over a few hours and result in adverse perinatal outcomes. BPP alone in severely premature fetuses is not a good test of fetal well-being, and other tests should be used to monitor these fetuses. It is important to emphasize, however, that at present, there is no single or optimal test to monitor these growth-restricted fetuses. Although the NST is part of the BPP, a reactive NST is rare in fetuses with early IUGR; therefore the subjective interpretation of HR monitoring remains an important tool to treat these fetuses. Further studies are needed to determine whether computed cardiotocography might become an acceptable diagnostic tool in these fetuses.

Growth-restricted fetuses between 25 and 29 weeks' gestation represent a group for whom optimal treatment can make a difference in survival, because for each week the fetus remains in utero, the mortality rate decreases by approximately 48%.[146] Fetuses with IUGR diagnosed in association with no medical complications in pregnancy undergo a series of changes well defined by Doppler ultrasound until fetal cardiac failure occurs, or until the fetus is delivered because of nonreassuring testing.[16] In this group of fetuses, Doppler ultrasound may play an important role for timing the delivery because changes can be predicted by Doppler study. On the other hand, in patients with preeclampsia, the sequential changes found by Doppler ultrasound are seen in only a few patients, because most of these fetuses are often delivered for maternal indication before the full range of changes occur on Doppler ultrasound. In this group of fetuses, therefore, Doppler ultrasound plays a less important role in regard to the timing of the delivery.

Fetuses with early-diagnosed, severe IUGR should have daily BPPs and NSTs at intervals more frequent than 8 hours (i.e., every 6 hours); and when the managing physician has concerns about fetal status, the HR should be monitored continuously. It is not known whether a combined Doppler result and BPP represents a better test than the BPP alone. Doppler ultrasound as reported, however, may play an important role in timing the delivery of IUGR fetuses when no maternal or fetal abnormality is detected.

In summary, a BPP alone is not a reliable test in the treatment of preterm IUGR fetuses because of high false-positive and false-negative results. The common notion that a good BPP provides reassurance, or at least 24 hours' notice of impending fetal decline, is not applicable in severely preterm, growth-restricted fetuses who weigh less than 1000 g.

CONCLUSION

Doppler ultrasound plays an important role in assessment of fetuses at risk for IUGR. Doppler ultrasound is also used to monitor fetuses at risk for anemia and follow up on those requiring in utero transfusion. Biophysical profile plays an important role in assessing fetal well-being in women with high-risk factors for stillbirth. These important tests need to be carefully performed and interpreted in conjunction with clinical factors to optimize obstetric care.

References

1. Alfirevic Z, Neilson JP. Doppler ultrasonography in high-risk pregnancies: systematic review with meta-analysis. Am J Obstet Gynecol 1995;172:1379-1387.
2. Almstrom H, Axelsson O, Cnattingius S, et al. Comparison of umbilical-artery velocimetry and cardiotocography for surveillance of small-for-gestational-age fetuses. Lancet 1992;340:936-940.
3. FitzGerald DE, Drumm JE. Non-invasive measurement of human fetal circulation using ultrasound: a new method. BMJ 1977;2:1450-1451.
4. American College of Obstetricians and Gynecologists. Utility of antepartum umbilical artery Doppler velocimetry in intrauterine growth restriction. (No 188, Oct 1997; replaces No 116, Nov 1992.) ACOG Committee on Obstetric Practice. Int J Gynaecol Obstet 1997;59:269-270.
5. American College of Obstetricians and Gynecologists. ACOG Practice Bulletin No 75. Management of alloimmunization. Obstet Gynecol 2006;108:457-464.
6. Mari G, Deter RL, Carpenter RL, et al. Noninvasive diagnosis by Doppler ultrasonography of fetal anemia due to maternal red-cell alloimmunization. Collaborative Group for Doppler Assessment of the Blood Velocity in Anemic Fetuses. N Engl J Med 2000;342:9-14.

7. Oepkes D, Seaward PG, Vandenbussche FP, et al. Doppler ultrasonography versus amniocentesis to predict fetal anemia. N Engl J Med 2006;355:156-164.

8. Zimmerman R, Carpenter Jr RJ, Durig P, Mari G. Longitudinal measurement of peak systolic velocity in the fetal middle cerebral artery for monitoring pregnancies complicated by red cell alloimmunisation: a prospective multicentre trial with intention-to-treat. BJOG 2002;109:746-752.

Fetal Circulation

9. Chacko AW, Reynolds SR. Embryonic development in the human of the sphincter of the ductus venosus. Anat Rec 1953;115:151-173.

10. Kiserud T. The ductus venosus. Semin Perinatol 2001;25:11-20.

11. Kiserud T, Ebbing C, Kessler J, Rasmussen S. Fetal cardiac output, distribution to the placenta and impact of placental compromise. Ultrasound Obstet Gynecol 2006;28:126-136.

12. Kiserud T, Rasmussen S, Skulstad S. Blood flow and the degree of shunting through the ductus venosus in the human fetus. Am J Obstet Gynecol 2000;182:147-153.

13. Cosmi E, Ambrosini G, D'Antona D, et al. Doppler, cardiotocography, and biophysical profile changes in growth-restricted fetuses. Obstet Gynecol 2005;106:1240-1245.

Intrauterine Growth Restriction

14. Mari G, Hanif F. Intrauterine growth restriction: how to manage and when to deliver. Clin Obstet Gynecol 2007;50:497-509.

15. Assali NS, Nuwayhid B, Brinkman 3rd CR. Placental insufficiency: problems of etiology, diagnosis and management. Eur J Obstet Gynecol Reprod Biol 1975;5:87-91.

16. Mari G, Hanif F, Kruger M. Sequence of cardiovascular changes in IUGR in pregnancies with and without preeclampsia. Prenat Diagn 2008;28:377-383.

17. Mari G, Abuhamad AZ, Cosmi E, et al. Middle cerebral artery peak systolic velocity: technique and variability. J Ultrasound Med 2005;24:425-430.

18. Arduini D, Rizzo G, Romanini C. Changes of pulsatility index from fetal vessels preceding the onset of late decelerations in growth-retarded fetuses. Obstet Gynecol 1992;79:605-610.

19. Detti L, Mari G, Akiyama M, et al. Longitudinal assessment of the middle cerebral artery peak systolic velocity in healthy fetuses and in fetuses at risk for anemia. Am J Obstet Gynecol 2002;187:937-939.

20. Fu J, Olofsson P. Fetal ductus venosus, middle cerebral artery and umbilical artery flow responses to uterine contractions in growth-restricted human pregnancies. Ultrasound Obstet Gynecol 2007;30:867-873.

21. Kingdom J, Huppertz B, Seaward G, Kaufmann P. Development of the placental villous tree and its consequences for fetal growth. Eur J Obstet Gynecol Reprod Biol 2000;92:35-43.

22. Mari G, Hanif F, Kruger M, et al. Middle cerebral artery peak systolic velocity: a new Doppler parameter in the assessment of growth-restricted fetuses. Ultrasound Obstet Gynecol 2007;29:310-316.

23. Mari G, Hanif F, Drennan K, Kruger M. Staging of intrauterine growth-restricted fetuses. J Ultrasound Med 2007;26:1469-1477; quiz 1479.

24. Pardi G, Cetin I, Marconi AM, et al. Diagnostic value of blood sampling in fetuses with growth retardation. N Engl J Med 1993;328:692-696.

25. Trudinger BJ, Giles WB, Cook CM, et al. Fetal umbilical artery flow velocity waveforms and placental resistance: clinical significance. Br J Obstet Gynaecol 1985;92:23-30.

26. Mari G, Deter RL. Middle cerebral artery flow velocity waveforms in normal and small-for-gestational-age fetuses. Am J Obstet Gynecol 1992;166:1262-1270.

27. Kaminopetros P, Higueras MT, Nicolaides KH. Doppler study of uterine artery blood flow: comparison of findings in the first and second trimesters of pregnancy. Fetal Diagn Ther 1991;6:58-64.

28. Khong TY, De Wolf F, Robertson WB, Brosens I. Inadequate maternal vascular response to placentation in pregnancies complicated by pre-eclampsia and by small-for-gestational age infants. Br J Obstet Gynaecol 1986;93:1049-1059.

29. Lin S, Shimizu I, Suehara N, et al. Uterine artery Doppler velocimetry in relation to trophoblast migration into the myometrium of the placental bed. Obstet Gynecol 1995;85:760-765.

30. Valcamonico A, Danti L, Frusca T, et al. Absent end-diastolic velocity in umbilical artery: risk of neonatal morbidity and brain damage. Am J Obstet Gynecol 1994;170:796-801.

31. Mari G. Doppler ultrasonography in obstetrics: from the diagnosis of fetal anemia to the treatment of intrauterine growth-restricted fetuses. Am J Obstet Gynecol 2009;200:613 e1-e9.

32. Cnossen JS, Morris RK, ter Riet G, et al. Use of uterine artery Doppler ultrasonography to predict pre-eclampsia and intrauterine growth restriction: a systematic review and bivariable meta-analysis. CMAJ 2008;178:701-711.

33. Campbell S, Diaz-Recasens J, Griffin DR, et al. New Doppler technique for assessing uteroplacental blood flow. Lancet 1983;1:675-677.

34. Maulik D, Yarlagadda AP, Youngblood JP, Willoughby L. Components of variability of umbilical arterial Doppler velocimetry: a prospective analysis. Am J Obstet Gynecol 1989;160:1406-1409; discussion 1409-1412.

35. Stuart B, Drumm J, FitzGerald DE, Duignan NM. Fetal blood velocity waveforms in normal pregnancy. Br J Obstet Gynaecol 1980;87:780-785.

36. Thompson RS, Trudinger BJ, Cook CM, Giles WB. Umbilical artery velocity waveforms: normal reference values for A/B ratio and Pourcelot ratio. Br J Obstet Gynaecol 1988;95:589-591.

37. Trudinger BJ, Stevens D, Connelly A, et al. Umbilical artery flow velocity waveforms and placental resistance: the effects of embolization of the umbilical circulation. Am J Obstet Gynecol 1987;157:1443-1448.

38. Devoe LD, Gardner P, Dear C, Faircloth D. The significance of increasing umbilical artery systolic-diastolic ratios in third-trimester pregnancy. Obstet Gynecol 1992;80:684-687.

39. Fleischer A, Schulman H, Farmakides G, et al. Umbilical artery velocity waveforms and intrauterine growth retardation. Am J Obstet Gynecol 1985;151:502-505.

40. Gudmundsson S, Marsal K. Umbilical and uteroplacental blood flow velocity waveforms in pregnancies with fetal growth retardation. Eur J Obstet Gynecol Reprod Biol 1988;27:187-196.

41. Rochelson BL, Schulman H, Fleischer A, et al. The clinical significance of Doppler umbilical artery velocimetry in the small for gestational age fetus. Am J Obstet Gynecol 1987;156:1223-1226.

42. Trudinger BJ, Cook CM, Giles WB, et al. Fetal umbilical artery velocity waveforms and subsequent neonatal outcome. Br J Obstet Gynaecol 1991;98:378-384.

43. Westergaard HB, Langhoff-Roos J, Lingman G, et al. A critical appraisal of the use of umbilical artery Doppler ultrasound in high-risk pregnancies: use of meta-analyses in evidence-based obstetrics. Ultrasound Obstet Gynecol 2001;17:466-476.

44. Mari G, Moise Jr KJ, Deter RL, et al. Doppler assessment of the pulsatility index of the middle cerebral artery during constriction of the fetal ductus arteriosus after indomethacin therapy. Am J Obstet Gynecol 1989;161:1528-1531.

45. Dobbing J, Sands J. Timing of neuroblast multiplication in developing human brain. Nature 1970;226:639-640.

46. Cohn HE, Sacks EJ, Heymann MA, Rudolph AM. Cardiovascular responses to hypoxemia and acidemia in fetal lambs. Am J Obstet Gynecol 1974;120:817-824.

47. Wladimiroff JW, Tonge HM, Stewart PA. Doppler ultrasound assessment of cerebral blood flow in the human fetus. Br J Obstet Gynaecol 1986;93:471-475.

48. Richardson BS, Rurak D, Patrick JE, et al. Cerebral oxidative metabolism during sustained hypoxaemia in fetal sheep. J Dev Physiol 1989;11:37-43.

49. Mari G, Wasserstrum N. Flow velocity waveforms of the fetal circulation preceding fetal death in a case of lupus anticoagulant. Am J Obstet Gynecol 1991;164:776-778.

50. Vyas S, Nicolaides KH, Bower S, Campbell S. Middle cerebral artery flow velocity waveforms in fetal hypoxaemia. Br J Obstet Gynaecol 1990;97:797-803.

51. Chandran R, Serra Serra V, Sellers SM, Redman CW. Fetal middle cerebral artery flow velocity waveforms: a terminal pattern—case report. Br J Obstet Gynaecol 1991;98:937-938.

52. Respondek M, Woch A, Kaczmarek P, Borowski D. Reversal of diastolic flow in the middle cerebral artery of the fetus during the second half of pregnancy. Ultrasound Obstet Gynecol 1997;9:324-329.

53. Sepulveda W, Shennan AH, Peek MJ. Reverse end-diastolic flow in the middle cerebral artery: an agonal pattern in the human fetus. Am J Obstet Gynecol 1996;174:1645-1647.

54. Hanif F, Drennan K, Mari G. Variables that affect the middle cerebral artery peak systolic velocity in fetuses with anemia and intrauterine growth restriction. Am J Perinatol 2007;24:501-505.

55. Eik-Nes SH, Marsal K, Brubakk AO, et al. Ultrasonic measurement of human fetal blood flow. J Biomed Eng 1982;4:28-36.

56. Lingman G, Marsal K. Fetal central blood circulation in the third trimester of normal pregnancy: a longitudinal study. II. Aortic blood velocity waveform. Early Hum Dev 1986;13:151-159.

57. Mari G. Arterial blood flow velocity waveforms of the pelvis and lower extremities in normal and growth-retarded fetuses. Am J Obstet Gynecol 1991;165:143-151.

58. Abuhamad AZ, Mari G, Bogdan D, Evans 3rd AT. Doppler flow velocimetry of the splenic artery in the human fetus: is it a marker of chronic hypoxia? Am J Obstet Gynecol 1995;172:820-825.

59. Finne PH, Halvorsen S. Regulation of erythropoiesis in the fetus and newborn. Arch Dis Child 1972;47:683-687.

60. Fischer JW. Control of erythropoietin production. Exp Biol Med 1984;173:289-305.

61. Abuhamad AZ, Mari G, Cortina RM, et al. Superior mesenteric artery Doppler velocimetry and ultrasonographic assessment of fetal bowel in gastroschisis: a prospective longitudinal study. Am J Obstet Gynecol 1997;176:985-990.

62. Rhee E, Detti L, Mari G. Superior mesenteric artery flow velocity waveforms in small for gestational age fetuses. J Matern Fetal Med 1998;7:120-123.

63. Mari G, Uerpairojkit B, Abuhamad AZ, Copel JA. Adrenal artery velocity waveforms in the appropriate and small-for-gestational-age fetus. Ultrasound Obstet Gynecol 1996;8:82-86.

64. Mari G, Kirshon B, Abuhamad A. Fetal renal artery flow velocity waveforms in normal pregnancies and pregnancies complicated by polyhydramnios and oligohydramnios. Obstet Gynecol 1993;81: 560-564.

65. Vyas S, Nicolaides KH, Campbell S. Renal artery flow-velocity waveforms in normal and hypoxemic fetuses. Am J Obstet Gynecol 1989;161:168-172.

66. Uerpairojkit B, Chan L, Reece AE, et al. Cerebellar Doppler velocimetry in the appropriate- and small-for-gestational-age fetus. Obstet Gynecol 1996;87:989-993.

67. Gudmundsson S, Tulzer G, Huhta JC, Marsal K. Venous Doppler in the fetus with absent end-diastolic flow in the umbilical artery. Ultrasound Obstet Gynecol 1996;7:262-267.

68. Nakai Y, Miyazaki Y, Matsuoka Y, et al. Pulsatile umbilical venous flow and its clinical significance. Br J Obstet Gynaecol 1992;99: 977-980.

69. Edelstone DI, Rudolph AM, Heymann MA. Liver and ductus venosus blood flows in fetal lambs in utero. Circ Res 1978;42: 426-433.

70. Rudolph AM. Distribution and regulation of blood flow in the fetal and neonatal lamb. Circ Res 1985;57:811-821.

71. Mari G, Uerpairojkit B, Copel JA. Abdominal venous system in the normal fetus. Obstet Gynecol 1995;86:729-733.

72. Van Splunder IP, Huisman TW, Stijnen T, Wladimiroff JW. Presence of pulsations and reproducibility of waveform recording in the umbilical and left portal vein in normal pregnancies. Ultrasound Obstet Gynecol 1994;4:49-53.

73. Reed KL, Appleton CP, Anderson CF, et al. Doppler studies of vena cava flows in human fetuses: insights into normal and abnormal cardiac physiology. Circulation 1990;81:498-505.

74. Rizzo G, Arduini D, Romanini C. Inferior vena cava flow velocity waveforms in appropriate- and small-for-gestational-age fetuses. Am J Obstet Gynecol 1992;166:1271-1280.

75. Kiserud T, Eik-Nes SH, Blaas HG, Hellevik LR. Ultrasonographic velocimetry of the fetal ductus venosus. Lancet 1991;338:1412-1414.

76. Rizzo G, Arduini D, Romanini C. Umbilical vein pulsations: a physiologic finding in early gestation. Am J Obstet Gynecol 1992; 167:675-677.

77. Picconi JL, Hanif F, Drennan K, Mari G. The transitional phase of ductus venosus reversed flow in severely premature IUGR fetuses. Am J Perinatol 2008;25:199-203.

78. Picconi JL, Kruger M, Mari G. Ductus venosus S-wave/isovolumetric A-wave (SIA) index and A-wave reversed flow in severely premature growth-restricted fetuses. J Ultrasound Med 2008;27:1283-1289.

79. Rizzo G, Arduini D, Romanini C, Mancuso S. Doppler echocardiographic assessment of atrioventricular velocity waveforms in normal and small-for-gestational-age fetuses. Br J Obstet Gynaecol 1988; 95:65-69.

80. Hecher K, Campbell S, Snijders R, Nicolaides K. Reference ranges for fetal venous and atrioventricular blood flow parameters. Ultrasound Obstet Gynecol 1994;4:381-390.

81. Carceller-Blanchard AM, Fouron JC. Determinants of the Doppler flow velocity profile through the mitral valve of the human fetus. Br Heart J 1993;70:457-460.

82. Hata T, Hata K, Takamiya O, et al. Fetal ventricular relaxation assessed by Doppler echocardiography. J Cardiovasc Ultrasonogr 1988;7:207-213.

83. Reed KL, Anderson CF, Shenker L. Changes in intracardiac Doppler blood flow velocities in fetuses with absent umbilical artery diastolic flow. Am J Obstet Gynecol 1987;157:774-779.

84. Shapiro I, Degani S, Leibovitz Z, et al. Fetal cardiac measurements derived by transvaginal and transabdominal cross-sectional echocardiography from 14 weeks of gestation to term. Ultrasound Obstet Gynecol 1998;12:404-418.

85. Mari G, Deter RL, Hanif F, et al. Sequence of cardiovascular changes occurring in severe IUGR fetuses. Part II. Ultrasound Obstet Gynecol 2006;28:390.

86. Kenny JF, Plappert T, Doubilet P, et al. Changes in intracardiac blood flow velocities and right and left ventricular stroke volumes with gestational age in the normal human fetus: a prospective Doppler echocardiographic study. Circulation 1986;74:1208-1216.

87. Machado MV, Chita SC, Allan LD. Acceleration time in the aorta and pulmonary artery measured by Doppler echocardiography in the midtrimester normal human fetus. Br Heart J 1987;58:15-18.

88. Kitabatake A, Inoue M, Asao M, et al. Noninvasive evaluation of pulmonary hypertension by a pulsed Doppler technique. Circulation 1983;68:302-309.

89. Al-Ghazali W, Chita SK, Chapman MG, Allan LD. Evidence of redistribution of cardiac output in asymmetrical growth retardation. Br J Obstet Gynaecol 1989;96:697-704.

90. Allan LD, Chita SK, Al-Ghazali W, et al. Doppler echocardiographic evaluation of the normal human fetal heart. Br Heart J 1987;57:528-533.

91. De Smedt MC, Visser GH, Meijboom EJ. Fetal cardiac output estimated by Doppler echocardiography during mid- and late gestation. Am J Cardiol 1987;60:338-342.

92. Shiraishi H, Silverman NH, Rudolph AM. Accuracy of right ventricular output estimated by Doppler echocardiography in the sheep fetus. Am J Obstet Gynecol 1993;168:947-953.

93. Moise Jr KJ, Mari G, Fisher DJ, et al. Acute fetal hemodynamic alterations after intrauterine transfusion for treatment of severe red blood cell alloimmunization. Am J Obstet Gynecol 1990;163:776-784.

94. Rizzo G, Nicolaides KH, Arduini D, Campbell S. Effects of intravascular fetal blood transfusion on fetal intracardiac Doppler velocity waveforms. Am J Obstet Gynecol 1990;163:1231-1238.

95. Gonzalez R, Medina L, Arriagada P, et al. Transdermal administration of a nitric oxide donor is not associated with changes in major fetal cardiac and systemic hemodynamic parameters. Am J Obstet Gynecol 1999;180:S3.

Prediction of Fetal Hematocrit

96. Mari G, Moise Jr KJ, Deter RL, Carpenter Jr RJ. Flow velocity waveforms of the umbilical and cerebral arteries before and after intravascular transfusion. Obstet Gynecol 1990;75:584-589.

97. Mari G, Moise Jr KJ, Deter RL, et al. Flow velocity waveforms of the vascular system in the anemic fetus before and after intravascular transfusion for severe red blood cell alloimmunization. Am J Obstet Gynecol 1990;162:1060-1064.

98. Mari G, Moise Jr KJ, Deter RL, Carpenter Jr RJ. Doppler assessment of renal blood flow velocity waveforms in the anemic fetus before and after intravascular transfusion for severe red cell alloimmunization. J Clin Ultrasound 1991;19:15-19.

99. Mari G, Rahman F, Olofsson P, et al. Increase of fetal hematocrit decreases the middle cerebral artery peak systolic velocity in pregnancies complicated by rhesus alloimmunization. J Matern Fetal Med 1997;6:206-208.

100. Stefos T, Cosmi E, Detti L, Mari G. Correction of fetal anemia on the middle cerebral artery peak systolic velocity. Obstet Gynecol 2002;99:211-215.

101. Mari G, Moise KJ, Kirshon B, et al. Middle cerebral artery pulsatility index and maximal velocity as indicators of fetal anemia. 37th Annual Meeting of Society for Gynecologic Investigation, 1990.

102. Mari G, Adrignolo A, Abuhamad A, et al. Doppler ultrasound in the management of the pregnancy complicated by fetal anemia. Am J Obstet Gynecol 1993;168:318.

103. Mari G, Adrignolo A, Abuhamad AZ, et al. Diagnosis of fetal anemia with Doppler ultrasound in the pregnancy complicated by

maternal blood group immunization. Ultrasound Obstet Gynecol 1995;5:400-405.

104. Mari G, Detti L, Oz U, et al. Accurate prediction of fetal hemoglobin by Doppler ultrasonography. Obstet Gynecol 2002;99:589-593.

105. Pereira L, Jenkins TM, Berghella V. Conventional management of maternal red cell alloimmunization compared with management by Doppler assessment of middle cerebral artery peak systolic velocity. Am J Obstet Gynecol 2003;189:1002-1006.

106. Van Dongen H, Klumper FJ, Sikkel E, et al. Non-invasive tests to predict fetal anemia in Kell-alloimmunized pregnancies. Ultrasound Obstet Gynecol 2005;25:341-345.

107. Cosmi E, Mari G, Delle Chiaie L, et al. Noninvasive diagnosis by Doppler ultrasonography of fetal anemia resulting from parvovirus infection. Am J Obstet Gynecol 2002;187:1290-1293.

108. Delle Chiaie L, Buck G, Grab D, Terinde R. Prediction of fetal anemia with Doppler measurement of the middle cerebral artery peak systolic velocity in pregnancies complicated by maternal blood group alloimmunization or parvovirus B19 infection. Ultrasound Obstet Gynecol 2001;18:232-236.

109. Senat MV, Loizeau S, Couderc S, et al. The value of middle cerebral artery peak systolic velocity in the diagnosis of fetal anemia after intrauterine death of one monochorionic twin. Am J Obstet Gynecol 2003;189:1320-1324.

110. Mari G, Detti L. Doppler ultrasound: application to fetal medicine. In: Fleischer AC, Manning FA, Jeanty P, Romero R, editors. Sonography in obstetrics and gynecology: principles and practice. New York: McGraw-Hill; 2001. p. 247-283.

111. Sueters M, Arabin B, Oepkes D. Doppler sonography for predicting fetal anemia caused by massive fetomaternal hemorrhage. Ultrasound Obstet Gynecol 2003;22:186-189.

112. Cosmi E, Dessole S, Uras L, et al. Middle cerebral artery peak systolic and ductus venosus velocity waveforms in the hydropic fetus. J Ultrasound Med 2005;24:209-213.

113. Hernandez-Andrade E, Scheier M, Dezerega V, et al. Fetal middle cerebral artery peak systolic velocity in the investigation of non-immune hydrops. Ultrasound Obstet Gynecol 2004;23:442-445.

Multiple Gestations

114. Gaziano EP, Knox H, Ferrera B, et al. Is it time to reassess the risk for the growth-retarded fetus with normal Doppler velocimetry of the umbilical artery? Am J Obstet Gynecol 1994;170:1734-1741; discussion 1741-1743.

115. Giles WB, Trudinger BJ, Cook CM, Connelly A. Umbilical artery flow velocity waveforms and twin pregnancy outcome. Obstet Gynecol 1988;72:894-897.

116. Divon MY, Girz BA, Sklar A, et al. Discordant twins: a prospective study of the diagnostic value of real-time ultrasonography combined with umbilical artery velocimetry. Am J Obstet Gynecol 1989;161:757-760.

117. Degani S, Gonen R, Shapiro I, et al. Doppler flow velocity waveforms in fetal surveillance of twins: a prospective longitudinal study. J Ultrasound Med 1992;11:537-541.

118. Hecher K, Ville Y, Nicolaides KH. Fetal arterial Doppler studies in twin-twin transfusion syndrome. J Ultrasound Med 1995;14:101-108.

119. Kontopoulos EV, Quintero RA, Chmait RH, et al. Percent absent end-diastolic velocity in the umbilical artery waveform as a predictor of intrauterine fetal demise of the donor twin after selective laser photocoagulation of communicating vessels in twin-twin transfusion syndrome. Ultrasound Obstet Gynecol 2007;30:35-39.

120. Quintero RA, Morales WJ, Allen MH, et al. Staging of twin-twin transfusion syndrome. J Perinatol 1999;19:550-555.

121. Mari G, Roberts A, Detti L, et al. Perinatal morbidity and mortality rates in severe twin-twin transfusion syndrome: results of the International Amnioreduction Registry. Am J Obstet Gynecol 2001;185:708-715.

122. Huhta JC, Moise KJ, Fisher DJ, et al. Detection and quantitation of constriction of the fetal ductus arteriosus by Doppler echocardiography. Circulation 1987;75:406-412.

123. Robyr R, Lewi L, Salomon LJ, et al. Prevalence and management of late fetal complications following successful selective laser coagulation of chorionic plate anastomoses in twin-to-twin transfusion syndrome. Am J Obstet Gynecol 2006;194:796-803.

Indomethacin and Ductus Arteriosus

124. Rasanen J, Debbs RH, Wood DC, et al. The effects of maternal indomethacin therapy on human fetal branch pulmonary arterial vascular impedance. Ultrasound Obstet Gynecol 1999;13:112-116.

125. American College of Obstetricians and Gynecologists. ACOG Practice Bulletin. Antepartum fetal surveillance. (No 9, Oct 1999; replaces Tech Bull No 188, Jan 1994.) Clinical management guidelines for obstetrician-gynecologists. Int J Gynaecol Obstet 2000;68:175-185.

Biophysical Profile Scoring

126. Manning FA, Platt LD, Sipos L. Antepartum fetal evaluation: development of a fetal biophysical profile. Am J Obstet Gynecol 1980;136:787-795.

127. Morrison I. Perinatal mortality: basic considerations. Semin Perinatol 1985;9:144-150.

128. Manning FA, Morrison I, Lange IR, et al. Fetal biophysical profile scoring: selective use of the nonstress test. Am J Obstet Gynecol 1987;156:709-712.

129. Chamberlain PF, Manning FA, Morrison I, et al. Ultrasound evaluation of amniotic fluid volume. I. The relationship of marginal and decreased amniotic fluid volumes to perinatal outcome. Am J Obstet Gynecol 1984;150:245-249.

130. Patrick JE, Dalton KJ, Dawes GS. Breathing patterns before death in fetal lambs. Am J Obstet Gynecol 1976;125:73-78.

131. Romero R, Chervenak FA, Berkowitz RL, Hobbins JC. Intrauterine fetal tachypnea. Am J Obstet Gynecol 1982;144:356-357.

132. Manning FA, Baskett TF, Morrison I, Lange I. Fetal biophysical profile scoring: a prospective study in 1,184 high-risk patients. Am J Obstet Gynecol 1981;140:289-294.

133. Phelan JP, Ahn MO, Smith CV, et al. Amniotic fluid index measurements during pregnancy. J Reprod Med 1987;32:601-604.

134. Manning FA, Harman CR, Morrison I, et al. Fetal assessment based on fetal biophysical profile scoring. IV. An analysis of perinatal morbidity and mortality. Am J Obstet Gynecol 1990;162:703-709.

135. Magann EF, Doherty DA, Field K, et al. Biophysical profile with amniotic fluid volume assessments. Obstet Gynecol 2004;104:5-10.

136. Jansen AH, Chernick V. Fetal breathing and development of control of breathing. J Appl Physiol 1991;70:1431-1446.

137. Kurjak A, Andonotopo W, Hafner T, et al. Normal standards for fetal neurobehavioral developments: longitudinal quantification by four-dimensional sonography. J Perinat Med 2006;34:56-65.

138. Kim SY, Khandelwal M, Gaughan JP, et al. Is the intrapartum biophysical profile useful? Obstet Gynecol 2003;102:471-476.

139. Odibo AO, Quinones JN, Lawrence-Cleary K, et al. What antepartum fetal test should guide the timing of delivery of the preterm growth-restricted fetus? A decision-analysis. Am J Obstet Gynecol 2004;191:1477-1482.

140. Clark SL, Sabey P, Jolley K. Nonstress testing with acoustic stimulation and amniotic fluid volume assessment: 5973 tests without unexpected fetal death. Am J Obstet Gynecol 1989;160:694-697.

141. Nageotte MP, Towers CV, Asrat T, Freeman RK. Perinatal outcome with the modified biophysical profile. Am J Obstet Gynecol 1994;170:1672-1676.

142. Seeds AE. Current concepts of amniotic fluid dynamics. Am J Obstet Gynecol 1980;138:575-586.

143. Rutherford SE, Phelan JP, Smith CV, Jacobs N. The four-quadrant assessment of amniotic fluid volume: an adjunct to antepartum fetal heart rate testing. Obstet Gynecol 1987;70:353-356.

144. Miller DA, Rabello YA, Paul RH. The modified biophysical profile: antepartum testing in the 1990s. Am J Obstet Gynecol 1996;174:812-817.

145. Baschat AA, Gembruch U, Harman CR. The sequence of changes in Doppler and biophysical parameters as severe fetal growth restriction worsens. Ultrasound Obstet Gynecol 2001;18:571-577.

146. Mari G, Hanif F, Treadwell MC, Kruger M. Gestational age at delivery and Doppler waveforms in very preterm intrauterine growth-restricted fetuses as predictors of perinatal mortality. J Ultrasound Med 2007;26:555-559; quiz 560-562.

147. Manning FA, Martin Jr CB, Murata Y, et al. Breathing movements before death in the primate fetus (Macaca mulatta). Am J Obstet Gynecol 1979;135:71-76.

CHAPTER 44

Sonographic Evaluation of the Placenta

Thomas D. Shipp

Chapter Outline

*T*he use of ultrasound to evaluate the placenta is routine among the majority of pregnant American women because they have at least one ultrasound examination during pregnancy. A wide range of pregnancy complications result from abnormal placental development, including preeclampsia, intrauterine growth restriction (IUGR), and abruption. Other placental abnormalities, such as placenta previa, percreta, or vasa previa, may cause major maternal and fetal complications. Timely recognition of these abnormalities can lead to improved management of pregnancy and delivery. Thus, careful examinations of the placenta by ultrasound can contribute directly to enhanced patient care and improved outcomes.

PLACENTAL DEVELOPMENT

The early developing embryo is surrounded by amnion and chorion. Villi cover the entire surface of the chorion up to about 8 weeks of gestation (Fig. 44-1). The villi, which are the basic structures of the placenta, initially form by 4 or 5 weeks' gestation. The villi next to the **decidua capsularis** degenerate, forming the **chorion laeve.** The villi contiguous with the **decidua basalis** become the **chorion frondosum** and later the placenta. The fetal side of the placenta consists of the **chorionic plate** and **chorionic villi**. The maternal side consists of the decidua basalis, which open up into large cisterns, the **intervillous spaces.** The fetal villi are immersed in maternal blood located in the intervillous spaces. Anchoring villi develop from the chorionic plate.[1] These attach to the decidua basalis, holding the placenta in place.[2,3] By the end of pregnancy, the villi have a surface area of 12 to 14 square meters.[4]

Placental Appearance

The placenta in the first and second trimesters is slightly more echogenic than the surrounding myometrium (Fig. 44-2, *A*). The attachment site, or base of the placenta, should be clearly delineated from the underlying myometrium. The edges of the placenta usually have a small sinus, the **marginal sinus of the placenta** (Fig. 44-2, *B*), where intervillous blood drains into the maternal venous circulation. This structure should not be confused with placental separation. As the placenta matures, areas of echogenicity within the placenta are visualized (Fig. 44-2, *D* and *E*). In cases of **placental infarction,** there may be hypoechoic lesions with echogenic borders.

Placental lakes (venous lakes) occur in up to 5% of pregnancies[5-9] (Fig. 44-2, *C;* **Video 44-1**). They represent areas of intervillous spaces devoid of placental villous trees. They can be seen as hypoechoic structures in the placenta. Moving blood flow can be seen in these areas. They may have irregular shapes or a narrow, cleftlike appearance and may change in appearance over time.

Placental Size

Placental length is approximately six times its maximal width at 18 to 20 weeks' gestation. The mean thickness of the placenta in millimeters in the first half of pregnancy closely approximates the gestational age in weeks.[10]

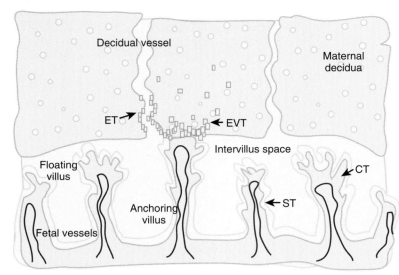

FIGURE 44-1. Human placenta microarchitecture. Fetal derivatives in the placenta consist of fetal vessels and placental cotyledons (villi). Villi consist of fetal vessels surrounded by **cytotrophoblast** cells *(CT)*. Covering the cytotrophoblast cells is a multinucleated cellular layer called the **syncytiotrophoblast** *(ST)*. Anchoring villi are in direct contact with the maternal uterine lining, called the **decidua.** The decidua is traversed by maternal vasculature. Blood from these vessels empties into the intervillous space and bathes the placental villi. Note that maternal and fetal blood vessels are separated by trophoblast, villous stroma, and fetal vascular endothelium. Cytotrophoblast cells from anchoring villae can change into an invasive phenotype called extravillous cytotrophoblast cells *(EVT)*. EVT invade deeply into the maternal decidua. Some EVT, called endovascular trophoblast cells *(ET)*, embed within the walls of the maternal vasculature. (From Comiskey M, Warner CM, Schust DJ: MHC molecules of the preimplantation embryo and trophoblast. In: Mor G, ed. Immunology of Pregnancy. Austin/New York: Landes Bioscience, 2006.)

FIGURE 44-2. Normal appearance of placenta. A, At 18 weeks, note the uniformly echogenic appearance of the placenta and a uterine contraction deviating the placenta. **B,** Note **marginal sinus of placenta** *(arrow)*, a circumferential venous drainage point into the maternal uterine veins that should not be mistaken for placental separation. **C, Placental lake** *(arrow)* at 20 weeks. Calipers denote length of placenta. **D** and **E,** Note the increasing echogenicity in the placenta as it matures. *(D and E from Burton GJ, Jauniaux E. Sonographic, stereological and Doppler flow velocimetric assessments of placental maturity. Br J Obstet Gynaecol 1995;102:818-825.)*

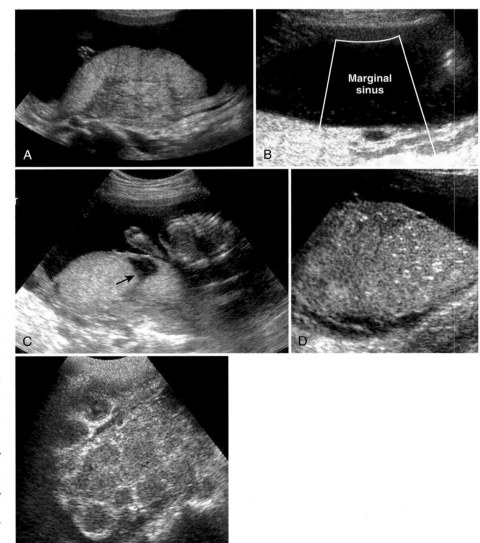

If the placenta thickness is greater than 4 cm (40 mm) before 24 weeks, an abnormality should be suspected. These abnormalities include **ischemic-thrombotic damage, intraplacental hemorrhage, chorioangioma,** and **fetal hydrops** (Fig. 44-3).

Given the variable shape of the placenta, calculating a volume from two-dimensional (2-D) imaging can be complicated. Multiplanar volume calculation involves sequential sections of the placenta at intervals such as 1.0 mm. The margins are manually traced, and a volume is calculated.[11] Most current studies appraising the use of three-dimensional (3-D) sonography have used the VOCAL (Virtual Organ Computer-aided AnaLysis) method,[11] in which the 3-D volume in question is rotated and the area of interest traced at its margin, after which a volume is calculated (Fig. 44-4).

Placental volume approximation in the first trimester holds promise as an important part of early pregnancy evaluation. Uterine artery Doppler analysis can provide some information regarding IUGR and maternal hypertension, but it is insufficient as a sole indicator of trophoblast invasion, in part because it is typically performed late in the second trimester. Small placental volumes in the first trimester presage abnormal uterine artery perfusion.[12] Uterine artery Doppler ultrasound combined with assessment of placental volume may identify pregnant women at risk for hypertension, abruption, or IUGR.[13,14] First-trimester placental volumes correlate with pregnancy-associated plasma protein A (PAPP-A) and free beta-human chorionic gonadotropin (f-β-hCG) levels,[15] suggesting the potential introduction of placental volumes in the first trimester with maternal serum screening for aneuploidy.[15] The first-trimester **placental volume quotient** (placental volume/crown-rump length) is low for aneuploid fetuses, with 53% having a quotient less than 10th centile.[16] For twins, the placental volume is 83%, and for triplets, 76%, that of singletons, for a given gestational age.[17]

The placenta dramatically increases in size until approximately 15 to 17 weeks' gestation. From this

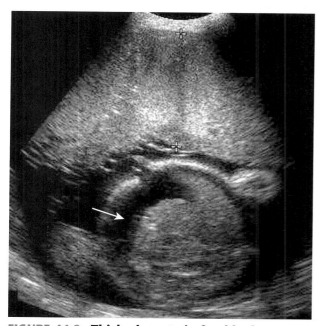

FIGURE 44-3. Thick placenta in fetal hydrops. Note the ascites *(arrow).*

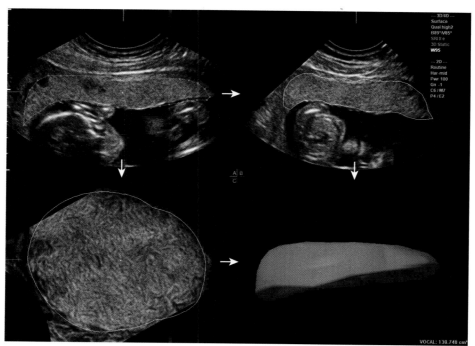

FIGURE 44-4. Three-dimensional assessment of placental volume in second trimester.

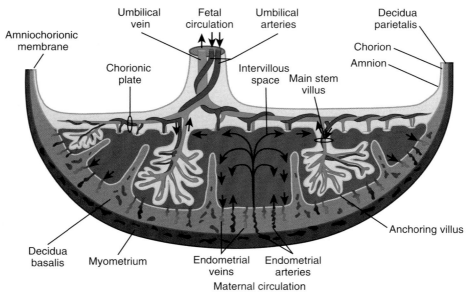

FIGURE 44-5. Schematic drawing of placental vasculature.

point, there is a fourfold increase in placental size until delivery, whereas the fetus has a 50-fold increase in size until delivery.[18] Midtrimester placental volume is associated with maternal nutritional status, birth weight, and pregnancy outcome.[19-23]

Placental Vascularity and Doppler Ultrasound

The human placenta is a discoidal, villous, hemochorial structure. Nutrients are exchanged over many villi. Surrounding the villi are the **intervillous spaces,** which are bathed in maternal blood. The villi are sproutlike projections from the chorionic plate into the intervillous space. The villi are directly connected to the fetal vascular system, whereas the maternal blood emanates from the developing spiral arteries to the intervillous spaces to contact directly the trophoblasts of the villi[24] (Fig. 44-5). Maternal blood flow of the intervillous space depends on flow from the spiral arteries. Maternal vascular disease (e.g., hypertension) can directly affect the pregnancy by limiting this blood flow.[25]

Intervillous blood flow begins early in the first trimester.[26-28] Color Doppler ultrasound has been used to detect this intervillous and spiral artery flow by 12 weeks' gestation, but the flow, if any, that occurs before this time is not well understood.[29] Before 12 weeks, the presence of intervillous blood flow by gray-scale imaging may indicate failed pregnancy.[30]

Color and power Doppler sonography have been used to identify blood flow in intraplacental villous arteries.[31] A decrease in the number of detectable intraplacental villous arteries is associated with IUGR.[32] Three-dimensional power Doppler ultrasound provides a better appreciation of placental vascularity and pathophysiol-

ogy by assessing placental flow and documenting the amount of flow in a given area. Because of its low variability between sampling sites in varied parts of the placenta, 3-D imaging may have a future role in assessing flow in high-risk pregnancies (e.g., hypertension, IUGR).[33]

Amnion-Chorion Separation

The amnion normally "fuses" with the chorion early in the second trimester. Failure of the amnion and chorion to fuse after 17 weeks is a rare complication of pregnancy, associated with multiple abnormalities. Previous amniocentesis is a risk factor for amnion-chorion separation.[34] Associated factors may include IUGR, preterm delivery, oligohydramnios, placental abruption, and Down syndrome[35] (Fig. 44-6).

PLACENTA PREVIA

The term "placenta previa" refers to a placenta that is "previous" to the fetus in the birth canal. The incidence at delivery is approximately 0.5% of all pregnancies.[36] **Bleeding** in the second and third trimesters is the hallmark of placenta previa. This bleeding can be life threatening to the mother and fetus. With expectant management and cesarean delivery, both maternal and perinatal mortality have decreased over the past 40 years.[37,38] Accurate diagnosis of placenta previa is vital to improve the outcome for mother and neonate.

The differentiation of placental positions has historically been performed by digital assessment of the lower uterine segment and placenta through the cervix. Using this potentially hazardous method of evaluation,

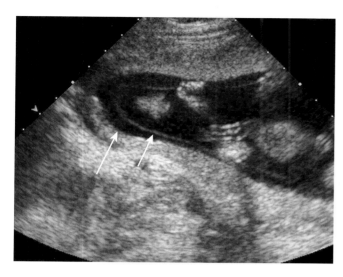

FIGURE 44-6. Chorioamniotic separation in second trimester. Amnion *(short arrow)* is separated from the chorion *(long arrow).*

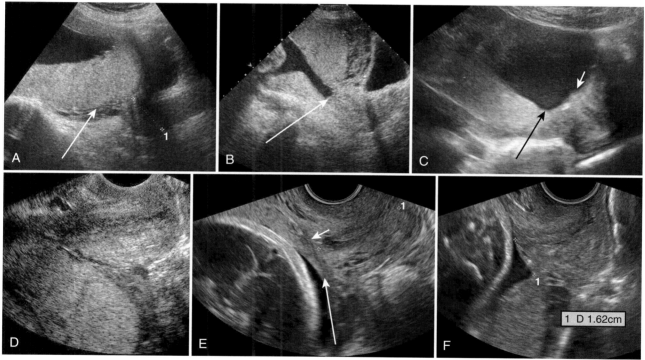

FIGURE 44-7. Placental position. Transabdominal sonography **(A-C)** and transvaginal sonography **(C-E)** can be used to determine placental position. If the position is unclear transabdominally, vaginal sonography should be used. **A,** Complete placenta previa *(arrow).* The maternal cervix is demarcated by the calipers. **B,** Marginal placenta previa. The internal cervical os is indicated by the arrow. **C,** Low placenta. The long arrow indicates the placental edge and the short arrow indicates the internal cervical os. **D,** Complete placenta previa. **E,** Complete placenta previa. The placental tip *(long arrow)* crosses the os *(short arrow).* **F,** Low placenta. The tip of the placenta is 1.6 cm from the internal os.

placental position was classified as complete placenta previa, partial placenta previa, incomplete placenta previa, marginal placenta previa, low-lying placenta, and placenta distant from the internal cervical os. These classifications do not directly apply to the ultrasound examination of placental position relative to the cervix. The use of ultrasound to evaluate the position of the placenta in the uterus has both improved knowledge of the placenta within the uterus and simplified terminology with respect to placental position (Fig. 44-7). **Complete placenta previa** describes the situation in which the internal cervical os is totally covered by the placenta. **Marginal placenta previa** denotes placental tissue at the edge of or encroaching on the internal cervical os. A **low placenta** is one in which the placental edge is within 2 cm, but not covering any portion, of the internal cervical os. The terms "incomplete placenta previa" and "partial placenta previa" have no place in the current sonographic assessment of placental position and should be used only by a clinician performing a digital examination when a "double setup" is necessary to determine where the leading edge of the placenta lies.

Transabdominal scanning can be used to visualize the internal cervical os and to determine the relation of the placenta to the cervix in most cases. Factors that can adversely affect the visualization of the cervix include prior abdominal surgery, obesity, deep or low position of the fetal head or presenting part, overfilled or underfilled maternal bladder, or uterine contractions. Transvaginal sonography is safe[39] and accurate in depicting the internal cervical os. The proximity of the cervix to the vaginal probe allows higher-frequency probes to be used, with better resolution and thus better visualization of the internal cervical os. With improved resolution, clinicians can accurately determine the position of the leading placental edge to the internal cervical os. The use of transvaginal sonography has been shown to change the assessment of the placental location in 25% of cases when the placenta is within 2 cm of the internal cervical os, as identified transabdominally.[40] A leading placental edge greater than 2 cm from the internal cervical os is associated with vaginal delivery, and distances less than 2 cm are associated with bleeding, leading to cesarean delivery.[41,42]

Although placenta previa can occur in nulliparas, risk factors include number of prior cesarean deliveries (odds ratio: 4.5 for one; 44.9 for four[43]), increasing parity independent of number of prior cesarean deliveries,[44] and increasing maternal age.[45]

Early in the second trimester, the placenta occupies a relatively large portion of the uterine cavity and often is positioned near the cervix. As the uterus grows, a lesser proportion of placentas are located near the internal cervical os. This relative change in placental position is best understood by the placental migration theory.[46] This theory of "dynamic placentation" suggests that as the uterus develops, the placenta is "drawn away" from the internal cervical os. It is unclear whether the primary mechanism is disproportionate development of the lower uterine segment so that the placenta, although it does not detach from the uterine wall, comes to lie more distant from the internal cervical os. This theory would also be consistent with complete central placenta previas that do not resolve at a rate approaching that of other low-lying placentas, because the expansion of the lower uterine segment would not lead to the resolution of this type of placenta previa.

If the placenta overlaps the cervix by less than 2 cm, more than 88% of patients deliver vaginally.[47] A rate of migration (in the second and third trimesters) away from the internal os of 3.0 to 5.4 mm per week is also associated with vaginal delivery, whereas a placental-internal os distance of less than 2 cm or a pattern of migration of 0.3 to 0.6 mm weekly are associated with interventional cesarean delivery and a higher rate of peripartum complications.[47,48]

The prediction of a placenta previa at delivery is best when the placenta overlaps the internal cervical os by 1.4 cm at 10 to 16 weeks' gestation,[49] or 2 cm at 20 to 23 weeks.[50] Mustafa et al.[51] demonstrated that if the placenta overlaps by 2.3 cm at 11 to 14 weeks, the probability of a placenta previa at term is 8%, with a sensitivity of 83% and a specificity of 86%.[51] Aside from a complete central placenta previa, given the current data, it is still difficult to predict precisely which patients will have resolution of their low placenta; therefore, further ultrasound examinations are required to assess placental position if a low placenta is identified early in gestation.

For women with a low placenta, the description of the leading edge of the placenta in the early third trimester as "thin" (≤1 cm in thickness and/or angle of placental edge <45 degrees) or "thick" (any other type of placenta) can be predictive of delivery complications. Antepartum hemorrhage is more common with thick-edged placentas, as is the rate of cesarean delivery, placenta accreta, low birth weight, and earlier gestational age at delivery.[52] Interestingly, a more recent study performed in the first and second trimesters suggested that a thin-edged placenta with a smaller angle was more predictive of placenta previa.[53] Although not ready for clinical implementation, this parameter may help identify patients who can be reassured early in pregnancy that they will not have a placenta previa at delivery.

PLACENTA ACCRETA

The normal placenta invades the inner third of the myometrium. At delivery, the placenta separates at the decidual plane, with an abrupt cessation of intraplacental flow as the myometrium contracts.[54] A placenta that is abnormally adherent to the uterine wall after delivery is termed **placenta accreta. Placenta increta** occurs if the placenta invades the myometrium more deeply, and **placenta percreta** refers to a placenta that at least in part protrudes through the uterine serosa. Placenta accreta, increta, and percreta are serious complications of pregnancy associated with maternal blood loss, need for hysterectomy, and retained products of conception. With ultrasound, placenta accreta can be identified antenatally so that delivery plans can be made prospectively, improving the outcome for mother and child.

Although placenta accreta (or increta or percreta) can occur in any pregnancy, important risk factors include prior uterine surgery (with risk increasing with increasing number of prior cesarean deliveries), placenta previa, unexplained elevated maternal serum alpha-fetoprotein (MS-AFP), increased maternal cell-free placental lactogen, and advancing maternal age.[55-58] A woman with no placenta previa and no prior history of cesarean section has a baseline risk of 0.26% for placenta accreta. This increases almost linearly with number of prior cesarean sections, to 10% in patients with four or more.[59] Women with a placenta previa and an unscarred uterus have a 5% risk of clinical placenta accreta. With a placenta previa and one previous cesarean section, the risk of placenta accreta is 24%; this risk increases to 67% with a placenta previa and four or more cesarean deliveries.[59]

Several sonographic signs are associated with placenta accreta. The presence of a coexisting **placenta previa** in the majority of cases makes it particularly likely that the adherent portion of the placenta will be low in the uterus, in the region of a prior cesarean section scar. This simple fact makes the evaluation of these placentas much more straightforward with the transvaginal ultrasound probe. Sonographic findings of placenta accreta include loss of the normal hypoechoic retroplacental-myometrial interface, thinning or disruption of the hyperechoic subvesicular uterine serosa, presence of focal exophytic masses, and numerous placental lakes[60-63] (Fig. 44-8).

The color Doppler ultrasound findings suggestive of placenta previa accreta include diffuse lacunar blood flow throughout the placenta, dilated vascular channels between the placenta and bladder or cervix, absence of the normal subplacental venous flow, and the demonstration of vessels crossing the placental-myometrial disruption site.[64,65] Three-dimensional sonography may also be helpful for evaluation of vascular anatomy in the setting of a placenta accreta.[66,67] The gray-scale and color Doppler sonographic findings described for placenta accreta are also present, but more exaggerated, in placenta increta/percreta (Fig. 44-9; **Videos 44-2** and **44-3**). Three-dimensional color and power Doppler ultrasound is helpful to demonstrate the extensive torturous vascularity seen with such placentas. Greatly increased vascular lacunae with turbulent or "tornado" blood flow increases the likelihood of placenta increta/percreta.[68]

As in many aspects of obstetric sonography, early diagnosis is preferable. In women with a history of cesarean delivery, a gestational sac in the lower half of the uterus, at or before 10 weeks' gestation, is associated with

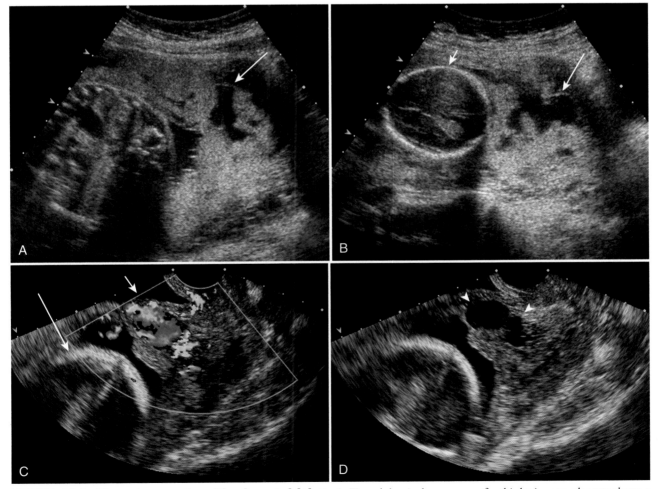

FIGURE 44-8. Placenta accreta with placental lakes. A, Transabdominal sonogram of a third-trimester placenta shows a placental (venous) lake *(arrow).* **B,** In a different patient, transabdominal sonogram of second-trimester placenta shows multiple placental lakes *(long arrow); short arrow,* fetal head. **C,** In another patient, transvaginal sonogram of second-trimester placenta shows intense color flow within and below the placenta; *long arrow,* fetal head; *short arrow,* maternal bladder. **D,** In the same patient as **C,** multiple placental lakes are visualized *(arrowheads).*

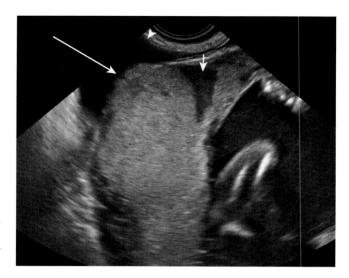

FIGURE 44-9. Placenta percreta. Transvaginal sonogram of a third-trimester placenta shows loss of the hypoechoic border between the placenta and the myometrium, with protrusion of the placenta *(long arrow)* into the maternal bladder *(arrowhead); short arrow,* placental lake.

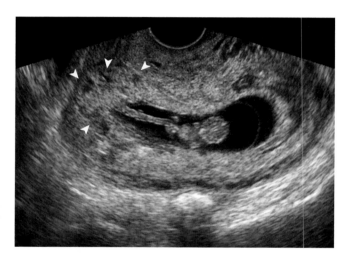

FIGURE 44-10. First-trimester placenta accreta. The umbilical cord insertion is low in the uterus; arrowheads indicate multiple small placental lakes. This patient had a prior cesarean delivery and subsequently was shown to have a placental previa accreta.

placenta accreta,[69] as are first-trimester placental lacunae[70,71] (Fig. 44-10). When the diagnosis is unclear or nonspecific findings are present, magnetic resonance imaging (MRI) may be helpful,[72-76] particularly when the placenta is posterior over an area of prior uterine scar, such as from myomectomy (Fig. 44-11).

Information about placenta accreta and its variants is indispensable for delivery management. Accurate prenatal diagnosis allows uterine conservation and avoidance of massive blood loss at delivery. Strategies include preoperative placement of internal iliac artery balloon catheters and ultrasound-guided fundal classic cesarean section to deliver the fetus above the upper margin of the placenta.

PLACENTAL ABRUPTION

Placental abruption is one of the worrisome causes of vaginal bleeding in the latter part of pregnancy because it contributes to perinatal mortality. Patients typically present with third-trimester vaginal bleeding associated with abdominal or uterine pain and labor. The incidence is approximately 0.5% of pregnancies. History of prior abruption, hypertension, prolonged rupture of membranes, IUGR, chorioamnionitis, polyhydramnios, maternal thrombophilias, maternal substance use (tobacco, alcohol, cocaine), maternal trauma, and advanced maternal age are all risk factors for placental abruption.[77-79] The diagnosis of placental abruption is typically made based on clinical findings; the retroplacental clot is frequently isoechoic to the placenta or myometrium and cannot always be identified sonographically.

A **subplacental hematoma** between the placenta and uterine wall is a placental abruption (Fig. 44-12). This should be differentiated from a **subchorionic hematoma,** in which the hematoma is underneath the chorion, not the placenta. Although a subchorionic hematoma can occur anytime during pregnancy, it is more common in the first half of pregnancy, and its appearance will change as the hematoma organizes (Fig. 44-13, *A*). A **preplacental hematoma** is a rare condition likely caused

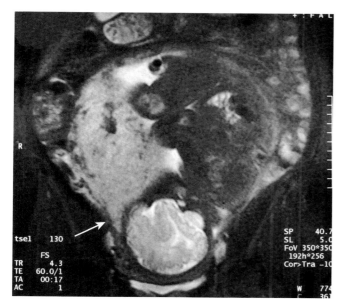

FIGURE 44-11. Placenta accreta. Coronal T2-weighted MR image shows an absent myometrial-placental interface in a posterolateral location *(arrow)* surrounded by normal myometrial-placental interface in a patient with previous posterior myomectomy. This region was not well evaluated with ultrasound. *(From Levine D. Placenta accreta: evaluation with color Doppler, power Doppler and fast MRI. Radiology 1997;205:773.)*

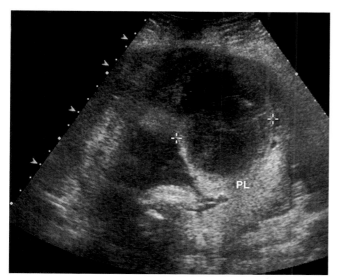

FIGURE 44-12. Placental abruption. Transabdominal sonogram of the placenta *(PL)* with a hematoma *(calipers)* lifting the placenta away from the uterine wall.

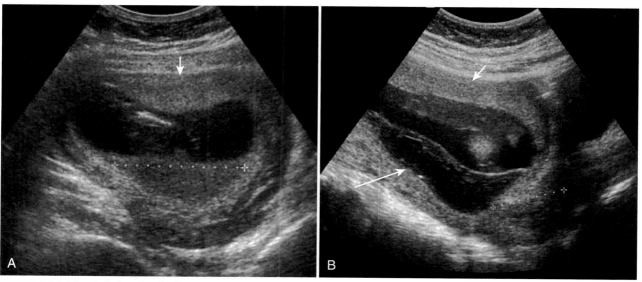

FIGURE 44-13. Subchorionic hematoma. A, Transabdominal transverse view of the uterus in the second trimester shows acute subchorionic hematoma *(calipers)*. The anterior placenta is shown by the short arrow. **B,** Transabdominal midsagittal view of the same patient later in pregnancy demonstrates the subchorionic hematoma *(long arrow)* more hypoechoic and located overlying the cervix *(calipers)*; *short arrow*, placenta.

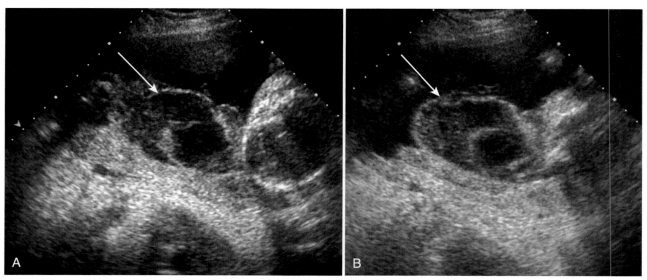

FIGURE 44-14. Preplacental hematoma. A and B, Transabdominal sonograms early in the third trimester demonstrate a hematoma on the fetal side of the placenta *(arrow)*. The fetus had severe growth restriction and died within 2 days of the ultrasound examination.

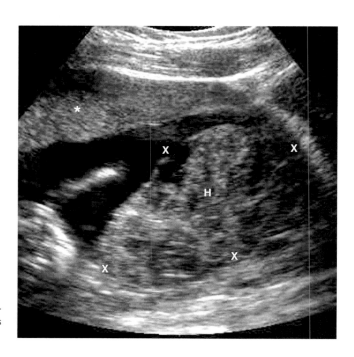

FIGURE 44-15. Large hematoma. Transabdominal sonogram shows large hematoma *(H, calipers)*. The placenta (*) is anterior.

by bleeding from fetal vessels and located on the fetal surface of the placenta under the chorion (Fig. 44-14). Because preplacental hematomas likely result from the accumulation of fetal blood, prognosis may be poorer.[80] When massive, these hematomas are sometimes termed **Breus mole.** Preplacental hematomas may be associated with maternal hypertension.[81]

An acute hematoma has an echogenicity similar to that of the placenta, making sonographic visualization difficult. As the hematoma organizes, it becomes more hypoechoic (Fig. 44-13, *B*) and can approach the echogenicity of the myometrium. An indirect sign of the presence of a hematoma is apparent thickening of the placenta, which is associated with worse outcomes.[82,83]

Even though placental abruption remains a clinical diagnosis, ultrasound can play an important role. Larger hematomas are expected to be seen (Fig. 44-15), and these are more likely to be clinically important. Glantz and Purnell[84] reported that the identification of placental abruption by ultrasound had a sensitivity, specificity, positive predictive value, and negative predictive value of 24%, 96%, 88%, and 53%, respectively. They

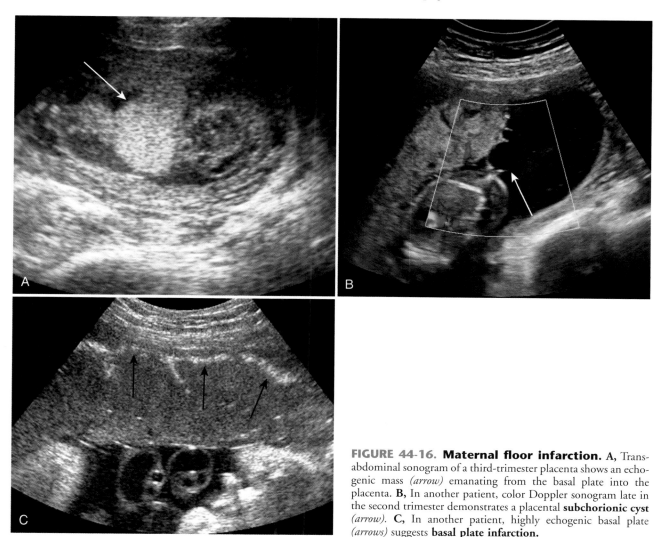

FIGURE 44-16. Maternal floor infarction. A, Transabdominal sonogram of a third-trimester placenta shows an echogenic mass *(arrow)* emanating from the basal plate into the placenta. **B,** In another patient, color Doppler sonogram late in the second trimester demonstrates a placental **subchorionic cyst** *(arrow).* **C,** In another patient, highly echogenic basal plate *(arrows)* suggests **basal plate infarction.**

determined that if a hematoma was identified by sonography, there was an increased risk of preterm delivery, low birth weight, and neonatal intensive care unit admission. Increased size of hematoma and percentage of placental involvement are associated with increased fetal mortality.[85]

PLACENTAL INFARCTION

Placental infarctions can occur focally or throughout the placenta and are thought to have a vascular etiology. **Maternal floor infarction** is a diffuse entity overtaking the villi with a fibrinoid deposition at the maternal surface and basal plate, reaching into the placental substance. The presence of this fibrin surrounding the villi obstructs nutrient exchange from mother to fetus. Both abnormalities are associated with oligohydramnios, umbilical artery Doppler abnormalities, IUGR, central nervous system injury, and fetal demise. Maternal floor infarction tends to recur in subsequent pregnancies.[24,86-88]

Although peripheral infarctions are common at term, infarctions larger than 3 cm or involving more than 5% of the placenta are associated with increased perinatal morbidity. Both maternal and fetal thrombophilias can lead to placental infarctions.[89]

The sonographic findings of maternal floor infarction include a hyperechoic placental mass (Fig. 44-16, *A*) or placental thickening. Hyperechoic areas of the placenta are especially prominent along the maternal surface of the placenta and can stretch into the placental substance itself. These can be a normal finding, especially with mature placentas. Hyperechoic placental masses may be associated with central hypoechoic spaces as they organize. **Subchorionic cysts** are also commonly present with maternal floor infarction (Fig. 44-16, *B*). The hyperechoic mass seen with maternal floor infarction resembles that seen with placental chorioangiomas.[90]

Placental infarctions caused by maternal vascular disease often result in uteroplacental ischemia and infarction of the villi. These appear as echogenic, rimmed cystic lesions within the placenta, not necessarily at the

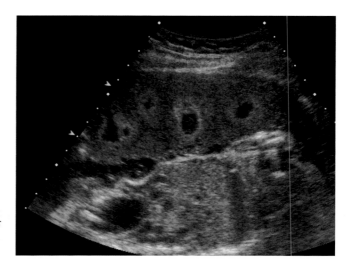

FIGURE 44-17. Placental infarctions in patient with severe preeclampsia. Transabdominal sonogram of a third-trimester placenta demonstrates multiple hyperechoic bordered cysts with sonolucent cores.

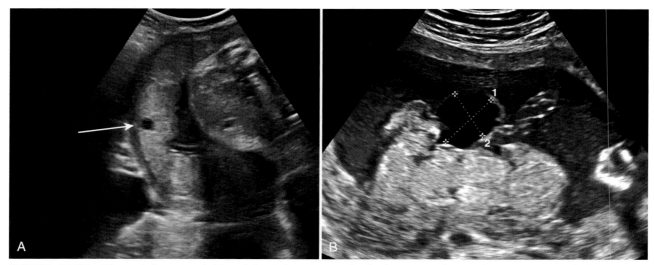

FIGURE 44-18. Placental cysts. A, Transabdominal sonogram of a third-trimester placenta demonstrates a small placental cyst. **B,** Transabdominal sonogram of a second-trimester placenta with a surface cyst *(calipers)* located near the umbilical cord insertion.

maternal side of the placenta or basal plate (Fig. 44-17; **Video 44-4**). When identified early in gestation, anticoagulation with heparin may improve outcome.[91]

PLACENTAL MASSES

Solid-appearing placental masses include chorioangioma, **subamniotic hematoma, subchorionic hematoma,** and **placental hemorrhage.** These masses should be differentiated from fluid-filled placental regions of placental cysts and venous lakes. As just discussed, placental infarctions may also have a masslike appearance.

Subchorionic placental cysts on the fetal surface of the placenta are predominantly innocuous findings on prenatal sonography, similar to cysts in the substance of the placenta (Fig. 44-18). Most fetuses whose placentas

contain these cysts have normal outcomes. Larger cysts (>4.5 cm) are associated with IUGR. Maternal floor infarction may also be associated with placental cysts.[92,93]

The most common benign tumor of the placenta is the **chorioangioma,** occurring in approximately 1% of pregnancies (Fig. 44-19). Although most are asymptomatic, large chorioangiomas can lead to high-output fetal cardiac failure, anemia, hydrops, and death.[94] Chorioangiomas appear as well-circumscribed solid tumors in the placenta. They can range from hypoechoic to hyperechoic compared to the echogenicity of the placenta. A threshold of 5 cm in diameter typically portends a high risk for adverse outcome.[95,96] Use of color or power Doppler ultrasound is helpful to identify increased blood flow within the solid mass, thereby distinguishing the mass as a chorioangioma.[97,98] Blood flow is not consistently demonstrable, especially with smaller chorioangiomas;

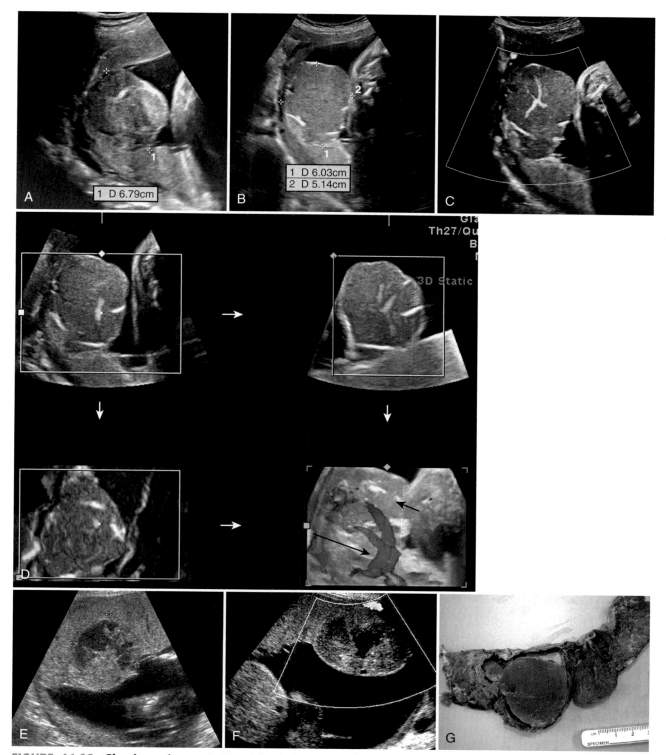

FIGURE 44-19. Chorioangioma. A, Transabdominal sonogram shows a heterogeneous placental mass *(calipers).* **B,** In another patient, transabdominal sonogram of a more homogeneous and isoechoic placental mass *(calipers).* **C,** In a different patient, transabdominal color Doppler sonogram shows blood flow within the tumor. **D,** Same patient as **C;** 3-D color Doppler sonography demonstrates feeding vessel *(long arrow)* and vasculature *(short arrow)* in the placental tumor. **E** and **F,** Gray-scale and color Doppler sonograms show another patient with a small, hypovascular chorioangioma. **G,** Specimen.

those with low flow tend to have a better outcome, whereas chorioangiomas with extremely elevated flow usually are associated with adverse perinatal outcome. These pregnancies require close follow-up and surveillance for polyhydramnios and other signs of fetal hydrops.[99,100] Decreasing blood flow, as documented by color or power Doppler ultrasound, signals an improved prognosis.[100] Three-dimensional power Doppler can assist with the diagnosis of chorioangioma and can be used to quantitate blood flow to the tumor.[95]

In cases where the fetus is at risk for **hydrops,** in utero intervention improves perinatal outcomes. Interventions include injection of thrombogenic material,[101] microcoil embolization,[102] and endoscopic laser devascularization.[103]

Maternal **malignancies** rarely metastasize to the placenta. Malignant melanoma and adenocarcinoma of the breast, pancreas, and colon are most common.[104,105] These deposits are typically microscopic and do not interfere with placental function.

MESENCHYMAL DYSPLASIA OF THE PLACENTA

Mesenchymal dysplasia of the placenta resembles a partial hydatidiform mole both grossly and microscopically, with a thickened placenta and small cystic lesions. In contrast to partial moles, mesenchymal dysplasia of the placenta may be associated with a normal fetus, although IUGR is common. There is also an association with **Beckwith-Wiedemann syndrome**[106] (Fig. 44-20). The villi in these cases are cystic with dilated vasculature. The karyotype is usually normal.[107]

MOLAR GESTATIONS

Gestational trophoblastic disease consists of **complete mole** (Fig. 44-21) and **partial mole** and **choriocarcinoma.** These placental abnormalities are discussed in detail in Chapter 15.

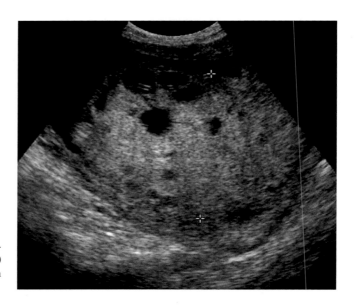

FIGURE 44-20. Mesenchymal dysplasia of placenta. Associated with Beckwith-Weidemann syndrome at 20 weeks' gestation. Note the enlarged placenta (8 cm, *calipers*) with multiple cystic spaces.

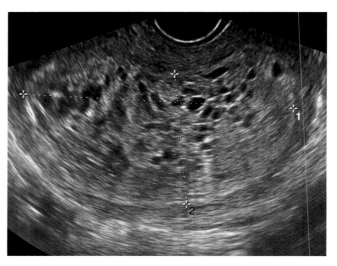

FIGURE 44-21. Molar pregnancy. Transvaginal sonogram in the late first trimester demonstrates a moderate amount of gestational tissue with multiple cystic spaces.

MORPHOLOGIC PLACENTAL ABNORMALITIES

There are a number of placental shape abnormalities, some quite rare.

Circumvallate Placenta

In circumvallate placenta the membranes of the chorion laeve, instead of inserting at the margin of the placental disc, insert more toward the center of the disc. The pathologist can identify fibrin at the margin along with evidence of bleeding. With a complete circumvallate placenta, a ring may constrict the chorion frondosum.[24]

Because of this placement, there is disproportionate folding of the placenta and fetal membranes. This results in the chorionic plate being smaller than the basal plate. Within the membrane fold hyalinized villi may be seen after being incorporated into the fold.

Circumvallate placenta has the sonographic appearance of a rolled edge of membranes at the placental edge inserting toward the center of the placental chorionic disc (Fig. 44-22; **Video 44-5**). Termed a **placental shelf**, this rolled edge of membranes can be thick and most often occupies only a small portion of the placenta. Circumvallate placentas can also be confused with **uterine synechiae** (Fig. 44-23, *A*), **uterine septum** (Fig. 44-23, *B*), and **amniotic bands.** Carefully identifying

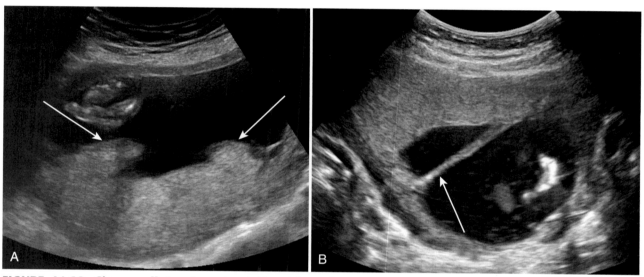

FIGURE 44-22. Circumvallate placenta. A, Transabdominal sonogram in the early third trimester shows rolled edges of the placenta *(arrows)*. **B,** Transabdominal sonogram in the second trimester shows a placental shelf *(arrow)*, which has echogenicity similar to the remainder of the placenta.

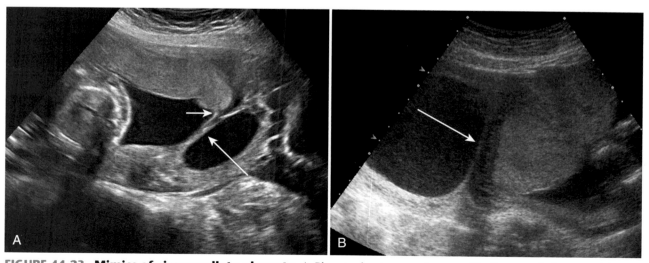

FIGURE 44-23. Mimics of circumvallate placenta. A, Placenta abutting a **uterine synechia** *(long arrow)* of myometrial tissue; *short arrow,* placental edge. **B,** Transabdominal sonogram of a second-trimester pregnancy with a **uterine septum** *(arrow).* The placenta partially inserts on the uterine septum.

the insertion of the membranes and determination of the echogenicity of the rolled edge of placenta, which should be similar to that of the placenta, should provide the correct diagnosis.

If a circumvallate placenta is identified, even if it seems to occupy only a small portion of the placenta, the rest of the placenta must be evaluated to determine whether the rolled edge of membranes involves the entire placenta. Complete circumvallate placentae are associated with adverse neonatal outcomes, including placental abruption, preterm delivery, oligohydramnios, IUGR, emergency cesarean delivery, Apgar scores less than 7, and perinatal death.[108,109] Fortunately, complete circumvallate placenta is rare, whereas partial circumvallate placentas are quite common and should be regarded as normal variants.

Evaluating second-trimester placental shelves to determine whether the sonographic finding persisted into the third trimester, Shen et al.[108] found an incidence of 11% for the identification of these shelves at the 13 to 16–week scan. Of note, none of the placental shelves occupied more than 25% of the placenta. Also, none of the partial circumvallate placentas could be sonographically appreciated in the third trimester. All neonates had a normal outcome. A recent large study of postdelivery placenta inspection yielded a complete circumvallate placenta incidence of 1.8%, none of which was detected antenatally.

Succenturiate Lobe

Succenturiate lobes, or **accessory lobes,** of the placenta can be a single lobe or multiple lobes in addition to the main placental lobe (Fig. 44-24). Their incidence is as high as 6%.[24] Given that placental tissue is present in the accessory lobe, there must be arterial and venous connections to the main portion of the placenta. One concern involves a retained placental accessory lobe after delivery, if not expected from the antenatal sonogram.

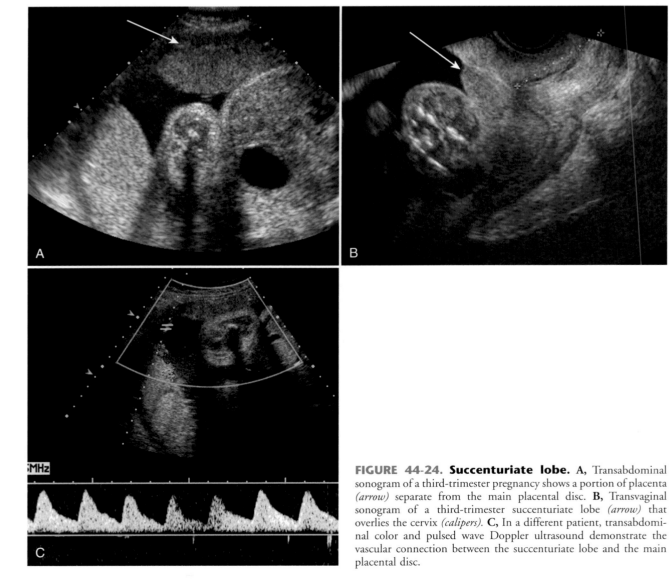

FIGURE 44-24. Succenturiate lobe. A, Transabdominal sonogram of a third-trimester pregnancy shows a portion of placenta *(arrow)* separate from the main placental disc. **B,** Transvaginal sonogram of a third-trimester succenturiate lobe *(arrow)* that overlies the cervix *(calipers)*. **C,** In a different patient, transabdominal color and pulsed wave Doppler ultrasound demonstrate the vascular connection between the succenturiate lobe and the main placental disc.

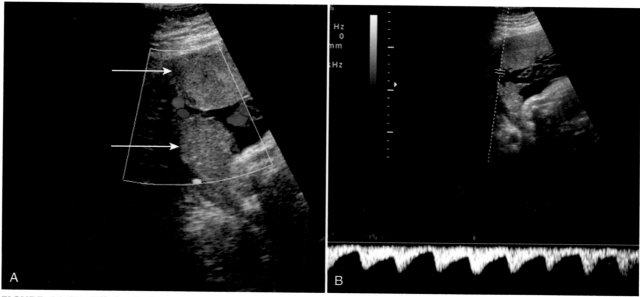

FIGURE 44-25. Bilobed placenta. A, Transabdominal sonogram of a third-trimester bilobed placenta. Both placental discs are of comparable size *(arrows).* **B,** Pulsed wave Doppler ultrasound demonstrates a fetal vascular connection between the lobes. The umbilical cord insertion inserts into the lower lobe.

Succenturiate lobes can also lie over the cervix as a variant of **placenta previa.**[106] Even more important is the concern over the location of the vascular connection between the main placenta and the succenturiate lobe. If the vessels lie in proximity to the cervix, a **vasa previa** may be present.

When a succenturiate lobe of the placenta is identified, it is imperative that the vascular connection between the succenturiate lobe and placenta be identified. This can be difficult at times because of poor visualization, especially later in pregnancy, and because the closest distance between succenturiate lobe and placenta is not always the route taken by the vessels. At a minimum, the internal cervical os should be evaluated to assess for fetal vessels.

Bilobed Placenta

Bilobed placentas consist of two similarly sized placental lobes separated by intervening membranes (Fig. 44-25). There must be some vascular connection between the lobes, and the umbilical cord may insert between the lobes in the membranes. Although rare, a bilobed placenta can be regarded similar to succenturiate lobes, with similar risks. Bilobed placentas may have more unprotected vessels, however, reinforcing the need for careful evaluation of the placental vasculature in such cases.

UMBILICAL CORD

Size and Appearance

Umbilical cord length varies, and a normal length has not been established. However, extremes of cord length are associated with abnormal outcome. **Short umbilical cords** are associated with conditions that impair fetal movement early in gestation, such as akinesia syndromes, aneuploidy, and extreme IUGR. **Excessive cord length** is associated with asphyxia or death resulting from a variety of situations that compromise cord flow, including excessive coiling, true knots, multiple loops of nuchal cord, and cord prolapse.

The potential importance of the **diameter** of the umbilical cord is unclear. In the first trimester, fetal size correlates with cord diameter, and small diameter may be a marker for pregnancy loss.[110] Also, data from multiple centers suggest that cord diameter may be a marker for chromosomal abnormalities when larger[111] or smaller than expected.[112] In the second and third trimesters, the largest contributor to the size of the umbilical cord is **Wharton's jelly.** A nomogram has been developed for the area of Wharton's jelly that correlate with fetal biometry up to 32 weeks' gestation.[113,114] In the second trimester, a larger-than-expected umbilical cord is associated with aneuploidy.[115] IUGR has been associated with thin cords, and diabetes, fetal macrosomia, placental abruption, and rhesus isoimmunization have been associated with thicker cords.[116] The associations between fetal umbilical cord size and fetal growth overlap too greatly to be useful screening tools.[117]

Information on the umbilical cord and its manner of **twisting** comes from the pathology literature. Left twists occur in 83%, right twists in 12%, and absent twists in 5% of umbilical cords in live-born singletons. For the umbilical cords that have a twist, ascertainment of the degree of twist has been reported antenatally. The **umbilical coiling index** is calculated by dividing the number of helices by the cord length in centimeters

(Fig. 44-26). The mean umbilical coiling index is 0.44 ± 0.11 antenatally and 0.28 ± 0.08 after delivery.[118] Umbilical coiling does not vary with respect to the amount of Wharton's jelly present.[119] Assessment of the degree of coiling in the second trimester does not correlate well with the umbilical coiling index at term.[120]

Absent umbilical cord twists are associated with single umbilical arteries, multiple gestations, fetal demise, preterm delivery, aneuploidy, and both marginal and velamentous umbilical cord insertions[121-123] (Fig. 44-27). Lower degrees of coiling are associated with lesser degrees of fetal growth.[124]

True knots of the umbilical cord occur in 1% to 2% of pregnancies. Although some are normal variants,[125] these knots may also be associated with increased fetal mortality. Sonographic features such as the "hanging noose sign" have been proposed to make this diagnosis

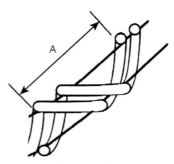

FIGURE 44-26. Umbilical coiling index. Defined as the distance *(A)* between the same umbilical artery making one turn around the umbilical vein. *(From Otsubo Y, Yoneyama Y, Suzuki S, et al. Sonographic evaluation of umbilical cord insertion with umbilical coiling index. J Clin Ultrasound 1999;27:341-344.)*

antenatally, with 2-D imaging as well as 3-D and 4-D sonography.[126,127] Although 3-D sonography may be helpful for suggesting the presence of a true knot of the umbilical cord, multiple loops of cord lying next to each other can mimic the presence of a knot.[128,129]

Cysts of the umbilical cord can be seen throughout pregnancy, occurring most frequently on the portion closest to the fetus (Fig. 44-28). Many cysts develop from the allantois and omphalomesenteric duct, or **pseudocysts** may develop through liquefaction of Wharton's jelly, giving the umbilical cord a hydropic appearance[130,131] (Fig. 44-29). All cord cysts are associated with both structural and chromosomal defects, so a detailed structural survey is required whenever a cyst is encountered.[132] However, cord cysts seen in the first trimester often resolve, without sequelae.[133] **Trisomies 13 and 18** are the most common chromosomal abnormalities associated with umbilical cord cysts,[131,134] and genitourinary and gastrointestinal anomalies are the most common structural defects.[135-138]

Vascular anomalies of the umbilical cord are associated with adverse fetal outcomes. **Umbilical artery aneurysms** are associated with vascular abnormalities, trisomy 18, and fetal demise.[131,139-141] **Spontaneous rupture** of the umbilical artery with a resultant umbilical cord hematoma has also been reported.[141]

Umbilical cord tumors are exceedingly rare. The most common is the umbilical cord **hemangioma,** which appears as a heterogeneous mass surrounded by multiple peripheral cystic areas. Cord hematomas are associated with an increased risk of fetal demise.[142,143]

Nuchal cord (cord around neck of fetus) is often seen in the second and third trimesters. Multiple tight loops of nuchal cord indenting the skin late in the third trimester should prompt a nonstress test.

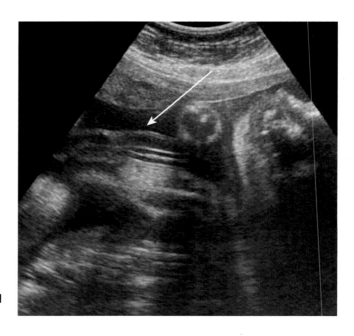

FIGURE 44-27. Uncoiled cord in second trimester.

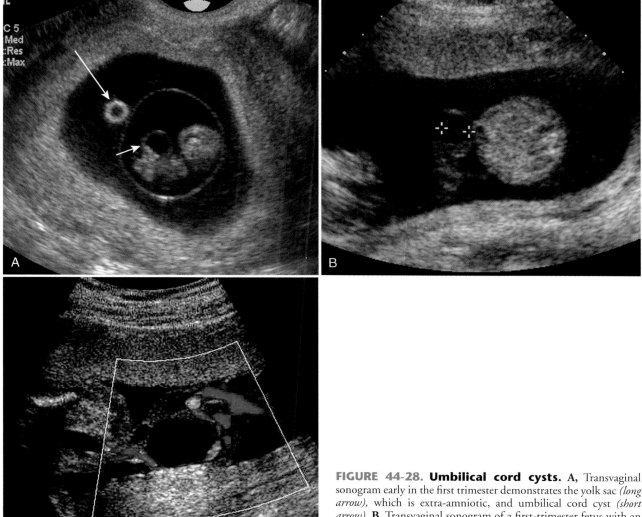

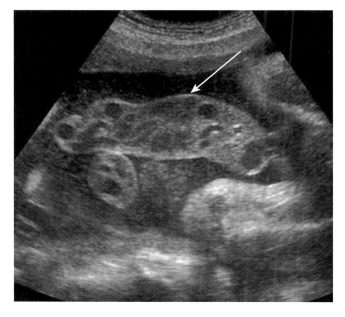

FIGURE 44-28. Umbilical cord cysts. A, Transvaginal sonogram early in the first trimester demonstrates the yolk sac *(long arrow)*, which is extra-amniotic, and umbilical cord cyst *(short arrow)*. **B,** Transvaginal sonogram of a first-trimester fetus with an umbilical cord cyst *(calipers)*, which is near the abdominal umbilical cord insertion site. **C,** Color Doppler sonogram with flow in the umbilical cord around the cyst.

FIGURE 44-29. Edematous cord. Transabdominal sonogram of a third-trimester fetus shows an edematous area *(arrow)* of cord near the abdominal umbilical cord insertion.

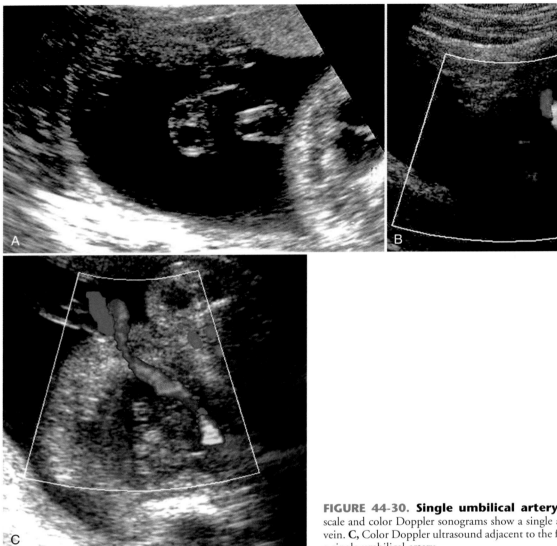

FIGURE 44-30. Single umbilical artery. A and **B,** Gray-scale and color Doppler sonograms show a single artery and a single vein. **C,** Color Doppler ultrasound adjacent to the fetal bladder shows a single umbilical artery.

The normal umbilical cord has three vessels; one vein carries oxygenated blood to the fetus, and two arteries carry deoxygenated blood from the fetus. In 1% to 2% of pregnancies, however, there is only a **single umbilical artery** (Fig. 44-30). The diagnosis is made either by examining a free loop of cord in the amniotic fluid or by assessing the umbilical arteries around the fetal bladder. Although associated with aneuploidy as well as renal and cardiac abnormalities, in isolation a single umbilical artery has no functional importance.

Insertion into the Placenta

The normal umbilical cord inserts into the central portion of the placenta. Identifying the placental umbilical cord insertion is important to recognize abnormalities of the umbilical cord vessels, as with gray-scale imaging and color or power Doppler sonography (Fig. 44-31).

Velamentous and Marginal Cord Insertions

A **velamentous umbilical cord insertion** refers to the situation where the umbilical cord inserts into the membranes and not the placental disc (Fig. 44-32). A **marginal cord insertion**, also known as a **battledore placenta,** occurs when the umbilical cord inserts into the very margin of the placenta (Fig. 44-33). Velamentous umbilical cord insertions occur in approximately 1% of singleton pregnancies; marginal cord insertions occur in approximately 7% of singletons. Both these cord insertions are more common in multiple gestations and are also associated with single umbilical arteries.[24]

Velamentous umbilical cord insertions are sonographically identified throughout the second and third trimesters of pregnancy with great reliability. Sepulveda et al.[144] identified the placental cord insertion in more than 99% of pregnancies, correctly identifying all

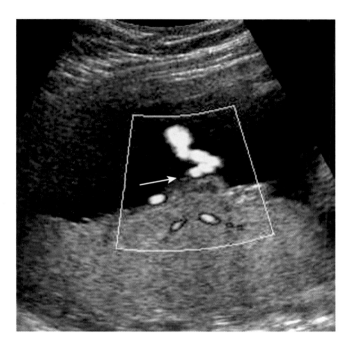

FIGURE 44-31. Normal cord insertion into placenta. Power Doppler sonogram shows central cord insertion *(arrow)* in a posterior placenta.

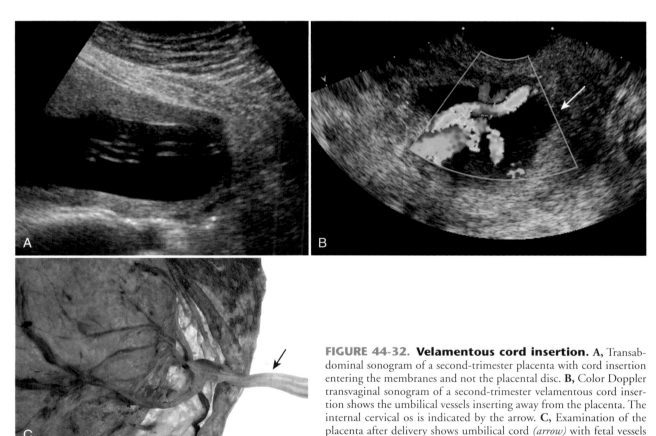

FIGURE 44-32. Velamentous cord insertion. A, Transabdominal sonogram of a second-trimester placenta with cord insertion entering the membranes and not the placental disc. **B,** Color Doppler transvaginal sonogram of a second-trimester velamentous cord insertion shows the umbilical vessels inserting away from the placenta. The internal cervical os is indicated by the arrow. **C,** Examination of the placenta after delivery shows umbilical cord *(arrow)* with fetal vessels coursing through the membranes into the placental disc.

velamentous cord insertions using both gray-scale and color Doppler sonography.[144] A velamentous cord insertion has been identified as early as 10 weeks' gestation[145] and can be routinely identified on the 11 to 14–week first-trimester scan.[146] Velamentous cord insertions are associated with IUGR, preterm delivery, congenital anomalies, low Apgar scores, neonatal death, and retained placenta after delivery.[144,147] Marginal umbilical cord insertions are not associated with IUGR or preterm delivery[148] but are associated with vasa previa.

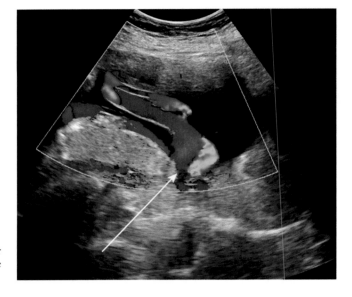

FIGURE 44-33. Marginal cord insertion. Color Doppler sonogram shows the umbilical cord inserting into the edge of the placenta *(arrow)*.

The insertion of the umbilical cord into the membranes leads to the unsupported coursing of the umbilical vessels to the placental disc and many complications. Wharton's jelly supports and protects the umbilical vessels in the umbilical cord. With the vessels in the membranes, no Wharton's jelly is present, leading to increased risk of compression or even rupture of these vessels. Intrapartum fetal heart rate patterns show more variable decelerations and no accelerations with velamentous cord insertions during the first and second stages of labor compared to controls.[147] Increasing length of the unsupported membrane vessels is associated with increasing rates of abnormal heart rate patterns, as is the umbilical cord insertion being in the lower portion rather than the middle or upper portion of the uterus.[147] Nonreassuring fetal heart rate patterns and emergency cesarean deliveries are more frequent with velamentous cord insertions in the lower third than in the middle or upper third of the uterus.[147]

Because velamentous cord insertions are typically located low in the uterus, transvaginal sonography can be critical to making this diagnosis.

Vasa Previa

Vasa previa is the situation where the umbilical cord vessels overlie the internal cervical os (Fig. 44-34; **Video 44-6**). Because these are fetal vessels, even a small amount of blood loss can lead to fetal death. High-risk situations that require specific exclusion of vasa previa include velamentous umbilical cord insertions in which the membranous fetal umbilical vessels can traverse the internal cervical os somewhere along their length. Marginal umbilical cord insertions, especially those with aberrant vessels within the membranes, also are associated with vasa previa.[149] Presence of bilobed placentas[150] or the more common succenturiate lobes[151] requires that a vasa previa be excluded, given the potential for a poor neonatal outcome. Prior low placenta, placenta previa, multiple gestations, and pregnancies resulting from in vitro fertilization are all associated with vasa previa.[149,151,152]

Once a vasa previa is diagnosed, obstetric management is critical to optimize outcome. Delivery at 35 to 36 weeks' gestation is recommended to obviate the risks of vessel rupture that can occur with labor or rupture of the membranes. If the patient has preterm labor, ruptured membranes, or bleeding before 35 weeks, delivery at the earlier gestational age should be considered.[152,153]

Vasa previa is diagnosed when a fetal vessel is identified overlying the internal cervical os. Although grayscale ultrasound can identify the vessel, color or power Doppler sonography can assist with visualizing the vessel. Pulsed wave Doppler ultrasound should confirm a fetal artery, by demonstrating the heart rate of the fetus rather than that of the pregnant woman. Three-dimensional sonography may assist with making the diagnosis of a vasa previa,[149,154] especially using 3-D power Doppler sonography to map out the aberrant vessels.[155] The clinician must be careful, however, especially when using color or power Doppler ultrasound, not to equate identification of the umbilical cord in the lower uterine segment or overlying the cervix with a vasa previa. The cord could be free floating in this area, termed a **funic presentation,** and not a vasa previa (Fig. 44-35). Careful attention to detail, using movement of the probe or follow-up sonography, may be necessary to reach the correct diagnosis.[156]

PLACENTA DURING LABOR AND POSTPARTUM

Third Stage of Labor

Ultrasound may have some role during the third stage of labor, the time from delivery of the neonate to delivery

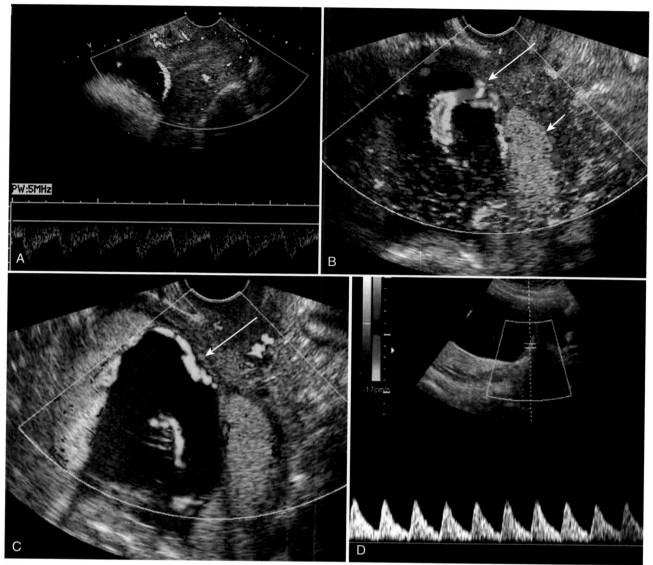

FIGURE 44-34. Vasa previa. A, Transvaginal sonogram of a vasa previa using color and pulsed wave Doppler ultrasound. The gate is at the level of the internal cervical os. A fetal arterial pulse wave is shown. **B,** In another patient, transvaginal color Doppler sonogram shows the umbilical cord inserting into the membranes, consistent with a **velamentous cord insertion.** Long arrow shows the cord insertion at the level of the internal cervical os; short arrow indicates placenta. **C,** In a different patient, transvaginal power Doppler sonogram shows vessels between two lobes of a **bilobed placenta;** arrow indicates internal cervical os. **D,** Transabdominal color and pulsed Doppler sonogram shows a low placenta with a fetal artery traversing the internal cervical os.

of the placenta. A prolonged third stage, with the placenta retained, has various etiologies. If the placenta does not separate, a placenta accreta could be present.[54] A prolonged third stage may also be caused by retention of a detached placenta from poor contractility or atony of the uterus, sometimes from infection. These abnormalities are treated differently, and ultrasound may help differentiate the various causes of a prolonged third stage of labor and lead to improved patient care.[157]

The mechanism of placental separation has been reported using gray-scale sonography.[158] Color Doppler ultrasound provides information on the phases of placental separation during the third stage of labor by specifically assessing blood flow between the myometrium

and the placenta.[159] The manner in which the placenta separates varies, based on prior cesarean delivery and a prolonged second stage of labor.[160]

Retained Products of Conception

Women with suspected retained products of conception (RPOC) typically present with abnormal bleeding. RPOC are most common after second-trimester spontaneous abortion, extreme preterm birth, medical termination of pregnancy, and unsuspected placenta accreta. RPOC are suggested when an echogenic endometrial mass is visualized within the uterine cavity (Fig. 44-36). This mass may extend into the myometrium[161] and can

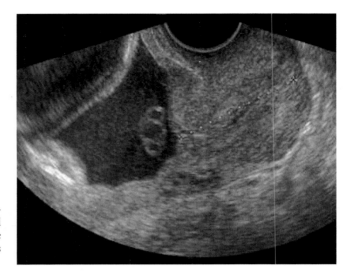

FIGURE 44-35. Funic presentation. Transvaginal ultrasound of a single loop of normal umbilical cord, free floating and overlying the internal cervical os. The cervix is indicated by the calipers. The three vessels of the umbilical cord are seen in cross section.

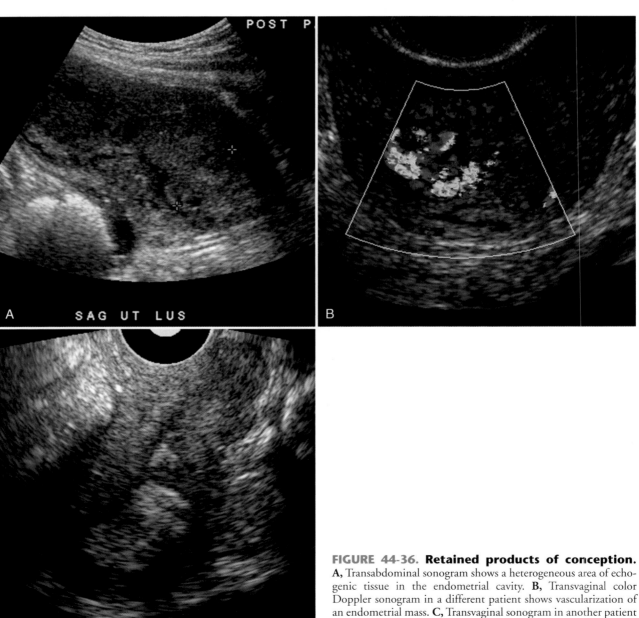

FIGURE 44-36. Retained products of conception.
A, Transabdominal sonogram shows a heterogeneous area of echogenic tissue in the endometrial cavity. **B,** Transvaginal color Doppler sonogram in a different patient shows vascularization of an endometrial mass. **C,** Transvaginal sonogram in another patient shows a calcified endometrial mass. In each case, the mass has retained products of conception.

be differentiated from blood clot when flow is demonstrated. However, lack of flow does not exclude RPOC. Care should be taken not to mistake vascularized RPOC for a uterine arteriovenous malformation, because prominent flow can be seen in RPOC.[161] Calcifications in the endometrial mass are highly suggestive of RPOC. These calcifications present normal placental maturation that occurred during pregnancy.

CONCLUSION

Multiple abnormalities associated with placental development and function can be identified by prenatal sonography. Sonographers and sonologists need to understand the basic anatomy and physiology of the placenta so that abnormal findings on prenatal sonography can be acknowledged, to achieve the best possible outcome for mother and neonate.

References

Placental Development

1. Pijnenborg R, Vercruysse L. Shifting concepts of the fetal-maternal interface: a historical perspective. Placenta 2008;29(Suppl A):S20-S25.
2. Moore KL. The developing human. 3rd ed. Philadelphia: Saunders; 1982.
3. Kanne JP, Lalani TA, Fligner CL. The placenta revisited: radiologic-pathologic correlation. Curr Probl Diagn Radiol 2005;34:238-255.
4. Jauniaux E, Poston L, Burton GJ. Placental-related diseases of pregnancy: involvement of oxidative stress and implications in human evolution. Hum Reprod Update 2006;12:747-755.
5. Fujikura T, Sho S. Placental cavities. Obstet Gynecol 1997;90:112-116.
6. Reis NS, Brizot ML, Schultz R, et al. Placental lakes on sonographic examination: correlation with obstetric outcome and pathologic findings. J Clin Ultrasound 2005;33:67-71.
7. Morikawa M, Cho K, Kataoka S, et al. Magnetic resonance image findings of placental lake: report of two cases. Prenat Diagn 2005;25:250-252.
8. Has R, Yuksel A, Gunay S, et al. Antenatal sonographic detection of an unusual placental lake under the cord insertion. Arch Gynecol Obstet 2005;271:59-61.
9. Thompson MO, Vines SK, Aquilina J, et al. Are placental lakes of any clinical significance? Placenta 2002;23:685-690.
10. Tongsong T, Boonyanurak P. Placental thickness in the first half of pregnancy. J Clin Ultrasound 2004;32:231-234.
11. Nowak PM, Nardozza LM, Araujo Junior E, et al. Comparison of placental volume in early pregnancy using multiplanar and VOCAL methods. Placenta 2008;29:241-245.
12. Hafner E, Metzenbauer M, Dillinger-Paller B, et al. Correlation of first trimester placental volume and second trimester uterine artery Doppler flow. Placenta 2001;22:729-734.
13. Schuchter K, Metzenbauer M, Hafner E, Philipp K. Uterine artery Doppler and placental volume in the first trimester in the prediction of pregnancy complications. Ultrasound Obstet Gynecol 2001;18:590-592.
14. Rizzo G, Capponi A, Cavicchioni O, et al. First trimester uterine Doppler and three-dimensional ultrasound placental volume calculation in predicting pre-eclampsia. Eur J Obstet Gynecol Reprod Biol 2008;138:147-151.
15. Metzenbauer M, Hafner E, Hoefinger D, et al. Three-dimensional ultrasound measurement of the placental volume in early pregnancy: method and correlation with biochemical placenta parameters. Placenta 2001;22:602-605.
16. Metzenbauer M, Hafner E, Schuchter K, Philipp K. First-trimester placental volume as a marker for chromosomal anomalies: preliminary results from an unselected population. Ultrasound Obstet Gynecol 2002;19:240-242.
17. Wegrzyn P, Fabio C, Peralta A, et al. Placental volume in twin and triplet pregnancies measured by three-dimensional ultrasound at 11 + 0 to 13 + 6 weeks of gestation. Ultrasound Obstet Gynecol 2006;27:647-651.
18. Hafner E, Schuchter K, van Leeuwen M, et al. Three-dimensional sonographic volumetry of the placenta and the fetus between weeks 15 and 17 of gestation. Ultrasound Obstet Gynecol 2001;18:116-120.
19. Thame M, Osmond C, Wilks RJ, et al. Blood pressure is related to placental volume and birth weight. Hypertension 2000;35:662-667.
20. Michailidis GD, Morris RW, Mamopoulos A, et al. The influence of maternal hematocrit on placental development from the first to the second trimesters of pregnancy. Ultrasound Obstet Gynecol 2002;20:351-355.
21. Thame M, Osmond C, Bennett F, et al. Fetal growth is directly related to maternal anthropometry and placental volume. Eur J Clin Nutr 2004;58:894-900.
22. Hafner E, Metzenbauer M, Hofinger D, et al. Comparison between three-dimensional placental volume at 12 weeks and uterine artery impedance/notching at 22 weeks in screening for pregnancy-induced hypertension, pre-eclampsia and fetal growth restriction in a low-risk population. Ultrasound Obstet Gynecol 2006;27:652-657.
23. Wolf H, Oosting H, Treffers PE. Second-trimester placental volume measurement by ultrasound: prediction of fetal outcome. Am J Obstet Gynecol 1989;160:121-126.
24. Benirschke K, Kaufman P, Baergen R. Pathology of the human placenta. 5th ed. New York: Springer; 2006.
25. Matijevic R, Kurjak A, Hafner T. Terminal parts of uteroplacental circulation in pregnancy: assessment by color/pulsed Doppler ultrasound. Ultrasound Rev Obstet Gynecol 2001;1:262-274.
26. Valentin L, Sladkevicius P, Laurini R, et al. Uteroplacental and luteal circulation in normal first-trimester pregnancies: Doppler ultrasonographic and morphologic study. Am J Obstet Gynecol 1996;174:768-775.
27. Craven CM, Ward K. Syncytiotrophoblastic fragments in first-trimester decidual veins: evidence of placental perfusion by the maternal circulation early in pregnancy. Am J Obstet Gynecol 1999;181:455-459.
28. Guimaraes Filho HA, da Costa LL, Araujo Junior E, et al. Placenta: angiogenesis and vascular assessment through three-dimensional power Doppler ultrasonography. Arch Gynecol Obstet 2008;277:195-200.
29. Carbillon L, Challier JC, Alouini S, et al. Uteroplacental circulation development: Doppler assessment and clinical importance. Placenta 2001;22:795-799.
30. Jauniaux E, Greenwold N, Hempstock J, Burton GJ. Comparison of ultrasonographic and Doppler mapping of the intervillous circulation in normal and abnormal early pregnancies. Fertil Steril 2003;79:100-106.
31. Campbell S. Placental vasculature as visualized by 3D power Doppler angiography and 3D color Doppler imaging. Ultrasound Obstet Gynecol 2007;30:917-920.
32. Mu J, Kanzaki T, Tomimatsu T, et al. Investigation of intraplacental villous arteries by Doppler flow imaging in growth-restricted fetuses. Am J Obstet Gynecol 2002;186:297-302.
33. Guiot C, Gaglioti P, Oberto M, et al. Is three-dimensional power Doppler ultrasound useful in the assessment of placental perfusion in normal and growth-restricted pregnancies? Ultrasound Obstet Gynecol 2008;31:171-176.
34. Levine D, Callen PW, Pender SG, et al. Chorioamniotic separation after second-trimester genetic amniocentesis: importance and frequency. Radiology 1998;209:175-181.
35. Bromley B, Shipp TD, Benacerraf BR. Amnion-chorion separation after 17 weeks' gestation. Obstet Gynecol 1999;94:1024-1026.

Placenta Previa

36. Mabie WC. Placenta previa. Clin Perinatol 1992;19:425-435.
37. Silver R, Depp R, Sabbagha RE, et al. Placenta previa: aggressive expectant management. Am J Obstet Gynecol 1984;150:15-22.
38. McShane PM, Heyl PS, Epstein MF. Maternal and perinatal morbidity resulting from placenta previa. Obstet Gynecol 1985;65:176-182.

39. Timor-Tritsch IE, Yunis RA. Confirming the safety of transvaginal sonography in patients suspected of placenta previa. Obstet Gynecol 1993;81:742-744.

40. Smith RS, Lauria MR, Comstock CH, et al. Transvaginal ultrasonography for all placentas that appear to be low-lying or over the internal cervical os. Ultrasound Obstet Gynecol 1997;9:22-24.

41. Oppenheimer LW, Farine D, Ritchie JW, et al. What is a low-lying placenta? Am J Obstet Gynecol 1991;165:1036-1038.

42. Bhide A, Prefumo F, Moore J, et al. Placental edge to internal os distance in the late third trimester and mode of delivery in placenta praevia. BJOG 2003;110:860-864.

43. Ananth CV, Smulian JC, Vintzileos AM. The association of placenta previa with history of cesarean delivery and abortion: a meta-analysis. Am J Obstet Gynecol 1997;177:1071-1078.

44. Gilliam M, Rosenberg D, Davis F. The likelihood of placenta previa with greater number of cesarean deliveries and higher parity. Obstet Gynecol 2002;99:976-980.

45. Faiz AS, Ananth CV. Etiology and risk factors for placenta previa: an overview and meta-analysis of observational studies. J Matern Fetal Neonatal Med 2003;13:175-190.

46. King DL. Placental migration demonstrated by ultrasonography: a hypothesis of dynamic placentation. Radiology 1973;109:167-170.

47. Oppenheimer L, Holmes P, Simpson N, Dabrowski A. Diagnosis of low-lying placenta: can migration in the third trimester predict outcome? Ultrasound Obstet Gynecol 2001;18:100-102.

48. Predanic M, Perni SC, Baergen RN, et al. A sonographic assessment of different patterns of placenta previa "migration" in the third trimester of pregnancy. J Ultrasound Med 2005;24:773-780.

49. Rosati P, Guariglia L. Clinical significance of placenta previa detected at early routine transvaginal scan. J Ultrasound Med 2000;19:581-585.

50. Becker RH, Vonk R, Mende BC, et al. The relevance of placental location at 20-23 gestational weeks for prediction of placenta previa at delivery: evaluation of 8650 cases. Ultrasound Obstet Gynecol 2001;17:496-501.

51. Mustafa SA, Brizot ML, Carvalho MH, et al. Transvaginal ultrasonography in predicting placenta previa at delivery: a longitudinal study. Ultrasound Obstet Gynecol 2002;20:356-359.

52. Ghourab S. Third-trimester transvaginal ultrasonography in placenta previa: does the shape of the lower placental edge predict clinical outcome? Ultrasound Obstet Gynecol 2001;18:103-108.

53. Shukunami K, Nishijima K, Kurokawa T, et al. A small-angled thin edge of the placenta predicts abnormal placentation at delivery. J Ultrasound Med 2005;24:331-335.

Placenta Accreta

54. Krapp M, Baschat AA, Hankeln M, Gembruch U. Gray scale and color Doppler sonography in the third stage of labor for early detection of failed placental separation. Ultrasound Obstet Gynecol 2000;15:138-142.

55. Zelop C, Nadel A, Frigoletto Jr FD, et al. Placenta accreta/percreta/increta: a cause of elevated maternal serum alpha-fetoprotein. Obstet Gynecol 1992;80:693-694.

56. Miura K, Miura S, Yamasaki K, et al. Increased level of cell-free placental mRNA in a subgroup of placenta previa that needs hysterectomy. Prenat Diagn 2008;28:805-809.

57. Wu S, Kocherginsky M, Hibbard JU. Abnormal placentation: twenty-year analysis. Am J Obstet Gynecol 2005;192:1458-1461.

58. Armstrong CA, Harding S, Matthews T, Dickinson JE. Is placenta accreta catching up with us? Aust NZ J Obstet Gynaecol 2004;44:210-213.

59. Clark SL, Koonings PP, Phelan JP. Placenta previa/accreta and prior cesarean section. Obstet Gynecol 1985;66:89-92.

60. Finberg HJ, Williams JW. Placenta accreta: prospective sonographic diagnosis in patients with placenta previa and prior cesarean section. J Ultrasound Med 1992;11:333-343.

61. Comstock CH, Love Jr JJ, Bronsteen RA, et al. Sonographic detection of placenta accreta in the second and third trimesters of pregnancy. Am J Obstet Gynecol 2004;190:1135-1140.

62. Yang JI, Lim YK, Kim HS, et al. Sonographic findings of placental lacunae and the prediction of adherent placenta in women with placenta previa totalis and prior cesarean section. Ultrasound Obstet Gynecol 2006;28:178-182.

63. Kerr de Mendonca L. Sonographic diagnosis of placenta accrete: presentation of six cases. J Ultrasound Med 1988;7:211-215.

64. Chou MM, Ho ES, Lee YH. Prenatal diagnosis of placenta previa accreta by transabdominal color Doppler ultrasound. Ultrasound Obstet Gynecol 2000;15:28-35.

65. Wong HS, Cheung YK, Strand L, et al. Specific sonographic features of placenta accreta: tissue interface disruption on gray-scale imaging and evidence of vessels crossing interface- disruption sites on Doppler imaging. Ultrasound Obstet Gynecol 2007;29:239-240.

66. Comstock CH. Antenatal diagnosis of placenta accreta: a review. Ultrasound Obstet Gynecol 2005;26:89-96.

67. Mazouni C, Gorincour G, Juhan V, Bretelle F. Placenta accreta: a review of current advances in prenatal diagnosis. Placenta 2007;28:599-603.

68. Chou MM, Tseng JJ, Hwang JI, et al. Sonographic appearance of tornado blood flow in placenta previa accreta/increta. Ultrasound Obstet Gynecol 2001;17:362-363.

69. Comstock CH, Lee W, Vettraino IM, Bronsteen RA. The early sonographic appearance of placenta accreta. J Ultrasound Med 2003;22:19-23; quiz 24-26.

70. Shih JC, Cheng WF, Shyu MK, et al. Power Doppler evidence of placenta accreta appearing in the first trimester. Ultrasound Obstet Gynecol 2002;19:623-625.

71. Chen YJ, Wang PH, Liu WM, et al. Placenta accreta diagnosed at 9 weeks' gestation. Ultrasound Obstet Gynecol 2002;19:620-622.

72. Taipale P, Orden MR, Berg M, et al. Prenatal diagnosis of placenta accreta and percreta with ultrasonography, color Doppler, and magnetic resonance imaging. Obstet Gynecol 2004;104:537-540.

73. Levine D, Hulka CA, Ludmir J, et al. Placenta accreta: evaluation with color Doppler US, power Doppler US, and MR imaging. Radiology 1997;205:773-776.

74. Warshak CR, Eskander R, Hull AD, et al. Accuracy of ultrasonography and magnetic resonance imaging in the diagnosis of placenta accreta. Obstet Gynecol 2006;108:573-581.

75. Masselli G, Brunelli R, Casciani E, et al. Magnetic resonance imaging in the evaluation of placental adhesive disorders: correlation with color Doppler ultrasound. Eur Radiol 2008;18:1292-1299.

76. Dwyer BK, Belogolovkin V, Tran L, et al. Prenatal diagnosis of placenta accreta: sonography or magnetic resonance imaging? J Ultrasound Med 2008;27:1275-1281.

Placental Abruption

77. Kramer MS, Usher RH, Pollack R, et al. Etiologic determinants of abruptio placentae. Obstet Gynecol 1997;89:221-226.

78. Tikkanen M, Nuutila M, Hiilesmaa V, et al. Clinical presentation and risk factors of placental abruption. Acta Obstet Gynecol Scand 2006;85:700-705.

79. Oyelese Y, Ananth CV. Placental abruption. Obstet Gynecol 2006;108:1005-1016.

80. Loi K, Tan KT. Massive pre-placental and subchorionic haematoma. Singapore Med J 2006;47:1084-1086.

81. Fisteag-Kiprono L, Foster K, McKenna D, Baptista M. Antenatal sonographic diagnosis of massive subchorionic hematoma: a case report. J Reprod Med 2005;50:219-221.

82. Kikutani M, Ishihara K, Araki T. Value of ultrasonography in the diagnosis of placental abruption. J Nippon Med Sch 2003;70:227-233.

83. Raio L, Ghezzi F, Cromi A, et al. The thick heterogeneous (jellylike) placenta: a strong predictor of adverse pregnancy outcome. Prenat Diagn 2004;24:182-188.

84. Glantz C, Purnell L. Clinical utility of sonography in the diagnosis and treatment of placental abruption. J Ultrasound Med 2002;21:837-840.

85. Nyberg DA, Mack LA, Benedetti TJ, et al. Placental abruption and placental hemorrhage: correlation of sonographic findings with fetal outcome. Radiology 1987;164:357-361.

Placental Infarction

86. Vernof KK, Benirschke K, Kephart GM, et al. Maternal floor infarction: relationship to X cells, major basic protein, and adverse perinatal outcome. Am J Obstet Gynecol 1992;167:1355-1363.

87. Adams-Chapman I, Vaucher YE, Bejar RF, et al. Maternal floor infarction of the placenta: association with central nervous system injury and adverse neurodevelopmental outcome. J Perinatol 2002;22:236-241.

88. Kumazaki K, Nakayama M, Sumida Y, et al. Placental features in preterm infants with periventricular leukomalacia. Pediatrics 2002;109:650-655.

89. Roberts D, Schwartz RS. Clotting and hemorrhage in the placenta: a delicate balance. N Engl J Med 2002;347:57-59.

90. Mandsager NT, Bendon R, Mostello D, et al. Maternal floor infarction of the placenta: prenatal diagnosis and clinical significance. Obstet Gynecol 1994;83:750-754.

91. Alkazaleh F, Viero S, Simchen M, et al. Ultrasound diagnosis of severe thrombotic placental damage in the second trimester: an observational study. Ultrasound Obstet Gynecol 2004;23:472-476.

92. Raga F, Ballester MJ, Osborne NG, Bonilla-Musoles F. Subchorionic placental cyst: a cause of fetal growth retardation—ultrasound and color-flow Doppler diagnosis and follow-up. J Natl Med Assoc 1996;88:285-288.

Placental Masses

93. Brown DL, DiSalvo DN, Frates MC, et al. Placental surface cysts detected on sonography: histologic and clinical correlation. J Ultrasound Med 2002;21:641-646.

94. Haak MC, Oosterhof H, Mouw RJ, et al. Pathophysiology and treatment of fetal anemia due to placental chorioangioma. Ultrasound Obstet Gynecol 1999;14:68-70.

95. Shih JC, Ko TL, Lin MC, et al. Quantitative three-dimensional power Doppler ultrasound predicts the outcome of placental chorioangioma. Ultrasound Obstet Gynecol 2004;24:202-206.

96. Taori K, Patil P, Attarde V, et al. Chorioangioma of placenta: sonographic features. J Clin Ultrasound 2008;36:113-115.

97. Prapas N, Liang RI, Hunter D, et al. Color Doppler imaging of placental masses: differential diagnosis and fetal outcome. Ultrasound Obstet Gynecol 2000;16:559-563.

98. Sepulveda W, Aviles G, Carstens E, et al. Prenatal diagnosis of solid placental masses: the value of color flow imaging. Ultrasound Obstet Gynecol 2000;16:554-558.

99. Jauniaux E, Ogle R. Color Doppler imaging in the diagnosis and management of chorioangiomas. Ultrasound Obstet Gynecol 2000;15:463-467.

100. Zalel Y, Gamzu R, Weiss Y, et al. Role of color Doppler imaging in diagnosing and managing pregnancies complicated by placental chorioangioma. J Clin Ultrasound 2002;30:264-269.

101. Nicolini U, Zuliani G, Caravelli E, et al. Alcohol injection: a new method of treating placental chorioangiomas. Lancet 1999;353:1674-1675.

102. Lau TK, Leung TY, Yu SC, et al. Prenatal treatment of chorioangioma by microcoil embolisation. BJOG 2003;110:70-73.

103. Quintero RA, Reich H, Romero R, et al. In utero endoscopic devascularization of a large chorioangioma. Ultrasound Obstet Gynecol 1996;8:48-52.

104. Eltorky M, Khare VK, Osborne P, Shanklin DR. Placental metastasis from maternal carcinoma: a report of three cases. J Reprod Med 1995;40:399-403.

105. Ferreira CM, Maceira JM, Coelho JM. Melanoma and pregnancy with placental metastases: report of a case. Am J Dermatopathol 1998;20:403-407.

Mesenchymal Dysplasia of the Placenta

106. Gibson BR, Muir-Padilla J, Champeaux A, Suarez ES. Mesenchymal dysplasia of the placenta. Placenta 2004;25:671-672.

107. Robertson M, Geerts LT, de Jong G, Wainwright H. Mesenchymal dysplasia in a monochorionic diamniotic twin pregnancy with review of the differential diagnosis of cystic changes in the placenta. J Ultrasound Med 2007;26:689-693.

Morphologic Placental Abnormalities

108. Shen O, Golomb E, Lavie O, et al. Placental shelf: a common, typically transient and benign finding on early second-trimester sonography. Ultrasound Obstet Gynecol 2007;29:192-194.

109. Suzuki S. Clinical significance of pregnancies with circumvallate placenta. J Obstet Gynaecol Res 2008;34:51-54.

Umbilical Cord

110. Ghezzi F, Raio L, Di Naro E, et al. First-trimester sonographic umbilical cord diameter and the growth of the human embryo. Ultrasound Obstet Gynecol 2001;18:348-351.

111. Ghezzi F, Raio L, Di Naro E, et al. First-trimester umbilical cord diameter: a novel marker of fetal aneuploidy. Ultrasound Obstet Gynecol 2002;19:235-239.

112. Rembouskos G, Cicero S, Papadopoulos V, et al. Umbilical cord diameter at 11-14 weeks of gestation: relation to chromosomal defects. Ultrasound Obstet Gynecol 2004;23:237-239.

113. Ghezzi F, Raio L, Di Naro E, et al. Nomogram of Wharton's jelly as depicted in the sonographic cross section of the umbilical cord. Ultrasound Obstet Gynecol 2001;18:121-125.

114. Togni FA, Araujo Junior E, Vasques FA, et al. The cross-sectional area of umbilical cord components in normal pregnancy. Int J Gynaecol Obstet 2007;96:156-161.

115. Predanic M, Perni SC, Chasen S, Chervenak FA. Fetal aneuploidy and umbilical cord thickness measured between 14 and 23 weeks' gestational age. J Ultrasound Med 2004;23:1177-1183.

116. Cromi A, Ghezzi F, Di Naro E, et al. Large cross-sectional area of the umbilical cord as a predictor of fetal macrosomia. Ultrasound Obstet Gynecol 2007;30:861-866.

117. Barbieri C, Cecatti JG, Krupa F, et al. Validation study of the capacity of the reference curves of ultrasonographic measurements of the umbilical cord to identify deviations in estimated fetal weight. Acta Obstet Gynecol Scand 2008;87:286-291.

118. Degani S, Lewinsky RM, Berger H, Spiegel D. Sonographic estimation of umbilical coiling index and correlation with Doppler flow characteristics. Obstet Gynecol 1995;86:990-993.

119. Predanic M, Perni SC. Absence of a relationship between umbilical cord thickness and coiling patterns. J Ultrasound Med 2005;24:1491-1496.

120. Qin Y, Lau TK, Rogers MS. Second-trimester ultrasonographic assessment of the umbilical coiling index. Ultrasound Obstet Gynecol 2002;20:458-463.

121. Lacro RV, Jones KL, Benirschke K. The umbilical cord twist: origin, direction, and relevance. Am J Obstet Gynecol 1987;157:833-838.

122. Otsubo Y, Yoneyama Y, Suzuki S, et al. Sonographic evaluation of umbilical cord insertion with umbilical coiling index. J Clin Ultrasound 1999;27:341-344.

123. Strong Jr TH, Elliott JP, Radin TG. Non-coiled umbilical blood vessels: a new marker for the fetus at risk. Obstet Gynecol 1993;81:409-411.

124. De Laat MW, van Alderen ED, Franx A, et al. The umbilical coiling index in complicated pregnancy. Eur J Obstet Gynecol Reprod Biol 2007;130:66-72.

125. Maher JT, Conti JA. A comparison of umbilical cord blood gas values between newborns with and without true knots. Obstet Gynecol 1996;88:863-866.

126. Ramon YCCL, Martinez RO. Prenatal diagnosis of true knot of the umbilical cord. Ultrasound Obstet Gynecol 2004;23:99-100.

127. Ramon y Cajal CL, Martinez RO. Four-dimensional ultrasonography of a true knot of the umbilical cord. Am J Obstet Gynecol 2006;195:896-898.

128. Hasbun J, Alcalde JL, Sepulveda W. Three-dimensional power Doppler sonography in the prenatal diagnosis of a true knot of the umbilical cord: value and limitations. J Ultrasound Med 2007;26:1215-1220.

129. Stempel LE. Beyond the pretty pictures: giving obstetricians just enough (umbilical) cord to hang themselves. Am J Obstet Gynecol 2006;195:888-890.

130. Kiran H, Kiran G, Kanber Y. Pseudocyst of the umbilical cord with mucoid degeneration of Wharton's jelly. Eur J Obstet Gynecol Reprod Biol 2003;111:91-93.

131. Shipp TD, Bromley B, Benacerraf BR. Sonographically detected abnormalities of the umbilical cord. Int J Gynaecol Obstet 1995;48:179-185.

132. Weissman A, Drugan A. Sonographic findings of the umbilical cord: implications for the risk of fetal chromosomal anomalies. Ultrasound Obstet Gynecol 2001;17:536-541.

133. Skibo LK, Lyons EA, Levi CS. First-trimester umbilical cord cysts. Radiology 1992;182:719-722.

134. Ghezzi F, Raio L, Di Naro E, et al. Single and multiple umbilical cord cysts in early gestation: two different entities. Ultrasound Obstet Gynecol 2003;21:215-219.

135. Tong SY, Lee JE, Kim SR, Lee SK. Umbilical cord cyst: a prenatal clue to bladder exstrophy. Prenat Diagn 2007;27:1177-1179.

136. Schiesser M, Lapaire O, Holzgreve W, Tercanli S. Umbilical cord edema associated with patent urachus. Ultrasound Obstet Gynecol 2003;22:646-647.

137. Emura T, Kanamori Y, Ito M, et al. Omphalocele associated with a large multilobular umbilical cord pseudocyst. Pediatr Surg Int 2004;20:636-639.

138. Sepulveda W. Beware of the umbilical cord "cyst." Ultrasound Obstet Gynecol 2003;21:213-214.

139. Berg C, Geipel A, Germer U, et al. Prenatal diagnosis of umbilical cord aneurysm in a fetus with trisomy 18. Ultrasound Obstet Gynecol 2001;17:79-81.

140. Sepulveda W, Corral E, Kottmann C, et al. Umbilical artery aneurysm: prenatal identification in three fetuses with trisomy 18. Ultrasound Obstet Gynecol 2003;21:292-296.

141. Shen O, Reinus C, Baranov A, Rabinowitz RR. Prenatal diagnosis of umbilical artery aneurysm: a potentially lethal anomaly. J Ultrasound Med 2007;26:251-253.

142. Daniel-Spiegel E, Weiner E, Gimburg G, Shalev E. The association of umbilical cord hemangioma with fetal vascular birthmarks. Prenat Diagn 2005;25:300-303.

143. Iyoob SD, Tsai A, Ruchelli ED, et al. Large umbilical cord hemangioma: sonographic features with surgical pathologic correlation. J Ultrasound Med 2006;25:1495-1498.

144. Sepulveda W, Rojas I, Robert JA, et al. Prenatal detection of velamentous insertion of the umbilical cord: a prospective color Doppler ultrasound study. Ultrasound Obstet Gynecol 2003;21:564-549.

145. Monteagudo A, Sfakianaki AK, Timor-Tritsch IE. Velamentous insertion of the cord in the first trimester. Ultrasound Obstet Gynecol 2000;16:498-499.

146. Sepulveda W. Velamentous insertion of the umbilical cord: a first-trimester sonographic screening study. J Ultrasound Med 2006;25:963-968; quiz 970.

147. Hasegawa J, Matsuoka R, Ichizuka K, et al. Velamentous cord insertion and atypical variable decelerations with no accelerations. Int J Gynaecol Obstet 2005;90:26-30.

148. Liu CC, Pretorius DH, Scioscia AL, Hull AD. Sonographic prenatal diagnosis of marginal placental cord insertion: clinical importance. J Ultrasound Med 2002;21:627-632.

149. Lee W, Lee VL, Kirk JS, et al. Vasa previa: prenatal diagnosis, natural evolution, and clinical outcome. Obstet Gynecol 2000;95:572-576.

150. Stafford IP, Neumann DE, Jarrell H. Abnormal placental structure and vasa previa: confirmation of the relationship. J Ultrasound Med 2004;23:1521-1522.

151. Baulies S, Maiz N, Munoz A, et al. Prenatal ultrasound diagnosis of vasa praevia and analysis of risk factors. Prenat Diagn 2007;27:595-599.

152. Oyelese Y, Spong C, Fernandez MA, McLaren RA. Second trimester low-lying placenta and in-vitro fertilization? Exclude vasa previa. J Matern Fetal Med 2000;9:370-372.

153. Catanzarite V, Maida C, Thomas W, et al. Prenatal sonographic diagnosis of vasa previa: ultrasound findings and obstetric outcome in ten cases. Ultrasound Obstet Gynecol 2001;18:109-115.

154. Oyelese Y, Chavez MR, Yeo L, et al. Three-dimensional sonographic diagnosis of vasa previa. Ultrasound Obstet Gynecol 2004;24:211-215.

155. Canterino JC, Mondestin-Sorrentino M, Muench MV, et al. Vasa previa: prenatal diagnosis and evaluation with 3-dimensional sonography and power angiography. J Ultrasound Med 2005;24:721-724; quiz 725.

156. Seince N, Carbillon L, Perrot N, Uzan M. Various Doppler sonographic appearances and challenges in prenatal diagnosis of vasa praevia. J Clin Ultrasound 2002;30:450-454.

Placenta during Labor and Postpartum

157. Herman A. Complicated third stage of labor: time to switch on the scanner. Ultrasound Obstet Gynecol 2000;15:89-95.

158. Herman A, Zimerman A, Arieli S, et al. Down-up sequential separation of the placenta. Ultrasound Obstet Gynecol 2002;19:278-281.

159. Krapp M, Katalinic A, Smrcek J, et al. Study of the third stage of labor by color Doppler sonography. Arch Gynecol Obstet 2003;267:202-204.

160. Mo A, Rogers MS. Sonographic examination of uteroplacental separation during the third stage of labor. Ultrasound Obstet Gynecol 2008;31:427-431.

161. Rufener SL, Adusumilli S, Weadock WJ, Caoili E. Sonography of uterine abnormalities in postpartum and postabortion patients: a potential pitfall of interpretation. J Ultrasound Med 2008;27:343-348.

CHAPTER 45

Cervical Ultrasound and Preterm Birth

Wendy L. Whittle, Katherine W. Fong, and Rory Windrim

Chapter Outline

PRETERM BIRTH

Preterm birth (PTB), defined as delivery before 37 weeks of gestation, occurs in 5% to 11% of all pregnancies, with a range as low as 4.5% in Ireland and as high as 15% in the United States, attributable to geographic, socioeconomic, and racial disparities.[1-3] PTB is the leading cause of neonatal morbidity and mortality not attributable to congenital anomalies or aneuploidy. If an infant is born preterm, the risk of death in the first year of life is 40-fold greater compared with an infant born at term.[1]

Immediate consequences of PTB include respiratory distress, intraventricular hemorrhage, sepsis, and retinopathy of prematurity.[1] In the long term, infants born preterm represent half the children with cerebral palsy, one third of those with abnormal vision, one quarter of those with chronic lung disease, and one fifth of children with mental retardation.[1,4,5] The morbidity of prematurity persists to adulthood, with an increased incidence of behavioral problems, lower levels of educational achievement, reduced rates of reproductive success (with incidence of both conception and live birth adversely affected), and an increased incidence of second-generation PTB.[6-8] The impact of prematurity extends beyond the individual and the family, with the average cost of a stay in a Canadian neonatal intensive care unit (NICU) about $9700, but in excess of $117,000 if the birth weight is less than 750 g.[1,9,10]

The risk of prematurity persists in subsequent pregnancies, with a twofold increased risk in the next pregnancy and up to 50% risk of PTB if the woman has experienced two or more prior PTBs.[1] Given the substantial and far-reaching impact of preterm birth, it is important to recognize patients at increased risk of **spontaneous preterm birth** (SPTB), such that therapeutic interventions can be implemented to improve neonatal outcome.

About 85% of preterm delivery occurs spontaneously and is traditionally classified as one of three discrete events: **preterm labor** (uterine activity with coordinated cervical effacement and dilation), **preterm premature ruptured membranes** (ruptured fetal membranes in the absence of uterine activity and cervical change), or **cervical incompetence** (cervical dilation in the absence of uterine activity).[1,11,12] Cervical incompetence can be further defined as either a **mechanical failure** of the cervix to remain closed against the increasing intrauterine expansion or as a **functional failure,** with premature activation of the events of cervical ripening (dilation and effacement) that normally occur at term.[11] Although categorized in this manner, spontaneous prematurity is best described along a continuum of biologic events leading to early delivery, given that the biochemical mediators that effect uterine contractions, fetal membrane disruption, and cervical ripening are similar: prostaglandins, the metallomatrix proteases and their inhibitors, and the families of proinflammatory and anti-inflammatory cytokines.[1,12] As such, the events of prematurity often overlap; in particular, cervical change can precede fetal membrane rupture and uterine contractions, although the cervix may not be functionally or mechanically incompetent.

Evaluation of the cervix has been used as a tool to predict SPTB based on the concept that the cervix acts as an anatomic marker of the underlying pathologic processes leading to a premature delivery. Digital examination of the cervix measures only the length from the external cervical os to the cervical-vaginal junction, not the intra-abdominal cervical-isthmus portion of the cervix. Therefore, digital examination underestimates cervical length by a mean difference of 12 mm in more than 80% of women in the second and third trimesters compared with sonography.[13] The traditional approach to evaluation of the cervix has been by sonographic visualization. This chapter reviews the techniques of uterine cervix sonography and its relationship with preterm birth prediction.

SONOGRAPHY OF THE UTERINE CERVIX

Sonographic visualization and appropriate measurements of the uterine cervix may facilitate the diagnosis and management of the patient at increased risk of SPTB. For this reason, evaluation of the maternal cervix is an integral part of the comprehensive obstetric ultrasound examination. There are three approaches to scanning the cervix: transabdominal, transperineal (translabial), and transvaginal. Each approach has advantages and limitations for different clinical scenarios.

Transabdominal Approach

Transabdominal sonography (TAS) of the cervix is performed during the standard second- and third-trimester obstetric ultrasound examinations and is used as a routine screening tool for cervical length. The examination usually requires a full urinary bladder (typically 45-60 mm in diameter) to create an acoustic window.[14-18] Longitudinal scanning is initiated in the midline of the lower abdomen, just above the symphysis pubis, using a transducer with a frequency of 3 MHz or higher.[14-18] When the **endocervical canal** comes into view, a slight adjustment or angulation of the transducer may be necessary to visualize the entire canal from the internal to external os (Fig. 45-1). Measurement of cervical length is affected by overdistention of the urinary bladder. Increased bladder pressure can compress the lower uterine segment and falsely elongate the cervix or mask cervical dilation.[17] Cervices less than 2 cm in length cannot be easily visualized against the vaginal and bladder tissue.[17]

In the second trimester, if the urinary bladder is empty, amniotic fluid can be used as an acoustic window

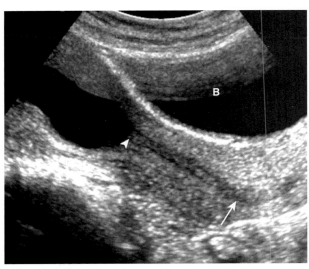

FIGURE 45-1. Normal cervix. Transabdominal full-bladder technique. Longitudinal midline image of the cervix. The cervical canal is seen from the internal os *(arrowhead)* to the external os *(arrow)*. B, Bladder.

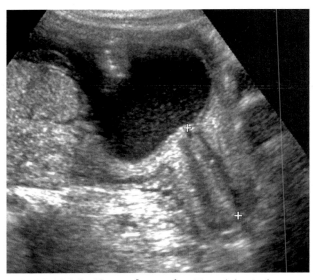

FIGURE 45-2. Normal cervix. Transabdominal empty-bladder technique. Longitudinal midline image of the cervix obtained by scanning through the amniotic fluid. The cervical canal is indicated by calipers.

to scan the cervix. Longitudinal scans are obtained with the transducer angled downward from just below the umbilicus. The cervix may assume a more vertical orientation and appear bulkier (Fig. 45-2). Difficulty in identifying the external os could contribute to error in cervical length measurement.

Visualization of the cervix can be difficult because of large maternal habitus or an engaged position of the fetal head. As the third trimester approaches, fetal and maternal size impairs visualization of the cervix in about 30% of patients.[14-18] Regardless of the gestational age, there is relatively poor reproducibility of transabdominal measurement of the cervix. TAS is a useful screening tool to identify patients at increased risk of SPTB but should not be used for the evaluation of patients previously determined to be at increased risk of SPTB.

Transperineal/Translabial Approach

Transperineal sonography is useful in patients for whom the cervix cannot be visualized by TAS or if vaginismus prevents the transvaginal approach. Scanning is performed with an empty urinary bladder. An abdominal transducer with a frequency of 3 MHz or higher can be used.[19-22] To minimize the risk of transmission of infection, the transducer is covered with plastic wrap or a glove and then lubricant gel. With the patient supine and hips abducted, the transducer is placed between the labia minora at the vaginal introitus. The ultrasound beam is oriented in a sagittal plane along the direction of the vagina. The vagina is seen in a vertical plane between the bladder and the rectum (Fig. 45-3). The cervix is oriented horizontally, at a right angle with the vagina. The full length of the cervical canal can be visualized in 86% to 96% of patients with this technique.[20,21] However, the region of the external os can be obscured by rectal gas or the symphysis pubis, and reproducibility of the measurements is poor.[23-25] As such, the transperineal approach is not used for measuring cervical length in the patient at increased risk of SPTB.

Transvaginal Sonography

Transvaginal sonography (TVS) of the cervix is the reference-standard technique for accurate determination of the dimensions and characteristics of the uterine cervix.[26,27] The examination is performed with an empty urinary bladder. A gynecologic table fitted with stirrups is preferred, although the examination can be carried out with the patient's hips elevated on a thick cushion or wedge. With the patient in a dorsal lithotomy position,

supine and hips abducted, an endovaginal transducer (5-MHz or higher frequency) is placed in the vagina and oriented in a longitudinal plane. The probe is inserted until the cervix comes into view. Usually, the transducer is inserted only 3 to 4 cm into the vagina to avoid contact with the cervix so that the images will have the cervix within the effective focal range of the transducer (Fig. 45-4). Depending on the position of the cervix in the vagina, the probe may need to be moved anteriorly, posteriorly, and/or laterally.[26,27]

To ensure measurement of the cervical length is reproducible, the following standardized criteria have been developed[28]:
1. The entire echogenic cervical canal should be seen.
2. The internal os should be flat or should have a V-shaped notch;

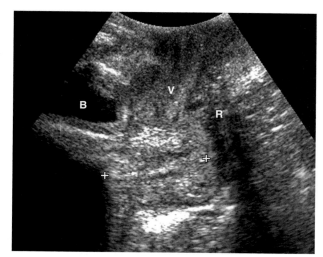

FIGURE 45-3. Transperineal scan of normal cervix. The cervix *(calipers)* is oriented horizontally, approximately perpendicular to the ultrasound beam. The vagina *(V)* is oriented in a nearly vertical plane. *B,* Bladder; *R,* rectum.

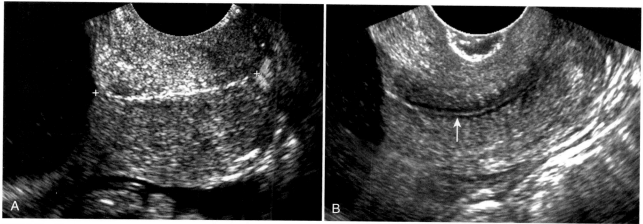

FIGURE 45-4. Transvaginal scan of normal cervix. A, Suggested placement of cursors for measuring cervical length. **B,** Normal cervical glandular area. The cervical canal is seen as an echogenic line *(arrow)* surrounded by a hypoechoic zone resulting from endocervical glands.

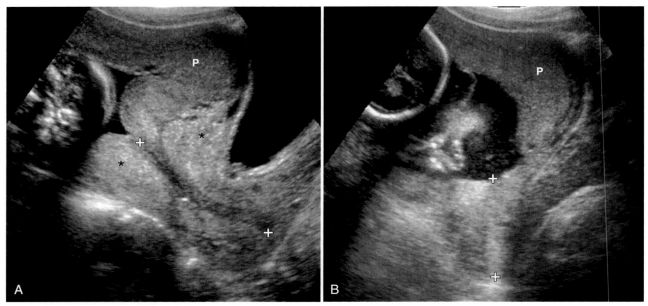

FIGURE 45-5. Uterine contractions. A, Transabdominal longitudinal image shows contraction (*) leading to a falsely elongated cervical canal *(calipers),* which measures 7.4 cm. **B,** After relaxation of the contraction, the cervix *(calipers)* measures 4.2 cm; *P,* placenta.

3. The external os should have a dimple or a triangular area of echodensity.
4. The distance from the surface of the anterior lip to the cervical canal should be equal to the distance from the posterior lip to the canal (a difference in the width of the anterior and posterior lips indicates too much pressure on the cervix, which could falsely increase the measurement).
5. The distance between the internal and external os should be measured over a minimum of 3 minutes with an average of three measurements.[26,29]

It is recommended that one first obtain a satisfactory image of the cervix, then withdraw the probe until the image is blurred, and finally, reapply only enough pressure to restore the image. This repositioning of the transducer avoids the error of falsely elongating the cervix with too much pressure of the probe on the cervix anteriorly. When the cervix appears curved, the cervical length should be measured as a sum of individual measurements rather than a line of "best fit," which underestimates the full length by up to 3 mm if the cervix is longer than 25 mm. Using these standard criteria, the intraobserver and interobserver variations are as low as 3.5 mm and 4.2 mm, respectively.[26,27]

The transvaginal technique is superior to the transabdominal technique. Higher-frequency transducers and closer proximity to the structures studied allow for better resolution. Potential complications of TVS include an increased risk of bleeding in the presence of placenta previa; induction of uterine activity in women with cervical shortening caused by cervical stimulation, and chorioamnionitis in the presence of ruptured membranes. However, Odibo et al.[30] did not demonstrate a relationship between chorioamnionitis or neonatal sepsis with sterile TVS after preterm premature rupture of membranes (PPROM).

To date, transvaginal assessment of cervical length by three-dimensional (3-D) sonography has been limited to the development of a normal distribution curve of cervical length through gestation. Overall, mean cervical length appears to be longer than the measurement by traditional 2-D scanning. However, there appears to be high intra/interobserver variability.[31] Currently, there are no reported studies of the relationship between 3-D TVS and SPTB prediction.

Technical Limitations and Pitfalls

The technical limitations and pitfalls associated with cervical sonography are outlined in Table 45-1. Uterine contractions can falsely elongate the cervix (Fig. 45-5) or cause pseudodilation (or hourglass appearance).

Normal Cervix

Sonographically, the cervix appears as a distinct, soft tissue structure containing midrange echoes. The **endocervical canal** often appears as an echogenic line surrounded by a hypoechoic zone attributed to the endocervical glands (see Fig. 45-4, *B*). Occasionally, the endocervical canal may appear hypoechoic and minimally dilated along its entire length. Benign **nabothian cysts** can be seen within the cervical soft tissues.

Numerous studies have evaluated **cervical length** in normal pregnancy. The typical cervix increases its length in the first trimester because of elaboration of the glandular content of the cervix.[27] Gramellini et al.[27] published a reference curve of cervical length through

TABLE 45-1. CERVICAL SONOGRAPHY: TECHNICAL LIMITATIONS AND PITFALLS

	TRANSABDOMINAL	TRANSPERINEAL	TRANSVAGINAL
Technical Factors			
Presenting part	++	–	–
Large maternal habitus	++	+	–
Limited field of view	–	+	++
Poor depth penetration*	–	–	+
Bowel gas	–	+	–
Gas in vagina	–	++	+
Pitfalls			
Overdistended bladder elongates cervix	+	–	–
Contractions	+	+	+
Cervical fibroid	+	+	+
Visualization of Internal os in Third Trimester			
	70%	86%	99.5%

*Caused by high-frequency transducer.

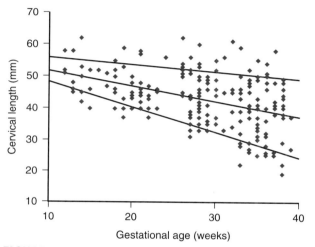

FIGURE 45-6. Relationship between cervical length and gestational age in normal pregnancy. Straight lines indicate 10th, 50th, and 90th percentiles. *(From Gramellini D, Fieni S, Molina E, et al. Transvaginal sonographic cervical length changes during normal pregnancy. J Ultrasound Med 2002;21:227-232.)*

gestation in both nulliparous and multiparous patients using TVS (Fig. 45-6). At about 20 weeks' gestation, at the fetal anatomic survey, the 10th, 50th, and 90th percentiles of cervical length are 40, 47, and 53 mm, respectively, regardless of parity. A progressive linear reduction in cervical length occurs over the 10th to 40th week of gestation.

"Short" Cervix

With the goal of understanding the relationship between cervical length and SPTB (delivery before 35 weeks' gestation), in 1996, Iams et al.[29] conducted a prospective, multicenter study in which an unselected general population of women with singleton pregnancies underwent TVS at 24 and 28 weeks' gestation. Cervical length at both examinations was comparable and normally

distributed, with a mean ±SD of 35.2 ± 8.3 mm at 24 weeks and 33.7 ± 8.5 mm at 28 weeks. A correlation between cervical length and the rate of SPTB was determined (Fig. 45-7); if the cervix was less than 26 mm (10th centile) or less than 13 mm (1st centile), risk of SPTB was increased by 6.49-fold and 13.99-fold, respectively, compared with the rate of SPTB if the cervix was at the 75th percentile length (40 mm) or greater.[29] Based on this landmark study, the definition of a **"short cervix" as less than 25 mm** (or <10th centile length at 24-28 weeks) was accepted (Fig. 45-8).

Since then, more than 50 studies of TVS evaluation of the cervix and the risk of SPTB have been published. In 2003, Honest et al.[32] conducted a meta-analysis of 46 studies (including >31,000 asymptomatic singleton patients) and concluded that the utility of TVS assessment of cervical length for the prediction of SPTB varies with the gestational age at assessment and the definition of SPTB (birth before gestational age <32 weeks, <34 weeks, or <37 weeks). To summarize, the earlier in gestation, the shorter the cervix, the greater is the risk of SPTB, with the best predictive value when cervical length measures less than 25 mm and SPTB is defined as delivery before 34 weeks' gestation (Table 45-2).

However, it should be recognized that the previous studies assessed cervical length at or before 28 weeks' gestation. Several reports have demonstrated no predictive value of TVS measurement of the cervix beyond 30 weeks of gestation for any definition of SPTB, likely because the cervix undergoes a gradual shortening process beyond this gestational age regardless of the timing of delivery.

The controversial aspect of TVS assessment of cervical length and the prediction of SPTB remains, that not all patients with a defined "short" cervix at any gestational age will deliver preterm. TVS is a reasonable tool for identifying patients who will deliver at or close to term with good negative predictive value. However, greater than 50% of patients with a cervical length less than

TABLE 45-2. PREDICTION OF SPONTANEOUS PRETERM BIRTH (SPTB) BASED ON GESTATIONAL AGE (GA) AT CERVICAL LENGTH MEASUREMENT (<25 MM)*

GA AT DELIVERY	GA at Measurement			
	<20 WEEKS	20-24 WEEKS	24-28 WEEKS	>28 WEEKS
<32 weeks	4.1 (1.6-10.1)	4.19 (2.6-6.7)	No data	No data
<34 weeks	6.2 (3.2-12.0)	4.40 (3.5-5.4)	4.0 (3.1-5.2)	No data
<37 weeks	8.7 (3.8-19.9)	25.6 (8.5-76.7)	3.1 (1.1-8.9)	No data

Modified from Honest H, Bachmann LM, Coomarasamy A, et al. Accuracy of cervical transvaginal sonography in predicting preterm birth: a systematic review. Ultrasound Obstet Gynecol 2003;22:305-322.
*Data presented as odds ratio ±95th percentile confidence intervals.

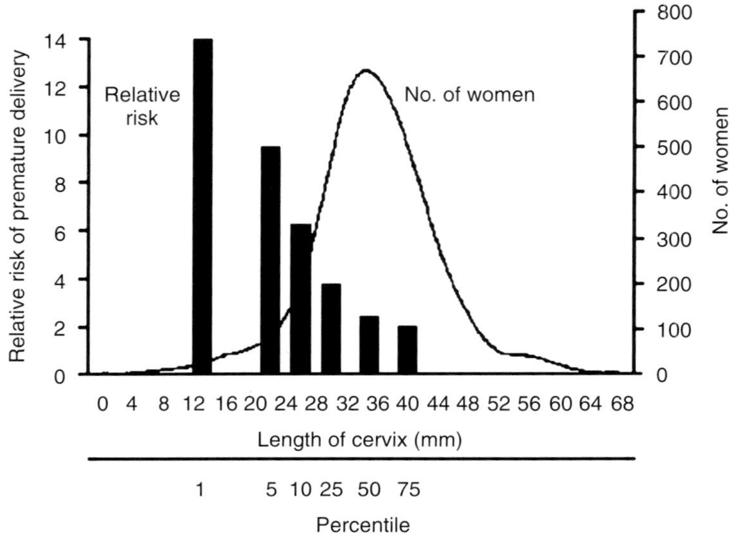

FIGURE 45-7. Cervical length and risk of preterm delivery percentile ranking. Transvaginal ultrasound cervical length percentile rank, at 24 weeks' gestation, and relative risk of preterm delivery before 35 weeks. *(From Iams JD, Goldenberg RL, Meis PJ, et al. The length of the cervix and the risk of spontaneous premature delivery. N Engl J Med 1996;334:567-572.)*

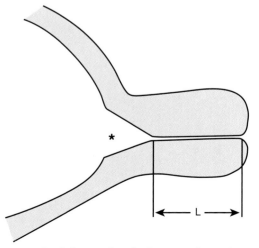

FIGURE 45-8. Schematic of abnormal cervix. Length of the closed cervical canal *(L)* and the presence or absence of funneling (*) should be reported.

25 mm measured at 20 weeks will deliver beyond 34 weeks' gestation.[29,32] Several studies have attempted to improve the predictive value of TVS by combining with other factors, including obstetric history and the concentration of fetal fibronectin in cervicovaginal secretions, to create a risk assessment formula.

PREDICTION OF SPONTANEOUS PRETERM BIRTH

Obstetric Factors

Celik et al.[33] presented a model to evaluate the ability of combinations of maternal demographics (age, race, weight, height, smoking status, history of cervical surgery, obstetric history) and cervical length between 20 and 24 weeks' gestation for prediction of SPTB in about

59,000 women with singleton pregnancies. The best prediction for SPTB was provided by cervical length alone, which was improved by adding obstetric history but not maternal characteristics. The estimated detection rates for extreme (<28 weeks), early (28-30 weeks), moderate (31-33 weeks), and mild (34-36 weeks) PTB by combining obstetric history and cervical length were 80.6%, 58.5%, 53.0%, and 28.6%, respectively, with a 10% false-positive rate. These data suggest that the combined screening model has better predictive value than either factor alone; similar findings in smaller-scale studies have been reported.[34]

Fetal fibronectin (FFN) is a glycoprotein that binds the amniochorion to the decidua and is released into cervicovaginal fluid in response to inflammation or separation of amniochorion from the decidua. In one study, 23% of symptomatic patients with FFN detected in the cervicovaginal fluid delivered within 7 days of the test, compared with 2% with a negative FFN, prompted several authors to evaluate the combination of short cervix and a positive FFN test in high-risk and low-risk patients.[35-38] In both low-risk women and women at increased risk for SPTB (based on maternal demographics and obstetric history), presence of FFN in the cervicovaginal secretions does not improve the ability to predict preterm birth, beyond that prediction available by ultrasound, because FFN positivity increases as cervical length decreases.[35-37]

Cervical Width and Funneling

The cervical width is obtained by measuring the anteroposterior (AP) diameter of the cervix at the midpoint between the internal and external cervical os. This dimension increases with gestational age, and nomograms exist for cervical width from 10 to 37 weeks' gestation.[39,40] In practice, this measurement is not widely used for diagnosis.

Much controversy surrounds the utility of measuring the **cervical "funnel,"** defined as the dilation of the internal os and the herniation of the fetal membranes into the cervical canal (Figs. 45-9 and 45-10; **Video 45-1**). To et al.[41] reported that **funneling** of the internal os was present in 4% of all pregnancies; the shorter the cervix, the greater the rate of funneling, with 98% prevalence if the length was less than 15 mm and only 1% if greater than 30 mm. The rate of SPTB was increased in pregnancies demonstrating cervical funneling. However, funneling did not provide any significant contribution to the prediction of SPTB when combined with cervical length.[42,43] As an isolated finding compared with cervical length, length measurements have a better predictive

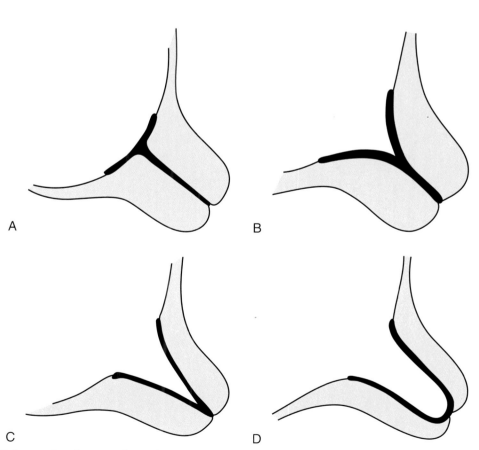

FIGURE 45-9. Schematic of normal cervix and cervical funnel shapes. A, The normal closed internal os and the cervical canal appear T shaped. **B, C,** and **D,** Different stages of funneling resemble the letters Y, V, and U.

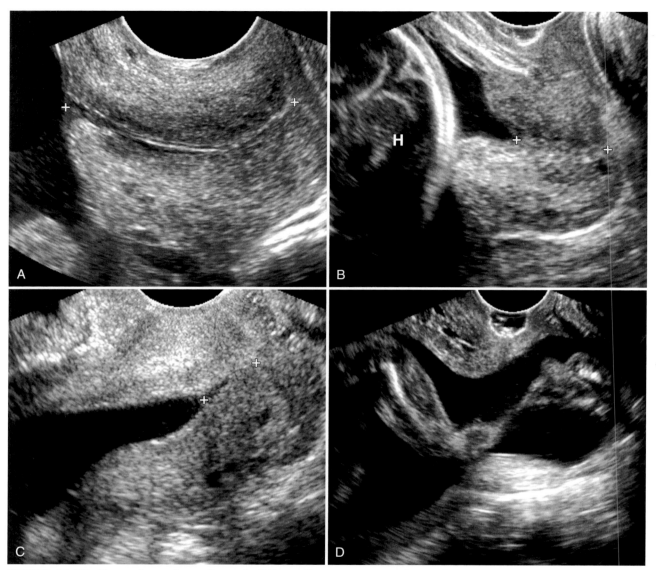

FIGURE 45-10. Normal cervix and cervical funneling. A, Transvaginal scan of normal cervix, showing a T-shaped closed internal os. **B, C, and D,** Transvaginal scan shows different stages of herniation of membranes, which resemble the letters Y, V, and U. Calipers denote closed cervical length. In **D,** with the U configuration, there is no closed cervix, and the fetal lower extremities are herniating into the cervix. *H,* Fetal head.

value than funneling. In addition, the shape or size of the funnel was not correlated to SPTB. As such, funneling is best reported as a categorical variable (present or absent) and best interpreted in the context of overall cervical length and obstetrical history.

Pseudodilation of the cervix, an apparent short and dilated cervix, is caused by contraction of the lower uterine segment during the ultrasound scan (Fig. 45-11). Pseudodilation can be distinguished from true cervical shortening by the following criteria[44]:

1. The cervical length is greater than 5 cm in total length.
2. A length of opposed cervical tissue can be seen distal to the dilated portion.

3. A rounded myometrium surrounds the dilated portion of the "cervix."

With repeat scanning after the contraction relaxes, the appearance will return to normal. Pseudodilation is not correlated with prediction of SPTB.

Rate of Cervical Change

In their meta-analysis, Honest et al.[32] correlated a single measurement of cervical length at a single time point in gestation with the risk of SPTB. However, the events of prematurity occur along a continuum and likely develop over an as-yet undefined and variable period. Therefore, **progressive shortening of the cervix** may be more important than a single abnormal cervical length measurement. A "short and shortening" cervical length may be a more effective tool for SPTB prediction than a "short but stable" cervical length. In a cohort of unselected patients, Naim et al.[45] demonstrated that if cervical length decreased on serial scans, the odds ratio (OR) for SPTB increased 6.8-fold per unit of change (one unit = decline of 10 mm per month). In women at increased risk of preterm birth, Owen at el.[46] reported that serial measurements up to 24 weeks' gestation significantly improved the prediction of SPTB compared

with a single cervical measurement at 16 to 18 weeks. Similarly, in women at increased risk of SPTB (based on obstetric history), if cervical length remained stable from 12 to 20 weeks and greater than 25 mm, all patients delivered at term.[47] For women in whom cervical length became serially shorter (ultimately <15 mm) and the decrease in length occurred before 20 weeks, each patient was offered and accepted a cervical cerclage, and all delivered after 30 weeks' gestation. Groom et al.[48] and Szychowski et al.[49] reported similar results. These studies suggest three important caveats, as follows:

1. Serial cervical assessment is important to predict SPTB;
2. Progressive cervical shortening in patients at increased risk begins before the typical timing of routine cervical assessment at the second-trimester fetal anatomic scan, advocating for initiation of serial cervical assessment early in the second trimester.
3. Serial cervical shortening in the second trimester may identify patients with true mechanical failure of the cervix, who may benefit from the placement of a cerclage to prevent SPTB.

Dynamic Cervical Change

A **dynamic cervix** is defined as having spontaneous shortening, lengthening, or funneling observed during real-time TVS[50] (Fig. 45-12). However, the value of a dynamic cervix for the prediction of SPTB has not been clearly defined. In asymptomatic women with a history of SPTB, the presence of dynamic cervical shortening did not improve the predictive value of absolute cervical length for SPTB, but it was associated with progressive cervical shortening.[51] However, patients with uterine contractions had a greater incidence of dynamic cervical

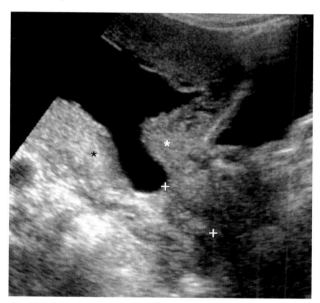

FIGURE 45-11. Pseudodilation caused by uterine contractions. Transabdominal longitudinal scan shows a lower uterine segment contraction *(asterisks)* leading to a false appearance of dilated cervical canal. The closed cervix *(calipers)* measures 3.5 cm.

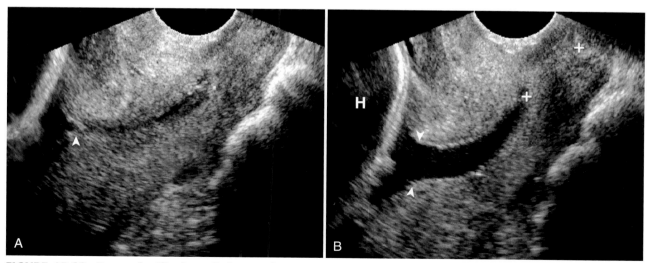

FIGURE 45-12. Dynamic dilation of the cervix, transvaginal ultrasound. A, Initially, the internal os is closed *(arrowhead).* **B,** Image obtained 30 seconds later shows funneling of the internal os *(arrowheads).* The residual closed cervix *(calipers)* measures 12 mm. *H,* Fetal head.

change than asymptomatic patients.[51] In both clinical scenarios, the **minimal closed cervical length,** not the "dynamic change," was the better predictor of SPTB.

Several noninvasive stress techniques have been suggested to elicit cervical change and improve the ability of TVS to predict cervical incompetence. These stressors include **transfundal pressure** (pressure applied at the fundus for 15 seconds that elicits >5 mm in cervical length shortening), standing, and coughing. Several small studies found that transfundal pressure was the most effective tool in cervical assessment and the most sensitive tool to predict progressive cervical shortening.[52,53]

Other Sonographic Features

Several sonographic features other than cervical length have been studied to predict SPTB, including canal dilation, absence of the glandular area along the length of the canal, and amniotic fluid debris. Each feature is associated with an increased risk of preterm birth independent of cervical length. **Cervical canal dilation** of 2 to 4 mm was associated with a 5.5-fold increased risk of

SPTB.[54] The **cervical glandular area** is a hypoechoic zone that runs along the length of the cervical canal (see Fig. 45-4, *B*). In 388 unselected women, an absent cervical glandular area at 21 to 24 weeks' gestation predicted SPTB before 35 weeks (odds ratio of 129), suggesting a strong association.[55]

"Sludge" or **debris** can be observed in the amniotic fluid immediately above the cervical canal (Fig. 45-13). Samples of the sludge in patients with impending preterm delivery have been aspirated under ultrasound guidance, and the microbiologic examination reveals clusters of inflammatory cells and bacteria. Presence of sludge is an independent risk factor for SPTB, preterm PROM, increased concentration of microbes within the amniotic fluid and histologic chorioamnionitis in asymptomatic patients at high risk for spontaneous preterm delivery. Furthermore, the combination of "sludge" and a short cervix conferred a greater risk for SPTB than a short cervix alone.[56,57]

CERVICAL ASSESSMENT IN SPECIFIC CLINICAL SCENARIOS

General Obstetric Population Screening

The disadvantages of routine general population screening are twofold: (1) a low sensitivity of the test and the low prevalence of preterm deliveries in a low-risk population, and (2) an effective tool for the prevention of SPTB for all patients determined to be at risk has not yet been determined. Women with no risk factors for SPTB (the general obstetric population) have a low prevalence of preterm birth of 4%, and in this low-risk group, Iams

---

ABNORMAL FINDINGS ON TRANSVAGINAL SONOGRAPHY (TVS)*

Shortest closed cervical length less than 25 mm
Presence of funneling
Presence of positive response to fundal pressure
Presence of amniotic fluid debris ("sludge")
Shortening of 8 to 10 mm since previous TVS

*Gestational age less than 30 weeks.

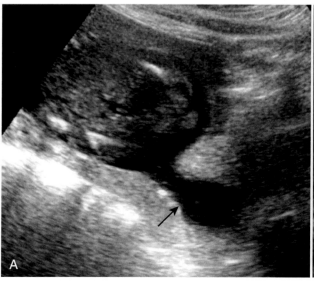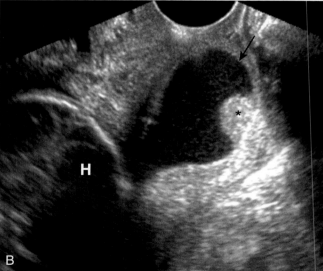

FIGURE 45-13. Dilated cervical canal. A, Transabdominal longitudinal scan shows an open cervical canal *(arrow).* This is an indication for further evaluation. **B,** Subsequent transvaginal scan demonstrates bulging amnion *(arrow)* into the proximal vagina; *H,* fetal head; asterisk indicates amniotic fluid "sludge" or potentially the mucus plug.

et al.[29] and more recent studies have failed to show a high sensitivity or positive predictive value for SPTB when the cervical length measurement was less than 25 mm at either 24 or 28 weeks' gestation.[29] Poor sensitivity of TVS cervical length assessment results in cervical length cutoff values being set at a very low level (<15 mm) in order to obtain acceptable specificity. Randomized controlled studies of cerclage placement in low-risk women identified with a "short cervix" have clearly demonstrated no benefit of the cerclage for the prolongation of pregnancy in this clinical scenario.[58] In 250 unselected women identified as having a cervix less than 25 mm at 20 to 24 weeks' gestation, progesterone therapy reduced but did not eliminate the rate of SPTB, from 32% to 19%, compared with placebo.[59] Antibiotic therapy and bed rest clearly have no effect on the rate of SPTB in women with a "short cervix."[1]

In summary, no intervention has been proven to decrease SPTB in the general obstetric population, and therefore TVS cervical assessment in women at low risk of preterm birth is not justified and not currently recommended as part of the routine evaluation. However, during TAS for routine fetal anatomy or other indications, if the closed cervical length is less than 25 mm before 28 weeks' gestation, or if other findings include a dilated cervical canal, a ballooned fluid-filled lower segment with no visible cervix, or a cord or fetal part in the canal, further evaluation of the cervix by TVS is indicated (see Fig. 45-13).

TAS FINDINGS THAT INDICATE TVS FOLLOW-UP

Closed cervical length less than 25 mm (<28 weeks)
Dilated cervical canal
Ballooned, fluid-filled lower segment with no visible cervix
Evidence of cord or fetal part in the canal

TAS, Transabdominal sonography; TVS, transvaginal sonography.

High-Risk Obstetric Population Screening

Prior Preterm Birth

Once a patient has experienced an SPTB, the risk of recurrence is increased twofold based on history alone. TVS assessment of cervical length has been suggested as a tool of surveillance to evaluate the risk of SPTB specific to the individual patient and to identify those at greatest risk. Iams et al.[29] reported that cervical length was more predictive of preterm birth when other risk factors were also present. For a cervical length less than 25 mm at 22 to 24 weeks of gestation in a woman with a previous preterm birth, the relative risk was approximately 10-fold greater than that of women in the unselected population. Berghella et al.[43] demonstrated that the risk of recurrent SPTB varies with the gestational age at the time of measurement and the total length of cervix, but is not affected by the number of previous preterm births or the gestational age at delivery of the previous PTB. The risk SPTB was decreased by 5.5% per week of gestation gained and by 6.0% per mm increase in cervical length. Most recently, Crane et al.[60] performed a systematic review of 14 studies involving 2258 asymptomatic high risk women. In women with previous SPTB, for cervical length <25 mm, the likelihood ratios for SPTB were 4.3 and 2.8, when gestational age at assessment was <20 weeks and 20-24 weeks respectively. Since then, Seaward et al.[61] found limited utility of cervical length after 24 weeks' gestation in 75 high-risk patients; cervical length less than 25 mm or less than 15 mm measured at 24 to 30 weeks did not predict SPTB (defined as either <32 or <35 weeks' gestation) or adverse perinatal outcome. As discussed previously, the rate of cervical change may be a better predictive tool to identify those at greatest (and conversely lower) risk.

Multiple Gestations

Twin and higher-order multiple gestations are at increased risk of SPTB; 50% of twin gestations deliver before 35 weeks of gestation, and the mean gestational age for a triplet gestation is 32 weeks. Several studies have attempted to define individual patient risk by using TVS assessment of the cervix. For the twin gestation, when measured at 20 to 22 weeks, both length less than 25 mm and presence of funneling were predictive of SPTB; but at 27 weeks, only length less than 25 mm predicted SPTB.[62-65] The likelihood ratio of SPTB for cervical length less than 25 mm was 5.4-fold, but if the cervix measured greater than 30 mm, rate of SPTB was as low as 4%. For the triplet gestation, using the same cutoff length of less than 25 mm, a positive predictive value of 83% for SPTB was reported when the cervix was measured at 14 to 20 weeks' gestation.[62-65]

Uterocervical Anomalies and Cervical Surgery

Previous cervical surgery (cone biopsy or laser excisional therapy) and a known uterine or cervical congenital anomaly (uterine didelphys, bicornuate uterus, or DES exposure in utero) are factors that significantly increase the risk of SPTB. Several authors have sought to determine if the cutoff cervical length value of less than 25 mm provides the best predictive for SPTB for women with known congenital uterine anomalies. As expected, women with a unicornuate uterus had the shortest mean cervical length and the highest rate of SPTB, compared with women with a bicornuate or septate uterus. However, the mean gestational age at delivery was typically greater than 30 weeks' gestation. Using a cervical length cutoff of 30 mm when measured after 20 weeks, rate of SPTB was increased by 13-fold; at 14 to 23 weeks, if the cervix was less than 25 mm, rate of SPTB was as high as 50%.[66] After cervical amputation by cone biopsy or laser excisional surgery (LEEP), the mean cervical length is shorter.[67] LEEP and cone biopsy therapy are associated with increased risk of SPTB by 3.45-fold, presumably from effects on cervical length and function. Again, a longer cervical cutoff of greater than 30 mm gave the best predictive value for identifying patients not at risk of SPTB, with a negative predictive value of 97%.

Preterm Premature Rupture of Membranes

Although OR for prediction of PPROM by TVS cervical assessment increases in relation to serial decreases in cervical length less than 20 mm, the positive and negative predictive values for PPROM specifically are low compared with the prediction of SPTB in general. TVS after PPROM can be performed without increased risk of chorioamnionitis or neonatal sepsis.[30] A cervical length less than 20 mm was associated with a latency period of less than 48 hours following PPROM.[30]

Polyhydramnios

Given that polyhydramnios is a risk factor for SPTB, presumably related to uterine distention triggering of uterine activity or mechanical cervical incompetence, one small study examined the relationship among the severity of polyhydramnios, cervical length, and SPTB.[68] A gradual shortening of cervical length was associated with advancing gestational age, but not the severity of the polyhydramnios. Cervical length less than 15 mm was associated with an earlier gestational age at delivery.

Fetal Therapy

Based on the assumption that cervical length is an anatomic marker of underlying pathologic processes that lead to SPTB, clinicians have sought to use the cervical length measurement to quantify risk in patients undergoing a fetal therapeutic intervention that in itself increases the risk of SPTB. A cervical length less than 30 mm at multipregnancy reduction from triplet to twin gestation (at <14 weeks) has a positive predictive value of 67% for delivery less than 33 weeks after the procedure.[69-71] Similarly, a cervical length less than 30 mm before laser treatment of twin-twin transfusion syndrome was associated with SPTB, independent of parity, intrauterine death of one fetus, disease severity, or volume of the amniotic fluid reduction as part of the procedure.[69-71]

Symptomatic Patients

A patient presenting with symptoms consistent with preterm labor (uterine contractility, vaginal discharge or bleeding) is considered at increased risk of SPTB, although two thirds of women admitted with the diagnosis of threatened preterm birth deliver at term.[1] Although cervical length has been used to identify those women who will deliver preterm, data are limited on the utility of TVS cervical length measurement in the symptomatic patient. Honest et al.[32] summarized the risk of SPTB before 34 weeks' gestation as follows: if the cervix measured less than 30 mm, risk increased by 1.98-fold if measured before 20 weeks and increased by 2.33-fold after 20 weeks. The presence of funneling, regardless of gestational age, increased the likelihood ratio to 4.7-fold. Alternatively, a TVS cervical length of longer than 30 mm makes the diagnosis of preterm labor extremely unlikely, with a negative predictive value of 98% to 99%. Assessment of FFN in the cervical-vaginal secretions does not improve the prediction of delivery provided by cervical length evaluation alone.[36] However, no study has examined the length of the cervix after 28 weeks' gestation in the symptomatic patient or evaluated the length of the cervix and the rate of SPTB after the symptoms have resolved. Extrapolation of the cervical length cutoff value of 25 mm should be used with caution in such patients.

Cervical Incompetence and Cervical Cerclage

Overall, cervical length has been evaluated as an anatomic marker of an underlying process leading to SPTB, regardless of the etiology: preterm labor, premature ruptured membranes, or cervical incompetence. Cervical length assessment may have its greatest value for the diagnosis of **cervical incompetence.** Failure of the cervix to remain closed, in the absence of uterine activity or membrane rupture, occurs in 0.5% to 1.0% of all pregnancies, with a recurrence risk of 30%.[1,11] **Functional failure** of the cervix is premature cervical ripening (shortening and dilation normally occurring at the end of gestation) and most often is related to urogenital or intrauterine infection or inflammation and thus has a low risk of recurrence. **Mechanical failure** of the cervix, defined as a defect in the structural integrity of the cervix, may result from traumatic injury to the cervix, including cervical laceration, amputation, conization, excessive cervical dilation before diagnostic curettage, or therapeutic abortion.[1] It may also be associated with diethylstilbestrol (DES) in utero or uterine malformations. Serial cervical shortening in the second trimester and a positive response to fundal pressure may be used to unmask specific cervical mechanical incompetence during pregnancy.[48,49,53]

These patients may benefit from the placement of a **cervical cerclage**, a suture used to reinforce the structural integrity of the cervical canal. Alternatively, some practitioners will place a cerclage prophylactically in any patient who has delivered preterm, because of presumed cervical incompetence. Sonography has been used in the operating room to guide the placement of cervical cerclage, especially when the cervix is short to ensure that the suture material is placed within the cervical tissue and does not encroach on bladder mucosa or rectum. Once in place, the cervical cerclage will appear as one or more echodense "dots" along the length of the cervical canal (Fig. 45-14). Postcerclage evaluation includes location of the sutures in relation to both the internal and the external cervical os and measurement of the length of the closed cervical canal both above and below the level of the suture line. Once the cerclage has been placed, cervical length assessment continues to have value in the prediction of SPTB. Several studies reported that if the residual total closed cervical length after cerclage placement was less than 15 mm, or if "funneling to stitch" (open canal to level of suture line) was present (Fig. 45-15), the patient was at significantly increased risk of delivery before 32 weeks' gestation, regardless of the indication for stitch placement.[61,72,73] Beyond 30 weeks, there was no predictive value of cervical assessment in women with a cerclage.

When the vaginal portion of the cervical tissue is absent or damaged (trachelectomy, cone biopsy, birth trauma), the placement of a cerclage in the vaginal component of the cervix is not possible. Alternatively, a cerclage can be placed at the level of the cervicouterine isthmus either by laparoscopy or laparotomy. On TVS assessment, the echodense dots of this "abdominal" cerclage will be visualized close to the bladder and adjacent to the lower uterine segment (Fig. 45-16).

MANAGEMENT PROTOCOLS FOR THE ABNORMAL CERVIX

Because of improved test characteristics in women at increased risk of SPTB, and because interventions such as bed rest, cerclage, and progesterone therapy may have a potential benefit in the high-risk patient, cervical length measurement is used as a screening test

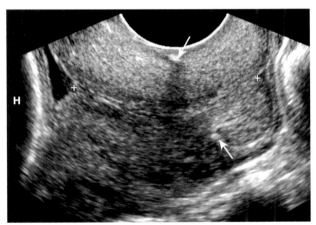

FIGURE 45-14. Cervical cerclage. Transvaginal scan demonstrates a closed cervix that measures 28 mm *(calipers)*. The cerclage sutures *(arrows)* appear hyperechoic. *H,* Fetal head.

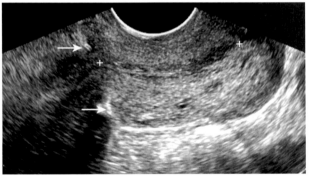

FIGURE 45-16. Abdominal cervical cerclage. Transvaginal longitudinal scan demonstrates hyperechoic sutures *(arrows)* at the internal os in this woman with a history of incompetent cervix. The cervix is closed and long, measuring 4.5 cm *(calipers)*.

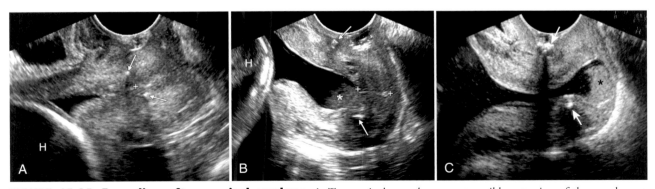

FIGURE 45-15. Funneling after cervical cerclage. A, Transvaginal scan demonstrates mild protrusion of the membranes. There is 10-mm closed cervix *(calipers)* above the sutures *(arrows)*. **B,** Transvaginal scan demonstrates protrusion of the membranes to the level of the sutures *(arrows)*. The residual closed cervix measures 10 mm *(calipers)*. **C,** Transvaginal scan demonstrates protrusion of the membranes beyond the sutures *(arrows)*. *H,* Fetal head; asterisk indicates amniotic fluid sludge.

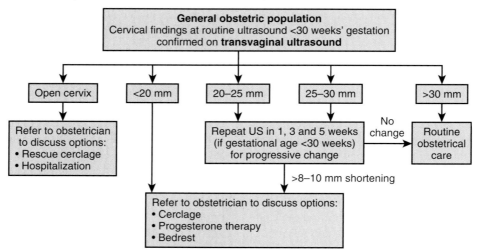

FIGURE 45-17. Management protocol: general obstetric population. Algorithm to guide response to cervical length measurements at transvaginal sonography (<30 weeks' gestation).

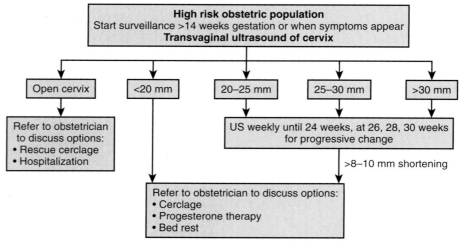

FIGURE 45-18. Management protocol: high-risk obstetric population. Algorithm to guide response to cervical length measurements at transvaginal sonography, with surveillance starting after 14 weeks' gestation or when symptoms appear.

in high-risk pregnancies. What remains to be determined is the frequency of evaluation, the gestational age of first evaluation, and the utility of the measurements after 30 weeks of gestation. Thus, whether a short cervix is identified by coincidence as part of a routine fetal ultrasound or as a targeted TVS of a patient identified to be at increased risk of SPTB, specific management protocols are suggested (Figs. 45-17 and 45-18).

CONCLUSION

Transvaginal sonography is the reference-standard approach for cervical assessment in pregnancy. Cervical length is used most often to predict spontaneous preterm birth. Cervical length should be taken in the context of maternal risk factors for SPTB (obstetric history, uterine contractions), gestational age, funneling, response to fundal pressure, previous measurement, presence of

cervical glandular area, and amniotic fluid debris. Cervical length should not be used as a screening tool for the general obstetric population but reserved for patients at increased risk of SPTB because of history, symptoms, or pregnancy complications or interventions. The cervical length cutoff of 25 mm at 20 to 28 weeks provides the best predictive values for SPTB before 34 weeks. A "short" (<25 mm) cervical length is not a diagnosis of impending SPTB, but rather a tool to quantify the increased risk of such an event.

References

Preterm Birth
1. Spong CY. Prediction and prevention of recurrent spontaneous preterm birth. Obstet Gynecol 2007;110:405-415.
2. Blondel B, Macfarlane A, Gissler M, et al. Preterm birth and multiple pregnancy in European countries participating in the PERISTAT project. BJOG 2006;113:528-535.
3. Kuehn BM. Groups take aim at US preterm birth rate. JAMA 2006;296:2907-2908.

4. Kramer MS, Demissie K, Yang H, et al. The contribution of mild and moderate preterm birth to infant mortality. Fetal and Infant Health Study Group of the Canadian Perinatal Surveillance System. JAMA 2000;284:843-849.

5. O'Shea TM, Klinepeter KL, Goldstein DJ, et al. Survival and developmental disability in infants with birth weights of 501 to 800 grams, born between 1979 and 1994. Pediatrics 1997;100:982-986.

6. Saigal S, Hoult LA, Streiner DL, et al. School difficulties at adolescence in a regional cohort of children who were extremely low birth weight. Pediatrics 2000;105:325-331.

7. Buck GM, Msall ME, Schisterman EF, et al. Extreme prematurity and school outcomes. Paediatr Perinat Epidemiol 2000;14:324-331.

8. Botting N, Powls A, Cooke RW, Marlow N. Attention deficit hyperactivity disorders and other psychiatric outcomes in very low birth-weight children at 12 years. J Child Psychol Psychiatry 1997;38:931-941.

9. Gilbert WM, Nesbitt TS, Danielsen B. The cost of prematurity: quantification by gestational age and birth weight. Obstet Gynecol 2003;102:488-492.

10. Petrou S, Mehta Z, Hockley C, et al. The impact of preterm birth on hospital inpatient admissions and costs during the first 5 years of life. Pediatrics 2003;112:1290-1297.

11. Golan A, Barnan R, Wexler S, Langer R, Bukovsky I, David MP. Incompetence of the uterine cervix. Obstet Gynecol Surv 1989;44:96-107.

12. Romero R, Espinoza J, Goncalves LF, et al. The role of inflammation and infection in preterm birth. Semin Reprod Med 2007;25:21-39.

13. Sonek JD, Iams JD, Blumenfeld M, et al. Measurement of cervical length in pregnancy: comparison between vaginal ultrasonography and digital examination. Obstet Gynecol 1990;76:172-175.

Sonography of the Cervix

14. Sarti DA, Sample WF, Hobel CJ, Staisch KJ. Ultrasonic visualization of a dilated cervix during pregnancy. Radiology 1979;130:417-420.

15. Bowie JD, Andreotti RF, Rosenberg ER. Sonographic appearance of the uterine cervix in pregnancy: the vertical cervix. AJR Am J Roentgenol 1983;140:737-740.

16. Ayers JW, DeGrood RM, Compton AA, et al. Sonographic evaluation of cervical length in pregnancy: diagnosis and management of preterm cervical effacement in patients at risk for premature delivery. Obstet Gynecol 1988;71:939-944.

17. Mason GC, Maresh MJ. Alterations in bladder volume and the ultrasound appearance of the cervix. Br J Obstet Gynaecol 1990;97:457-458.

18. Andersen HF. Transvaginal and transabdominal ultrasonography of the uterine cervix during pregnancy. J Clin Ultrasound 1991;19:77-83.

19. Jeanty P, d'Alton M, Romero R, Hobbins JC. Perineal scanning. Am J Perinatol 1986;3:289-295.

20. Mahony BS, Nyberg DA, Luthy DA, et al. Translabial ultrasound of the third-trimester uterine cervix: correlation with digital examination. J Ultrasound Med 1990;9:717-723.

21. Hertzberg BS, Bowie JD, Weber TM, et al. Sonography of the cervix during the third trimester of pregnancy: value of the transperineal approach. AJR Am J Roentgenol 1991;157:73-76.

22. Hertzberg BS, Kliewer MA, Baumeister LA, et al. Optimizing transperineal sonographic imaging of the cervix: the hip elevation technique. J Ultrasound Med 1994;13:933-936; quiz 1009-1010.

23. Kurtzman JT, Goldsmith LJ, Gall SA, Spinnato JA. Transvaginal versus transperineal ultrasonography: a blinded comparison in the assessment of cervical length at midgestation. Am J Obstet Gynecol 1998;179:852-857.

24. Owen J, Neely C, Northen A. Transperineal versus endovaginal ultrasonographic examination of the cervix in the midtrimester: a blinded comparison. Am J Obstet Gynecol 1999;181:780-783.

25. Okun N. Is transperineal ultrasonography of cervical length in pregnant women as accurate as endovaginal ultrasonography? A prospective, blinded comparison of level of agreement of two techniques. J Obstet Gynaecol Can 2001;23:592-596.

26. Kushnir O, Vigil DA, Izquierdo L, et al. Vaginal ultrasonographic assessment of cervical length changes during normal pregnancy. Am J Obstet Gynecol 1990;162:991-993.

27. Gramellini D, Fieni S, Molina E, et al. Transvaginal sonographic cervical length changes during normal pregnancy. J Ultrasound Med 2002;21:227-232; quiz 234-235.

28. Heath VC, Souka AP, Erasmus I, et al. Cervical length at 23 weeks of gestation: the value of Shirodkar suture for the short cervix. Ultrasound Obstet Gynecol 1998;12:318-322.

29. Iams JD, Goldenberg RL, Meis PJ, et al. The length of the cervix and the risk of spontaneous premature delivery. National Institute of Child Health and Human Development Maternal Fetal Medicine Unit Network. N Engl J Med 1996;334:567-572.

30. Odibo AO, Berghella V, Reddy U, et al. Does transvaginal ultrasound of the cervix predict preterm premature rupture of membranes in a high-risk population? Ultrasound Obstet Gynecol 2001;18:223-227.

31. Rovas L, Sladkevicius P, Strobel E, Valentin L. Reference data representative of normal findings at three-dimensional power Doppler ultrasound examination of the cervix from 17 to 41 gestational weeks. Ultrasound Obstet Gynecol 2006;28:761-767.

32. Honest H, Bachmann LM, Coomarasamy A, et al. Accuracy of cervical transvaginal sonography in predicting preterm birth: a systematic review. Ultrasound Obstet Gynecol 2003;22:305-322.

33. Celik E, To M, Gajewska K, et al. Cervical length and obstetric history predict spontaneous preterm birth: development and validation of a model to provide individualized risk assessment. Ultrasound Obstet Gynecol 2008;31:549-554.

34. To MS, Skentou CA, Royston P, et al. Prediction of patient-specific risk of early preterm delivery using maternal history and sonographic measurement of cervical length: a population-based prospective study. Ultrasound Obstet Gynecol 2006;27:362-367.

35. Schmitz T, Maillard F, Bessard-Bacquaert S, et al. Selective use of fetal fibronectin detection after cervical length measurement to predict spontaneous preterm delivery in women with preterm labor. Am J Obstet Gynecol 2006;194:138-143.

36. Heath VC, Daskalakis G, Zagaliki A, et al. Cervicovaginal fibronectin and cervical length at 23 weeks of gestation: relative risk of early preterm delivery. BJOG 2000;107:1276-1281.

37. Tsoi E, Akmal S, Geerts L, et al. Sonographic measurement of cervical length and fetal fibronectin testing in threatened preterm labor. Ultrasound Obstet Gynecol 2006;27:368-372.

38. Honest H, Bachmann LM, Gupta JK, et al. Accuracy of cervicovaginal fetal fibronectin test in predicting risk of spontaneous preterm birth: systematic review [see comment]. BMJ 2002;325:301.

39. Varma TR, Patel RH, Pillai U. Ultrasonic assessment of cervix in "at risk" patients. Acta Obstet Gynecol Scand 1986;65:147-152.

40. Smith CV, Anderson JC, Matamoros A, Rayburn WF. Transvaginal sonography of cervical width and length during pregnancy. J Ultrasound Med 1992;11:465-467.

41. To MS, Skentou C, Liao AW, et al. Cervical length and funneling at 23 weeks of gestation in the prediction of spontaneous early preterm delivery. Ultrasound Obstet Gynecol 2001;18:200-203.

42. Meijer-Hoogeveen M, Stoutenbeek P, Visser GH. Methods of sonographic cervical length measurement in pregnancy: a review of the literature. J Matern Fetal Neonatal Med 2006;19:755-762.

43. Berghella V, Roman A, Daskalakis C, et al. Gestational age at cervical length measurement and incidence of preterm birth. Obstet Gynecol 2007;110:311-317.

44. Karis JP, Hertzberg BS, Bowie JD. Sonographic diagnosis of premature cervical dilatation: potential pitfall due to lower uterine segment contractions. J Ultrasound Med 1991;10:83-87.

45. Naim A, Haberman S, Burgess T, et al. Changes in cervical length and the risk of preterm labor. Am J Obstet Gynecol 2002;186:887-889.

46. Owen J, Yost N, Berghella V, et al. Mid-trimester endovaginal sonography in women at high risk for spontaneous preterm birth. JAMA 2001;286:1340-1348.

47. Iqbal S, Kfouri J, Whittle WL, Windrim R. Early serial cervical length measurement as a toll to select candidates for cervical cerclage in a population of patients at increased risk for spontaneous preterm birth. Presented at Society for Obstetricians and Gynecologists of Canada Annual Meeting, 2007, Ottawa.

48. Groom KM, Shennan AH, Bennett PR. Ultrasound-indicated cervical cerclage: outcome depends on preoperative cervical length and presence of visible membranes at time of cerclage. Am J Obstet Gynecol 2002;187:445-449.

49. Szychowski JM, Owen J, Hankins G, et al. Timing of mid-trimester cervical length shortening in high-risk women. Ultrasound Obstet Gynecol 2009;33:70-75.

50. Wong G, Levine D, Ludmir J. Maternal postural challenge as a functional test for cervical incompetence. J Ultrasound Med 1997;16:169-175.

51. Pugatsch R, Elad D, Jaffa AJ, Eytan O. Analysis of cervical dynamics by ultrasound imaging. Ann NY Acad Sci 2007;1101:203-214.
52. Guzman ER, Rosenberg JC, Houlihan C, et al. A new method using vaginal ultrasound and transfundal pressure to evaluate the asymptomatic incompetent cervix. Obstet Gynecol 1994;83:248-252.
53. Guzman ER, Pisatowski DM, Vintzileos AM, et al. A comparison of ultrasonographically detected cervical changes in response to transfundal pressure, coughing, and standing in predicting cervical incompetence. Am J Obstet Gynecol 1997;177:660-665.
54. Hartmann K, Thorp Jr JM, McDonald TL, et al. Cervical dimensions and risk of preterm birth: a prospective cohort study. Obstet Gynecol 1999;93:504-509.
55. Pires CR, Moron AF, Mattar R, et al. Cervical gland area as an ultrasonographic marker for preterm delivery. Int J Gynaecol Obstet 2006;93:214-219.
56. Bujold E, Pasquier JC, Simoneau J, et al. Intra-amniotic sludge, short cervix, and risk of preterm delivery. J Obstet Gynaecol Can 2006; 28:198-202.
57. Espinoza J, Goncalves LF, Romero R, et al. The prevalence and clinical significance of amniotic fluid "sludge" in patients with preterm labor and intact membranes. Ultrasound Obstet Gynecol 2005;25: 346-352.

Cervical Assessment in Specific Clinical Scenarios

58. Pramod R, Okun N, McKay D, et al. Cerclage for the short cervix demonstrated by transvaginal ultrasound: current practice and opinion. J Obstet Gynaecol Can 2004;26:564-570.
59. Fonseca EB, Celik E, Parra M, et al. Progesterone and the risk of preterm birth among women with a short cervix. N Engl J Med 2007;357:462-469.
60. Crane JM, Hutchens D. Use of transvaginal ultrasonography to predict preterm birth in women with a history of preterm birth. Ultrasound Obstet Gynecol 2008;32:640-645.
61. Seaward A, Kfouri J, Dodd J, et al. Does transvaginal ultrasound assessment of the total cervical length and/or "funnelling to the stitch" predict preterm birth in women with a cervical cerclage in situ? Presented at Society for Maternal Fetal Medicine 2008 Annual Meeting.
62. Maslovitz S, Hartoov J, Wolman I, et al. Cervical length in the early second trimester for detection of triplet pregnancies at risk for preterm birth. J Ultrasound Med 2004;23:1187-1191.

63. Vayssiere C, Favre R, Audibert F, et al. Cervical assessment at 22 and 27 weeks for the prediction of spontaneous birth before 34 weeks in twin pregnancies: is transvaginal sonography more accurate than digital examination? Ultrasound Obstet Gynecol 2005;26:707-712.
64. Vayssiere C, Favre R, Audibert F, et al. Cervical length and funneling at 22 and 27 weeks to predict spontaneous birth before 32 weeks in twin pregnancies: a French prospective multicenter study. Am J Obstet Gynecol 2002;187:1596-1604.
65. Guzman ER, Walters C, O'Reilly-Green C, et al. Use of cervical ultrasonography in prediction of spontaneous preterm birth in triplet gestations. Am J Obstet Gynecol 2000;183:1108-1113.
66. Airoldi J, Berghella V, Sehdev H, Ludmir J. Transvaginal ultrasonography of the cervix to predict preterm birth in women with uterine anomalies. Obstet Gynecol 2005;106:553-556.
67. Crane JM, Delaney T, Hutchens D. Transvaginal ultrasonography in the prediction of preterm birth after treatment for cervical intraepithelial neoplasia. Obstet Gynecol 2006;107:37-44.
68. Hershkovitz R, Sheiner E, Maymon E, et al. Cervical length assessment in women with idiopathic polyhydramnios. Ultrasound Obstet Gynecol 2006;28:775-778.
69. Fait G, Har-Toov J, Gull I, et al. Cervical length, multifetal pregnancy reduction, and prediction of preterm birth. J Clin Ultrasound 2005; 33:329-332.
70. Robyr R, Boulvain M, Lewi L, et al. Cervical length as a prognostic factor for preterm delivery in twin-to-twin transfusion syndrome treated by fetoscopic laser coagulation of chorionic plate anastomoses. Ultrasound Obstet Gynecol 2005;25:37-41.
71. Rebarber A, Carreno CA, Lipkind H, et al. Cervical length after multifetal pregnancy reduction in remaining twin gestations. Am J Obstet Gynecol 2001;185:1113-1117.
72. Scheib S, Visintine JF, Miroshnichenko G, et al. Is cerclage height associated with the incidence of preterm birth in women with an ultrasound-indicated cerclage? Am J Obstet Gynecol 2009;200: e12-e5.
73. O'Brien JM, Hill AL, Barton JR. Funneling to the stitch: an informative ultrasonographic finding after cervical cerclage. Ultrasound Obstet Gynecol 2002;20:252-255.

CHAPTER 46

Ultrasound-Guided Invasive Fetal Procedures

Benjamin Hamar

Chapter Outline

$\mathcal{U}$ltrasound has made dramatic progress since its infancy and has evolved into an indispensable tool in the care of high-risk pregnancies. Advances in genetics and perinatology have increased the information available in the care of the fetus. Advances in aneuploidy risk assessment now allow karyotype analysis earlier in the pregnancy. Outcomes for fetuses with treatable anomalies have been improved through in utero diagnostic and therapeutic techniques. Ultrasound is crucial in the evaluation and delivery of these therapies to the fetus.

AMNIOCENTESIS

Indications and Complications

Amniocentesis was first described in the 1950s and later used to obtain amniocytes for fetal karyotype. Since then, other indications for amniocentesis have included prenatal genetic diagnosis of specific disorders, evaluation for neural tube defects,[1] evaluation for infection,[2] determination of fetal lung indices,[3] determination of degree of fetal anemia,[4] and therapeutic amniocentesis for polyhydramnios.[5]

Amniocentesis has been used for the infusion of a dye such as indigo carmine to evaluate for rupture of membranes.[6] Methylene blue, another dye, has been associated with increased risk for jejunal hypoplasia and hemolytic anemia in exposed fetuses and should not be used.[7-9] Also, amniocentesis with infusion of fluids **(amnioinfusion)** has been used in pregnancies complicated by oligohydramnios to improve visualization or for therapeutic reasons (e.g., before placement of shunts in obstructive uropathy, or intrapartum to prevent fetal heart rate decelerations).[10]

The amniotic fluid contains amniocytes and fetal epithelial cells. The cells obtained through amniocentesis may be tested directly or grown in culture for a variety of biochemical and genetic tests. In general, amniocentesis results are available 10 to 14 days after the procedure. When information is needed sooner, **fluorescence in situ hybridization** (FISH) can be performed for specific analyses (e.g., trisomy 21, 18, or 13).

The rate of **miscarriage** after amniocentesis is reported as approximately 0.5%.[11,12] However, these data were based on earlier studies with less modern techniques. The only randomized controlled trial was performed in the 1980s and showed a relative risk of 2.3 for pregnancy loss after amniocentesis.[13] More recent studies have shown no statistical increase in the rate of miscarriage with second-trimester amniocentesis;[14-16] others have shown a procedure-associated increase in miscarriage of 1 in 769 and 1 in 1667 pregnancies.[17,18] Factors that increase the risk for miscarriage include withdrawal of bloody or discolored fluid and vaginal bleeding in the current pregnancy.[19,20] Transplacental passage of the needle initially seemed to increase the rate of pregnancy loss,[13] but subsequent work has shown no increase in loss rates with this approach.[19,21,22] **Leakage of amniotic fluid** may occur after a genetic amniocentesis, although favorable pregnancy outcomes are seen in more than 90% of these women with expectant management.[23,24] Amniotic fluid culture fails in approximately 0.1% of cases.[12] Outcome studies of infants after amniocentesis show no long-term sequelae.[25]

Amniocentesis for **genetic testing** is generally performed between 15 and 20 weeks' gestational age. Earlier amniocentesis is associated with increased miscarriage rates and birth defects.[26] Amniocentesis has been described in women with a variety of chronic viral infections; however, caution should be exercised in these women because of concerns over vertical transmission.[27-29] Amniocentesis is compared with chorionic villus sampling in Table 46-1.

Amniocentesis for fetal lung maturity is performed in the third trimester if elective delivery before term is being considered.[30] Different biochemical tests (including lecithin/sphingomyelin ratio and phosphatidylglycerol and foam stability index) are available to assess surfactant phospholipids secreted by the fetal lungs into the amniotic fluid to predict the risk for respiratory distress syndrome. However, with corticosteroids to accelerate fetal lung maturity and ultrasound for accurate dating,

amniocentesis for fetal lung maturity is no longer as frequently performed, with its cost-effectiveness questioned.[31] Complications of third-trimester amniocentesis include **infection**, **bleeding**, **rupture of membranes**, and **preterm labor.** Fetal distress is quoted as a risk, but a retrospective study reported no cases of urgent delivery for fetal distress.[32]

Technique

The abdomen is prepared with antiseptic solution (povidone-iodine [Betadine] or chlorhexidine). The transducer is sterilely draped to facilitate real-time imaging of needle trajectory. Most often, a 22-gauge needle is used for genetic amniocentesis, although a larger needle (e.g., 20 gauge) may be used for therapeutic amniocentesis later in gestation (Fig. 46-1; **Video 46-1**). A 3.5-inch-long spinal needle is usually adequate,

TABLE 46-1. COMPARISON OF AMNIOCENTESIS AND CHORIONIC VILLUS SAMPLING (CVS)

	AMNIOCENTESIS	CVS
Indication	Karyotype, genetic testing, biochemical tests, infection, lung maturity, fluid instillation, amnioreduction	Karyotype, genetic testing, biochemical tests
Gestational age	≥15 weeks	10-13 weeks
Miscarriage risk*	0.3%	1%
FISH possible?	Yes	Yes
Time to diagnosis	2 weeks	1 week

*See text for discussion of comparison in risks.

FISH, Fluorescence in situ hybridization.

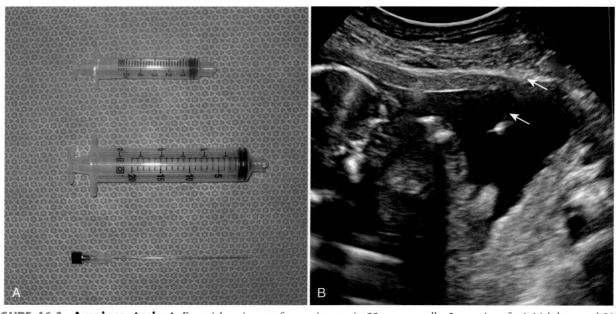

FIGURE 46-1. Amniocentesis. A, Essential equipment for amniocentesis: 22-gauge needle, 5-cc syringe for initial draw, and 20-cc syringe for sample collection. **B,** Transverse ultrasound image of amniocentesis at 17 weeks' gestation. Needle *(arrows)* can be seen entering the amniotic fluid.

although for obese patients and difficult needle trajectories, a 5- or 7-inch needle may be required. If possible, the placenta is avoided. Once in the amniotic fluid cavity, the stylet is removed and a syringe (with or without connector tubing) attached to the needle. Fetal cardiac activity is documented before the patient leaves the ultrasound suite. $Rh_0(D)$ immune globulin (RhoGAM) should be given for Rh-negative mothers after amniocentesis.

Midtrimester **diagnostic amniocentesis** is the most common amniocentesis procedure. A 3-cc or 5-cc syringe is used to withdraw the initial 1 to 2 mL of fluid and is discarded. This minimizes the risk of maternal contamination of the specimen. A new syringe is connected and a sample obtained. For midtrimester **genetic amniocentesis**, 1 mL per gestational week is obtained. Additional fluid may be required for special studies.

When amniocentesis is performed in multiple gestations, care must be taken to sample each fetus separately.[33] If the distinction between two sacs is unclear, blue dye can be injected after sampling fluid from the first sac. Aspiration of fluid from the second sac is then performed from a different site, and fluid without contrast material should be obtained.

Therapeutic amniocentesis involves the removal of a substantial amount of amniotic fluid. This may be performed for polyhydramnios that causes preterm contractions or maternal respiratory compromise.[34] Additionally, it may be used in the management of **twin-twin transfusion syndrome** (TTTS).[35] Amniocentesis is performed as previously described, except a 20-gauge needle is used and connected through extension tubing to a vacuum bottle to withdraw amniotic fluid. Fluid may be withdrawn (1-2 L) to achieve a normal amount of in utero amniotic fluid. Fetal monitoring for bradycardia and distress during the amniocentesis and after the procedure is important because abruption can result from decompression of the uterine cavity.[36] **Serial amnioreduction** has been shown to be equivalent to septostomy in the management of TTTS.[37] **Laser photocoagulation** using fetoscopy has been performed since the 1990s,[38,39] and recent meta-analyses have shown superior outcomes to TTTS managed with amnioreduction or septostomy.[35,40]

Fluid instillation into the amniotic cavity is performed with warm sterile saline. The amniocentesis needle is guided into the intra-amniotic space with ultrasound. Care should be taken to ensure the tip is in the fluid space, and not a loop of cord. This is done with color Doppler ultrasound during the procedure and with aspiration after needle placement.

CHORIONIC VILLUS SAMPLING

Indications and Complications

Chorionic villus sampling (CVS) was first described in the 1960s as a means to obtain genetic diagnosis.[41] The approach was initially transcervical, but transabdominal approaches were described later.[42] The technique initially involved blind aspiration, endoscopic direct-vision biopsy, ultrasound-guided needle aspiration or biopsy forceps, or a combination of ultrasound-guided endoscopy.[43] The indications for testing include fetal karyotype analysis, evaluation for fetal gene status in individuals at risk for certain heritable conditions, and biochemical tests of fetal cells for evaluation of disease status. The CVS procedure is usually performed at 10 to 13 weeks' gestational age. In the era of early aneuploidy risk assessment, the rate of diagnostic testing has stayed the same or decreased somewhat, but the number of women electing first trimester diagnostic testing has increased.[44,45]

The chorion is composed of an outer trophoblast layer containing syncytiotrophoblast and cytotrophoblast, as well as an inner mesenchymal layer. Once the biopsy is obtained, the specimen is carefully washed and maternal decidua microscopically dissected away from the fetal villi. The CVS specimen can then be tested with FISH, direct cytogenetic analysis, or cultured villi for a number of conditions.[46,47]

The U.S. Collaborative study on CVS and other large registries have found that a successful genetic diagnosis can be obtained in 99.7% of cases, with a false-positive rate of only 11 per 10,000 pregnancies.[48,49] There were no diagnostic errors involving trisomy 13, 18, or 21 in these studies.[48] Maternal cell contamination occurs in 0.8% to 2.2% of cases.[48,50] **Confined placental mosaicism** is seen in 0.7% to 1.6% of cases[48-50] and may be caused by meiotic errors with subsequent "trisomy rescue" or by mitotic errors in the developing morula.[51] Trisomy rescue can lead to uniparental disomy, and further studies may be indicated if the mosaicism is found to be confined to the placenta. Confined placental mosaicism also can lead to decreased placental function and adverse perinatal outcomes.[52]

The risk for pregnancy loss with CVS and the miscarriage rate compared with amniocentesis are somewhat controversial. The background rate of pregnancy loss at the time of CVS is approximately 1% greater than at amniocentesis, so direct head-to-head comparisons and retrospective studies may not generate a representative comparison.[53] There is a learning curve, with higher loss rates seen with less experienced practitioners and programs.[54] The largest series have shown fetal loss rates of 1% to 5%.[55-60] Odibo et al.[58] compared women who had CVS to women presenting for care at a similar gestational age and detected no significant difference in fetal loss rates.

A variety of studies have examined the difference in loss rates between CVS and amniocentesis (see Table 46-1). These studies have significant heterogeneity with regard to classification of pregnancy loss (e.g., loss within weeks of procedure, loss before 24 weeks, loss before 28 weeks). The most rigorous studies are prospective studies that recruit women before 10 weeks who are interested in diagnostic testing and randomize them to CVS or amniocentesis. The Canadian Collaborative CVS-Amniocentesis Clinical Trial group recruited women at less than 12 weeks' gestational age and randomized them to CVS in the first trimester or amniocentesis at 15 to 17 weeks' gestational age. No significant differences were seen in fetal loss rates.[61] A U.S. study found no significant difference in loss rate between CVS and amniocentesis.[62] A Danish study that randomized women to transabdominal CVS, transcervical CVS, or amniocentesis found no difference between transabdominal CVS and amniocentesis. There was a significant increase in the miscarriage rate between amniocentesis and transcervical CVS, but this group was less experienced with transcervical CVS.[63] The Medical Research Council's randomized controlled study of amniocentesis versus CVS found a 4.6% increased rate of pregnancy loss in the CVS group. However, this trial used 31 centers, and the significant heterogeneity in experience with CVS may have explained the increased risk for the CVS group.[64] Caughey et al.[59] compared CVS, amniocentesis, and control groups of women at similar gestational ages who declined intervention and found no significant differences in the adjusted loss rates between CVS and amniocentesis in the most recent period.

Studies comparing early amniocentesis to CVS have found similar or higher rates of pregnancy loss and higher rates of clubfoot in the early-amniocentesis group.[55,65-67] Although early reports suggested an increased risk for pregnancy loss with a transabdominal approach, later reports suggest no difference in loss rates between transabdominal and transcervical approaches.[68-72]

Case reports of limb reduction defects (e.g., oromandibular-limb hypogenesis syndrome) have involved women who underwent CVS.[73] These defects are usually seen in 1 in 175,000 births and were seen in 5 of 289 infants born to mothers undergoing CVS at one center.[73] The underlying etiology was thought to be a vascular accident, and a gestational age–related susceptibility was postulated. A large, international population registry showed no increase rate in these defects compared with the general population.[74] A subsequent data analysis found that the risk of limb reduction defects by week was comparable to the general population, except at 8 weeks' gestational age, when it was elevated with CVS.[75] It is generally thought that CVS performed after 10 weeks does not increase the risk for limb reduction defects.

In pregnancies with normal karyotype after CVS, risk for adverse outcomes or malformations is not increased.[76] Women who undergo CVS have no increased risk of other sequelae of uteroplacental insufficiency or hypertension in pregnancy.[77]

The CVS procedure may be performed in twins, and the loss rate is not substantially different from that of twin amniocentesis. However, care must be taken to ensure that both placentas are sampled.[78]

Technique

The CVS procedure can be performed through a transabdominal or transvaginal approach. In general, the placental location dictates the approach: fundal and anterior placentas lead to a transabdominal approach, and posterior and low placentas necessitate a transcervical approach. A full bladder can aid in optimal positioning of the uterus. RhoGAM should be given for Rh-negative mothers following CVS.

Transabdominal Approach

The equipment and guidance are similar to amniocentesis. The abdomen is prepared with antiseptic solution (Betadine or chlorhexidine). The skin is infiltrated with a local anesthetic (e.g., 1% lidocaine). The ultrasound transducer is sterilely draped to facilitate real-time sonographic guidance. An 18- or 20-gauge needle is advanced into the placenta and the stylet removed (Fig. 46-2). A 20-cc syringe with about 2 mL of cell-transport medium is connected to the needle. The needle is guided back and forth through the placenta while suction is intermittently applied to the syringe. Some practitioners use a device to hold the syringe and aid in this pumping action. The needle is withdrawn, and the remainder of the cell-transport medium aliquot is drawn through the needle to clear any villi lodged in the needle. The specimen is examined under a dissecting microscope for adequacy. In general, the cytogenetic examination requires at least 15 mg of villi. Inadequate specimen size may necessitate a repeat pass with a new needle. Fetal cardiac activity is documented before the patient leaves the ultrasound suite.

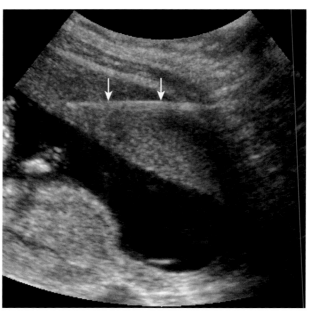

FIGURE 46-2. Transabdominal chorionic villus sampling. Transverse image of needle (arrows) entering the placenta.

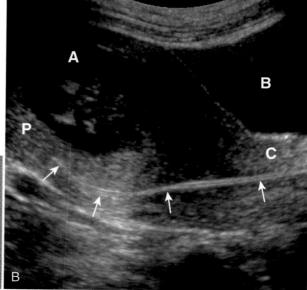

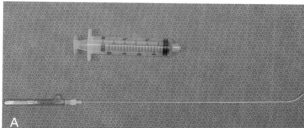

FIGURE 46-3. Transcervical chorionic villus sampling (CVS). A, Equipment for transcervical CVS: Cook Chorion Villus Sampling Set and 20-cc syringe for sample collection. **B,** Sagittal ultrasound image of transcervical CVS shows catheter *(arrows)* passing through cervix *(C)* and into placenta *(P)*. Note full bladder *(B)* and amniotic cavity *(A)*.

Transcervical Approach

A speculum is inserted into the vagina and the cervix cleansed with antiseptic solution (Betadine or chlorhexidine). A 5.7-Fr flexible CVS cannula with a rigid metal introducer is guided into the placenta under ultrasound guidance (Fig. 46-3). A curve may be introduced into the shape of the cannula before introduction, to accommodate the uterine curvature and placental location. In rare cases, a tenaculum may be needed to position the cervix optimally. The introducer is withdrawn and a 20-cc syringe with about 2 mL of cell-transport medium connected to the cannula. Suction is intermittently applied to the cannula as it is slowly withdrawn from the placenta. Once withdrawn from the placenta, continuous suction is applied as the cannula is withdrawn from the uterus and cervix. The remainder of the cell-transport medium aliquot is drawn through the cannula to clear any residual villi. The specimen is examined as for transabdominal CVS, with fetal cardiac activity documented before the patient leaves.

CORDOCENTESIS AND PERCUTANEOUS UMBILICAL BLOOD SAMPLING

Indications and Complications

Cordocentesis and percutaneous umbilical blood sampling (PUBS) were first described in the 1970s and evolved into the ultrasound-guided procedure currently used.[79] **Cordocentesis** has been used for the diagnosis of hemoglobinopathies, evaluation of fetal infection,[80] clarification of mosaicism and other chromosomal abnormalities found by CVS or amniocentesis,[81] and acquisition of fetal DNA for a rapid karyotype.[82] PUBS has been used to evaluate and treat a number of fetal conditions, including thrombocytopenia idiopathic or neonatal alloimmune), anemia, cardiac arrhythmias, and hypothyroidism and hyperthyroidism. The technique has also been used for feticide.[83] **Fetal cardiocentesis** is used for diagnostic and therapeutic purposes as well as for feticide, but the complications are greater than for cordocentesis.[84]

The management of several conditions has evolved over recent decades. In fetuses at risk for **thrombocytopenia**, PUBS was initially used for the diagnosis and treatment of significant fetal thrombocytopenia but was found to substantially increase the fetal loss rate.[85] Also, PUBS did not reduce the risk for fetal intracranial hemorrhage. Consequently, PUBS is seldom used in the management of women at high risk for fetal thrombocytopenia.[86-88] The management of **red cell alloimmunization** has evolved from serial amniocentesis to identify fetuses at high risk for moderate to severe anemia,[4] to using middle cerebral artery (MCA) Doppler ultrasound evaluation to determine the need for PUBS. This allows for fewer PUBS procedures, with those performed typically timed to the need for in utero transfusions.[89,90] MCA Doppler ultrasound can help time a second fetal transfusion procedure,[91] but subsequent transfusions are better predicted by estimating the decrease in fetal hematocrit over time[92] (see Chapter 43).

Cordocentesis has a 1% to 1.6% risk of fetal loss.[93-97] The fetal risks need to be interpreted knowing that these fetuses are at particularly high background risk for fetal loss and adverse outcomes. Ghidini, et al.[97] performed a meta-analysis that excluded cases with pathologic fetal conditions and determined that the loss rate in a "low risk" population undergoing fetal blood sampling was approximately 1.4%. A more recent study found that procedure-related complications of 3.1% and procedure-related loss rates of 1.6%.[93] Other complications of cordocentesis include fetal bradycardia (4%-12%), bleeding at puncture site (20%-40%), hematomas (17%), infection (1%), abruption (rare), fetomaternal hemorrhage (40%), and preterm contractions (7%).[93,95,97,98] Complications are more common with arterial than venous puncture.[96]

Technique

Cordocentesis or PUBS is usually performed in a setting that allows maternal sedation and intervention for fetal distress after 24 weeks, most often an operating room for labor and delivery. The patient is prepped and sterilely draped and the uterus displaced slightly to the left with appropriate maternal wedging. The ultrasound transducer is draped with a sterile sheath to allow guidance on the sterile field. The patient is often given conscious sedation for comfort and to minimize maternal movement during the procedure. Local anesthetic with lidocaine may be used for patient comfort. Ultrasound guidance may be provided by a second provider or by the operator using a freehand technique. A 20- to 22-gauge needle is typically used, and most often the umbilical vein is targeted at the **placental cord insertion** (Fig. 46-4). Other approaches include the **umbilical vein at the fetal cord insertion**, the **intrahepatic vein** (Fig. 46-5), or a **free loop of cord.** The needle position is confirmed by obtaining a blood specimen, ultrasound observation of the needle in the vein, and sonographic streaming within the umbilical vein after injection of saline. Heparinized syringes are used for fetal blood sampling, and values for hemoglobin/hematocrit, platelets, and mean corpuscular volume (MCV) are obtained. The fetal MCV is higher than the maternal value and can help confirm fetal origin of the blood sample.

Depending on the insertion site and indication for cordocentesis, fetal paralysis can be considered with vecuronium (0.1 mg/kg estimated fetal weight)[99] or atracurium besylate (0.4 mg/kg estimated fetal weight).[100] Fetal cardiac activity is documented throughout the procedure.

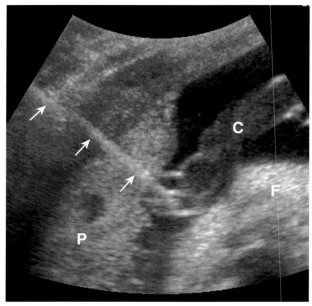

FIGURE 46-4. Cordocentesis. Transverse ultrasound image shows needle *(arrows)* traversing placenta *(P)* and entering placental cord insertion. Note loop of umbilical cord *(C)* and fetus *(F)*.

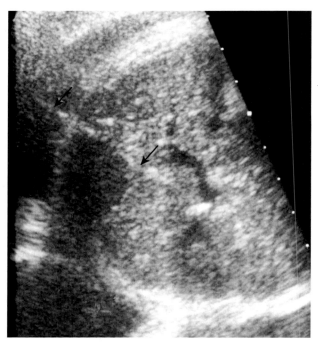

FIGURE 46-5. Fetal blood sampling in intrahepatic portion of umbilical vein. Arrows point to the position of the 20-gauge needle in the intrahepatic portion of the umbilical vein.

$$\text{Volume}_{\text{transfused}}(\text{mL}) = \text{Volume}_{\text{fetoplacental unit}}(\text{mL}) \times \left[\frac{\text{Hematocrit}_{\text{final}} - \text{Hematocrit}_{\text{initial}}}{\text{Hematocrit}_{\text{transfused blood}}} \right]$$

Fetal Transfusion

If fetal transfusion is required, a T-connector tubing is often employed for ease of transfusion. The volume to be transfused can be calculated by using the above formula[101]:

The fetoplacental volume can be estimated as $1.046 + $ fetal weight in grams $\times 0.14$.[101] Either maternal cells or donated O-negative, washed, leukocyte-reduced blood is used for transfusion. Maternal cells may be consumed less rapidly than anonymous donation, but timing and pregnancy-associated anemia limit its use.[102] A posttransfusion sample is obtained to evaluate the effects of the procedure. Future transfusions are scheduled based on fetal Doppler assessment,[91] or by estimating a 0.7% decrease in the hematocrit per day and scheduling transfusion for estimated hematocrits of 20 to 22 mL/dL.[103]

If the cordocentesis or transfusion is being performed for reasons other than Rh(D) isoimmunization, in a Rh(D)-negative mother, RhoGAM should be administered after the procedure.

FETAL REDUCTION

Indications and Complications

As assisted reproductive technologies increase in availability and use, the rate of higher-order multiple gestations has increased dramatically. Risks for adverse perinatal outcomes and prematurity increase with increasing number of gestations.[104] Even with the efforts of the reproductive endocrinology community to limit the numbers of higher-order multiples, a substantial number of these pregnancies still occur.[105] Since initially described,[106] fetal reduction has become more widely available and used in the management of higher-order multiple gestations and can improve the associated risks.[107]

The decision to pursue a fetal reduction raises difficult ethical and medical questions for couples. The decision is made to improve fetal outcomes, achieve a desired number of gestations in the pregnancy, and for other considerations. In most cases, triplets or higher-order multiples are reduced to a twin pregnancy. However, reductions resulting in a singleton as the target have been used with maternal medical conditions or by patient preference.[108,109]

Compared to spontaneous twin pregnancies, higher-order pregnancies reduced to twins do not appear to be substantially different in regard to pregnancy loss, birth before 34 weeks, stillbirth, or neonatal death.[110] Conversely, pregnancies continued as a triplet pregnancy had higher rates of miscarriage, delivery before 36 weeks, very low birth weight (<1500 g), and neonatal death compared to pregnancies reduced to twins.[110]

Fetal loss rate with fetal reduction depends on the starting and finishing number. Recent data suggest that pregnancies with three or more fetuses that end with twins have a 5.3% loss rate, compared to a 3.8% loss rate in pregnancies reduced to a singleton. Reduction to a singleton had significant improvements in the gestational age at delivery.[111]

Other complications of fetal reduction include infection, bleeding, and discomfort at the injection site. If potassium chloride is used and injected into the maternal circulation, maternal cardiac arrhythmias are possible.

Technique

Selection of the fetus(es) for reduction takes into account avoidance of the presenting fetus (if possible) and selecting the fetus(es) with lagging growth, evidence of increased nuchal translucency, or other evidence of abnormality. CVS is possible before reduction and does not appear to affect the risk for complications with the reduction.[112] If multiple fetuses are reduced in higher-order multiples, usually no more than two fetal reductions per session are performed. The procedure is usually performed between 10 and 12 weeks' gestational age. If there are fetuses with a monochorionic component, these fetuses are either reduced together or left alone.

The maternal abdomen is prepped and sterilely draped. The ultrasound transducer is draped with a sterile sheath. A local anesthetic is sometimes administered. Under ultrasound guidance, a 20- or 22-gauge needle is advanced into the fetal thorax. Confirmation of the needle tip in the fetus is essential. A small volume (1-2 mL) of a 2 mEq/mL solution of potassium chloride is injected. Cessation of fetal cardiac motion is often immediate but may take several minutes if the injection is not intracardiac, and patience can avoid the need for additional injection. Once fetal cardiac motion has stopped, the fetus is monitored with ultrasound for 1 minute to ensure cardiac cessation. The stylet is replaced and the needle withdrawn. Cardiac activity in the surviving fetus(es) is documented before the patient leaves the ultrasound suite. RhoGAM should be given for Rh-negative mothers following any invasive diagnostic or therapeutic fetal test.

OTHER PROCEDURES

Ultrasound has been used to guide various procedures for diagnostic and therapeutic purposes. Pleural effusions and macrocystic fetal chest masses such as congenital cystic adenoid malformations have been treated with serial **in utero thoracentesis**[113] (Fig. 46-6) and **thoracoamniotic shunt** for continuous drainage of fluid to permit lung development.[114,115]

In fetuses with obstructive uropathy, ultrasound-guided aspiration of the bladder has been used in the

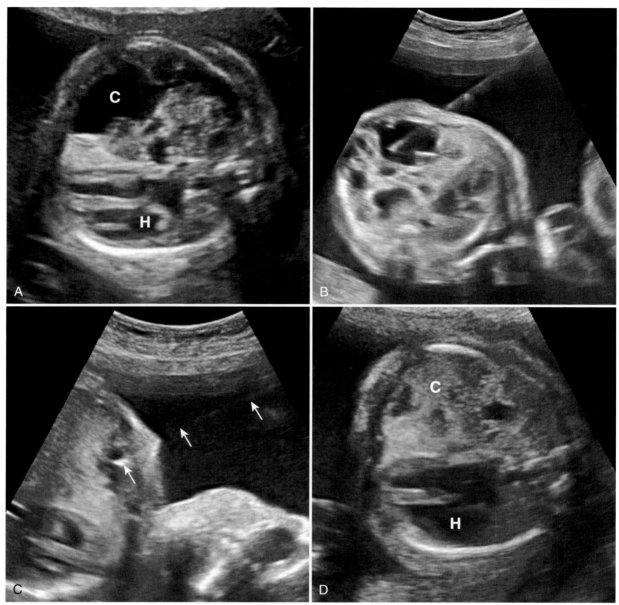

FIGURE 46-6. Drainage of macrocystic congenital cystic adenoid malformation (CCAM) at 22 weeks. **A,** Transverse image of right-sided macrocystic CCAM *(C)*, causing hydrops. The heart *(H)* is displaced to the far left, and the CCAM occupies much of the thoracic cavity. **B,** Transverse image during aspiration of the CCAM. Note the needle in the largest cystic component. **C,** Toward the end of the procedure, the needle *(arrows)* is in the residual fluid pocket. **D,** Transverse ultrasound image after aspiration. CCAM *(C)* has been somewhat decompressed, and the heart *(H)* is less compressed, although still displaced.

diagnosis and evaluation of fetal renal function.[116] Sequential evaluation of the fetal bladder aspirate has been shown to improve evaluation of fetal renal function, and threshold values for sodium, chloride, protein, calcium, osmolality, and beta-2-microglobulin have been established.[117] In fetuses deemed to have a good prognosis for preserved renal function, **vesicoamniotic shunts** are placed for drainage of the fetal bladder[118] (Fig. 46-7). The evaluation of fetuses for potential shunt placement is detailed in Chapter 39.

In fetuses with ascites, ultrasound-guided drainage has been used for diagnostic purposes[119] (Fig. 46-8). Ultrasound has guided in utero biopsies of the skin,[120] liver,[121]

and muscle[122] for diagnostic purposes. **Cephalocentesis** for the management of hydrocephalus was associated with higher rates of procedure-related fetal death and adverse outcomes in survivors.[123] More recently, cephalocentesis has been used to assist in the delivery of a nonviable fetus with hydrocephalus to permit vaginal delivery.[124]

Drainage Technique

The technique for ultrasound-guided drainage is similar to that of amniocentesis. Instead of accessing the amniotic cavity, however, the fluid cavity of interest is

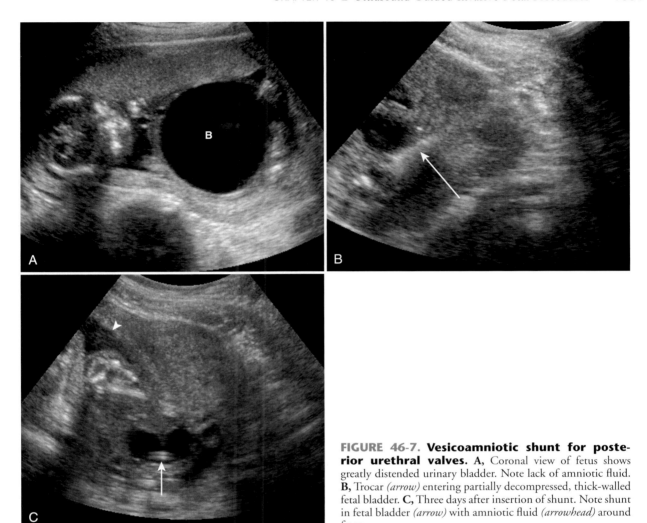

FIGURE 46-7. Vesicoamniotic shunt for posterior urethral valves. A, Coronal view of fetus shows greatly distended urinary bladder. Note lack of amniotic fluid. **B,** Trocar *(arrow)* entering partially decompressed, thick-walled fetal bladder. **C,** Three days after insertion of shunt. Note shunt in fetal bladder *(arrow)* with amniotic fluid *(arrowhead)* around fetus.

targeted. Depending on the tissue and gestational age, a 20-gauge needle is usually required. A longer spinal needle (5 or 7 inch) is often helpful because of the distances required for the trajectories to access the fetal structures.

Shunt Placement

A variety of catheter sets are available for in utero shunts. Our group uses the Rocket KCH Bladder Drain catheter (Rocket Medical, Hingham, Mass). The introducer has a central channel for passage of the shunt and a side channel for diagnostic and therapeutic purposes. The procedure is usually done in an operating room to allow for adequate maternal analgesia; some level of conscious sedation and local anesthesia is usually adequate. A stab incision on the skin with an 11 blade is made to facilitate the passage of the trocar. Under ultrasound guidance, the trocar is advanced into the cavity, such as the pleural space (large pleural effusion) or bladder (obstructive uropathy). In the case of fetal obstructive uropathy with bladder drainage (see Fig. 46-7), care should be taken to

avoid the umbilical vessels. Fluid may be instilled in the amniotic cavity through the introducer's side channel or with a separate amniocentesis to aid in visualization. Placing a separate amniocentesis needle allows continued infusion of fluid during the procedure.

Once the introducer is in the fetal cavity, the trocar is removed, the shunt is passed down the central channel, and the first "pigtail" is fed into the fetal cavity. The introducer tip is then withdrawn into the amniotic cavity and the remaining shunt deployed. The two "pigtails" keep the shunt in place, and the metallic markers on each end help confirm shunt placement. The shunt is compatible with magnetic resonance imaging (MRI). Follow-up is important because the shunts can migrate over time and become displaced.

Fetal Surgery

Ultrasound has been used as an adjunct to fetoscopy during fetal surgery and other fetoscopic techniques.[125] Ultrasound has been used in the surgical planning and postprocedure evaluation for **laser photocoagulation** in

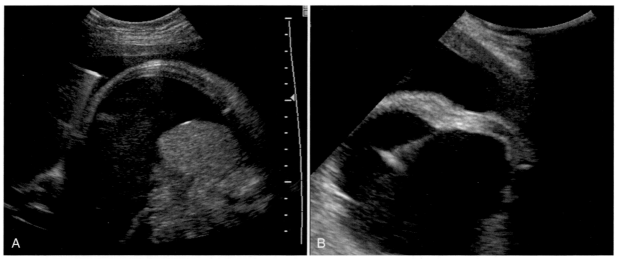

FIGURE 46-8. Drainage of fetal ascites. A, Note massive ascites and polyhydramnios. Needle is in amniotic fluid cavity for initial amniocentesis. **B,** Needle is in peritoneal cavity for paracentesis.

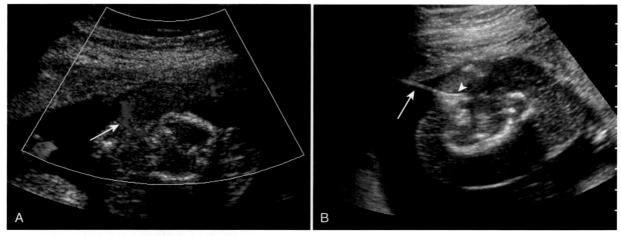

FIGURE 46-9. Thermal ablation of acardiac twin. A, Color Doppler sonogram demonstrates the edematous acardiac twin, with a short umbilical cord and a single umbilical artery entering the torso of the acardiac twin. **B,** The electrode (*arrow* in amniotic fluid and *arrowhead* in body of acardiac twin) is seen in the region of the umbilical artery in the acardiac twin during thermal ablation procedure.

monochorionic twins with TTTS[126] or in acardiac twins (Fig. 46-9).

CONCLUSION

Ultrasound-guided in utero procedures have evolved from their experimental infancy into an indispensable diagnostic and therapeutic tool in the evaluation and management of the fetus. Combined with advances in genetics and medicine, many new approaches and procedures are now available for fetal diagnosis and therapy. As with any procedure, the risks and benefits and the impact on the care of the pregnancy must be taken into account when considering whether or when to perform

these procedures. Performance of complex fetal diagnostic and therapeutic procedures should be reserved for centers with expertise in their use.

References

Amniocentesis

1. Wald N, Cuckle H, Nanchahal K. Amniotic fluid acetylcholinesterase measurement in the prenatal diagnosis of open neural tube defects. Second Report of the Collaborative Acetylcholinesterase Study. Prenat Diagn 1989;9:813-829.
2. Buhimschi CS, Bhandari V, Hamar BD, et al. Proteomic profiling of the amniotic fluid to detect inflammation, infection, and neonatal sepsis. PLoS Med 2007;4:e18.
3. Gluck L, Kulovich MV, Borer Jr RC. Estimates of fetal lung maturity. Clin Perinatol 1974;1:125-139.
4. Liley AW. Liquor amnil analysis in the management of the pregnancy complicated by resus sensitization. Am J Obstet Gynecol 1961;82:1359-1370.

5. Jauniaux E, Holmes A, Hyett J, et al. Rapid and radical amniodrain-age in the treatment of severe twin-twin transfusion syndrome. Prenat Diagn 2001;21:471-476.
6. Fujimoto S, Kishida T, Sagawa T, et al. Clinical usefulness of the dye-injection method for diagnosing premature rupture of the mem-branes in equivocal cases. J Obstet Gynaecol 1995;21:215-220.
7. Cragan JD. Teratogen update: methylene blue. Teratology 1999; 60:42-48.
8. Nicolini U, Monni G. Intestinal obstruction in babies exposed in utero to methylene blue. Lancet 1990;336:1258-1259.
9. Van der Pol JG, Wolf H, Boer K, et al. Jejunal atresia related to the use of methylene blue in genetic amniocentesis in twins. Br J Obstet Gynaecol 1992;99:141-143.
10. Gramellini D, Fieni S, Kaihura C, et al. Antepartum amnioinfusion: a review. J Matern Fetal Neonatal Med 2003;14:291-296.
11. Centers for Disease Control and Prevention. Chorionic villus sam-pling and amniocentesis: recommendations for prenatal counseling. MMWR Recomm Rep 1995;44:1-12.
12. Invasive prenatal testing for aneuploidy. ACOG Pract Bull No 88. Obstet Gynecol 2007;110:1459-1467.
13. Tabor A, Philip J, Madsen M, et al. Randomised controlled trial of genetic amniocentesis in 4606 low-risk women. Lancet 1986;1: 1287-1293.
14. Towner D, Currier RJ, Lorey FW, et al. Miscarriage risk from amniocentesis performed for abnormal maternal serum screening. Am J Obstet Gynecol 2007;196:608 e1-e5; discussion e5.
15. Mazza V, Pati M, Bertucci E, et al. Age-specific risk of fetal loss post second trimester amniocentesis: analysis of 5043 cases. Prenat Diagn 2007;27:180-183.
16. Tongsong T, Wanapirak C, Sirivatanapa P, et al. Amniocentesis-related fetal loss: a cohort study. Obstet Gynecol 1998;92:64-67.
17. Odibo AO, Gray DL, Dicke JM, et al. Revisiting the fetal loss rate after second-trimester genetic amniocentesis: a single center's 16-year experience. Obstet Gynecol 2008;111:589-595.
18. Eddleman KA, Malone FD, Sullivan L, et al. Pregnancy loss rates after midtrimester amniocentesis. Obstet Gynecol 2006;108:1067-1072.
19. Kong CW, Leung TN, Leung TY, et al. Risk factors for procedure-related fetal losses after mid-trimester genetic amniocentesis. Prenat Diagn 2006;26:925-930.
20. Antsaklis A, Papantoniou N, Xygakis A, et al. Genetic amniocentesis in women 20-34 years old: associated risks. Prenat Diagn 2000;20: 247-250.
21. Giorlandino C, Mobili L, Bilancioni E, et al. Transplacental amnio-centesis: is it really a higher-risk procedure? Prenat Diagn 1994;14: 803-806.
22. Bombard AT, Powers JF, Carter S, et al. Procedure-related fetal losses in transplacental versus nontransplacental genetic amniocen-tesis. Am J Obstet Gynecol 1995;172:868-872.
23. Borgida AF, Mills AA, Feldman DM, et al. Outcome of pregnancies complicated by ruptured membranes after genetic amniocentesis. Am J Obstet Gynecol 2000;183:937-939.
24. Devlieger R, Millar LK, Bryant-Greenwood G, et al. Fetal mem-brane healing after spontaneous and iatrogenic membrane rupture: a review of current evidence. Am J Obstet Gynecol 2006;195: 1512-1520.
25. Baird PA, Yee IM, Sadovnick AD. Population-based study of long-term outcomes after amniocentesis. Lancet 1994;344:1134-1136.
26. Randomised trial to assess safety and fetal outcome of early and midtrimester amniocentesis. The Canadian Early and Mid-trimester Amniocentesis Trial (CEMAT) Group. Lancet 1998;351:242-247.
27. Alexander JM, Ramus R, Jackson G, et al. Risk of hepatitis B trans-mission after amniocentesis in chronic hepatitis B carriers. Infect Dis Obstet Gynecol 1999;7:283-286.
28. Davies G, Wilson RD, Desilets V, et al. Amniocentesis and women with hepatitis B, hepatitis C, or human immunodeficiency virus. J Obstet Gynaecol Can 2003;25:145-152.
29. Somigliana E, Bucceri AM, Tibaldi C, et al. Early invasive diagnostic techniques in pregnant women who are infected with the HIV: a multicenter case series. Am J Obstet Gynecol 2005;193:437-442.
30. Assessment of fetal lung maturity. ACOG Educ Bull No 230. Int J Gynaecol Obstet 1997;56:191-198.
31. Luo G, Norwitz ER. Revisiting amniocentesis for fetal lung maturity after 36 weeks' gestation. Rev Obstet Gynecol 2008;1:61-68.
32. Gordon MC, Narula K, O'Shaughnessy R, Barth Jr WH. Complica-tions of third-trimester amniocentesis using continuous ultrasound guidance. Obstet Gynecol 2002;99:255-259.
33. Weisz B, Rodeck CH. Invasive diagnostic procedures in twin preg-nancies. Prenat Diagn 2005;25:751-758.
34. Moise Jr KJ. Polyhydramnios. Clin Obstet Gynecol 1997;40:266-279.
35. Roberts D, Gates S, Kilby M, Neilson JP. Interventions for twin-twin transfusion syndrome: a Cochrane review. Ultrasound Obstet Gynecol 2008;31:701-711.
36. Leung WC, Jouannic JM, Hyett J, et al. Procedure-related complica-tions of rapid amniodrainage in the treatment of polyhydramnios. Ultrasound Obstet Gynecol 2004;23:154-158.
37. Moise Jr KJ, Dorman K, Lamvu G, et al. A randomized trial of amnioreduction versus septostomy in the treatment of twin-twin transfusion syndrome. Am J Obstet Gynecol 2005;193:701-707.
38. De Lia JE, Cruikshank DP, Keye Jr WR. Fetoscopic neodymium:YAG laser occlusion of placental vessels in severe twin-twin transfusion syndrome. Obstet Gynecol 1990;75:1046-1053.
39. De Lia JE, Kuhlmann RS, Harstad TW, Cruikshank DP. Fetoscopic laser ablation of placental vessels in severe previable twin-twin trans-fusion syndrome. Am J Obstet Gynecol 1995;172:1202-1208; dis-cussion 1208-1211.
40. Rossi AC, D'Addario V. Laser therapy and serial amnioreduction as treatment for twin-twin transfusion syndrome: a metaanalysis and review of literature. Am J Obstet Gynecol 2008;198:147-152.

Chorionic Villus Sampling
41. Hahneman N, Mohr J. Genetic diagnosis in the embryo by means of biopsy from extra-embryonic membrane. Bull Eur Soc Hum Genet 1968;2:23-29.
42. Smidt-Jensen S, Hahnemann N. Transabdominal fine needle biopsy from chorionic villi in the first trimester. Prenat Diagn 1984;4: 163-169.
43. Rodeck CH, Morsman JM. First-trimester chorion biopsy. Br Med Bull 1983;39:338-342.
44. Norton ME, Hopkins LM, Pena S, et al. First-trimester combined screening: experience with an instant results approach. Am J Obstet Gynecol 2007;196:606 e1-e5; discussion e5.
45. Chasen ST, McCullough LB, Chervenak FA. Is nuchal translucency screening associated with different rates of invasive testing in an older obstetric population? Am J Obstet Gynecol 2004;190:769-774.
46. Van den Berg C, Van Opstal D, Brandenburg H, et al. Accuracy of abnormal karyotypes after the analysis of both short- and long-term culture of chorionic villi. Prenat Diagn 2000;20:956-969.
47. Aina-Mumuney A, Wood ED, Corson VL, et al. Clinical conse-quences of an increasing trend of preferential use of cultured villi for molecular diagnosis by CVS. Prenat Diagn 2008;28:332-334.
48. Ledbetter DH, Zachary JM, Simpson JL, et al. Cytogenetic results from the U.S. Collaborative Study on CVS. Prenat Diagn 1992; 12:317-345.
49. Hahnemann JM, Vejerslev LO. Accuracy of cytogenetic findings on chorionic villus sampling (CVS): diagnostic consequences of CVS mosaicism and non-mosaic discrepancy in centres contributing to EUCROMIC 1986–1992. Prenat Diagn 1997;17:801-820.
50. Brun JL, Mangione R, Gangbo F, et al. Feasibility, accuracy and safety of chorionic villus sampling: a report of 10,741 cases. Prenat Diagn 2003;23:295-301.
51. Wolstenholme J. Confined placental mosaicism for trisomies 2, 3, 7, 8, 9, 16, and 22: their incidence, likely origins, and mechanisms for cell lineage compartmentalization. Prenat Diagn 1996;16:511-524.
52. Stetten G, Escallon CS, South ST, et al. Reevaluating confined placental mosaicism. Am J Med Genet A 2004;131:232-239.
53. Wapner RJ. Invasive prenatal diagnostic techniques. Semin Perinatol 2005;29:401-404.
54. World Health Organization Special Report: Risk evaluation in cho-rionic villus sampling. Prenat Diagn 1986;6:451-456.
55. Philip J, Silver RK, Wilson RD, et al. Late first-trimester invasive prenatal diagnosis: results of an international randomized trial. Obstet Gynecol 2004;103:1164-1173.
56. Williams 3rd J, Wang BB, Rubin CH, et al. Chorionic villus sam-pling: experience with 3016 cases performed by a single operator. Obstet Gynecol 1992;80:1023-1029.

57. Brambati B, Tului L, Cislaghi C, Alberti E. First 10,000 chorionic villus samplings performed on singleton pregnancies by a single operator. Prenat Diagn 1998;18:255-266.

58. Odibo AO, Dicke JM, Gray DL, et al. Evaluating the rate and risk factors for fetal loss after chorionic villus sampling. Obstet Gynecol 2008;112:813-819.

59. Caughey AB, Hopkins LM, Norton ME. Chorionic villus sampling compared with amniocentesis and the difference in the rate of pregnancy loss. Obstet Gynecol 2006;108:612-616.

60. Papp C, Beke A, Mezei G, et al. Chorionic villus sampling: a 15-year experience. Fetal Diagn Ther 2002;17:218-227.

61. Lippman A, Tomkins DJ, Shime J, Hamerton JL. Canadian multicentre randomized clinical trial of chorion villus sampling and amniocentesis. Final report. Prenat Diagn 1992;12:385-408.

62. Rhoads GG, Jackson LG, Schlesselman SE, et al. The safety and efficacy of chorionic villus sampling for early prenatal diagnosis of cytogenetic abnormalities. N Engl J Med 1989;320:609-617.

63. Smidt-Jensen S, Permin M, Philip J, et al. Randomised comparison of amniocentesis and transabdominal and transcervical chorionic villus sampling. Lancet 1992;340:1237-1244.

64. Medical Research Council European Trial of Chorion Villus Sampling. MRC Working Party on the Evaluation of Chorion Villus Sampling. Lancet 1991;337:1491-1499.

65. Cederholm M, Axelsson O. A prospective comparative study on transabdominal chorionic villus sampling and amniocentesis performed at 10-13 weeks' gestation. Prenat Diagn 1997;17:311-317.

66. Sundberg K, Bang J, Smidt-Jensen S, et al. Randomised study of risk of fetal loss related to early amniocentesis versus chorionic villus sampling. Lancet 1997;350:697-703.

67. Nicolaides K, Brizot Mde L, Patel F, Snijders R. Comparison of chorionic villus sampling and amniocentesis for fetal karyotyping at 10-13 weeks' gestation. Lancet 1994;344:435-439.

68. Jackson LG, Zachary JM, Fowler SE, et al. A randomized comparison of transcervical and transabdominal chorionic-villus sampling. The U.S. National Institute of Child Health and Human Development Chorionic-Villus Sampling and Amniocentesis Study Group. N Engl J Med 1992;327:594-598.

69. Silver RK, MacGregor SN, Muhlbach LH, et al. A comparison of pregnancy loss between transcervical and transabdominal chorionic villus sampling. Obstet Gynecol 1994;83:657-660.

70. Chueh JT, Goldberg JD, Wohlferd MM, Golbus MS. Comparison of transcervical and transabdominal chorionic villus sampling loss rates in nine thousand cases from a single center. Am J Obstet Gynecol 1995;173:1277-1282.

71. Brambati B, Terzian E, Tognoni G. Randomized clinical trial of transabdominal versus transcervical chorionic villus sampling methods. Prenat Diagn 1991;11:285-293.

72. Bovicelli L, Rizzo N, Montacuti V, Morandi R. Transabdominal versus transcervical routes for chorionic villus sampling. Lancet 1986;2:290.

73. Firth HV, Boyd PA, Chamberlain P, et al. Severe limb abnormalities after chorion villus sampling at 56-66 days' gestation. Lancet 1991;337:762-763.

74. Froster UG, Jackson L. Limb defects and chorionic villus sampling: results from an international registry, 1992-94. Lancet 1996;347:489-494.

75. Evaluation of chorionic villus sampling safety: WHO/PAHO consultation on CVS. Prenat Diagn 1999;19:97-99.

76. Schaap AH, van der Pol HG, Boer K, et al. Long-term follow-up of infants after transcervical chorionic villus sampling and after amniocentesis to compare congenital abnormalities and health status. Prenat Diagn 2002;22:598-604.

77. Adusumalli J, Han CS, Beckham S, et al. Chorionic villus sampling and risk for hypertensive disorders of pregnancy. Am J Obstet Gynecol 2007;196:591 e1-e7; discussion e7.

78. Wapner RJ, Johnson A, Davis G, et al. Prenatal diagnosis in twin gestations: a comparison between second-trimester amniocentesis and first-trimester chorionic villus sampling. Obstet Gynecol 1993; 82:49-56.

Cordocentesis and Percutaneous Umbilical Blood Sampling

79. Daffos F, Capella-Pavlovsky M, Forestier F. A new procedure for fetal blood sampling in utero: preliminary results of fifty-three cases. Am J Obstet Gynecol 1983;146:985-987.

80. Schild RL, Bald R, Plath H, et al. Intrauterine management of fetal parvovirus B19 infection. Ultrasound Obstet Gynecol 1999;13:161-166.

81. Shalev E, Zalel Y, Weiner E, et al. The role of cordocentesis in assessment of mosaicism found in amniotic fluid cell culture. Acta Obstet Gynecol Scand 1994;73:119-122.

82. Tharapel SA, Dev VG, Shulman LP, Tharapel AT. Prenatal karyotyping using fetal blood obtained by cordocentesis: rapid and accurate results within 24 hours. Ann Genet 1998;41:69-72.

83. Bhide A, Sairam S, Hollis B, Thilaganathan B. Comparison of feticide carried out by cordocentesis versus cardiac puncture. Ultrasound Obstet Gynecol 2002;20:230-232.

84. Sarno Jr AP, Wilson RD. Fetal cardiocentesis: a review of indications, risks, applications and technique. Fetal Diagn Ther 2008;23:237-244.

85. Paidas MJ, Berkowitz RL, Lynch L, et al. Alloimmune thrombocytopenia: fetal and neonatal losses related to cordocentesis. Am J Obstet Gynecol 1995;172:475-479.

86. Peleg D, Hunter SK. Perinatal management of women with immune thrombocytopenic purpura: survey of United States perinatologists. Am J Obstet Gynecol 1999;180:645-649.

87. Silver RM, Porter TF, Branch DW, et al. Neonatal alloimmune thrombocytopenia: antenatal management. Am J Obstet Gynecol 2000;182:1233-1238.

88. Payne SD, Resnik R, Moore TR, et al. Maternal characteristics and risk of severe neonatal thrombocytopenia and intracranial hemorrhage in pregnancies complicated by autoimmune thrombocytopenia. Am J Obstet Gynecol 1997;177:149-155.

89. Mari G, Deter RL, Carpenter RL, et al. Noninvasive diagnosis by Doppler ultrasonography of fetal anemia due to maternal red-cell alloimmunization. Collaborative Group for Doppler Assessment of the Blood Velocity in Anemic Fetuses. N Engl J Med 2000;342:9-14.

90. Mari G, Adrignolo A, Abuhamad AZ, et al. Diagnosis of fetal anemia with Doppler ultrasound in the pregnancy complicated by maternal blood group immunization. Ultrasound Obstet Gynecol 1995;5:400-405.

91. Detti L, Oz U, Guney I, et al. Doppler ultrasound velocimetry for timing the second intrauterine transfusion in fetuses with anemia from red cell alloimmunization. Am J Obstet Gynecol 2001;185:1048-1051.

92. Scheier M, Hernandez-Andrade E, Fonseca EB, Nicolaides KH. Prediction of severe fetal anemia in red blood cell alloimmunization after previous intrauterine transfusions. Am J Obstet Gynecol 2006;195:1550-1556.

93. Van Kamp IL, Klumper FJ, Oepkes D, et al. Complications of intrauterine intravascular transfusion for fetal anemia due to maternal red-cell alloimmunization. Am J Obstet Gynecol 2005;192:171-177.

94. Tongsong T, Wanapirak C, Kunavikatikul C, et al. Fetal loss rate associated with cordocentesis at midgestation. Am J Obstet Gynecol 2001;184:719-723.

95. Tongsong T, Wanapirak C, Kunavikatikul C, et al. Cordocentesis at 16-24 weeks of gestation: experience of 1,320 cases. Prenat Diagn 2000;20:224-228.

96. Weiner CP, Okamura K. Diagnostic fetal blood sampling-technique related losses. Fetal Diagn Ther 1996;11:169-175.

97. Ghidini A, Sepulveda W, Lockwood CJ, Romero R. Complications of fetal blood sampling. Am J Obstet Gynecol 1993;168:1339-1344.

98. Liao C, Wei J, Li Q, et al. Efficacy and safety of cordocentesis for prenatal diagnosis. Int J Gynaecol Obstet 2006;93:13-17.

99. Daffos F, Forestier F, Mac Aleese J, et al. Fetal curarization for prenatal magnetic resonance imaging. Prenat Diagn 1988;8:312-314.

100. Bernstein HH, Chitkara U, Plosker H, et al. Use of atracurium besylate to arrest fetal activity during intrauterine intravascular transfusions. Obstet Gynecol 1988;72:813-816.

101. Mandelbrot L, Daffos F, Forestier F, et al. Assessment of fetal blood volume for computer-assisted management of in utero transfusion. Fetal Ther 1988;3:60-66.

102. El-Azeem SA, Samuels P, Rose RL, et al. The effect of the source of transfused blood on the rate of consumption of transfused red blood cells in pregnancies affected by red blood cell alloimmunization. Am J Obstet Gynecol 1997;177:753-757.

103. Mari G, Zimmermann R, Moise Jr KJ, Deter RL. Correlation between middle cerebral artery peak systolic velocity and fetal hemoglobin after 2 previous intrauterine transfusions. Am J Obstet Gynecol 2005;193:1117-1120.

Fetal Reduction

104. Elliott JP. High-order multiple gestations. Semin Perinatol 2005; 29:305-311.
105. El-Toukhy T, Khalaf Y, Braude P. IVF results: optimize not maximize. Am J Obstet Gynecol 2006;194:322-331.
106. Berkowitz RL, Lynch L, Chitkara U, et al. Selective reduction of multifetal pregnancies in the first trimester. N Engl J Med 1988; 318:1043-1047.
107. Evans MI, Britt DW. Fetal reduction. Semin Perinatol 2005;29: 321-329.
108. Evans MI, Kaufman MI, Urban AJ, et al. Fetal reduction from twins to a singleton: a reasonable consideration? Obstet Gynecol 2004;104: 102-109.
109. Stone J, Belogolovkin V, Matho A, et al. Evolving trends in 2000 cases of multifetal pregnancy reduction: a single-center experience. Am J Obstet Gynecol 2007;197:394 e1-e4.
110. Dodd J, Crowther C. Multifetal pregnancy reduction of triplet and higher-order multiple pregnancies to twins. Fertil Steril 2004;81: 1420-1422.
111. Stone J, Ferrara L, Kamrath J, et al. Contemporary outcomes with the latest 1000 cases of multifetal pregnancy reduction (MPR). Am J Obstet Gynecol 2008;199:406 e1-e4.
112. Ferrara L, Gandhi M, Litton C, et al. Chorionic villus sampling and the risk of adverse outcome in patients undergoing multifetal pregnancy reduction. Am J Obstet Gynecol 2008;199:408 e1-e4.

Other Procedures

113. Obwegeser R, Deutinger J, Bernaschek G. Fetal pulmonary cyst treated by repeated thoracocentesis. Am J Obstet Gynecol 1993;169: 1622-1624.
114. Picone O, Benachi A, Mandelbrot L, et al. Thoracoamniotic shunting for fetal pleural effusions with hydrops. Am J Obstet Gynecol 2004;191:2047-2050.
115. Wilson RD, Baxter JK, Johnson MP, et al. Thoracoamniotic shunts: fetal treatment of pleural effusions and congenital cystic adenomatoid malformations. Fetal Diagn Ther 2004;19:413-420.
116. Nicolini U, Fisk NM, Rodeck CH, Beacham J. Fetal urine biochemistry: an index of renal maturation and dysfunction. Br J Obstet Gynaecol 1992;99:46-50.
117. Johnson MP, Corsi P, Bradfield W, et al. Sequential urinalysis improves evaluation of fetal renal function in obstructive uropathy. Am J Obstet Gynecol 1995;173:59-65.
118. Wilson RD, Johnson MP. Prenatal ultrasound guided percutaneous shunts for obstructive uropathy and thoracic disease. Semin Pediatr Surg 2003;12:182-189.
119. Chen FY, Chen M, Shih JC, et al. Meconium peritonitis presenting as isolated massive fetal ascites. Prenat Diagn 2004;24:930-931.
120. Holbrook KA, Smith LT, Elias S. Prenatal diagnosis of genetic skin disease using fetal skin biopsy samples. Arch Dermatol 1993;129: 1437-1454.
121. Murotsuki J, Uehara S, Okamura K, et al. Fetal liver biopsy for prenatal diagnosis of carbamoyl phosphate synthetase deficiency. Am J Perinatol 1994;11:160-162.
122. Ladwig D, Mowat D, Tobias V, et al. In utero fetal muscle biopsy in the diagnosis of Duchenne muscular dystrophy. Aust NZ J Obstet Gynaecol 2002;42:79-82.
123. Manning FA, Harrison MR, Rodeck C. Catheter shunts for fetal hydronephrosis and hydrocephalus. Report of the International Fetal Surgery Registry. N Engl J Med 1986;315:336-340.
124. Chasen ST, Chervenak FA, McCullough LB. The role of cephalocentesis in modern obstetrics. Am J Obstet Gynecol 2001;185:734-736.
125. Young BK, Stephenson CD, Mackenzie AP, et al. Combined sonographic and endoscopic umbilical cord occlusion in twin and triplet gestations. J Perinat Med 2005;33:530-533.
126. Habli M, Livingston J, Harmon J, et al. The outcome of twin-twin transfusion syndrome complicated with placental insufficiency. Am J Obstet Gynecol 2008;199:424 e1-e6.

Part V

Pediatric Sonography

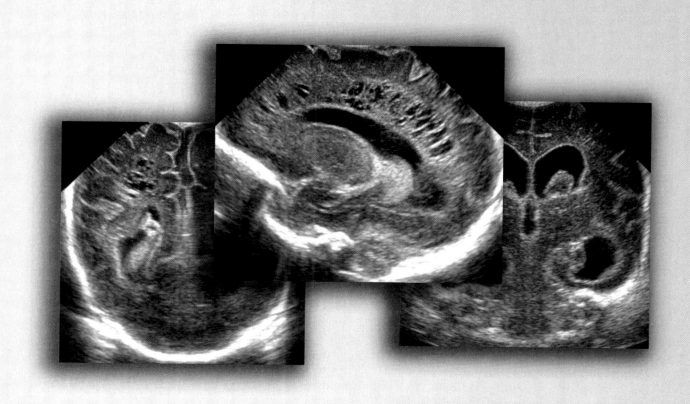

CHAPTER 47

Neonatal and Infant Brain Imaging

Carol M. Rumack and Julia A. Drose

Chapter Outline

*N*eonatal sonography of the brain is now an essential part of newborn care, particularly in high-risk and unstable premature infants.[1,2] Current ultrasound (US) technology allows for rapid evaluation of infants in the intensive care nursery with virtually no risk.[3] The advantages of sonography over computed tomography (CT) or magnetic resonance imaging (MRI) include portability, lower cost, speed, no ionizing radiation, and no sedation. Screening of premature infants for intracranial hemorrhage has proven highly sensitive and specific.

Ultrasound is essential to the neonatal evaluation and follow-up of hydrocephalus and periventricular leukomalacia (PVL). Prenatal US and MRI diagnosis[4] of

central nervous system malformations, infection, or masses are now followed up by ultrasound in the neonatal period. When major anomalies are present, associated anomalies may need evaluation by neonatal MRI. CT is not typically used in the premature infant because of the instability of the infant and the lack of good gray/white matter differentiation from the high water content in the newborn brain. CT is used infrequently for term infants, typically after a history of birth trauma.

Ultrasound can be useful for the follow-up of ventricular shunt therapy or possible complications. Color and spectral Doppler ultrasound of cranial blood flow may prove valuable, particularly for cystic lesions when the differential diagnosis includes a vascular lesion, or for possible subdural hematomas, and to separate normal vascular structures from clot. Doppler ultrasound is also useful in infants receiving extracorporeal membrane oxygenation or when decreased blood flow is a risk for infarction.[5-7] Sonography has been described in the evaluation of normal cranial sutures, which may allow diagnosis of craniosynostosis or a lacunar skull in myelomeningocele patients.[8,9]

EQUIPMENT

In the premature infant, a 7.5-MHz or higher transducer is recommended to obtain the highest resolution possible. A 5-MHz transducer may be necessary to allow for adequate sound penetration of a larger infant head.[10] Electronic phased array transducers with a 120-degree sector angle and multifocal zone capabilities are generally used for imaging through the anterior fontanelle. **Small-footprint, linear array, high-frequency transducers** (up to 12 MHz) can provide quality images for scanning of near-field pathology through the anterior fontanelle. These transducers are best for subdural hematomas, meningitis, superior sagittal sinus thrombosis, and cerebral edema, and in some cases, migrational abnormalities,[11] or when scanning over the mastoid fontanelle, posterior fontanelle, and foramen magnum.[12] The squamosal portion of the temporal bone is thin but may require a 5-MHz transducer if not imaged through the mastoid fontanelle. The multifocal zone capability provides excellent resolution throughout the field of view, but requires a cooperative patient because the frame rate is slowed significantly. **Compound imaging,** allowing for multiple angles of insonation, is also useful when imaging through small spaces such as the fontanelles. Video clip capabilities are invaluable in an uncooperative infant or when documenting motion, such as blood flow.[6]

Several formats are available to record permanent copies of the ultrasound examinations. Digital storage, allowing postprocessing of images, can improve quality. It has become useful to save video clips of a complex examination for later review, to prevent repeating an examination if there is a questionable finding on the individual images. Clips can greatly improve the understanding of the pathology. Areas of increased or decreased echogenicity may be extremely subtle on single images, but they become much more apparent when integrated with cine or video that captures real-time ultrasound findings and the relationship to normal structures.

SONOGRAPHIC TECHNIQUE

Currently, most brain sonographic examinations are performed through the **anterior fontanelle** in both the coronal and the sagittal plane. It is increasing apparent, however, that the posterior fossa is much better evaluated through the **posterior and mastoid fontanelles.** Cerebellar hemorrhage may be missed without the posterior fossa views. Posterior fossa malformations may not be well understood without these highly detailed views of the cerebellum, 4th ventricle, and cisterna magna.[13-15] Good skin-to-transducer coupling can be achieved by an acoustic coupling gel. Occasionally, a standoff pad can be useful to evaluate superficial abnormalities such as subdural hemorrhage, but a higher-resolution transducer is a better option to evaluate the near field in detail.

It is very important to use color Doppler ultrasound imaging to evaluate **fluid collections** because some cystic areas are actually vessels.[16] If extracerebral fluid collections are expected, they are better evaluated with CT or MRI. Axial scanning has been used extensively in utero, particularly for accurate measurements of fetal ventricular dimensions. In the newborn, axial scanning is used in evaluation of the posterior fossa through the mastoid fontanelle and to evaluate the circle of Willis with color Doppler ultrasound.[6,10,12,17-19] The posterior scanning techniques are the best approach to evaluate the occipital horns for ventricular clot. The posterior fossa views from the mastoid fontanelle are extremely important in the evaluation of cerebellar hemorrhage or posterior fossa anomalies, which are quite common. The foramen magnum approach may be useful when evaluating the upper spinal canal, as in patients with a Chiari malformation.

The anterior fontanelle remains open until approximately 2 years of age but is suitable for scanning only until about 12 to 14 months. The smaller the fontanelle, the smaller is the acoustic window and the more difficult the examination will be.[10,17]

Every effort should be made to maintain normal body temperature in premature infants when performing ultrasound. Their small size results in a high surface-to-volume ratio and rapid heat loss when they are exposed. Overhead warming lamps, blankets, and warmed coupling gel should be routinely used. If the infant is in an Isolette, heat loss may be minimized by using access side holes as an entry site for the transducer.

Handwashing and cleansing of the transducer between patients are of paramount importance to avoid the spread of infection in the intensive care nursery. Simple cleansing of the transducer head with a manufacturer-approved disinfectant should be adequate. A transducer should never be autoclaved because this will destroy it. When absolute sterility is required, such as during operative sonography, the transducer can be placed inside a sterile surgical glove or sterile transducer cover with coupling gel. Sterile aqueous gel or saline solution can be used as a coupler outside the sterile cover.

Standard brain scanning includes sagittal and coronal planes through the anterior fontanelle and should also routinely include at least two axial views: through the

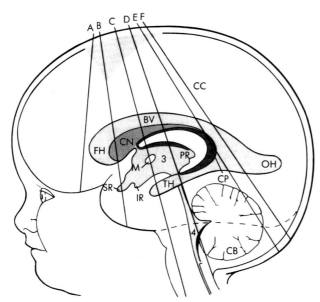

FIGURE 47-1. Coronal brain ultrasound planes through anterior fontanelle. *A* through *F* correspond to front to back. *CC,* Cerebral cortex; *BV,* body of lateral ventricle; *FH,* frontal horn; *OH,* occipital horn; *CN,* caudate nucleus; *M,* massa intermedia; *PR,* pineal recess; *3,* third ventricle; *TH,* temporal horn; *SR,* supraoptic recess; *IR,* infundibular recess; *CP,* choroid plexus; *4,* fourth ventricle; *CB,* cerebellum. *(From Rumack CM, Manco-Johnson ML. Perinatal and infant brain imaging: role of ultrasound and computed tomography. St Louis, 1984, Mosby.)*

posterior fontanelle and the mastoid fontanelle. Coronal images acquired through the posterior fontanelle may be useful as well, to compare ventricular size. Magnified views are essential to study near-field pathology. Whenever possible, the transducer should be held firmly between the thumb and index finger, and the lateral aspect of the hand should rest on the infant's head for stability. Video clips should be obtained routinely for any abnormality to improve ultrasound diagnosis, avoid repeating a scan on an unstable newborn, and allow review of complex images and prompt diagnosis without delaying the patient workflow.

Coronal Imaging

Coronal images are obtained by placing the scan head of the transducer transversely across the anterior fontanelle (Fig. 47-1). The plane of the ultrasound beam should then sweep in an anterior-to-posterior direction, completely through the brain. Care must be taken to maintain symmetrical imaging of each half of the brain and skull. An initial sweep of the brain to obtain parallel alignment of the thick glomus of the choroid plexus in each trigone is a good method to obtain symmetry. At least six standard coronal images should be obtained during this anterior to posterior sweep.[17]

The most anterior image is acquired just **anterior to the frontal horns** of the lateral ventricles[20] (Fig. 47-2, *A*). Visualization of the anterior cranial fossa is obtained,

CORONAL BRAIN SCANS: NORMAL STRUCTURES

MIDLINE STRUCTURES
Interhemispheric fissure
Cingulate sulcus
Corpus callosum
Cavum septi pellucidi
Cavum vergae (when present)
Third ventricle
Fourth ventricle
Brainstem
Vermis of cerebellum

PARAMEDIAN STRUCTURES
Frontal lobe
Parietal lobe
Occipital lobe
Frontal horn of lateral ventricle
Body of lateral ventricle
Temporal horn of lateral ventricle
Trigone of lateral ventricle
Choroid plexus
Glomus of choroid plexus
Caudate nucleus
Internal capsule
Thalamus
Lentiform nucleus
Tentorium cerebelli
Cerebellar hemisphere
Sylvian fissure
Cisterna magna

including the frontal lobes of the cerebral cortex with the orbits deep to the floor of the skull base.

Moving posteriorly, the **frontal horns of the lateral ventricles** appear as symmetrical, anechoic, comma-shaped structures with the hypoechoic caudate heads within the concave lateral border (Fig. 47-2, *B*). Structures visualized from superior to inferior in the midline include the interhemispheric fissure; cingulate sulcus; genu and anterior body of the corpus callosum, and septum pellucidum between the ventricles. Moving laterally from the midline, the caudate nucleus is separated from the putamen by the internal capsule. Lateral to the putamen, the sylvian fissure is echogenic because it contains the **middle cerebral artery** (MCA). The sylvian fissure separates the frontal from the temporal lobe. Inferiorly, the internal carotid arteries bifurcate to form the echogenic anterior and middle cerebral arteries.

Progressing farther posteriorly to the level **above the midbrain,** the **body of the lateral ventricles** is seen on either side of the cavum septi pellucidi (Fig. 47-2, *C*). Below this, the thalami lie on either side of the third ventricle, which is usually too thin to visualize in normal infants. Deep to the thalami, the brainstem begins to be visualized. Lateral to the midline, the thalami are separated from the lentiform nuclei (caudate and putamen) by the internal capsule. Lateral to the lentiform nuclei is

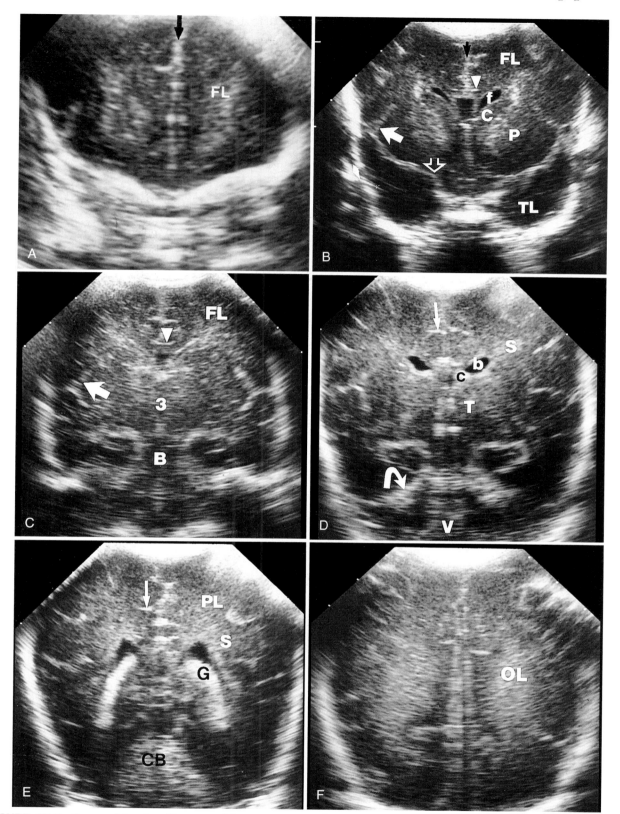

FIGURE 47-2. Coronal brain ultrasound images: normal full-term infant. Anterior to posterior corresponds to sections *A* to *F* in Figure 47-1. **A,** *FL,* Frontal lobes; *black arrow,* interhemispheric fissure. **B,** *P,* Putamen; *C,* caudate nucleus; *f,* frontal horns of lateral ventricles; *TL,* temporal lobe; *arrowhead,* corpus callosum; *closed arrow,* sylvian fissure; *open arrow,* bifurcation of internal carotid artery. (On images **A** and **B** black arrow represents interhemispheric fissure.) **C,** *B,* Brainstem; *3,* location of third ventricle (third and fourth ventricles are difficult to see in normal patients on coronal cuts). **D,** *S,* Centrum semiovale; *b,* body of lateral ventricle; *c,* choroid plexus; *T,* thalamus; *V,* vermis of cerebellum; *curved arrow,* tentorium cerebelli; *straight white arrow,* cingulate sulcus. **E,** *PL,* Parietal lobe; *G,* glomus of choroid plexus; *CB,* cerebellum. **F,** *OL,* Occipital lobe. (*B and C from Rumack CR, Horgan JG, Hay TC, et al.* Pocket atlas of pediatric ultrasound. *Philadelphia, 1990, Lippincott-Raven.*)

the deep white matter region of brain called the **centrum semiovale.** Again, the sylvian fissures are seen.

A slightly more posterior transducer angulation results in a plane that includes the **cerebellum.** The body of the lateral ventricles becomes somewhat more rounded as the size of the caudate nucleus decreases once posterior to the foramen of Monro (Fig. 47-2, *D*). At this level in the midline, the body of the corpus callosum is deep to the cingulate sulcus, and the third ventricle is located between the anterior portions of the thalami. Echogenic material visualized in the floor of the lateral ventricles is the **choroid plexus.** Echogenic choroid plexus is also seen in the roof of the third ventricle, resulting in three echogenic foci of choroid. The thalami are now more prominent on either side of the third ventricle. Midline structures are unchanged, except that deep to the thalami, the tentorium covering the cerebellum is visualized. Below this, in the posterior fossa, the **vermis** is the echogenic structure in the midline surrounded by the more hypoechoic cerebellar hemispheres. When the septum pellucidum is cystic posteriorly, it is called the **cavum vergae.** Because the cystic center of the septum pellucidum closes from posterior to anterior as the brain matures, late-gestation neonates often have only the more anterior cavum septi pellucidi. The lentiform nuclei may no longer be seen at this level. The **temporal horns** of the lateral ventricles may be seen lateral and inferior to the thalami, but are usually not seen unless there is hydrocephalus.

Further posteriorly, the **trigone** or **atrium of the lateral ventricles** and **occipital horns** are visualized (Fig. 47-2, *E*). The extensive echogenic glomus of the choroid plexus nearly obscures the lumen of the cerebrospinal fluid (CSF)–filled ventricle at the trigone. In the midline—the visualized portion of the corpus callosum deep to the cingulate sulcus—is the splenium. Inferiorly, the cerebellum is separated from the occipital cortex by the tentorium cerebelli.

The most posterior section visualizes predominantly **occipital lobe cortex** and the most posterior aspect of the occipital horns of the lateral ventricles that do not contain choroid plexus (Fig. 47-2, *F*). This section is angled posterior to the cerebellum.

Normal premature brain ultrasound images in the same planes are shown in Figure 47-3. The lateral ventricles are slightly larger; the cavum septi pellucidi extends back to become the cavum vergae between the lateral ventricle bodies and occipital horns (Fig. 47-3, *B-E*). There are only a few sulci, and the sylvian fissures are wider and may appear boxlike rather than as thin fissures.

Sagittal Imaging

The sagittal images are obtained by placing the transducer longitudinally across the anterior fontanelle and angling it to each side (Fig. 47-4). The **midline** is first identified through the interhemispheric fissure by recognition of the curving line of the corpus callosum above the cystic cavum septi pellucidi and cavum vergae, the third and fourth ventricles, and the highly echogenic cerebellar vermis (Fig. 47-5). The cingulate sulcus lies parallel to and above the corpus callosum. In this view, the size of cerebellar vermis has been used to assess gestational age.[21] The degree of sulcal development can be used as well. Shallow angulation to each side of about 10 degrees will show the normally small **lateral ventricles** (Fig. 47-6, *A*). The ventricles are not located in a perfectly straight plane anterior to posterior. The transducer must be angled so that the anterior portion of the sector is directed more medially and the posterior portion more laterally, to include the entire lateral ventricle in a single image.[17]

SAGITTAL BRAIN SCANS: NORMAL STRUCTURES

MIDLINE STRUCTURES
Frontal lobe
Parietal lobe
Occipital lobe
Cingulate sulcus
Pericallosal artery
Corpus callosum
Cavum septi pellucidi
Cavum vergae*
Cavum velum interpositum*
Third ventricle
Fourth ventricle
Tentorium
Choroid plexus, third ventricle
Aqueduct
Occipitoparietal fissure
Brainstem
Vermis of cerebellum

PARAMEDIAN STRUCTURES
Frontal lobe
Parietal lobe
Occipital lobe
Frontal horn of lateral ventricle
Body of lateral ventricle
Atrium of lateral ventricle (trigone)
Temporal horn of lateral ventricle
Occipital horn of lateral ventricle
Choroid plexus
Caudate nucleus
Thalamus
Caudothalamic groove
Cerebellum

*Not always present.

Above the lateral ventricle is the cerebral cortex, and below it is the cerebellar hemisphere. The caudate nucleus and the thalamus are within the arms of the ventricle (Fig. 47-6, *B*). The **caudothalamic groove** at the junction of these two structures is an important area to recognize, because this is the most common site of

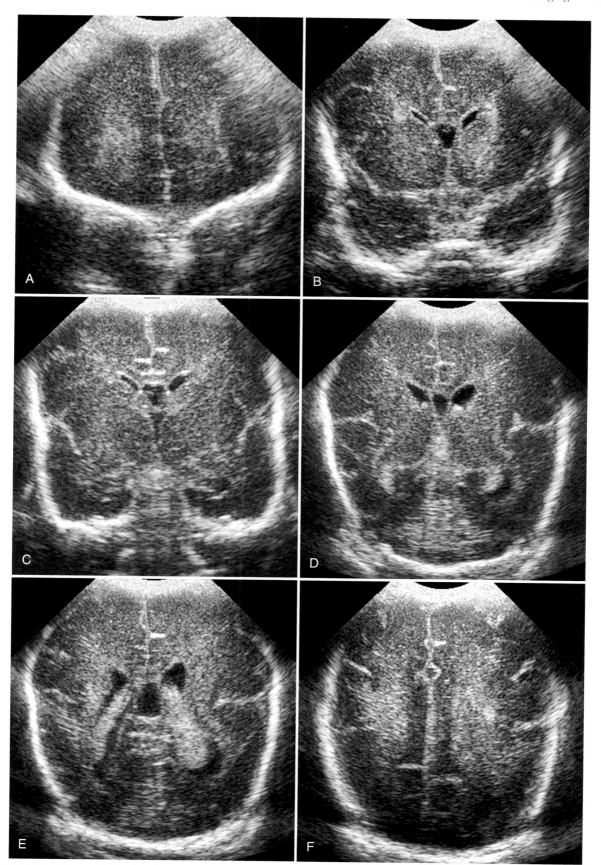

FIGURE 47-3. Coronal brain ultrasound images: normal premature newborn infant. Note cavum septi pellucidi extends posteriorly and becomes cavum vergae. Sylvian fissures are wider.

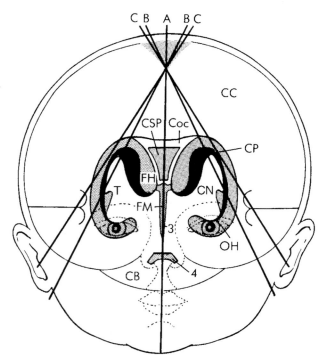

FIGURE 47-4. Sagittal planes used in brain scanning through anterior fontanelle. *A* to *C* correspond to midline to lateral. *CB,* Cerebellum; *CC,* cerebral cortex; *Coc,* corpus callosum; *CN,* caudate nucleus; *CP,* choroid plexus; *CSP,* cavum septi pellucidi; *FH,* frontal horn; *FM,* foramen of Monro; *OH,* occipital horn; *T,* temporal horn; *3,* third ventricle; *4,* fourth ventricle. (*Modified from Rumack CM, Manco-Johnson ML. Perinatal and infant brain imaging: role of ultrasound and computed tomography. St Louis, 1984, Mosby.*)

germinal matrix hemorrhage in the subependymal region of the ventricle.

More pronounced lateral angulation will demonstrate the peripheral aspect of the ventricles and the more lateral **cerebral hemisphere**, including the temporal lobes (Fig. 47-6, *C*) where the middle cerebral artery branches extend toward the ventricle.

Sagittal sonography almost always reveals a normal hyperechoic **peritrigonal blush** just posterior and superior to the ventricular trigones on parasagittal views (Fig. 47-6, *B*). It is caused by the interface of numerous parallel fibers that are almost perpendicular to the longitudinal angle of the ultrasound beam passing through the anterior fontanelle. A similar area of increased echogenicity is not seen on sonograms obtained through the posterior fontanelle, because with that angulation, the long axis of the ultrasound beam and the fiber tracts are almost parallel. Sonographic-pathologic correlations demonstrate the normal peritrigonal hyperechogenicity or "blush."[22]

Posterior Fontanelle Imaging

The posterior fontanelle is a very useful view to evaluate the occipitals horns for the diagnosis of intraventricular hemorrhage. The posterior fontanelle lies in the midline at the junction of the lambdoid and sagittal sutures; it is open only until about 3 months of age[23] (Fig. 47-7). The transducer should be angled slightly off midline with the anterior portion of the probe directed slightly medially, to demonstrate the lateral ventricular trigone with its

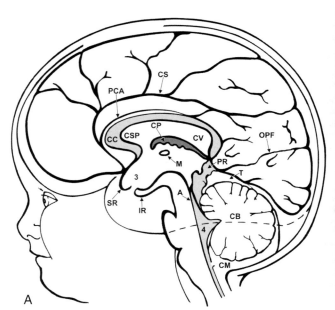
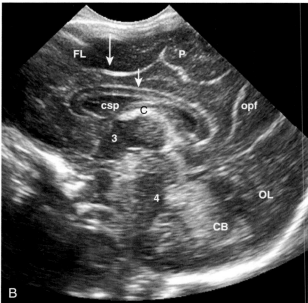

FIGURE 47-5. Normal midline sagittal anatomy. A, Schematic drawing. *CC,* Corpus callosum; *CSP,* cavum septi pellucidi; *CP,* choroid plexus; *CV,* cavum vergae; *PR,* pineal recess; *SR,* supraoptic recess; *IR,* infundibular recess; *3,* third ventricle; *4,* fourth ventricle; *A,* aqueduct; *CB,* cerebellum (vermis); *CM,* cisterna magna; *PCA,* pericallosal artery; *CS,* cingulate sulcus; *M,* massa intermedia; *T,* tentorium; *OPF,* occipitoparietal fissure. B, Normal midline sagittal ultrasound brain scan. *FL,* Frontal lobe; *P,* parietal lobe; *OL,* occipital lobe; *short arrow,* corpus callosum; *csp,* cavum septi pellucidi; *3,* third ventricle; *4,* fourth ventricle; *CB,* cerebellar vermis; *long arrow,* cingulate sulcus. *opf,* occipitoparietal fissure.

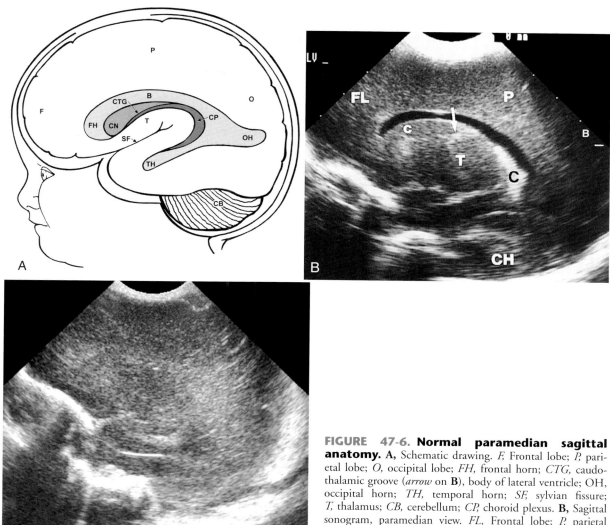

FIGURE 47-6. Normal paramedian sagittal anatomy. A, Schematic drawing. *F,* Frontal lobe; *P,* parietal lobe; *O,* occipital lobe; *FH,* frontal horn; *CTG,* caudothalamic groove (*arrow* on **B**), body of lateral ventricle; *OH,* occipital horn; *TH,* temporal horn; *SF,* sylvian fissure; *T,* thalamus; *CB,* cerebellum; *CP,* choroid plexus. **B,** Sagittal sonogram, paramedian view. *FL,* Frontal lobe; *P,* parietal lobe; *T,* thalamus; *c,* caudate nucleus; *C,* choroid plexus; *CH,* cerebellar hemisphere; *B,* peritrigonal blush. **C,** Parasagittal sonogram of cerebral cortex.

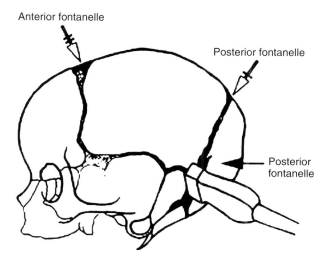

FIGURE 47-7. Acoustic windows: anterior, posterior, and mastoid fontanelles. (*Modified from Di Salvo DN. A new view of the neonatal brain: clinical utility of supplemental neurologic US imaging windows. Radiographics 2001;21:943-955.*)

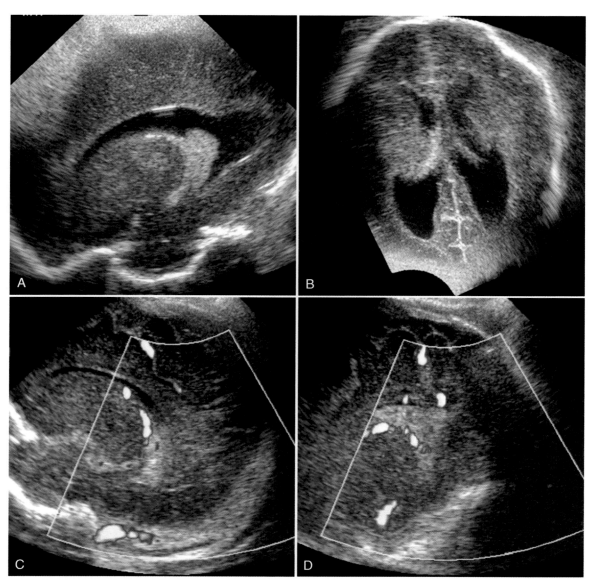

FIGURE 47-8. Occipital horn: posterior fontanelle images. A, Occipital horn with lobular choroid, sagittal plane. **B,** Occipital horns, axial plane (turned 90 degrees clockwise). **C** and **D,** Choroid plexus on color Doppler sonography is vascular; clot can be separated by the lack of vascular flow. Motion may suggest flow, so careful imaging is needed.

occipital horn in the near field (Fig. 47-8). The choroid glomus will be seen with extensions into the ventricular body and temporal horn. The occipital horn does not contain choroid plexus and should be completely anechoic. Angling the transducer into the left and right parasagittal planes will display each occipital horn. These planes are extremely useful for detecting dependently layering clot and clot attached to the choroid plexus. Inverted coronal images of both occipital horns can be obtained for comparison of ventricular size and echogenicity (Fig. 47-8, *B*).

Mastoid Fontanelle Imaging

The mastoid fontanelle allows assessment of the brainstem and posterior fossa, which are not well demonstrated in the standard planes through the anterior fontanelle. The ultrasound transducer is placed about 1 cm behind the helix of the ear and 1 cm above the tragus. The mastoid fontanelle is located at the junction of the squamosal, lambdoidal and occipital sutures (see Fig. 47-7). Posterior fossa axial images, with the anterior portion of the transducer angled slightly cephalad, will demonstrate the fourth ventricle, posterior cerebellar vermis, cerebellar hemispheres, and the cisterna magna. These axial images should be displayed with the top of the head to the left. A rotated display may be useful occasionally to relate the anatomy to standard axial views from other modalities (Fig. 47-9). The radiating folia or surface folds of the cerebellum are quite echogenic compared to the cerebellar hemispheric parenchyma. Behind the fourth ventricle is the echogenic

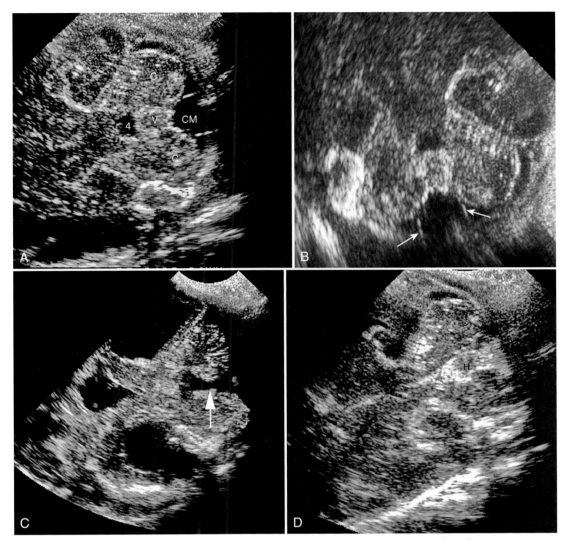

FIGURE 47-9. Mastoid fontanelle images at fourth ventricle level in posterior fossa. A, Normal cerebellar hemispheres *(C)*, cerebellar vermis *(V)*, fourth ventricle *(4)*, and cisterna magna *(CM)*. **B,** Normal cisterna magna septa extend straight and parallel through the subarachnoid space *(arrows)* and may be a remnant of Blake's pouch cysts. (**A** turned 90 degrees into standard axial imaging format.) **C,** Low posterior fossa view through the vallecula *(arrow)* between the cerebellar hemispheres in a newborn with posthemorrhagic hydrocephalus. **D,** Foramen of Magendie, which connects the fourth ventricle and the cisterna magna, is enlarged and contains intraventricular hemorrhage *(H)*.

midline vermis, which appears much less echogenic in the axial view compared to midline sagittal scans. When angled axial images are obtained through the lower parts of the cerebellum below the fourth ventricle, the (normally thin) **vallecula** may be seen in the midline as a space between the cerebellar hemispheres (Fig. 47-9, *C*), particularly in the presence of hydrocephalus. In steeply angled axial scans, the **foramen of Magendie** can be seen in the midline as a thin sonolucent line between the cerebellar hemispheres extending from and the fourth ventricle to the cisterna magna (Fig. 47-9, *D*). It should not be mistaken for a Dandy-Walker variant. The presence of an intact vermis on higher images and the marked caudal angulation required to see the vallecula allow differentiation of this normal variant.[14,15,18] Color Doppler ultrasound in this view allows evaluation of flow in

the transverse and straight sinuses to exclude venous thrombosis.[24]

A slightly higher axial scan should include the thalami, midbrain, third ventricle, aqueduct of Sylvius, and quadrigeminal plate cistern, with the transducer angled from the standard axial plane and placed cephalad to the external auricle (Fig. 47-10). At this level, the thalami are hypoechoic, inverted, heart-shaped structures. The midbrain, including the cerebral peduncles and corpora quadrigemina, consists of paired hypoechoic lenticular structures just caudal to the thalami. The third ventricle is usually a thin cleft, barely visible between the thalami. The aqueduct is usually a thin echogenic line but may occasionally be a thin slit in the midbrain. The quadrigeminal cistern is echogenic and surrounds the midbrain.

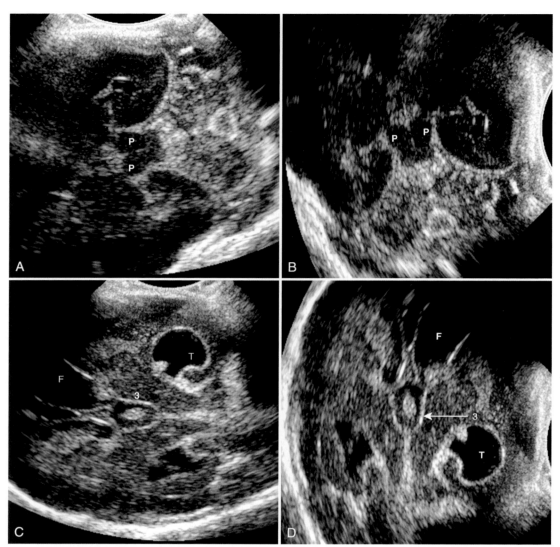

FIGURE 47-10. Mastoid fontanelle images of posterior fossa, midbrain level above fourth ventricle.
A, Normal axial plane of the superior cerebellum posteriorly and the cerebral pedicles anteriorly *(P)*. **B,** Normal, turned 90 degrees to match axial view in other modalities. **C** and **D,** Posthemorrhagic hydrocephalus. *F,* Frontal horn; *3,* third ventricle with *arrow* to clot in third ventricle; *T,* temporal horn.

THREE-DIMENSIONAL ULTRASOUND

Three-dimensional (3-D) ultrasound may be a useful adjunct to standard two-dimensional (2-D) imaging of the neonatal brain.[25] A volume of brain can be acquired in a few seconds, and then computer displays of three octagonal slices at any angle can be reconstructed, in addition to coronal, sagittal, and axial planes. Brain lesions can be tracked in three views at once, which can better identify the position in the brain and the most likely diagnosis (Fig. 47-11). Some authors recommend 3-D volume measurement of the ventricles;[26,27] the standard method is still a qualitative assessment based on typical normal ventricles of different age groups.

STANDARDIZED REPORTS

Standardized Views for Display

Brain anatomy images should be displayed in a consistent manner so that comparisons can be easily made. At our institution, routine images are always shown with the infant's face on the left. Labels on sagittal scans should be "left" or "right." Labeling "L to R" is confusing and should not be necessary; the person scanning should always know which side off midline is being scanned, and the physician interpreting the scan certainly needs the correct side labeled as well. Video clips are more difficult and might be best done separately on the left and right, in addition to a full sweep through the entire brain from side to side.

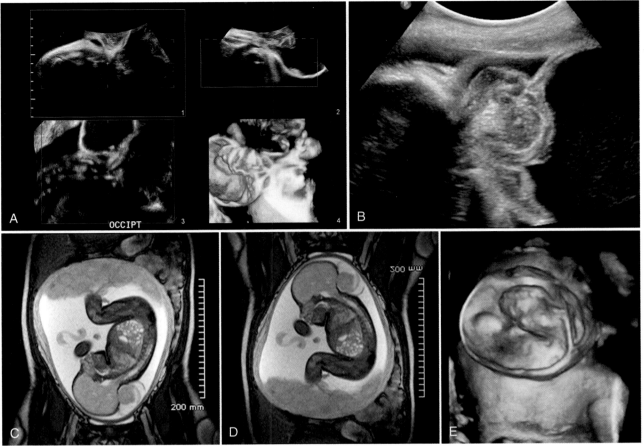

FIGURE 47-11. **Fetal encephalocele. A,** Three-dimensional (3-D) ultrasound orthogonal views shown simultaneously with a volume-rendered *(gold)* image. **B,** Magnified view of encephalocele alone. **C** and **D,** Fetal T2-weighted MRI and same image flipped to head up, facing left, shows encephalocele with cystic and solid components. **E,** Posterior, volume-rendered 3-D ultrasound shows a magnified view of the encephalocele. A large amount of brain has extended out of the skull into the large, cystic cerebrospinal fluid.

Using the American College of Radiology (ACR) Practice Guideline for the Performance of Neurosonography in Neonates and Infants,[28] there are specific questions to answer. Developing a template for reports is a useful task to pursue to ensure you do not forget what needs to be covered. Be careful not to make the template so completely normal that you forget to change sections where that patient is abnormal. Setting defaults that require you to approve the normal or change to an abnormal dictation is much safer, to remind you to look at each of these anatomic areas as you dictate.

ULTRASOUND OF THE BRAIN: STANDARD REPORT TEMPLATE

The ventricular size and configuration are
    <normal>.
The corpus callosum is <present> <above the
    cavum septum pellucidi and/or cavum vergae>.
There is <no hemorrhage in the caudothalamic
    groove or in the ventricular system>.
The cerebellar vermis, fourth ventricle, and
    cerebellar hemispheres <appear normal>.

DEVELOPMENTAL ANATOMY

Brain Sulcal Development and Subarachnoid Spaces

In the very premature infant, the brain sulci are not fully developed and the brain appears quite smooth[29,30] (Fig. 47-12). The first sulcus to form is the primitive, almost square, **sylvian fissure,** best seen on coronal images[31] (see Fig. 47-3, *C*). Sulcal development, best evaluated on midline sagittal images, then extends to the **calcarine fissure** as a simple straight line in the fifth gestational month (20 weeks).[32] By 24 to 25 weeks' gestation, the **occipitoparietal fissure** is present, but no actual sulci (Fig. 47-13, *A*). By 28 weeks, the **callosomarginal sulcus** over the corpus callosum and a simple linear **cingulate sulcus** superior and parallel to the corpus callosum are seen (Fig. 47-13, *B*). By 30 weeks, the cingulate sulcus is also branched (Fig. 47-13, *C*). Between 33 and 40 weeks' gestation, sulci bend, branch, and anastomose so that a full-term infant has many peripheral branches over the brain surface (Fig. 47-13, *D*). The **subarachnoid spaces** are prominent in the very

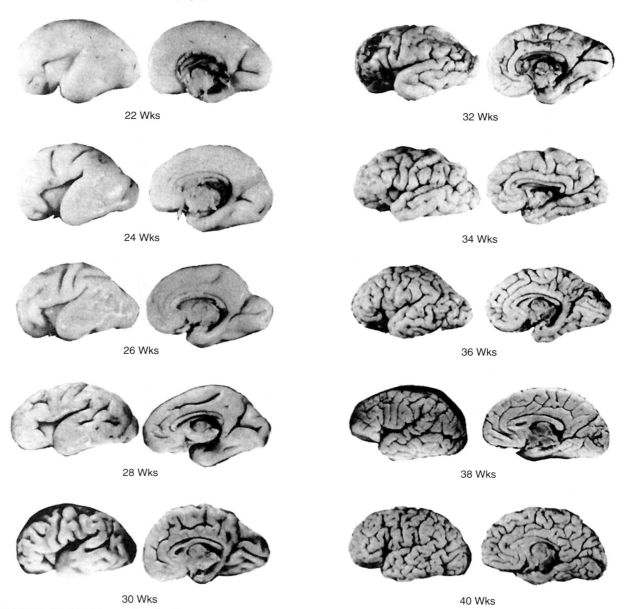

22 Wks

24 Wks

26 Wks

28 Wks

30 Wks

32 Wks

34 Wks

36 Wks

38 Wks

40 Wks

FIGURE 47-12. Normal sulcal pattern development. At 22 to 40 weeks' gestation. *(From Dorovini-Zis K, Dolman CL. Gestational development of brain. Arch Pathol Lab Med 1977;101:192-195.)*

premature infant, causing the sylvian fissure to be almost square, whereas later, after infolding of the insula (opercularization), it becomes a narrow, echogenic fissure filled with middle cerebral artery branches.[30,33]

Although not used routinely, measurement of the subarachnoid space on a magnified view of the brain can be done from the triangular sagittal sinus to the surface of the cortex. Armstrong et al.[34] report this space is normally less than 3.5 mm in 95% of preterm infants before 36 weeks' gestation. Closer to term, the values tended to be at the higher end of the range, increasing weekly.

Cavum Septi Pellucidi and Cavum Vergae

There is one continuous cystic midline structure in the septum pellucidum during fetal life. The septum

contains the cavum septi pellucidi anterior to the foramen of Monro (Fig. 47-13; see also Fig. 47-3) and the cavum vergae posteriorly. Both parts are normally present early in gestation, but they close from back to front, starting at approximately 6 months' gestation (Fig. 47-14). By full term, closure has occurred posteriorly in 97% of infants so that there is only a cavum septi pellucidi at birth. By 3 to 6 months after birth, this septum is completely closed in 85% of infants, although in some, the septum remains open into adulthood.[35] In fetal brain imaging, Callen et al.[36] reported that the columns of the **fornix** can be mistaken for the cavum septi pellucidi. On axial views below the frontal horns, the fornix appears as a cystic structure with a central linear echo. Absence of the corpus callosum may be missed on diagnosis because the fornices will be present and simulate the cavum between the two frontal horns. Careful evaluation of the

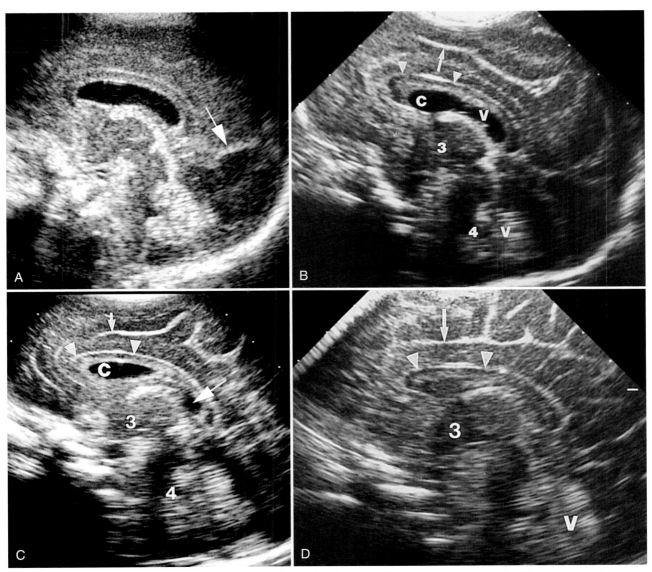

FIGURE 47-13. Normal premature infant brain. Sagittal images at 25 to 40 weeks' gestation. **A, 25 weeks.** No sulci; corpus callosum lies above completely cystic cavum septi pellucidi and cavum vergae. *Arrow,* Occipitoparietal fissure. **B, 27 weeks.** Cingulate sulcus *(arrow)* is just developed, and cavum septi pellucidi *(C)* and cavum vergae *(V)* are readily visible. **C, 30 weeks.** Cingulate sulcus *(short arrow)* has a few branches. *Long arrow,* Cavum velum interpositum. **D, 40 weeks.** Cingulate sulcus *(arrow)* has many branches. The septum pellucidum is no longer cystic. *V,* Cerebellar vermis; *3,* third ventricle; *4,* fourth ventricle; *arrowheads,* corpus callosum.

inferior position of the fornices below the frontal horns will avoid this error.

Cavum Veli Interpositi

The cavum of the velum interpositum represents a potential space above the choroid in the roof of the third ventricle and below the columns of the fornices.[2,37] It may appear as an anechoic, inverted, helmetlike space just inferior and posterior to the splenium in the pineal region (see Fig. 47-13, *C*). Blasi et al.[38] describe the prenatal diagnosis of the cavum veli interpositi on 2-D and 3-D ultrasound with color flow Doppler. Careful study of the anatomic location of the cystic structure, its size, and changes over time is required to be certain this is a normal variant, not an arachnoid cyst with mass

effect or associated anomaly of the corpus callosum. Chen et al.[37] reports that 21% of neonates have a cavum velum interpositum on sonography. By 2 years of age, this cystic structure is an uncommon finding and thus is thought to be a normal stage of brain development. Rarely, a cyst is found in this area that causes compression of other structures.

Frontal Horn Variants

A few newborns have cysts exactly parallel (not above or below) and adjacent to the frontal horns (Fig. 47-15). These cysts are typically bilateral and have septations between the cyst and the frontal horns. Frontal horn cysts, also called **coarctation of the frontal horn**[39] and **connatal cysts,**[40] are caused by folding of the frontal horn on itself, resulting in kinking (seen as a septation). Typical normal frontal horns are directly lateral to the cavum septi pellucidi on coronal images, below the corpus callosum. The frontal horns are relatively thin compared to the occipital horns.

Choroid Plexus and Variants

The choroid plexus is the site of CSF production in the ventricles (Fig. 47-16). The largest portion of the choroid plexus is the **glomus,** a highly echogenic structure attached to the trigone of each lateral ventricle. The choroid tapers as it extends anteriorly to the foramen of Monro and continues from each lateral ventricle into and along the roof of the third ventricle. The choroid

plexus tapers laterally as it extends into the temporal horn of the lateral ventricle. The choroid plexus does not extend into the frontal or occipital horn. Choroid plexus is also present in the roof of the fourth ventricle. Small cysts in the choroid plexus are common and in fact are usually small vessels.

The glomus of the choroid plexus is often doubled and thus appears **lobulated** (Fig. 47-17). Some authors have termed this appearance a **"split" choroid plexus.**[41] It may be mistaken for clot adhering to the choroid plexus. Color Doppler ultrasound will differentiate the normal highly vascular choroid from similarly echogenic, but avascular, clot (see Fig. 47-8, *C*). Coronal views may also show a flattened or truncated choroid plexus at the level

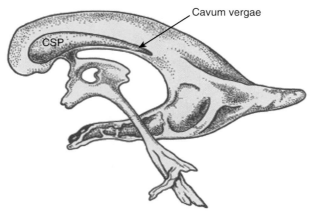

FIGURE 47-14. Cavum septi pellucidi (CSP). Arrow indicates cavum vergae projecting on the medial surface of the lateral ventricles. *(From Rumack CM, Manco-Johnson ML. Perinatal and infant brain imaging: role of ultrasound and computed tomography. St Louis, 1984, Mosby.)*

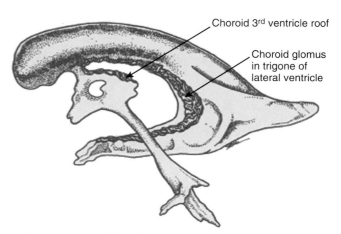

FIGURE 47-16. Choroid plexus. Drawing shows choroid plexus as it courses through the third and lateral ventricles *(arrows)*. *(From Rumack CM, Manco-Johnson ML. Perinatal and infant brain imaging: role of ultrasound and computed tomography. St Louis, 1984, Mosby.)*

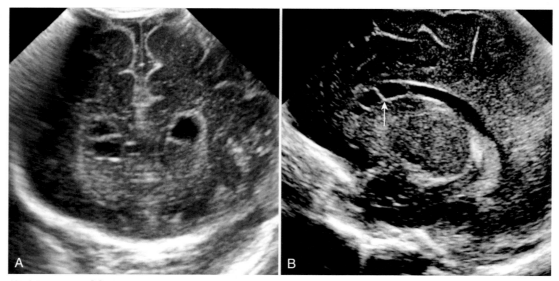

FIGURE 47-15. Frontal horn cysts. A and **B,** Coronal and sagittal sonograms show uncommon normal cystic variants, also called frontal horn coarctation or connatal cysts. Frontal horn cysts appear to be septations in the ventricles *(arrow)* but are thought to be caused by folding of the frontal horn on itself.

of the thickest portion at the trigone, probably related to the angle of the transducer to the choroid.[41] If there is a large ventricle, the choroid will normally "dangle," or hang down toward the dependent ventricle, when the infant is lying on its side (Fig. 47-17, *C*). Look carefully at choroid cysts, and turn on color Doppler ultrasound; many "choroid cysts" are actually vessels to the choroid.

PITFALLS IN NEUROSONOGRAPHY

Peritrigonal blush
Choroid plexus shapes affected by position
   Normal choroid plexus: split, lobulated, or
     truncated
   Dangling choroid (in hydrocephalus)
   Normal choroidal vessels vs. choroid plexus cyst
   Normal choroid plexus vs. hemorrhage around
     the choroid
Asymmetrical normal-sized ventricles
Dandy-Walker malformation in fetal imaging

Germinal Matrix

The germinal matrix develops deep to the ependyma and consists of loosely organized, proliferating cells that give rise to the neurons and glia of the cerebral cortex and basal ganglia (Fig. 47-18). Its vascular bed is the most richly perfused region of the developing brain. Vessels in this region form an immature vascular rete of fine capillaries, extremely thin-walled veins, and larger irregular vessels.[42] The capillary network is best developed on the periphery of the germinal matrix and becomes less well developed toward the central glioblastic mass. Although the germinal matrix is not visualized on sonography, it is important as the typical anatomic site over the caudate nucleus where germinal matrix hemorrhage occurs in premature infants.

Early in gestation, the germinal matrix forms the entire wall of the ventricular system. After the third month of gestation, the germinal matrix regresses, first around the third ventricle, then around the temporal and occipital

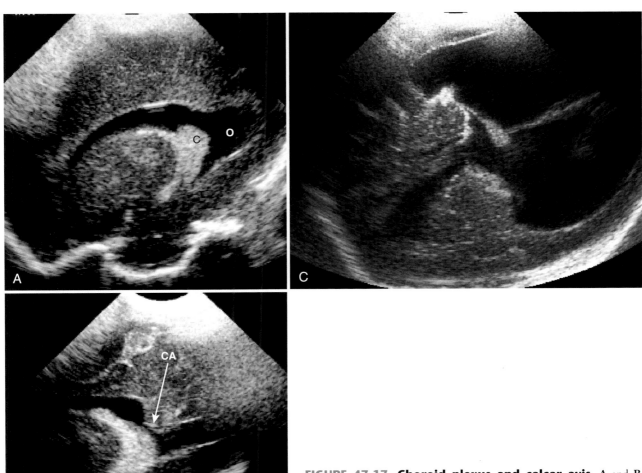

FIGURE 47-17. Choroid plexus and calcar avis. A and **B,** Posterior fontanelle views of lateral ventricle. **A,** Normal choroid plexus glomus *(c)* does not extend into the occipital horn *(O)*. **B,** Calcar avis *(CA)* can be averaged into the occipital horn and imitate hemorrhage. Note continuity with the adjacent brain identifies this structure. **C,** Axial view of two lateral ventricles shows "dangling" choroid plexus hanging down into the lower ventricle in this newborn with hydrocephalus from aqueductal stenosis (same patient as Fig. 47-40).

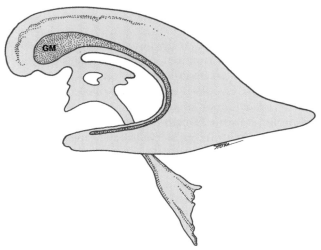

FIGURE 47-18. Germinal matrix. Drawing shows germinal matrix *(GM)* at 30 to 32 weeks' gestation, with largest amount near the caudate nucleus. *(From Rumack CM, Manco-Johnson ML. Perinatal and infant brain imaging: role of ultrasound and computed tomography. St Louis, 1984, Mosby.)*

horns and trigone. By 24 weeks' gestation, the germinal matrix persists only over the head of the caudate nucleus and to a lesser extent over the body of the caudate. By 32 weeks' gestation, it is unusual to see germinal matrix hemorrhage because these cells migrate out to the cerebral cortex. This regression continues until 40 weeks' gestation, when the germinal matrix ceases to exist as a discrete structure, and the immature vascular rete has been remodeled to form adult vascular patterns.

Calcar Avis

On posterior fontanelle views, a normal gyrus, the calcar avis, frequently protrudes into the medial aspect of the lateral ventricle at the junction of the trigone and occipital horn (see Fig. 47-17, *B*). It can be recognized due to a central echogenic sulcus (**calcarine fissure**), its continuity with the adjacent brain, and normal vascularity on color Doppler ultrasound.[41] The calcar avis is seen when the occipital horn is cut slightly off center and catches that portion of brain. Although this normal brain gyrus may mimic intraventricular clot, slightly turning the transducer will show its continuity with the brain.

Cerebellar Vermis

Because the cerebellum develops late in gestation, a mistaken fetal diagnosis of cerebellar vermian hypoplasia is occasionally made. If axial scans are done below the normal level of the 4th ventricle, the vallecula between the cerebellar hemispheres may be mistaken for a Dandy-Walker variant. Pseudoabsence of the inferior vermis[41] or pseudo–vermian hypoplasia can be appreciated on axial views through the posterior fossa. There may appear to be a small or absent cerebellar vermis and a wide communication between the fourth ventricle and cisterna magna. Slightly more superior axial views will show the normal cerebellar vermis. This appearance has caused the mistaken fetal diagnosis of a Dandy-Walker malformation, particularly since the cerebellum is not fully formed normally and still growing at birth. The appearance of a missing or hypoplastic vermis can be evaluated carefully by moving the transducer superiorly to catch the normal vermis. The cerebellar vallecula is a variably sized subarachnoid space below and not continuous with the fourth ventricle. The foramen of Magendie is thinner than the vermian cleft in a Dandy-Walker variant[18] (see Fig. 47-9).

Evaluation of posterior fossa anatomic developmental stages has greatly improved with MRI of the fetal brain and may be necessary to diagnose a Dandy-Walker malformation confidently. Without confirming findings, however, this diagnosis should be approached cautiously because it may be a normal variant.[43-45]

Cisterna Magna

Cisterna magna septa are typically seen inferior and posterior to the cerebellar vermis, usually straight and parallel (see Fig. 47-9). These septa arise at the cerebellovermian angle and continue to the occipital bone. Robinson and Goldstein[46] propose that these septa are a remnant of Blake's pouch cysts and thus a marker of normal cerebellar development.[47,48]

CONGENITAL BRAIN MALFORMATIONS

Congenital brain malformations are the most common anomalies in humans.[42,49,50] Malformations can be classified based on brain development and the types of anomalies that result when development is altered.

Brain development can be divided into three stages.[51] **Cytogenesis** involves the formation of cells from molecules. **Histogenesis** is the formation of cells into tissues and involves neuronal proliferation and differentiation. **Organogenesis** is the formation of tissues into organs.

Organogenesis can be subdivided into further stages[52] (Fig. 47-19). The first stage, **neural tube formation and closure**, occurs at 3 to 4 weeks' gestation. The neural plate folds in on itself, fusing dorsally and giving rise to the earliest recognizable brain and spinal cord. In the next stage, **segmentation and diverticulation** of the forebrain occur at approximately 5 to 6 weeks. The single central fetal ventricle separates into two lateral ventricles, and the brain divides into two cerebral hemispheres. Anterior diverticulation results in the formation of the olfactory bulbs, optic vesicles, and the induction of facial development. The pituitary and pineal gland also develop by diverticulation from the ventricle at this stage.

CONGENITAL BRAIN MALFORMATIONS

DISORDERS OF ORGANOGENESIS
Disorders of Neural Tube Closure
Chiari malformations
Agenesis of the corpus callosum
Lipoma of the corpus callosum
Dandy-Walker malformation/variant
Posterior fossa arachnoid cyst
Teratoma

Disorders of Diverticulation and Cleavage
Septo-optic dysplasia
Holoprosencephaly (alobar, semilobar, lobar)

Disorders of Sulcation/Cellular Migration
Lissencephaly
Schizencephaly
Heterotopias
Pachymicrogyria or polymicrogyria

DISORDERS OF SIZE

DISORDERS OF MYELINATION

DESTRUCTIVE LESIONS

DISORDERS OF HISTOGENESIS
Neurocutaneous Syndromes (Phakomatoses)
Tuberous Sclerosis
Neurofibromatosis

Congenital Vascular Malformations

DISORDERS OF CYTOGENESIS
Congenital neoplasms

Modified from DeMyer classification of anomalies.[22-24]

STAGES OF BRAIN DEVELOPMENT*

Cytogenesis: Development of molecules into cells.
Histogenesis: Development of cells into tissues.
Organogenesis: Development of tissues into organs.
   Neural tube closure (dorsal induction: 3-4 weeks' gestation)
   Diverticulation (ventral induction: 5-6 weeks' gestation)
   Neuronal proliferation (8-16 weeks' gestation)
   Neuronal migration (24 weeks' gestation to years)
   Organization (6 months' gestation to years after birth)
   Myelination (birth to years after birth)

Modified from Volpe JJ. *Neurology of the newborn.* 5th ed. Philadelphia, 2008, Saunders-Elsevier.
   *Stages overlap in time but may be individually abnormal.

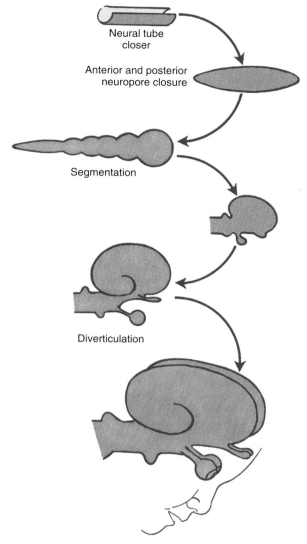

FIGURE 47-19. Stages of organogenesis. The neural tube closes at 3 to 4 weeks' gestation, including closure of the anterior and posterior neuropores. At 5 to 6 weeks, the brain segments and five types of diverticula form. First, the paired olfactory tracts, optic tracts, and cerebral ventricles develop, then the unpaired pineal and pituitary. Neural proliferation, migration, organization, and myelination occur after these stages. (*From DeMyer W. Classification of cerebral malformations. Birth Defects Orig Artic Ser 1971;7:78-93.*)

Neuronal proliferation and migration occur at 8 to 24 weeks' gestation. Tremendous cellular proliferation is necessary to provide a growing brain with the necessary building blocks to form properly. Finally, millions of cells must migrate into the organized functional structure that is recognized as a normal brain. The germinal matrix is a source of many of the migrating cells and eventually disappears as they migrate out. **Myelination** occurs from approximately the second trimester to adulthood but is most active from directly after birth until approximately 2 years of age.[49,50] Migration and myelination defects are best evaluated by MRI and well described by Barkovich.[31] MRI has greatly increased our understanding of brain development, and many genetic and environmental factors may interfere with normal development.

Destructive lesions can occur at any point in brain development. Congenital malformations of the brain are often diagnosed in utero, and neonatal sonographic imaging may be needed to confirm or further evaluate the prenatal diagnosis. In most cases, MRI may be required to clarify the ultrasound findings. CT is rarely able to add value in premature infants because contrast of normal structures is obscured by large amounts of normal brain water. In general, MRI is preferred because it best demonstrates sulcal patterns, migrational anomalies, and abnormal myelination. Disorders of cerebellar growth and development are now better understood with major advances in fetal MR neuroimaging and with major advances in genetics. Limperopoulos and du Plessis[53] discuss cerebellar development in a detailed review. Patel and Barkovich[54] describe a revised classification of cerebellar malformations that updates molecular biology findings with recent MRI discoveries.

DISORDERS OF NEURAL TUBE CLOSURE

Chiari Malformations

There are three classic Chiari malformations. **Chiari I** malformation is simply the downward displacement of the cerebellar tonsils, without displacement of the fourth ventricle or medulla. **Chiari II** malformation is the most common and of greatest clinical importance because of its almost universal association with myelomeningocele. **Chiari III** malformation is a high cervical encephalomeningocele in which the medulla, fourth ventricle, and virtually the entire cerebellum reside.

Classic sonographic findings of the Chiari II malformation involve the entire brain. Present theories propose that a failure in neural tube closure results in a small posterior fossa.[31,55] In early brain development, abnormal neural tube closure may result in a spinal defect such as a myelomeningocele. This decompresses the ventricles and leads to underdevelopment of the posterior fossa bony structures. The intracranial findings are the result of the small posterior fossa.[56-59] The tentorial attachment is low, and the combined effect causes compression of the upper cerebellum by the tentorium. The inferior cerebellum is compressed and displaced into the foramen magnum. The cerebellar tonsils and vermis herniate into the spinal canal through an enlarged foramen magnum. The pons and medulla are inferiorly displaced, as is the elongated fourth ventricle (Figs. 47-20 and 47-21; **Video 47-1**).

CHIARI II MALFORMATION: SONOGRAPHIC FINDINGS

Anterior and inferior pointed frontal horns
    Batwing configuration
Enlarged lateral ventricles with occipital horns
    larger than frontal horns
    Colpocephaly
Third ventricle appearing only slightly enlarged
    Enlarged massa intermedia fills third ventricle.
Elongation and caudal displacement of fourth
    ventricle, pons, medulla, and vermis
Nonvisualized fourth ventricle because of
    compression
Partial absence of septum pellucidum
Interhemispheric fissure
    Wide, especially after shunting
    Interdigitation of gyri causes serrated appearance.

There is usually marked **enlargement of the massa intermedia** on the coronal and midline sagittal ultrasound images. Although the third ventricle is often enlarged and the aqueduct is kinked, the enlarged massa intermedia often fills the third ventricle, causing it to appear only slightly larger than normal. The fourth ventricle is often not visualized because it is thin, elongated, compressed, and displaced into the upper spinal canal. The frontal horns are typically small and pointed, with the posterior horns of the lateral ventricles often disproportionately large, in a configuration similar to fetal ventricles called **colpocephaly.** The corpus callosum is usually absent. If only partial absence of the corpus callosum occurs, the ventricles may not be parallel, as typical of complete agenesis. The **anterior and inferior pointing of the frontal horns** has often been referred to as a **"bat wing"** configuration (Figs. 47-20 to 47-24; **Videos 47-2** and **47-3**). The septum pellucidum may be completely or partially absent (Fig. 47-24). The interhemispheric fissure usually appears to be widened on coronal images, particularly after shunting (Fig. 47-22). There may also be **gyral interdigitation** (Fig. 47-23). The posterior fossa is usually small, and the tentorium appears relatively low and hypoplastic. Hydrocephalus resulting from the Chiari II malformation is frequently mild in utero and becomes more severe at birth after repair of the myelomeningocele and the tethered cord **(Video 47-4).** When CSF circulation can no longer decompress into the myelomeningocele after the repair, hydrocephalus typically worsens. Neonatal screening for hydrocephalus will be best done routinely about 2 days after the myelomeningocele repair, as the ventricles may appear undilated before this event. Ultrasound diagnosis of **craniolacunia** (lacuna skull, lückenschädel) may be seen on sonography. Lacunar skull is a dysplasia that is often present at birth in the Chiari II malformation. The lacunar skull has a wavy, irregular appearance of the

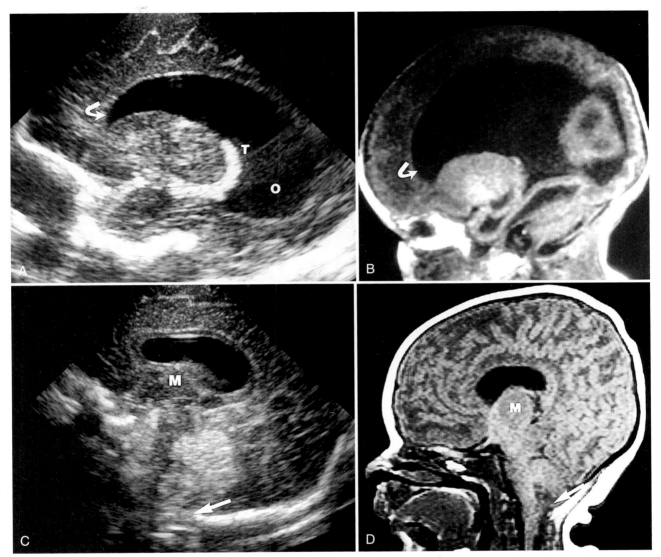

FIGURE 47-20. Chiari II malformation. A, Lateral parasagittal sonogram, and **B,** MR image, show pointing of frontal horn *(curved arrow)* and colpocephaly; *O,* occipital horn; *T,* trigone of lateral ventricle. **C,** Midline sagittal sonogram, and **D,** midline sagittal MR image, show enlargement of massa intermedia *(M)* and tonsillar herniation through foramen magnum *(arrow). (From Rumack CM, Manco-Johnson ML.* Perinatal and infant brain imaging: role of ultrasound and computed tomography. *St Louis, 1984, Mosby.)*

inner calvarium.[9] Craniolacunia will disappear over the first year of life even without shunting.

Routine prenatal screening for maternal serum alpha-fetoprotein (MS-AFP), which is elevated with neural tube defects, and the widespread use of sonography in pregnancy allow for the prenatal diagnosis of most Chiari malformations[60] (see Fig. 47-22). Because of its classic appearance, the Chiari II brain malformation is often recognized in utero and alerts the sonographer to look closely for a myelomeningocele. In less than 2% of myelomeningoceles, the neural tube defect is covered by skin, so there is no elevation of MS-AFP and there may be no Chiari II malformation (Fig. 47-25). Sonography or CT is reliable for follow-up of shunting procedures. MRI may be necessary to evaluate infants with symptoms suggesting brainstem compression because this may require decompression of the foramen magnum.

Agenesis of Corpus Callosum

The corpus callosum forms broad bands of connecting fibers between the cerebral hemispheres. Development of the corpus callosum occurs between the eighth and 20th week of gestation, beginning ventral and extending dorsal.[31,61,62] MR images from early fetuses show that the genu and anterior body develop first, and development proceeds both anteriorly to the rostrum and posteriorly to develop the splenium.[31,63] Therefore, depending on the timing of the intrauterine insult, development may be partially arrested, or complete agenesis may occur. If partial, the genu is usually present, and the dorsal splenium or the anterior rostrum is absent. Because an insult causing anomalies of the corpus callosum must occur early in development (8-20 weeks' gestation), other central nervous system (CNS) anomalies occur in up to

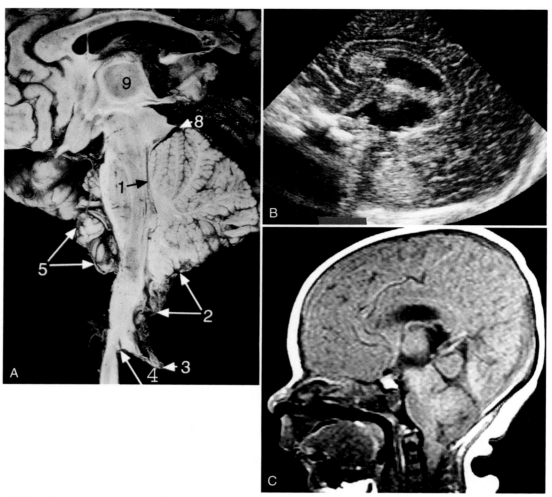

FIGURE 47-21. Classic Chiari II malformation. Midline sagittal images show large massa intermedia *(9)* and tonsillar herniation *(2)*. **A,** Pathology specimen; *1,* compressed fourth ventricle. **B,** Sonogram. **C,** MR image. *(From Osborn AG. Diagnostic neuroradiology. St Louis, 1994, Mosby.)*

80% of cases.[27,63] These associated anomalies include **Chiari II** and **Dandy-Walker** malformations, **holoprosencephaly, encephaloceles, lipomas, arachnoid cysts, migrational abnormalities,** and **Aicardi syndrome** (female infants with agenesis of the corpus callosum, ocular abnormalities, and infantile spasms). If the corpus callosum is absent, MRI will be valuable either in utero or at birth to delineate associated findings that may cause a poor prognosis and change patient management.[31,64,65] Isolated agenesis of the corpus callosum may have a normal prognosis. However, Barkovich[31] reports symptomatic patients with absence of the corpus callosum typically present with seizures, microcephaly, delayed development, mental retardation or hypothalamic dysfunction.

The key diagnostic clues to agenesis of the corpus callosum on sonography are the widely spaced, parallel-oriented lateral ventricles that have extremely narrow, often slitlike frontal horns[62] (Fig. 47-26). Coronally, the frontal horns and ventricular bodies have sharply angled, lateral peaks. There may be relative enlargement of the

occipital horns (colpocephaly) and often, enlarged temporal horns (Fig. 47-27). **Probst bundles,** longitudinal callosal fibers that failed to decussate or cross to the other cerebral hemisphere, bulge into the ventricles along the superomedial aspect of the lateral ventricles (see Figs. 47-23 and 47-25). These are best seen on coronal images as the concave medial border to the lateral ventricles. There is no septum pellucidum. The third ventricle is dilated and elevated; its roof extends superiorly between the lateral ventricles and into the interhemispheric fissure and may be associated with a dorsal midline cyst (Fig. 47-28). The medial cerebral sulci are typically radially arranged, perpendicular to the expected course of the corpus callosum, causing a **"sunburst" sign** on sagittal midline images (Fig. 47-29). The pericallosal sulcus is missing, and the cingulate sulcus is absent or present only as unconnected segments. Because agenesis of the corpus callosum has additional brain anomalies in more than 75% of patients, further evaluation with postnatal MRI is indicated. **Cerebellar hypoplasia, gyral anomalies,** and **heterotopia** are seen most often on fetal MRI.[27]

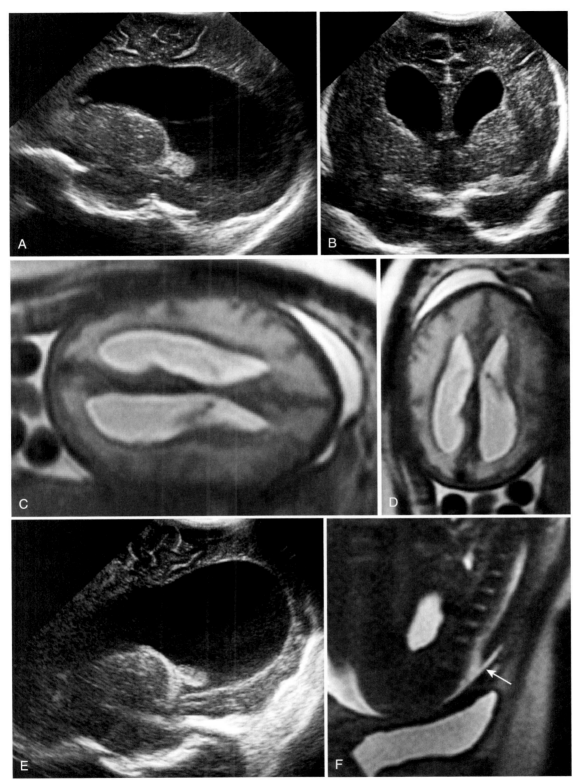

FIGURE 47-22. Chiari II malformation: neonatal ultrasound and fetal MRI comparison. A and **B,** Sagittal and coronal sonograms show typical pointed frontal horns with large occipital horns (called **colpocephaly**), but these frontal horns are not as thin as when the entire corpus callosum is absent. Low-level echoes from intraventricular hemorrhage during birth. Fetal ultrasound did not visualize the spinal defect because of a breech position. **C** to **F,** Fetal T2-weighted MR scans. **C,** Axial view, and **D,** axial view turned 90 degrees, show typical pointed frontal horns and hydrocephalus. **E,** Posterior fontanelle view of the huge occipital horn at birth shows the unusually large shape more clearly than the axial views, which only demonstrate the lateral width and do not display as well the posterior dilation laterally. **F,** Sagittal view shows the small spinal defect *(arrow)* missed on fetal ultrasound.

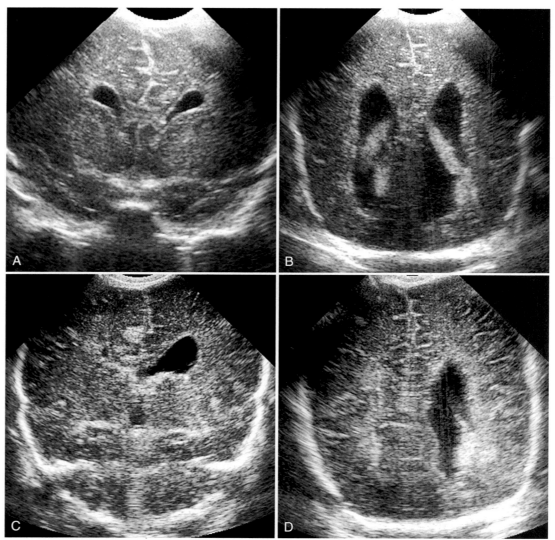

FIGURE 47-23. Chiari II and absent corpus callosum. A and **B,** Anterior and posterior coronal ultrasound scans show widely separated ventricles and thin frontal horns typical of absence of the corpus callosum, with pointing of the ventricles seen in both anomalies. Gyral interdigitation is best seen before shunting in this patient. **C** and **D,** Anterior and posterior coronal ultrasound scans show Chiari II after ventriculoperitoneal shunting for hydrocephalus. The right lateral ventricle is much smaller, typical of the side with the shunt. Interhemispheric widening is present often after shunts are placed.

AGENESIS OF CORPUS CALLOSUM: SONOGRAPHIC FINDINGS

Absent corpus callosum
Absent cingulate gyrus and sulcus
Radial arrangement of medial sulci above third
  ventricle ("sunburst" sign)
Widely spaced, parallel lateral ventricles
Extremely narrow frontal horns (slitlike)
Concave or straight medial borders secondary to
  Probst bundles
Colpocephaly (dilated atria and occipital horns)
Elevated third ventricle extending between lateral
  ventricles, continuous with interhemispheric
  fissure, with or without dorsal cyst
Absent septum pellucidum

Corpus Callosum Lipoma

Maldevelopment of embryonic neural crest tissues may result in lipomas of the interhemispheric fissure. These lipomas have no mass effect and thus do not require surgery. Corpus callosum lipomas account for 30% to 50% of intracranial lipomas and are associated with dysgenesis of the corpus callosum[31,61] (Fig. 47-30).

Dandy-Walker Malformation

Dandy-Walker malformation presents as a dilated fourth ventricle in direct communication with the cisterna magna (Fig. 47-31, *A* and *B*). The posterior fossa is enlarged, with elevation of the tentorium cerebelli, straight sinus, and torcula herophili at the venous sinus

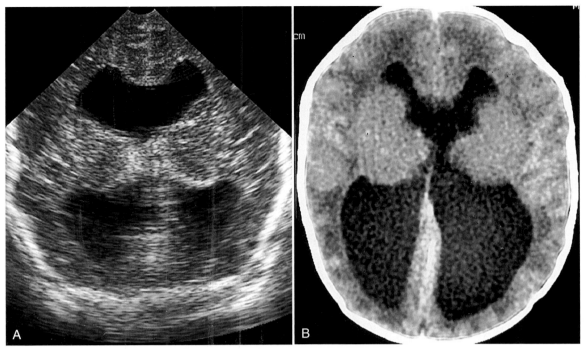

FIGURE 47-24. Chiari II and absence of septum pellucidum. A, Coronal sonogram, and **B,** CT scan, show continuity between frontal horns resulting from absence of the septum pellucidum.

confluence. The vermis of the cerebellum is hypoplastic to absent, and the cerebellar hemispheres are variably hypoplastic and displaced laterally by the enlarged fourth ventricle. The brainstem may be compressed anteriorly or hypoplastic. **Generalized obstructive hydrocephalus** occurs in up to 80% of cases. If there is also agenesis of the corpus callosum (Fig. 47-31, *C-F*), colpocephaly (fetal-like ventricles) is typically present.[10,61,66]

DANDY-WALKER MALFORMATION: SONOGRAPHIC FINDINGS

Enlarged fourth ventricle connects to Dandy-Walker cyst posteriorly
Large posterior fossa
Hypoplastic cerebellar vermis
Hypoplastic cerebellar hemispheres displaced laterally by fourth ventricle
Small brainstem
Hydrocephalus of ventricles (80%)
  Obstruction above and below fourth ventricle
Absent corpus callosum (70%)

The etiology of Dandy-Walker malformation is not definitively known. Theories include agenesis of the foramina of Luschka and Magendie in the first trimester, malformation of the roof of the fourth ventricle, and delayed opening of the foramen of Magendie.[31,61] The prenatal diagnosis of Dandy-Walker malformation, with differentiation from Dandy-Walker variant, a posterior fossa arachnoid cyst, and mega cisterna magna, is usually possible. Some severe cases may be diagnosed early, but typically, Dandy-Walker malformation is diagnosed after 17 weeks' gestation, when the inferior vermis has normally completely formed.[40,67-71]

The Dandy-Walker malformation is associated with other CNS anomalies in up to 70% of cases. These include partial or complete agenesis of the corpus callosum, encephalocele, holoprosencephaly, microcephaly, gray matter heterotopia, and gyral malformations. Chromosomal abnormalities are described in up to 20% to 50% of cases and include trisomy 13, 18, and 21. Other associated anomalies include: gastrointestinal, genitourinary, cardiac, musculoskeletal, and pulmonary malformations, including congenital diaphragmatic hernia and cystic hygroma.[59,66,67,71-73]

Therapy for the Dandy-Walker malformation includes ventriculoperitoneal shunting, which will decompress the lateral ventricles but may not decompress the posterior fossa cyst (see Fig. 47-30, *C*). The cyst may require a separate shunt for decompression. Sonography can be used to follow these procedures until the infant is approximately 18 months of age, but this method is rarely used after the first few months of life.

In **Dandy-Walker variant,** there again is variable hypoplasia of the posterior inferior vermis and communication between the fourth ventricle and cisterna magna (Fig. 47-32). The fourth ventricle is slightly to moderately enlarged. In the Dandy-Walker variant, the posterior fossa is normal in size, and although the vermis is small,

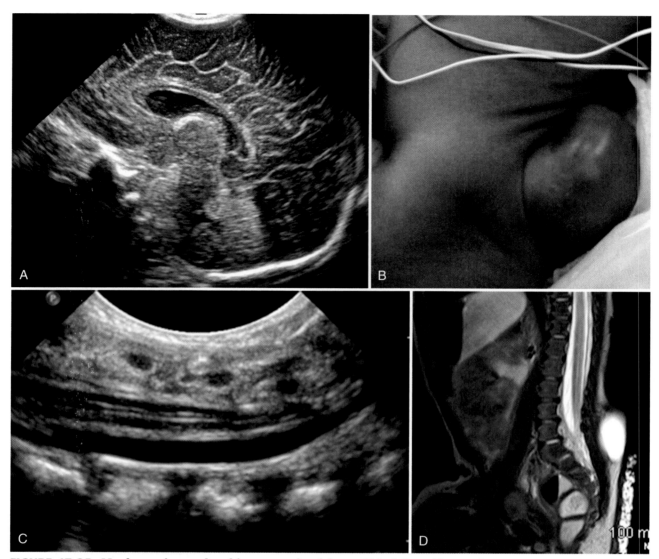

FIGURE 47-25. Myelomeningocele, skin covered, with no Chiari II malformation. A, Midline sagittal brain ultrasound, and **B,** photograph, of myelomeningocele. **C,** Sagittal spine ultrasound, and **D,** T2-weighted MRI, show tethered cord extending almost to the sacrum. With 98% of myelomeningoceles having a Chiari II malformation, only 2% are skin covered and may not have a Chiari malformation.

the cerebellar hemispheres are normal. There is no associated hydrocephalus. Mastoid fontanelle views should be taken in this setting through the fourth ventricle so that the normal foramen of Magendie and vallecula, which may be enlarged with hydrocephalus, are not mistaken for a Dandy-Walker variant (see Fig. 47-9, C). The Dandy-Walker variant typically has vermian hypoplasia, an enlarged 4th ventricle, a large aqueduct, and a large third ventricle.[18] Chromosomal abnormalities occur in up to 30% of these infants. Associated CNS or extra-CNS anomalies may impact the outcome of the infant more than the Dandy-Walker variant.[31,61,66,68,70]

Two differential diagnoses of posterior fossa cystic lesions mimic Dandy-Walker syndrome. A **mega cisterna magna** is a normal variant with no mass effect that is not associated with the development of hydrocephalus and has a normal cerebellar vermis, fourth ventricle, and

cerebellar hemisphere[61] (Fig. 47-33). A **posterior fossa subarachnoid cyst** can be differentiated from Dandy-Walker malformation or variant by the lack of communication of the cyst with the fourth ventricle. The normal fourth ventricle, vermis, and cerebellum are displaced by the arachnoid cyst.[69,72]

Complete agenesis of the cerebellar vermis without hydrocephalus occurs in **Joubert's syndrome,** with

POSTERIOR FOSSA CYSTIC LESIONS

Dandy-Walker syndrome
Mega cisterna magna
   Normal variant
Posterior fossa subarachnoid cyst
   Cyst does not connect with the fourth ventricle.

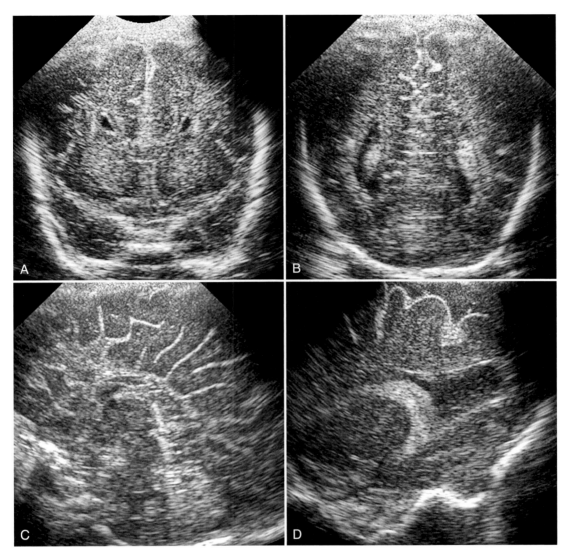

FIGURE 47-26. Agenesis of the corpus callosum, isolated anomaly. A, Tiny frontal horns are widely separated. **B,** Starburst sulci radiate above the third ventricle. **C** and **D,** Occipital horns are larger than frontal horns and widely separated.

associated symptoms including episodic hyperpnea, ataxia, abnormal eye movements, and mental retardation.[31,61] This anomaly is thought to be caused by the inability of the posterior fossa axons to cross the midline.[74] There is a Meckel-like syndrome with Dandy-Walker malformation, polycystic kidneys, hepatic fibrosis, and hand and genital anomalies. True **Meckel-Gruber syndrome** includes an encephalocele, renal cystic dysplasia, short limbs, and polydactyly.[73]

DISORDERS OF DIVERTICULATION AND CLEAVAGE: HOLOPROSENCEPHALY

Holoprosencephaly results from a failure of diverticulation when the primitive prosencephalon does not divide into the telencephalon and the diencephalon between the fourth and eighth weeks of gestation. The telencephalon normally develops into the cerebral hemispheres, ventricles, putamen, and caudate nuclei. The diencephalon becomes the third ventricle, thalami, hypothalamus, and lateral globus pallidus. Holoprosencephaly represents a spectrum of malformations that form a continuum from most severe, with no separation of the telencephalon into hemispheres (**alobar** holoprosencephaly), to least severe, with partial separation of the dorsal aspects of the brain (**lobar** holoprosencephaly). The septum pellucidum is absent in all forms of holoprosencephaly (Fig. 47-34).

Septo-optic Dysplasia

Some consider the mildest form of lobar holoprosencephaly to be **septo-optic dysplasia**, with absence of the septum pellucidum and optic nerve hypoplasia (Fig. 47-35; **Video 47-5**). About two thirds of these infants

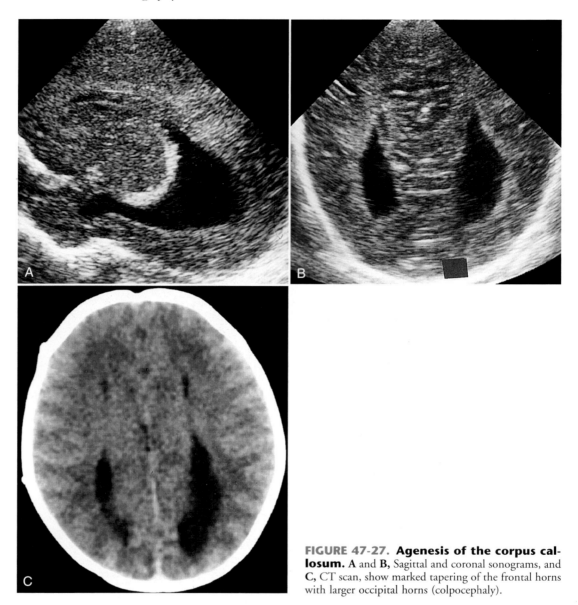

FIGURE 47-27. Agenesis of the corpus callosum. A and **B,** Sagittal and coronal sonograms, and **C,** CT scan, show marked tapering of the frontal horns with larger occipital horns (colpocephaly).

have hypothalamic-pituitary dysfunction. They may have visual symptoms and growth restriction. Besides presenting with holoprosencephaly, callosal agenesis, and Chiari I malformations, other associations suggest septo-optic dysplasia may occur from destructive processes that cause schizencephaly and chronic severe hydrocephalus.[31] Intermediate severity between alobar and lobar is **semi-lobar** holoprosencephaly, with fusion of the cortex and ventricle anteriorly but variable separation posteriorly; facial anomalies are mild or absent. Anomalies of the face and calvarium accompany and help predict the severity of the brain malformation, because the face develops at the same time as the brain during diverticulation. Cases of holoprosencephaly are usually suspected as a result of the accompanying facial anomalies, with more severe facial anomalies predicting more severe intracranial

anomalies. Holoprosencephaly is most frequently seen in **trisomy 13 and 18 syndromes** and can also be caused by **teratogens,** the most common mechanism in **infants of diabetic mothers.**[31,73-77]

Alobar Holoprosencephaly

Alobar holoprosencephaly is the most severe form of this disorder. Infants with this defect usually die within the first months of life or are stillborn. Facial features may include **cebocephaly** (Fig. 47-36, *D*), **cyclopia,** and **ethmocephaly** (cyclopia or hypotelorism with a midline proboscis above the eyes).[76] The brain surrounds a single midline horseshoe- or crescent-shaped ventricle with a surrounding thin, primitive cerebral cortex[72] (Fig. 47-36). The hemispheres are fused as a pancake-like

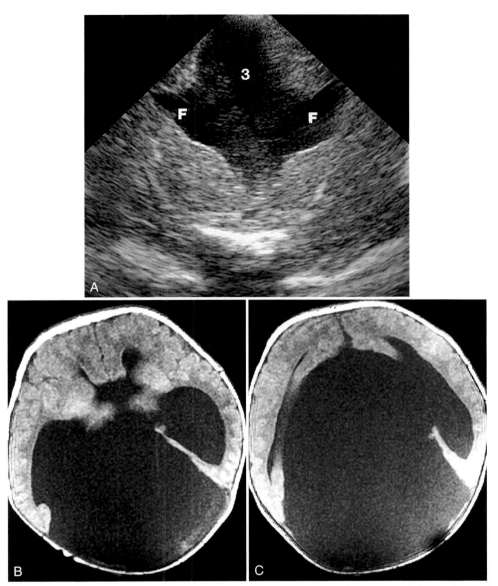

FIGURE 47-28. Agenesis of corpus callosum (ACC) with elevation of third ventricle and continuation into a large dorsal cyst. A, Coronal sonogram, and **B** and **C,** CT scans, show widely separated frontal horns, a large third ventricle that extends superiorly as a dorsal cyst between the lateral ventricles. ACC often has associated cysts. A central dorsal cyst extending above the midline is a classic appearance of ACC.

mass of tissue in the most anterior portion of the calvarium. Only in holoprosencephaly will the splenium of the corpus callosum be the only segment present.[31] The thalami are fused, and there is no falx, corpus callosum, or interhemispheric fissure between them. Midline, moderately echogenic, fused thalami are seen anterior to the fused, hyperechogenic choroid plexus. The third ventricle is usually absent, so the large, single, central holoventricle communicates inferiorly with the aqueduct and may also connect posteriorly with a dorsal cyst.[78] Pachygyria may be seen. Posterior fossa structures may be normal.

ALOBAR HOLOPROSENCEPHALY: SONOGRAPHIC FINDINGS

Single midline crescent-shaped ventricle
Thin layer of cerebral cortex
No falx
No interhemispheric fissure
No corpus callosum
Fused thalami and basal ganglia
Fused echogenic choroid plexus
Absent third ventricle
Large dorsal cyst

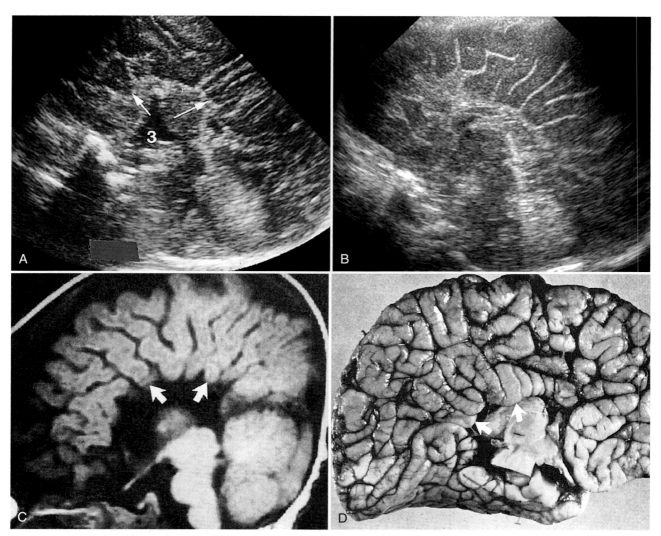

FIGURE 47-29. "Sunburst" or radial arrangement of sulci in agenesis of corpus callosum. A and **B,** Midline sagittal sonograms. **C,** Midline sagittal MR image. **D,** Sagittal pathologic specimen. Third ventricle *(3)* is elevated and lacks the normal parallel corpus callosum and cingulate sulcus. Arrows indicate radial array of sulci. *(**C** from Osborn AG. Diagnostic neuroradiology. St. Louis, 1994, Mosby;* **D** *from Friede R. Developmental neuropathology. 2nd ed. New York, 1975, Springer-Verlag.)*

Semilobar Holoprosencephaly

In semilobar holoprosencephaly, more brain parenchyma is present, but the single ventricle persists. There may be separate occipital and temporal horns. A small portion of the falx and interhemispheric fissure develops in the occipital cortex posteriorly. The splenium and genu of the corpus callosum are often formed and may be seen on midline sagittal sections. The thalami are partially separated, and the third ventricle is rudimentary. Facial anomalies are less severe than in alobar holoprosencephaly, usually with only mild hypotelorism and median or lateral cleft lip.

Lobar Holoprosencephaly

Lobar holoprosencephaly is the least severe form of this disorder. There is almost complete separation of hemispheres, with development of a falx and interhemispheric fissure, but these may be shallow anteriorly, and the frontal lobes are fused. The septum pellucidum is absent. The anterior horns of the lateral ventricles are fused and square shaped, but the occipital horns are separated. Temporal horns may be present. The third ventricle is usually present, separating the thalami. The splenium and body of the corpus callosum are often present, with absence of the genu and rostrum. Facial anomalies are mild and similar to the semilobar form or absent.

DISORDERS OF SULCATION AND CELLULAR MIGRATION

Schizencephaly

Believed to be caused by a primary neuronal migration malformation in utero, schizencephaly has been reported

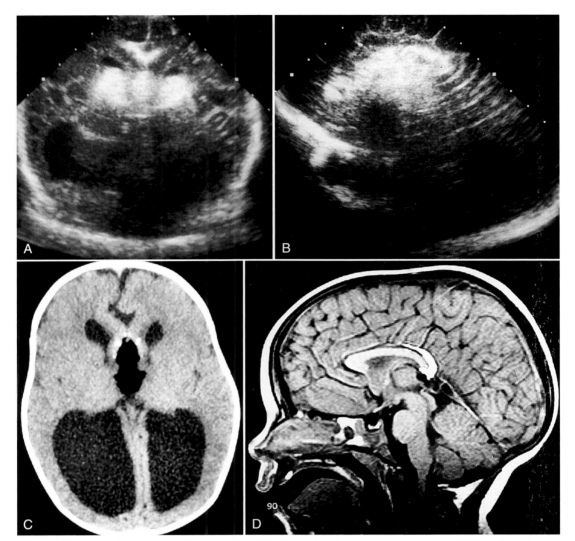

FIGURE 47-30. Lipoma of corpus callosum. A and **B,** Coronal and sagittal sonograms show highly echogenic fat surrounded by calcification; both are causing major acoustic shadowing. **C,** CT scan shows black central fat surrounded by white flecks of calcium. **D,** Sagittal MR scan shows fat (bright white on T1-weighted image) extending over the corpus callosum.

in familial cases and in early prenatal injury from drug abuse and abdominal trauma.[79] It causes gray matter–lined clefts that extend through the entire hemisphere, from the ependymal lining of the lateral ventricles to the pial covering of the cortex. The clefts may be bilateral or unilateral (Fig. 47-37, *A* and *B*). There may be wide openings of the clefts (**open-lip** schizencephaly). In some cases the cleft is closed (**closed-lip** schizencephaly) (Fig. 47-37, *C* and *D*) and may require MRI for diagnosis, because gray matter–white matter differentiation is not well demonstrated on sonography. Most of these patients develop seizures, hemiparesis, and variable developmental delay. The severity is related to the amount of brain involved. Some patients have blindness, thought to be associated with absence of the septum pellucidum and associated optic nerve hypoplasia, which may be associated. This is thought to be an acquired septo-optic dysplasia. There are genetic cases from the EMX2 Homeobox gene[31] and other patients with possible in utero injury

during the second trimester. **Cytomegalovirus** has been reported to cause schizencephaly in some patients.[80,81] In patients with unilateral involvement, recent reports show functional reorganization of the motor area so that the unaffected hemisphere takes over function.[82]

Lissencephaly

Complete lack of sulcal formation caused by lissencephaly is a difficult diagnosis on ultrasound. Some have studied the lack of opercularization in lissencephaly.[30,33]

DESTRUCTIVE LESIONS

Porencephalic Cyst

Before 26 weeks' gestation, focal brain destruction will typically heal with dysplastic gray matter and result

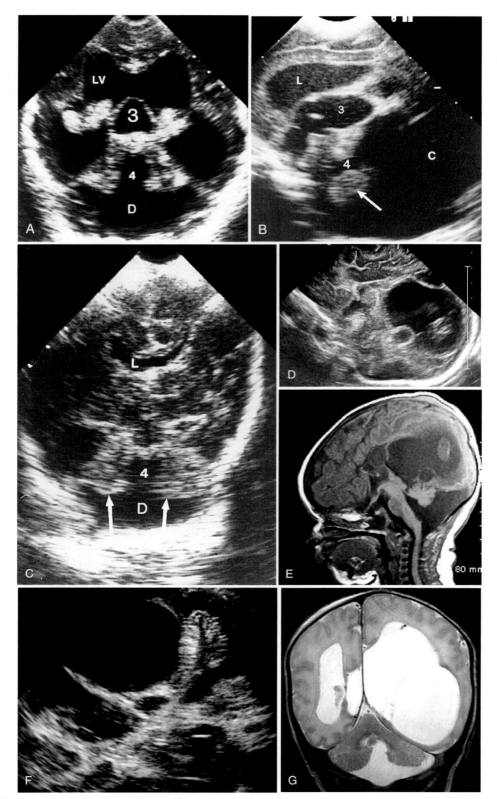

FIGURE 47-31. Dandy-Walker malformation: classic isolated malformation. A and **B,** Coronal and sagittal sonograms. *C,* Dandy-Walker posterior fossa cyst; *3,* third ventricle; *4,* fourth ventricle; *L* and *LV,* dilated lateral ventricles. Internal echoes in the ventricles represent blood in the cerebrospinal fluid. **C,** Coronal ultrasound shows Dandy-Walker malformation after ventriculoperitoneal shunt. Lateral and third ventricles have decompressed, but Dandy Walker cyst *(D)* remains dilated. Frequently, posterior fossa cysts require additional shunts for decompression. **D** to **G,** Fetal brain infection caused ventriculitis and hydrocephalus in term infant with absence of the corpus callosum, classic cerebellar vermian hypoplasia, and a posterior fossa cyst continuous with the fourth ventricle; septations in the temporal horn also caused a temporal lobe cyst. **D,** Sagittal ultrasound; **E,** sagittal T1-weighted MRI; **F,** axial ultrasound; **G,** coronal T2-weighted MRI.

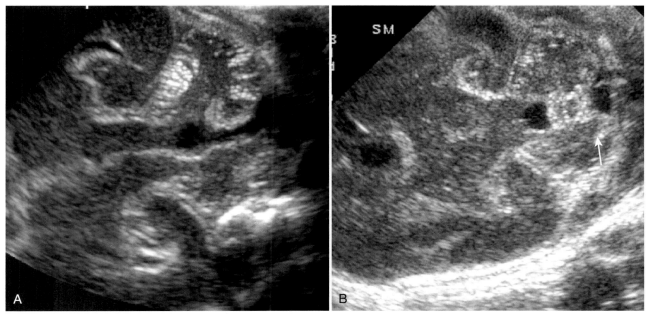

FIGURE 47-32. Dandy-Walker variant compared to normal posterior fossa. A, Axial posterior fossa ultrasound shows a wide continuity between the fourth ventricle and the cisterna magna, where the cerebellar vermis is hypoplastic and separated behind the fourth ventricle. **B,** Normal axial ultrasound of fourth ventricle covered by echogenic cerebellar vermis.

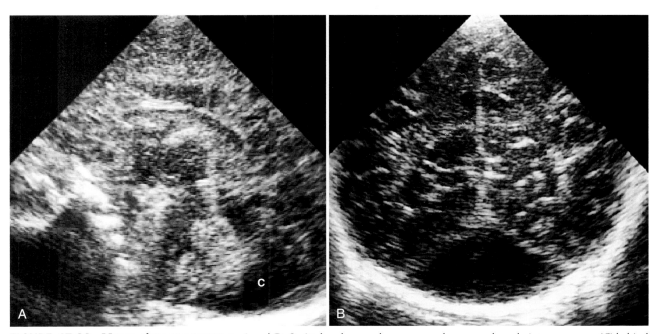

FIGURE 47-33. Mega cisterna magna. A and **B,** Sagittal and coronal sonograms show an enlarged cisterna magna *(C)* behind the vermis on **A** and below the tentorium on **B,** with no communication to the fourth ventricle and no hydrocephalus.

in schizencephaly, usually associated with migrational defects.[42] After 26 weeks' gestation, a porencephalic cyst will develop in an area of normally developed brain that has been damaged and heals with scarring because of a lining of gliotic white matter. By definition, porencephalic cysts always connect with the ventricular system but do not extend to the surface cortex. They usually occur after birth secondary to intraparenchymal hemorrhage (IPH), infection (focal vasculitis, abscess), or trauma.

Hydranencephaly

Classically, hydranencephaly is believed to be caused by bilateral occlusion of the internal carotid arteries during fetal development, but it may result from any of several

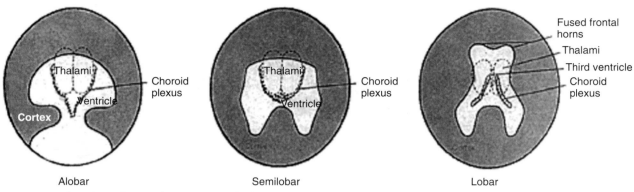

FIGURE 47-34. Holoprosencephaly. Three common types are alobar (most severe), semilobar, and lobar.

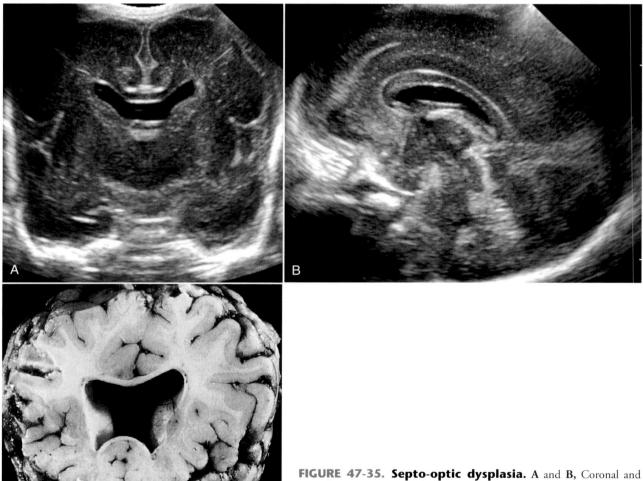

FIGURE 47-35. Septo-optic dysplasia. A and B, Coronal and sagittal sonograms; C, pathology specimen. Although the cavum septum pellucidum is absent, the corpus callosum is present.

intracranial destructive processes (Fig. 47-38). Hydran-encephaly is the severest form of porencephaly in that there is almost total destruction of the cerebral cortex.[83,84] These infants may appear surprisingly normal at birth but are developmentally delayed from an early age and frequently die within the first year of life.

The sonographic findings include a calvarium filled with CSF, but little else (Fig. 47-38). Structures that receive their blood supply from the posterior cerebral artery and vertebral artery, such as the thalamus, cerebellum, brainstem, and posterior choroid plexus, are spared and are usually identifiable. Blood flow will not be

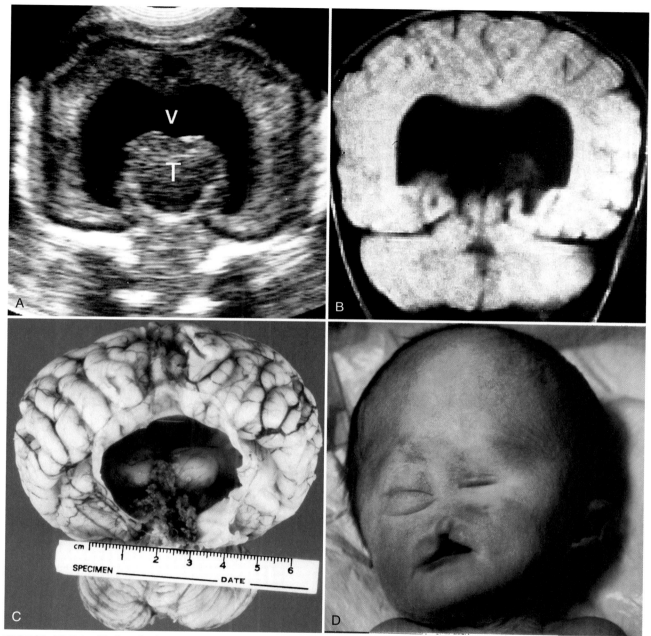

FIGURE 47-36. Alobar holoprosencephaly. A, Coronal sonogram shows single central ventricle *(V)* and fused thalami *(T)*. No falx or interhemispheric fissure is present. **B,** MR image, and **C,** pathology specimen, show single central ventricle and fused thalami. **D,** Autopsy specimen shows **cebocephaly** (severe hypotelorism and malformed nose).

appreciated by color or spectral Doppler in the carotid arteries. An incomplete or complete falx may be identifiable even in utero. The presence of the falx helps differentiate this lesion from alobar holoprosencephaly, in which the falx does not form. It can be difficult to differentiate hydranencephaly from severe hydrocephalus, but a thin rim of cortex should be visualized by sonography in hydrocephalus.[83,84] If there is an enlarging head circumference, ventriculoperitoneal shunting may be indicated, regardless of the actual diagnosis to control growth.

Cystic Encephalomalacia

Encephalomalacia is an area of focal brain damage that pathologically has astrocytic proliferation and glial septations. In diffuse brain damage, there may be large areas of cystic encephalomalacia (Fig. 47-39). The location of the damage depends on the type of insult. Typically, there is no connection to the ventricular system. In neonates, infection or anoxia can cause widespread damage, whereas a thrombus may cause focal damage.

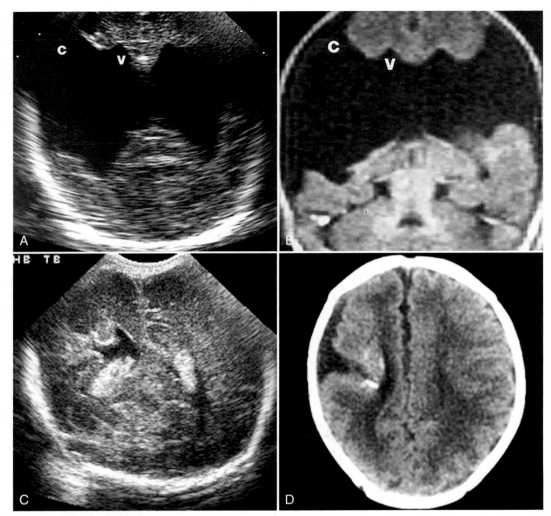

FIGURE 47-37. Schizencephaly. A, Coronal sonogram, and **B,** coronal MR image, of open-lip schizencephaly show bilateral clefts *(c)* with wide openings to the ventricular *(v)* system. **C,** Sonogram, and **D,** CT image, show closed-lip schizencephaly with calcification from in utero infection.

Metabolic Disorders

A wide range of abnormalities are seen on neonatal brain ultrasound in metabolic disorders,[85] including cysts, calcifications, structural brain abnormalities, and white matter echogenicity.

HYDROCEPHALUS

Hydrocephalus occurs in 5% to 25% per 10,000 births and results from an imbalance between CSF production and its drainage by the arachnoid villi. Three mechanisms account for the development of hydrocephalus: obstruction to CSF outflow, decreased CSF absorption, or CSF overproduction (e.g., choroid plexus tumor).

Cerebrospinal Fluid Production and Circulation

Cerebrospinal fluid provides a chemically controlled protective environment that continually bathes and circulates around the CNS. Although mainly produced by the choroid plexus, CSF it is also produced by the ventricular ependyma, the intracranial subarachnoid lining, and the spinal subarachnoid lining. CSF normally flows from the lateral ventricles, through the foramina of Monro, third ventricle, aqueduct of Sylvius, fourth ventricle, lateral foramina of Luschka or medial foramen of Magendie, and into the basal cisterns. From there, a small quantity circulates down into the spinal subarachnoid space. CSF flows upward around the brain anteriorly and posteriorly to reach the vertex, where it is resorbed by the arachnoid granulations into the superior sagittal sinus.

Diagnosis

Hydrocephalus often can be diagnosed in utero by 15 weeks' gestation.[86-88] The size of the atrium of the ventricle and the glomus of the choroid plexus remains constant in the second and third trimesters in the transaxial plane. In utero an upper limit of 10 mm for

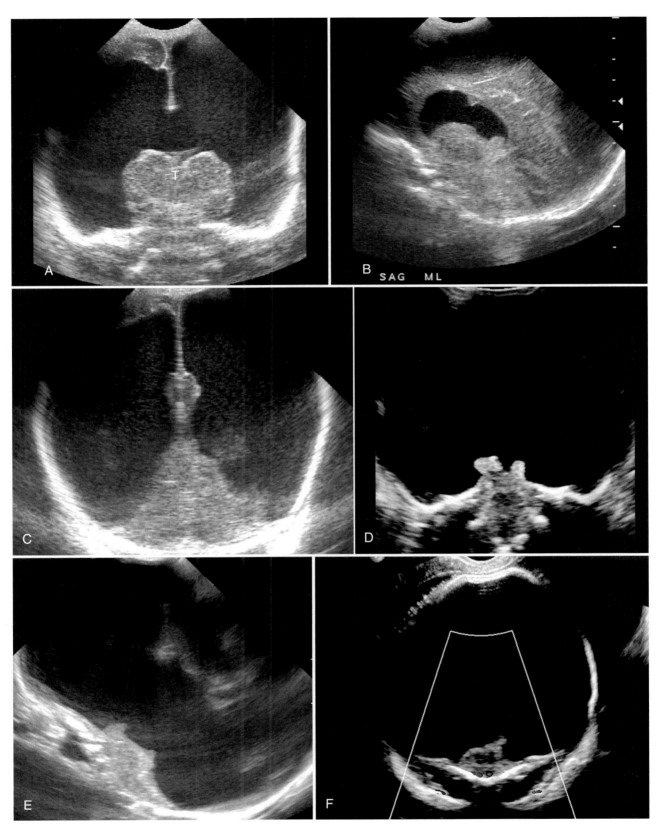

FIGURE 47-38. Hydranencephaly in two full-term newborns. A, Coronal anterior; **B,** midline sagittal; and **C,** coronal posterior sonograms. Note that only anechoic cerebrospinal fluid is seen above thalamus *(T)*, which at first looks like holoprosencephaly, but the definitive diagnosis is made because there is a falx seen in the midline on all three views. Note the echogenic falx on the midline view. **D, E,** and **F,** Coronal, sagittal, and color Doppler ultrasound views show a thin remnant of cerebral cortex posteriorly. Thalami are absent; only remnants of brainstem persist. **F,** Color Doppler image shows complete absence of the normal anterior and middle cerebral arteries. Both patients had difficulty with temperature control and swallowing at birth. Facial features were unremarkable.

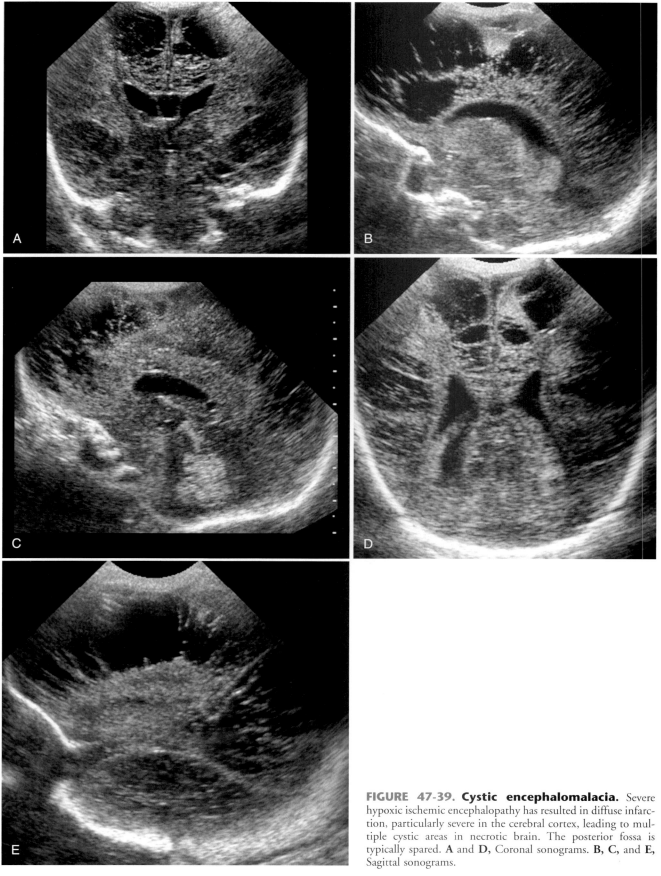

FIGURE 47-39. Cystic encephalomalacia. Severe hypoxic ischemic encephalopathy has resulted in diffuse infarction, particularly severe in the cerebral cortex, leading to multiple cystic areas in necrotic brain. The posterior fossa is typically spared. **A** and **D**, Coronal sonograms. **B, C,** and **E,** Sagittal sonograms.

the ventricular atrium has been established and well reviewed.[89-91] Once hydrocephalus is recognized, close inspection for spinal dysraphism and other CNS or extra-CNS anomalies is warranted because these findings will affect outcome. Chromosome evaluation is necessary if other anomalies are recognized.[92] Hydrocephalus diagnosed in utero has a variable course, making counseling of the family difficult. Often, especially if other severe anomalies or chromosome abnormalities are diagnosed, the family chooses to terminate the pregnancy. Signs of the Chiari II malformation should be especially sought because this is associated with a myelomeningocele in almost 100% of cases.

Neonatal hydrocephalus is easily recognized by routine coronal and sagittal imaging.[8,89-91] Ventricular size is slightly larger in newborns than in older children. Progression of hydrocephalus can best be estimated by comparison with previous studies. Sonography is also helpful in following ventricular decompression in patients shunted for hydrocephalus. In following ventricular size in cases of hydrocephalus, care must be taken so that changes in ultrasound sector depth do not result in apparent enlargement or decompression of the ventricles related to magnification differences when different depth scales are used. Failure to do so may result in a false impression of changing hydrocephalus.

Level of Obstruction

Asymmetry of the lateral ventricles can cause a ventricle to be slightly larger as a normal variant. The entire ventricular system should be evaluated to identify the level at which a transition occurs from a large to a small ventricle.[93] Dilation of the lateral and third ventricles indicates an aqueduct of Sylvius obstruction, most often caused by intraventricular hemorrhage (IVH) and often a linked recessive trait. The rare case of isolated dilation of the fourth ventricle also requires ventricular system evaluation. Dilation of all ventricles should lead to an extraventricular source.

Doppler ultrasound has been used to evaluate neonatal hydrocephalus in a few cases to assess (indirectly) intracranial pressure and help determine the need for shunt placement.[94] Taylor et al.[95] report the use of sonographic contrast agents in neonatal hydrocephalus. In animal models, injecting contrast through ventricular catheters allowed direct visualization of ventricular patency. Although currently experimental, this may be an excellent method to study hydrocephalus in patients with catheters.

Etiology

Hydrocephalus can result from **intraventricular obstruction,** when CSF flow is obstructed within the ventricular system, or from **extraventricular obstruction** to CSF circulation, which occurs within the subarachnoid spaces

and cisterns or is secondary to decreased CSF absorption at the arachnoid villi in the sagittal sinus. **Overproduction** of CSF from a choroid plexus papilloma is an unusual cause. Other causes include venous obstruction or vascular malformations; vein of Galen malformation often obstructs. The most common causes of **intraventricular obstructive hydrocephalus** (IVOH) include infection or hemorrhage (causing obstruction to the exiting foramina of the third or fourth ventricle), congenital anomalies (e.g., aqueductal stenosis (Fig. 47-40), Dandy-Walker malformation) (see Fig. 47-31), and tumors. Aqueductal stenosis presents in males from an X-linked gene (L1-CAM) and may be diagnosed by about 18 weeks of gestation with hydrocephalus and adducted thumbs.[96] The most common causes of **extraventricular obstructive hydrocephalus** (EVOH) are hemorrhage and infection with fibrosis at the basal cisterns, incisura, convexity cisterns, or parasagittal region.

CAUSES OF HYDROCEPHALUS

INTRAVENTRICULAR OBSTRUCTION
Posthemorrhagic
   Aqueductal obstruction
   Fourth ventricle obstruction
Posterior fossa subdural hematoma
Chiari II malformation
Dandy-Walker malformation
Aqueductal stenosis
Postinfectious scarring
Vein of Galen malformation
Tumor or cyst

EXTRAVENTRICULAR OBSTRUCTION
Posthemorrhagic scarring
Postinfectious scarring
Achondroplasia
Absence or hypoplasia of arachnoid granulations
Venous obstruction

OVERPRODUCTION OF CSF
Choroid plexus papilloma

CSF, Cerebrospinal fluid.

Ventricular enlargement does not always mean obstruction. Severe cases of **hypoxic-ischemic injury** result in large ventricles due to brain atrophy 2 to 4 weeks after the insult rather than obstructive hydrocephalus. One rare cause of ventricular enlargement is **glutaric aciduria type 1.**[97] These patients actually have macrocephaly at birth or within the first few weeks of life. Cystlike bilateral widening of the sylvian fissures may be the first sign, followed by progressive frontotemporal subarachnoid and ventricular enlargement, thought to be caused by atrophy. If glutaric aciduria is

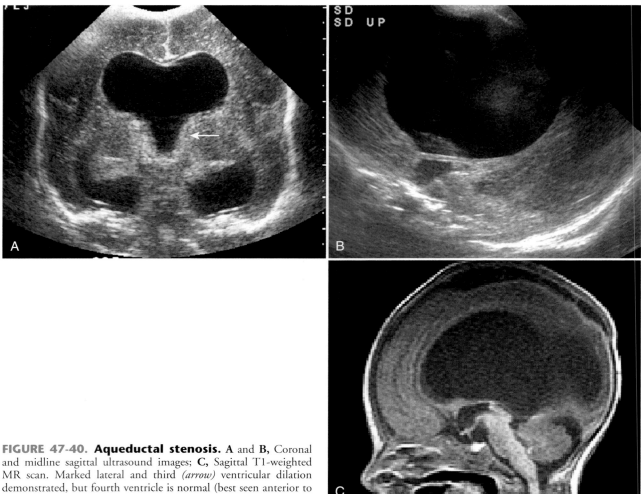

FIGURE 47-40. Aqueductal stenosis. A and **B,** Coronal and midline sagittal ultrasound images; **C,** Sagittal T1-weighted MR scan. Marked lateral and third *(arrow)* ventricular dilation demonstrated, but fourth ventricle is normal (best seen anterior to the cerebellar vermis on sagittal MRI).

diagnosed in early infancy, rigorous dietary control may allow normal neurologic development. Some believe the cystic changes represent focal areas of edema causing the macrocephaly and later atrophy as the head size becomes smaller, apparently from brain destruction. It is essential to recognize this pattern and test for glutaric aciduria.

HYPOXIC-ISCHEMIC EVENTS

Hypoxic-ischemic events in the neonate can be divided into maternal causes and causes attributable to the neonate. **Maternal causes** include chronic cardiac or pulmonary lung disease, placental insufficiency, shock, placental abruption, and cardiorespiratory arrest, all of which can cause severe birth asphyxia. An uncommon cause is maternal cocaine use.[98] Some **therapeutic maneuvers** in these extremely sick, hypoxic neonates have also been associated with an increased risk for germinal matrix hemorrhage (GMH) secondary to increased

venous obstruction.[99] Increased venous pressure has been demonstrated in infants breathing out of sequence with a mechanical ventilator, during endotracheal tube suctioning, and with high peak inspiratory pressure.[100] Tension pneumothorax, exchange transfusions, rapid infusions of colloid, and myocardial injury caused by asphyxia are other factors that may greatly affect hemodynamics and venous pressure.[100-102]

Arterial Watershed Determines Regional Pattern of Brain Damage

The sonographic findings are varied depending on the cause and the age of the neonate when the hypoxic-ischemic event occurs, because the watershed areas of the brain change in location during the last trimester[51,103] (Table 47-1). In premature infants the watershed is in the immediate periventricular region, and thus **germinal matrix hemorrhage (GMH)** and **periventricular leukomalacia (PVL)** are common pathologic findings. In full-term infants, damage tends to occur more in the

TABLE 47-1. PATTERNS OF HYPOXIC-ISCHEMIC INJURY IN NEWBORNS

HYPOTENSION	PREMATURE INFANT	TERM INFANT
Mild to moderate	Periventricular ICH or PVL	Parasagittal cortical or subcortical injury
Severe	Deep gray matter Brainstem and cerebellar infarct	Lateral thalamus Posterior putamen hippocampus Corticospinal and sensorimotor tracts

PVL, Periventricular leukomalacia; *ICH*, intracranial hemorrhage.

TABLE 47-2. GRADES OF GERMINAL MATRIX HEMORRHAGE

GRADE	TYPE/DESCRIPTION
I	Subependymal hemorrhage
II	Intraventricular extension without hydrocephalus
III	Intraventricular hemorrhage with hydrocephalus
IV	Intraparenchymal hemorrhage with or without hydrocephalus

cortical or subcortical regions, because the watershed moves to these areas more toward the brain surface, resulting in **parasagittal infarction** regions in term infants.[104] How to study hypoxic-ischemic encephalopathy (HIE) depends on the brain maturity and stability of the newborn infant. Findings at MRI may complement ultrasound and may more often predict noncystic white matter lesions.[105-109]

Lack of autoregulation of cerebral blood pressure, which typically occurs in premature infants and less often in asphyxiated full-term infants, will cause cerebral perfusion to be directly affected by hypertensive or hypotensive episodes. This pressure-passive system can result in sudden focal hemorrhage or with hypotension, diffuse or focal infarction.

The neurologic manifestations of brain injury in the premature infant range from the less severe motility and cognitive deficits to major spastic motor deficits, including spastic diplegia and spastic quadriplegia with more profound intellectual deficits. In the full-term infant the hypoxic-ischemic events may manifest as seizures, movement disorders including arching and fisting, altered tone, absent suck, and depending on the severity, intellectual deficits.

Germinal Matrix Hemorrhage

Germinal matrix hemorrhage (GMH) may lead to **intraventricular hemorrhage, hydrocephalus,** and **porencephaly.** GMH is a common event occurring primarily in premature infants less than 32 weeks' gestational age. Although the incidence once was as high as 55%, most nurseries have experienced a significant drop in GMH. Recent reports of GMH and intraventricular hemorrhage now range from 10% to 25% in very-low-birthweight infants (<1000 g) in most neonatal intensive care units.[110,111] Infants at greatest risk are those at gestational ages of less than 30 weeks, with birth weight less than 1500 g, or both.[112]

Multiple factors have been studied as causes for GMH. Although no single cause has been identified, common

associations include prematurity with complications such as hypoxia, hypertension, hypercapnia, hypernatremia, rapid volume increase, and pneumothorax.[100-102] Full-term infants rarely experience this type of hemorrhage.

Germinal matrix hemorrhage may occur in subependymal (SEH), intraventricular (IVH), or intraparenchymal (IPH) regions.[113] However, GMH originates predominantly as hemorrhage in the germinal matrix below the subependymal layer and may be contained by the ependyma or may rupture into the ventricular system or less often into the adjacent parenchyma (Fig. 47-41). The **germinal matrix** is a fine network of blood vessels and primitive neural tissue that lines the ventricular system in the subependymal layer during fetal life. As the fetus matures, the germinal matrix regresses toward the foramen of Monro so that, by full term, only a small amount of germinal matrix is present in the caudothalamic groove between the thalamus and the caudate nucleus. This fine network of blood vessels is highly susceptible to pressure and metabolic changes, which can lead to rupture of the vessels. The germinal matrix is rarely a site of hemorrhage after 32 weeks' gestation because it has almost disappeared.

The classification of GMH most widely used was proposed by Burstein et al.[113] Other systems are used as well, but the **anatomic description** of exactly where the brain damage occurs is more important than the classification. The key causes of poor neurologic outcome relate to hydrocephalus and parenchymal extension into the descending white matter tracts (Table 47-2).

Sonography is the most effective method for detecting this hemorrhage in the newborn period and for follow-up in the subsequent weeks. Most hemorrhage (90%) occurs in the first 7 days of life, but only one third of these occur in the first 24 hours.[114] The optimal cost-effective timing to screen premature infants is at 1 to 2 weeks of age, to identify patients with significant hemorrhage as well as those developing hydrocephalus.[115] Small subependymal hemorrhages (grade I) might be missed when screening late if they resolve quickly, but these have not proven clinically important. A late screen for periventricular leukomalacia (PVL) should performed at 1 month to search for the cystic changes of PVL,[116,117] because the clinical course or first brain ultrasound will

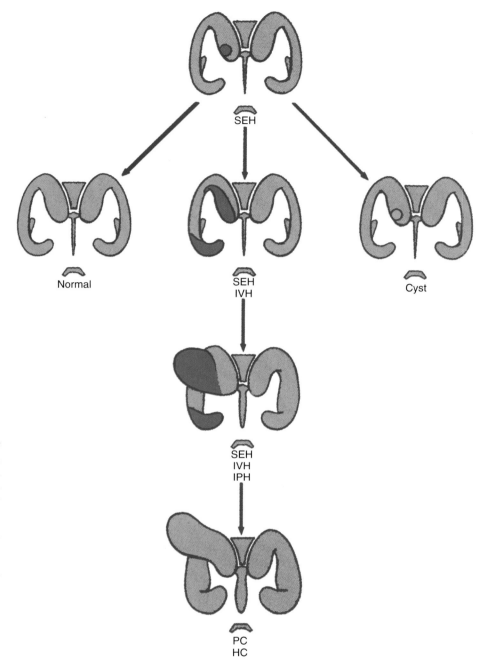

SEH

Normal

SEH
IVH

Cyst

SEH
IVH
IPH

PC
HC

FIGURE 47-41. Sequelae of subependymal hemorrhage (SEH). SEH may resolve, leaving a normal scan; may resolve, leaving a small subependymal cyst; or may progress, rupturing into the ventricle, causing intraventricular hemorrhage *(IVH),* or extending into the parenchyma, causing intraparenchymal hemorrhage *(IPH).* Hydrocephalus *(HC)* and porencephaly *(PC)* are common sequelae of SEH. *(From Rumack CM, Manco-Johnson ML.* Perinatal and infant brain imaging: role of ultrasound and computed tomography. *St Louis, 1984, Mosby.)*

not predict the later development of hydrocephalus or PVL. These predictors of the most severe neurologic outcome (PVL and ventricular enlargement) may be missed if the late screen is not done. An examination should be performed earlier if required by the patient's condition.

Severe grades of hemorrhage with hydrocephalus (grade III) and intraparenchymal hemorrhage (grade IV) have stabilized at about 11%, according to a large, outcome study of very-low-birth-weight (VLBW) infants (<1500 g).[118] Many factors have contributed to this decreased incidence of hemorrhage including increased use of antenatal steroids[119,120] and improved neonatal

OPTIMAL BRAIN ULTRASOUND SCREENING IN PREMATURE INFANTS*

First Scan: 10 to 14 Days
For germinal matrix hemorrhage
For posthemorrhagic hydrocephalus

Second Scan: 4 Weeks of Age†
For periventricular leukomalacia (PVL)
For ventricular enlargement

*Less than 30 weeks' gestation or less than 1500 g.
†Cystic PVL lesions coalesce, leaving only thin white matter after 4 weeks.

respiratory care, such as surfactant therapy. Because pneumothoraces have been associated with a higher incidence of GMH, the effective use of high-frequency ventilators, oscillators, and surfactant, which decrease pressure to the lung, are also likely causes for the decreasing incidence of GMH.

Complications of subependymal and intraventricular hemorrhage are intraventricular obstructive hydrocephalus (IVOH), usually at the foramina of Monro or the sylvian aqueduct, and extraventricular obstructive hydrocephalus (EVOH), at the arachnoid granulations. Complications of intraparenchymal hemorrhage are permanent areas of damaged brain that can become necrotic, leading to porencephalic cysts.

Subependymal Hemorrhage (Grade I Hemorrhage)

On sonographic examination, acute subependymal hemorrhage (SEH) presents as a homogeneous, moderately to highly echogenic mass (Fig. 47-42). The echogenic clot often causes focal hemorrhage in the caudothalamic groove. The choroid plexus is normally quite thick at the trigone of the lateral ventricle and tapers progressively anteriorly, descending between the head of the caudate and the thalamus just above the foramen of Monro. SEH may appear as a bulge in the choroid plexus. As the hematoma ages, the clot becomes less echogenic, with its center becoming sonolucent (Fig. 47-43; **Video 47-6**). The aging of the clot can often be followed on ultrasound for weeks to months (as on MRI), depending on its initial size. The clot retracts, and necrosis occurs with complete resolution of hemorrhage or occasionally development of a **subependymal cyst.** It may persist as a linear echo adjacent to the ependyma. Hemorrhage in the brain becomes isodense on CT about 2 to 3 weeks after the event.

Intraventricular Hemorrhage (Grade II Hemorrhage)

When SEH bursts into the lateral ventricle, intraventricular hemorrhage (IVH) presents as hyperechoic clot that fills a portion of the ventricular system or all of a ventricle when the clot forms a cast of the ventricle (Fig. 47-44). The clot itself may obscure the ventricle due to complete filling of the lumen. The normally thick, echogenic choroid plexus may appear asymmetrically thick and may be difficult to define within the ventricle separate from the densely echogenic hemorrhage. As the clot matures, it becomes echolucent centrally and more well defined and separable from the more echogenic choroid plexus. Low-level echoes from debris floating in a ventricle may occur in IVH as the clot breaks apart (Fig. 47-45). Use of the posterior fontanelle or axial views will increase the detection of IVH in normal-sized ventricles, because at times there are only small clots or **CSF-blood fluid levels** in the occipital horn[12] (Fig. 47-46).

SIGNS OF INTRAVENTRICULAR HEMORRHAGE

Hyperechoic material fills portion of ventricular system.
Clot forms a cast of the ventricle.
  May obscure ventricle because lumen completely filled
Thick, echogenic choroid plexus
Echolucent centrally later, as clot matures
Low-level echoes floating in a ventricle
Cerebrospinal fluid–blood fluid levels

Blood in the third or fourth ventricle may be missed and is much more clearly diagnosed on posterior fossa ultrasound with mastoid views. If the blood extends into the cisterna magna, there is an increased risk for posthemorrhagic hydrocephalus[121,122] (Fig. 47-47; **Video 47-7**). **Cisterna magna clot** is a better predictor of posthemorrhagic hydrocephalus than initial hydrocephalus. Early-onset IVH, in the first 6 hours of life, is uncommon and has been associated with a higher risk for both cognitive and motor impairment, including cerebral palsy.[123]

Intraventricular Hemorrhage with Hydrocephalus (Grade III Hemorrhage)

Because IVH causes hydrocephalus, the clot and then the choroid plexus may be better defined (Fig. 47-48). Echogenic clot may be adherent to ventricular walls or may become dependent within the ventricle. A change in the head position while scanning will demonstrate clot movement in some cases (Fig. 47-49). Posterior fontanelle images may show IVH in the occipital horn in subtler cases. As with SEH, in time the echogenic clot will become more echolucent centrally and may eventually resolve. A **chemical ventriculitis** as a response to blood in the CSF typically causes thickening and increased echogenicity of the subependymal lining of the ventricle.[124] Posthemorrhagic hydrocephalus may require shunting if it is progressive. Follow-up scans should be obtained weekly unless the head grows rapidly or another crisis intervenes. Typically, the most severe degree of hydrocephalus occurs after several weeks. As the blood clears from the ventricles, particularly with a block at the aqueduct, the ventricular size may return to normal. In one series, posthemorrhagic ventricular dilation required surgical treatment with a ventriculoperitoneal reservoir or shunt in only 34% of very low birth weight (VLBW) infants with hydrocephalus.[125] Occasionally, a **trapped fourth ventricle** may be caused by obstruction of both the aqueduct and the outlets of the fourth ventricle.[24] In these cases a ventriculoperitoneal shunt will decompress only the lateral and third ventricles.

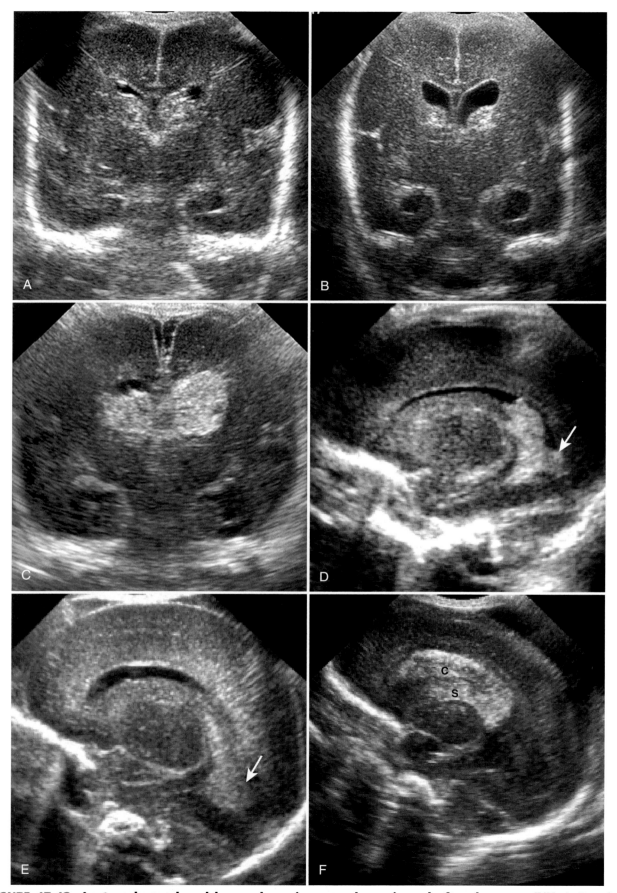

FIGURE 47-42. Acute subependymal hemorrhage is very echogenic and often becomes IVH. A, B, and C, Highly echogenic SEH may appear isolated on coronal scans. **D** and **E**, Sagittal scans show intraventricular clot in the occipital horn *(arrows)*, or **F**, clot *(C)* extending into the frontal horn and body above the subependymal hemorrhage *(S)*.

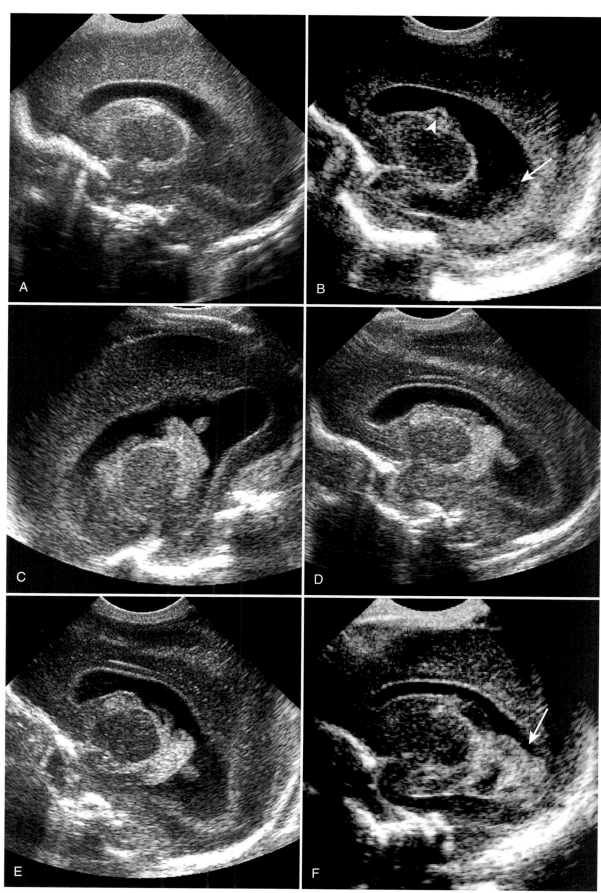

FIGURE 47-43. Aging of subependymal hemorrhage: sagittal sonograms. Subependymal and intraventricular hemorrhage become sonolucent centrally over several days with low-level echoes *(arrow* in **F)** settling into the occipital horn. **A** and **D,** Acute hemorrhage. **B, C, E,** and **F,** One week after initial hemorrhage. *(Arrowhead* in **B,** subependymal cyst; *arrow,* clot on choroid plexus in occipital horn.) Hemorrhage in the brain will often still be visible on ultrasound or MRI for weeks to months but will become isodense on CT in about 2 weeks.

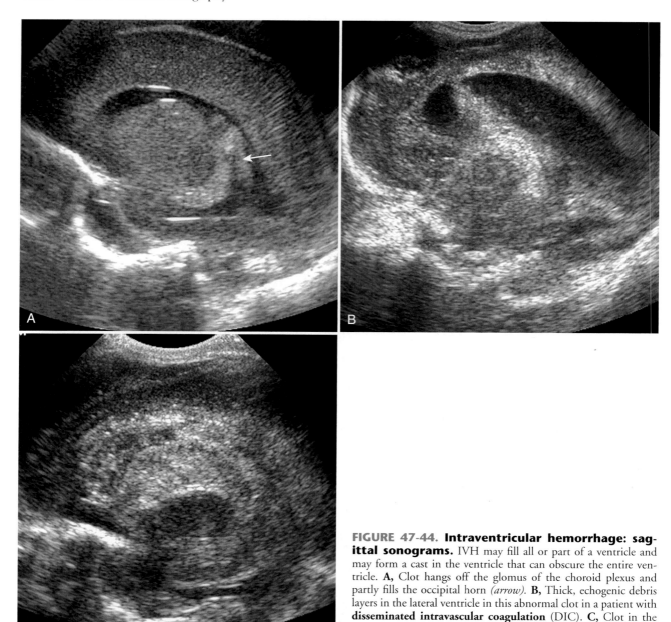

FIGURE 47-44. Intraventricular hemorrhage: sagittal sonograms. IVH may fill all or part of a ventricle and may form a cast in the ventricle that can obscure the entire ventricle. **A,** Clot hangs off the glomus of the choroid plexus and partly fills the occipital horn *(arrow).* **B,** Thick, echogenic debris layers in the lateral ventricle in this abnormal clot in a patient with **disseminated intravascular coagulation** (DIC). **C,** Clot in the frontal horn, body, and temporal horn forms a cast of echogenic material in the lateral ventricle.

Intraparenchymal Hemorrhage (Grade IV Hemorrhage)

Intraparenchymal hemorrhage (IPH) is usually in the cerebral cortex and located in the frontal or parietal lobes, because it often extends from the subependymal layer over the **caudothalamic groove** (Fig. 47-50; **Video 47-8**). However, our experience in posterior fossa imaging through the mastoid fontanelle has made it clear that cerebellar hemorrhage occurs more often than previously reported. Studies suggest that IPH is caused by hemorrhagic venous infarction.[100,101] Taylor[102] has shown obstruction of terminal veins by SEH or IVH is often

seen with secondary IPH or periventricular white matter hemorrhage. **Periventricular hemorrhagic infarction** (PHI) is believed to be venous infarction secondary to a large SEH compressing subependymal veins. These focal periventricular white matter infarcts may be frontal to parieto-occipital and are asymmetrical, usually unilateral, and if bilateral, asymmetrical in size.[126] Infants with parenchymal hemorrhage associated with GMH typically develop hemiparesis, and if there is periventricular hyperintensity, they may develop cerebral palsy.[127-132] It is thought that this hyperintensity may relate to pressure from hydrocephalus. This is in contrast to infants with periventricular echogenicity and minimal or no IVH,

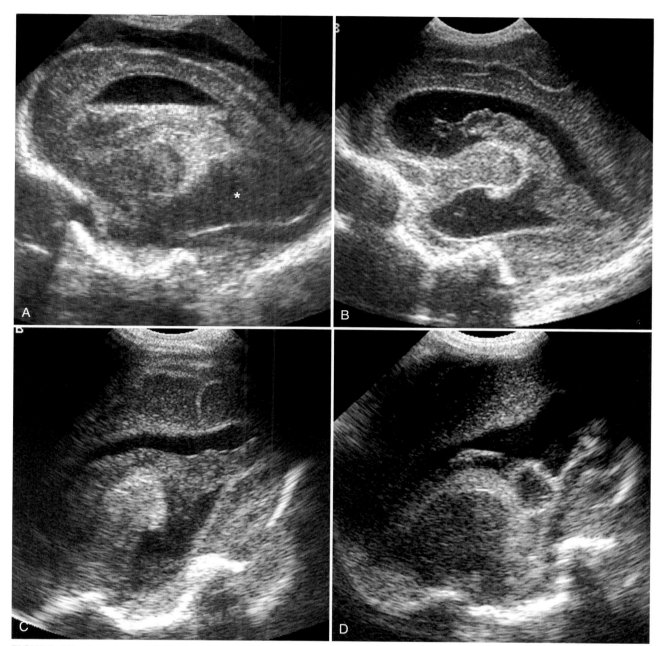

FIGURE 47-45. Intraventricular hemorrhage: sagittal sonograms. Late IVH may show low-level echoes, fluid-fluid levels, and clot fragments in the occipital horn. **A,** Cerebrospinal fluid–echogenic blood fluid level in patient with DIC after placental abruption. *Asterisk,* abnormal hypoechoic clot from DIC. **B** and **C,** Debris in lateral ventricle and clot fragments extend into the occipital horn. **D,** Occipital horn angled inferiorly in this posterior fontanelle view. Clot on the choroid is becoming sonolucent centrally.

who are at much higher risk for PVL. These infarcts typically cause spastic hemiparesis.[31,112,127] In IPH the venous infarction caused by the initial SEH leads to intraparenchymal damage. Later, necrosis may lead to porencephaly in this region.

Acutely, IPH appears as an echogenic homogeneous mass extending into the brain parenchyma. As the clot retracts, the edges form an echogenic rim around the center, which becomes sonolucent. The clot may move to a dependent position, and by 2 to 3 months after the injury, an area of **porencephaly** (if there is communication with the ventricle) or encephalomalacia develops (Fig. 47-51).

Unusual types and sites of IPH, acute cystic changes, midline shift, and downward extension of hemorrhage into the thalamus may result from hemorrhage into PVL, secondary to infarction or thromboembolism, from a bleeding diathesis (e.g., vitamin K deficiency), hemophilia, alloimmune thrombocytopenia or Rh immune incompatibility (Fig. 47-52), and hypernatremia.[133-135]

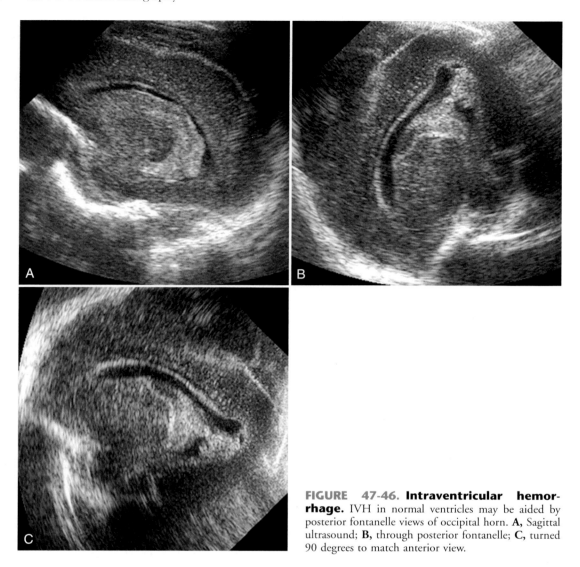

FIGURE 47-46. Intraventricular hemor-rhage. IVH in normal ventricles may be aided by posterior fontanelle views of occipital horn. **A,** Sagittal ultrasound; **B,** through posterior fontanelle; **C,** turned 90 degrees to match anterior view.

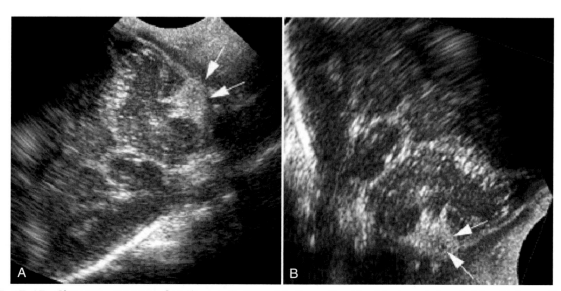

FIGURE 47-47. Cisterna magna clot (*arrows*). A good indicator for risk of hydrocephalus. **A,** Mastoid fontanelle view of posterior fossa. **B,** Turned 90 degrees into standard format.

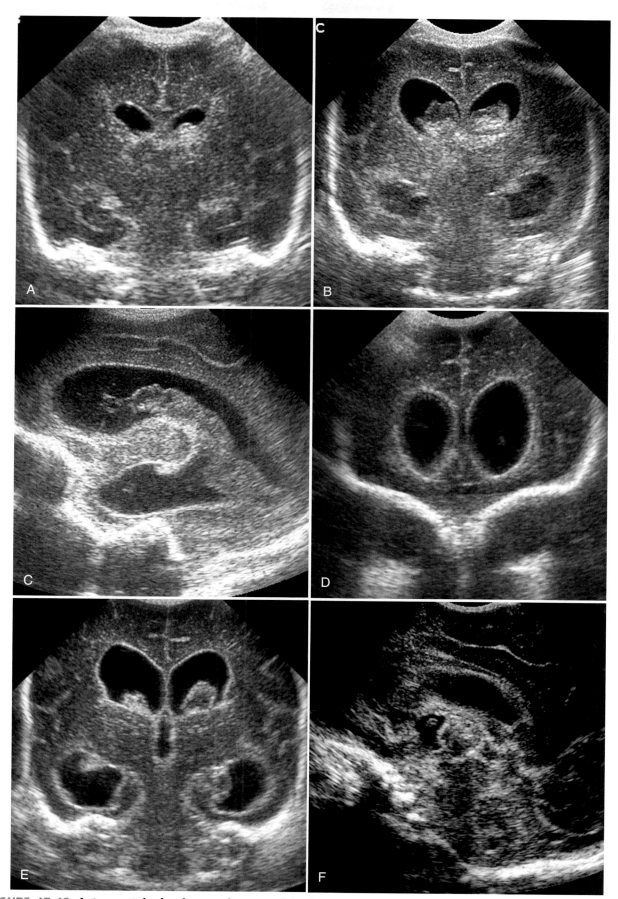

FIGURE 47-48. Intraventricular hemorrhage and hydrocephalus. **A** and **B,** Coronal sonograms show aging clot has become less echogenic than choroid. **D** and **E,** Coronal sonograms, and **F,** sagittal sonogram, show progressive hydrocephalus. The ventricular walls have become very echogenic, caused by a chemical ventriculitis from blood. The lateral and third ventricles are enlarged, and there is a clot in the back of the third ventricle causing aqueductal obstruction. Typically, the clot resolves, and the hydrocephalus may improve at that time.

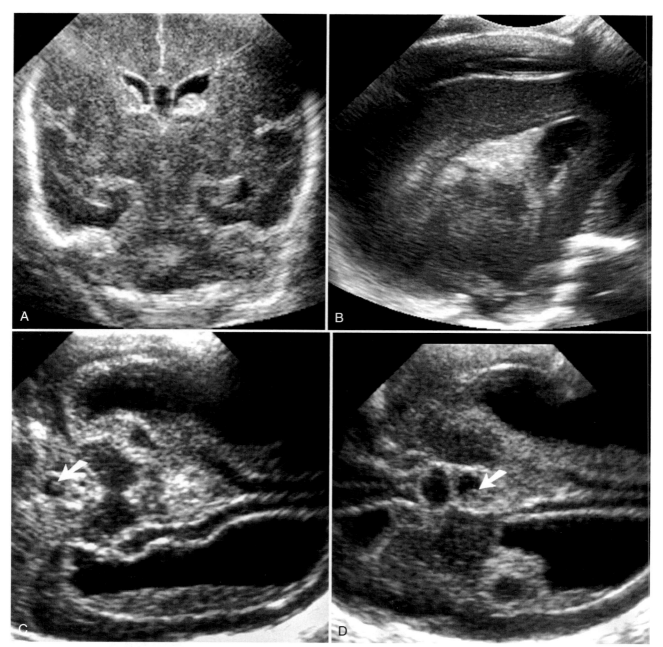

FIGURE 47-49. Intraventricular hemorrhage. Chronic IVH clot may change with position, particularly as it starts to dissolve and becomes more sonolucent. **A,** Coronal; **B,** sagittal; **C** and **D,** axial. Sonograms show clot settling dependently *(arrows)* in the third and lateral ventricles.

Hemophilia has been associated with intracranial hemorrhage. A review of 102 newborns with hemorrhage in 33 publications found 65% intracranial and 35% extracranial.[136] Spontaneous IPH has been reported in term infants but was associated with signs of trauma or venous compression.[137]

Extracorporeal membrane oxygenation (ECMO) complications include IPH secondary to infarction, ischemia, and thromboembolism. GMH or IVH is less common after ECMO because premature infants are at high risk for these types of hemorrhage and thus almost never undergo this procedure. These complications may be from the hypoxic brain damage secondary to the underlying lung disease, even before initiation of ECMO therapy. The complications from ECMO are also caused by heparinization and transient hypertension.[138]

Ultrasound is used for daily evaluation of the newborn receiving ECMO. The portability and ease of use in the critically ill infant without the need for transport are the main advantages. Sonography can alert the clinician to intracranial hemorrhage and the option to stop ECMO therapy.[138-140]

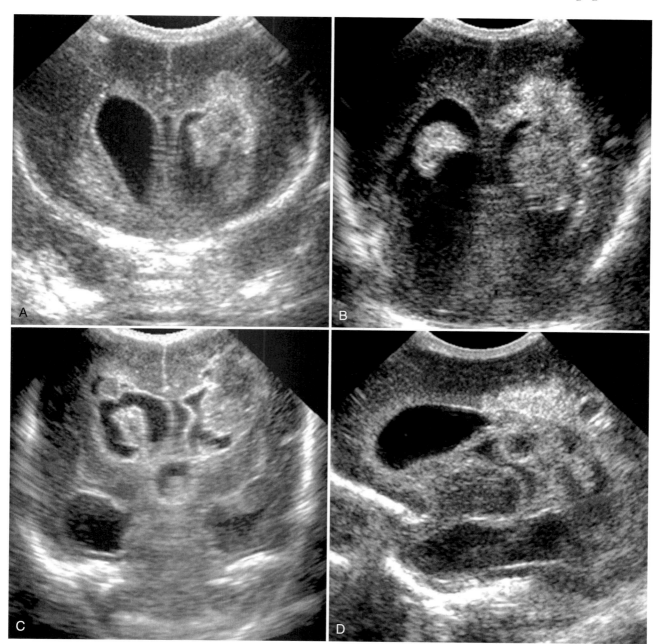

FIGURE 47-50. Intraparenchymal hemorrhage is uncommon (grade IV hemorrhage). Parietal cortex hemorrhage may involve the motor area, causing contralateral hemiparesis. Coronal (**A, B, C**) and sagittal (**D**) sonograms.

Cerebellar Hemorrhage

Cerebellar hemorrhage has been diagnosed more frequently with special sonographic views through the mastoid fontanelle and from MR evaluation of disrupted cerebellar development.[141-146] **Posterior fossa hemorrhage** is a reported complication of a traumatic delivery in full-term infants, in ECMO therapy, or with a coagulopathy. However, cerebellar hemorrhage can occur in premature infants because there is germinal matrix in the fourth ventricle (Fig. 47-53). Mastoid fontanelle imaging is now routinely used to visualize the cerebellum in the optimum focal zone to allow cerebellar hemorrhage to

be seen and the posterior fossa fully evaluated. Cerebellar hemorrhage occurs more often than previously thought, when only anterior fontanelle imaging was done. Resolution of cerebellar hemorrhage into a cyst in the posterior fossa may allow easier diagnosis; the normal echogenic cerebellum may obscure hemorrhage when acute.

Merrill et al.[147] reported 13 cerebellar hemorrhages in 525 infants under 1500 g, occurring in the first week of life in unstable neonates with acidosis or hypotension requiring intensive resuscitation, but not always associated with supratentorial hemorrhage. On follow-up to 2 years, four infants had cognitive deficits and developmental delay without signs of motor abnormalities. Three

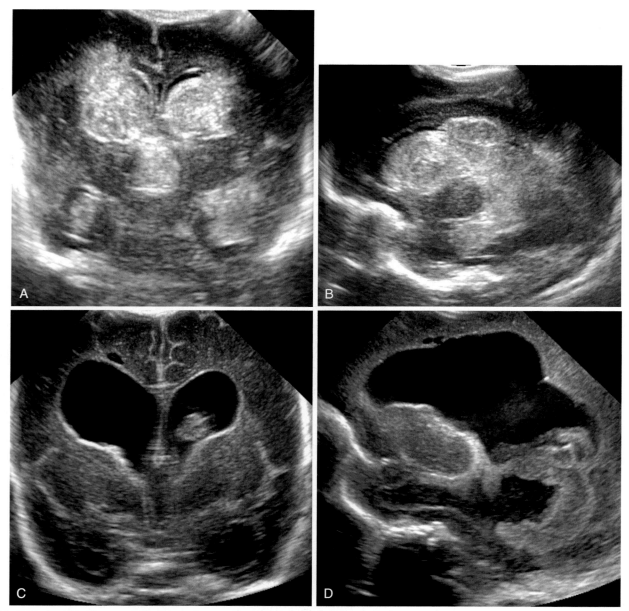

FIGURE 47-51. Porencephaly and posthemorrhagic hydrocephalus. Placental abruption has led to DIC and IVH (grade IV). **A** and **B,** Coronal and sagittal sonograms show right parietal **intraparenchymal hemorrhage** (IPH) above the lateral ventricle and IVH in the bodies and temporal horns of the lateral ventricles and third ventricle. **C** and **D,** Coronal and sagittal sonograms show IPH becoming **porencephaly** at 1 month. Right IPH clot above the body of the lateral ventricle has progressed to necrosis; clot is gone, leaving a cystic cavity formed continuous with the lateral ventricle.

cases of prenatally diagnosed posterior fossa cysts were found to result from hemorrhage. These were initially thought to be congenital posterior fossa arachnoid cysts but were recognized because of debris in the cysts and hemosiderin on MRI. In neonates, cerebellar hemorrhage has rarely required surgical intervention, although older children may require emergency drainage.[148,149]

Subarachnoid Hemorrhage

The presence of enlarged interhemispheric and sylvian fissures with thickened sulci and increased echogenicity can suggest the diagnosis of subarachnoid hemorrhage (SAH).[140] Subarachnoid hemorrhage may occur in neonates who have experienced asphyxia, trauma, or disseminated intravascular coagulation (DIC) and may be the only hemorrhage in full-term infants who are not at risk for GMH. Cisternal SAH has been found after IVH but can be a difficult diagnosis on ultrasound. Posterior fossa views may aid in making the diagnosis (Fig. 47-54). Spread of blood from the ventricular system into the spinal subarachnoid space after GMH is common and can be seen within 24 hours of the initial, severe ICH in premature infants.[122]

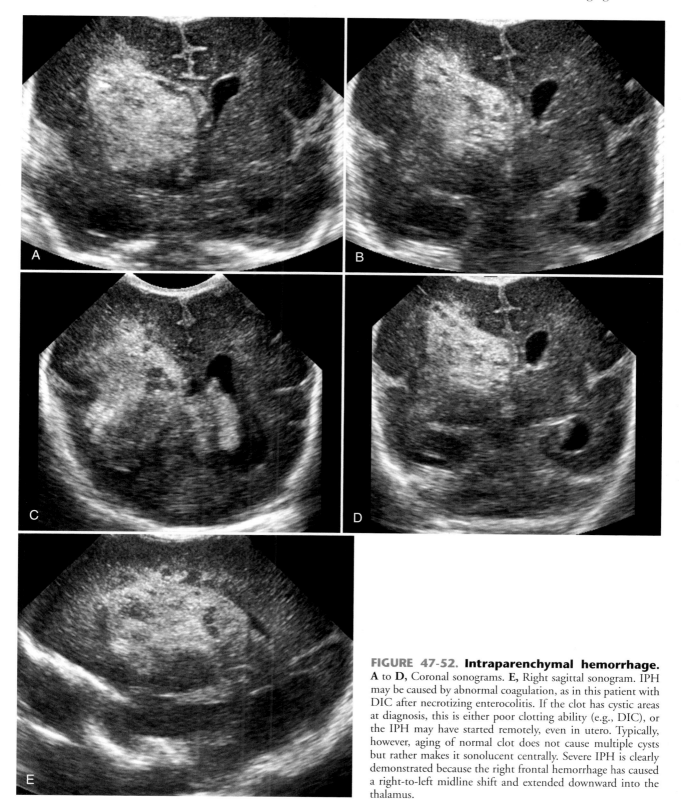

FIGURE 47-52. Intraparenchymal hemorrhage.
A to **D,** Coronal sonograms. **E,** Right sagittal sonogram. IPH may be caused by abnormal coagulation, as in this patient with DIC after necrotizing enterocolitis. If the clot has cystic areas at diagnosis, this is either poor clotting ability (e.g., DIC), or the IPH may have started remotely, even in utero. Typically, however, aging of normal clot does not cause multiple cysts but rather makes it sonolucent centrally. Severe IPH is clearly demonstrated because the right frontal hemorrhage has caused a right-to-left midline shift and extended downward into the thalamus.

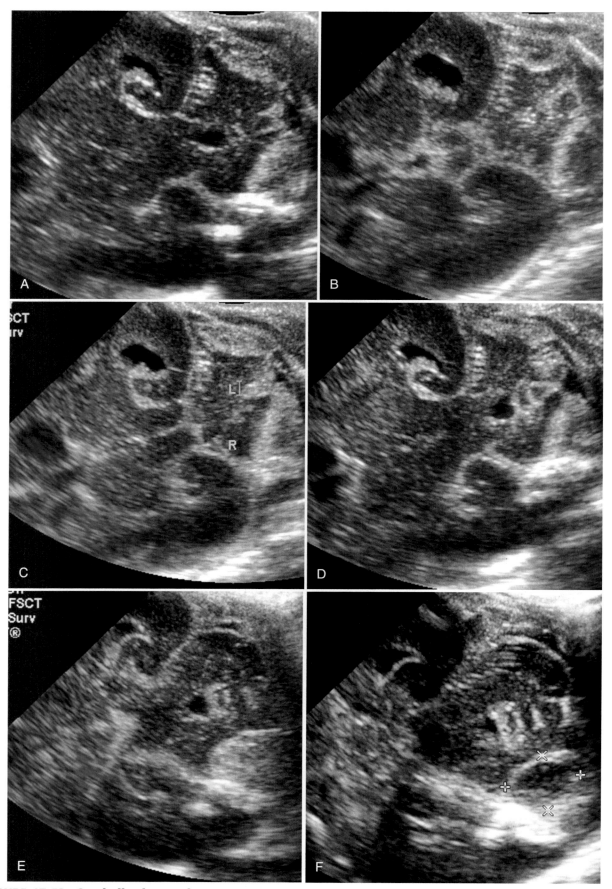

FIGURE 47-53. Cerebellar hemorrhage spectrum. A, B, and **C,** Axial posterior fossa sonograms. Acute hemorrhage may be subtle or missed because of normal hyperechoic cerebellum, but only the central vermis is normally echogenic. **D,** Punctate hemorrhage. **E,** Centrally sonolucent bilateral hemorrhage is subacute. **F,** Chronic cerebellar hemorrhage becomes centrally sonolucent lesions over 1 or 2 weeks; chronic cystic changes are easier to diagnose. (**A, B,** and **E,** Same patient; **C** and **F,** different patient).

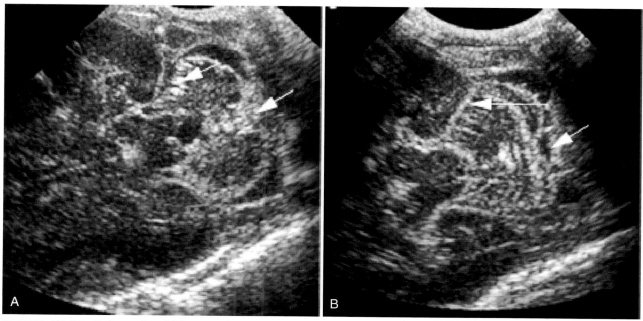

FIGURE 47-54. Subarachnoid hemorrhage. A, Cerebellar, and **B,** midbrain, axial sonograms show blood *(short arrows)* in the subarachnoid spaces and cisterna magna. Increased echogenicity of cerebellar folia *(long arrow)* may be normal in the near field on mastoid fontanelle scans (note fourth ventricle blood on **B**).

Hemorrhage is easily demonstrated on CT or MRI, so when SAH occurs alone in term infants, it is better to screen with these modalities.

Cerebral Edema and Infarction

Periventricular Leukomalacia

Periventricular leukomalacia, the principal ischemic lesion of the premature infant, is infarction and necrosis of the periventricular white matter. In some cases, there is a history of cardiorespiratory compromise, resulting in hypotension and severe hypoxia and ischemia. The pathogenesis of PVL has been found to relate to three major factors: (1) the immature vasculature in the periventricular watershed; (2) the absence of vascular autoregulation in premature infants, particularly in the cerebral white matter; and (3) the maturation-dependent vulnerability of the oligodendroglial precursor cell damaged in PVL. These cells are extremely vulnerable to attack by free radicals generated in the ischemia-reperfusion sequence.[112]

The prevalence of PVL in the very low birth weight infant (<1000 g) was previously reported as 25% to 40%.[102] Later, Ment et al.[110] reported that PVL incidence decreased to 7%. Also, however, with increasing survival rates of very low birth weight infants, **cerebral palsy** has increased and is closely associated with PVL. Because more infants are surviving with PVL than in the past, it becomes even more important to diagnose this lesion accurately and improve the ability to treat the patient and change the outcome. The cystic changes of PVL are more often visualized on ultrasound, and noncystic white matter damage is better seen on MRI.[150]

In PVL the white matter most affected is in the arterial border zones at the level of the optic radiations adjacent to the trigones of the lateral ventricles and the frontal cerebral white matter near the foramina of Monro. The prevalence of PVL has been noted to increase with the duration of survival in premature infants, raising the possibility of cumulative postnatal insults, including circulatory compromise, patent ductus arteriosus, apneic spells, and sepsis.[112,113,151,152]

Maternal chorioamnionitis has been associated with PVL, possibly the result of vasoactive proteins being released into the fetal circulation, causing fluctuations in cerebral blood flow. Inflammatory responses to infection in the fetus or the neonate that activate astrocytes and microglia may cause PVL,[153,154] or these may represent a pathologic response to repair the tissue injury in PVL.[155] Proinflammatory cytokines found after chorioamnionitis correlate with PVL development.[156] Prevention of PVL may depend on treatment with maternal antibiotics or anticytokine agents and therapy with free-radical scavengers.[112]

Cystic PVL can been anticipated to follow a severe hemodynamic event in 56% of premature infants with PVL. Unexpected PVL (without a specific clinical neonatal event) has been reported in as many as 44% of cases.[157] This series of PVL patients had been treated for preterm delivery and often had maternal chorioamnionitis. It is proposed that the maternal infection predisposes to preterm delivery and PVL. Antenatal steroids have been shown to decrease the incidence of PVL and the incidence of IPH from GMH.[158-161]

Later neurologic problems from PVL include developmental delay and symmetrical spastic diplegia involving both legs, often noticeable by 6 months of age. Spastic diplegia occurs because the pyramidal tracts from the motor cortex that innervate the legs pass through the internal capsule and travel close to the lateral ventricular wall. Severe cases of PVL will also affect the arms, resulting in spastic quadriplegia and cause vision and intellectual deficits.[162-165] The prevalence of cerebral palsy has been evaluated in the French EPIPAGE cohort study of 2364 children between 22 and 32 weeks' gestation; 1954 (88%) were studied at 2 years of age. A retrospective review showed that 20% had cerebral palsy at 24 to 26 weeks' gestation, whereas only 4% had cerebral palsy at 32 weeks. On the ultrasound evaluation, 17% of children with IVH (grade III) and 25% with white matter damage had cerebral palsy based on findings of large ventricles, persistent periventricular echogenicity, and cystic PVL.[166]

Pathologically, the periventricular white matter undergoes coagulation necrosis, followed by phagocytosis of the necrotic tissue. This necrosis usually occurs in the white matter adjacent to the external angles of the lateral ventricles. This results in decreased myelination in these areas and focal dilated lateral ventricles. In more severe cases of PVL, cystic cavities develop.[40,162,164] Petechial hemorrhages can complicate PVL. In fact, hemorrhagic PVL has been shown to be much more common (64%) than thought when there is MRI and ultrasound correlation.[167]

The initial sonographic examination in PVL may be normal. Within 2 weeks of the initial insult, however, the periventricular white matter increases in echogenicity until it is greater than the adjacent choroid plexus. This increased echogenicity is usually caused by edema from infarction and may also result from hemorrhage[168] (Fig. 47-55). Two to 4 weeks after the insult, cystic changes may develop in the area of abnormal echogenic parenchyma (Fig. 47-56; **Video 47-9**). The cysts can be single or multiple and are parallel to the ventricular border in the deep white matter and often lateral and/or superior to the top of the ventricles. These cysts measure from millimeters to 1 to 2 cm in diameter. The cystic changes are usually bilateral and often symmetrical. One case has been reported to show cystic changes in the corpus callosum with later thinning, similar to pathologic reports of callosal PVL.[152,169] **Thinning of the corpus callosum** often follows PVL because of white matter necrosis and a decrease in crossing fibers. Pathologic studies suggest that sonography actually underestimates the incidence of PVL.[168,170] In 51 cases of postmortem-proven PVL, Adcock et al.[170] found that in 44% the neurosonogram failed to make the diagnosis for two main reasons: (1) most often the ultrasound examinations were

performed before 1 month of age and missed the cystic stage of PVL, and (2) the lesions were microcystic and not large enough to find on ultrasound. MRI may be the best method for PVL diagnosis when done at term age in the very low birth weight infants most at risk for PVL.[171,172] MRI shows parenchymal lesions of the white matter that predict motor outcome. **Diffusion tensor imaging** has been added to evaluate myelination in white matter not studied on ultrasound.[173] Delayed myelination, ventricular enlargement, and width of extracerebral spaces were not found to be good predictors of cerebral palsy.

On subsequent sonograms, the cystic lesions may enlarge or resolve.[164] Therefore, normal-appearing white matter on either ultrasound or CT examinations performed several weeks to months after the insult does not exclude the occurrence of PVL.[174] MRI becomes more sensitive than either CT or ultrasound for long-term follow-up of parenchymal injury, because when myelination progresses, **glial scarring** from damaged white matter can be diagnosed (Fig. 47-56), typically with thinning of the white matter adjacent to an enlarged ventricle where the cysts have coalesced and are no longer visible. Because the initial ultrasound examination is often normal in infants who have sustained a significant hypoxic-ischemic event, late sonograms should be obtained at about 4 weeks after birth to exclude evolving PVL. The characteristic distribution of cystic lesions that are clearly separate from the ventricle in PVL should distinguish them from the parenchymal hemorrhage that occurs in grade IV GMH. However, PVL and GMH can occur simultaneously.[175] Periventricular white matter damage can be studied with cranial ultrasound if technical factors include careful attention to focal areas of hyperechogenicity. Leijser et al.[176] divided white matter into **grade 0,** less echogenicity than choroid plexus; **grade 1,** same echogenicity as choroid plexus; and **grade 2,** brighter than choroid plexus. Only severe (grade 2) predicted a poor neurologic outcome. MRI added more detail on extent of severe white matter disease.

Diffuse Cerebral Edema

Diffuse cerebral edema with or without SAH is a common result of hypoxic-ischemic events in full-term infants. Initially, the brain edema will cause slitlike ventricles in a diffusely echogenic brain with poorly defined sulci. This echogenicity may cause **silhouetting of the sulci** so that the sulci seem to disappear (Fig. 47-57). The brain parenchyma appears echogenic in the distribution of the injury, and the sulci are difficult to appreciate because of surrounding echogenic edematous brain. The mechanism of the increased echogenicity of the brain parenchyma from cerebral edema is not understood completely. One possibility is that the increased intracellular fluid causes more interfaces, which accounts for the hyperechoic appearance.

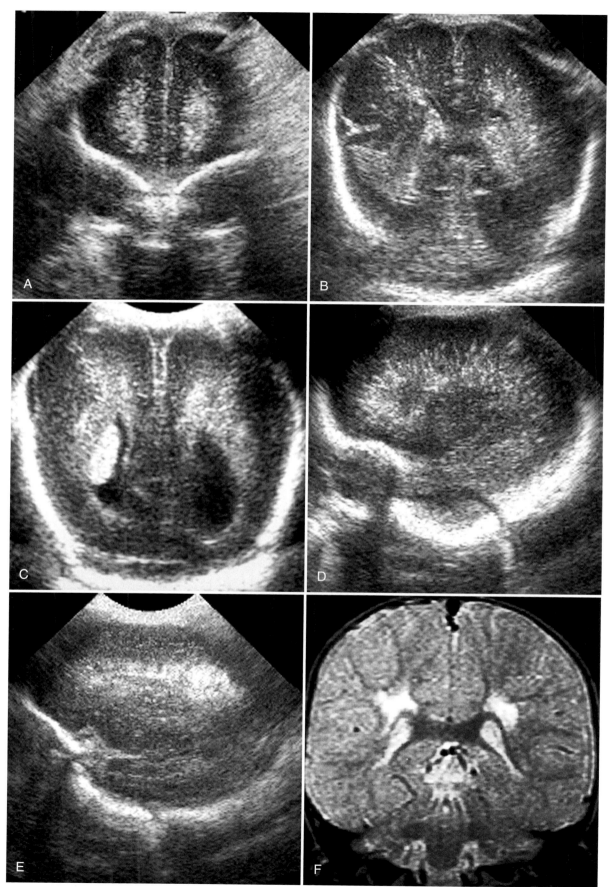

FIGURE 47-55. Early periventricular leukomalacia can be echogenic. A, B, and C, Coronal sonograms; D and E, sagittal sonograms. Increased echogenicity early is uncommon and may indicate hemorrhage with edema. F, Same patient as C; later T2-weighted MR image. Focal ventricular enlargement may develop later from loss of white matter adjacent to ventricles. White matter is thin near the large ventricle as myelination develops.

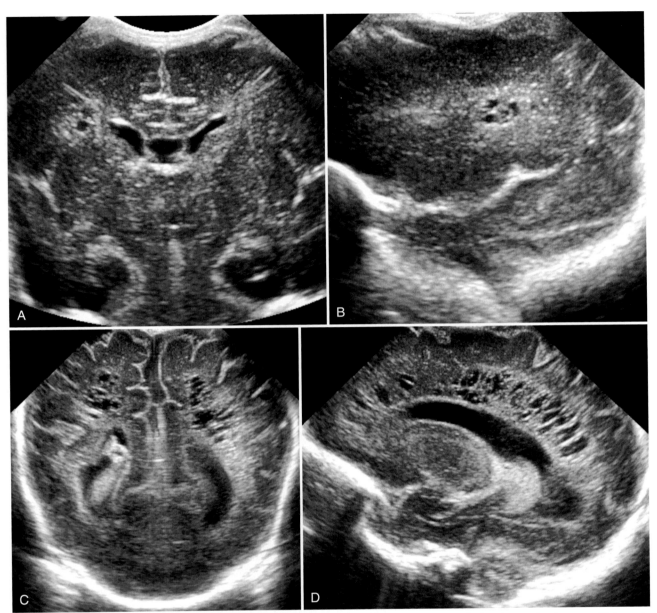

FIGURE 47-56. Periventricular leukomalacia (PVL). Cystic changes of PVL (late findings) may develop even if the early scan at 10 days is normal. **A** and **B,** Coronal and sagittal sonograms at 1 month show only right frontal focal cystic changes. **C** and **D,** Coronal and sagittal sonograms on a second patient show extensive cystic PVL above the lateral ventricles at 1 month after birth, which is the usual age of diagnosis.

Color Doppler ultrasound evaluation of severely asphyxiated infants has demonstrated earlier and at times more focal abnormalities than on gray scale alone. Investigators have used Doppler sonography to classify brain edema[177] or to predict outcome.[178] Outcome of children with significantly abnormal cerebral blood flow was noted in 47 patients, from newborns to 4 years of age. However, loss or reversal of diastolic flow did not necessarily imply a lethal outcome. Survival was associated with prompt and effective treatment.[179] A few studies show MRI changes early in neonatal life from asphyxia, but most neonatologists resist moving a very unstable

newborn for MR scanning If the ischemic event was severe enough to lead to infarction, diffuse brain volume loss occurs within 2 weeks, with ventricular enlargement secondary to atrophy.[31] Enlarged extra-axial fluid spaces also develop as a consequence of the atrophic changes. The head circumference is very helpful to distinguish diffuse atrophy from hydrocephalus, because the head circumference is normal to small in patients who have undergone diffuse brain atrophy. Depending on the type of insult, generalized brain atrophy or focal areas of porencephaly or encephalomalacia may occur. With **acute near-total intrauterine asphyxia** in the newborn,

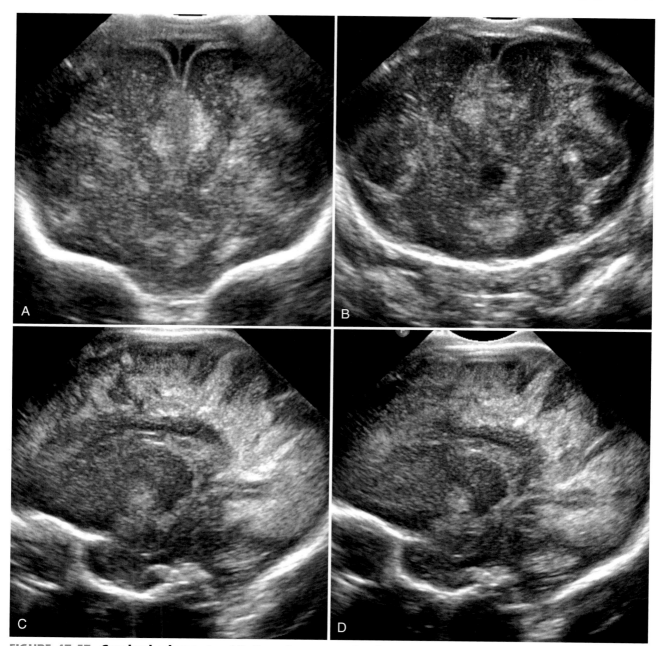

FIGURE 47-57. Cerebral edema. A and **B,** Coronal sonograms; **C** and **D,** sagittal sonograms. Severe cerebral edema has caused silhouetting of the sulci from acute, near-total intrauterine asphyxia after placental abruption. Diffuse increased echogenicity from edema obscures sulci. Ventricles are slitlike because of the severe edema.

an unusual pattern of basal ganglia damage with sparing of the cerebral cortex and white matter has been reported. This may be difficult to diagnose with ultrasound if it is not hemorrhagic until late changes of atrophy develop[31] (Fig. 47-58).

Sonography can detect these complications of hypoxic-ischemic events, but MRI is more sensitive to the full extent of the insult near the cortical surface.[31,180-183] To optimize ultrasound imaging of the term neonatal brain, Daneman et al.[184] used higher frequencies (8-17 MHz) with multiple focal planes in near-field, midfield, and far-field magnified views with spectral and color Doppler ultrasound, searching for abnormal resistive indices (RIs) on spectral Doppler ultrasound. They also emphasized the need to obtain the ultrasound within 2 hours of MRI for an accurate comparison. Special features to be evaluated on every ultrasound in neonates with hypoxic-ischemic insult should include gray matter–white matter differentiation and focal abnormal echogenicity in cerebral cortex and deeper structures. Doppler ultrasound with RIs to look for flow fluctuations in RI and flow in the dural sinuses is valuable.

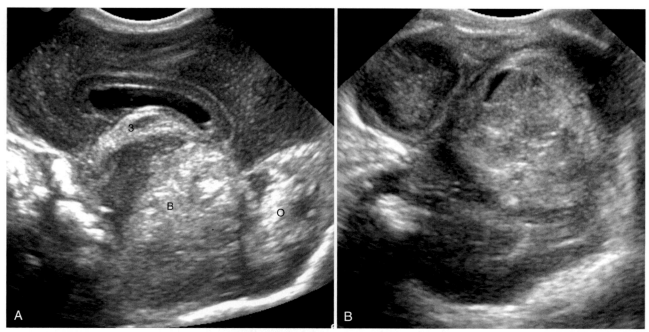

FIGURE 47-58. Brainstem and cerebellar hemorrhage. A and **B,** Sagittal and axial sonograms show highly echogenic hemorrhage in the brainstem *(B),* cerebellar vermis and hemispheres, and posteriorly in the occipital cortex *(O),* after acute, near-total intrauterine asphyxia. Clot is also seen in the third ventricle *(3)* just below the cavum septi pellucidi.

Focal Infarction

Cerebral infarction in the neonate, aside from PVL, is uncommon. Risk factors are prematurity, severe birth asphyxia, congenital heart disease (resulting in a left-to-right shunt), meningitis, emboli (from the placenta or systemic circulation), polycythemia, hypernatremia, and trauma.[133,185,186] Symptoms can vary, ranging from asymptomatic to seizures with lethargy and coma. The middle cerebral artery distribution is the most frequent site, although the anterior and posterior circulations have also been affected.[49] Single areas of infarction are more frequently seen in full-term infants, whereas premature infants often demonstrate multiple sites of injury. Cerebral blood flow evaluation with color and or power Doppler sonography may be the most sensitive test available in the unstable neonate when diffusion-weighted MRI cannot be used to identify the earliest signs of stroke.[187-192]

Cerebellar infarction is much less common than cerebral infarction. However, six cases were reported in 3 years at Hammersmith Hospital in London, diagnosed by MRI in patients at several years of age who were born prematurely.[193] All these patients also had IVH, and thus cerebellar damage was likely a result of diffuse ischemic injury. Only one of the six patients was diagnosed on sonography as having cerebellar damage. Because the vermis is so echogenic, edema or hemorrhage can be a difficult diagnosis in this region (see Fig. 47-53). Cerebellar infarction was also diagnosed with MRI in 13 patients with severe cerebral palsy who had cerebellar hemispheric and vermian damage.[194] Now that we are more routinely evaluating the posterior fossa in detail, we may become more aware of cerebellar infarction at the time of the injury in premature infants.[195]

On sonography, the infarcted brain parenchyma demonstrates specific findings within the first 2 weeks (Fig. 47-59). These include echogenic parenchyma, lack of arterial pulsation, lack of blood flow appreciated by pulsed or color Doppler sonography, mass effect from edema, arterial territorial distribution of injury, decreased sulcal definition, and increased pulsation in the periphery of the infarcted section.[196-199] After 2 weeks, the echogenic lesions begin to show cystic changes, and ipsilateral ventricular enlargement from evolving atrophy (hydrocephalus ex vacuo), as well as a gradual return of arterial pulsations in the major branches from proximal to peripheral distribution. Using color Doppler imaging, Taylor[197,198] demonstrated **luxury perfusion** within

---

CEREBRAL INFARCTION: SONOGRAPHIC SIGNS

Echogenic parenchyma
Lack of arterial pulsation at real-time examination
Lack of a vascular waveform on pulsed Doppler
Lack of flow on color Doppler
Mass effect from edema
Arterial territorial distribution of injury
Decreased sulcal definition
Increased pulsation in periphery of infarcted section
Early collateral arterial vessels within hours of insult

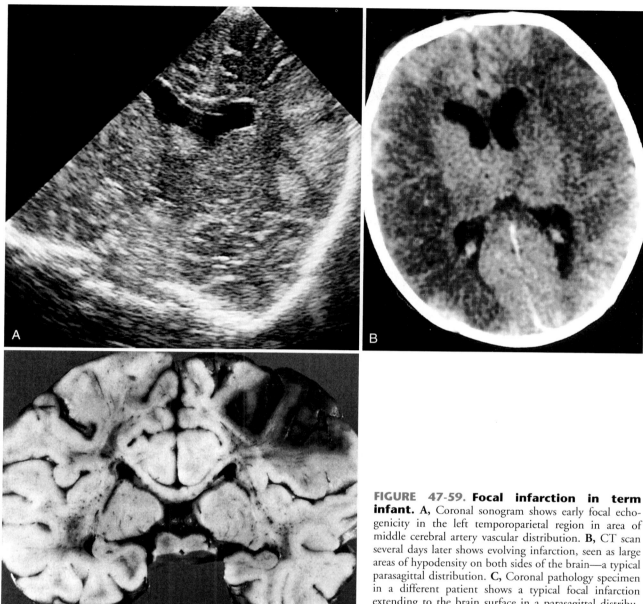

FIGURE 47-59. Focal infarction in term infant. A, Coronal sonogram shows early focal echogenicity in the left temporoparietal region in area of middle cerebral artery vascular distribution. **B,** CT scan several days later shows evolving infarction, seen as large areas of hypodensity on both sides of the brain—a typical parasagittal distribution. **C,** Coronal pathology specimen in a different patient shows a typical focal infarction extending to the brain surface in a parasagittal distribution. *(From Friede R. Developmental neuropathology. 2nd ed. New York, 1975, Springer-Verlag.)*

hours of a focal vascular insult, both experimentally and in newborn infants.[199] Power Doppler may be more sensitive than color Doppler in detecting the increase in the size and number of vessels seen with luxury perfusion.[196]

Basal Ganglia Vasculopathy

 Linear branching echogenicity in the lenticulostriate arteries of the thalamus and basal ganglia are uncommon but have been described in intrauterine viral infections (rubella, CMV, syphilis) **(Video 47-10),** neonatal asphyxia, nonimmune hydrops, fetal alcohol syndrome, and trisomies 13 and 21. Coley et al.[200] reported that hypoxic-ischemic conditions accounted for 30 of 63

cases. An interesting correlation by Denbow at al.[201] showed that the twin-twin transfusion syndrome had multiple signs of focal infarction as well as lenticulostriate vasculopathy. On sonography, these echogenic vessels develop at a mean age of 1 month and appear to be a marker for more diffuse brain injury; some found an increased risk for poor neurologic outcome.[202,203]

Hyperechoic Caudate Nuclei

Bilateral hyperechoic foci in the caudate nuclei develop in the characteristic location of GMH but are atypical in that they are sharply marginated, teardrop shaped, bilateral, and symmetrical (Fig. 47-60). Schlesinger

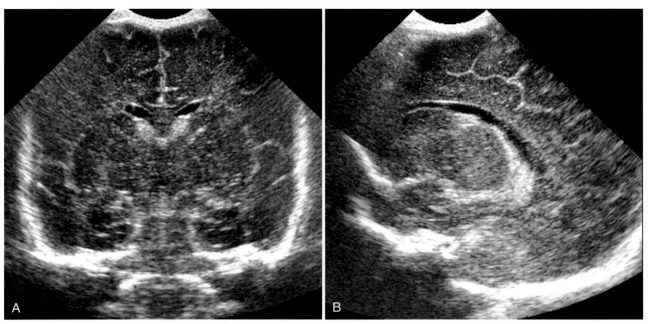

FIGURE 47-60. Hyperechoic caudate nucleus (bilateral). A and **B,** Coronal and sagittal sonograms show echogenic caudate nuclei that did not appear abnormal until the premature infant was about 1 month of age (postulated to be remote ischemic damage).

et al.[204] reported that five of nine infants had ischemia and two were normal in this area, based on MRI and histopathologic review. Hyperechoic caudate nuclei seem to occur late, usually after the first week of life, when most GMH occurs.

POSTTRAUMATIC INJURY

Subdural and Epidural Hematomas

Subdural and epidural hemorrhage can be a difficult diagnosis on sonography compared with CT or MRI.[10,205] On sonographic examination, these hematomas present as unilateral or bilateral hypoechoic fluid collections surrounding the brain parenchyma (Fig. 47-61). Subdural hematomas are uncommon in newborns and not necessarily indicative of birth trauma, since 13 of 26 affected infants diagnosed on CT had a history of trauma.[206] Fortunately, surgery is rarely required. Small amounts of fluid may be difficult to detect secondary to the near-field artifact inherent in every transducer. However, this is less of a problem if a high-frequency transducer (10-12 MHz) is used. With a lower-frequency transducer, interposing an acoustic gel pad between the transducer and the fontanelle can assist in eliminating the near-field artifact by moving it superiorly out of the brain. Magnified coronal sections with high-frequency linear transducers (at least 10-12 MHz) are best for appreciating the epidural and subdural collections in the supratentorial space. Imaging through the foramen magnum or posterior fontanelle can assist in diagnosing infratentorial extra-axial fluid collections.

Cheng Yu Chen[16] reported that color Doppler sonography distinguishes subarachnoid and subdural fluid and hemorrhage based on displacement of vessels on the brain surface (Fig. 47-62; see Chapter 48). It remains to be proven whether color Doppler can reliably predict atrophy with subarachnoid fluid collections from the excess fluid under pressure in subdural fluid collections. Doppler ultrasound may be useful in determining which patients may be simply observed and which require MRI for a more specific diagnosis of hemorrhage.

After the neonatal period, when birth trauma may cause hemorrhage, the presence of new subdural fluid collections should suggest preexisting meningitis (most often from *Haemophilus influenzae*) or nonaccidental trauma.[16,207] If an infant's head circumference increases abnormally fast after the first 2 weeks of life, a CT examination is usually performed to search for extra-axial fluid, because the most common cause is subdural hemorrhage, not hydrocephalus. If a sonographic examination is performed, the clinician should carefully search the near field with magnified views for extracerebral fluid and cerebral tears, as well as membranes seen in chronic subdural fluid collections.[16,208]

INFECTION

Congenital Infections

Congenital infections can have serious consequences for the developing fetus. Death of the fetus, congenital malformations, mental retardation or developmental delay, and spasticity or seizures may result from infection

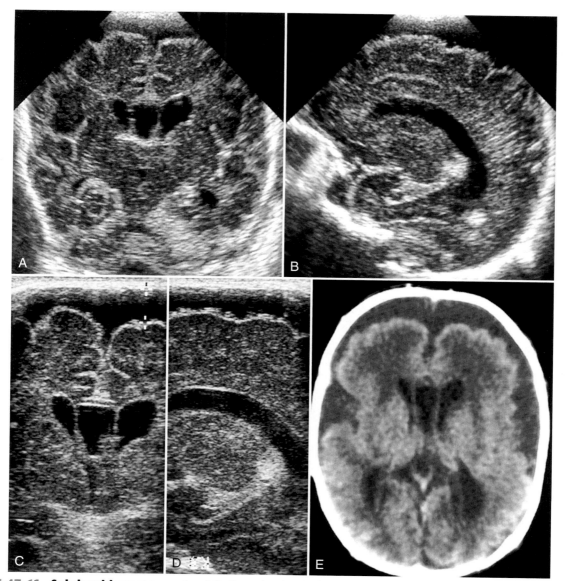

FIGURE 47-61. Subdural hematoma. A and **B,** Coronal and sagittal sonograms show fluid over the surface of the brain. Surface sulci are usually not imaged because the initial transducer artifact obscures the first 1 cm below the fontanelle. **C** and **D,** Magnified, high-resolution sonograms show sulci more clearly. **E,** CT scan shows extracerebral fluid.

at critical times during gestation.[209] Ultrasound plays an important role in identifying and following both antenatal and neonatal complications from congenital infections.[210]

The most frequent congenital infections are commonly referred to by the acronym TORCH. This refers to the infections *Toxoplasma gondii*, rubella, cytomegalovirus (CMV), and herpes simplex virus (HSV) type 2. The O stands for "other," such as syphilis. Syphilis causes acute meningitis, infrequently resulting in parenchymal lesions in the newborn.[211]

Cytomegalovirus and Toxoplasmosis

Of the TORCH group, congenital infection by CMV is the most common, occurring in approximately 1% of all

births.[209,212] CMV may be acquired at or after birth with little or no consequence, but prenatal infections may result in serious damage to the developing brain.[213,214] Toxoplasmosis is the second common congenital infection and is caused by the unicellular parasite *Toxoplasma gondii*.[209,215,216] Maternal infection is usually subclinical. Maternal immunity to CMV reduces the risk of CMV in utero, and vaccines are being considered.[217]

The severity of the infection with either CMV or toxoplasmosis depends on the timing of the infection during gestation. Earlier infection, before 20 to 24 weeks, results in more devastating outcomes: microcephaly, lissencephaly with abnormal myelination, a hypoplastic cerebellum, polymicrogyria and cortical dysplasias, porencephaly, and multicystic encephalomalacia.[218] CMV has been reported to cause schizencephaly in some

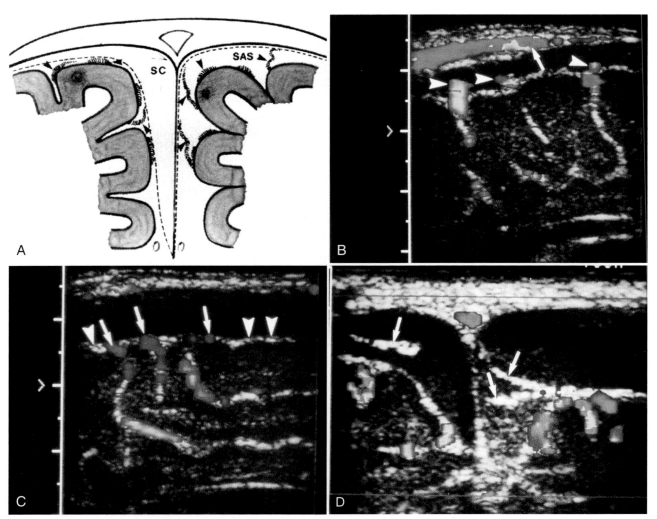

FIGURE 47-62. Subdural versus subarachnoid fluid collections. A, Drawing shows vessels are compressed onto the surface of the brain in subdural fluid collections *(SC)* and vessels cross the fluid in subarachnoid space *(SAS).* **B,** Color Doppler shows vessels crossing into subarachnoid fluid *(arrowheads).* **C,** Color Doppler image shows vessels compressed in subdural region *(arrows, arrowheads).* **D,** Color Doppler image shows "neomembrane" *(arrows)* formed in subdural fluid collections. *(From Chen CY, Chou TY, Zimmerman RA, et al. Pericerebral fluid collection: differentiation of enlarged subarachnoid spaces from subdural collections with color Doppler ultrasound. Radiology 1996;201:389-392.)*

patients[80,81] (see Fig. 47-37). Ventriculomegaly may result from brain volume loss. Later infection, after 24 weeks, will result in less severe neurologic damage. Perinatal or neonatal death is expected with the more severe and earlier insults. Mental retardation, developmental delay, spasticity, and seizures are all potential outcomes.

To differentiate CMV from toxoplasmosis, serum titers for antibodies against these organisms are useful.[219] Other differentiating criteria include the petechial skin lesions and hepatomegaly associated with CMV and chorioretinitis associated with toxoplasmosis. Intracranial calcifications have been described in both infections.[220,221] CMV classically causes periventricular calcifications (Figs. 47-63 and 47-64; **Video 47-10**). Toxoplasmosis causes more scattered calcifications with

a predilection for the basal ganglia. However, both patterns have been seen in either infection.[219-222] Resolution of intracranial calcification has been reported after treatment of congenital toxoplasmosis, consistent with improved neurologic outcome.[223]

Sonography can demonstrate the periventricular or scattered cerebral calcifications as echogenic foci with or without acoustic shadowing. In eight proven cases of CMV, Malinger et al.[218] reported periventricular hyperintensity in all cases, as well as calcification, ventriculomegaly, hypoplastic vermis, periventricular cysts, intraventricular adhesions, and echogenic vasculature in the basal ganglia **(Video 47-10).** Cerebellar calcification was seen in one patient.[218] The brain parenchyma may appear disorganized, with poorly defined sulci and corpus callosum. CT demonstrates the calcification

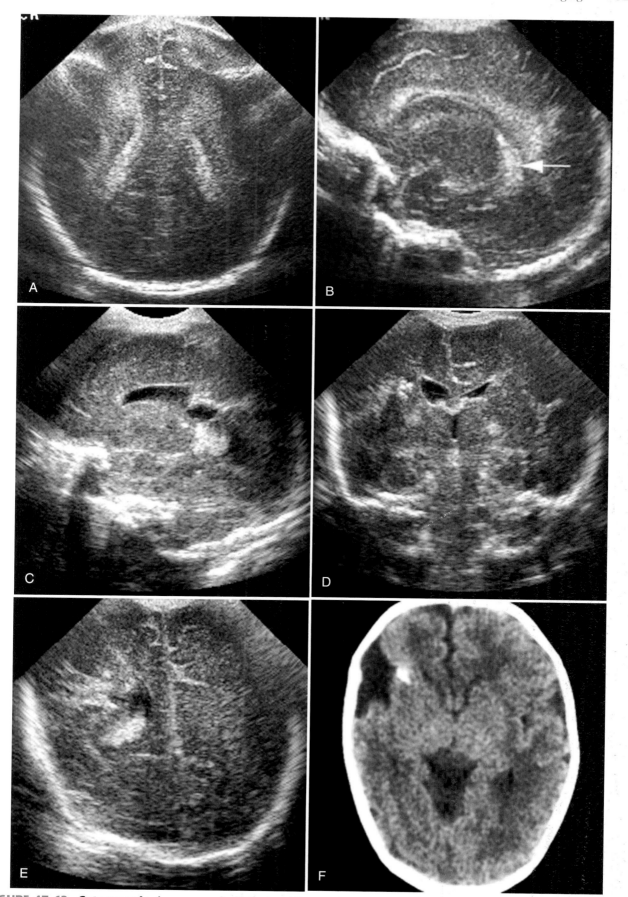

FIGURE 47-63. Cytomegalovirus encephalitis. A and **B,** Periventricular echogenicity and focal calcification *(arrow)* with little acoustic shadowing. **C, D,** and **E,** In another patient, focal calcifications on ultrasound; **F,** CT scan.

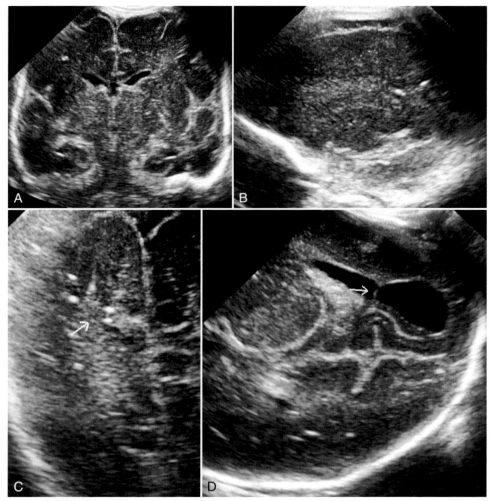

FIGURE 47-64. Cytomegalovirus infection. **A** and **C,** Coronal; **B,** sagittal; and **D,** posterior fontanelle views of the occipital horn show septations typical of postinfectious intraventricular damage. CMV calcifications and septations may be subtle and require magnified views to be certain of the diagnosis.

better, but MRI shows abnormal myelination or cortical dysplasias most reliably.[174]

Herpes Simplex Virus

Herpes simplex virus type 1 (HSV-1) or type 2 (HSV-2) may cause disease of the CNS, although HSV-2 is more common in the neonate, and HSV-1 occurs primarily in older children and adults.[209] HSV-2 may be acquired transplacentally or by vaginal exposure to herpetic genital lesions during birth. The resulting encephalitis is typically diffuse, resulting in loss of gray/white matter differentiation. (This differs from the temporal lobe disease seen in older children and adults with HSV-1.) Cystic encephalomalacia of periventricular white matter and hemorrhagic infarction with scattered parenchymal calcifications frequently result.[224] Relative sparing of the lower neural axis, including the basal ganglia, thalamus, cerebellum, and brainstem, is typical.[225,226] Infections acquired in utero may lead to microcephaly, intracranial calcifications, and retinal dysplasias.[227]

Rubella

Since the widespread availability of rubella vaccine after 1967, congenital rubella has fortunately become extremely uncommon in the Western world. Unfortunately, it remains a significant problem in many other parts of the world. Rubella is not known to cause cerebral malformations. Levene et al.[225] described a case of echogenic calcifications in the basal ganglia confirmed at autopsy. Subependymal cysts are also described.[228] Microcephaly, vasculopathy,[228] and massive calcification of the brain detectable on plain radiography have been described in an infant who died at 9 days of age.[226]

Neonatal Acquired Infections

Meningitis and Ventriculitis

Despite the development of antibiotics to treat bacterial infections in the latter half of the 20th century, bacterial meningitis remains a serious concern for infants and

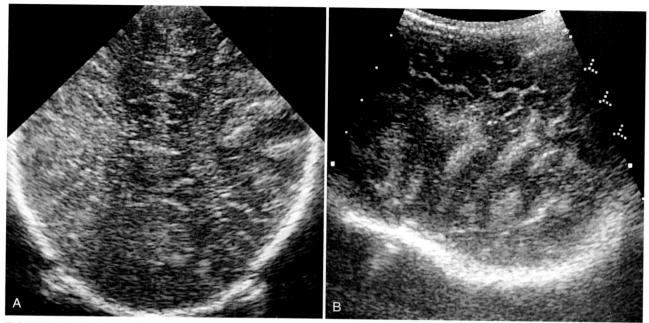

FIGURE 47-65. Group B streptococcal meningitis. A and **B,** Coronal and sagittal sonograms show diffusely echogenic sulci that appear thicker than normal.

children. During the first month of an infant's life, the two most common infections result from *Escherichia coli* and group B streptococci. Between 4 and 12 weeks, *E. coli* and *Streptococcus pneumoniae* are the most common, and from 3 months to 3 years, *Haemophilus influenzae* is most frequent. This is usually a clinical diagnosis; imaging is needed only to evaluate for complications or when the patient's clinical situation deteriorates.[31,228]

Complications of meningitis include subdural empyemas or fluid collections (see Figs. 47-61 and 47-62), cerebritis, abscess formation, and venous sinus thrombosis. Infarctions can occur from either arterial vasculitis or venous obstruction, as a result of venous sinus thrombosis. Sonography can identify these complications but is not specific. Areas of increased or decreased echogenicity of brain parenchyma or sulci may represent edema, cerebritis, or evolving infarction (Figs. 47-65 and 47-66).

Ventriculitis, another complication of meningitis seen in 60% to 95% of cases, is suggested by the sonographic findings of hydrocephalus, echogenic debris within the ventricles, increased echogenicity, or a shaggy ependymal lining or fibrous septa within the ventricles[124] (Fig. 47-67). Ultrasound is best for identifying intraventricular septa formation compared to CT or MRI. These septations can result in shunt failure or allow bacteria to escape antibiotic exposure. MRI and CT with enhancement are more sensitive for localizing the complications of infection, such as infarcts, venous sinus thrombosis, and extra-axial fluid collections.[209]

INTRACRANIAL MASSES

Brain Tumors

Only 11% of children with brain neoplasms present before 2 years of age. Tumors that do present before 2 years are usually congenital. Brain tumors can be difficult to diagnosis in the neonate. If the neoplasm causes hydrocephalus, signs and symptoms of increased intracranial pressure, such as enlarging head size, vomiting, or behavioral alteration. may be recognized. More specific signs and symptoms depend on the location of the tumor, such as cranial nerve findings or pituitary gland and hypothalamic functions. MRI or CT is generally the imaging modality of choice in these infants.[229] However, with nonspecific signs and symptoms, including an enlarging head from hydrocephalus, ultrasound may be the first imaging performed. Sonography can delineate the tumor site and size and evaluate cystic and solid components.

Tumors may present initially because of hemorrhage into the tumor. In fact, because hemorrhage is so much more common than tumor in newborns, it may be extremely difficult to differentiate a simple hematoma from a tumor; both can be quite echogenic. We have seen at least three cases of congenital tumor presenting as hemorrhage. Any hemorrhage presenting in unusual circumstances or in an unusual location should be investigated by contrast-enhanced CT or MRI, searching for an occult tumor.[10] For unusual hemorrhage, follow-up

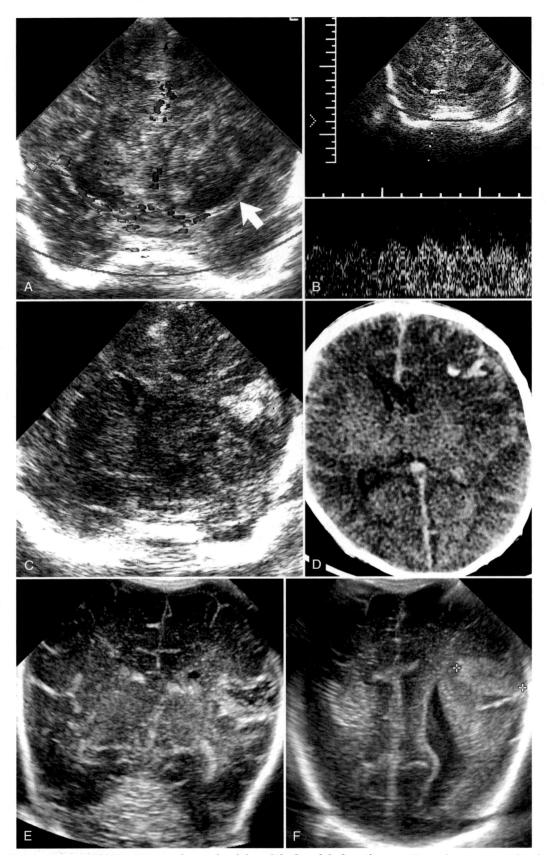

FIGURE 47-66. Group B streptococcal meningitis with focal infarction. A, Coronal sonogram with color Doppler shows lack of flow in the left middle cerebral artery (MCA, *arrow*); gray scale alone showed symmetrical, increased echogenicity. **B,** Pulsed Doppler image in the right MCA (opposite side) shows greatly increased diastolic flow. **C,** Coronal sonogram, and **D,** CT scan, later show hemorrhage into an infarction with midline shift from left to right. **E** and **F,** Coronal anterior and posterior sonograms show left MCA focal echogenic infarct, etiology unknown, in another premature infant at 2 weeks after birth.

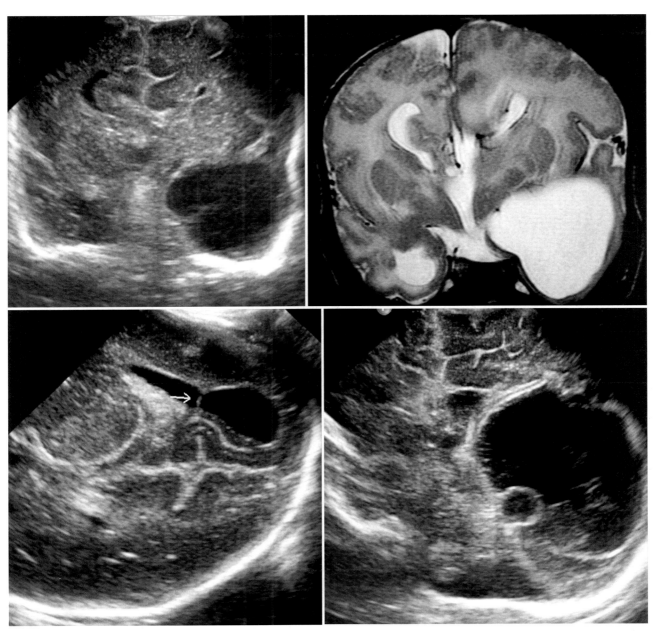

FIGURE 47-67. Antenatal infection: ventriculitis. Term infant with diffusely echogenic cerebral cortex and hydrocephalus. Septations have isolated the left temporal horn into a cystic mass, in addition to absence of the corpus callosum and vermian hypoplasia from a Dandy-Walker malformation.

scans are also helpful because clotting from the hemorrhage will resolve over time, allowing the tumor to be visualized.

Spectral and color Doppler imaging can identify vascular components of the tumor. Follow-up with MRI or CT is then performed to evaluate the full extent of the neoplasm, assist with differential diagnosis, and evaluate for therapeutic approaches. Differentiating the histologic type of the neoplasm is not possible, but localizing the tumor usually allows a differential diagnosis.

Tumor location in infants less than 1 year of age differs from that in older children and differs by

series.[31,229-232] **Supratentorial neoplasms** are more common than infratentorial tumors by approximately 2.5:1. **Teratomas** are now the most frequent neoplasms reported in the first year of life. **Astrocytomas** (astrocytic gliomas) are second in most series, usually arising from the optic chiasm and nerves or the hypothalamus (Figs. 47-68 and 47-69). Other neoplasms include **atypical teratomas or rhabdoid tumors** (rather than medulloblastomas) **primitive neuroectodermal tumors** (PNETs), **ependymomas,**[233-238] and **choroid plexus papillomas** (Fig. 47-70). Sporadic cases of oligodendrogliomas, hemangioblastomas, hemangiomas, dermoid

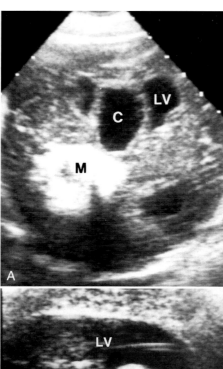

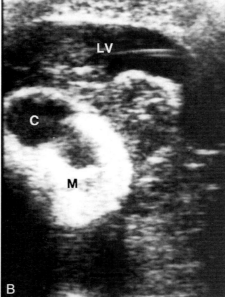

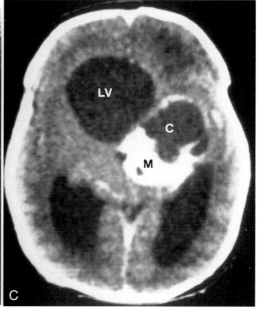

FIGURE 47-68. Astrocytic glioma (astrocytoma). A and B, Coronal and sagittal scans show echogenic mass (M) with cystic component (C) extending superiorly between lateral ventricles (LV). C, Axial enhanced CT scan. (Courtesy T. Stoeker, MD, Roanoke, Va)

COMMON BRAIN TUMORS IN FIRST YEAR OF LIFE

Teratomas
Suprasellar astrocytomas (hypothalamic)
Teratomas/rhabdoid tumors
Ependymomas
Choroid plexus tumors

---

cysts, lipomas, primary neuroblastoma, teratomas, and meningiomas have been reported.[239] A few cases of diffuse neonatal hemangiomatosis have been reported, with numerous hemangiomas of the brain, skin, spinal cord, liver, and heart. Although these may cause conges-

tive heart failure, the greatest risk is bleeding into the lesions and possible DIC. These infants do not usually live long enough for steroid therapy to cause involution of the lesions, which typically helps in neonatal hemangiomas.[240]

The ultrasound appearances of brain tumors are variable and nonspecific, but many are hyperechoic. Insufficient data are available on the ultrasound evaluation of neoplasms because most are evaluated with MRI or CT.

Cystic Intracranial Lesions

Cystic intracranial lesions are quite common, and ultrasound is the best method for evaluating such lesions

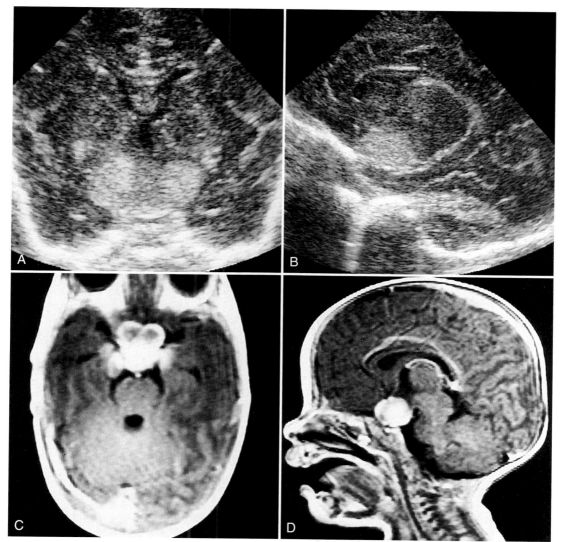

FIGURE 47-69. Optic glioma. A and **B,** Coronal and sagittal sonograms show midline echogenic mass. **C,** CT scan, and **D,** sagittal T1-weighted MR image, with contrast, show enhancement of midline optic glioma.

(short of surgical proof). Fortunately, most cystic masses of the brain are quite benign, so it is important to recognize them for what they are[31] (Table 47-3). Epelman et al.[40] describe the differential diagnosis of intracranial cystic lesions on ultrasound, CT, and MRI.[39,241,242] First, it is important to recognize the **normal cystic structures** and the variants discussed earlier under Developmental Anatomy, including the cavum septi pellucidi and vergae, cavum velum interpositum, frontal horn cysts, and the cisterna magna. Second, a normal variant, a large or **mega cisterna magna,** is not a true cyst (see Fig. 47-33).

Arachnoid Cysts

Arachnoid cysts are the most common true cysts of the brain but make up only 1% of all space-occupying lesions in children.[31] Arachnoid cysts are CSF-containing

TABLE 47-3. CYSTIC BRAIN LESIONS

CATEGORY	SPECIFIC LESIONS
Normal variants	Frontal horn cysts*
	Choroid plexus cysts
Congenital	Primary arachnoid cyst
	Dandy-Walker malformation
	Hydranencephaly
	Holoprosencephaly
Periventricular	Periventricular leukomalacia
	Subependymal cyst
	Porencephalic cyst
Neoplastic	Cerebellar astrocytoma (cystic type)
	Craniopharyngioma
	Teratoma
Inflammatory	Abscess
	Subdural empyema
Other	Secondary arachnoid cysts
	Vein of Galen malformation

*Also called connatal cysts or coarctation of the lateral ventricle.

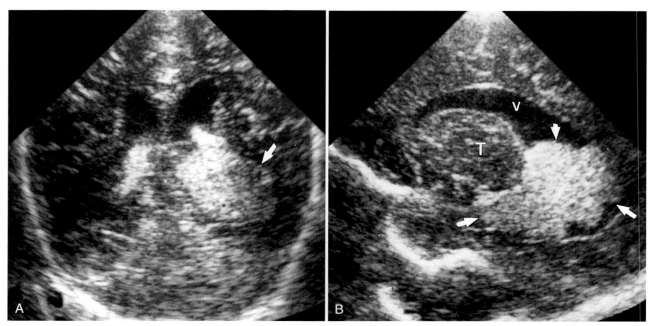

FIGURE 47-70. Choroid plexus papilloma *(arrows)* in left lateral ventricle. A and B, Coronal and sagittal sonograms; *T,* thalamus; *V,* lateral ventricle. *(Courtesy D. Pretorius, MD, University of California at San Diego.)*

spaces between two layers of arachnoid membrane. Primary and secondary cysts are believed to develop by different mechanisms. Primary cysts are believed to result from abnormal splitting of the arachnoid and from CSF collecting between the two layers. Secondary arachnoid cysts may develop by CSF trapped between arachnoid adhesions. Arachnoid cysts, particularly those in the midline, may grow and cause obstruction of the ventricular system.[31,243] These midline arachnoid cysts most often present with hydrocephalus in infancy. The ultrasound appearance of an arachnoid cyst is an anechoic area with discrete walls. Midline arachnoid cysts are frequently associated with other brain anomalies. With agenesis of the corpus callosum, midline cysts are frequently continuous with an elevated third ventricle. In alobar holoprosencephaly, a dorsal cyst may be continuous with the single central ventricle.

SITES OF ARACHNOID CYSTS*

Anterior portions of middle cranial fossa
Suprasellar region
Posterior fossa
Quadrigeminal region
Cerebral convexities
Interhemispheric fissure

*In decreasing order of frequency.

Porencephalic Cysts

Porencephalic cysts are a result of brain necrosis and cavitation, which is continuous with the ventricular system (see Fig. 47-51). These lesions are usually caused by brain parenchymal hemorrhage, infection, or surgery.[10]

Choroid Plexus Cysts

Choroid plexus cysts are common and usually asymptomatic.[244-247] Choroid cysts occur in all age groups and are found in 34% of fetuses and infants at autopsy.[207] However, prenatal and neonatal ultrasound reports have identified choroid cysts in only approximately 1% of the populations studied. They are distinctly different from and should not be confused with subependymal cysts. Choroid plexus cysts tend to be single and present as an isolated finding, not associated with other CNS or chromosomal abnormalities.[245] However, large (>10 mm) and multiple choroid cysts may be associated with chromosomal anomalies, particularly trisomy 18,[2] trisomy 21, and Aicardi syndrome.[248] Many other anomalies are typically present in these newborns.

A choroid plexus cyst appears as a cystic mass with well-defined walls within the plexus (Fig. 47-71). Choroid cysts vary in size from less than 4 mm to 7 mm and are usually unilateral, left greater than right, and situated in the dorsal aspect of the choroid plexus. Rare cases of symptomatic choroid cysts causing obstructive hydrocephalus have been reported but are probably related to some specific cause rather than a normal variant.[247,248] Some choroid plexus "cysts" are actually vessels in the choroid,[249] which can be recognized with color Doppler even in utero. Occasional choroid cysts develop after choroid plexus hemorrhage into the ventricle (Fig. 47-71).

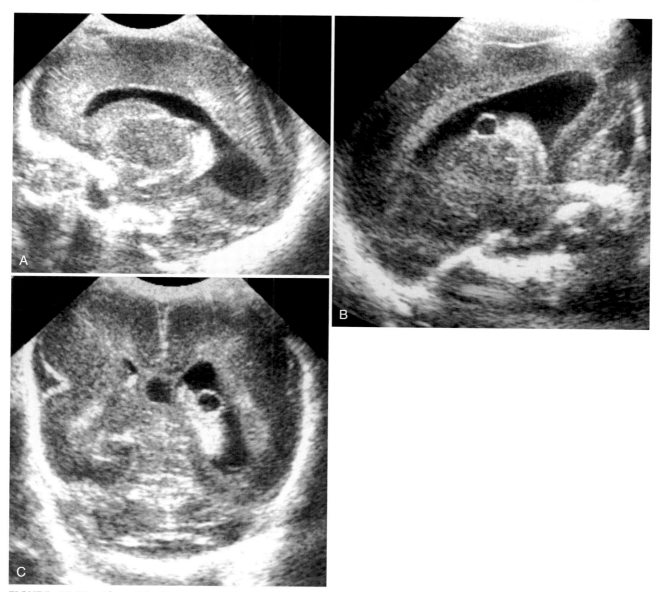

FIGURE 47-71. Choroid plexus cyst. A, Subacute hypoechoic choroid plexus hemorrhage. **B** and **C,** Choroid plexus cyst that developed after the hemorrhage.

Supratentorial Cystic Lesions in Periventricular Location

Many periventricular cysts are found in and around the normal ventricles (Fig. 47-72).

Frontal Horn Cysts

The frontal horn cysts that are attached directly lateral to the frontal horn have also been called **coarctation of the lateral ventricles** and **connatal cysts**[40] (see Fig. 47-15). Although these frontal horn cysts were previously thought to be postischemic, it is now believed that they form as a normal variant anterior to the foramen of Monro. The ventricle seems to have folded on itself, causing the wall to lie against the frontal horn.

Subependymal Cysts

Subependymal cysts present as discrete cysts in the lining of the ventricles (Fig. 47-73). These cysts most often result from the sequelae of GMH in premature infants.[250,251] Other causes include infection, including CMV and rubella, and the rare **cerebrohepatorenal (Zellweger) syndrome.**[73,252] Subependymal cysts can also be an isolated finding with no apparent predisposing event.[246] Cocaine exposure has been reported to significantly increase the incidence of subependymal cysts in premature infants.[253]

Periventricular Leukomalacia

Periventricular cysts also result from PVL (see Fig. 47-56). These cysts develop lateral and above the entire lateral ventricle, typically above the frontal horn and body of the ventricle.

Galenic Venous Malformations

Galenic venous malformations are frequently referred to as "vein of Galen aneurysms," but this is a misnomer because these are not true aneurysms. These abnormalities actually represent dilation of the vein of Galen caused by a vascular malformation that is fed by large arteries off the anterior or posterior cerebral artery circulation.[254] Infants with large shunts usually present in the first month of life with congestive heart failure.[255] In later childhood, smaller shunts present with seizure, cranial bruit, hydrocephalus, and cardiomegaly.

Sonographically, a galenic venous malformation appears as an anechoic cystic mass between the lateral ventricles (Fig. 47-74). It lies posterior to the foramen of Monro, superior to the third ventricle, and primarily in the midline.[256,257] These malformations are differentiated from other cystic masses by identification of a large feeding vessel. Spectral or color Doppler sonography can be used to identify blood flow filling the mass, thus confirming the diagnosis.[258] Hydrocephalus may or may not be present. Calcification may occur, especially if there is thrombosis in the malformation.[259] MRI and MR angiography may be valuable in planning treatment.[260] If treatment is considered with embolization, angiography may be required.[261]

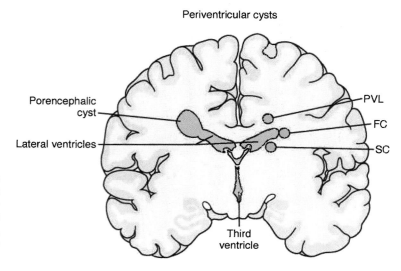

FIGURE 47-72. Periventricular cysts. These cysts include the normal-variant frontal horn cyst *(FC)*, the subependymal cyst *(SC)*, cystic periventricular leukomalacia *(PVL)*, and porencephalic cysts that communicate directly with the ventricle, caused by intraparenchymal hemorrhage or infection (cerebritis).

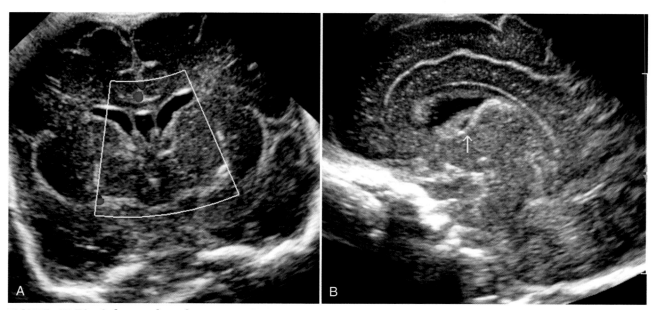

FIGURE 47-73. Subependymal cyst. A and **B,** Coronal and midline sagittal sonograms show cyst *(arrow),* which formed after cytomegalovirus antenatal infection in the region of the caudothalamic notch, where we typically expect to see germinal matrix hemorrhage. The cyst was present at birth.

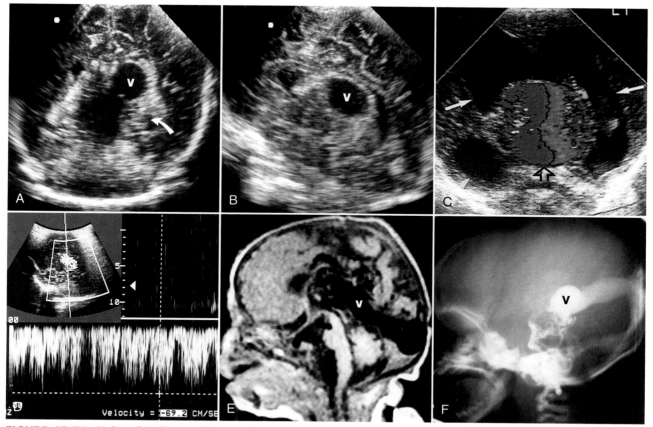

FIGURE 47-74. Vein of Galen malformation. A and **B,** Coronal and sagittal sonograms show enlarged vein of Galen *(V)* and straight sinus. Echogenic arterial feeding vessels below and anterior to dilated vein of Galen *(curved arrow).* **C** and **D,** Color Doppler and duplex Doppler ultrasound scans show turbulent flow, which clearly defines this cystic-appearing mass as vascular. **E,** Sagittal MR scan, and **F,** angiogram, in a different patient, show the echogenic region is a tortuous tangle of abnormal feeding vessels; cystic mass is dilated vein of Galen *(V).*

References

1. Barr LL. Neonatal cranial ultrasound. Radiol Clin North Am 1999;37:1127-1146, vi.
2. Benson JE, Bishop MR, Cohen HL. Intracranial neonatal neurosonography: an update. Ultrasound Q 2002;18:89-114.
3. DiPietro MA, Faix RG, Donn SM. Procedural hazards of neonatal ultrasonography. J Clin Ultrasound 1986;14:361-366.
4. Bulas D. Fetal magnetic resonance imaging as a complement to fetal ultrasonography. Ultrasound Q 2007;23:3-22.
5. Mitchell DG, Merton D, Desai H, et al. Neonatal brain: color Doppler imaging. Part II. Altered flow patterns from extracorporeal membrane oxygenation. Radiology 1988;167:307-310.
6. Cohen HL, Haller JO. Advances in perinatal neurosonography. AJR Am J Roentgenol 1994;163:801-810.
7. Bezinque SL, Slovis TL, Touchette AS, et al. Characterization of superior sagittal sinus blood flow velocity using color flow Doppler in neonates and infants. Pediatr Radiol 1995;25:175-179.
8. Soboleski D, McCloskey D, Mussari B, et al. Sonography of normal cranial sutures. AJR Am J Roentgenol 1997;168:819-821.
9. Coley BD. Ultrasound diagnosis of lückenschädel (lacunar skull). Pediatr Radiol 2000;30:82-84.

Equipment

10. Rumack CM, Manco-Johnson ML. Perinatal and infant brain imaging: role of ultrasound and computed tomography. St Louis: Mosby; 1984.
11. Thomson GD, Teele RL. High-frequency linear array transducers for neonatal cerebral sonography. AJR Am J Roentgenol 2001; 176:995-1001.

12. Anderson N, Allan R, Darlow B, Malpas T. Diagnosis of intraventricular hemorrhage in the newborn: value of sonography via the posterior fontanelle. AJR Am J Roentgenol 1994;163:893-896.

Sonographic Technique

13. Angtuaco TL. Navigating the neonatal brain through the base of the skull: an effective sonographic teaching tool. Ultrasound Q 2004;20: 38-44.
14. Enriquez G, Correa F, Aso C, et al. Mastoid fontanelle approach for sonographic imaging of the neonatal brain. Pediatr Radiol 2006; 36:532-540.
15. Correa F, Enriquez G, Rossello J, et al. Posterior fontanelle sonography: an acoustic window into the neonatal brain. AJNR Am J Neuroradiol 2004;25:1274-1282.
16. Chen CY, Chou TY, Zimmerman RA, et al. Pericerebral fluid collection: differentiation of enlarged subarachnoid spaces from subdural collections with color Doppler ultrasound. Radiology 1996; 201:389-392.
17. Pigadas A, Thompson JR, Grube GL. Normal infant brain anatomy: correlated real-time sonograms and brain specimens. AJR Am J Roentgenol 1981;137:815-820.
18. Di Salvo DN. A new view of the neonatal brain: clinical utility of supplemental neurologic US imaging windows. Radiographics 2001;21:943-955.
19. Luna JA, Goldstein RB. Sonographic visualization of neonatal posterior fossa abnormalities through the posterolateral fontanelle. AJR Am J Roentgenol 2000;174:561-567.
20. Rumack CR, Horgan JG, Hay TC, et al. Pocket atlas of pediatric ultrasound. Philadelphia: Lippincott-Raven; 1990.

21. Cuddihy SL, Anderson NG, Wells JE, Darlow BA. Cerebellar vermis diameter at cranial sonography for assessing gestational age in low-birth-weight infants. Pediatr Radiol 1999;29:589-594.

22. DiPietro MA, Brody BA, Teele RL. Peritrigonal echogenic "blush" on cranial sonography: pathologic correlates. AJR Am J Roentgenol 1986;146:1067-1072.

23. Buckley KM, Taylor GA, Estroff JA, et al. Use of the mastoid fontanelle for improved sonographic visualization of the neonatal midbrain and posterior fossa. AJR Am J Roentgenol 1997;168:1021-1025.

24. Taylor GA. Recent advances in neonatal cranial ultrasound and Doppler techniques. Clin Perinatol 1997;24:677-691.

Three-Dimensional Ultrasound

25. Salerno CC, Pretorius DH, Hilton SW, et al. Three-dimensional ultrasonographic imaging of the neonatal brain in high-risk neonates: preliminary study. J Ultrasound Med 2000;19:549-555.

26. Csutak R, Unterassinger L, Rohrmeister C, et al. Three-dimensional volume measurement of the lateral ventricles in preterm and term infants: evaluation of a standardised computer-assisted method in vivo. Pediatr Radiol 2003;33:104-109.

27. Glenn OA, Goldstein RB, Li KC, et al. Fetal magnetic resonance imaging in the evaluation of fetuses referred for sonographically suspected abnormalities of the corpus callosum. J Ultrasound Med 2005;24:791-804.

28. American College of Radiology. ACR practice guideline for the performance of neurosonography in neonates and infants. Revised 2009 (Res 18).

Developmental Anatomy

29. Dorovini-Zis K, Dolman CL. Gestational development of brain. Arch Pathol Lab Med 1977;101:192-195.

30. Ghai S, Fong KW, Toi A, et al. Prenatal ultrasound and MR imaging findings of lissencephaly: review of fetal cerebral sulcal development. Radiographics 2006;26:389-405.

31. Barkovich AJ. Pediatric neuroimaging. 4th ed. Philadelphia: Lippincott–Williams & Wilkins; 2005.

32. Worthen NJ, Gilbertson V, Lau C. Cortical sulcal development seen on sonography: relationship to gestational parameters. J Ultrasound Med 1986;5:153-156.

33. Govaert P, Swarte R, De Vos A, Lequin M. Sonographic appearance of the normal and abnormal insula of Reil. Dev Med Child Neurol 2004;46:610-616.

34. Armstrong DL, Bagnall C, Harding JE, Teele RL. Measurement of the subarachnoid space by ultrasound in preterm infants. Arch Dis Child Fetal Neonatal Ed 2002;86:F124-F126.

35. Shaw CM, Alvord Jr EC. Cava septi pellucidi et vergae: their normal and pathogical states. Brain 1969;92:213-223.

36. Callen PW, Callen AL, Glenn OA, Toi A. Columns of the fornix, not to be mistaken for the cavum septi pellucidi on prenatal sonography. J Ultrasound Med 2008;27:25-31.

37. Chen CY, Chen FH, Lee CC, et al. Sonographic characteristics of the cavum velum interpositum. AJNR Am J Neuroradiol 1998;19:1631-1635.

38. Blasi I, Henrich W, Argento C, Chaoui R. Prenatal diagnosis of a cavum veli interpositi. J Ultrasound Med 2009;28:683-687.

39. Rosenfeld DL, Schonfeld SM, Underberg-Davis S. Coarctation of the lateral ventricles: an alternative explanation for subependymal pseudocysts. Pediatr Radiol 1997;27:895-897.

40. Epelman M, Daneman A, Blaser SI, et al. Differential diagnosis of intracranial cystic lesions at head ultrasound: correlation with CT and MR imaging. Radiographics 2006;26:173-196.

41. Enriquez G, Correa F, Lucaya J, et al. Potential pitfalls in cranial sonography. Pediatr Radiol 2003;33:110-117.

42. Friede R. Developmental neuropathology. 2nd ed. New York: Springer Verlag; 1975.

43. Jaspan T. New concepts on posterior fossa malformations. Pediatr Radiol 2008;38(Suppl 3):409-414.

44. Adamsbaum C, Moutard ML, Andre C, et al. MRI of the fetal posterior fossa. Pediatr Radiol 2005;35:124-140.

45. Triulzi F, Parazzini C, Righini A. MRI of fetal and neonatal cerebellar development. Semin Fetal Neonatal Med 2005;10:411-420.

46. Robinson AJ, Goldstein R. The cisterna magna septa: vestigial remnants of Blake's pouch and a potential new marker for normal development of the rhombencephalon. J Ultrasound Med 2007;26:83-95.

47. Oh KY, Rassner UA, Frias Jr AE, Kennedy AM. The fetal posterior fossa: clinical correlation of findings on prenatal ultrasound and fetal magnetic resonance imaging. Ultrasound Q 2007;23:203-210.

48. Robinson AJ, Blaser S, Toi A, et al. The fetal cerebellar vermis: assessment for abnormal development by ultrasonography and magnetic resonance imaging. Ultrasound Q 2007;23:211-223.

Congenital Brain Malformations

49. Volpe JJ. Neurology of the newborn. 5th ed. Philadelphia: Saunders-Elsevier; 2008.

50. Gilles FH, Leviton A, Dooling EC. The developing human brain. Boston: John Wright–PSG; 1983.

51. Volpe JJ. Brain injury in premature infants: a complex amalgam of destructive and developmental disturbances. Lancet Neurol 2009; 8:110-124.

52. DeMyer W. Classification of cerebral malformations. Birth Defects Orig Artic Ser 1971;7:78-93.

53. Limperopoulos C, du Plessis AJ. Disorders of cerebellar growth and development. Curr Opin Pediatr 2006;18:621-627.

54. Patel S, Barkovich AJ. Analysis and classification of cerebellar malformations. AJNR Am J Neuroradiol 2002;23:1074-1087.

Disorders of Neural Tube Closure

55. McLone DG, Naidich TP. Developmental morphology of the subarachnoid space, brain vasculature, and contiguous structures, and the cause of the Chiari II malformation. AJNR Am J Neuroradiol 1992;13:463-482.

56. Naidich TP, Pudlowski RM, Naidich JB. Computed tomographic signs of Chiari II malformation. II. Midbrain and cerebellum. Radiology 1980;134:391-398.

57. Naidich TP, Pudlowski RM, Naidich JB. Computed tomographic signs of the Chiari II malformation. III. Ventricles and cisterns. Radiology 1980;134:657-663.

58. Zimmerman RD, Breckbill D, Dennis MW, Davis DO. Cranial CT findings in patients with meningomyelocele. AJR Am J Roentgenol 1979;132:623-629.

59. Fitz CR. Disorders of ventricles and CSF spaces. Semin Ultrasound CT MR 1988;9:216-230.

60. Babcook CJ, Goldstein RB, Barth RA, et al. Prevalence of ventriculomegaly in association with myelomeningocele: correlation with gestational age and severity of posterior fossa deformity. Radiology 1994;190:703-707.

61. Osborn AG. Diagnostic neuroradiolog. St Louis: Mosby; 1994.

62. Babcock DS. The normal, absent, and abnormal corpus callosum: sonographic findings. Radiology 1984;151:449-453.

63. Kier EL, Truwit CL. The normal and abnormal genu of the corpus callosum: an evolutionary, embryologic, anatomic, and MR analysis. AJNR Am J Neuroradiol 1996;17:1631-1641.

64. Goodyear PW, Bannister CM, Russell S, Rimmer S. Outcome in prenatally diagnosed fetal agenesis of the corpus callosum. Fetal Diagn Ther 2001;16:139-145.

65. d'Ercole C, Girard N, Cravello L, et al. Prenatal diagnosis of fetal corpus callosum agenesis by ultrasonography and magnetic resonance imaging. Prenat Diagn 1998;18:247-253.

66. Aletebi FA, Fung KF. Neurodevelopmental outcome after antenatal diagnosis of posterior fossa abnormalities. J Ultrasound Med 1999; 18:683-689.

67. Nyberg DA, Mahony BS, Hegge FN, et al. Enlarged cisterna magna and the Dandy-Walker malformation: factors associated with chromosome abnormalities. Obstet Gynecol 1991;77:436-442.

68. Bromley B, Nadel AS, Pauker S, et al. Closure of the cerebellar vermis: evaluation with second trimester ultrasound. Radiology 1994;193:761-763.

69. Estroff JA, Parad RB, Barnes PD, et al. Posterior fossa arachnoid cyst: an in utero mimicker of Dandy-Walker malformation. J Ultrasound Med 1995;14:787-790.

70. Chang MC, Russell SA, Callen PW, et al. Sonographic detection of inferior vermian agenesis in Dandy-Walker malformations: prognostic implications. Radiology 1994;193:765-770.

71. Keogan MT, DeAtkine AB, Hertzberg BS. Cerebellar vermian defects: antenatal sonographic appearance and clinical significance. J Ultrasound Med 1994;13:607-611.

72. Hart MN, Malamud N, Ellis WG. The Dandy-Walker syndrome: a clinicopathological study based on 28 cases. Neurology 1972;22:771-780.

73. Lachman RS, Taybi H. Taybi and Lachman's radiology of syndromes, metabolic disorders, and skeletal dysplasias. 5th ed. St Louis: Mosby-Elsevier; 2007.

74. Ball WS. Pediatric neuroradiology. Philadelphia: Lippincott-Raven; 1997.

Disorders of Diverticulation and Cleavage: Holoprosencephaly

75. Demyer W, Zeman W, Palmer CG. The face predicts the brain: diagnostic significance of median facial anomalies for holoprosencephaly (arhinencephaly). Pediatrics 1964;34:256-263.

76. Fitz CR. Holoprosencephaly and related entities. Neuroradiology 1983;25:225-238.

77. Stashinko EE, Clegg NJ, Kammann HA, et al. A retrospective survey of perinatal risk factors of 104 living children with holoprosencephaly. Am J Med Genet 2004;128A:114-119.

78. Altman NR, Altman DH, Sheldon JJ, Leborgne J. Holoprosencephaly classified by computed tomography. AJNR Am J Neuroradiol 1984;5:433-437.

Disorders of Sulcation and Cellular Migration

79. Oh KY, Kennedy AM, Frias Jr AE, Byrne JL. Fetal schizencephaly: pre- and postnatal imaging with a review of the clinical manifestations. Radiographics 2005;25:647-657.

80. Sener RN. Schizencephaly and congenital cytomegalovirus infection. J Neuroradiol 1998;25:151-152.

81. Iannetti P, Nigro G, Spalice A, et al. Cytomegalovirus infection and schizencephaly: case reports. Ann Neurol 1998;43:123-127.

82. Lee HK, Kim JS, Hwang YM, et al. Location of the primary motor cortex in schizencephaly. AJNR Am J Neuroradiol 1999;20:163-166.

Destructive Lesions

83. Pretorius DH, Russ PD, Rumack CM, et al. Diagnosis of brain neuropathology in utero. In: Naidich TP, Quencer RM, editors. Clinical neurosonography. Berlin: Springer-Verlag; 1987.

84. Diebler C, Dulac O. Pediatric neurology and neuroradiology. Berlin, Springer-Verlag; 1987.

85. Leijser LM, de Vries LS, Rutherford MA, et al. Cranial ultrasound in metabolic disorders presenting in the neonatal period: characteristic features and comparison with MR imaging. AJNR Am J Neuroradiol 2007;28:1223-1231

Hydrocephalus

86. Benacerraf BR, Shipp TD, Bromley B, Levine D. What does magnetic resonance imaging add to the prenatal sonographic diagnosis of ventriculomegaly? J Ultrasound Med 2007;26:1513-1522.

87. Lee CS, Hong SH, Wang KC, et al. Fetal ventriculomegaly: prognosis in cases in which prenatal neurosurgical consultation was sought. J Neurosurg 2006;105:265-270.

88. Levine D, Feldman HA, Tannus JF, et al. Frequency and cause of disagreements in diagnoses for fetuses referred for ventriculomegaly. Radiology 2008;247:516-527.

89. Farrell TA, Hertzberg BS, Kliewer MA, et al. Fetal lateral ventricles: reassessment of normal values for atrial diameter at ultrasound. Radiology 1994;193:409-411.

90. Filly RA, Goldstein RB. The fetal ventricular atrium: fourth down and 10 mm to go. Radiology 1994;193:315-317.

91. Alagappan R, Browning PD, Laorr A, McGahan JP. Distal lateral ventricular atrium: reevaluation of normal range. Radiology 1994;193:405-408.

92. Rosseau GL, McCullough DC, Joseph AL. Current prognosis in fetal ventriculomegaly. J Neurosurg 1992;77:551-555.

93. Rosenfeld DL, Lis E, DeMarco K. Transtentorial herniation of the fourth ventricle. Pediatr Radiol 1995;25:436-439.

94. Taylor GA, Madsen JR. Neonatal hydrocephalus: hemodynamic response to fontanelle compression—correlation with intracranial pressure and need for shunt placement. Radiology 1996;201:685-689.

95. Taylor GA, Soul JS, Dunning PS. Sonographic ventriculography: a new potential use for sonographic contrast agents in neonatal hydrocephalus. AJNR Am J Neuroradiol 1998;19:1931-1934.

96. Senat MV, Bernard JP, Delezoide A, et al. Prenatal diagnosis of hydrocephalus-stenosis of the aqueduct of Sylvius by ultrasound in the first trimester of pregnancy: report of two cases. Prenat Diagn 2001;21:1129-1132.

97. Forstner R, Hoffmann GF, Gassner I, et al. Glutaric aciduria type I: ultrasonographic demonstration of early signs. Pediatr Radiol 1999;29:138-143.

Hypoxic-Ischemic Events

98. Dogra VS, Shyken JM, Menon PA, et al. Neurosonographic abnormalities associated with maternal history of cocaine use in neonates of appropriate size for their gestational age. AJNR Am J Neuroradiol 1994;15:697-702.

99. Dean LM, Taylor GA. The intracranial venous system in infants: normal and abnormal findings on duplex and color Doppler sonography. AJR Am J Roentgenol 1995;164:151-156.

100. Taylor GA. New concepts in the pathogenesis of germinal matrix intraparenchymal hemorrhage in premature infants. AJNR Am J Neuroradiol 1997;18:231-232.

101. Ghazi-Birry HS, Brown WR, Moody DM, et al. Human germinal matrix: venous origin of hemorrhage and vascular characteristics. AJNR Am J Neuroradiol 1997;18:219-229.

102. Taylor GA. Effect of germinal matrix hemorrhage on terminal vein position and patency. Pediatr Radiol 1995;25(Suppl 1):37-40.

103. Chao CP, Zaleski CG, Patton AC. Neonatal hypoxic-ischemic encephalopathy: multimodality imaging findings. Radiographics 2006;26(Suppl 1):159-172.

104. Huang BY, Castillo M. Hypoxic-ischemic brain injury: imaging findings from birth to adulthood. Radiographics 2008;28:417-439; quiz 617.

105. Hintz SR, O'Shea M. Neuroimaging and neurodevelopmental outcomes in preterm infants. Semin Perinatol 2008;32:11-19.

106. Leijser LM, de Bruine FT, Steggerda SJ, et al. Brain imaging findings in very preterm infants throughout the neonatal period. Part I. Incidences and evolution of lesions, comparison between ultrasound and MRI. Early Hum Dev 2009;85:101-109.

107. Rutherford M, Srinivasan L, Dyet L, et al. Magnetic resonance imaging in perinatal brain injury: clinical presentation, lesions and outcome. Pediatr Radiol 2006;36:582-592.

108. Swarte R, Lequin M, Cherian P, et al. Imaging patterns of brain injury in term-birth asphyxia. Acta Paediatr 2009;98:586-592.

109. Liauw L, van der Grond J, van den Berg-Huysmans AA, et al. Hypoxic-ischemic encephalopathy: diagnostic value of conventional MR imaging pulse sequences in term-born neonates. Radiology 2008;247:204-122.

110. Ment LR, Schneider KC, Ainley MA, Allan WC. Adaptive mechanisms of developing brain: the neuroradiologic assessment of the preterm infant. Clin Perinatol 2000;27:303-323.

111. Paul DA, Pearlman SA, Finkelstein MS, Stefano JL. Cranial sonography in very-low-birth-weight infants: do all infants need to be screened? Clin Pediatr (Phila) 1999;38:503-509.

112. Volpe JJ. Neurobiology of periventricular leukomalacia in the premature infant. Pediatr Res 2001;50:553-562.

113. Burstein J, Papile LA, Burstein R. Intraventricular hemorrhage and hydrocephalus in premature newborns: a prospective study with CT. AJR Am J Roentgenol 1979;132:631-635.

114. Rumack CM, Manco-Johnson ML, Manco-Johnson MJ, et al. Timing and course of neonatal intracranial hemorrhage using real-time ultrasound. Radiology 1985;154:101-105.

115. Boal DK, Watterberg KL, Miles S, Gifford KL. Optimal cost-effective timing of cranial ultrasound screening in low-birth-weight infants. Pediatr Radiol 1995;25:425-428.

116. Townsend SF, Rumack CM, Thilo EH, et al. Late neurosonographic screening is important to the diagnosis of periventricular leukomalacia and ventricular enlargement in preterm infants. Pediatr Radiol 1999;29:347-352.

117. Perlman JM, Rollins N. Surveillance protocol for the detection of intracranial abnormalities in premature neonates. Arch Pediatr Adolesc Med 2000;154:822-826.

118. Lemons JA, Bauer CR, Oh W, et al. Very low birth weight outcomes of the National Institute of Child Health and Human Development Neonatal Research Network, January 1995 through December 1996. Pediatrics 2001;107:E1.

119. Shankaran S, Bauer C, Bain R, et al. Antenatal steroids to reduce the risk of intracranial hemorrahge in the neonate. In Report of the Consensus Development Conference on the Effects of Corticosteroids for Fetal Maturation on Perinatal Outcomes, 1994, NIH 95-3784.

120. Maher JE. Effects of corticosteroid therapy in the very premature infant. In Report of the Consensus Development Conference on the

Effects of Corticosteroids for Fetal Maturation on Perinatal Outcomes, 1994, NIH 95-3784.

121. Cramer BC, Walsh EA. Cisterna magna clot and subsequent posthemorrhagic hydrocephalus. Pediatr Radiol 2001;31:153-159.

122. Rudas G, Varga E, Meder U, et al. Changes in echogenicity of spinal subarachnoid space associated with intracranial hemorrhage: new observations. Pediatr Radiol 2000;30:739-742.

123. Vohr B, Allan WC, Scott DT, et al. Early-onset intraventricular hemorrhage in preterm neonates: incidence of neurodevelopmental handicap. Semin Perinatol 1999;23:212-217.

124. Rypens E, Avni EF, Dussaussois L, et al. Hyperechoic thickened ependyma: sonographic demonstration and significance in neonates. Pediatr Radiol 1994;24:550-553.

125. Murphy BP, Inder TE, Rooks V, et al. Posthaemorrhagic ventricular dilatation in the premature infant: natural history and predictors of outcome. Arch Dis Child Fetal Neonatal Ed 2002;87:F37-F41.

126. De Vries LS, Rademaker KJ, Groenendaal F, et al. Correlation between neonatal cranial ultrasound, MRI in infancy and neurodevelopmental outcome in infants with a large intraventricular haemorrhage with or without unilateral parenchymal involvement. Neuropediatrics 1998;29:180-188.

127. Bass WT, Jones MA, White LE, et al. Ultrasonographic differential diagnosis and neurodevelopmental outcome of cerebral white matter lesions in premature infants. J Perinatol 1999;19:330-336.

128. Bassan H, Limperopoulos C, Visconti K, et al. Neurodevelopmental outcome in survivors of periventricular hemorrhagic infarction. Pediatrics 2007;120:785-792.

129. O'Shea TM, Kuban KC, Allred EN, et al. Neonatal cranial ultrasound lesions and developmental delays at 2 years of age among extremely low gestational age children. Pediatrics 2008;122:e662-e669.

130. Bassan H, Benson CB, Limperopoulos C, et al. Ultrasonographic features and severity scoring of periventricular hemorrhagic infarction in relation to risk factors and outcome. Pediatrics 2006;117:2111-2118.

131. Wood NS, Costeloe K, Gibson AT, et al. The EPICure study: associations and antecedents of neurological and developmental disability at 30 months of age following extremely preterm birth. Arch Dis Child Fetal Neonatal Ed 2005;90:F134-F140.

132. Kobayashi S, Fujimoto S, Fukuda S, et al. Periventricular leukomalacia with late-onset circulatory dysfunction of premature infants: correlation with severity of magnetic resonance imaging findings and neurological outcomes. Tohoku J Exp Med 2006;210:333-339.

133. Korkmaz A, Yigit S, Firat M, Oran O. Cranial MRI in neonatal hypernatraemic dehydration. Pediatr Radiol 2000;30:323-325.

134. Mocharla R, Schexnayder SM, Glasier CM. Fatal cerebral edema and intracranial hemorrhage associated with hypernatremic dehydration. Pediatr Radiol 1997;27:785-787.

135. Dean LM, McLeary M, Taylor GA. Cerebral hemorrhage in alloimmune thrombocytopenia. Pediatr Radiol 1995;25:444-445.

136. Kulkarni R, Lusher JM. Intracranial and extracranial hemorrhages in newborns with hemophilia: a review of the literature. J Pediatr Hematol Oncol 1999;21:289-295.

137. Huang AH, Robertson RL. Spontaneous superficial parenchymal and leptomeningeal hemorrhage in term neonates. AJNR Am J Neuroradiol 2004;25:469-475.

138. Jarjour IT, Ahdab-Barmada M. Cerebrovascular lesions in infants and children dying after extracorporeal membrane oxygenation. Pediatr Neurol 1994;10:13-19.

139. Bulas DI, Taylor GA, O'Donnell RM, et al. Intracranial abnormalities in infants treated with extracorporeal membrane oxygenation: update on sonographic and CT findings. AJNR Am J Neuroradiol 1996;17:287-294.

140. Kazam E, Rudelli R, Monte W, et al. Sonographic diagnosis of cisternal subarachnoid hemorrhage in the premature infant. AJNR Am J Neuroradiol 1994;15:1009-1020.

141. Messerschmidt A, Brugger PC, Boltshauser E, et al. Disruption of cerebellar development: potential complication of extreme prematurity. AJNR Am J Neuroradiol 2005;26:1659-1667.

142. Steggerda SJ, Leijser LM, Wiggers-de Bruine FT, et al. Cerebellar injury in preterm infants: incidence and findings on ultrasound and MR images. Radiology 2009;252:190-199.

143. Messerschmidt A, Fuiko R, Prayer D, et al. Disrupted cerebellar development in preterm infants is associated with impaired neurodevelopmental outcome. Eur J Pediatr 2008;167:1141-1147.

144. Muller H, Beedgen B, Schenk JP, et al. Intracerebellar hemorrhage in premature infants: sonographic detection and outcome. J Perinat Med 2007;35:67-70.

145. Limperopoulos C, Bassan H, Gauvreau K, et al. Does cerebellar injury in premature infants contribute to the high prevalence of long-term cognitive, learning, and behavioral disability in survivors? Pediatrics 2007;120:584-593.

146. Limperopoulos C, Benson CB, Bassan H, et al. Cerebellar hemorrhage in the preterm infant: ultrasonographic findings and risk factors. Pediatrics 2005;116:717-724.

147. Merrill JD, Piecuch RE, Fell SC, et al. A new pattern of cerebellar hemorrhages in preterm infants. Pediatrics 1998;102:E62.

148. Folkerth RD, McLaughlin ME, Levine D. Organizing posterior fossa hematomas simulating developmental cysts on prenatal imaging: report of 3 cases. J Ultrasound Med 2001;20:1233-1240.

149. Chadduck WM, Duong DH, Kast JM, Donahue DJ. Pediatric cerebellar hemorrhages. Childs Nerv Syst 1995;11:579-583.

150. Mirmiran M, Barnes PD, Keller K, et al. Neonatal brain magnetic resonance imaging before discharge is better than serial cranial ultrasound in predicting cerebral palsy in very low birth weight preterm infants. Pediatrics 2004;114:992-998.

151. Silveira RC, Procianoy RS, Dill JC, da Costa CS. Periventricular leukomalacia in very low birth weight preterm neonates with high risk for neonatal sepsis. J Pediatr (Rio J) 2008;84:211-216.

152. Veyrac C, Couture A, Saguintaah M, Baud C. Brain ultrasonography in the premature infant. Pediatr Radiol 2006;36:626-635.

153. Gibbs RS. The relationship between infections and adverse pregnancy outcomes: an overview. Ann Periodontol 2001;6:153-163.

154. Bracci R, Buonocore G. Chorioamnionitis: a risk factor for fetal and neonatal morbidity. Biol Neonate 2003;83:85-96.

155. Rezaie P, Dean A. Periventricular leukomalacia, inflammation and white matter lesions within the developing nervous system. Neuropathology 2002;22:106-132.

156. Vigneswaran R. Infection and preterm birth: evidence of a common causal relationship with bronchopulmonary dysplasia and cerebral palsy. J Paediatr Child Health 2000;36:293-296.

157. Batton DG, Kirtley X, Swails T. Unexpected versus anticipated cystic periventricular leukomalacia. Am J Perinatol 2003;20:33-40.

158. Leviton A, Dammann O, Allred EN, et al. Antenatal corticosteroids and cranial ultrasonographic abnormalities. Am J Obstet Gynecol 1999;181:1007-1017.

159. Verma U, Tejani N, Klein S, et al. Obstetric antecedents of intraventricular hemorrhage and periventricular leukomalacia in the low-birth-weight neonate. Am J Obstet Gynecol 1997;176:275-281.

160. Perlman JM. White matter injury in the preterm infant: an important determination of abnormal neurodevelopment outcome. Early Hum Dev 1998;53:99-120.

161. Cooke RW. Trends in incidence of cranial ultrasound lesions and cerebral palsy in very low birthweight infants 1982-93. Arch Dis Child Fetal Neonatal Ed 1999;80:F115-F117.

162. Stannard MW, Jimenez JF. Sonographic recognition of multiple cystic encephalomalacia. AJR Am J Roentgenol 1983;141:1321-1324.

163. Schellinger D, Grant EG, Richardson JD. Cystic periventricular leukomalacia: sonographic and CT findings. AJNR Am J Neuroradiol 1984;5:439-445.

164. Dubowitz LM, Bydder GM, Mushin J. Developmental sequence of periventricular leukomalacia: correlation of ultrasound, clinical, and nuclear magnetic resonance functions. Arch Dis Child 1985;60:349-355.

165. Melhem ER, Hoon Jr AH, Ferrucci Jr JT, et al. Periventricular leukomalacia: relationship between lateral ventricular volume on brain MR images and severity of cognitive and motor impairment. Radiology 2000;214:199-204.

166. Ancel PY, Livinec F, Larroque B, et al. Cerebral palsy among very preterm children in relation to gestational age and neonatal ultrasound abnormalities: the EPIPAGE cohort study. Pediatrics 2006;117:828-835.

167. Sie LT, van der Knaap MS, van Wezel-Meijler G, et al. Early MR features of hypoxic-ischemic brain injury in neonates with periventricular densities on sonograms. AJNR Am J Neuroradiol 2000;21:852-861.

168. Carson SC, Hertzberg BS, Bowie JD, Burger PC. Value of sonography in the diagnosis of intracranial hemorrhage and periventricular leukomalacia: a postmortem study of 35 cases. AJR Am J Roentgenol 1990;155:595-601.

169. Coley BD, Hogan MJ. Cystic periventricular leukomalacia of the corpus callosum. Pediatr Radiol 1997;27:583-585.

170. Adcock LM, Moore PJ, Schlesinger AE, Armstrong DL. Correlation of ultrasound with postmortem neuropathologic studies in neonates. Pediatr Neurol 1998;19:263-271.

171. Valkama AM, Paakko EL, Vainionpaa LK, et al. Magnetic resonance imaging at term and neuromotor outcome in preterm infants. Acta Paediatr 2000;89:348-355.

172. Aida N, Nishimura G, Hachiya Y, et al. MR imaging of perinatal brain damage: comparison of clinical outcome with initial and follow-up MR findings. AJNR Am J Neuroradiol 1998;19:1909-1921.

173. Ferriero DM. Neonatal brain injury. N Engl J Med 2004;351: 1985-1995.

174. Skranes JS, Nilsen G, Smevik O, et al. Cerebral magnetic resonance imaging (MRI) of very low birth weight infants at one year of corrected age. Pediatr Radiol 1992;22:406-409.

175. De Vries LS, Dubowitz LM, Pennock JM, Bydder GM. Extensive cystic leucomalacia: correlation of cranial ultrasound, magnetic resonance imaging and clinical findings in sequential studies. Clin Radiol 1989;40:158-166.

176. Leijser LM, Liauw L, Veen S, et al. Comparing brain white matter on sequential cranial ultrasound and MRI in very preterm infants. Neuroradiology 2008;50:799-811.

177. Deeg KH, Rupprecht T, Zeilinger G. Doppler sonographic classification of brain edema in infants. Pediatr Radiol 1990;20:509-514.

178. Stark JE, Seibert JJ. Cerebral artery Doppler ultrasonography for prediction of outcome after perinatal asphyxia. J Ultrasound Med 1994;13:595-600.

179. Chiu NC, Shen EY, Ho CS. Outcome in children with significantly abnormal cerebral blood flow detected by Doppler ultrasonography: focus on the survivors. J Neuroimaging 2003;13:53-56.

180. Connolly B, Kelehan P, O'Brien N, et al. The echogenic thalamus in hypoxic ischaemic encephalopathy. Pediatr Radiol 1994;24:268-271.

181. Volpe JJ. Value of MR in definition of the neuropathology of cerebral palsy in vivo. AJNR Am J Neuroradiol 1992;13:79-83.

182. Truwit CL, Barkovich AJ, Koch TK, Ferriero DM. Cerebral palsy: MR findings in 40 patients. AJNR Am J Neuroradiol 1992;13: 67-78.

183. Barkovich AJ, Sargent SK. Profound asphyxia in the premature infant: imaging findings. AJNR Am J Neuroradiol 1995;16:1837-1846.

184. Daneman A, Epelman M, Blaser S, Jarrin JR. Imaging of the brain in full-term neonates: does sonography still play a role? Pediatr Radiol 2006;36:636-646.

185. Han BK, Lee M, Yoon HK. Cranial ultrasound and CT findings in infants with hypernatremic dehydration. Pediatr Radiol 1997;27: 739-742.

186. Triulzi F, Parazzini C, Righini A. Patterns of damage in the mature neonatal brain. Pediatr Radiol 2006;36:608-620.

187. Mader I, Schoning M, Klose U, Kuker W. Neonatal cerebral infarction diagnosed by diffusion-weighted MRI: pseudonormalization occurs early. Stroke 2002;33:1142-1145.

188. Huppi PS, Murphy B, Maier SE, et al. Microstructural brain development after perinatal cerebral white matter injury assessed by diffusion tensor magnetic resonance imaging. Pediatrics 2001;107: 455-460.

189. Seibert JJ, Avva R, Hronas TN, et al. Use of power Doppler in pediatric neurosonography: a pictorial essay. Radiographics 1998;18:879-890.

190. Blankenberg FG, Loh NN, Norbash AM, et al. Impaired cerebrovascular autoregulation after hypoxic-ischemic injury in extremely low-birth-weight neonates: detection with power and pulsed wave Doppler ultrasound. Radiology 1997;205:563-568.

191. Allison JW, Faddis LA, Kinder DL, et al. Intracranial resistive index (RI) values in normal term infants during the first day of life. Pediatr Radiol 2000;30:618-620.

192. Nishimaki S, Iwasaki S, Minamisawa S, et al. Blood flow velocities in the anterior cerebral artery and basilar artery in asphyxiated infants. J Ultrasound Med 2008;27:955-960.

193. Mercuri E, He J, Curati WL, et al. Cerebellar infarction and atrophy in infants and children with a history of premature birth. Pediatr Radiol 1997;27:139-143.

194. Johnsen SD, Tarby TJ, Lewis KS, et al. Cerebellar infarction: an unrecognized complication of very low birthweight. J Child Neurol 2002;17:320-324.

195. Bulas DI, Vezina GL. Preterm anoxic injury: radiologic evaluation. Radiol Clin North Am 1999;37:1147-1161.

196. Steventon DM, John PR. Power Doppler ultrasound appearances of neonatal ischaemic brain injury. Pediatr Radiol 1997;27:147-149.

197. Taylor GA. Alterations in regional cerebral blood flow in neonatal stroke: preliminary findings with color Doppler sonography. Pediatr Radiol 1994;24:111-115.

198. Taylor GA. Regional cerebral blood flow estimates in newborn lamb using amplitude-mode color Doppler ultrasound. Pediatr Radiol 1996;26:282-286.

199. Taylor GA, Trescher WA, Traystman RJ, Johnston MV. Acute experimental neuronal injury in the newborn lamb: ultrasound characterization and demonstration of hemodynamic effects. Pediatr Radiol 1993;23:268-275.

200. Coley BD, Rusin JA, Boue DR. Importance of hypoxic/ischemic conditions in the development of cerebral lenticulostriate vasculopathy. Pediatr Radiol 2000;30:846-855.

201. Denbow ML, Battin MR, Cowan F, et al. Neonatal cranial ultrasonographic findings in preterm twins complicated by severe fetofetal transfusion syndrome. Am J Obstet Gynecol 1998;178:479-483.

202. Chamnanvanakij S, Rogers CG, Luppino C, et al. Linear hyperechogenicity within the basal ganglia and thalamus of preterm infants. Pediatr Neurol 2000;23:129-133.

203. Wang HS, Kuo MF, Chang TC. Sonographic lenticulostriate vasculopathy in infants: some associations and a hypothesis. AJNR Am J Neuroradiol 1995;16:97-102.

204. Schlesinger AE, Shackelford GD, Adcock LM. Hyperechoic caudate nuclei: a potential mimic of germinal matrix hemorrhage. Pediatr Radiol 1998;28:297-302.

Posttraumatic Injury

205. Huang LT, Lui CC. Tentorial hemorrhage associated with vacuum extraction in a newborn. Pediatr Radiol 1995;25(Suppl 1):230-231.

206. Chamnanvanakij S, Rollins N, Perlman JM. Subdural hematoma in term infants. Pediatr Neurol 2002;26:301-304.

207. Kleinman PK. Diagnostic imaging in infant abuse. AJR Am J Roentgenol 1990;155:703-712.

208. Jaspan T, Narborough G, Punt JA, Lowe J. Cerebral contusional tears as a marker of child abuse: detection by cranial sonography. Pediatr Radiol 1992;22:237-245.

Infection

209. Shaw DW, Cohen WA. Viral infections of the CNS in children: imaging features. AJR Am J Roentgenol 1993;160:125-133.

210. Lequin MH, Vermeulen JR, van Elburg RM, et al. Bacillus cereus meningoencephalitis in preterm infants: neuroimaging characteristics. AJNR Am J Neuroradiol 2005;26:2137-2143.

211. Filippi L, Serafini L, Dani C, et al. Congenital syphilis: unique clinical presentation in three preterm newborns. J Perinat Med 2004;32:90-94.

212. Benoist G, Salomon LJ, Mohlo M, et al. Cytomegalovirus-related fetal brain lesions: comparison between targeted ultrasound examination and magnetic resonance imaging. Ultrasound Obstet Gynecol 2008;32:900-905.

213. Ancora G, Lanari M, Lazzarotto T, et al. Cranial ultrasound scanning and prediction of outcome in newborns with congenital cytomegalovirus infection. J Pediatr 2007;150:157-161.

214. De Vries LS, Gunardi H, Barth PG, et al. The spectrum of cranial ultrasound and magnetic resonance imaging abnormalities in congenital cytomegalovirus infection. Neuropediatrics 2004;35:113-119.

215. Nowakowska D, Respondek-Liberska M, et al. Too late prenatal diagnosis of fetal toxoplasmosis: a case report. Fetal Diagn Ther 2005;20:190-193.

216. Moinuddin A, McKinstry RC, Martin KA, Neil JJ. Intracranial hemorrhage progressing to porencephaly as a result of congenitally acquired cytomegalovirus infection: an illustrative report. Prenat Diagn 2003;23:797-800.

217. Fowler KB, Stagno S, Pass RF. Maternal immunity and prevention of congenital cytomegalovirus infection. JAMA 2003;289:1008-1011.

218. Malinger G, Lev D, Zahalka N, et al. Fetal cytomegalovirus infection of the brain: the spectrum of sonographic findings. AJNR Am J Neuroradiol 2003;24:28-32.

219. Virkola K, Lappalainen M, Valanne L, Koskiniemi M. Radiological signs in newborns exposed to primary *Toxoplasma* infection in utero. Pediatr Radiol 1997;27:133-138.

220. Graham D, Guidi SM, Sanders RC. Sonographic features of in utero periventricular calcification due to cytomegalovirus infection. J Ultrasound Med 1982;1:171-172.

221. Molloy PM, Lowman RM. The lack of specificity of neonatal intracranial paraventricular calcifications. Radiology 1963;80:98-102.

222. Shaw CM, Alvord Jr EC. Subependymal germinolysis. Arch Neurol 1974;31:374-381.

223. Patel DV, Holfels EM, Vogel NP, et al. Resolution of intracranial calcifications in infants with treated congenital toxoplasmosis. Radiology 1996;199:433-440.

224. Gray PH, Tudehope DI, Masel J. Cystic encephalomalacia and intrauterine herpes simplex virus infection. Pediatr Radiol 1992; 22:529-532.

225. Levene MI, Williams JL, Fawer CL. Ultrasound of the infant brain. London: Spastics International Medical Publications; 1985.

226. Harwood-Nash DC, Reilly BJ, Turnbull I. Massive calcification of the brain in a newborn infant. Am J Roentgenol Radium Ther Nucl Med 1970;108:528-532.

227. George R, Andronikou S, du Plessis J, et al. Central nervous system manifestations of HIV infection in children. Pediatr Radiol 2009; 39:575-585.

228. Ben-Ami T, Yousefzadeh D, Backus M, et al. Lenticulostriate vasculopathy in infants with infections of the central nervous system: sonographic and Doppler findings. Pediatr Radiol 1990;20:575-579.

Intracranial Masses

229. Ball WS. Pediatric neuroradiology. In: RSNA Special Course in Neuroradiology. Part I, 1994. p. 113-126.

230. Jooma R, Kendall BE. Intracranial tumours in the first year of life. Neuroradiology 1982;23:267-274.

231. Ambrosino MM, Hernanz-Schulman M, Genieser NB, et al. Brain tumors in infants less than a year of age. Pediatr Radiol 1988;19: 6-8.

232. Jooma R, Hayward RD, Grant DN. Intracranial neoplasms during the first year of life: analysis of one hundred consecutive cases. Neurosurgery 1984;14:31-41.

233. Chow PP, Horgan JG, Burns PN, et al. Choroid plexus papilloma: detection by real-time and Doppler sonography. AJNR Am J Neuroradiol 1986;7:168-170.

234. Han BK, Babcock DS, Oestreich AE. Sonography of brain tumors in infants. AJR Am J Roentgenol 1984;143:31-36.

235. Smith WL, Menezes A, Franken EA. Cranial ultrasound in the diagnosis of malignant brain tumors. J Clin Ultrasound 1983;11: 97-100.

236. Schellhas KP, Siebert RC, Heithoff KB, Franciosi RA. Congenital choroid plexus papilloma of the third ventricle: diagnosis with real-time sonography and MR imaging. AJNR Am J Neuroradiol 1988;9: 797-798.

237. Hopper KD, Foley LC, Nieves NL, Smirniotopoulos JG. The interventricular extension of choroid plexus papillomas. AJNR Am J Neuroradiol 1987;8:469-472.

238. Shkolnik A. B-mode scanning of the infant brain: a new approach—case report: craniopharyngioma. J Clin Ultrasound 1975;3:229-231.

239. Mazewski CM, Hudgins RJ, Reisner A, Geyer JR. Neonatal brain tumors: a review. Semin Perinatol 1999;23:286-298.

240. Balaci E, Sumner TE, Auringer ST, Cox TD. Diffuse neonatal hemangiomatosis with extensive involvement of the brain and cervical spinal cord. Pediatr Radiol 1999;29:441-443.

241. Pal BR, Preston PR, Morgan ME, et al. Frontal horn thin-walled cysts in preterm neonates are benign. Arch Dis Child Fetal Neonatal Ed 2001;85:F187-F193.

242. Malinger G, Lev D, Ben Sira L, et al. Congenital periventricular pseudocysts: prenatal sonographic appearance and clinical implications. Ultrasound Obstet Gynecol 2002;20:447-451.

243. Chuang S, Harwood-Nash D. Tumors and cysts. Neuroradiology 1986;28:463-475.

244. Fakhry J, Schechter A, Tenner MS, Reale M. Cysts of the choroid plexus in neonates: documentation and review of the literature. J Ultrasound Med 1985;4:561-563.

245. Riebel T, Nasir R, Weber K. Choroid plexus cysts: a normal finding on ultrasound. Pediatr Radiol 1992;22:410-412.

246. Shuangshoti S, Netsky MG. Neuroepithelial (colloid) cysts of the nervous system. Neurology 1966;16:887-903.

247. Giorgi C. Symptomatic cyst of the choroid plexus of the lateral ventricle. Neurosurgery 1979;5:53-56.

248. Naeini RM, Yoo JH, Hunter JV. Spectrum of choroid plexus lesions in children. AJR Am J Roentgenol 2009;192:32-40.

249. Kurjak A, Schulman H, Predanic A, et al. Fetal choroid plexus vascularization assessed by color flow ultrasonography. J Ultrasound Med 1994;13:841-844.

250. Shackelford GD, Fulling KH, Glasier CM. Cysts of the subependymal germinal matrix: sonographic demonstration with pathologic correlation. Radiology 1983;149:117-121.

251. Larcos G, Gruenewald SM, Lui K. Neonatal subependymal cysts detected by sonography: prevalence, sonographic findings, and clinical significance. AJR Am J Roentgenol 1994;162:953-956.

252. Russel IM, van Sonderen L, van Straaten HL, Barth PG. Subependymal germinolytic cysts in Zellweger syndrome. Pediatr Radiol 1995;25:254-245.

253. Smith LM, Qureshi N, Renslo R, Sinow RM. Prenatal cocaine exposure and cranial sonographic findings in preterm infants. J Clin Ultrasound 2001;29:72-77.

254. Litvak J, Yahr MD, Ransohoff J. Aneurysms of the great vein of Galen and midline cerebral arteriovenous anomalies. J Neurosurg 1960;17:945-954.

255. Long DM, Seljeskog EL, Chou SN, French LA. Giant arteriovenous malformations of infancy and childhood. J Neurosurg 1974;40: 304-312.

256. Soto G, Daneman A, Hellman J. Doppler evaluation of cerebral arteries in a Galenic vein malformation. J Ultrasound Med 1985;4: 673-675.

257. Tessler FN, Dion J, Vinuela F, et al. Cranial arteriovenous malformations in neonates: color Doppler imaging with angiographic correlation. AJR Am J Roentgenol 1989;153:1027-1030.

258. Westra SJ, Curran JG, Duckwiler GR, et al. Pediatric intracranial vascular malformations: evaluation of treatment results with color Doppler ultrasound. Work in progress. Radiology 1993;186:775-783.

259. Chapman S, Hockley AD. Calcification of an aneurysm of the vein of Galen. Pediatr Radiol 1989;19:541-542.

260. Jones BV, Ball WS, Tomsick TA, et al. Vein of Galen aneurysmal malformation: diagnosis and treatment of 13 children with extended clinical follow-up. AJNR Am J Neuroradiol 2002;23: 1717-1724.

261. Hurst RW, Kagetsu NJ, Berenstein A. Angiographic findings in two cases of aneurysmal malformation of vein of Galen prior to spontaneous thrombosis: therapeutic implications. AJNR Am J Neuroradiol 1992;13:1446-1450.

CHAPTER 48

Doppler Sonography of the Neonatal and Infant Brain

George A. Taylor

Chapter Outline

*C*ontinuous and pulsed wave or spectral Doppler techniques have been in use for many years in the monitoring of intracranial hemodynamics in the newborn.[1-3] Although early Doppler studies were useful in attempting to understand the pathophysiology of cerebrovascular injury, they were limited by the inability to image the actual vessels. The introduction of color flow Doppler technology made identification of the origin of the Doppler signal and its orientation to the transducer easier to achieve. Further improvements in color sensitivity and transducer design now allow routine imaging of the intracranial vasculature in newborns, including the identification of flow in submillimeter arteries and in the main venous drainage pathways of the brain.[4] The extended dynamic range and increased sensitivity of power-mode Doppler (amplitude-mode color or color flow Doppler energy) can be used to improve depiction of low-velocity and low-amplitude flow. Although not used as part of the routine screening examination of asymptomatic premature infants, cranial Doppler sonography can be a helpful diagnostic and problem-solving tool in a variety of clinical situations.

SONOGRAPHIC TECHNIQUE

Transcranial Approaches

Three different scanning approaches to the neonatal brain have worked well, each with its own advantages.[5-9] The **anterior fontanelle approach** is the most common

and easiest to use. The basilar, internal carotid, and anterior cerebral arteries, as well as the internal cerebral veins, vein of Galen, and the superior sagittal and straight sinus, can be routinely visualized on sagittal scans near the midline (Fig. 48-1, *A* and *C*). The inferior sagittal sinus is difficult to resolve as a separate vessel because its course is often superimposed on the posterior portion of the pericallosal artery. The smaller thalamostriate arteries and opercular branches of the middle cerebral artery may be seen on angled sagittal images (Fig. 48-1, *B*).

On **coronal scans** through the anterior fontanelle, the supraclinoid internal carotid arteries, M1 segments of the middle cerebral arteries, thalamostriate arteries, A1 segments of the anterior cerebral arteries, and the cavernous sinus can almost always be visualized on anteriorly angled scans (Fig. 48-2). Paired terminal and internal cerebral veins, thalamostriate arteries, the basilar artery, straight sinus, and transverse sinuses can be seen on more posteriorly angled scans. A major drawback of the coronal plane is the near perpendicular angle between the middle cerebral arteries and the ultrasound beam, such that measured frequency shifts from flowing red blood cells approach zero.

The **temporal bone approach** is best for the middle cerebral artery because it is parallel to flow. The transducer is placed in axial orientation approximately 1 cm anterior and superior to the tragus of the ear. Using the thin temporal bone as an acoustic window, adequate penetration for imaging and Doppler studies can be achieved in most full-term neonates. This approach allows visualization of the major branches of the circle

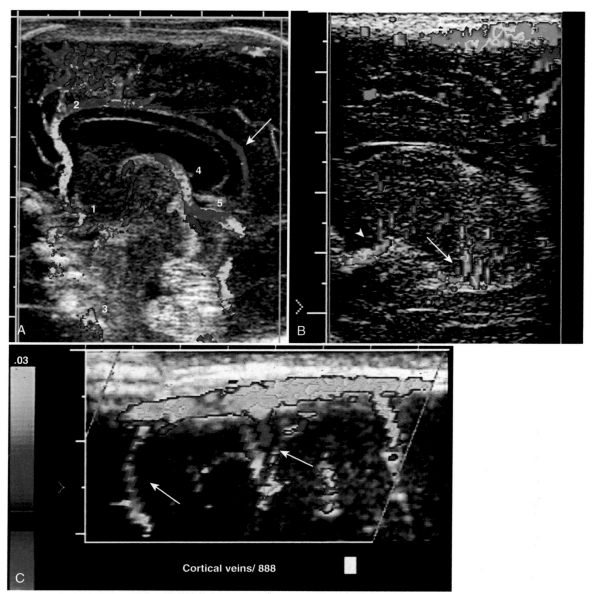

FIGURE 48-1. Normal sagittal color flow Doppler sonogram of cerebral arteries and veins. A, Sagittal midline scan with infant facing left shows *1,* the internal carotid artery; *2,* pericallosal artery; *3,* basilar artery; *4,* vein of Galen; and *5,* straight sinus. The inferior sagittal sinus and distal pericallosal artery *(arrow)* are often superimposed and cannot be resolved as separate vessels. **B,** Angled sagittal scan shows anterior and posterior thalamostriate arteries coursing through basal ganglia *(arrowhead)* and thalamus *(arrow).* **C,** Close-up sagittal view of superior sagittal sinus shows flow in small cortical veins *(arrows)* draining into sinus.

of Willis (Fig. 48-3). In most premature infants, both middle cerebral arteries can be easily insonated from one side of the head.

The **posterolateral (mastoid) fontanelle approach** is an angled axial scan. This portal is located approximately 1 cm behind and superior to the concha of the ear. It is the preferred approach for imaging flow in the transverse venous sinuses, and the torcular herophili in selected patients (Fig. 48-4).

Additional images of the posterior fossa circulation may be obtained using the **foramen magnum approach.** The patient is placed in lateral recumbent position with the head gently flexed, similar to the positioning for a lumbar puncture. The transducer is placed in the midline,

just inferior to the occipital protuberance, and angled cephalad in either sagittal or axial orientation. The cerebellar venous arcade, cerebellar arteries, and basilar artery can be depicted in most patients (Fig. 48-5).

Doppler Optimization

For the best visualization of the intracranial vascular system, the image should be electronically magnified and the color region of interest restricted to enhance color sensitivity and frame rate. Color gain should be adjusted to maximize vascular signal and minimize tissue motion artifacts, and the lowest bandpass filter should be used to maximize low-flow sensitivity necessary for

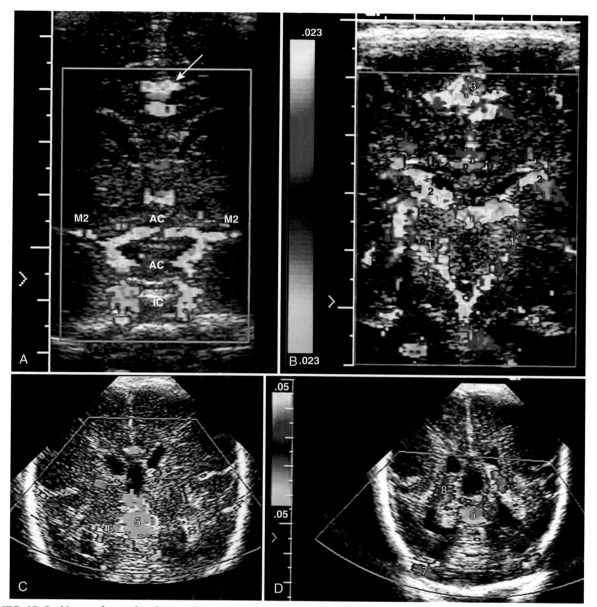

FIGURE 48-2. Normal cerebral arteries and veins, coronal view. A, Coronal scan anterior to caudate head shows paired internal cerebral arteries (IC), M1 and M2 segments of the middle cerebral arteries, and anterior cerebral arteries (AC). Pericallosal artery *(arrow)* is seen in the interhemispheric fissure *(3)*. **B,** Coronal scan at the level of caudate head shows *1,* thalamostriate arteries; *2,* terminal veins; *3,* sagittal sinus; and pericallosal artery. **C,** Coronal scan through posterior third ventricle shows *5,* straight sinus, and *6,* basal veins of Rosenthal. **D,** Posteriorly angled scan through atria of lateral ventricles shows *5,* straight sinus; *7,* transverse sinuses; and *8,* choroidal vessels.

evaluating venous structures. A 7 to 15–MHz linear transducer is recommended for examining the superficially located superior sagittal sinus. Visualization of the smaller arterial branches of the middle and anterior cerebral arteries can also be accomplished in the majority of normal premature and full-term infants, but often requires higher-frequency (7 or 10 MHz) vector or sector transducers capable of detecting lower velocity and amplitude signal. The use of power Doppler sonography is recommended when directional information is of secondary importance and detection of flow is primary.

DOPPLER OPTIMIZATION

Electronically magnify image.
Restrict color region of interest to enhance color sensitivity and frame rate.
Adjust color gain to maximize vascular signal and minimize tissue artifact.
Use lowest bandpass filter to maximize low-flow sensitivity and evaluate venous structures.
Use 7-MHz linear transducer for superior sagittal sinus.
Use power-mode Doppler for smallest vessels when flow direction is not needed.

For specific vessel evaluation, spectral or duplex pulsed wave Doppler imaging can be performed using 3.5 to 15–MHz probes, depending on the depth and location of the target vessel. Spectral Doppler imaging is essential for the evaluation of intracranial hemodynamics in both the arterial and the venous system.

Safety Considerations

During pulsed wave and color flow Doppler examinations, signal is obtained by imparting energy into tissues. Although intracranial Doppler ultrasound is safe, biologic effects may be identified in the future. Thus, Doppler exposure should be time limited, and the signal intensity should be maximized by increasing gain and not transducer power output settings. The U.S. Food and Drug Administration (FDA) has revised its approach to ultrasound safety. In doing so, it set a new overall upper limit of 720 mW/cm^2 maximum in situ spatial peak, temporal average intensity (I_{SPTA}) intensities, an eightfold increase in ultrasound intensity for fetal and

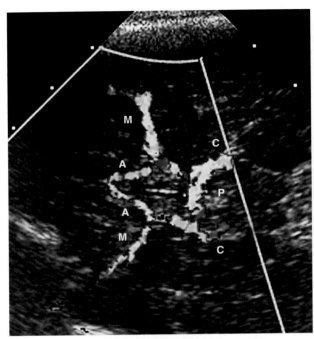

FIGURE 48-3. Normal middle cerebral artery and circle of Willis, axial view. Axial scan obtained through left temporal bone shows major branches of the circle of Willis. The A1 segment of the left and right anterior cerebral artery (A); the middle cerebral arteries (M); posterior communicating arteries (P); and posterior cerebral arteries (C).

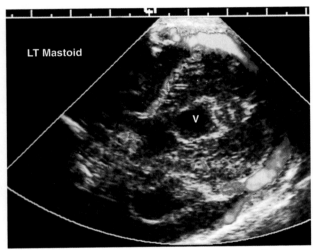

FIGURE 48-4. Normal transverse sinus flow on power Doppler ultrasound. Angled axial amplitude-mode color flow Doppler image through mastoid fontanelle shows flow in both transverse sinuses. Note dilated fourth ventricle (V).

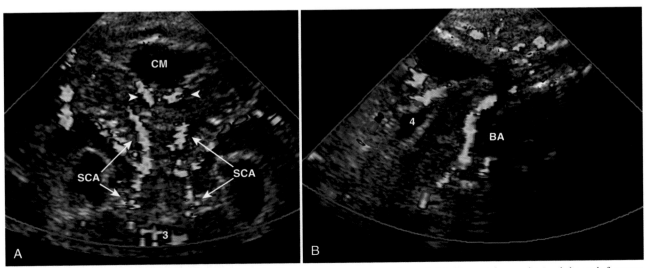

FIGURE 48-5. Normal posterior fossa vessels, foramen magnum view. A, Midline axial scan obtained through foramen magnum shows branches of the superior cerebellar arteries (SCA), and portions of the cerebellar venous arcade (arrowheads). **B,** Midline sagittal scan shows basilar artery (BA), along anterior surface of pons, and fourth ventricle (4).

neonatal intracranial applications.[10] These new guidelines place much more responsibility on the operator to understand and limit the two most important determinants of ultrasound energy output during examinations, the mechanical index (MI) and thermal index (TI). The ALARA principle (as low as reasonably achievable) should be followed to limit energy exposure to tissues.[11,12]

Doppler Measurements

The **resistive index** (RI), instantaneous peak systolic and end diastolic velocities, and mean blood flow velocity over time (time-averaged velocity) are the most common spectral Doppler measures for monitoring intracranial hemodynamics. The easiest and most reproducible are measures of **pulsatility** (Fig. 48-6). These measures are relatively insensitive to differences in angle of insonation and correlate well with acute changes in intracerebral perfusion pressure.[13] However, many factors other than cerebrovascular resistance may affect RI in an intracranial vessel[14-16] (Fig. 48-7 and Table 48-1).

These factors modify RI through the following mechanism. With **increasing filter settings,** lower velocities are not depicted, resulting in a falsely elevated RI. Transducer pressure on the anterior fontanelle may transiently increase intracranial pressure, which in turn preferentially reduces flow during diastole and increases RI. In infants with a symptomatic **patent ductus arteriosus,** resistance to flow in the cerebrovascular bed is higher than pulmonary vascular resistance. This results in shunting of blood away from the brain during diastole and an elevated intracranial RI. During **tachycardia**, the arterial pressure wave has less time to dissipate before another systolic ejection occurs. Intracranial RI is artificially lower because diastolic velocities are measured at middiastole, when velocities are higher, rather than during end diastole. **Left ventricular dysfunction** (decreased cardiac output) results in a decreased systolic pressure wave, lowered systolic velocities, and a reduced RI.

The RI is only a weak predictor of cerebrovascular resistance under most physiologic conditions.[17] Mean blood flow velocity measures are the most informative indices of **cerebral blood flow** (CBF). Although accurate placement of the sample volume and angle of insonation are required, a strong correlation has been demonstrated between mean blood flow velocity and changes in global CBF under a variety of clinical and experimental conditions[17-20] (Fig. 48-8).

NORMAL HEMODYNAMICS

Normal Arterial Blood Flow Patterns

Arterial hemodynamics in the cerebral circulation are affected by normal maturational events in the healthy newborn. The resistive index in the **anterior cerebral artery** decreases from a mean of 0.78 (range, 0.5-1.0) in **preterm infants** to a mean of 0.71 (range, 0.6-0.8) in full-term newborns.[2,3,21-23] This trend is associated with increasing diastolic flow velocities and may be related to

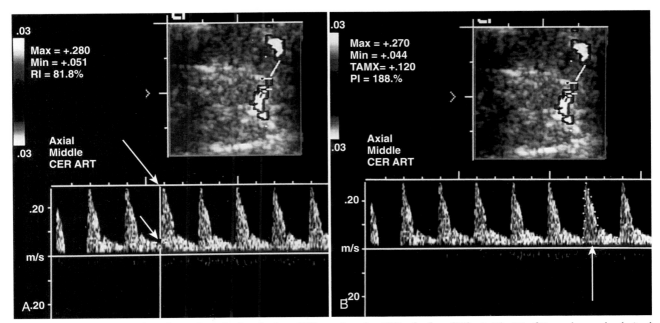

FIGURE 48-6. Determination of resistive index (RI) and pulsatility index (PI). A, The RI of Pourcelot can be derived by placing the Doppler cursor at peak systolic velocity, Vs, or maximum velocity *(long arrow),* and at end diastolic velocity, Ved, or minimum velocity *(short arrow).* The RI is calculated as Vs-Ved/Vs. **B,** The PI of Gosling is derived by tracing the outer envelope of a single cardiac cycle *(arrow)* and calculating the time-averaged maximum velocity envelope (TAMX). The PI is calculated as Vs-Ved/TAMX.

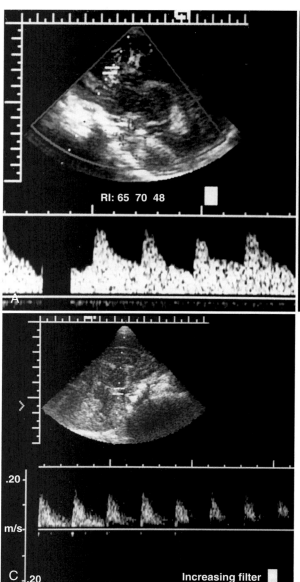

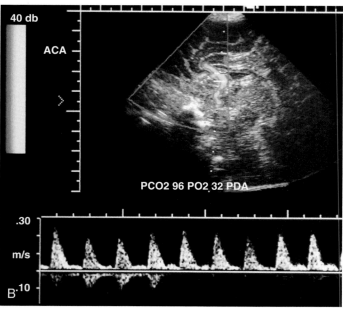

FIGURE 48-7. Factors affecting intracranial resistive index (RI). A, High variability in pulsatility of flow related to left ventricular dysfunction. Doppler tracing from the anterior cerebral artery in an infant with congenital heart disease. B, High pulsatility with absent diastolic flow in infant with symptomatic patent ductus arteriosus (PDA). C, Progressively higher wall filter settings show what appears to be absent flow during diastole as the filter cuts out lower flow.

TABLE 48-1. FACTORS THAT CHANGE RESISTIVE INDEX (RI)

FACTOR	EFFECT ON RI
High-pass filter settings	Increased
Scanning pressure	Increased
Patent ductus arteriosus	Increased
Elevated heart rate	Decreased
Decreased cardiac output	Decreased

peripheral changes in cerebrovascular resistance or to changes proximal to the site of recording, such as a closing ductus arteriosus and a diminishing left-to-right shunt. In **full-term infants,** RI may also change over the first few days of life.[2] In a study of 476 normal newborns weighing over 2500 g at birth, anterior cerebral artery RI decreased from a mean of 70.6 ± 7 (range, 51-87) to 68.3 ± 6 (range, 51-83) within the first 24 hours.[24]

Table 48-2 provides the range of published peak systolic and end diastolic velocities and RI values in several intracranial arteries. Although the range of normal values is broad, no great variability should be seen in the individual patient. Changes of more than 50% from baseline values should be considered abnormal. There are no consistent differences in instantaneous blood flow velocity or pulsatility of flow among the major branches of the circle of Willis or between right-sided and left-sided structures.

Normal Venous Blood Flow Patterns

Venous blood flow is continuous in smaller intracerebral veins such as the terminal and internal cerebral veins.[25]

Cardiac pulsations of variable amplitude are common in more central venous structures, such as the vein of Galen and the sagittal and transverse sinuses (Fig. 48-9). High-amplitude or sawtooth patterns of pulsatility are not normal and may be seen in infants with **elevated right-sided heart pressures** or **tricuspid regurgitation** (Fig. 48-10). Although respiratory changes are not usually observed during normal quiet respiration, marked changes in velocity can occur during **forceful crying** as a result of rapid changes in intrathoracic pressure.[8,25,26]

Table 48-3 provides ranges for mean blood flow velocities in several intracranial veins and sinuses.

INTENSIVE CARE THERAPIES AND CEREBRAL HEMODYNAMICS

Mechanical Ventilation

Cerebral hemodynamics can be greatly affected by mechanical ventilation. Changes in venous return to the heart caused by **breathing out of synchrony** with the ventilator may result in significant beat-to-beat variability in arterial waveforms.[27]

Similarly, **high peak inspiratory pressures** can impede venous return to the heart and result in reversal of flow in the intracranial veins. Treatment with

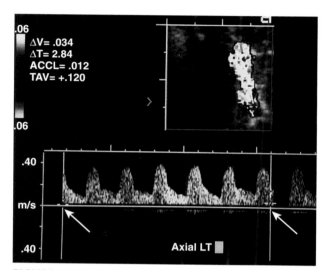

FIGURE 48-8. Determination of mean blood flow velocity. Angle-corrected Doppler tracing obtained from the middle cerebral artery. Cursors are placed at the beginning and end of a continuous Doppler tracing *(arrows)*. The time-averaged mean blood flow velocity *(TAV)* is calculated by integrating all instantaneous mean blood flow velocities between both cursors. In this example, the TAV measured 0.12 cm/sec.

TABLE 48-2. RANGE OF ARTERIAL BLOOD FLOW VELOCITIES IN FULL-TERM INFANTS*

ARTERY	PEAK SYSTOLIC VELOCITY (cm/sec)	END DIASTOLIC VELOCITY (cm/sec)	RESISTIVE INDEX
Internal carotid	12-80	3-20	0.5-0.8
Basilar	30-80	5-20	0.6-0.8
Middle cerebral	20-70	8-20	0.6-0.8
Anterior cerebral	12-35	6-20	0.6-0.8
Posterior cerebral	20-60	8-25	0.6-0.8

*Values modified from references 2 and 21 to 23.

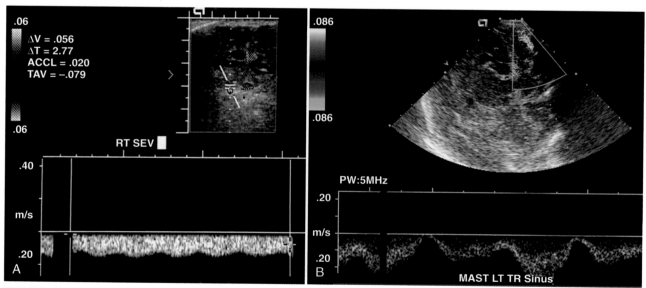

FIGURE 48-9. Normal referred cardiac pulsations in veins. A, Low-amplitude pulsatility from referred cardiac pulsations in a Doppler tracing from terminal vein in a normal full-term infant. **B,** Normal, higher-amplitude and variable cardiac pulsations in transverse sinus in 37-week infant.

high-frequency ventilation exerts its effects on both arterial and venous hemodynamics in the form of short-amplitude oscillations at approximately 15 cycles per second[9,28] (Fig. 48-11). **Endotracheal suctioning** has been associated with marked increases in mean arterial blood pressure and arterial blood flow velocities in premature infants and has been attributed to the relative pressure-passive cerebral circulation (lack of autoregulation) in these patients.[29] Treatment with **inhaled nitric oxide** has also been reported to decrease cerebral blood flow velocities in newborns with pulmonary hypertension who experience an acute improvement in pulmonary hemodynamics and gas exchange at the onset of therapy.[30]

Extracorporeal Membrane Oxygenation

Extracorporeal membrane oxygenation (ECMO) may be used for the treatment of infants with severe respiratory failure who have not responded to maximal conventional

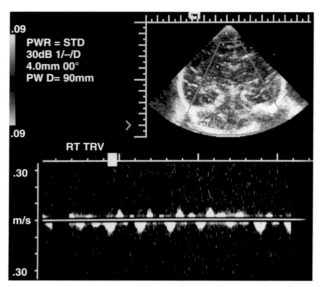

FIGURE 48-10. Exaggerated venous pulsations from tricuspid regurgitation. Doppler tracing from transverse sinus shows an abnormal sawtooth pattern of flow caused by referred right atrial pulsations.

TABLE 48-3. MEAN VENOUS BLOOD FLOW VELOCITIES IN FULL-TERM NEWBORNS

VESSEL	MEAN TAV* (cm/sec)
Terminal veins	3.0 ± 0.3
Internal cerebral veins	3.3 ± 0.3
Vein of Galen	4.3 ± 0.7
Straight sinus	5.9 ± 1.0
Superior sagittal sinus	9.2 ± 1.1
Inferior sagittal sinus	3.5 ± 0.3

Values modified from Taylor GA. Intracranial venous system in the newborn: evaluation of normal anatomy and flow characteristics with color Doppler ultrasound. Radiology 1992;183:449-452.
*Time-averaged mean blood flow velocity (±standard error of the mean).

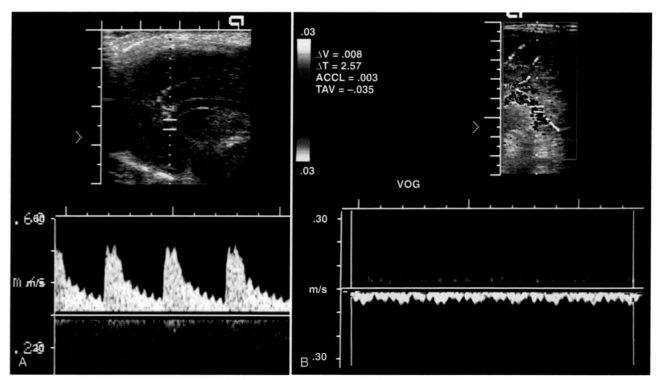

FIGURE 48-11. Effect of high-frequency ventilation on arterial and venous hemodynamics. A, Anterior cerebral artery; **B,** vein of Galen. Pulsed wave Doppler tracings in a premature infant receiving high-frequency ventilation shows superimposed 15-Hz oscillations in flow.

ventilatory support. ECMO is also used for postoperative support in patients with temporary cardiac failure after surgical repair of congenital heart lesions. During venoarterial ECMO, infants undergo cannulation and ligation of the right common carotid artery and jugular vein for vascular access and are placed on **nonpulsatile partial cardiopulmonary bypass.** This results in significant alterations in intracranial hemodynamics[31,32] (Fig. 48-12). As the amount of flow through the ECMO bypass circuit increases, arterial pulsatility decreases proportionately and may disappear altogether, especially in association with severe cardiac dysfunction.[33] During bypass, flow to the right middle cerebral artery is typically achieved by shunting blood from the left internal carotid and A1 segment of the anterior cerebral artery across the anterior communicating artery. Flow then proceeds in retrograde fashion along the left A1 segment to the left middle cerebral artery[4] (Fig. 48-13).

Alterations in venous drainage may also occur during ECMO bypass as a result of jugular vein ligation and may be associated with altered hemodynamics in the right middle cerebral artery and a higher overall risk of hemorrhagic infarction[30,34] (Fig. 48-14).

DIFFUSE NEURONAL INJURY

Asphyxia

The hemodynamic changes associated with asphyxia depend on the severity of the insult, ongoing hypercapnia and hypoxemia, and the time from injury. Infants with mild degrees of asphyxia will have normal cerebral hemodynamics throughout the event. In the setting of

severe or prolonged asphyxia, tissue hypoxic injury results in the excessive release or diminished reuptake of endogenous excitatory amino acids, such as glutamate and aspartate. This in turn results in the production of intracellular nitric oxide and subsequent cerebral vasodilation.[35] As a consequence, **increased mean blood flow velocities** and **decreased arterial pulsatility** may be seen on spectral Doppler imaging after the first 12 hours of life and lasting several days after the initial insult[36,37] (Fig. 48-15). This reflects the impaired autoregulation and elevated cerebral blood flow associated with diffuse hypoxic brain injury. In asphyxiated infants, an **extremely low RI** (<60) in the first few days of life is associated with severe subsequent neurodevelopmental delay.[38] Persistent hypoxia or hypercapnia will also contribute to generalized vasodilation and abnormal Doppler spectra, and fluctuation of systolic velocities may be caused by asphyxia-related cardiac ischemia.[39,40]

Cerebral Edema

Cerebral edema often accompanies hypoxic-ischemic brain injury. Edema begins during the course of hypoxia-ischemia and appears to be related to the formation of idiogenic osmoles (H^+ ions and lactate) within cells, combined with cellular energy failure and loss of

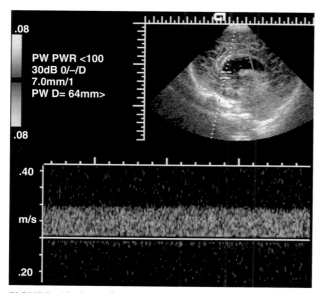

FIGURE 48-12. Absent arterial pulsatility during extracorporeal membrane oxygenation (ECMO). Continuous nonpulsatile flow on pulsed wave Doppler tracing from the anterior cerebral artery in an infant with congenital heart disease and severe cardiac dysfunction.

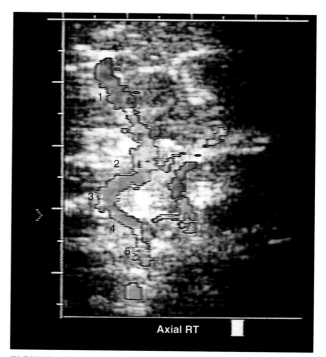

FIGURE 48-13. Collateral flow through circle of Willis during ECMO. Left axial scan shows antegrade flow in left middle cerebral artery *(1)* and A1 segment, left anterior cerebral artery *(2).* Flow to right middle cerebral artery *(5)* is by retrograde flow through A1 segment, right anterior cerebral artery *(4),* and anterior communicating artery *(3).* Compare with normal appearance in Figure 48-3. *(From Taylor GA: Current concepts in neonatal cranial Doppler sonography. Ultrasound Q 1992;4:223-244.)*

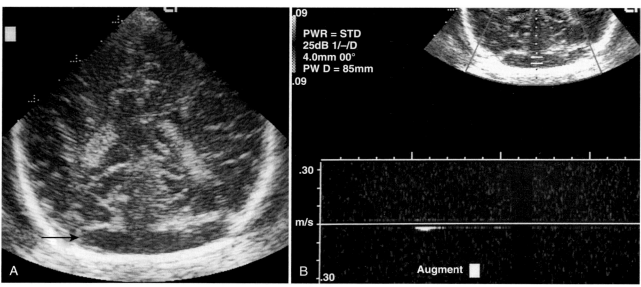

FIGURE 48-14. Partial venous obstruction during ECMO. A, Posteriorly angled coronal scan shows dilated sinus confluence *(arrow).* **B,** Flow only detectable during augmentation by gentle compression and release of left internal jugular vein. Infant developed signs of superior vena cava obstruction on day 3 of ECMO. *(From Taylor GA, Walker LK: Intracranial venous system in newborns treated with extracorporeal membrane oxygenation: Doppler US evaluation after ligation of the right jugular vein. Radiology 1992;183:452-456.)*

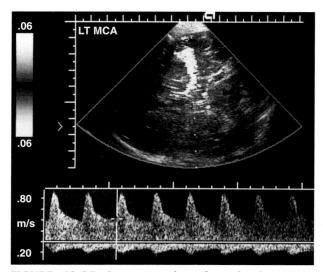

FIGURE 48-15. Severe perinatal asphyxia. Middle cerebral artery Doppler shows elevated flow during diastole and a reduced pulsatility of flow (RI, 54).

transcellular ionic gradients. The more severe the brain injury, the more extensive and prolonged is the associated edema.[41] As cerebral edema worsens, cerebrovascular resistance increases, resulting in dampening of diastolic blood flow velocities. Pulsed wave Doppler imaging typically shows progressive elevation of the RI and reversal of diastolic flow in the intracranial arteries.[40,42]

Brain Death

Eventually, flow during systole becomes diminished and present only during a brief portion of the cardiac cycle.

This represents **nonviable brain blood flow**[42] (Fig. 48-16). Although absence of intracranial flow by Doppler techniques is a reliable sign of absent cortical function, the presence of flow does not guarantee functional integrity, and brain death may be seen in the presence of preserved intracranial blood flow.[43,44]

INTRACRANIAL HEMORRHAGE AND STROKE

The periventricular white matter is drained primarily by the medullary veins into the terminal and internal cerebral veins. Obstruction of these small veins by germinal matrix hemorrhage (GMH) and subsequent venous hypertension may play an important role in the pathogenesis of periventricular hemorrhagic infarction in the preterm infant.[45,46] Color flow Doppler imaging may be used to show initial displacement, gradual encasement, and **obstruction of the terminal veins** by an enlarging GMH (Fig. 48-17). In one study, displacement or occlusion of the terminal vein could be demonstrated in 50% of GMHs and in 92% of periventricular white matter hemorrhages.[47] This finding may be useful in the early prediction of infants at risk for worsening intracranial hemorrhage.

Not all cerebral infarcts show alterations in regional blood flow. However, decreased arterial pulsations, increased size and number of visible vessels, and increased mean blood flow velocities can be demonstrated in the tissues surrounding larger cerebral infarcts[48,49] (Fig. 48-18). This pattern of vasodilation has been well described on computed tomography (CT) and angiog-

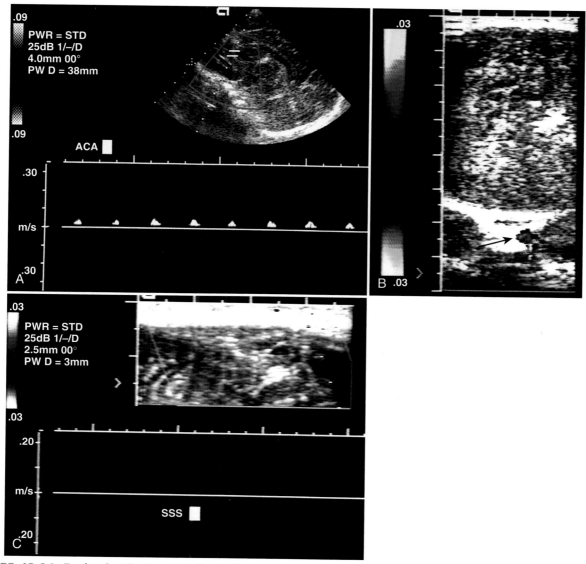

FIGURE 48-16. Brain death. Nonviable brain blood flow in an infant with diffuse cerebral edema. **A,** Pulsed wave Doppler tracing from anterior cerebral artery shows very low flow velocities during peak systole and absence of flow during diastole. **B,** Coronal color Doppler scan shows flow only in extracranial portion of left internal carotid artery *(arrow)*. **C,** Pulsed Doppler of superior sagittal sinus with low-velocity settings shows no venous flow.

raphy and is thought to be caused by the uncoupling of cerebral blood flow from local metabolic demands and is known as **luxury perfusion.**[50,51]

HYDROCEPHALUS

As the intracranial pressure (ICP) rises, arterial flow tends to be more affected during diastole than during systole, resulting in an elevated pulsatility of flow. Seibert et al.[13] showed that **increasing RI** correlates well with intracranial pressure elevation in an animal model of acute hydrocephalus. Also, a significant decrease in pulsatility follows ventricular tapping and shunting in infants with hydrocephalus.[13,52] However, elevated ICP may not always be present in infants with ventricular

dilation, and the RI may be well within the normal range. Doppler examination of the anterior or middle cerebral artery during fontanelle compression may be useful in the early identification of infants with abnormal intracranial compliance before development of increased ICP, as shown by elevated baseline RI.[53]

Taylor and Madsen[54] directly measured changes in ICP and intracranial RI before and after ventricular drainage procedures.[55] These studies showed that the change in RI during fontanelle compression is a strong predictor of ICP and can help predict the need for shunt placement. This technique has also been used successfully to evaluate intracranial compliance in young children with **craniosynostosis** before surgical repair.[56]

According to the Monro-Kellie hypothesis, the volume of brain, cerebrospinal fluid (CSF), blood, and other

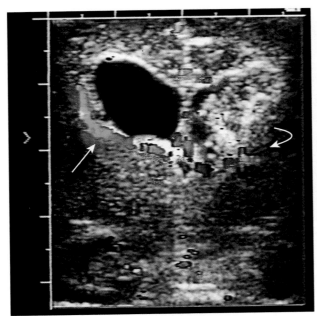

FIGURE 48-17. Grade IV intracranial hemorrhage with obstruction of terminal vein. Flow in left subependymal vein *(curved arrow)* is obliterated by hematoma. Flow in normal right subependymal vein *(straight arrow)* is shown.

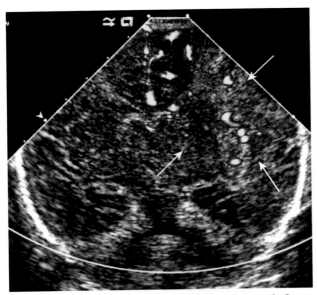

FIGURE 48-18. Left middle cerebral artery infarct with luxury perfusion in full-term infant. Coronal amplitude-mode Doppler image shows greatly increased blood flow to infarcted, echogenic area *(arrows)*, consistent with luxury perfusion. Note transfalcine herniation of left hemisphere.

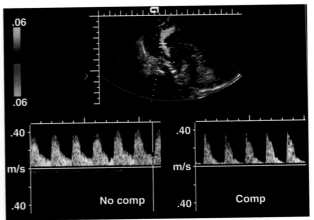

FIGURE 48-19. Effect of increased fontanelle pressure on RI in infant with hydrocephalus. Pulsed wave Doppler tracing of the anterior cerebral artery with transducer held lightly over anterior fontanelle *(No comp)* shows an RI of 0.69. Repeat tracing obtained a few seconds later with transducer firmly held over fontanelle *(Comp)*. RI has increased to 0.99, indicating abnormal intracranial compliance. *Comp,* compression.

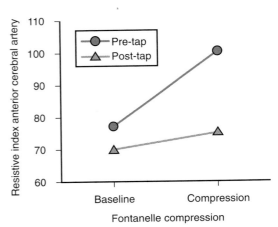

FIGURE 48-20. Shunted hydrocephalus less sensitive to pressure effects on fontanelle. Graph of serial resistive index (RI) determinations in an infant with hydrocephalus before and after shunt shows greatly diminished hemodynamic response to fontanelle compression after ventricular drainage. Note similar RI without fontanelle compression.

intracranial components is constant.[57] During graded fontanelle compression in normal infants, CSF or blood can be readily displaced to compensate for the small increase in volume delivered by compression of the anterior fontanelle, causing no increase in ICP. In infants with hydrocephalus, however, the increase in intracranial volume with fontanelle compression is translated into a transient increase in ICP and an **acute increase in arterial pulsatility** (Fig. 48-19). Serial examinations using this technique can follow an individual infant's ability to compensate for minor changes in intracranial volume, providing a noninvasive, indirect measure of intracranial compliance[58] (Fig. 48-20).

Color flow Doppler techniques may also be helpful in evaluating CSF dynamics in these infants. Winkler[59] showed that Doppler examination of the ventricular system during cranial or abdominal compression may induce CSF movement that is detectable with color flow or duplex Doppler imaging.[59] These dynamic techniques can be used to demonstrate obstruction at the foramina of Monro and aqueduct of Sylvius (Fig. 48-21).

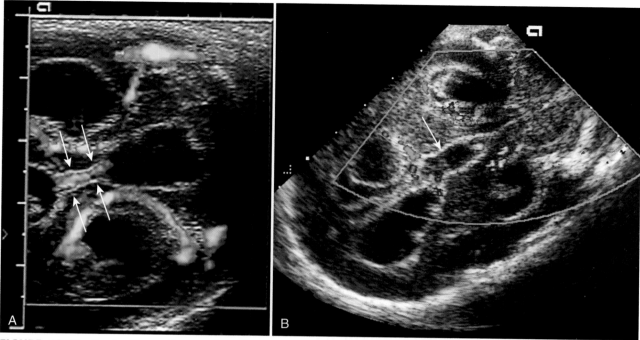

FIGURE 48-21. Evaluation of aqueductal patency. Angled axial power Doppler sonogram turned 90 degrees for ease of visualization. **A, Extraventricular obstructive "communicating" hydrocephalus.** Patent aqueduct of Sylvius shows color signal *(arrows)* in the third ventricle caused by normal retrograde flow of cerebrospinal fluid from the fourth ventricle obtained immediately after manual compression and rapid release of fontanelle. **B, Intraventricular hemorrhage causing hydrocephalus.** Clot obstructs the outlet of third ventricle *(arrow)* and allows no retrograde flow during rapid release of fontanelle compression.

VASCULAR MALFORMATIONS

Vein of Galen malformation is the most common intracranial vascular malformation presenting in the neonatal period. Color flow Doppler imaging is useful in detecting these lesions and in distinguishing the two most common types.[60] The **choroidal type** is characterized by multiple abnormal feeding vessels arising in the midbrain, with venous drainage by an aneurysmally dilated vein of Galen and straight sinus (Fig. 48-22). The **infundibular type** is an arteriovenous fistula with one or few arterial feeders draining directly into the vein of Galen. Spectral Doppler imaging typically shows arterialization of venous flow and increased flow velocities, with reduced pulsatility of the arterial feeders. Blood flow in the more peripheral portions of brain may show diminished or absent flow as a result of a "vascular steal" phenomenon away from the normal cerebral circulation through the low-resistance malformation.[61] Color flow Doppler imaging can also been used to monitor and quantify the hemodynamic effects of interventional procedures, such as transcatheter embolization.[62]

INTRACRANIAL TUMORS

Neonatal intracranial tumors are uncommon, and experience with Doppler characterization of these lesions is limited.[63] Doppler sonography may be helpful in characterizing the degree of intratumoral vascularity and in identifying its vascular supply[64] (Fig. 48-23).

NEAR-FIELD STRUCTURES

Differentiation of Subarachnoid from Subdural Fluid Collections

Color flow Doppler ultrasound using high-frequency linear transducers can be used to characterize extracerebral fluid collections as **subarachnoid, subdural,** or **combined.** Because superficial cortical blood vessels lie within the pia-arachnoid, fluid in this subarachnoid space surrounds and lifts the cortical vessels away from the brain surface (Fig. 48-24). Fluid in the subdural space pushes cortical vessels toward the brain surface and is separated from these vessels by a thin membrane (Fig. 48-25). Correlation with magnetic resonance imaging and CT suggests that color flow Doppler imaging is reliable in making this differentiation.[65] However, cortical veins drain into the superior sagittal sinus through emissary veins that course through the extra-axial spaces and can be mistaken for vessels in the subarachnoid space.[66]

Venous Thrombosis

Thrombosis of the intracranial venous sinuses occurs in the neonate as the result of dehydration and as a

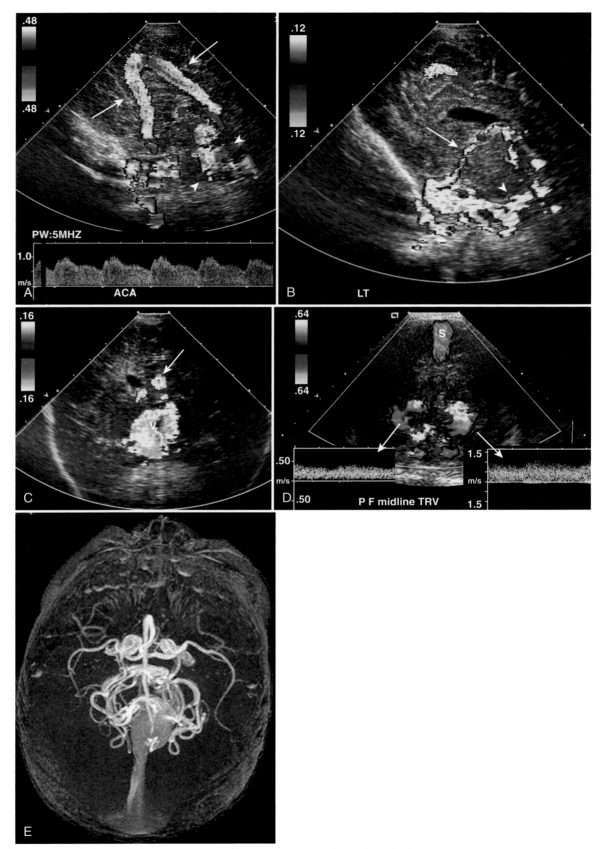

FIGURE 48-22. Vein of Galen aneurysm, choroidal type. A and **B,** Sagittal, and **C,** coronal, color flow Doppler images show large vein of Galen aneurysm *(V)* and dilated pericallosal artery *(arrow).* **D,** Pulsed wave Doppler tracing of the basilar artery shows greatly elevated flow velocities with dampened pulsatility. **E,** Axial time-of-flight magnetic resonance angiography confirms findings.

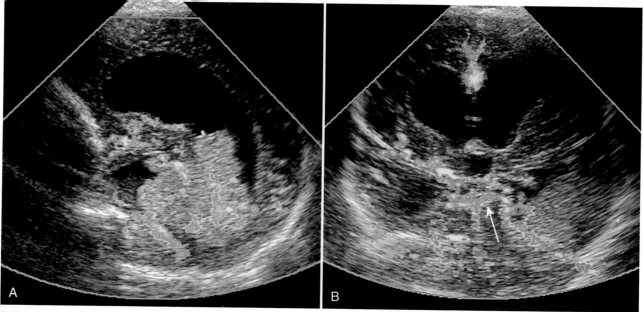

FIGURE 48-23. Choroid plexus papilloma in 6-week-old infant. A, Angled sagittal, and **B,** coronal, color amplitude (power) Doppler images show increased tumor vascularity within the echogenic mass, with arterial supply arising from a branch of the basilar artery *(arrow)*.

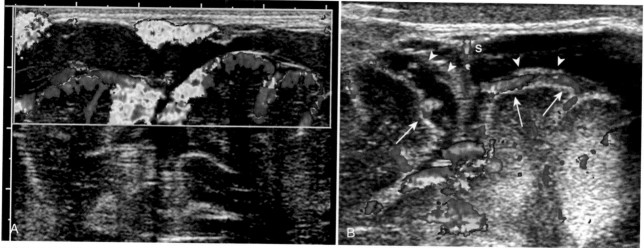

FIGURE 48-24. Subdural and subarachnoid effusions. A, Magnified coronal color Doppler image of interhemispheric fissure in 2-week infant. Large bilateral echogenic subdural effusions from meningitis compress the superficial cortical vessels onto the cortical surface. **B,** Coronal color Doppler image of interhemispheric fissure in 1-month-old infant. Large left and small right hypoechoic chronic subdural hematomas from nonaccidental trauma lie above the echogenic subarachnoid fluid. The cortical surface is compressed by the echogenic subarachnoid fluid, which surrounds superficial cortical vessels *(arrows)* separated from the relatively lucent subdural fluid by echogenic and thickened pia-arachnoid *(arrowheads)*. Note the echogenic subcortical white matter and superior sagittal sinus.

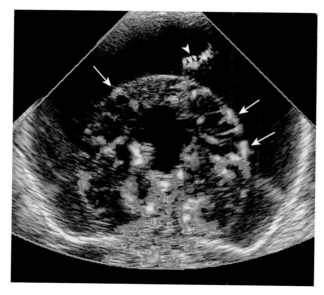

FIGURE 48-25. Large subdural effusion. After ventriculo-peritoneal shunt placement in 3-week-old infant with holoprosen-cephaly. Coronal power Doppler image shows cortical vessels compressed against brain surface *(arrows)* and single emissary vein within subdural fluid *(arrowhead)*.

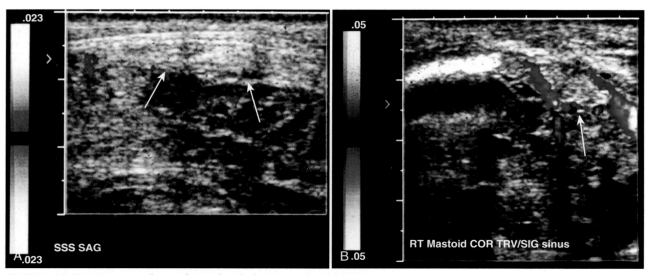

FIGURE 48-26. Venous sinus thrombosis in 6-week-old infant. A, No flow is present within the superior sagittal sinus *(arrows).* Coronal color amplitude Doppler image. **B,** Mastoid view of transverse sinus shows clot partially occluding flow in sinus *(arrow).*

complication of meningitis. Color flow Doppler ultrasound can be used as a noninvasive tool for initial identification and monitoring of these infants[13,67,68] (Fig. 48-26).

References

1. Bada HS, Hajjar W, Chua C, Sumner DS. Noninvasive diagnosis of neonatal asphyxia and intraventricular hemorrhage by Doppler ultrasound. J Pediatr 1979;95:775-779.
2. Archer LN, Evans DH, Levene MI. Doppler ultrasound examination of the anterior cerebral arteries of normal newborn infants: the effect of postnatal age. Early Hum Dev 1985;10:255-260.
3. Grant EG, White EM, Schellinger D, et al. Cranial duplex sonography of the infant. Radiology 1987;163:177-185.
4. Taylor G. Current concepts in neonatal cranial Doppler sonography. Ultrasound Q 1992:223-244.

Sonographic Technique

5. Wong WS, Tsuruda JS, Liberman RL, et al. Color Doppler imaging of intracranial vessels in the neonate. AJR Am J Roentgenol 1989;152:1065-1070.
6. Mitchell DG, Merton D, Needleman L, et al. Neonatal brain: color Doppler imaging. Part I. Technique and vascular anatomy. Radiology 1988;167:303-306.
7. Mitchell DG, Merton DA, Mirsky PJ, Needleman L. Circle of Willis in newborns: color Doppler imaging of 53 healthy full-term infants. Radiology 1989;172:201-205.
8. Taylor GA. Intracranial venous system in the newborn: evaluation of normal anatomy and flow characteristics with color Doppler ultrasound. Radiology 1992;183:449-452.
9. Dean LM, Taylor GA. The intracranial venous system in infants: normal and abnormal findings on duplex and color Doppler sonography. AJR Am J Roentgenol 1995;164:151-156.
10. Diagnostic ultrasound guidance for 1993. Revised 501(k). Rockville, Md: US Food and Drug Administration; 1993.
11. American Institute of Ultrasound in Medicine. Neurosonography in neonates and young children. In *AIUM practice guidelines.* Laurel, Md, 2004.
12. Barnett SB, Maulik D. Guidelines and recommendations for safe use of Doppler ultrasound in perinatal applications. J Matern Fetal Med 2001;10:75-84.
13. Seibert JJ, McCowan TC, Chadduck WM, et al. Duplex pulsed Doppler ultrasound versus intracranial pressure in the neonate: clinical and experimental studies. Radiology 1989;171:155-159.

14. Perlman JM, Hill A, Volpe JJ. The effect of patent ductus arteriosus on flow velocity in the anterior cerebral arteries: ductal steal in the premature newborn infant. J Pediatr 1981;99:767-771.
15. Taylor GA. Effect of scanning pressure on intracranial hemodynamics during transfontanellar duplex ultrasound. Radiology 1992;185:763-766.
16. Taylor GA, Martin GR, Short BL. Cardiac determinants of cerebral blood flow during extracorporeal membrane oxygenation. Invest Radiol 1989;24:511-516.
17. Taylor GA, Short BL, Walker LK, Traystman RJ. Intracranial blood flow: quantification with duplex Doppler and color Doppler flow ultrasound. Radiology 1990;176:231-236.
18. Greisen G, Johansen K, Ellison PH, et al. Cerebral blood flow in the newborn infant: comparison of Doppler ultrasound and [133]xenon clearance. J Pediatr 1984;104:411-418.
19. Hansen NB, Stonestreet BS, Rosenkrantz TS, Oh W. Validity of Doppler measurements of anterior cerebral artery blood flow velocity: correlation with brain blood flow in piglets. Pediatrics 1983;72:526-531.
20. Lundell BP, Lindstrom DP, Arnold TG. Neonatal cerebral blood flow velocity. I. An in vitro validation of the pulsed Doppler technique. Acta Paediatr Scand 1984;73:810-815.

Normal Hemodynamics

21. Horgan JG, Rumack CM, Hay T, et al. Absolute intracranial blood-flow velocities evaluated by duplex Doppler sonography in asymptomatic preterm and term neonates. AJR Am J Roentgenol 1989;152:1059-1064.
22. Allison JW, Faddis LA, Kinder DL, et al. Intracranial resistive index (RI) values in normal term infants during the first day of life. Pediatr Radiol 2000;30:618-620.
23. Raju TN, Zikos E. Regional cerebral blood velocity in infants: a real-time transcranial and fontanellar pulsed Doppler study. J Ultrasound Med 1987;6:497-507.
24. Agoestina T, Humphrey JH, Taylor GA, et al. Safety of one 52-mumol (50,000 IU) oral dose of vitamin A administered to neonates. Bull WHO 1994;72:859-868.
25. Winkler P, Helmke K. Duplex-scanning of the deep venous drainage in the evaluation of blood flow velocity of the cerebral vascular system in infants. Pediatr Radiol 1989;19:79-90.
26. Cowan F, Thoresen M. Changes in superior sagittal sinus blood velocities due to postural alterations and pressure on the head of the newborn infant. Pediatrics 1985;75:1038-1047.

Intensive Care Therapies and Cerebral Hemodynamics

27. Rennie JM, South M, Morley CJ. Cerebral blood flow velocity variability in infants receiving assisted ventilation. Arch Dis Child 1987;62:1247-1251.

28. Laubscher B, van Melle G, Fawer CL, et al. Haemodynamic changes during high frequency oscillation for respiratory distress syndrome. Arch Dis Child Fetal Neonatal Ed 1996;74:F172-F176.

29. Perlman JM, Volpe JJ. Suctioning in the preterm infant: effects on cerebral blood flow velocity, intracranial pressure, and arterial blood pressure. Pediatrics 1983;72:329-334.

30. Day R. Cerebral blood flow velocity acutely decreases in newborns who respond to inhaled nitric oxide. Am J Perinatol 2000:185-194.

31. Taylor GA, Short BL, Glass P, Ichord R. Cerebral hemodynamics in infants undergoing extracorporeal membrane oxygenation: further observations. Radiology 1988;168:163-167.

32. Mitchell DG, Merton D, Desai H, et al. Neonatal brain: color Doppler imaging. Part II. Altered flow patterns from extracorporeal membrane oxygenation. Radiology 1988;167:307-310.

33. Taylor GA, Walker LK. Intracranial venous system in newborns treated with extracorporeal membrane oxygenation: Doppler US evaluation after ligation of the right jugular vein. Radiology 1992;183:453-456.

34. Weber TR, Kountzman B. The effects of venous occlusion on cerebral blood flow characteristics during ECMO. J Pediatr Surg 1996;31:1124-1127.

Diffuse Neuronal Injury

35. Taylor GA, Trescher WH, Johnston MV, Traystman RJ. Experimental neuronal injury in the newborn lamb: a comparison of N-methyl-D-aspartic acid receptor blockade and nitric oxide synthesis inhibition on lesion size and cerebral hyperemia. Pediatr Res 1995;38:644-651.

36. Van Bel F, van de Bor M, Stijnen T, et al. Cerebral blood flow velocity pattern in healthy and asphyxiated newborns: a controlled study. Eur J Pediatr 1987;146:461-467.

37. Ilves P, Lintrop M, Metsvaht T, et al. Cerebral blood-flow velocities in predicting outcome of asphyxiated newborn infants. Acta Paediatr 2004;93:523-528.

38. Stark JE, Seibert JJ. Cerebral artery Doppler ultrasonography for prediction of outcome after perinatal asphyxia. J Ultrasound Med 1994;13:595-600.

39. Van Bel F, van de Bor M, Baan J, Ruys JH. The influence of abnormal blood gases on cerebral blood flow velocity in the preterm newborn. Neuropediatrics 1988;19:27-32.

40. Deeg KH, Rupprecht T, Zeilinger G. Doppler sonographic classification of brain edema in infants. Pediatr Radiol 1990;20:509-514.

41. Vannucci RC. Mechanisms of perinatal hypoxic-ischemic brain damage. Semin Perinatol 1993;17:330-337.

42. McMenamin JB, Volpe JJ. Doppler ultrasonography in the determination of neonatal brain death. Ann Neurol 1983;14:302-307.

43. Glasier CM, Seibert JJ, Chadduck WM, et al. Brain death in infants: evaluation with Doppler US. Radiology 1989;172:377-380.

44. Taekuchi K, Iinuma K, Satoh H, et al. Report on the criteria for the determination of brain death in children. Part II. Determination of brain death in children in Japan. JMAJ 2002:336-357.

Intracranial Hemorrhage and Stroke

45. Ghazi-Birry HS, Brown WR, Moody DM, et al. Human germinal matrix: venous origin of hemorrhage and vascular characteristics. AJNR Am J Neuroradiol 1997;18:219-229.

46. Volpe JJ. Edward B. Neuhauser lecture. Current concepts of brain injury in the premature infant. AJR Am J Roentgenol 1989;153:243-251.

47. Taylor GA. Effect of germinal matrix hemorrhage on terminal vein position and patency. Pediatr Radiol 1995;25(Suppl. 1):37-40.

48. Hernanz-Schulman M, Cohen W, Genieser NB. Sonography of cerebral infarction in infancy. AJR Am J Roentgenol 1988;150:897-902.

49. Taylor GA. Alterations in regional cerebral blood flow in neonatal stroke: preliminary findings with color Doppler sonography. Pediatr Radiol 1994;24:111-115.

50. Savoiardo M. CT Scanning. In: Barnett H, Stein B, Mohr J, et al, editors. Stroke: pathophysiology, diagnosis and management. New York: Churchill Livingstone; 1986. p. 189-219.

51. Taylor GA, Trescher WA, Traystman RJ, Johnston MV. Acute experimental neuronal injury in the newborn lamb: ultrasound characterization and demonstration of hemodynamic effects. Pediatr Radiol 1993;23:268-275.

Hydrocephalus

52. Bada HS, Miller JE, Menke JA, et al. Intracranial pressure and cerebral arterial pulsatile flow measurement in neonatal intraventricular hemorrhage. J Pediatr 1982;100:291-296.

53. Taylor GA, Phillips MD, Ichord RN, et al. Intracranial compliance in infants: evaluation with Doppler ultrasound. Radiology 1994;191:787-791.

54. Taylor GA, Madsen JR. Neonatal hydrocephalus: hemodynamic response to fontanelle compression—correlation with intracranial pressure and need for shunt placement. Radiology 1996;201:685-689.

55. Westra SJ, Lazareff J, Curran JG, et al. Transcranial Doppler ultrasonography to evaluate need for cerebrospinal fluid drainage in hydrocephalic children. J Ultrasound Med 1998;17:561-569.

56. Westra SJ, Stotland MA, Lazareff J, et al. Perioperative transcranial Doppler ultrasound to evaluate intracranial compliance in young children undergoing craniosynostosis repair surgery. Radiology 2001;218:816-823.

57. Bruce DA, Berman WA, Schut L. Cerebrospinal fluid pressure monitoring in children: physiology, pathology and clinical usefulness. Adv Pediatr 1977;24:233-240.

58. De Oliveira RS, Machado HR. Transcranial color-coded Doppler ultrasonography for evaluation of children with hydrocephalus. Neurosurg Focus 2003;15:ECP3.

59. Winkler P. Colour-coded echographic flow imaging and spectral analysis of cerebrospinal fluid (CSF) in infants. Part II. CSF dynamics. Pediatr Radiol 1992;22:31-42.

Vascular Malfomations

60. Tessler FN, Dion J, Vinuela F, et al. Cranial arteriovenous malformations in neonates: color Doppler imaging with angiographic correlation. AJR Am J Roentgenol 1989;153:1027-1030.

61. Soto G, Daneman A, Hellman J. Doppler evaluation of cerebral arteries in a galenic vein malformation. J Ultrasound Med 1985;4:673-675.

62. Westra SJ, Curran JG, Duckwiler GR, et al. Pediatric intracranial vascular malformations: evaluation of treatment results with color Doppler ultrasound. Work in progress. Radiology 1993;186:775-783.

Intracranial Tumors

63. Chow PP, Horgan JG, Burns PN, et al. Choroid plexus papilloma: detection by real-time and Doppler sonography. AJNR Am J Neuroradiol 1986;7:168-170.

64. Simanovsky N, Taylor GA. Sonography of brain tumors in infants and young children. Pediatr Radiol 2001;31:392-398.

Near-Field Structures

65. Chen CY, Chou TY, Zimmerman RA, et al. Pericerebral fluid collection: differentiation of enlarged subarachnoid spaces from subdural collections with color Doppler ultrasound. Radiology 1996;201:389-392.

66. Amodio J, Spektor V, Pramanik B, et al. Spontaneous development of bilateral subdural hematomas in an infant with benign infantile hydrocephalus: color Doppler assessment of vessels traversing extra-axial spaces. Pediatr Radiol 2005;35:1113-1117.

67. Yikilmaz A, Taylor GA. Sonographic findings in bacterial meningitis in neonates and young infants. Pediatr Radiol 2008;38:129-137.

68. Bezinque SL, Slovis TL, Touchette AS, et al. Characterization of superior sagittal sinus blood flow velocity using color flow Doppler in neonates and infants. Pediatr Radiol 1995;25:175-179.

CHAPTER 49

Doppler Sonography of the Brain in Children

Dorothy I. Bulas and Joanna J. Seibert

Chapter Outline

uplex Doppler sonography with color flow imaging through the anterior fontanelle is simple and has proved useful in evaluating abnormalities of cerebral blood flow in the neonate and young child.[1-4] Once the fontanelle closes, transcranial Doppler (TCD) sonography can still be performed noninvasively using a 2 to 2.5–MHz pulsed wave Doppler transducer through the thin temporal bone, the orbits, or the foramen magnum. This technique, introduced by Aaslid[5] in the early 1980s, can be used to measure the velocity and pulsatility of blood flow within the intracranial arteries of the circle of Willis and the vertebrobasilar system. TCD sonography has become essential in the management of children with sickle cell anemia and has proved to be a valuable adjunct in the evaluation of various intracranial pathologies in children, including vasospasm, vascular malformations, and brain death, as well as the assessment of cerebral hemodynamics after trauma, migraine, and stroke.

Two types of TCD sonographic equipment are currently available: **nonimaging** (TCD) and **imaging** (TCDI). Continuous wave and nonimaging pulsed wave Doppler techniques insonate specific vessels using strict criteria for vessel identification based on the depth and direction of flow for intracranial vessels through the temporal bone.[6,7] This blinded technique requires meticulous skill and ability to maintain the mental image of the circle of Willis. Advantages include the small, portable size of units designed specifically for TCD sonography, the low price, Doppler sensitivity, and superior window maneuverability with small transducer size. Limitations include the need for intensive training, difficulty in finding vessels, and lack of units available in radiology departments. The development of duplex Doppler

sonography with color imaging using 2 to 2.5–MHz transducers has increased the utility of TCD sonography using the transtemporal approach. Advantages of this technique include quick vessel identification, a shorter learning curve, and availability of units in most radiology departments. This technique allows positive vessel identification, resulting in easier, more reliable and reproducible information.[8-10] With training and experience, both techniques are reliable and reproducible between operators.[11,12]

SONOGRAPHIC TECHNIQUE

The **anterior fontanelle** typically remains open through the first year of life. Once closed, three cranial windows (in addition to burr holes and surgical defects) can be used routinely to insonate the intracranial circulation: the **temporal bone**, **orbit**, and **foramen magnum**.[13] The **transtemporal approach** is through the thin suprazygomatic portion of the temporal bone using a 2 to 2.5–MHz transducer. The transtemporal window is usually found on the temporal bone cephalad to the zygomatic arch and anterior to the ear. The intracranial anatomic landmark in this plane is the heart-shaped cerebral **peduncles** (Fig. 49-1, *A*). Just anterior to the peduncles is the star-shaped, echogenic interpeduncular or suprasellar **cistern**. Anteriorly and laterally from this basilar cistern lies the echogenic fissure for the **middle cerebral artery** (MCA). Color Doppler sonographic imaging (Fig. 49-1, *B*) and spectral analysis (Figs. 49-1, *C*, and 49-2, *A*) of this vessel will show flow toward the transducer. Insonating the vessel deeper toward the

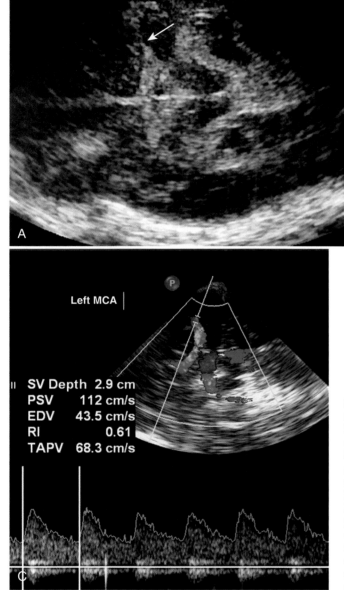

SV Depth 2.9 cm
PSV   112 cm/s
EDV   43.5 cm/s
RI   0.61
TAPV   68.3 cm/s

Left MCA

FIGURE 49-1. Temporal window. A, Transtemporal transcranial Doppler (TCD) sonogram with normal landmarks. Note the heart-shaped cerebral peduncles with the echogenic suprasellar cistern. Anteriorly and laterally from this basilar cistern is the echogenic fissure for the middle cerebral artery (MCA, *arrow*). **B,** Transtemporal color flow Doppler sonogram shows the circle of Willis anterior to the landmark of the heart-shaped cerebral peduncles. Flow directed toward the transducer *(red)* is the MCA in the middle cerebral fissure just anterior to the cerebral peduncles. Flow in the anterior cerebral artery (ACA) on that side *(blue)* is away from the transducer *(cursor)*. Flow is also seen in the MCA on the opposite side *(blue)* as it courses away from the transducer. **C,** Normal spectral Doppler ultrasound waveform in the right MCA with flow directed toward transducer. The posterior cerebral arteries are coursing around the cerebral peduncles.

midline directs the operator into the bifurcation of the A1 segment of the **anterior cerebral artery** (ACA) and the MCA. Spectral analysis at this bifurcation landmark will show bidirectional flow—flow toward the transducer in the MCA and flow in the ACA away from the transducer (Fig. 49-2, *B*). As the cursor is moved more medial anteriorly, flow is seen entirely in the ACA away from the transducer (Fig. 49-2, *C*). The MCA should be studied from its most peripheral location to the point of bifurcation, and the ACA studied as medially as possible. The **distal internal cerebral artery** (ICA) is inferior to the bifurcation. The flow may be dampened from the angle of insonation, with flow directed toward the

transducer (Fig. 49-2, *D*). The **posterior cerebral artery** (PCA) can be visualized as it circles around the cerebral peduncles. Flow in this vessel may be away or toward the transducer (Fig. 49-2, *E*). At times, the MCA, the ACA, and the PCA on the opposite side may also be evaluated.

The vertebral and basilar arteries can be studied through the **foramen magnum** with a 2-MHz transducer. The patient lies on one side or prone, and the head is bowed slightly so the chin touches the chest, causing a gap between the cranium and the atlas to enlarge. The transducer is placed midline in the nape of the neck and angled through the foramen magnum

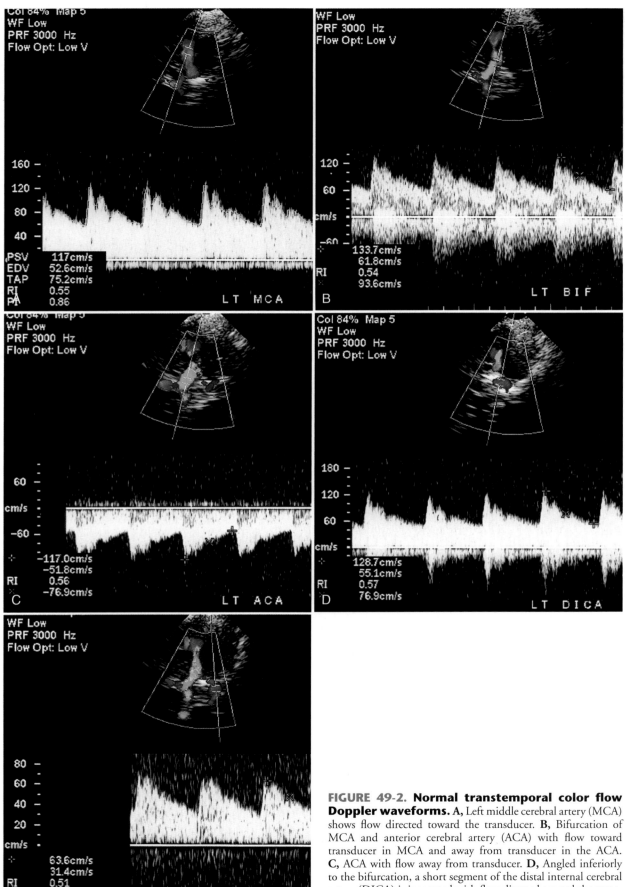

FIGURE 49-2. Normal transtemporal color flow Doppler waveforms. A, Left middle cerebral artery (MCA) shows flow directed toward the transducer. **B,** Bifurcation of MCA and anterior cerebral artery (ACA) with flow toward transducer in MCA and away from transducer in the ACA. **C,** ACA with flow away from transducer. **D,** Angled inferiorly to the bifurcation, a short segment of the distal internal cerebral artery (DICA) is insonated with flow directed toward the transducer. **E,** Posterior cerebral artery (PCA) with flow directed toward the transducer.

toward the eye. The normal landmark is the rounded hypoechoic **medulla** just anterior to the echogenic **clivus** (Fig. 49-3, *A*). The vertebral arteries appear in a V-shaped manner as they rise to the medullopontine junction to form the basilar artery between the hypoechoic medulla-pons junction and the echogenic clivus (Fig. 49-3, *B*). From this posterior view, flow in the vertebral and basilar arteries should be directed away from the transducer (Fig. 49-3, *C* and *D*).

The **ophthalmic artery** (OA) is evaluated **through the orbit** with the eyes closed using a 3-, 5-, or 7.5-MHz transducer on its lowest power setting (Fig. 49-4). Flow in the OA should be toward the transducer. The ophthalmic artery enters the optic foramen to lie lateral and slightly inferior to the optic nerve. It then usually crosses superior to the optic nerve and proceeds anteriorly on the medial side of the orbit. The central retinal artery branch of the OA is the easiest branch interrogated by color flow Doppler imaging, just posterior to the retina. Because visualization of this central retinal artery entails directing sound waves through the lens, the lowest power setting must be used. U.S. Food and Drug Administration (FDA) guidelines suggest limiting spatial peak temporal average (SPTA) to 17 mW/cm^2 for orbital imaging.[14,15] However, a large OA branch proceeds along the nasal or medial wall of the orbit. Because interrogating this vessel does not involve directing the sound beam through the lens, a higher power setting may be used for this branch.

On spectral analysis of the waveform, the maximum, minimum, and mean velocities including **time average mean of the maximum velocity** (TAMMX), sometimes called the **time average peak velocity** (TAP), can be measured in centimeters per second. At least two readings should be made for each vessel. The highest velocity obtained may be taken as the truest velocity, because it is believed to be the velocity obtained at the best insonating angle to the vessel.[16]

Angle correction cannot be performed with the non-imaging technique. Although angle correction is possible with the imaging technique because of visualization of the vessel course, published velocities typically have not been angle-corrected. Thus, it is important to remember that angle-corrected velocity measurements obtained with the imaging technique may be more accurate than non-angle-corrected velocity measurements. In clinical applications such as assessing stroke risk in children with sickle cell anemia, guidelines regarding normal versus abnormal/conditional velocities were validated in large clinical trials using nonduplex equipment that were not angle-corrected.[17-21] Angle correction can significantly increase velocities in vessels that are not coursing directly toward the transducer.[22] While angle correction has been suggested as a way to correct for variations between the imaging and nonimaging examination, the lack of published data for angle-corrected velocities currently limits this approach.[11,12,23] Because the MCA, ACA, and OA usually course almost directly toward or away from the transducer, angle correction is less of an issue in these

vessels. ACA and PCA velocities are more variable because of their tortuous course.

An index of pulsatility, either the Gosling **pulsatility index** (PI) (systolic velocity minus diastolic velocity divided by mean velocity) or Pourcelot **resistive index** (RI) (systolic velocity minus diastolic velocity divided by systolic velocity), can also be measured. Both these pulsatility indices, either the RI or the PI, are ratios that minimize the effect of vessel angulation. Because the RI is a ratio, it may be expressed as a whole number (50), representing a percentage (%), or as a fraction (0.5).

Age-dependent reference values are available for velocities and resistive indices of the various intracranial vessels. Normal mean velocity in the MCA in adults ranges from 50 to 80 cm/sec; in the ACA, 35 to 60 cm/sec; in the PCA, 30 to 50 cm/sec; and in the basilar artery, 25 to 50 cm/sec. Peak systolic velocities up to 150 cm/sec have been described in patients with sickle cell disease secondary to anemia.[24,25] The velocity in the OA is normally about one-fourth the velocity in the MCA. The velocity in the PCA and vertebral and basilar arteries should be about one-half the velocity in the MCA. Normal RI after fontanelle closure should be 0.50 to 0.59, except in the OA, which has a higher RI, usually 0.70 to 0.79, and less diastolic flow because it supplies a muscular bed[13] (see Fig. 49-3, *B*). An increase in diastolic flow will result in a decrease in the RI, whereas a decrease in diastolic flow will result in an increase in the RI. As intracranial pressure increases above mean arterial pressure, diastolic flow may become reversed, demonstrating an RI of greater than 1.[26]

ULTRASOUND DOSAGE: POWER SETTINGS

The American Institute of Ultrasound and Medicine (AIUM) and the federal guidelines of the spatial peak, temporal average intensity (I$_{SPTA}$) for the pediatric head should not exceed 94 mW/cm^2. For evaluating vessels in the eye, the limit is 17 mW/cm^2.[27] The power settings of transducers of various manufacturers are different for each piece of equipment and each probe.[28] Depending on the manufacturer and transducer, energy levels may be within the guidelines only on the low power setting. However, when the transtemporal approach is used, at least 65% (and likely more) of the energy is attenuated by the skull. These higher settings may therefore be used in the transtemporal approach, but should not be exceeded when insonating the eye or foramen magnum.[29]

PITFALLS IN DOPPLER INVESTIGATIONS

There are numerous pitfalls when performing a TCD sonographic examination in children.[12,30,31] Low wall filter adjustments, high Doppler ultrasound frequency,

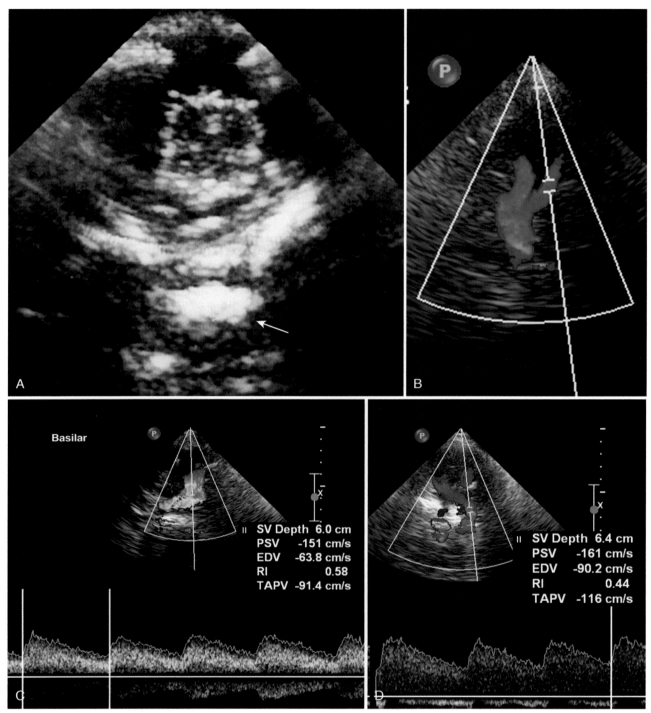

FIGURE 49-3. Occipital view through foramen magnum. A, Normal landmark in the foramen magnum view shows rounded medulla just anterior to the very echogenic clivus *(arrow).* **B,** With color flow Doppler imaging, the V-shaped vertebral arteries *(blue)* join to form the basilar artery at the medulla-pons junction. Cursor is on the left vertebral artery. **C** and **D,** Spectral Doppler ultrasound waveforms in the basilar artery show flow away from the transducer.

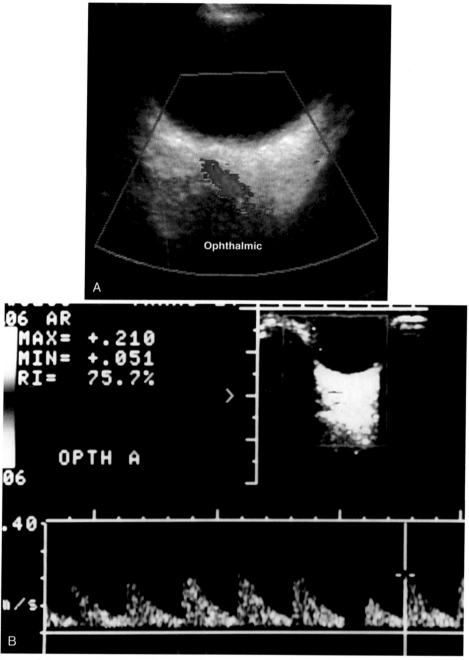

FIGURE 49-4. Normal transcranial Doppler (TCD) sonography through eye. A, Color flow Doppler sonogram visualizing the ophthalmic artery (OA) posterior to the globe with flow directed toward the transducer *(red)*. **B,** Normal waveform of OA with 0.75 resistive index (RI).

and critical assessment of velocity spectral analysis are crucial for accurate interpretation of the data.[10] Although the clinician can assume a patent circle of Willis in children, one artery should not be used to represent the entire cerebral circulation.

INDICATIONS FOR TRANSCRANIAL SONOGRAPHIC DOPPLER IMAGING

Vasospasm

In adults, TCD ultrasound has proved to be valuable in diagnosing vasospasm that may occur after subarachnoid hemorrhage secondary to rupture of an intracranial aneurysm or other pathology.[32,33] Patients with persistent severe vasospasm may develop permanent deficits from cerebral infarction. The vasospasm typically develops in the first 2 days after the hemorrhage, gradually increases for a week, then peaking between 11 and 17 days before gradually decreasing. TCD sonography has become an important tool in detecting vasospasm before the patient develops ischemic neurologic deficits or infarct and is highly specific in diagnosing vasospasm (98%-100%).[34,35]

TRANSCRANIAL DOPPLER SONOGRAPHY IN ADULTS

ESTABLISHED INDICATIONS
Detection of severe (>65%) stenosis in a major basal intracranial artery.
Evaluation of patterns and extent of collateral circulation in patients with known severe stenosis (occlusion).
Evaluation and follow-up of patients with vasospasm or vasoconstriction, especially after subarachnoid hemorrhage.
Detection of arteriovenous malformations and posttreatment evaluation.
Confirmation of the clinical diagnosis of brain death.

POTENTIAL APPLICATIONS
Monitoring of patients during cerebral endarterectomy, cardiopulmonary bypass, and other cerebrovascular or cardiovascular interventional and surgical procedures.
Evaluation of patients with dilated vasculopathies, such as fusiform aneurysms.
Assessment of autoregulation and the physiologic and pharmacologic responses of the cerebral arteries.
Evaluation of patients with migraine headaches.
Enhancement of thrombolytic activity of certain drugs.

In these cases, blood flow velocity increases because of a decrease in the luminal cross-sectional area of the affected vessels. Thus, TCD can be used to guide optimal timing of therapy and is useful in following the effects of therapies (Fig. 49-5). When a hemodynamically significant vasospasm of clinical concern is suggested, emergency cerebral angiography with balloon dilation angioplasty or intra-arterial infusion of vasodilating agents may be helpful.[36] Serial TCD studies showing reduction in velocities indicate the appropriate time to withdraw therapy, minimizing complications and shortening intensive care unit stay. TCD is most accurate in predicting vasospasm of the MCA. TCD cannot be used to assess the ACA beyond its A1 segment and is limited in the evaluation of the distal branches of the MCA.

Mean MCA velocities of 100 to 140 cm/sec correlate with **mild vasospasm** demonstrated by angiography. **Moderate vasospasm** is defined as velocities of 140 to 200 cm/sec, and **severe vasospasm,** greater than 200 cm/sec. A steep increase (>25 cm/sec/day) in velocity in the first few days after subarachnoid hemorrhage is associated with a worse prognosis. Sources of error in the detection of vasospasm by TCD sonography (vs. arteriography) include missing peripheral vasospasm, presence of increased **intracranial pressure** (ICP), and low volume flow.[7] Thus, TCD values should always be combined with clinical and laboratory data.[37,38]

Migraine Headaches

Adults with vascular headaches have been evaluated by TCD ultrasound.[7] Thie et al.[39] found a significant increase in mean velocity in migraine patients compared to controls during headache-free periods. Patients with common migraines had decreased intracranial velocities

---

INDICATIONS FOR TRANSCRANIAL DOPPLER SONOGRAPHY IN CHILDREN

Evaluation of children with various vasculopathies, such as sickle cell disease and moyamoya.
Evaluation of children with arteriovenous malformations.
Follow-up of children with hydrocephalus and subdural effusions.
Evaluation of children with asphyxia, cerebral edema, and their treatment, including hyperventilation therapy.
Confirmation of the diagnosis of clinical brain death.
Monitoring of children during cerebrovascular and cardiovascular interventional and surgical procedures.

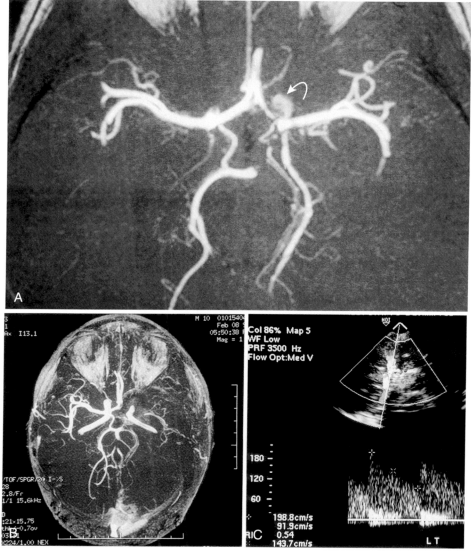

FIGURE 49-5. Vasospasm with aneurysm. A, Ten-year-old boy presents with acute headache. Magnetic resonance angiography (MRA) demonstrates narrow supraclinoid carotid, narrow A1 segment, and small left bifurcation aneurysm *(arrow)*. **B,** After clipping of aneurysm, susceptibility metal artifact limits MRA evaluation of the left proximal M1 segment. **C,** On day 15, transcranial Doppler (TCD) sonography demonstrates an increase in mean velocities to 144 cm/sec, consistent with moderate vasospasm. Patient did well after medical management.

and increased pulsatility during headache attacks, whereas symptomatic patients with classic migraines demonstrated an increase in velocities and a decrease in pulsatility.[40] Thus, TCD sonography may assist in the differential diagnosis of headaches of unknown etiology and could prove useful in therapeutic interventions.

Some headaches caused by increased ICP may demonstrate abnormal pulsatility. Wang et al.[41] evaluated the utility of TCD sonography in pediatric headache. In children with isolated headaches, TCD sensitivity and specificity in detecting intracranial lesions was 75% and 99.7%, respectively.

Sleep Apnea

Several studies have demonstrated changes in MCA velocities in children with **sleep-disordered breathing** (SDB) a spectrum of upper airway obstruction ranging from primary snoring to obstructive sleep apnea. Increases in MCA blood flow velocity have been documented in children with mild SDB.[42] An association between nocturnal oxyhemoglobin desaturation and central nervous system event risk in sickle cell disease has been described as well.[43] In a group of children with sleep-disordered breathing followed after adenotonsillectomy, MCA velocities decreased (suggesting a normalization of MCA

TABLE 49-1. FACTORS THAT CHANGE CEREBRAL DOPPLER INDICES

	RESISTIVE INDEX	SYSTOLIC VELOCITY
Intracranial Abnormalities		
Intracranial bleed	Increased	Beat-to-beat variation, risk factor for IVH
Periventricular leukomalacia	Increased	
Asphyxia	Decreased initially	
Brain edema	Increased	
Hydrocephalus	Increased, reverses after drainage	
Subdural	Increased	
Brain death	Increased	Decreased, reverse diastolic
ECMO	Decreased	
Vascular malformations	Decreased	Increased, turbulence
Extracranial Abnormalities		
Pco_2	Inverse relationship	
Heart rate	Inverse relationship	
Shock		Decreased systolic/diastolic
Patent ductus arteriosus	Increased	
Pneumothorax	Increased	
Cardiac ischemia	Increased	
Gastrointestinal bleed	Increased	
Polycythemia, hyperviscosity	Increased	Decreased
Anemia	Increased	
Drugs		
Indomethacin	Increased	Decreased
Maternal cocaine		Increased
Exogenous surfactant		Increased

IVH, Intraventricular hemorrhage; *ECMO*, extracorporeal membrane oxygenation; *Pco₂*, carbon dioxide partial pressure (tension).

velocities) with a resultant increase in mean overnight oxyhemoglobin saturation postoperatively. These children demonstrated an improvement in processing speed and visual attention postoperatively as well.[44]

Hydrocephalus

The ability to differentiate between **ventriculomegaly** and **hydrocephalus** (increasing ventriculomegaly and increasing intracranial pressure [ICP]) can be difficult. When hydrocephalus develops, ICP increases, resulting in a decrease in diastolic flow. Stable ventriculomegaly should have normal pulsatility, thus an elevated RI in cases where ventricular size is increased may imply the need for a shunt. Hill and Volpe[45] first described a decrease in diastolic/systolic flow ratio in 11 hydrocephalic infants. Because of its noninvasive and repeatable nature, Doppler sonography has been increasingly used to assess changes in cerebral hemodynamics in hydrocephalus through the anterior fontanelle in infants and transcranially through the temporal bone in older children.[4,46,47] There is agreement that a direct correlation exists between the ICP (from experimental fontanometric and direct measurement evidence) and the RI. The increasing RI has been predominantly caused by a reduction in the end diastolic velocity.[47,48] The two pulsatility indices most often applied in hydrocephalic patients have been the Pourcelot Resistive Index and Gosling Pulsatility Index. Both ratios minimize the error in estimating true velocity caused by a varying angle of insonation. This is particularly important in hydrocephalus because vascular anatomy can be significantly distorted by ventricular enlargement, and a small angle of insonation cannot be assumed.[49] Difficulties with using the RI to determine hydrocephalus have occurred because of two major issues, as follows[50]:

1. Many other intracranial and extracranial factors can change the RI other than increased ICP (Table 49-1). Therefore the RI must be correlated closely with the clinical condition of the patient (e.g., Pco_2, heart rate, presence of PDA).
2. There is a wide range of normal RI values: 0.65 to 0.85 in the neonate; 0.60 to 0.70 in the child before fontanelle closure; and 0.50 to 0.60 in older children and adults through temporal window after fontanelle closure.[13]

Goh et al.[47] used an RI of greater than 0.8 as a sign of increased ICP in the neonate and an RI of greater than 0.65 in children. Because of varying normal values and overlapping normal and abnormal values, RI is most useful on an individual basis following a patient's course to determine whether clinical changes and ventricular dilation are secondary to increased pressure or atrophy (Figs. 49-6 to 49-9).

Transcranial Doppler sonography has been useful for predicting **shunt malfunction.** Any increase in RI could be considered significant in terms of shunt malfunction. False-normal values may be the result of CSF fluid tracking along the shunt. Excessive thickness of the skull may prevent TCD ultrasound from being obtained successfully in some of these patients.[51,52]

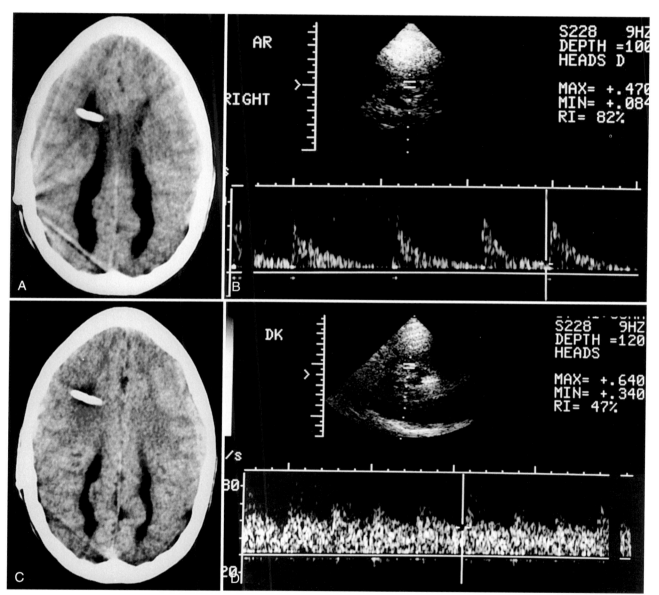

FIGURE 49-6. Shunt dysfunction in an 8-year-old. A, Computed tomography (CT) scan shows mildly dilated ventricles. **B,** TCD image through the temporal window shows an increased resistive index (RI) of 0.82 in the MCA. **C,** CT scan postshunt revision shows decrease in ventricular size. **D,** TCD image of the MCA demonstrates a decrease in RI to 0.47, now in the normal range (after age 2 years with fontanelle closure, normal RI is 0.5). *(From Seibert JJ, Glasier CM, Leithiser RE Jr, et al. Transcranial Doppler using standard duplex equipment in children. Ultrasound Q 1990;8:167-196.)*

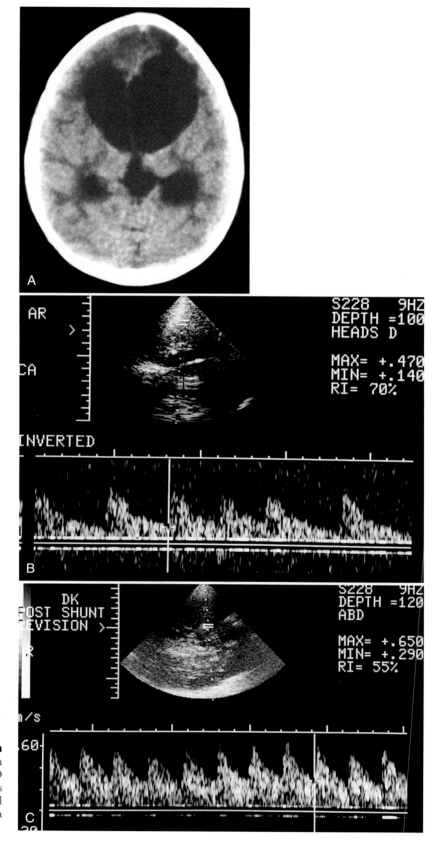

FIGURE 49-7. Shunt malfunction in a 3-year-old child. A, Hydrocephalus with increasing signs of shunt malfunction. **B,** TCD sonogram through the temporal window shows an elevated RI of 0.7 in the middle cerebral artery. **C,** TCD postshunt revision shows a normal RI of 0.55.

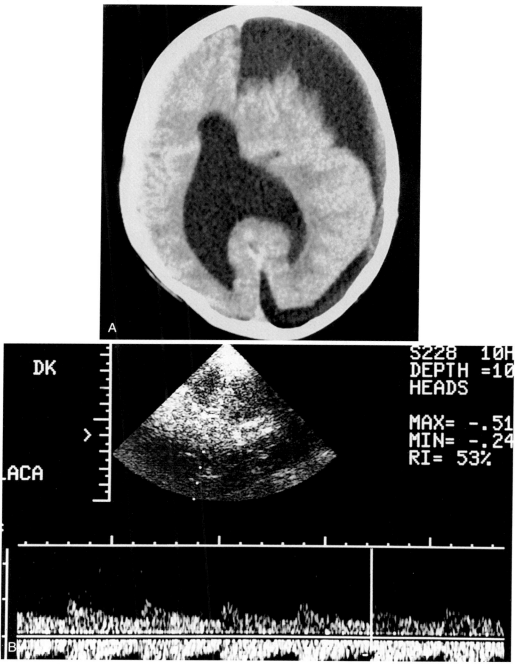

FIGURE 49-8. Atrophy. A, CT scan shows extra-axial fluid on the left and dilated ventricles in 9-year-old child with increasing seizure activity. **B,** Normal bifurcation landmark on Doppler imaging with flow toward the transducer in the middle cerebral artery (above the line) and flow away from the transducer in the anterior cerebral artery (below the line). The RI is 0.53, which is normal at age 9 years in this patient with atrophy. *(From Seibert JJ, Glasier CM, Leithiser RE Jr, et al. Transcranial Doppler using standard duplex equipment in children. Ultrasound Q 1990;8:167-196.)*

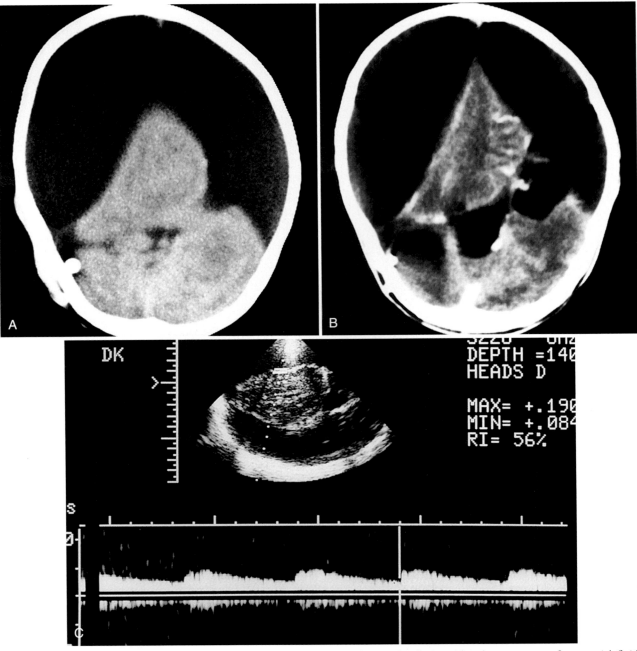

FIGURE 49-9. Atrophy. A, CT scan at age 7 years demonstrates a dysmorphic brain with a large amount of extra-axial fluid. **B,** Repeat CT scan at age 10 years for increasing seizures shows increasing ventricular dilation. **C,** TCD sonogram through temporal window shows a normal RI of 0.56, which is consistent with atrophy. *(From Seibert JJ, Glasier CM, Leithiser RE Jr, et al. Transcranial Doppler using standard duplex equipment in children. Ultrasound Q 1990;8:167-196.)*

Vascular Malformations

Intracranial Doppler imaging is particularly useful for detecting vascular malformations in the unstable neonate.[3,53] The vascular malformation may be imaged with color or power Doppler ultrasound. Spectral analysis of the involved vessels will show high velocity, with low pressure and low pulsatility caused by increased diastolic flow. These hemodynamic qualities result in higher-than-normal mean and peak systolic velocities, in conjunction with turbulence and lower-than-normal RIs (Fig. 49-10). TCD sonography can correctly diagnose **arteriovenous malformation** (AVM) with a sensitivity of 87% to 95%.[45-56] Because magnetic resonance imaging (MRI) affords an even higher sensitivity than TCD ultrasound in diagnostic screening, Doppler imaging is used more often to quantitate the hemodynamics of AVMs and to monitor the effects of surgical or

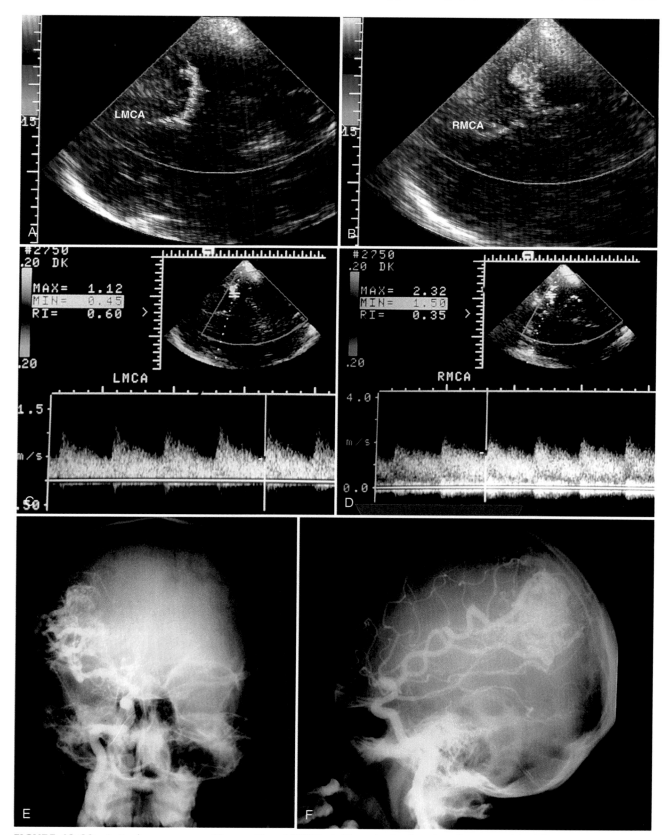

FIGURE 49-10. Arteriovenous malformation (AVM). A, Normal color flow Doppler image of the left middle cerebral artery (MCA). **B,** Increased number of vessels in the region of AVM at the right MCA. **C,** TCD spectral Doppler sonogram of left MCA shows normal maximum velocity of 112 cm/sec. **D,** Velocity on the right is increased, with a maximum velocity of 232 cm/sec. **E** and **F,** Anteroposterior and lateral views of an arteriogram in this teenager confirms the presence of a large AVM.

endoluminal interventions.[57] After surgical or embolization treatment, the decrease in systolic velocity and increase in RI in the feeding arteries can be followed.

Transcranial Doppler ultrasound has also been used to assess other vascular anomalies, such as **Sturge-Weber syndrome** and **dural arteriovenous fistulas.**[58,59] In a series of patients with Sturge-Weber syndrome, decreased arterial flow velocity and increased pulsatility index was noted on the affected side, suggesting chronic hypoperfusion of the tissue to that region.

Asphyxia

Transcranial Doppler sonography has been useful in the evaluation of hypoxic-ischemic brain injury. Asphyxia may result in impairment of cerebral autoregulation, producing an increase in diastolic blood flow and a decrease in cerebrovascular resistance.[2] Intracranial Doppler imaging in the neonate has been particularly helpful in predicting significant hypoxic-ischemic brain injury.[1,60-63] Archer et al.[62] found 100% sensitivity of a low RI caused by increased diastolic flow in the ACA and MCA and an adverse neurologic outcome when performed within the first 48 hours of the insult in the neonate. Stark and Seibert[60] reported 10 of 13 neonates with an initially low RI who later developed severe neurodevelopmental handicaps. The finding of increased diastolic flow can also be useful in evaluating the older child after head injury or cardiac arrest to predict significant cerebral injury before computed tomography (CT) findings (Fig. 49-11).

Cerebral Edema and Hyperventilation Therapy

Head trauma initiates several pathologic processes that may result in significant changes in cerebral hemodynamics. Diagnosis of these abnormalities can be crucial for the appropriate management of such cases. After a significant cerebral hypoxic insult, vasodilation may initially occur with a resultant increase in diastolic flow velocity and a reduced RI during this early hyperemic phase. As ICP increases, however, the diastolic flow velocity begins to decrease, and the systolic peak velocity becomes spiky.[2] As cerebral edema develops, there is further loss of forward diastolic flow, and RI increases.[48] Continuous or intermittent sequential TCD readings after a cerebral insult have been helpful in evaluating the presence of edema and the course of treatment[64] (Fig. 49-12).

Treatment for cerebral edema includes hyperventilation. An inverse relationship exists between carbon dioxide partial pressure (P_{CO_2}) and the RI. The higher the P_{CO_2}, the greater the vasodilation, the greater the diastolic flow, and the lower is the RI. When the P_{CO_2} is reduced, vasoconstriction results, with decreased diastolic flow and increased RI. Thus, CO_2 reactivity can be measured using the RI. The cerebral blood flow increases 4% per mm Hg rise in P_{CO_2}.[1,48,63,65] The absence of change in the RI as the patient's hyperventilation is increased is described as an absent "CO_2 reactivity test" and is a sign of severe brain injury.[65] Because of this, RI can be used to monitor hyperventilation therapy in cerebral edema associated with head trauma.[2,66] As hyperventilation decreases the P_{CO_2}, the RI should increase with the concomitant vasoconstriction of cerebral vessels. The clinician must take into account, however, that increasing cerebral edema will also increase the RI. Therefore, this measurement should be closely correlated with other clinical and laboratory findings. For example, hyperventilation treatment in a patient who has an increasing RI in the face of no change in ICP suggests that the treatment is causing too much cerebral vasoconstriction. In this scenario the patient may benefit from a decrease in the hyperventilation.

Brain Death

Establishing brain death can be problematic, and quick identification may be useful in the case of organ transplant donation. Neurologic examination, electroencephalography (EEG), brainstem-evoked potentials, and nuclear blood flow studies can be used at times to establish brain death. TCD sonography, another noninvasive tool, can be repeated as often as required and is portable, inexpensive, and easy to perform. For patients in phenobarbital coma in which EEG is not diagnostic, TCD ultrasound is particularly helpful in demonstrating the severity of cerebrovascular compromise.[67-69]

After a severe asphyxiating event, an initial drop in RI may be caused by vasodilation from loss of autoregulation. As cerebral edema develops, there is loss of forward diastolic flow, followed by reversal of diastolic flow. This results in an increase in RI, eventually measuring greater than 1 as diastolic flow reverses. Cessation of cerebral blood flow then occurs at the microcirculation level. The larger vessels will distend, then constrict, and eventually thrombose or collapse. As ICP increases above mean arterial pressure, arrest of cerebral circulation results in a decrease in antegrade systolic velocity. Small, early systolic spikes and complete cessation of antegrade flow then develops. Eventually, no systolic or diastolic flow can be detected[68,70] (Fig. 49-13).

SONOGRAPHIC CRITERIA FOR BRAIN DEATH AFTER FONTANELLE CLOSURE

- Sustained reversal of diastolic flow
- Small, early systolic spikes
- No flow in middle cerebral artery, with reversal of diastolic flow in extracranial internal cerebral artery
- Mean velocity in middle cerebral artery less than 10 cm/sec for more than 30 minutes

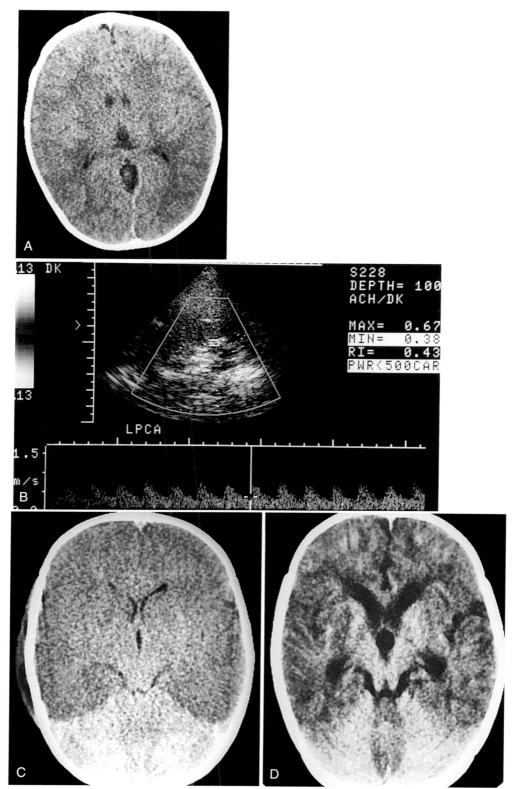

FIGURE 49-11. Asphyxia. A, One-year-old child after a respiratory arrest demonstrates mild cerebral edema on CT scan. **B,** However, the RI in the left posterior cerebral artery is abnormally low on spectral Doppler ultrasound evaluation, measuring 0.43, consistent with loss of autoregulation (normal range is 0.5 to 0.6). **C,** CT scan 2 days later shows severe cerebral edema. **D,** CT scan 1 month later shows marked atrophy.

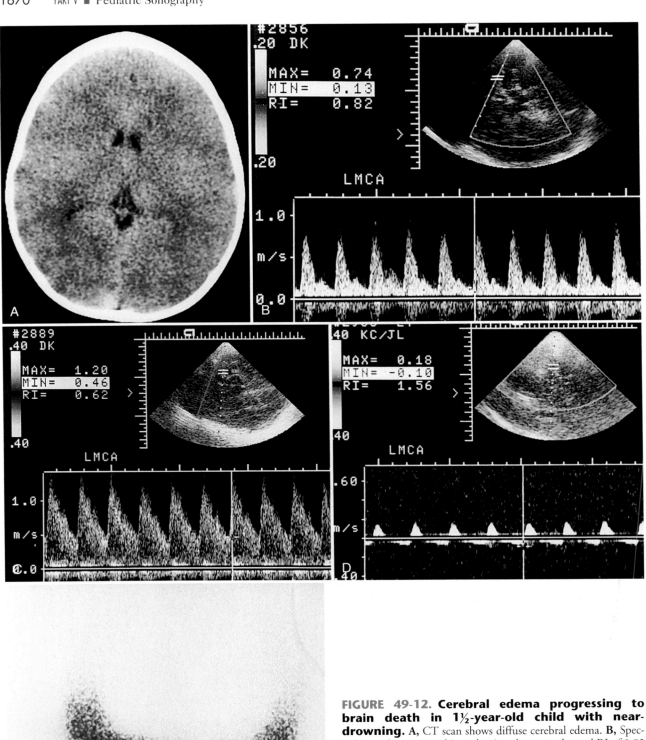

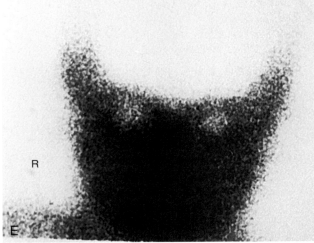

FIGURE 49-12. **Cerebral edema progressing to brain death in 1½-year-old child with near-drowning. A,** CT scan shows diffuse cerebral edema. **B,** Spectral Doppler sonographic evaluation shows an elevated RI of 0.82 from middle cerebral artery (MCA). **C,** Spectral Doppler sonographic evaluation of the MCA 2 days later shows that RI has decreased to a more normal range of 0.62 with treatment. **D,** However, MCA Doppler evaluation 4 days later shows decreased velocity and reversal of diastolic flow, with RI of 1.56, consistent with greatly diminished cerebral perfusion. **E,** ^{99m}Tc-DTPA brain scan at this time shows no cerebral perfusion, consistent with brain death. *(From Seibert JJ. Doppler evaluation of cerebral circulation. In Dieckmann RA, Fiser DHB, Selbst SM, editors. Illustrated textbook of pediatric emergency and critical care procedures. St Louis, 1997, Mosby–Year Book.)*

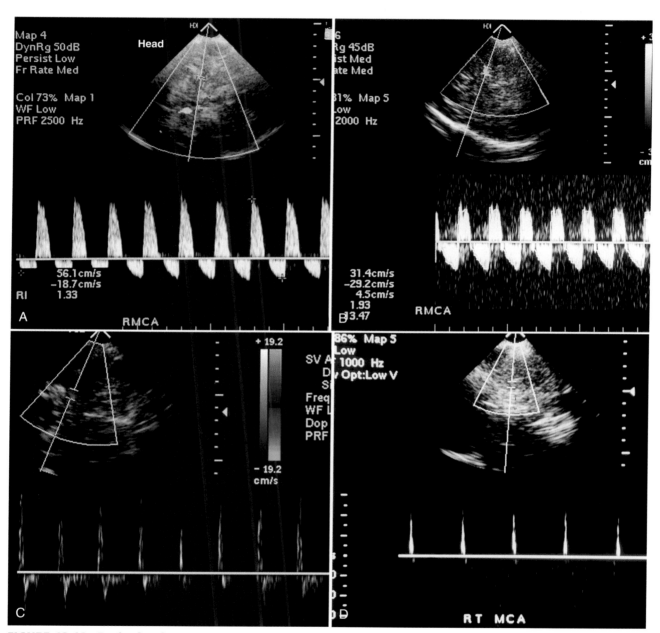

FIGURE 49-13. Brain death. Patterns of pediatric TCD spectral Doppler waveforms in impending brain death. **A,** Moderate reversal of diastolic flow, with elevated RI of 1.3. **B,** Significant reversal of diastolic flow (RI 1.9), with reversed diastolic velocity area almost equal to systolic velocity area. **C** and **D,** Brief systolic forward flow with diminished peak velocity.

Continued

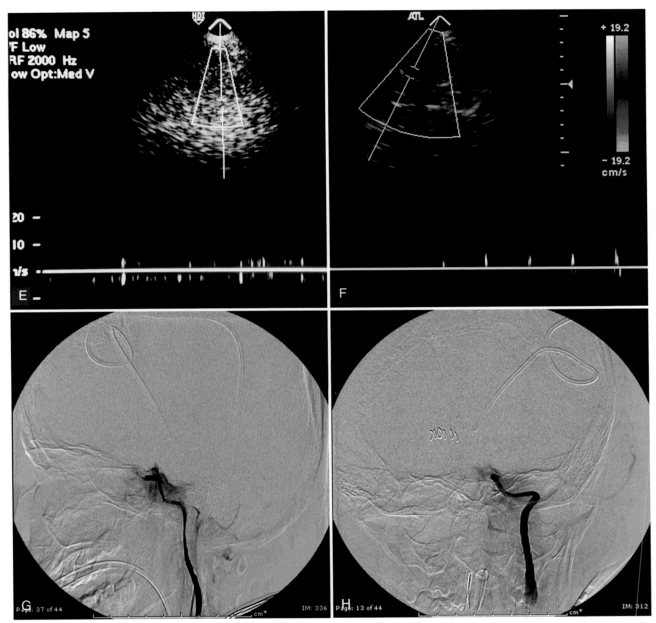

FIGURE 49-13, cont'd. E and **F,** No discernible systolic or diastolic flow. **G** and **H,** Lateral and anteroposterior projections of a carotid arteriogram in a 13 year old status post motor vehicle accident demonstrates lack of intracranial circulation confirming brain death.

There is some concern as to the reliability of TCD sonography in assessing infant brain death. Again, many factors can increase the RI above 1 in the neonate, most often increased ICP with or without hydrocephalus and a patent ductus arteriosus (PDA)[4,71] (see Table 49-1). In neonates, low RI has been described in patients clinically dead, whereas infants with high RIs have survived.[71,72] A greatly elevated RI (1-2) in a term infant with no evidence of hydrocephalus or a PDA strongly suggests brain death.[73]

After fontanelle closure, sustained reversal of diastolic flow can be characteristic of essentially absent effective cerebral blood flow in the adult and older child[72,74] (Figs. 49-14 and 49-15). In two independent studies of a total of 91 comatose patients, Petty et al.[70] and Feri et al.[75] found a TCD waveform of absent or complete reversed diastolic flow or small, early systolic spikes in at least two intracranial arteries in all 43 brain-dead patients, but in none of other patients with coma (age range, 2-88 years). Bulas et al.[76] reported a study in 19 children (age 4-14 years) who sustained severe closed-head injury. All seven children with complete retrograde diastolic flow on the initial examination met brain death criteria within

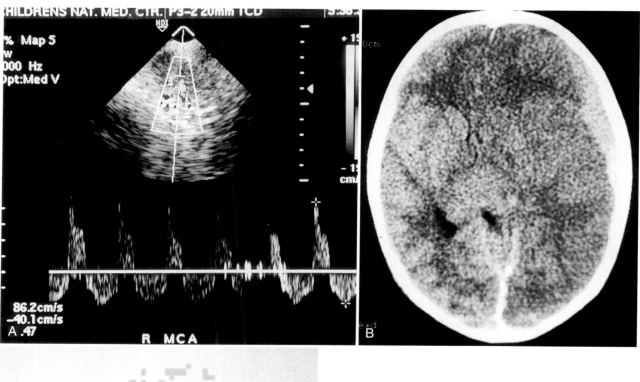

FIGURE 49-14. **Brain death from head trauma in 3-year-old boy. A,** TCD spectral waveform of the right MCA demonstrates reversal of diastolic flow with an RI of 1.5. **B,** CT demonstrates a left subdural hematoma with subfalcine herniation. **C,** ^{99m}Tc-DTPA brain scan the following day was consistent with brain death.

24 hours of that study. Feri et al.[75] and Shiogai et al.[74] described three unstable patients who briefly showed diastolic reversal followed by a forward diastolic flow in the same waveform who improved; but of the patients Feri observed, none with complete reversal of diastolic flow survived. Shiogai reported one 80-year-old survivor at 1 month, with Glasgow Coma Scale of 8 and complete reversal of diastolic flow in the MCA, who sustained forward diastolic flow in the PCA.

A few pediatric cases of mild diastolic reversed flow demonstrate recovery of forward diastolic flow and brainstem function. Kirkham et al.[67] therefore suggested using a **direction of flow index** (DFI = 1 − Maximum

diastolic velocity area/Maximum systolic velocity area).[67] All children with substantial diastolic reversed flow and a time average velocity of less than 10 cm/sec over a 30-minute period died. Some investigators have advocated continuous TCD monitoring. Powers et al.[68] showed that a mean velocity in the MCA of less than 10 cm/sec for longer than 30 minutes was not compatible with survival. Qian et al.[77] found that in children, reversed diastolic flow, small systolic forward flow, or a DFI less than 0.8 in the MCA for more than 2 hours was a reliable indicator to confirm brain death. Undetectable flow in the brain has also been described in brain death.[74-78] The occurrence of undetectable MCA flow,

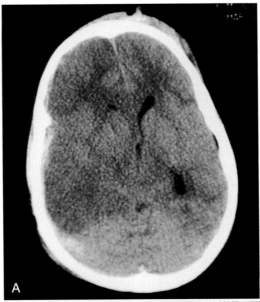

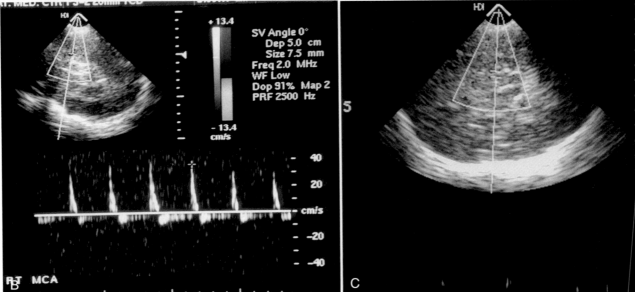

FIGURE 49-15. Brain death from head trauma in 6-year-old child after motor vehicle accident. A, CT image demonstrates a small, right subdural hematoma and diffuse edema with mild subfalcine herniation. **B,** TCD sonogram the following day demonstrates mild reversal of diastolic flow (RI 1.1) of the right middle cerebral artery (MCA). **C,** No flow was noted in the left MCA.

however, could sometimes be caused by technical factors. The use of contrast agents may improve the level of confidence when no flow is encountered.

Some investigators have studied simultaneously both the extracranial and the intracranial carotid circulation in their evaluation of brain death. Feri et al.[75] described three waveform patterns in the MCA as well as in the extracranial internal carotid and vertebral arteries as **specific for brain death:** (1) diastolic reverse flow without systolic forward flow, (2) brief systolic forward flow, and (3) undetectable flow. Absence of MCA flow on TCD sonography, with a simultaneous recording of complete reversal of diastolic flow in the extracranial internal

carotid artery, was a reliable sign of cerebral circulatory arrest. Some investigators have studied only the extracranial carotid circulation in the neck. Jalili et al.[79] reported 100% specificity for brain death with bilateral reversal of diastolic flow in the internal carotid artery of children with brain death.

The ease of performing TCD sonography and the ability to repeat the study as often as necessary also assist in proving the **absence of brain death,** particularly when a patient has taken sedative drugs (Fig. 49-16). It is important to remember that the TCD examination should never be used in isolation because the arrest of supratentorial flow is not synonymous with

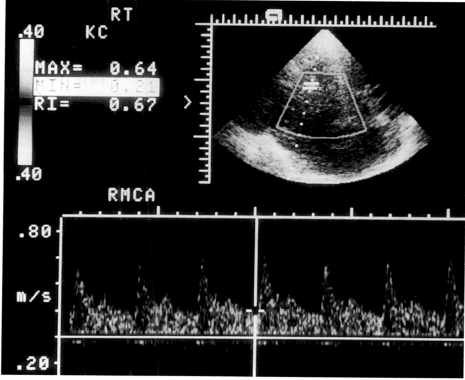

FIGURE 49-16. Coma, not brain death. Teenager in status epilepticus with flat electroencephalogram in phenobarbital coma with carbon dioxide tension (Pco_2) of 27 mm Hg. TCD spectral waveform shows antegrade diastolic flow in the right MCA with slightly elevated RI of 0.67 but no evidence of brain death. Patient recovered without sequelae.

brain death. Rather, the data should help indicate the severity of cerebrovascular arrest and is a useful confirmatory test.[80]

INTRAOPERATIVE NEURORADIOLOGIC PROCEDURES

Intraoperative TCD monitoring of the velocity in the MCA during **carotid endarterectomy** is an accepted clinical application in adults.[81] Intraoperative complications of carotid endarterectomy relate mainly to ischemia during cross-clamping, hyperemic phenomena, or embolization of atheromatous or gaseous materials. Hyperemic phenomena secondary to ischemia are depicted by a sudden increase in flow velocity. Solid or gaseous microemboli as small as 30 to 50 μm can be documented by TCD sonography as high-amplitude spikes on spectral waveform and a characteristic auditory "chirping" sound.[82] Ischemia during cross-clamping is a classic complication occurring in up to 10% of patients that is caused by incompetent intracranial collateral circulation, mainly the anterior and posterior communicating arteries and the leptomeningeal vessels. TCD ultrasound can be used to assess the effect of carotid cross-clamping on the MCA in both children and adults (Fig. 49-17).

Transcranial Doppler monitoring during **cardiopulmonary bypass** (CPB) for cardiac surgery has also been studied. TCD sonography can demonstrate **emboli showers** that occur during aortic cannulation, cardiac manipulation, or other surgical maneuvers.[83-85] Doppler ultrasound has been used to monitor flow patterns during cardiopulmonary bypass and a decrease in mean velocity with increasing hypothermia has been noted.[86] Profound hypothermic circulatory arrest and profound hypothermia with continuous low-flow cardiopulmonary bypass are used to facilitate repair of complex congenital heart lesions. Extended periods of profound hypothermic arrest may impair cerebral function and metabolism and produce ischemic brain injury. TCD sonography has enabled the noninvasive intraoperative monitoring of cerebral perfusion when using either circulatory arrest or low-flow bypass. Future TCD studies may help to develop improved modes of cerebral protection during repair of complex congenital heart lesions.[86-88]

Transcranial Doppler sonography has also been used during diagnostic and therapeutic neuroangiographic and surgical procedures.[88] It has shown that asymptomatic **microemboli** enter the cerebral circulation in large numbers during "routine" carotid angiography as well as pediatric scoliosis surgery. High rates of microemboli may be related to the presence of right-to-left cardiac shunts.[89] Intraoperative guidance using contrast agents

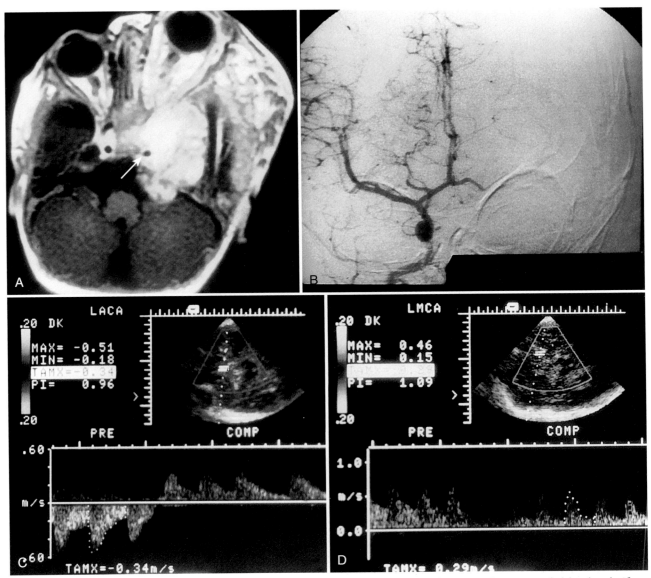

FIGURE 49-17. Plexiform neurofibroma. A, Left internal carotid artery *(arrow)* is patent but surrounded by the plexiform neurofibroma on MRI. **B,** Compression of left carotid artery at arteriography shows cross-filling from right side into left anterior cerebral artery (ACA). **C,** TCD spectral waveform at time of compression also shows good filling of left ACA from right side (reverse flow in the left ACA). **D,** Good filling of left middle cerebral artery.

and three-dimensional (3-D) TCD ultrasound has been investigated to improve the demonstration of vascular anatomy.

STROKE IN SICKLE CELL PATIENTS

In children with sickle cell disease, anemia decreases viscosity and increases flow rate, but exceptionally high velocities are primarily the consequence of luminal narrowing. **Cerebral infarction** secondary to occlusive vasculopathy is a major complication of patients with sickle cell disease, with a prevalence ranging from 5.5%[90] to 17%.[91] The stenotic lesions typically involve large vessels in the intracranial internal, middle, and anterior cerebral

artery circulation and progress for months and years before symptoms develop. Prevention of stroke symptoms by hypertransfusion therapy is possible in patients at risk.[16] Bone marrow transplantation has also proved curative in young patients with symptomatic sickle cell disease and has led to stabilization of nervous system vasculopathy, as documented by MRI.[92] TCD sonography has proved to be a safe, reliable, and cost-effective screening method for children at risk.

Adams et al.[93,94] first showed the effectiveness of non-imaging Doppler sonographic imaging in screening for cerebrovascular disease in sickle cell disease.[16,24,25] Using the transtemporal and suboccipital approach, Adams et al.[93] screened 190 asymptomatic sickle cell patients and found in clinical follow-up that a mean flow velocity

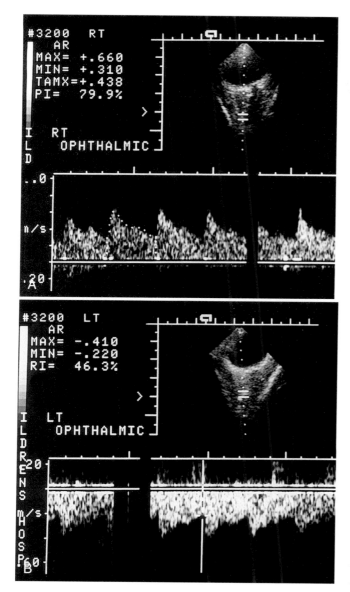

FIGURE 49-18. Abnormal ophthalmic artery (OA) flow in 16-year-old boy with sickle cell disease. Patient had his first left cerebrovascular accident (CVA, stroke) at age 7 years. Spectral Doppler ultrasound waveforms through the eye show increased diastolic flow in both OAs. **A,** Increased velocity in the right OA with maximum velocity of 66 cm/sec; **B,** reversed flow in the left OA.

in the MCA of 170 cm/sec or greater indicated a patient at risk for development of cerebrovascular accident (CVA, stroke). Comparing TCD to cerebral angiography in 33 neurologically symptomatic patients, the authors then found **five criteria for cerebrovascular disease:** (1) mean velocity of 190 cm/sec, (2) low velocity in the MCA (<70 cm/sec), (3) MCA ratio (lower or higher) of 0.5 or less, (4) ACA/MCA ratio greater than 1.2 on the same side, and (5) inability to detect an MCA in the presence of a demonstrated ultrasound window.[94]

Using duplex Doppler imaging, magnetic resonance angiography (MRA), and MRI, Seibert et al.[95] initially described five indicators of cerebrovascular disease in sickle cell patients: (1) maximum velocity in the OA of more than 35 cm/sec (Fig. 49-18); (2) mean velocity in the MCA of more than 170 cm/sec (Fig. 49-19); (3) RI in the OA less than 0.6 (Fig. 49-20); (4) velocity in the OA greater than that of the ipsilateral MCA; and (5)

maximum velocity in the PCA or the vertebral or basilar arteries greater than maximum velocity in the MCA. An 8-year follow-up of 27 neurologically symptomatic and 90 asymptomatic sickle cell patients showed all five original TCD indicators of disease were still significant.[96] Four additional factors were also significant: (1) turbulence, (2) PCA or ACA visualized without seeing the MCA (Figs. 49-21 to 49-23), (3) any RI less than 0.3, and (4) maximum MCA velocity greater than 200 cm/sec (Fig. 49-24). The sensitivity of Doppler ultrasound as a predictor of stroke was 94% with a specificity of 51%.

Siegel et al.[97] compared transtemporal TCD using duplex equipment to neurologic examination and also found a maximum flow in the MCA of greater than 200 cm/sec or less than 100 cm/sec (including no flow) as significant for disease. Verlhac et al.[98] studied sickle cell patients with duplex Doppler imaging with a 3-MHz

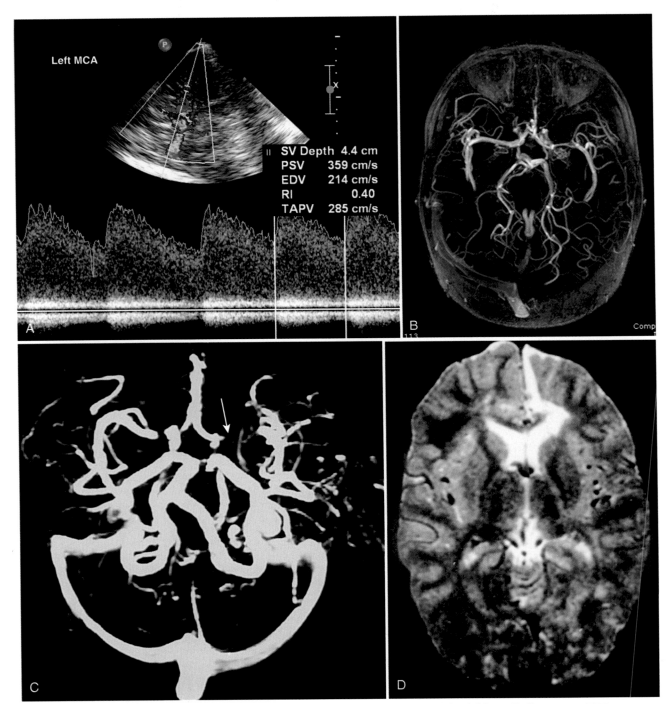

FIGURE 49-19. Middle cerebral artery (MCA) stenosis in 9-year-old with sickle cell disease. A, TCD sonogram demonstrates extremely elevated velocities in the left MCA, including a peak systolic velocity (PSV) of 359 cm/sec and time average maximum mean velocity (TAPV) of 285 cm/sec. **B,** MRA 3-D time-of-flight images of the circle of Willis demonstrate diffuse narrowing of the left MCA, with multiple small vessels suggestive of moyamoya disease. **C,** Reformatted maximum-intensity projection (MIP) image of the same patient confirms narrowing of the left MCA *(arrow).* **D,** Axial fast spin-echo (FSE) T2-weighted MR image demonstrates volume loss of the left basal ganglia and left hemispheric white matter, with signal voids secondary to multiple collaterals.

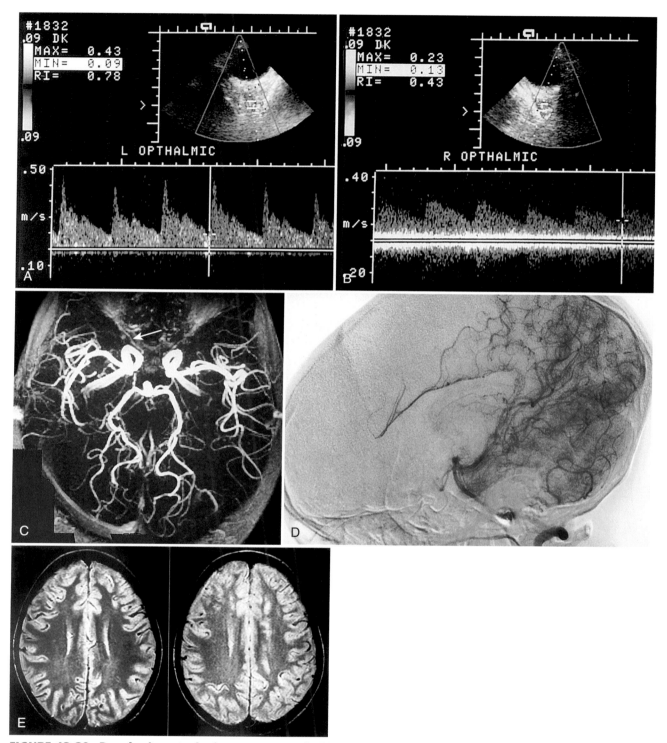

FIGURE 49-20. Developing stroke in asymptomatic 13-year-old boy with sickle cell anemia. A, TCD sonogram through the left eye shows relatively normal ophthalmic waveform with normal RI of 0.78, but increased flow with a maximum velocity of 43 cm/sec. **B,** TCD sonogram through the right eye shows more abnormal waveform with increased diastolic flow in the right ophthalmic artery (OA) with a low RI of 0.43. **C,** Collapsed image from axial 3-D time-of-flight MR angiogram shows absent anterior cerebral arteries (ACAs) bilaterally with prominent right OA *(arrow).* **D,** Vertebral arteriogram demonstrates retrograde filling of the ACA. **E,** Initial image (on left) obtained at time of MRA is normal. Six months later, patient had acute stroke, and second MR angiogram now shows bilateral, spotty, hyperintense areas in the ACA distribution. Both images are axial proton density weighted.

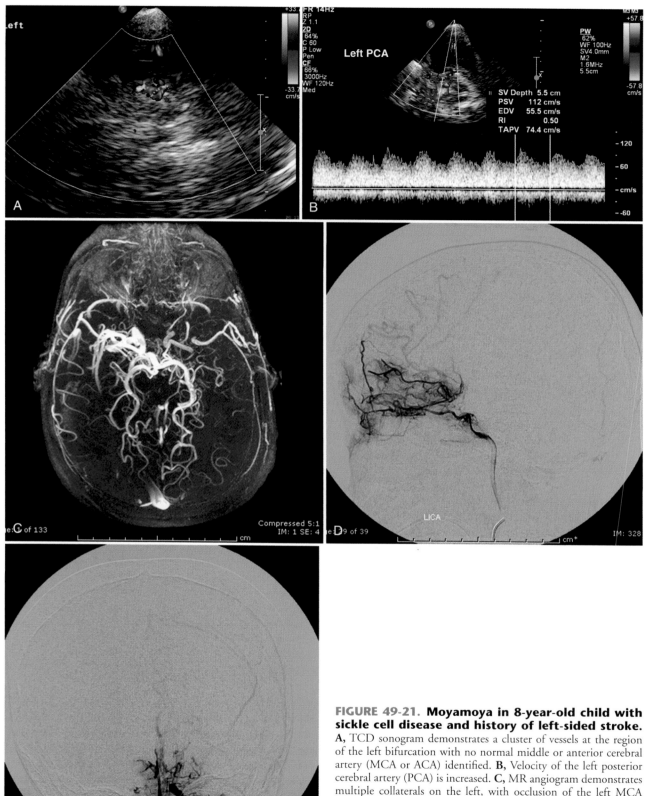

FIGURE 49-21. Moyamoya in 8-year-old child with sickle cell disease and history of left-sided stroke. **A,** TCD sonogram demonstrates a cluster of vessels at the region of the left bifurcation with no normal middle or anterior cerebral artery (MCA or ACA) identified. **B,** Velocity of the left posterior cerebral artery (PCA) is increased. **C,** MR angiogram demonstrates multiple collaterals on the left, with occlusion of the left MCA and ACA, as well as the right ACA. The PCAs and the pericallosal and middle meningeal arteries are enlarged. **D** and **E,** Lateral and anteroposterior projections of left carotid arteriogram demonstrates complete occlusion of the left internal carotid artery beyond the ophthalmic artery.

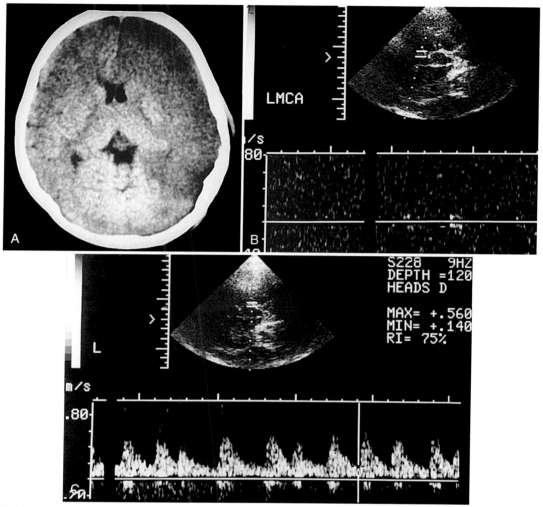

FIGURE 49-22. Acute stroke in 3-year-old child with sickle cell disease after CVA. A, CT scan shows low density in the distribution of the left anterior and middle cerebral artery (ACA and MCA). **B,** TCD sonogram through the temporal bone on the left demonstrates no flow in the ACA or MCA. **C,** Flow could be obtained through the temporal window in the posterior cerebral artery on the left as it circled the cerebral peduncle. *(From Seibert JJ, Glasier CM, Leithiser RE Jr, et al. Transcranial Doppler using standard duplex equipment in children. Ultrasound Q 1990;8:167-196.)*

CEREBROVASCULAR DISEASE: INDICATIONS IN CHILDREN

1. Maximum velocity, OA ≥35 cm/sec
2. Mean velocity, MCA ≥170 cm/sec
3. RI in OA ≤0.6
4. Velocity in OA greater than velocity in MCA (ipsilateral)
5. Maximum velocity in PCA, vertebral, or basilar arteries greater than or equal to MCA velocity
6. Turbulence
7. PCA or ACA visualized without MCA
8. Any RI <0.3
9. Maximum peak systolic MCA velocity ≥200 cm/sec

OA, Ophthalmic artery; *MCA,* middle cerebral artery; *RI,* resistive index; *PCA,* posterior cerebral artery; *ACA,* anterior cerebral artery.

transducer transtemporally and suboccipitally, as well as with MRA and MRI. Arteriography was performed in patients with suspected stenosis on TCD sonography. They found that patients with a mean velocity greater than 190 cm/sec had stenosis on arteriography. Kogutt et al.[99] also evaluated symptomatic sickle cell patients with duplex Doppler imaging, MRI, and MRA and found 91% sensitivity and 22% specificity of TCD using MRA as the standard. Abnormal TCD values were (1) maximum and mean velocity (V_{max} and V_{mean}) greater than 2 standard deviations (SD) from normal values reported by Adams et al.[93,94] in sickle cell patients: V_{max} MCA greater than 168 ± –38 cm/sec and V_{mean} MCA 115 ± –31 cm/sec, and V_{max} ACA 138 ± 34 cm/sec and V_{mean} ACA 94 ±cm/sec; (2) RI less than 40; and (3) V_{max} MCA less than V_{max} ACA (Fig. 49-25).

Screening sickle cell patients with the nonimaging pulsed Doppler ultrasound technique involves scanning

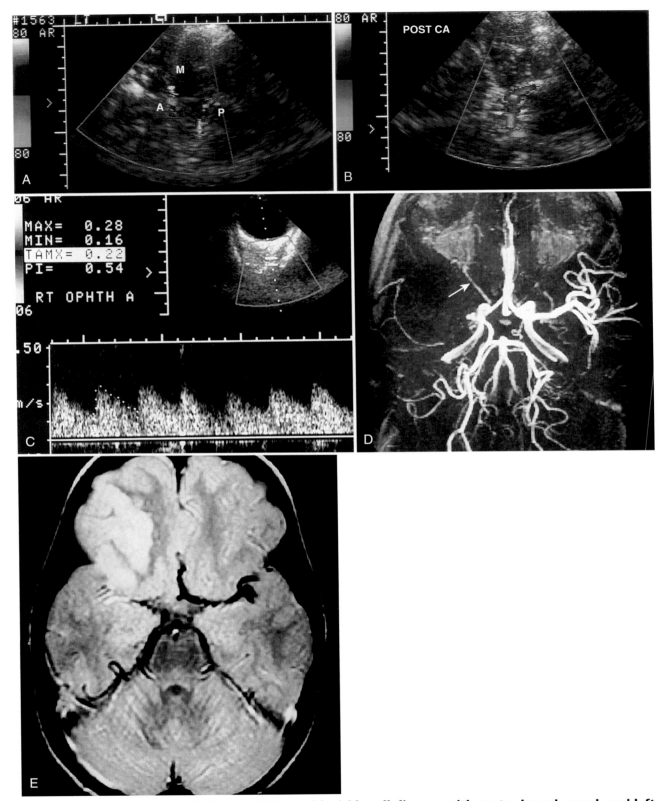

FIGURE 49-23. Acute stroke in 3-year-old boy with sickle cell disease, with acute slurred speech and left-sided weakness. A, Normal TCD color flow through temporal bone of left middle cerebral artery (MCA, *M*), left anterior cerebral artery (ACA, *A*), and left posterior cerebral artery (PCA, *P*). **B,** Right temporal TCD sonogram shows no right MCA, normal right PCA *(orange),* and normal left PCA *(blue).* **C,** Doppler waveform of the right ophthalmic artery (OA) shows increased diastolic flow. **D,** Axial collapsed image from 3-D time-of-flight MR angiogram shows absent flow in the right MCA and a prominent right OA *(arrow).* **E,** Axial proton-density-weighted image (2500/30, with three-fourths signal averaged) shows absent M1 segment of the right MCA and hyperintense area in the right frontal lobe, compatible with acute infarction. *(From Seibert JJ, Miller SF, Kirby RS, et al. Cerebrovascular disease in symptomatic and asymptomatic patients with sickle cell anemia: screening with duplex transcranial Doppler US—correlation with MR imaging and MR angiography. Radiology 1993;189:457-466.)*

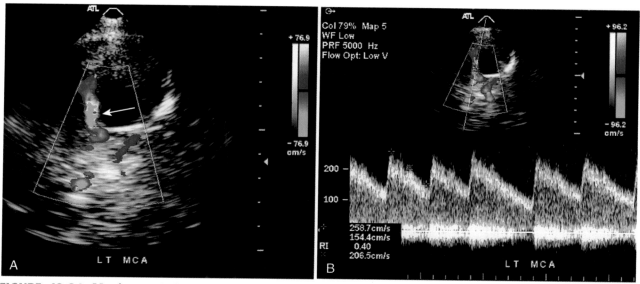

FIGURE 49-24. Maximum MCA velocity greater than 200 cm/sec indicates cerebrovascular disease in 4-year-old girl with sickle cell disease. A, Color Doppler imaging demonstrates a region of aliasing *(arrow)* at the proximal left MCA. **B,** Doppler waveform confirms the presence of abnormally high mean and peak velocities (TAMX, 206 cm/sec; PSV, 259 cm/ sec), which stratify into the "high" stroke risk category. The child started receiving transfusion therapy.

the patient transtemporally to evaluate the MCA, bifurcation, distal ICA, ACA, and PCA. The OA can be evaluated through the orbit. The basilar and vertebral arteries can be evaluated from the occipital approach. The peak systolic velocity (PSV), end diastolic velocity, time average maximum mean (TAMM) velocities, and RI of each of these vessels should be measured at least twice. The MCA should be tracked from the peripheral branch to the bifurcation with velocities obtained every 2 mm. Optimizing the tracing is crucial in identifying regions of stenosis.[100] Color Doppler flow imaging can also be used to screen sickle cell patients. This technique is faster to learn, allows for quicker vessel identification, and improves gate placement (see Fig. 49-24). Because probes tend to be larger, however, optimizing the tracing may be more difficult and can result in slightly lower velocities than those obtained by nonimaging methods.[17-19]

The Stroke Prevention Trial in Sickle Cell Anemia (STOP) study led by Robert Adams showed that regular transfusion of children at risk for stroke, as determined by Doppler sonography, could prevent CVA.[16,100-102] Adams studied 130 children age 2 to 16 years at 14 medical centers who were at risk to develop stroke, with mean velocity in the MCA greater than 200 cm/sec. Half received blood transfusions every 3 to 4 weeks, enough to lower sickle cell hemoglobin to below 30%. After 1 year, the transfusions lowered the stroke risk by 90%. Although only one transfusion patient had a stroke, 10 nontransfusion children sustained a CVA (Table 49-2).

Patients with a mean velocity greater than 200 cm/sec or a PSV greater than 250 cm/sec in the MCA on two examinations are now being recommended for hypertransfusion therapy to prevent stroke[103] (see Fig. 49-24). Correlation with MRI and MRA findings are useful as well. Pegelow et al.[104] found that children with abnormal TCD and MRI were at higher risk for developing a new silent infarct or stroke than those whose initial MRI was normal.[105]

When assigning the risk of stroke based on TAMM velocities, it is important to consider how velocities may differ with the specific equipment used compared to those obtained with nonduplex equipment in the initial STOP studies. Studies have evaluated the differences in technique, nonimaging TCD versus imaging TCDI. Non-angle-corrected velocities obtained with Acuson and ATL TCDI equipment are approximately 10% lower in the MCA than those obtained with Nicolet (Vascular, Madison, Wis) nonduplex equipment.[17-19] Other studies show no significant difference in TAMM velocity measurements obtained with General Electric TCDI equipment compared with Nicolet nonduplex equipment.[20,21] The reasons for these differing results are likely multifactorial. Centers should be aware of these potential differences when performing the STOP protocol and consider performing their own comparison studies when using imaging equipment. It is important to optimize instrument settings (volume size, gain, waveform display) and perform exams carefully so that the highest mean velocity is documented in the MCA and ICA. Closer attention to technique can reduce the differences between velocity data acquired with different ultrasound machines. A 10% lower cutoff point for TAMM velocities may be appropriate depending on the

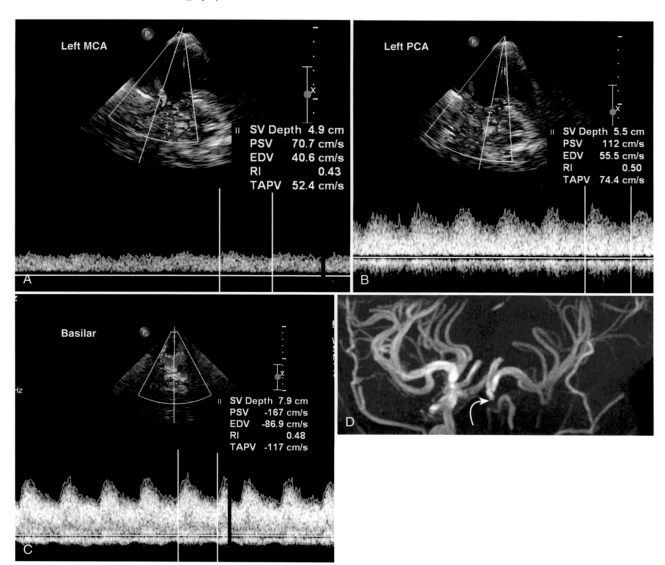

FIGURE 49-25. Low middle cerebral artery (MCA) velocity in 8-year-old child with sickle cell disease. Occluded distal internal cerebral artery (DICA) with collateralization from the posterior cerebral artery (PCA) and basilar artery. **A,** TCD sonogram demonstrates abnormally low velocities in the left MCA (TAMX, 70.7 cm/sec) with decreased pulsatility (RI 0.43). No flow was documented in the left DICA. **B** and **C,** Velocities in PCA and basilar artery are higher than in left MCA. **D,** Coronal reformatted MR angiograms demonstrate occlusion of the left DICA (arrow).

TABLE 49-2. STOP STROKE RISK CATEGORIES

CATEGORY	DEFINITION
Low	<170 cm/sec TAMX
Conditional	170-199 cm/sec TAMX
Abnormal	≥200 cm/sec TAMX or >250 cm/sec PSV

STOP, Stroke Prevention Trial in Sickle Cell Anemia; *TAMX,* Time-averaged maximum mean velocity, *PSV,* peak systolic velocity.

protocol and machine used.[12] Reviewing the STOP data, Jones et al.[103] reported that a PSV with velocities greater than 250 cm/sec may be another useful value to use when assessing stroke risk in sickle cell patients.[12,103]

Although **angle correction** with TCDI may be a way to correct for lower velocities obtained by TCDI compared with nonimaging TCD, this technique has not yet been validated and may overestimate stroke risk in children with sickle cell disease.[23] Therefore, angle correction currently should not be used when performing and interpreting TCDI for stroke risk assessment in pediatric

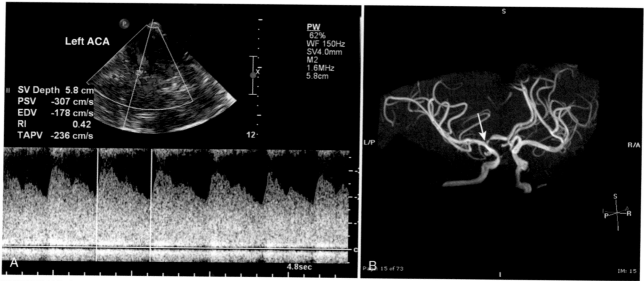

FIGURE 49-26. Anterior cerebral artery (ACA) stenosis in 11-year-old child with sickle cell disease. A, TCD sonogram demonstrates abnormally elevated left ACA velocities. **B,** 3-D time-of-flight reformatted MR angiogram demonstrates stenosis at the origin of the A1 segment of the left ACA *(arrow)*.

sickle cell disease.[11,12] The STOP velocity criteria apply only to children with sickle cell anemia who have not had a previous stroke. Children with conditional velocities should be rescreened within 3 to 6 months, and those with normal studies may be rescreened yearly.[100] Elevated ACA velocity, although not part of the STOP criteria, also suggests an increased stroke risk (Fig. 49-26). Kwiatkowski et al.[106] found that an elevated ACA velocity (≥170 cm/sec) was associated with an increased risk of stroke ($p = 0.0013$). In subjects with normal ICA-MCA velocities and elevated ACA velocity, the risk of stroke was greater than tenfold, whereas the risk more than doubled with those who had both elevated ACA and elevated ICA-MCA velocities.

The natural history of TCD velocities in sickle cell patients continues to be studied.[107-109] Optimal management for children with abnormal velocities remains problematic, with no consensus regarding long-term management in children with persistently abnormal velocities. The side effects of prolonged transfusion therapy have clinicians searching for other methods of improving stroke risk, including the use of hydroxy-carbamide (hydroxyurea) therapy and bone marrow transplant.[92,110-112]

The management of children with conditional velocities is also being studied. Many remain in the conditional range for years or eventually normalize, but up to 23% of this cohort convert over time to abnormal velocities[107,108] (Fig. 49-27). Protocols using less invasive therapies such as hydroxycarbamide (e.g., hydroxyurea therapy) in children with conditional velocities show promise and suggest that following these patients with TCD may be useful to assess treatment response.[110-112]

CONTRAST ENHANCEMENT

Visualization of normal or pathologic flow with TCD sonography can be obstructed by insufficient temporal bone windows, unfavorable insonation angles, or low flow velocities. In adult studies, echocontrast agents such as galactose microbubble suspensions have been used in an attempt to increase the applications of transcranial studies.[113-115] These contrast agents have been shown to facilitate visualization of vessel patency, stenosis, occlusion, and collateral flow.[116-118] Small-caliber arteries and vessels that run at unfavorable angles may be identified.[119] Velocities obtained using this method provide reliable data regarding stenosis and occlusion. Comparisons with digital subtraction angiography have been favorable.[113,119,120]

Indications for echo-enhancing agents include depiction of vessel anatomy of tumors, vascular malformations, and stenosis. In the evaluation of brain death, it may improve the level of confidence of documenting low flow. Limitations of this technique include short duration of some of the contrast agents, blooming artifact, and limited availability for pediatric studies in the United States.

Tissue plasminogen activator (TPA) activity has been shown to be enhanced with ultrasound. TCD sonography can identify residual blood flow signals around thrombi and, by delivering mechanical pressure waves, expose more thrombus surface to circulating TPA. The CLOTBUST international multicenter trial showed that ultrasound can enhance the thrombolytic activity of a drug. Clinical recovery from stroke with recanalization 2 hours after TPA bolus was seen in 25%

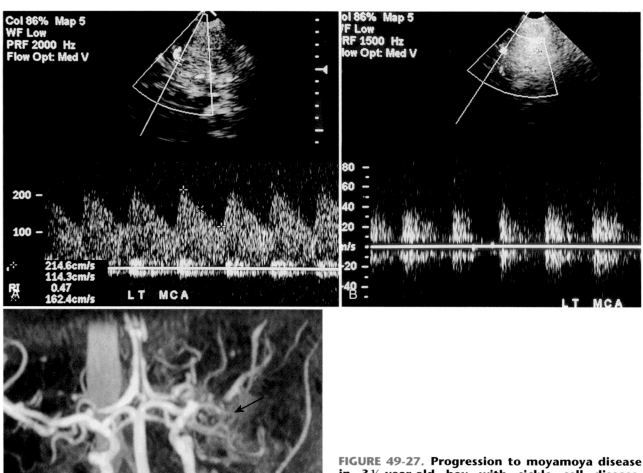

FIGURE 49-27. Progression to moyamoya disease in 3½-year-old boy with sickle cell disease. **A,** Patient had high normal velocities of the left middle cerebral artery (MCA). MRA performed 2 months later was normal. **B,** At 1-year follow-up screening, abnormally low flow in the left MCA (<40 cm/sec) is noted. **C,** MRA at this time demonstrates moyamoya changes with complete occlusion of the left A1 and M1 segments.

of patients treated with TPA and TCD compared with 8% who received TPA alone ($p = 0.02$). Current ongoing clinical trials include Phase II studies of 2-MHz TCD ultrasound with contrast agents or microbubbles.[121,122] Future applications using contrast agents may include evaluating perfusion of brain tumors after chemotherapy and radiation.

Doppler ultrasound has been provided an improved spatially oriented display of image position. Contrast-enhanced three-dimensional power Doppler (CE3DPD) sonography has also been shown to improve identification of vessels. Using CE3DPD on adults with inadequate windows, Postert et al.[119] noted clear 3-D visualization of most major intracranial vascular segments. The addition of contrast resulted in a more sensitive ultrasonic tool than unenhanced 3-D reconstructions. These studies were found to be easy to perform and interpret, increasing the level of operator diagnostic confidence.[123]

References

1. Raju TN. Cranial Doppler applications in neonatal critical care. Crit Care Clin 1992;8:93-111.
2. Saliba EM, Laugier J. Doppler assessment of the cerebral circulation in pediatric intensive care. Crit Care Clin 1992;8:79-92.
3. Taylor GA. Current concepts in neonatal cranial Doppler sonography. Ultrasound Q 1992;4:223-244.
4. Seibert JJ, McCowan TC, Chadduck WM, et al. Duplex pulsed Doppler US versus intracranial pressure in the neonate: clinical and experimental studies. Radiology 1989;171:155-159.
5. Aaslid R. Transcranial Doppler sonography. J Neurosurg 1982;57:769-774.
6. Lupetin AR, Davis DA, Beckman I, Dash N. Transcranial Doppler sonography. Part 1. Principles, technique, and normal appearances. Radiographics 1995;15:179-191.
7. Katz ML, Comerota AJ. Transcranial Doppler: a review of technique, interpretation and clinical applications. Ultrasound Q 1991; 8:241-265.
8. Byrd SM. An overview of transcranial Doppler color flow imaging: a technique comparison. Ultrasound Q 1996;13:197-210.
9. Rosendahl T, Muller C, Wagner W, et al. Transcranial imaging: a new angle on transcranial Doppler video. J Color Flow Imaging 1995;5:58.

10. Fujioka KA, Douville CM. Transcranial Doppler: anatomy and free hand examination techniques. New York: Raven Press; 1992.
11. McCarville MB. Comparison of duplex and nonduplex transcranial Doppler ultrasonography. Ultrasound Q 2008;24:167-171.
12. Bulas D. Screening children for sickle cell vasculopathy: guidelines for transcranial Doppler evaluation. Pediatr Radiol 2005;35:235-241.

Sonographic Technique
13. Seibert JJ, Glasier CM, Leithiser Jr RE, et al. Transcranial Doppler using standard duplex equipment in children. Ultrasound Q 1990;8:167-176.
14. Erickson SJ, Hendrix LE, Massaro BM, et al. Color Doppler flow imaging of the normal and abnormal orbit. Radiology 1989;173:511-516.
15. Baxter GM, Williamson TH. Color Doppler imaging of the eye: normal ranges, reproducibility, and observer variation. J Ultrasound Med 1995;14:91-96.
16. Adams R, McKie V, Nichols F, et al. The use of transcranial ultrasonography to predict stroke in sickle cell disease. N Engl J Med 1992;326:605-610.
17. Bulas DI, Jones A, Seibert JJ, et al. Transcranial Doppler (TCD) screening for stroke prevention in sickle cell anemia: pitfalls in technique variation. Pediatr Radiol 2000;30:733-738.
18. Jones AM, Seibert JJ, Nichols FT, et al. Comparison of transcranial color Doppler imaging (TCDI) and transcranial Doppler (TCD) in children with sickle-cell anemia. Pediatr Radiol 2001;31:461-469.
19. McCarville MB, Li C, Xiong X, Wang W. Comparison of transcranial Doppler sonography with and without imaging in the evaluation of children with sickle cell anemia. AJR Am J Roentgenol 2004;183:1117-1122.
20. Neish AS, Blews DE, Simms CA, et al. Screening for stroke in sickle cell anemia: comparison of transcranial Doppler imaging and nonimaging US techniques. Radiology 2002;222:709-714.
21. Malouf Jr AJ, Hamrick-Turner JE, Doherty MC, et al. Implementation of the STOP protocol for Stroke Prevention in Sickle Cell Anemia by using duplex power Doppler imaging. Radiology 2001;219:359-365.
22. Fujioka KA, Gates DT, Spencer MP. A comparison of transcranial color Doppler imaging and standard static pulsed wave doppler in the assessment of intracranial hemodynamics. J Vasc Tech 1994;18:29.
23. Krejza J, Rudzinski W, Pawlak MA, et al. Angle-corrected imaging transcranial Doppler sonography versus imaging and nonimaging transcranial Doppler sonography in children with sickle cell disease. AJNR Am J Neuroradiol 2007;28:1613-1618.
24. Adams RJ, Nichols FT, McKie VC, et al. Transcranial Doppler: Influence of hematocrit in children with sickle cell anemia without stroke. J Cardiovasc Tech 1989;8:97-101.
25. Adams RJ, Nichols 3rd FT, Aaslid R, et al. Cerebral vessel stenosis in sickle cell disease: criteria for detection by transcranial Doppler. Am J Pediatr Hematol Oncol 1990;12:277-282.
26. Chadduck WM, Seibert JJ. Intracranial duplex Doppler: practical uses in pediatric neurology and neurosurgery. J Child Neurol 1989;4(Suppl):77-86.

Ultrasound Dosage: Power Settings
27. Lizzi R, Mortimer A, Carstensen E, et al. Bioeffects considerations for the safety of diagnostic ultrasound. J Ultrasound 1988;7(Suppl):1.
28. Rabe H, Grohs B, Schmidt RM, et al. Acoustic power measurements of Doppler ultrasound devices used for perinatal and infant examinations. Pediatr Radiol 1990;20:277-281.
29. Aaslid R. Transcranial Doppler sonography. New York: Springer-Verlag; 1986.

Pitfalls in Doppler Investigations
30. Winkler P, Helmke K. Major pitfalls in Doppler investigations with particular reference to the cerebral vascular system. Part I. Sources of error, resulting pitfalls and measures to prevent errors. Pediatr Radiol 1990;20:219-228.
31. Winkler P, Helmke K, Mahl M. Major pitfalls in Doppler investigations. Part II. Low flow velocities and colour Doppler applications. Pediatr Radiol 1990;20:304-310.

Indications for Transcranial Doppler Sonography
32. Kincaid MS. Transcranial Doppler ultrasonography: a diagnostic tool of increasing utility. Curr Opin Anaesthesiol 2008;21:552-559.

33. Rigamonti A, Ackery A, Baker AJ. Transcranial Doppler monitoring in subarachnoid hemorrhage: a critical tool in critical care. Can J Anaesth 2008;55:112-123.
34. Lennihan L, Petty GW, Mohr JP, et al. Transcranial Doppler detection of anterior cerebral artery vasospasm (abstract). Stroke 1989;20:151.
35. Sloan MA, Haley Jr EC, Kassell NF, et al. Sensitivity and specificity of transcranial Doppler ultrasonography in the diagnosis of vasospasm following subarachnoid hemorrhage. Neurology 1989;39:1514-1518.
36. Topcuoglu MA, Pryor JC, Ogilvy CS, Kistler JP. Cerebral vasospasm following subarachnoid hemorrhage. Curr Treat Options Cardiovasc Med 2002;4:373-384.
37. Lysakowski C, Walder B, Costanza MC, Tramer MR. Transcranial Doppler versus angiography in patients with vasospasm due to a ruptured cerebral aneurysm: a systematic review. Stroke 2001;32:2292-2298.
38. Kincaid MS, Souter MJ, Treggiari MM, et al. Accuracy of transcranial Doppler ultrasonography and single-photon emission computed tomography in the diagnosis of angiographically demonstrated cerebral vasospasm. J Neurosurg 2009;110:67-72.
39. Thie A, Fuhlendorf A, Spitzer K, Kunze K. Transcranial Doppler evaluation of common and classic migraine. Part I. Ultrasonic features during the headache-free period. Headache 1990;30:201-208.
40. Thie A, Fuhlendorf A, Spitzer K, Kunze K. Transcranial Doppler evaluation of common and classic migraine. Part II. Ultrasonic features during attacks. Headache 1990;30:209-215.
41. Wang HS, Kuo MF, Huang SC, et al. Transcranial ultrasound diagnosis of intracranial lesions in children with headaches. Pediatr Neurol 2002;26:43-46.
42. Hill C, Hogan AM, Onugha N, et al. Increased CBF velocity in children with mild sleep-disordered breathing: a possible association with abnormal neuropsychological function. Pediatrics 2006;118:1100.
43. Kirkham FJ, Hewes DK, Prengler M, et al. Nocturnal hypoxaemia and central nervous system events in sickle-cell disease. Lancet 2001;357:1656-1659.
44. Hogan AM, Hill CM, Harrison D, Kirkham FJ. Cerebral blood flow velocity and cognition in children before and after adenotonsillectomy. Pediatrics 2008;122:75-82.
45. Hill A, Volpe JJ. Decrease in pulsatile flow in the anterior cerebral arteries in infantile hydrocephalus. Pediatrics 1982;69:4-7.
46. Goh D, Minns RA. Intracranial pressure and cerebral arterial flow velocity indices in childhood hydrocephalus: current review. Childs Nerv Syst 1995;11:392-396.
47. Goh D, Minns RA, Hendry GM, et al. Cerebrovascular resistive index assessed by duplex Doppler sonography and its relationship to intracranial pressure in infantile hydrocephalus. Pediatr Radiol 1992;22:246-250.
48. Klingelhofer J, Conrad B, Benecke R, et al. Evaluation of intracranial pressure from transcranial Doppler studies in cerebral disease. J Neurol 1988;235:159-162.
49. Finn JP, Quinn MW, Hall-Craggs MA, Kendall BE. Impact of vessel distortion on transcranial Doppler velocity measurements: correlation with magnetic resonance imaging. J Neurosurg 1990;73:572-575.
50. Hanlo PW, Gooskens RH, Nijhuis IJ, et al. Value of transcranial Doppler indices in predicting raised ICP in infantile hydrocephalus: a study with review of the literature. Childs Nerv Syst 1995;11:595-603.
51. Rodriguez-Nunez A, Somoza-Martin M, Gomez-Lado C, et al. Therapeutic criteria in communicating childhood hydrocephalus. J Neurosurg Sci 2008;52:17-21.
52. Pople IK. Doppler flow velocities in children with controlled hydrocephalus: reference values for the diagnosis of blocked cerebrospinal fluid shunts. Childs Nerv Syst 1992;8:124-125.
53. Westra SJ, Curran JG, Duckwiler GR, et al. Pediatric intracranial vascular malformations: evaluation of treatment results with color Doppler US. Work in progress. Radiology 1993;186:775-783.
54. Grolimund P, Seiler RW, Aaslid R, et al. Evaluation of cerebrovascular disease by combined extracranial and transcranial Doppler sonography. Experience in 1,039 patients. Stroke 1987;18:1018-1024.
55. Lindegaard KF, Aaslid R, Nornes H. Cerebral arteriovenous malformations. In: Aaslid R, editor. Transcranial Doppler sonography. New York: Springer-Verlag; 1986. p. 86-105.

56. Lindegaard KF, Grolimund P, Aaslid R, Nornes H. Evaluation of cerebral AVMs using transcranial Doppler ultrasound. J Neurosurg 1986;65:335-344.

57. Petty GW, Massaro AR, Tatemichi TK, et al. Transcranial Doppler ultrasonographic changes after treatment for arteriovenous malformations. Stroke 1990;21:260-266.

58. Jordan LC, Wityk RJ, Dowling MM, et al. Transcranial Doppler ultrasound in children with Sturge-Weber syndrome. J Child Neurol 2008;23:137-143.

59. Duan YY, Zhou XY, Liu X, et al. Carotid and transcranial color-coded duplex ultrasonography for the diagnosis of dural arteriovenous fistulas. Cerebrovasc Dis 2008;25:304-310.

60. Stark JE, Seibert JJ. Cerebral artery Doppler ultrasonography for prediction of outcome after perinatal asphyxia. J Ultrasound Med 1994;13:595-600.

61. Gray PH, Tudehope DI, Masel JP, et al. Perinatal hypoxic-ischaemic brain injury: prediction of outcome. Dev Med Child Neurol 1993;35:965-973.

62. Archer LN, Levene MI, Evans DH. Cerebral artery Doppler ultrasonography for prediction of outcome after perinatal asphyxia. Lancet 1986;2:1116-1118.

63. Raju TN. Cerebral Doppler studies in the fetus and newborn infant. J Pediatr 1991;119:165-174.

64. Bellner J, Romner B, Reinstrup P, et al. Transcranial Doppler sonography pulsatility index (PI) reflects intracranial pressure (ICP). Surg Neurol 2004;62:45-51.

65. Bode H. Pediatric applications of transcranial Doppler sonography. New York: Springer-Verlag; 1988.

66. Newell DW, Seiler RW, Aaslid R. Head injury and cerebral circulatory arrest. In: Newell DW, Aaslid R, editors. Transcranial Doppler. New York: Raven Press; 1992. p. 109-121.

67. Kirkham FJ, Neville BG, Gosling RG. Diagnosis of brain death by transcranial Doppler sonography. Arch Dis Child 1989;64:889-890.

68. Powers AD, Graeber MC, Smith RR. Transcranial Doppler ultrasonography in the determination of brain death. Neurosurgery 1989;24:884-889.

69. Valentin A, Karnik R, Winkler WB, et al. Transcranial Doppler for early identification of potential organ transplant donors. Wien Klin Wochenschr 1997;109:836-839.

70. Petty GW, Wiebers DO, Meissner I. Transcranial Doppler ultrasonography: clinical applications in cerebrovascular disease. Mayo Clin Proc 1990;65:1350-1364.

71. Chiu NC, Shen EY, Lee BS. Reversal of diastolic cerebral blood flow in infants without brain death. Pediatr Neurol 1994;11:337-340.

72. Ducrocq X, Hassler W, Moritake K, et al. Consensus opinion on diagnosis of cerebral circulatory arrest using Doppler-sonography: Task Force Group on cerebral death of the Neurosonology Research Group of the World Federation of Neurology. J Neurol Sci 1998;159:145-150.

73. Glasier CM, Seibert JJ, Chadduck WM, et al. Brain death in infants: evaluation with Doppler ultrasound. Radiology 1989;172:377-380.

74. Shiogai T, Sato E, Tokitsu M, et al. Transcranial Doppler monitoring in severe brain damage: relationships between intracranial haemodynamics, brain dysfunction and outcome. Neurol Res 1990;12:205-213.

75. Feri M, Ralli L, Felici M, et al. Transcranial Doppler and brain death diagnosis. Crit Care Med 1994;22:1120-1126.

76. Bulas D, Chadduck WM, Vezina GL. Pediatric closed head injury: evaluation with transcranial Doppler Ultrasound. Eighty-First Scientific Assembly and Annual Meeting, Chicago: Radiological Society of North America; 1995.

77. Qian SY, Fan XM, Yin HH. Transcranial Doppler assessment of brain death in children. Singapore Med J 1998;39:247-250.

78. Hassler W, Steinmetz H, Gawlowski J. Transcranial Doppler ultrasonography in raised intracranial pressure and in intracranial circulatory arrest. J Neurosurg 1988;68:745-751.

79. Jalili M, Crade M, Davis AL. Carotid blood-flow velocity changes detected by Doppler ultrasound in determination of brain death in children: a preliminary report. Clin Pediatr 1994;33:669-674.

80. Wang K, Yuan Y, Xu ZQ, et al. Benefits of combination of electroencephalography, short latency somatosensory evoked potentials, and transcranial Doppler techniques for confirming brain death. J Zhejiang Univ Sci B 2008;9:916-920.

Intraoperative Neuroradiologic Procedures

81. Lupetin AR, Davis DA, Beckman I, Dash N. Transcranial Doppler sonography. Part 2. Evaluation of intracranial and extracranial abnormalities and procedural monitoring. Radiographics 1995;15:193-209.

82. Albin MS, Bunegin L, Garcia C, McKay W. The transcranial Doppler can image microaggregates of intracranial air and particulate matter. J Neurosurg Anesthesiol 1989;1:134-135.

83. Pugsley W. The use of Doppler ultrasound in the assessment of microemboli during cardiac surgery. Perfusion 1986;4:115.

84. Jordan Jr WD, Voellinger DC, Doblar DD, et al. Microemboli detected by transcranial Doppler monitoring in patients during carotid angioplasty versus carotid endarterectomy. Cardiovasc Surg 1999;7:33-38.

85. Dagirmanjian A, Davis DA, Rothfus WE, et al. Silent cerebral microemboli occurring during carotid angiography: frequency as determined with Doppler sonography. AJR Am J Roentgenol 1993;161:1037-1040.

86. Burrows FA. Transcranial Doppler monitoring of cerebral perfusion during cardiopulmonary bypass. Ann Thorac Surg 1993;56:1482-1484.

87. Williams GD, Ramamoorthy C. Brain monitoring and protection during pediatric cardiac surgery. Semin Cardiothorac Vasc Anesth 2007;11:23-33.

88. Abdul-Khaliq H, Uhlig R, Bottcher W, et al. Factors influencing the change in cerebral hemodynamics in pediatric patients during and after corrective cardiac surgery of congenital heart diseases by means of full-flow cardiopulmonary bypass. Perfusion 2002;17:179-185.

89. Rodriguez RA, Letts M, Jarvis J, et al. Cerebral microembolization during pediatric scoliosis surgery: a transcranial Doppler study. J Pediatr Orthop 2001;21:532-536.

Stroke in Sickle Cell Patients

90. Powars D, Wilson B, Imbus C, et al. The natural history of stroke in sickle cell disease. Am J Med 1978;65:461-471.

91. Huttenlocher PR, Moohr JW, Johns L, Brown FD. Cerebral blood flow in sickle cell cerebrovascular disease. Pediatrics 1984;73:615-621.

92. Walters MC, Patience M, Leisenring W, et al. Bone marrow transplantation for sickle cell disease. N Engl J Med 1996;335:369-376.

93. Adams RJ, Aaslid R, el Gammal T, et al. Detection of cerebral vasculopathy in sickle cell disease using transcranial Doppler ultrasonography and magnetic resonance imaging: case report. Stroke 1988;19:518-520.

94. Adams RJ, Nichols FT, Figueroa R, et al. Transcranial Doppler correlation with cerebral angiography in sickle cell disease. Stroke 1992;23:1073-1077.

95. Seibert JJ, Miller SF, Kirby RS, et al. Cerebrovascular disease in symptomatic and asymptomatic patients with sickle cell anemia: screening with duplex transcranial Doppler ultrasound: correlation with MR imaging and MR angiography. Radiology 1993;189:457-466.

96. Seibert JJ, Glasier CM, Kirby RS, et al. Transcranial Doppler, MRA, and MRI as a screening examination for cerebrovascular disease in patients with sickle cell anemia: an 8-year study. Pediatr Radiol 1998;28:138-142.

97. Siegel MJ, Luker GD, Glauser TA, DeBaun MR. Cerebral infarction in sickle cell disease: transcranial Doppler ultrasound versus neurologic examination. Radiology 1995;197:191-194.

98. Verlhac S, Bernaudin F, Tortrat D, et al. Detection of cerebrovascular disease in patients with sickle cell disease using transcranial Doppler sonography: correlation with MRI, MRA and conventional angiography. Pediatr Radiol 1995;25(Suppl. 1):14-19.

99. Kogutt MS, Goldwag SS, Gupta KL, et al. Correlation of transcranial Doppler ultrasonography with MRI and MRA in the evaluation of sickle cell disease patients with prior stroke. Pediatr Radiol 1994;24:204-206.

100. Nichols FT, Jones AM, Adams RJ. Stroke prevention in sickle cell disease (STOP) study guidelines for transcranial Doppler testing. J Neuroimaging 2001;11:354-362.

101. Adams RJ, McKie VC, Hsu L, et al. Prevention of a first stroke by transfusions in children with sickle cell anemia and abnormal results on transcranial Doppler ultrasonography. N Engl J Med 1998;339:5-11.

102. Adams RJ, McKie VC, Brambilla D, et al. Stroke prevention trial in sickle cell anemia. Control Clin Trials 1998;19:110-129.

103. Jones A, Granger S, Brambilla D, et al. Can peak systolic velocities be used for prediction of stroke in sickle cell anemia? Pediatr Radiol 2005;35:66-72.

104. Pegelow CH, Wang W, Granger S, et al. Silent infarcts in children with sickle cell anemia and abnormal cerebral artery velocity. Arch Neurol 2001;58:2017-2021.

105. Wang WC, Gallagher DM, Pegelow CH, et al. Multicenter comparison of magnetic resonance imaging and transcranial Doppler ultrasonography in the evaluation of the central nervous system in children with sickle cell disease. J Pediatr Hematol Oncol 2000; 22:335-339.

106. Kwiatkowski JL, Granger S, Brambilla DJ, et al. Elevated blood flow velocity in the anterior cerebral artery and stroke risk in sickle cell disease: extended analysis from the STOP trial. Br J Haematol 2006;134:333-339.

107. Hankins JS, Fortner GL, McCarville MB, et al. The natural history of conditional transcranial Doppler flow velocities in children with sickle cell anaemia. Br J Haematol 2008;142:94-99.

108. Adams RJ, Brambilla DJ, Granger S, et al. Stroke and conversion to high risk in children screened with transcranial Doppler ultrasound during the STOP study. Blood 2004;103:3689-3694.

109. McCarville MB, Goodin GS, Fortner G, et al. Evaluation of a comprehensive transcranial Doppler screening program for children with sickle cell anemia. Pediatr Blood Cancer 2008;50:818-821.

110. Bernaudin F, Verlhac S, Coic L, et al. Long-term follow-up of pediatric sickle cell disease patients with abnormal high velocities on transcranial Doppler. Pediatr Radiol 2005;35:242-248.

111. Zimmerman SA, Schultz WH, Burgett S, et al. Hydroxyurea therapy lowers transcranial Doppler flow velocities in children with sickle cell anemia. Blood 2007;110:1043-1047.

112. Kratovil T, Bulas D, Driscoll MC, et al. Hydroxyurea therapy lowers TCD velocities in children with sickle cell disease. Pediatr Blood Cancer 2006;47:894-900.

Contrast Enhancement

113. Bazzocchi M, Quaia E, Zuiani C, Moroldo M. Transcranial Doppler: state of the art. Eur J Radiol 1998;27(Suppl. 2):141-148.

114. Totaro R, Marini C, Sacco S, et al. Contrast-enhanced transcranial Doppler sonography in patients with acute cerebrovascular diseases. Funct Neurol 2001;16:11-16.

115. Postert T, Federlein J, Przuntek H, Buttner T. Insufficient and absent acoustic temporal bone window: potential and limitations of transcranial contrast-enhanced color-coded sonography and contrast-enhanced power-based sonography. Ultrasound Med Biol 1997;23:857-862.

116. Griewing B, Schminke U, Motsch L, et al. Transcranial duplex sonography of middle cerebral artery stenosis: a comparison of colour-coding techniques—frequency- or power-based Doppler and contrast enhancement. Neuroradiology 1998;40:490-495.

117. Droste DW, Llull JB, Pezzoli C, et al. SonoVue (BR1), a new long-acting echocontrast agent, improves transcranial colour-coded duplex ultrasonic imaging. Cerebrovasc Dis 2002;14:27-32.

118. Droste DW, Jurgens R, Weber S, et al. Benefit of echocontrast-enhanced transcranial color-coded duplex ultrasound in the assessment of intracranial collateral pathways. Stroke 2000;31:920-923.

119. Postert T, Braun B, Pfundtner N, et al. Echo contrast-enhanced three-dimensional power Doppler of intracranial arteries. Ultrasound Med Biol 1998;24:953-962.

120. Gerriets T, Seidel G, Fiss I, et al. Contrast-enhanced transcranial color-coded duplex sonography: efficiency and validity. Neurology 1999;52:1133-1137.

121. Tsivgoulis G, Alexandrov AV. Ultrasound-enhanced thrombolysis in acute ischemic stroke: potential, failures, and safety. Neurotherapeutics 2007;4:420-427.

122. Alexandrov AV. Ultrasound enhanced thrombolysis for stroke. Int J Stroke 2006;1:26-29.

123. Seibert JJ. Doppler evaluation of cerebral circulation. In: Dieckmann RA, Fiser DHB, Selbst SM, editors. Illustrated textbook of pediatric emergency and critical care procedures. St Louis: Mosby–Year Book; 1997.

CHAPTER 50

The Pediatric Head and Neck

Beth M. Kline-Fath

Chapter Outline

NORMAL CERVICAL ANATOMY

The goal in pediatric imaging is to perform a study with the lowest possible radiation exposure and the least sedation necessary.[1-4] Sonography, given a lack of ionizing radiation and its noninvasive approach, should be considered as the initial imaging modality in a child with a neck lesion.[5] Sonography is also cost-effective, widely available, and portable, as needed.[6-9] Transducers with frequencies of 7.5 to 10 MHz are excellent for examination of the neck. Ultrasound can illustrate normal cervical anatomy, identify vascular structures with color Doppler flow imaging, and delineate pathology with regard to location, size, and presence of calcification.[8-10] Sonography is also excellent at distinguishing solid from cystic lesions; cystic masses are common pediatric neck lesions.[7,10]

Limitations of ultrasound technique include the inability to evaluate bone, small field of view, and degree of soft tissue contrast.[7] Because of these limitations, magnetic resonance imaging (MRI) and computed tomography (CT) are excellent adjunct modalities that can provide additional soft tissue and bone detail and further delineate extent of disease.[5,11,12]

Imaging of the head and neck can be confusing without an organized approach. The soft tissues of the neck can be separated into boundaries of the superficial and deep spaces.[13-15] The **superficial fascia** is primarily composed of subcutaneous fat. The platysma muscle, subcutaneous lymph nodes, and nerves lie within the superficial space. The **deep cervical fascia,** encircled by the superficial tissues, contains the major structures of the neck (Fig. 50-1). The deep cervical fascia includes superficial, middle, and deep layers (Fig. 50-2).

Simplifying the deep cervical fascial anatomy is best achieved by dividing the neck into suprahyoid and infrahyoid locations.[13,14] The **suprahyoid space** includes the areas of the neck between the skull base and hyoid bone.[13] The **infrahyoid space** is the area of the neck between the hyoid bone and clavicles.[14] Some deep fascial planes and lesions extend within both the infrahyoid and the suprahyoid space. These spaces and lesions are described as "lacking definition by the hyoid." Using this organization, with the knowledge of the normal anatomic elements in each space, the appropriate differential diagnosis for a mass can be proposed.[15]

SUPRAHYOID SPACE

The suprahyoid space includes the superficial, middle, and deep layers of the deep cervical fascia (Fig. 50-3). The superficial layer envelops three spaces. The **parotid space** includes the parotid gland, intraparotid facial nerve, retromandibular vein, lymph nodes, and external carotid artery. The **masticator space** includes muscles of mastication and posterior body of the mandible. The **submandibular space** includes the sublingual and submandibular glands, as well as the adjacent lymph nodes, muscles of the tongue, and hypoglossal nerve.

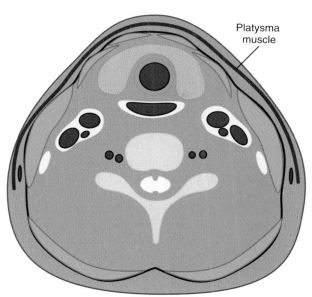

FIGURE 50-1. **Superficial and deep cervical boundaries.** Axial image of the neck at the level of the thyroid demonstrates the platysma muscle, which separates the peripheral superficial from central deep cervical fascial layers.

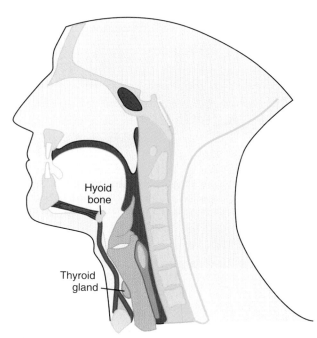

FIGURE 50-2. **Deep cervical fascial layers.** Sagittal image of the neck separates the deep cervical fascia into three boundaries: superficial *(blue)*, middle *(orange)*, and deep *(yellow)*.

The middle territory of the suprahyoid space lies between fascial layers and includes the **parapharyngeal** and **pharyngeal** spaces. This middle layer, which includes lymphoid tissue, minor salivary glands, and fat encircling the pharynx, is difficult to visualize with ultrasound and is not discussed separately. The **carotid space** is formed from fibers of the middle and deep layers of cervical fascia. The **retropharyngeal space** is contained

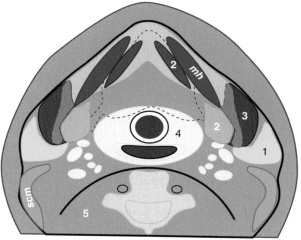

FIGURE 50-3. **Deep cervical fascial layers of suprahyoid neck, axial image.** The parotid, masticator, and submandibular spaces represent the superficial layer. *1,* Parotid gland. *2,* Submandibular space contains the sublingual *(brown)* and submandibular *(orange)* glands. *3,* Masticator space contains the masseter muscle. *4,* Middle layer. *5,* Deep fascial layer. *mh,* Mylohyoid muscle; *scm,* sternocleidomastoid muscle.

by layers of the middle cervical space anteriorly and deep cervical layers posteriorly. However, because the retropharyngeal space and **prevertebral** layer, a deep cervical space, cannot be separated, it is easiest to consider these layers together in the deep cervical facial layer as the retropharyngeal space. The carotid space and retropharyngeal space extend above and below the hyoid and are discussed later.

Parotid and Submandibular Spaces

Because the parotid and submandibular areas primarily contain salivary tissue and thus have similar pathology, these two spaces are considered together. The major salivary glands that occupy these spaces include the parotid glands, the submandibular glands, and the sublingual glands.

Normal Anatomy

The **parotid gland** is the largest salivary gland. This encapsulated gland, containing lymphoid tissue, vessels, and nerves, wraps around the angle of the mandible anterior to the mastoid tip (Fig. 50-4). Most parotid tissue lies superficial to the masseter muscle. In 20% of patients, an **accessory** parotid gland, which is a nodule of salivary tissue separate from the main parotid, can be identified on the masseter muscle.[16] The parotid gland contains acini that drain through **Stensen's duct,** a structure that extends anteriorly to exit above the upper second molar.[17] The duct lies approximately 1 cm below the inferior margin of the zygomatic arch.[18] The **facial nerve** travels within the parotid gland, lying lateral to the retromandibular vein and posterior belly of the digastric muscle, which is the muscle deep to the mastoid tip. The facial nerve acts a boundary to divide the parotid gland into superficial and deep components. The **deep lobe** of the parotid, which accounts for 20% of the gland, lies adjacent to the parapharyngeal space and beneath the angle of the mandible.

Imaging of the parotid should be obtained with the highest-frequency transducer. Usually, linear transducers of 5 to 12 MHz are used. The entire gland should be evaluated in two perpendicular planes. Because the facial nerve is poorly delineated on ultrasound, the **retromandibular vein,** which lies directly deep to the nerve and lateral to the external carotid artery, is an excellent landmark to separate the superficial and deep lobes.[18,19] Typically, the deep lobe can only be partially visualized, concealed by acoustic shadowing of the mandibular ramus. On sonography, the parotid gland is generally homogeneous and hyperechoic with regard to the adjacent muscle (Fig. 50-5). The degree of echogenicity of the gland depends on the amount of intraglandular fatty tissue; the greater the fat content, the higher the echogenicity. Normal intraparotid ducts may be visualized as linear reflective structures. Stensen's duct is usually not visible in the absence of dilation. In the parotid parenchyma, normal lymph nodes may be observed. Most nodes are identified as upper or lower pole, are oval in shape, measure 5 to 6 mm in the short axis, and appear hypoechoic with a hyperechoic central hilum.[18]

The submandibular space contains both the submandibular glands and the sublingual glands. The submandibular glands lie within the posterior submandibular space: whereas, the sublingual are anterior (Fig. 50-6).

The **submandibular glands** are bordered by the mandible laterally and the mylohyoid muscle superiorly and medially. A small portion of the gland may pass posterior to the mylohyoid muscle to lie within the sublingual area. The space anterior to the submandibular gland

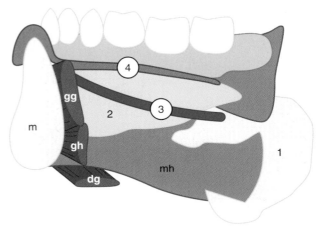

FIGURE 50-4. Diagram of parotid space. *1,* Parotid gland; *2,* Stensen's duct; *3,* masseter muscle; *4,* angle of mandible; *5,* mastoid; *6,* posterior belly of digastric muscle. Arrow points between the retromandibular vein *(open circle)* and external carotid artery *(partly solid circle),* demarcating superficial and deep lobes. Lenticular tan structure with asterisk is the facial nerve.

FIGURE 50-6. Normal submandibular space. Sagittal diagram shows submandibular gland *(1),* sublingual gland *(2),* submandibular (Wharton's) duct *(3),* sublingual duct *(4),* mylohyoid muscle *(mh),* genioglossus muscle *(gg),* geniohyoid muscle *(gh),* anterior belly of digastric muscle *(dg),* and mandible *(m).*

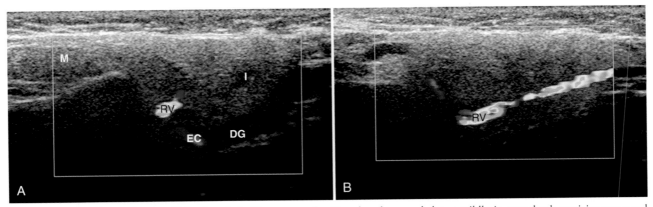

FIGURE 50-5. Normal parotid gland. A, Transverse color Doppler ultrasound shows mildly increased echogenicity compared to adjacent masseter muscle *(M).* Deep and superficial portions of the gland are separated by the retromandibular vein *(RV)* found lateral to the external carotid artery *(EC)* and posterior belly of the digastric muscle *(DG).* Small, hypoechoic intraparotid lesion is consistent with normal lymph node *(L).* **B,** Longitudinal color Doppler sonogram shows normal parotid displaying homogeneous hyperechoic texture and retromandibular vein *(RV).*

contains lymph nodes. The torturous facial artery typically crosses the parenchyma laterally. The anterior facial vein can often be identified along the anterosuperior aspect of the gland.[20] Medially, the lingual artery and vein may be evident. **Wharton's duct,** the excretory duct for the gland, extends along the mylohyoid and medial part of the sublingual gland to its orifice on the floor of the mouth. On sonography, the submandibular glands should be examined submental in two perpendicular planes, usually long and transverse, with a high-frequency linear transducer. The glands are triangular in shape, homogeneous, and more echogenic than muscle but less echogenic than the parotids[21] (Fig. 50-7). On high-resolution sonography, **fine linear streaks** can be observed, representing intraglandular ductules. Wharton's duct may be visualized as a thin echogenic wall, medial to the sublingual gland.[22] With movement of the patient's tongue, the duct may also be visible.[22]

The **sublingual gland** lies on the mylohyoid muscle between the mandible and genioglossus muscle. In addition to the gland, the sublingual area includes the submandibular duct and sublingual vessels, which lie medial to the gland. Scanning of the gland should be performed with a high-frequency linear transducer submental in two perpendicular planes with the patient supine and the head retroflexed.[23] A standoff pad can be helpful in accessing the anatomy. On transverse imaging the gland is oval, whereas on long sections the gland has a lentiform shape (Fig. 50-8). The echogenicity of the sublingual gland is similar to the parotid and submandibular glands.[23]

Inflammatory Lesions

Most salivary gland pathology in children is caused by inflammatory lesions. Inflammatory causes can be acute or chronic. The acute form may be secondary to viral or bacterial etiologies. The chronic form includes a long differential diagnosis (e.g., HIV, Sjögren's, sialoadenitis, sarcoidosis, other granulomatous processes).

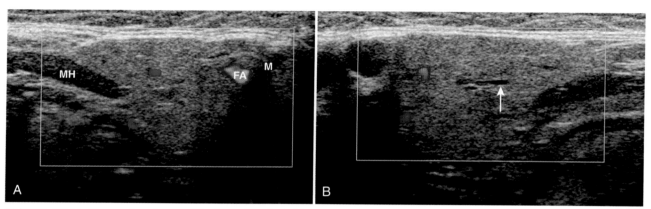

FIGURE 50-7. Normal submandibular gland. A, Transverse color Doppler scan shows homogeneous triangular gland with mandible *(M)* laterally and mylohyoid muscle *(MH)* medially. Facial artery *(FA)* is also present laterally along the gland. **B,** Longitudinal color Doppler imaging shows central linear structure without color *(arrow)*, representing nondilated Wharton's duct.

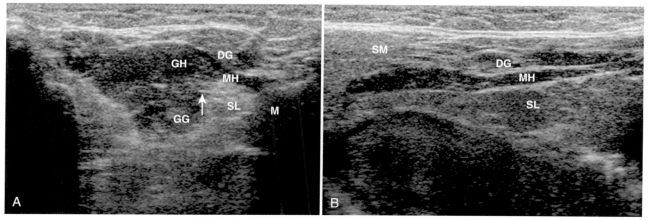

FIGURE 50-8. Normal sublingual gland. A, Transverse image shows triangular homogeneous sublingual glands laterally adjacent to mandible. *Arrow,* Wharton's duct; *SL,* sublingual gland; *M,* mandible; *DG,* anterior belly of digastric muscle; *MH,* mylohyoid; *GH,* geniohyoid; *GG,* genioglossus. **B,** Longitudinal ultrasound shows the submandibular gland *(SM)* posteriorly and the lenticular homogeneous sublingual gland *(SL).*

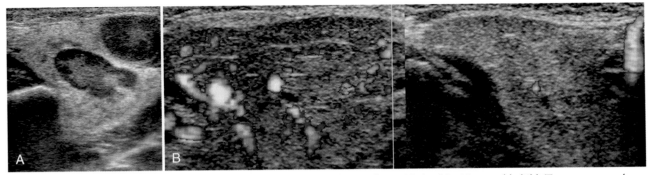

FIGURE 50-9. Viral salivary gland infection. A, Mononucleosis of parotid gland in 10-year-old child. Transverse scan shows a swollen, mildly inhomogeneous parotid with enlarged intraparotid lymph nodes. **B,** Color Doppler comparison sonograms of the submandibular glands show decreased echogenicity and increased vascularity in the left and normal appearance of the right.

Acute Salivary Gland Inflammation. In children, **viral** salivary gland infections are the most common cause of acute inflammation.[24] Endemic viruses, including mumps, mononucleosis, and cytomegalovirus (CMV), are the most common viral etiologies, causing painful unilateral or bilateral swelling of the salivary tissue. In 85% of cases, the parotid gland is involved. Although it declined with the advent of immunization, **mumps** is still the most common cause of parotitis.[17] Mumps, a highly contagious worldwide infection spread by airborne droplets, is typically encountered in the winter and spring and primarily affects children under age 15 years.[24] The incubation period for this virus is 14 to 21 days, but the infection is contagious 3 days before the onset of swelling until the resolution of the swelling.[25] With ultrasound, viral salivary infections show a diffusely enlarged gland that may have a normal, heterogeneous and/or hypoechoic echotexture with increased vascularity[26] (Fig. 50-9).

Bacterial infection is rare in children and primarily affects the parotid gland. *Staphylococcus aureus* is the most common etiology.[17,21,24,27] Children under age 1 year, especially premature infants (35%-40% cases) and immunosuppressed patients, are particularly vulnerable.[28] Infection is typically unilateral and associated with fever, dehydration, and gland pain and edema. Proposed etiologies include infection in the mouth or stasis of salivary flow through the ducts.[24] Using ultrasound, the parotid gland appears heterogeneous in echotexture with discrete, hypoechoic nodules representing enlarged intraparotid lymph nodes[17-19] (Fig. 50-10). Adjacent cervical lymphadenopathy is common. In patients with uncomplicated adenitis, treatment is primarily supportive with administration of intravenous (IV) antibiotics.[26] In the presence of severe dehydration and especially in neonates 7 to 14 days old with bacterial infection, an abscess may develop. These collections typically appear hypoechoic or anechoic with posterior acoustic enhancement and occasionally a hyperechoic halo[18] (Fig. 50-11). Internal debris may be noted, and in some cases, hyperechoic foci consistent with gas bubbles. Ultrasound-guided

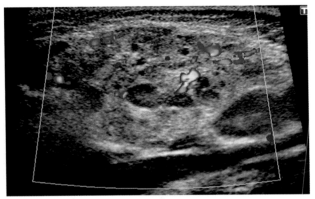

FIGURE 50-10. Bacterial parotid infection. Swollen, heterogeneous hypervascular parotid gland contains multiple areas of round, decreased echogenicity. Note adjacent lymphadenopathy.

drainage is useful when abscess is present. Recurrence is uncommon.

Sialolithiasis is uncommon in children, with 90% in the submandibular gland and 10% in the parotid.[18,24,26] In 25% of patients, stones are often multiple and intraglandular or intraductal in location.[29] Submandibular glands are prone to calculi because of the alkaline nature and high viscosity of their secretions. Wharton's duct is long with an upward course and thus also has a higher propensity for stone formation. Clinically, recurrent swelling during eating and superimposed infection may result from partial or complete obstruction of the duct by a stone. Sonography is as sensitive as 94% in the detection of salivary calculi.[30] Features include hyperechoic foci with acoustic shadowing representing stones (Fig. 50-12). With duct occlusion, hypoechoic tubular areas are typically consistent with dilated ducts.[18,31] About 50% of patients have inflammation of the gland in conjunction with the calculus,[18] and the gland will demonstrate a heterogeneous architecture. Although 80% of submandibular and 60% of parotid stones are radiopaque on x-ray examination, when more

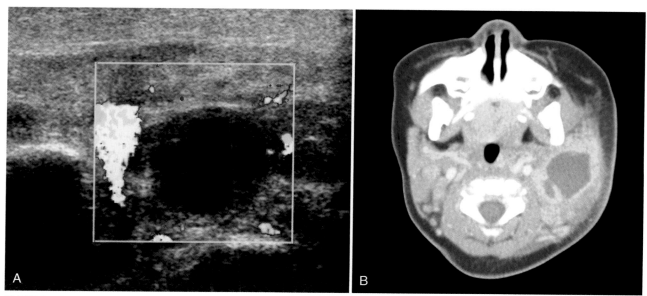

FIGURE 50-11. Parotid abscess. A, Two-month-old infant developed swelling along the left ear. Sonogram of the parotid area demonstrates round, well-defined, hypoechoic mass without internal blood flow centered within the deep parotid. **B,** Contrast CT 2 days later because of lack of response to IV antibiotics demonstrates a large, round, hypoattenuated lesion with partial enhancing peripheral wall within inflamed left parotid.

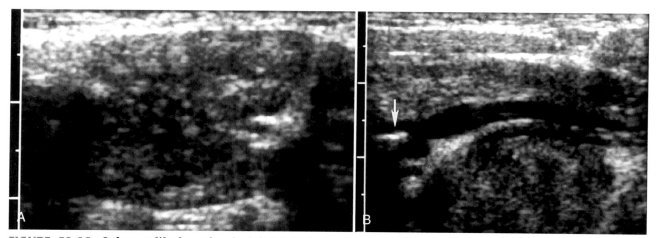

FIGURE 50-12. Submandibular gland sialolithiasis. A, Enlarged submandibular gland. **B,** Dilated submandibular duct secondary to obstructing stone *(arrow)*.

information is needed beyond ultrasound, a CT scan provides the best detail.[32]

Nodal enlargement in the parotid is often present in association with neck adenopathy caused by infection or neoplasm. **Parinaud oculoglandular syndrome** involves conjunctivitis and ipsilateral intraparotid or periauricular adenopathy and can result from *Chlamydia* infection or cat-scratch disease.[33] In the submandibular space, sonography is useful to differentiate nodal from glandular disease.[34]

Chronic Inflammatory Disease. Juvenile (recurrent) parotitis is the most common cause of parotid swelling in childhood in developed countries.[27] This disorder presents with intermittent pain, fever, and unilateral or bilateral parotid swelling. The submandibular and

sublingual glands are not affected, and there is no known etiology for recurrent parotitis. Differential diagnosis includes mumps or suppurative parotitis, which is excluded by lack of pus from the parotid duct.[35] Age at presentation is typically 3 to 6 years, and the episodes tend to cease near puberty or in late adolescence.[36] Boys are more often affected.[36,37] Some patients acquire superimposed acute infection, typically with *Streptococcus viridans*.[35,36] Although sialography was previously the prime modality for diagnosis, by demonstrating punctate or globular areas of sialectasis, ultrasound is now the favored imaging approach.[36] In the majority of patients, sonography demonstrates enlarged parotid glands containing multiple round, hypoechoic areas measuring 2 to 4 mm in diameter, likely representing peripheral sialectasis and

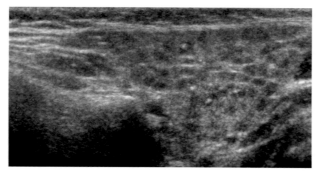

FIGURE 50-13. Juvenile parotitis. Five-year-old boy with recurrent parotitis demonstrates inhomogeneous enlarged gland with multiple small, round areas of decreased echogenicity.

lymphocytic infiltration[38] (Fig. 50-13). Some glands may be hypervascular, secondary to acute inflammation.[37] Treatment is generally supportive with analgesics and antibiotic administration.

Chronic sialadenitis is caused by an inflammatory process that damages the acini, altering the drainage system of the gland. The etiology may be infectious or noninfectious. Clinically, patients present with gland swelling and pain, particularly postprandial.

Infectious etiologies include granulomatous diseases such as **mycobacteriosis, actinomycosis,** and **histoplasmosis.** Primary tuberculosis of the salivary gland is rare; however, nontuberculous salivary gland infection, typically secondary to *Mycobacterium avium-intracellulare,* is more common, usually presenting between 16 and 36 months of age. It is important to remember that tuberculosis, mycobacteriosis, and actinomycosis can mimic neoplasm because as the disease progresses, the lesions may appear as hypoechoic masses with poorly defined margins. On color Doppler sonography, these infectious lesions, unlike neoplasm, shows no color flow. Complications with actinomycosis and mycobacteria include draining sinuses or fistula. Treatment is typically with antimicrobial therapy, although surgery may be necessary.

The most common **noninfectious** salivary gland inflammatory processes include autoimmune disease, sarcoid, and recurrent sialolithiasis. **Sjögren's syndrome** is an autoimmune disorder that results in inflammation and destruction of the exocrine glands, primarily lacrimal and salivary tissue.[39] These patients are usually monitored with ultrasound because of increased risk for lymphoma. **Sarcoid** is an idiopathic granulomatous disease that is uncommon in children. Parotid involvement, noted in 30% of patients, may be the only initial finding. **Heerfordt's disease** is the combination of parotid involvement, uveitis, and facial paralysis.[26,29] Calcified hypoechoic lesions may be present. Treatment is primarily with steroids.

Patients with chronic sialadenitis on sonography often demonstrate a heterogeneous gland with small, punctate, echogenic areas or with multiple hypoechoic areas[21] (Fig. 50-14). Punctate areas are believed to represent mucus

in the dilated ducts or walls of the dilated ducts. The hypoechoic areas likely represent edema and sialectasis, as noted on sialography. Increased vascularity can be demonstrated in areas of abnormal echotecture.[40] On imaging, findings may be bilateral and associated with intraglandular or adjacent lymph node involvement.

Human immunodeficiency virus (HIV) infection is the prime cause of immunodeficiency in infants and children.[41] HIV can affect all salivary glands, but primarily infects the parotid. The patient may demonstrate bilateral parotid swelling and lung disease from lymphocytic interstitial pneumonitis.[21] Infection is characterized by benign lymphoepithelial lesions, consisting of lymphoid hyperplasia accompanied by an intranodal cyst lined by epithelial cells.[41,42] Bilateral cystic enlargement of the parotid glands is pathognomonic for HIV infection but can be difficult to differentiate from recurrent parotitis, Sjögren's syndrome, lymphoma, and Warthin's tumor.[32,41] The most common sonographic appearance in 70% of cases is an enlarged gland with small, hypoechoic areas without acoustic enhancement and thick septations consistent with lymphoid infiltration[21,43,44] (Fig. 50-15). In 30%, there are large, anechoic areas, consistent with lymphoepithelial cysts replacing the gland. From 40% to 70% of HIV patients have associated symmetrical cervical adenopathy and enlarged adenoids.[45] Benign lymphoepithelial lesions can range from simple cysts to mixed masses with solid component.[43] When the parotid gland is abnormal, patient prognosis is better overall.[46,47]

Neoplasms

Tumors of the salivary glands account for only 1% of all pediatric tumors.[48] About 8% of primary tumors of the head and neck in children originate within the salivary glands;[21] 90% to 95% occur in the parotid and the rest in the submandibular and sublingual glands.[17] Most masses of the salivary gland are benign and have a vascular etiology.[26,46] About 60% of salivary gland tumors have been attributed to hemangioma and 27% to lymphangiomas or lymphatic malformations.[48] Only 13% were noted to be solid salivary tumors.[48] Pediatric epithelial salivary tumors tend to occur in children older than 10 years, and 23% to 50% are malignant in children.[24,26,48,49] Most malignant tumors are lower grade, although children younger than 10 years tend to have a higher-grade tumor.[26] The most common presentation for a salivary gland mass is a painless, slow-growing mass.

In children, sonography is the first step, especially for superficial lesions. With ultrasound, 95% of space-occupying lesions in the salivary glands can be delineated, and 90% are appropriately categorized as benign or malignant.[31] Sonography can easily distinguish focal from diffuse lesions, assess vascularity, and distinguish solid from cystic masses.[21] For further definition of a lesion; however, most believe MRI is the method of

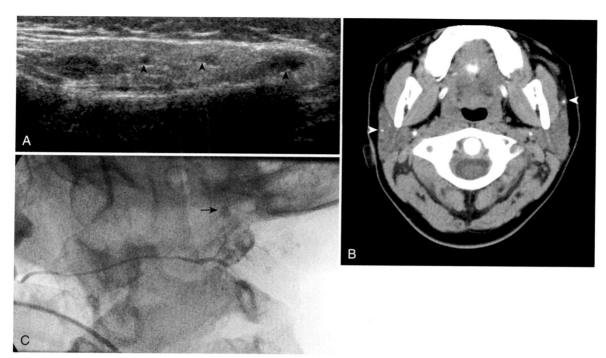

FIGURE 50-14. Chronic parotid sialadenitis secondary to sialolithiasis. A, Parotid contains round areas of decreased echogenicity typical of dilated ducts and small areas of increased echogenicity consistent with mucus and small calculi *(arrowheads).* **B,** CT shows multiple calculi in the right and left parotid *(arrowheads)* and inhomogeneous density of the right parotid. **C,** Sialogram excludes stone obstructing Stensen's duct but shows pooling in peripheral dilated ducts, sialectasis *(arrow).*

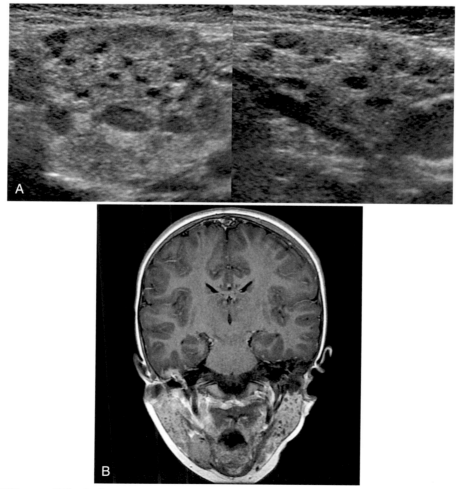

FIGURE 50-15. HIV parotitis. A, Comparison transverse images of the right and left parotid glands enlarged with small, hypoechoic areas. **B,** Coronal postgadolinium T1-weighted MR image demonstrates multiple lymphoepithelial cysts within enlarged, enhancing parotid tissue bilaterally.

choice because it provides precise information on extent and nature of the mass as well as presence of perineural invasion.[21,32]

Vascular Masses

Infantile **hemangiomas** are the most common vascular lesions in infancy and childhood.[49] These high-flow masses are benign neoplasms composed of proliferating endothelial cells.[49,50] Hemangiomas represent 60% of head and neck neoplasms and 60% of all salivary gland neoplasms.[51,52] Hemangiomas occur three times more often in girls than boys.[51,53] Most present as a painless, compressible, growing mass, and half have a bluish or red stain in the skin superficial to the lesion.[49,54] Hemangiomas are common in premature infants, usually evident shortly after birth, but 95% of these lesions present during the first 6 months.[54,55] These lesions typically undergo a phase of proliferation at 0 to 1 year, peak in size, then undergo spontaneous, slow involution at 1 to 7 years of age.[49,50] About 80% of salivary gland masses arise in the parotid, and 18% are present in submandibular tissue.[26] On ultrasound, the lesions are infiltrative or well circumscribed, usually hypoechoic relative to the parotid, and may involve all or part of the gland (Fig. 50-16). In the proliferative phase, on color Doppler sonography, there is a high vessel density,[29,56] with both increased arteries and increased veins (Fig. 50-17). Arterial Doppler waveforms and spectral Doppler demonstrate high flow velocity and low resistive index (RI) with broadening of the spectrum.[43,52] Because most infantile hemangiomas spontaneously regress, medical management with corticosteroids or surgical therapy is used only when symptoms warrant.[49,53,57]

Lymphatic malformations or **lymphangiomas** are part of a spectrum of anomalies in development now included in an entity termed **vascular malformations.** These lesions may involve the parotid gland or may infiltrate the submandibular space. However, on ultrasound, if a lymphatic malformation is present within the parotid, the gland typically contains cystic spaces, with or without solid elements and septations[17] (Fig. 50-18).

Salivary Gland Masses

Pleomorphic adenomas, also referred to as **benign mixed-cell tumors,** contain both mesenchymal and epithelial cell lines. These neoplasms are the most common benign salivary gland tumor in childhood and occur in all pediatric age groups (median, 15 years).[24,31] Most present as a solitary, hard, painless, slow-growing mass.[58] From 60% to 90% of these lesions originate in the parotid gland and 10% to 30% in the submandibular gland.[18,21] When arising from parotid tissue, the lesions may originate within the deep or the superficial lobe. These lesions can recur (1%-50%) as multiple masses[58] or rarely can develop late metastatic deposits.[30,58] On sonography, the lesion appears lobulated, well defined, and hypoechoic or isoechoic (with respect to normal salivary tissue) (Fig. 50-19). Cystic areas and hyperechoic shadowing foci representing small calcifications may be noted.[17] Typically, pleomorphic adenomas demonstrate peripheral vascularity with a hypovascular center[19,32,40] (Fig. 50-20). Treatment includes surgical resection with facial nerve–sparing techniques.

Warthin's tumor, also referred to as papillary cystadenoma lymphomatosum or **adenolymphoma,** is the second most common benign salivary gland neoplasm of children and solely identified in the parotid gland.[59] The lesion contains a double layer of epithelial cells resting on a dense lymphoid stroma and is believed to result from incorporation of lymphatic elements and

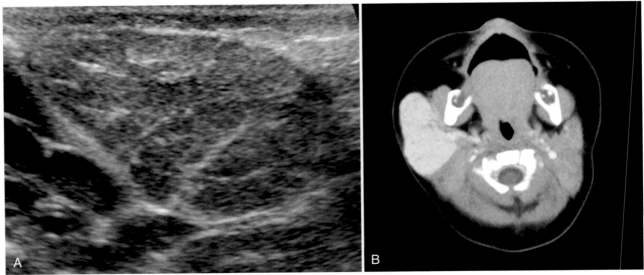

FIGURE 50-16. Parotid hemangioma. A, Enlarged hypoechoic parotid gland with a few internal linear striations. **B,** CT scan demonstrates intense homogeneous enhancement of the right parotid mass.

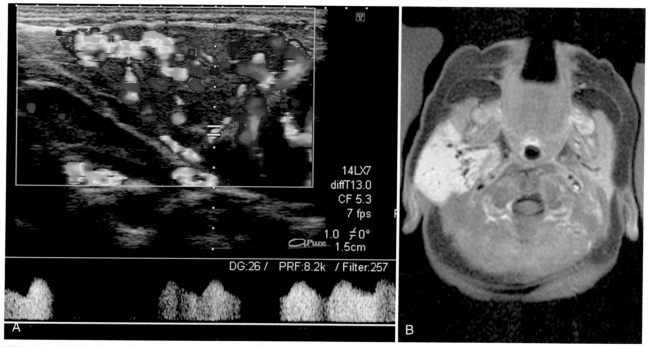

FIGURE 50-17. Parotid hemangioma. A, Color Doppler sonogram shows high vessel density with low arterial resistance. **B,** T1-weighted postgadolinium MR scan shows intensely enhancing right parotid with multiple dark, round areas centrally, consistent with flow voids in multiple enlarged vessels.

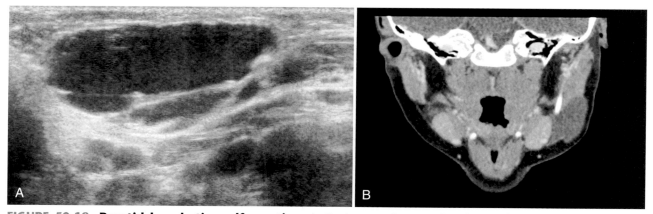

FIGURE 50-18. Parotid lymphatic malformation. A, Cystic septated mass within the superficial parotid. **B,** Coronal CT shows the cystic lesion lateral to and inseparable from the normal enhancing left parotid.

heterotopic ductal epithelium within the parotid lymph nodes. Typically, the lesion presents as a painless, solitary, slow-growing mass. In up to 10% of cases the lesion may be bilateral. Ultrasound findings include an oval, hypoechoic, well-defined mass containing multiple microcystic or anechoic areas, given the high propensity for cystic change.[18,19,59] With color and Doppler sonography, the tumor typically is hypervascular. Diagnosis of Warthin's tumor may be supported by intense uptake of the lesion by technetium 99m scintigraphy.[17,18] Treatment is surgical resection; however, recurrence is possible from multifocality.

Mucoepidermoid carcinoma, the most common malignant salivary gland neoplasm in children, consists of cords, sheets, or cystic spaces lined by squamous and mucous cells.[17,21] Of the malignant salivary gland lesions, 60% are diagnosed as mucoepidermoid carcinomas, and about 50% arise from the parotid.[21] Clinically, these lesions may be tender, may grow rapidly, and may cause facial nerve paralysis.[18,49] Ultrasound characteristics depend on histologic grade. Lower-grade lesions may be homogeneous in echotexture and well defined, whereas high-grade lesions appear irregular, poorly defined, with hypoechoic heterogeneous internal architecture. Doppler ultrasound is not reliable to differentiate benign from malignant lesions. However, increased intratumoral RI and high peak systolic flow velocity (PSV, >60 cm/sec) should increase suspicion for malignancy.[40] Sonography

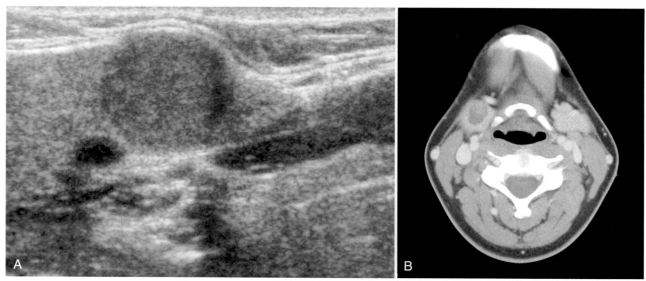

FIGURE 50-19. Submandibular pleomorphic adenoma. A, Submandibular gland containing a well-defined hypoechoic mass. **B,** CT scan shows a well-defined low-density lesion centered within the right submandibular gland.

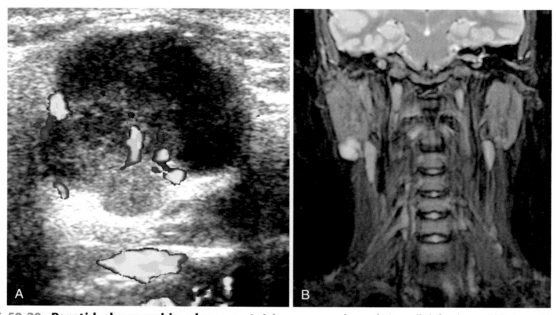

FIGURE 50-20. Parotid pleomorphic adenoma. A, Inhomogeneous, hypoechoic, well-defined parotid lesion with relatively hypovascular center. **B,** Coronal T2-weighted MR image shows well-defined, hyperintense lesion in the inferior right parotid.

should also be performed in the area of the lesion to assess for metastatic-appearing lymph nodes. Wide surgical resection of low-grade lesions is the therapy of choice. In the presence of high-grade neoplasm, resection of the lesion, lymph node dissections, and radiotherapy may be required.

Other Masses

Neurofibromas are benign tumors of the nerve sheath. They may arise along any nerve, including the facial nerve within the parotid. Multiple or plexiform neurofibromas are typical in patients with neurofibromatosis type 1.[60] Sonography demonstrates multiple hypoechoic areas within the gland.

Lipomas represent 1% of parotid tumors; 57% of lipomas in the parotid area arise within the gland.[29] These lesions are compressible, oval, and well defined. On ultrasound, lipomas contain striped or feathered internal echoes devoid of color and Doppler flow.[31]

Lingual thyroid may appear as a homogeneous solid mass in the midline dorsum of the tongue. In 70% of cases, this ectopic tissue is the only functioning thyroid tissue.[61]

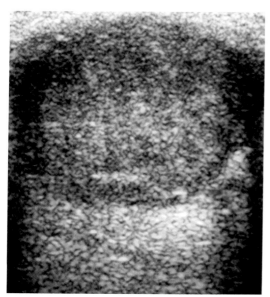

FIGURE 50-21. **Papillary thyroid cancer metastasis to parotid.** Well-defined mass with punctate hyperechoic areas within the mass, typical of thyroid metastasis.

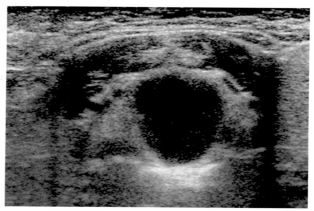

FIGURE 50-22. **Ranulae.** Well-defined anechoic lesion with acoustic enhancement centered between the sublingual glands in the floor of the mouth.

DIFFERENTIAL DIAGNOSIS OF SUPRAHYOID CYSTIC LESIONS

PAROTID SPACE
Branchial type I
Parotid retention cyst
Tumors
  Warthin's
  Malignant
Lymph node necrosis
Lymphatic malformation

SUBMANDIBULAR SPACE
Branchial type II
Ranulae
Dermoid/epidermoid
Thyroglossal duct cyst
Vallecular cyst
Lymph node necrosis
Lymphatic malformation

Rhabdomyosarcoma occurs 40% of the time in the head and neck and can arise from any muscle. This is the second most common salivary gland area malignancy in the pediatric population.[48] Salivary gland involvement is frequently by direct extension.[60]

Primary lymphoma of the salivary glands is termed **MALToma,** denoting origin from mucosa-associated lymphoid tissue. Patients with Sjögren's syndrome and other autoimmune disease, including HIV, are at risk for primary lymphoma. Secondary involvement of lymphoma is rare, but more common in the parotid.[62] Ultrasound demonstrates a focal mass or diffuse infiltration with an enlarged gland. Lesions may consist of multiple small, hypoechoic nodules or an irregularly shaped, heterogeneous mass without calcification or cystic degeneration.[62] A reported case of submandibular gland involvement by MALToma showed hypoechoic compartments surrounded by hyperechoic lines, creating a tortoiseshell appearance.[63] Increased color and Doppler flow is typical.

Leukemic infiltration is rare, presenting similar to lymphoma on ultrasound.

Metastatic disease is rare in children but would include neuroblastoma, squamous cell carcinoma, melanoma, and thyroid cancer[43,64] (Fig. 50-21).

Suprahyoid Cystic Lesions

In the parotid space, **type 1 branchial cysts** are most common. Simple cysts of the salivary glands are rare and likely caused by **mucous retention.** On ultrasound, the lesions are well defined, anechoic, with posterior acoustic enhancement and no internal blood flow.[18,64]

In the submandibular space laterally, **branchial type 2 cysts** can be identified posterior to the submandibular gland. **Lymphatic malformations** may also extend into the space. **Ranulae** (sublingual cysts) are mucous retention cysts resulting from obstruction of the sublingual gland or duct. They present paramidline, in the area of the sublingual gland, as a painless swelling along the floor of the mouth. When large, sublingual cysts can extend below the level of the mylohyoid muscle, termed "plunging ranulae."[26,29] Rarely, the lesions are bilateral, and some large lesions extend into the parapharyngeal space. Imaging of a simple ranula on ultrasound demonstrates a unilocular cyst (Fig. 50-22). If infected, the lesion may show internal debris, poorly defined borders, and adjacent inflammation. These lesions are managed with intraoral marsupialization or surgical resection.

Midline lesions in the suprahyoid area include **dermoid** or **epidermoid** tumors and **thyroglossal duct cysts.** A **cyst of the vallecula** results from retained

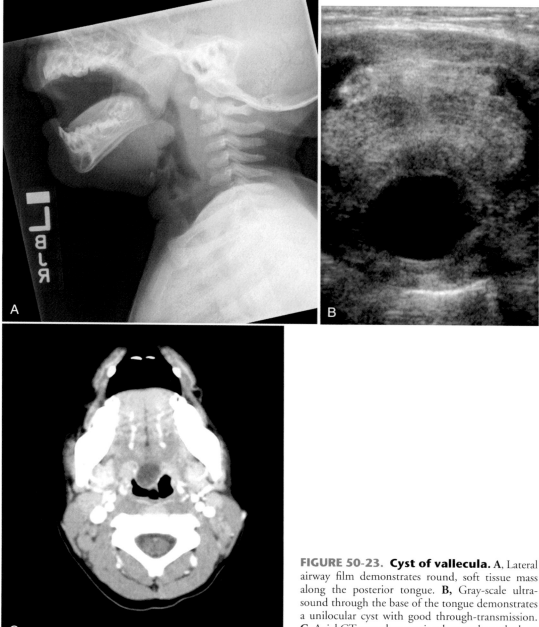

FIGURE 50-23. Cyst of vallecula. A, Lateral airway film demonstrates round, soft tissue mass along the posterior tongue. **B,** Gray-scale ultrasound through the base of the tongue demonstrates a unilocular cyst with good through-transmission. **C,** Axial CT scan shows a simple cyst along the base of the tongue at the level of the vallecula.

secretions in the mucous glands of the pharyngeal wall.[65] These cysts can be congenital or acquired and can cause upper airway obstruction, resulting in death.[66,67] The lesions are midline and on sonography appear as a hypoechoic cystic mass, behind and below the tongue[68] (Fig. 50-23).

Masticator Space

Ultrasound is helpful in evaluating pathology in the masticator space as well as excluding parotid gland involvement. The two most common soft tissue masses to consider in the masticator space are **sarcomas** and **vascular malformations.** It is important to remember that the masseter and pterygoid muscles are often involved in venous malformations.[69] An uncommon homogeneous mass to consider is benign hypertrophy of the masseter muscle.[64] However, tumor infiltration of the muscle from leukemia or lymphoma can mimic hypertrophy; thus clinical correlation is essential (Fig. 50-24). In the presence of trauma, a hematoma appearing as a hypoechoic area may be demonstrated. Inflammatory masses also may develop, including secondary or primary myositis or osteomyelitis of the mandible, often in the presence of an infected tooth. Cellulitis and soft tissue abscesses may accompany these infections[21,70] (Fig. 50-25).

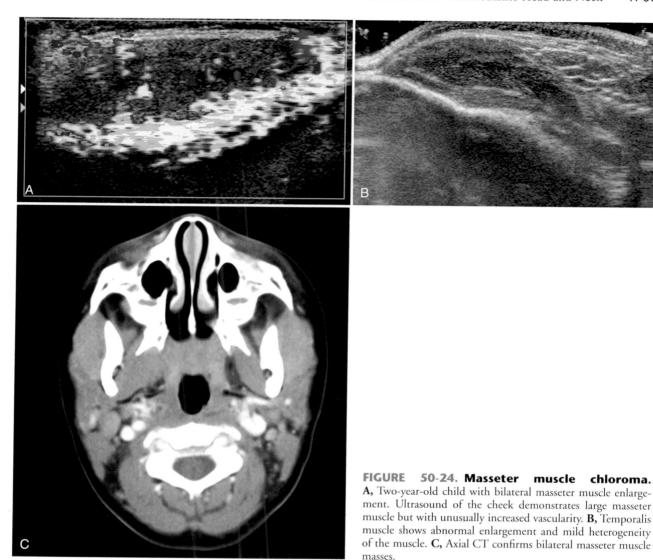

FIGURE 50-24. Masseter muscle chloroma.
A, Two-year-old child with bilateral masseter muscle enlargement. Ultrasound of the cheek demonstrates large masseter muscle but with unusually increased vascularity. **B,** Temporalis muscle shows abnormal enlargement and mild heterogeneity of the muscle. **C,** Axial CT confirms bilateral masseter muscle masses.

INFRAHYOID SPACE

The infrahyoid deep cervical fascia is split into superficial, middle, and deep compartments[14,29] (Fig. 50-26). The superficial layer at this level is the **suprasternal space,** lying above the sternum and anterior to the sternothyroid and sternohyoid muscles. The **visceral space** is delineated by the middle layer of deep cervical fascia. The visceral space contains the thyroid, parathyroid, trachea, esophagus, paraesophageal lymph nodes, and recurrent laryngeal nerve.

Visceral Space

Normal Thyroid Anatomy

The thyroid gland originates as an outpouching in the foramen cecum at the base of the tongue. The tissue descends by the seventh week of gestation to lie anterior to the larynx and upper trachea.[71,72] The common carotid arteries and internal jugular veins are present on the lateral edges, and the cervical esophagus is midline or to the left of the trachea. The thyroid gland contains two lobes and is connected by an **isthmus.** In 50% of patients, a **pyramidal lobe** extends superiorly from the isthmus.[73] Four parathyroid glands lie along the posterior surface of the thyroid lobes.

Ultrasound is performed with the patient supine and neck slightly hyperextended. A high-frequency linear array transducer (10-15 MHz) is necessary.[73,74] A stand-off pad may be helpful in older patients. Longitudinal and transverse imaging should be performed of the entire thyroid tissue. Doppler imaging may be considered in the examination of masses or nodules. Adjacent neck structures should be imaged, especially the jugular chain and supraclavicular nodes.

On ultrasound, the normal thyroid gland is homogeneous and hyperechoic compared to adjacent muscle

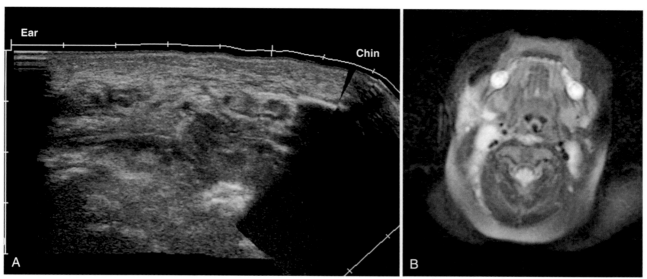

FIGURE 50-25. Masseter myositis caused by staphylococcus. A, Panoramic gray-scale ultrasound of the cheek shows heterogeneous echotexture and poorly defined planes between the masseter muscle and adjacent soft tissues. **B,** Axial T2-weighted fat-saturated MR image demonstrates enlargement and abnormal hyperintense T2 signal of the right masseter and adjacent soft tissues.

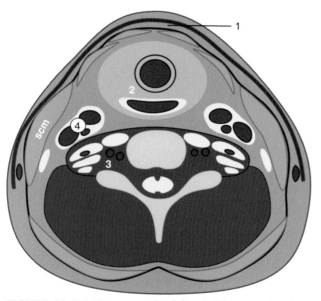

FIGURE 50-26. Deep cervical fascial layers of infrahyoid space. Axial diagram: *1,* superficial; *2,* middle (visceral); *3,* deep; *4,* carotid; *5,* sternocleidomastoid muscle *(scm).*

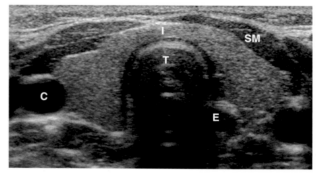

FIGURE 50-27. Normal thyroid. Transverse sonogram of the thyroid gland demonstrates homogeneous, increased echotexture compared to the sternohyoid and sternothyroid *(SM)* muscles. Normal right lobe, left lobe, and isthmus *(I)* identified. Trachea *(T)* is midline and esophagus *(E)* posterior to left lobe. Common carotid artery *(C)* is present along the peripheral margin.

(Fig. 50-27). The lobes of tissue are triangular on transverse and elliptical on sagittal images. The size of the thyroid gland changes with age; Tables 50-1 and 50-2 list normal values.[75,76]

Congenital Thyroid Lesions

Although some congenital thyroid lesions extend into both the suprahyoid and the infrahyoid space, the pathology is inherent to the thyroid.

Because untreated hypothyroidism can result in severe mental retardation and delayed bone development, there is a nationwide program in the United States for neonatal screening. **Congenital hypothyroidism** is present in 1 per 4000 infants and is twice as common in girls as in boys.[73,77] Causes include agenesis, dysgenesis, and goiter from inborn error of metabolism, maternal thyrotoxicosis, or maternal ingestion of iodine, antithyroid medication, or lithium.[40,73] About 85% of cases are caused by **dysgenesis,** either hypoplasia or ectopia.[77] Sonography is the best imaging modality because it correctly defines the normal thyroid gland, which may be classified as large, normal, small, or absent. Large glands are typically goitrous. Normal-sized glands in children with congenital hypothyroidism have been observed in patients with pseudohypoparathyroidism or Down syndrome.[77] Rarely (0.2% of cases), **thyroid hemiagenesis** can occur, with failure of development in both lobes, the left being absent in 60% of cases[77,78] (Fig. 50-28). On ultrasound, if no thyroid gland can be identified, imaging should be performed superiorly in the midline to the base of the tongue because tissue may be present anywhere along the embryologic descent. **Ectopic tissue** is lingual and thus suprahyoid in 90% of cases, lying close to the hyoid bone and deep to the muscles of the tongue.[78] Ultrasound imaging in the neonate with ectopic thyroid typically shows a well-defined ovoid structure equal in echotexture to normal thyroid tissue and hyperemic on color Doppler (Fig. 50-29). In older children treated for hypothyroidism in the presence of ectopic tissue, the gland may appear hypoechoic with no vascularity.[79] Some children with ectopic tissue are euthyroid and present with a mass at the base of the tongue. It is important to

identify this tissue as thyroid because removal in the absence of other thyroid tissue will result in a hypothyroid individual. When ultrasound is unable to identify ectopic thyroid tissue, a nuclear medicine scan, given the high sensitivity, may be employed[79,80] (Fig. 50-30).

Thyroglossal duct cyst (TDC), representing 70% of all congenital neck masses, is the most common midline cyst and developmental anomaly identified by ultrasound.[43,78,81] The anatomy of the thyroglossal duct follows the pathway of embryology from the foramen cecum of the tongue, along the inferior and posterior surface of the midline hyoid, to the pyramidal lobe of the thyroid. Persistence of the duct, which is lined by secretory epithelium, results in cyst or sinus formation. The majority of TDCs are present adjacent to the hyoid bone as an asymptomatic mass,[57,82] although they can be located at any point of descent. Anatomically, most are located midline or parasagittal, particularly to the left of midline. If a cyst is suprahyoid, the lesion will elevate

TABLE 50-1. NORMAL DIMENSIONS OF THE THYROID GLAND*

	NO. SUBJECTS (MALE/FEMALE)	THICKNESS (cm)†	WIDTH (cm)†
	Corrected Gestational Weeks		
30-33	5 (4:1)	0.8 ± 0.1	1.1 ± 0.3
33-37	19 (13:6)	1.1 ± 0.3‡	1.4 ± 0.3§
	Height (cm)		
45-50	42 (20:22)	1.4 ± 0.2‡	1.7 ± 0.2‡
50-70	42 (27:15)	1.4 ± 0.1	1.8 ± 0.2
70-90	8 (6:2)	1.4 ± 0.1	1.9 ± 0.1
90-100	8 (3:5)	1.4 ± 0.1	1.8 ± 0.2
100-110	34 (12:22)	1.5 ± 0.3	2.1 ± 0.3
110-120	35 (20:15)	1.7 ± 0.3	2.3 ± 0.3
120-130	45 (23:22)	1.8 ± 0.4	2.4 ± 0.3
130-140	36 (21:15)	1.9 ± 0.5	2.7 ± 0.2
140-150	42 (20:22)	2.1 ± 0.4	2.8 ± 0.3
150-160	59 (25:34)	2.2 ± 0.4	2.8 ± 0.4
160-170	16 (14:2)	2.4 ± 0.4	3.0 ± 0.4

Compared with 30-33 weeks: ‡p <0.01; §p <0.05.
*As a function of corrected gestational weeks in premature neonates and as a function of height from neonates to adolescence.
†Mean ±1 standard deviation.
From Ueda D, Mitamura R, Suzuki N, et al. Sonographic imaging of the thyroid gland in congenital hypothyroidism. Pediatr Radiol 1992;22:102-105.

TABLE 50-2. VOLUME OF THYROID GLAND AND THICKNESS OF EACH LOBE*

HEIGHT (cm)	NO. SUBJECTS	VOLUME (cm)	RLT (cm)†	LLT (cm)†
≤99	16	2.3 ± 0.7	0.8 ± 0.17	0.8 ± 0.18
100-109	34	3.3 ± 1.0	0.8 ± 0.19	0.8 ± 0.21
110-119	35	4.1 ± 1.1	0.9 ± 0.17	0.9 ± 0.19
120-129	45	4.9 ± 1.1	0.9 ± 0.18	0.9 ± 0.20
130-139	36	6.3 ± 2.0	0.9 ± 0.25	1.0 ± 0.25
140-149	42	7.4 ± 2.2	1.0 ± 0.23	1.0 ± 0.23
150-159	59	8.5 ± 2.3	1.1 ± 0.23	1.0 ± 0.24
≥160	20	10.9 ± 2.5	1.2 ± 0.24	1.2 ± 0.25

*As a function of body height.
†Mean ±1 standard deviation; *RLT*, right lobe thickness; *LLT*, left lobe thickness.
From Ueda D. Normal volume of the thyroid gland in children. J Clin Ultrasound 1998;18:455-462.

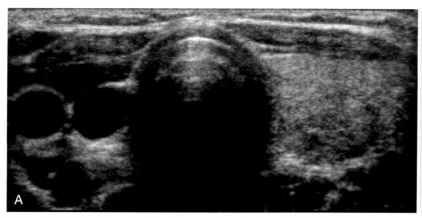
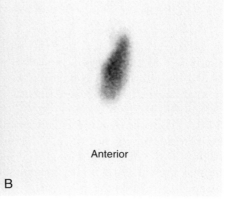

Anterior

FIGURE 50-28. Thyroid hemiagenesis. A, Normal left lobe of the thyroid is identified, but the right lobe is absent. Note that the right carotid and jugular vessels lie in the anatomic area of the right lobe. **B,** Iodine-123 nuclear medicine scan confirms presence of only a left thyroid lobe.

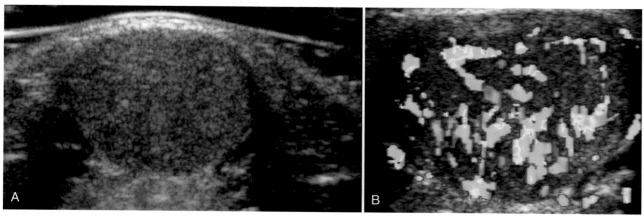

FIGURE 50-29. Ectopic thyroid. A, Submental mass in 3-month-old infant known to be hypothyroid. Ultrasound at site of lump shows homogeneous soft tissue mass equal in echotexture to normal thyroid. **B,** Color Doppler sonogram of the lesion demonstrates intense vascularity.

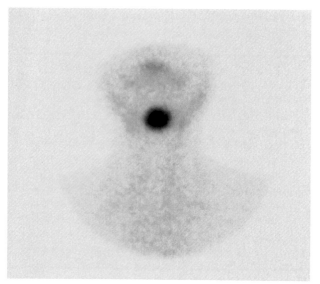

FIGURE 50-30. Ectopic thyroid. Anterior image of ^{99m}Tc-pertechnetate scan confirms lingual thyroid and lack of normal anatomic thyroid tissue.

with tongue movement.[43] Congenital fistulas in association with TDC are infrequent but can occur after inflammation.[83]

The classic sonographic appearance of TDC is noted in less than half of cases and includes a thin-walled, anechoic unilocular lesion. Typically, however, TDCs, caused by high protein content rather than inflammation, are hypoechoic or heterogeneous, some appearing pseudosolid and mimicking ectopic tissue[83-85] (Fig. 50-31). Posterior acoustic enhancement is present in most cysts, and absence of color Doppler flow can be helpful in the diagnosis. However, demonstration of a normal thyroid gland while imaging TDCs is recommended to exclude the diagnosis of ectopic tissue. Up to one third of patients with TDC will develop superimposed infection and demonstrate imaging findings of thick walls, internal septation, and heterogeneous

echotexture from debris[83,86] (Fig. 50-32). There is a 1% increased risk of cancer, primarily papillary, and calcification or a soft tissue mass in the presence of a cyst should raise suspicion.[69,81,87] Therapy is surgical resection with the Sistrunk procedure, which involves excision of cyst, remnant tract, and part of the hyoid bone.[88]

Differential diagnosis for cystic lesions in the infrahyoid space includes thyroglossal duct cyst, dermoid, epidermoid, branchial cyst, lymphatic malformation, laryngocele, necrotic adenopathy, teratoma, and thymic cyst.

DIFFERENTIAL DIAGNOSIS FOR INFRAHYOID CYSTIC LESIONS

MIDLINE
Thyroglossal duct cyst
Dermoid/epidermoid

LATERAL
Branchial cyst
Lymphatic malformation
Laryngocele
Thyroglossal duct cyst
Adenopathy, necrotic
Teratoma
Thymic cyst

Inflammatory Thyroid Disease

Acute bacterial infection of the thyroid is rare because the gland is highly resistant to infection.[89,90] If present, infection is usually caused by staphylococci, streptococci, or anaerobic bacteria. On sonography, the gland demonstrates heterogeneous, poorly defined echotexture. If the left lobe of the thyroid is abnormal, a congenital piriform sinus, type III or IV branchial apparatus remnant, should be considered[89-91] (Fig. 50-33). These patients usually present between age 2 and 12 years with

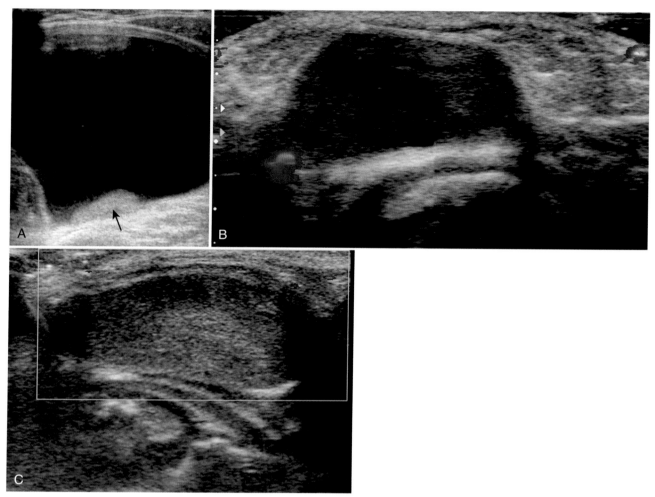

FIGURE 50-31. **Thyroglossal duct cyst. A,** Large, left paramidline, infrahyoid unilocular cystic mass with small, ectopic thyroid tissue posteriorly *(arrow).* **B,** Elliptical lesion in midline anterior to the trachea shows internal heterogeneous echotexture with good through-transmission and lack of color flow. **C,** Color Doppler sonogram shows avascular, solid-appearing lesion, infrahyoid left parasagittal, with subtle through-transmission.

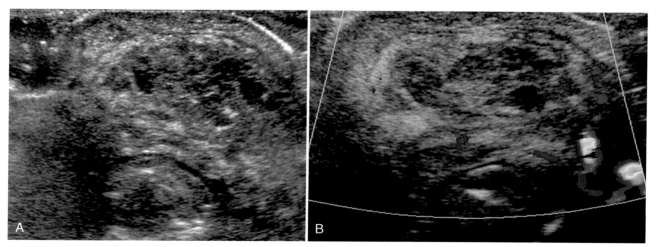

FIGURE 50-32. **Infected thyroglossal duct cyst. A,** Complex midline lesion anterior to the trachea shows heterogeneous echotexture with internal septations and thick wall. **B,** Color Doppler ultrasound demonstrates vascularity around the periphery of the complex mass.

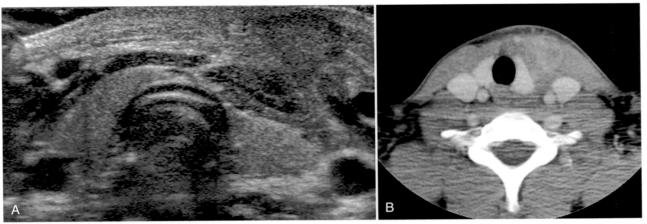

FIGURE 50-33. Type IV branchial sinus abscess. A, Hypoechoic, poorly defined collection in left anterior neck distorting muscle and soft tissue planes and inseparable, compressing the left thyroid gland. **B,** Axial CT scan at same level demonstrates inhomogeneously enhancing phlegmon adjacent to left lobe of thyroid.

fever, sore throat, and swelling in the lower neck. On ultrasound, the left lobe of the thyroid gland may be heterogeneous. If an abscess has developed, typically a focal hypoechoic lesion is surrounded by hyperemia in the left perithyroid area.[73,78,89,90]

Hashimoto's thyroiditis is the most common cause of thyroid disease in children and adolescents.[64] It is an autoimmune disorder caused by circulating antibodies. Injury to the gland results in a diffuse lymphocytic and plasma cell infiltration. The process is more common in girls than boys, with a family history of thyroid disease in one fourth of cases.[77,92] Clinically, the patient presents with painless enlargement of the thyroid. Although in the acute phase the patient may be hyperthyroid, most patients are hypothyroid at presentation. Hashimoto's thyroiditis may be associated with several syndromes (e.g., Turner, Noonan, Down) and has been described in patients with juvenile diabetes, receiving phenytoin therapy, and with Hodgkin's disease.[73] On ultrasound, the gland is enlarged with lobular margins and contains coarse septations and multiple hypoechoic micronodules measuring 1 to 6 mm in diameter[78] (Fig. 50-34). Normal, increased, or deceased color Doppler waveforms may be present. Adjacent cervical adenopathy is often noted. The majority of these patients have spontaneous resolution of symptoms.

De Quervain's thyroiditis, also known as **focal thyroiditis,** is an uncommon form of subacute thyroiditis likely caused by a viral infection.[71] Granulomatous inflammation of the gland results in thyromegaly and heterogeneous echogenicity.

Graves' disease is an autoimmune disease caused by thyroid-stimulated immunoglobulin binding to the thyroid-stimulating hormone (TSH) receptor, increasing the production of thyroid hormone. There is frequently a family history. It is more common in girls (5:1 female/male ratio) and has a peak incidence in adolescence, ages 11 to 15 years.[73,77] Children present with an

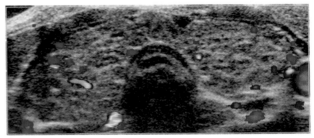

FIGURE 50-34. Hashimoto's thyroiditis. Thyroid imaging with color Doppler ultrasound shows lobular enlargement, coarse pattern with multiple hypoechoic areas, and mildly increased vascularity.

enlarged thyroid gland, exophthalmos, and hyperthyroidism. Fetuses and neonates born to mothers with Graves' disease are also at risk for transient thyroid dysfunction and goiter because of transfer of thyroid-stimulating immunoglobulins.[77,92] During ultrasound examination, patients with Graves' disease demonstrate enlargement of the gland, which appears heterogeneous and diffusely hypoechoic. Doppler imaging demonstrates intense hypervascularity, also known as "thyroid inferno"[78] (Fig. 50-35). Doppler waveform shows increased PSV and decreased RI.[93]

Neoplasm and Common Thyroid Masses

Thyroid nodules in pediatrics are uncommon; with an incidence of 1.5%.[94] Most children present with an asymptomatic palpable nodule in the presence of normal thyroid function.[95] In a child or adolescent, a solitary nodule should be approached with suspicion because there is a 33% risk of malignancy.[92] Ultrasound and radionuclide scintigraphy are the primary methods of imaging thyroid nodules. Fine-needle aspiration (FNA), especially with ultrasound guidance, may be helpful and

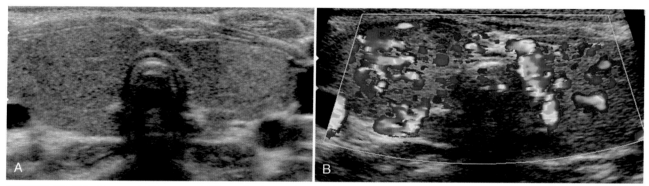

FIGURE 50-35. Graves' disease. A, Thyroid is hypoechoic and swollen, right lobe greater than left. **B,** Color Doppler ultrasound demonstrates "thyroid inferno."

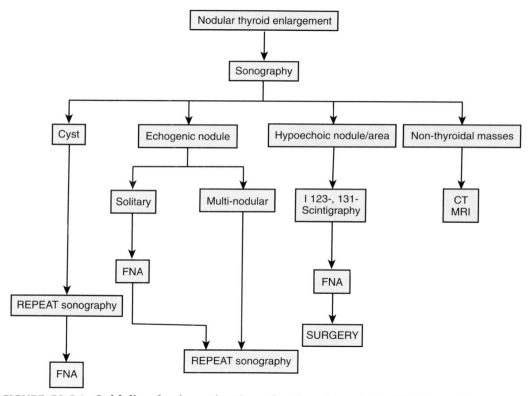

FIGURE 50-36. Guideline for investigation of a thyroid nodule. *FNA,* Fine-needle aspiration.

has 80% to 95% accuracy for defining pathology in pediatric cases.[94-96] If FNA is not diagnostic, surgical excision may be required. Figure 50-36 provides a simple guideline for management of thyroid lesions.[71]

A **pseudonodule** of the thyroid can be produced by uncalcified cricoid cartilage. On sagittal imaging, the cricoid can appear as a round or oval mass, similar in echotexture to the normal thyroid and posteromedial to the gland.[97]

Although uncommon, **hemorrhage** within the thyroid, related to direct or indirect trauma, can mimic a nodule. The hematoma on sonography typically appears heterogeneous and hypoechoic (Fig. 50-37). At

ultrasound, color Doppler flow imaging may be helpful to evaluate for injury to adjacent vessels.[98]

Follicular adenomas, the most common benign lesions of the thyroid, arise from an overproliferation of follicular cells (hyperplasia).[78,94] Lesions may be solitary or multinodular, are round and well defined, and have decreased, increased, or honeycomb echotexture. About 60% of adenomas demonstrate a peripheral, 1-to 2-mm hypoechoic halo caused by a fibrous capsule and peripheral blood vessels best delineated with color Doppler sonography[78,99] (Fig. 50-38). Many of these masses contain cystic areas resulting from hemorrhage or necrosis. Nuclear medicine studies show variable uptake, with

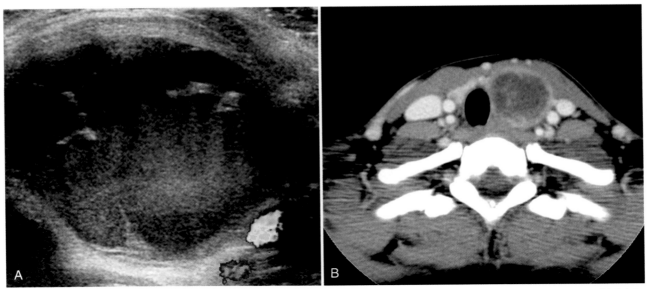

FIGURE 50-37. Thyroid hematoma. A, Teenage girl was elbowed in the left neck and developed a lump. Imaging of left lobe of thyroid demonstrates heterogeneous, well-defined, round avascular lesion. **B,** Axial CT scan shows hematoma replacing most of the left lobe.

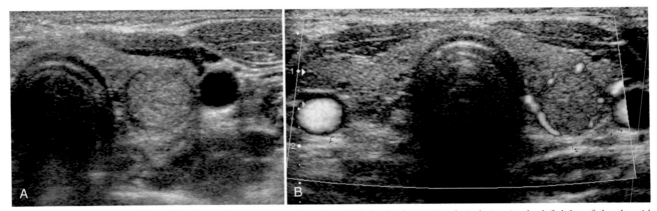

FIGURE 50-38. Thyroid follicular adenoma. A, Round, well-defined, almost-isoechoic lesion in the left lobe of the thyroid demonstrates a peripheral halo of decreased echogenicity. **B,** Color Doppler sonogram of mass demonstrates peripheral vascularity.

some follicular adenomas demonstrating intense activity. Despite benign imaging characteristics, these lesions can be difficult to differentiate from malignancy.[73]

Degenerative cysts are likely the result of necrosis within benign thyroid nodules. Most of these lesions are complex with mixed echotexture, thick irregular wall, septations, and in some cases, fluid-fluid levels from previous hemorrhage. Bright, echogenic internal areas result from colloid material, sometimes creating **comet-tail artifacts**[73,74] (Fig. 50-39). Calcifications in degenerative lesions may create echogenic foci of acoustic shadowing or peripheral eggshell calcifications. Doppler sonography typically shows peripheral vascularity, and nuclear medicine studies demonstrate variable uptake. Because malignancy may present as a cystic mass, close follow-up imaging and surgical diagnosis are typically indicated.[92,100]

Multinodular (adenomatous) goiter in children is uncommon but typically is diagnosed in adolescent girls near puberty.[101] In adults the etiology has been linked to iodine deficiency. In children, genetic susceptibility is more common.[102] Multinodular goiter has been described in patients with renal cystic disease, polydactyly, Hashimoto's thyroiditis, McCune-Albright syndrome, and previous radiation therapy.[101] At presentation, children are typically euthyroid and clinically are diagnosed with a palpable nodule or nodules. On ultrasound, the nodules show variable heterogeneity with macronodular or micronodular formation (Fig. 50-40). Some may become cystic because of necrosis or hemorrhage.[101] Continued ultrasound monitoring of these patients is warranted given the increased risk for nonmedullary cancer.[102]

Cancer of the thyroid before age 15 years represents 1.5% of all malignancies.[78,93] Among girls 15 to 19 years

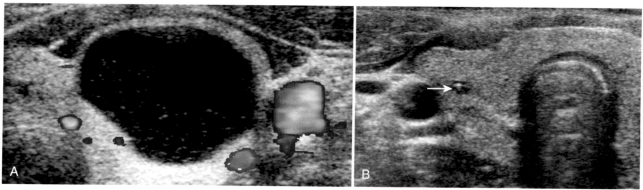

FIGURE 50-39. Thyroid degenerative (colloid) cyst. A, Avascular, well-defined, round, hypoechoic lesion with internal echoes but good through-transmission. **B,** Hypoechoic lesion in right lobe of thyroid demonstrates comet-tail artifact *(arrow).*

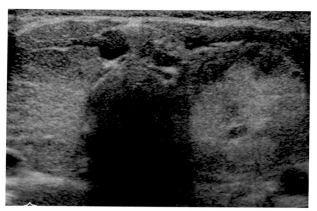

FIGURE 50-40. Multinodular goiter. Thyroid demonstrates heterogeneous hyperechogenic nodule within the left lobe and small, hypoechoic lesions in the isthmus. Enlarged and heterogeneous right lobe also noted.

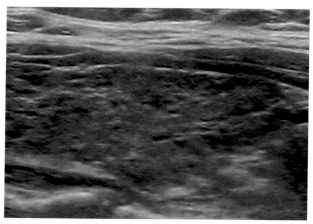

FIGURE 50-41. Multinodular gland from radiation. Right lobe of the thyroid shows multinodular architecture after neck radiation for Ewing's sarcoma.

of age, thyroid cancer is the second most common malignancy.[103] Factors that increase of risk of malignancy include genetic predisposition and radiation exposure, especially in patients with bone marrow transplant.[73] The irradiated thyroid can show a spectrum of abnormalities, from cysts to benign or malignant nodules (Fig. 50-41). Incidence of thyroid cancer after irradiation may increase more than 20-fold, and mean latency period is about 15 years.[96] Risk factors in the presence of radiation include female gender, younger age at irradiation, and longer time since irradiation.[104] Clinically, patients with thyroid cancer present with a palpable nodule or cervical adenopathy and rarely, hoarseness or pain. **Papillary cancer,** the most common pediatric thyroid neoplasm, represents 80% of all cases and can be multicentric in 20% of cases (Fig. 50-42). Metastatic disease with papillary tumor is through the lymphatics. **Follicular cancer** represents 17% of thyroid cancers and metastasizes through the bloodstream. **Medullary cancers,** the remaining 2% to 3%, secrete calcitonin and are typically diagnosed in patients with a strong family history or features of multiple endocrine neoplasia type II (MEN II). At presentation, children with medullary cancer are

usually at an advanced tumor stage, with lymph node involvement in 50% to 80% and metastasis to the lung in 6% to 18%.[78,96,105]

With sonography, it can be difficult to differentiate benign from malignant thyroid masses. Helpful differentiating ultrasound criteria for malignancy include predominantly solid lesion; presence of calcification, especially microcalcifications; hypoechogenicity; irregular margins; large height/width ratio; absence of peripheral halo; intranodular vascularity; and associated abnormal lymph nodes.[106-110] In their study of thyroid lesions in children, however, Lyshchik et al.[103] found that for nodules 15 mm or less in size, the most helpful sonographic findings to support malignancy were irregular tumor outline, subcapsular location, and increased intranodular vascularity. On the other hand, masses larger than 15 mm were difficult to diagnose with sonography, with the only reliable criterion being hypoechogenicity. On sonography, round laminated calcifications can be seen in 35% of papillary cancers. Follicular cancers often mimic adenomas.[99] Adjacent lymph nodes should always be inspected and, in the presence of calcification, are a concern for metastatic disease.

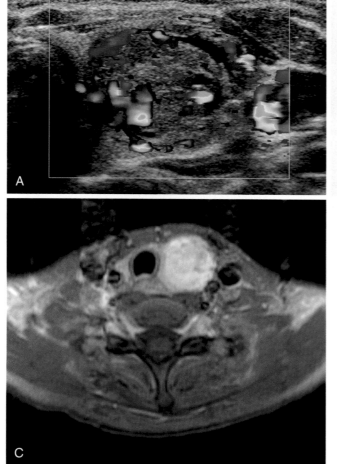

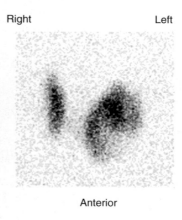

Right   Left

Anterior

B

FIGURE 50-42. **Thyroid cancer, papillary type.** A, Large, subcapsular heterogeneous mass with intranodular vascularity. B, ^{99m}Tc-pertechnetate scan demonstrates cold area in left lobe inferiorly at site of mass. C, Axial T1-weighted postgadolinium MR image shows heterogeneously enhancing mass in left lobe of the thyroid.

MALIGNANT THYROID NODULE: SONOGRAPHIC CHARACTERISTICS

Predominantly solid lesion
Presence of calcification, especially
  microcalcifications
Hypoechogenicity
Irregular margins
Large height/width ratio
Absence of peripheral halo
Intranodular vascularity
Associated abnormal lymph nodes

Nuclear medicine has been used to guide therapy because "cold" nodules on scintigraphy are suspicious for malignancy. Although "hot" nodules on nuclear medicine are usually not malignant, exceptions occur[56,92] (Fig. 50-43). Solid nodules in children should be biopsied and surgically excised to exclude malignancy. In general, thyroid neoplasms (excluding the medullary type) have a good prognosis, with 10-year survival greater than 95% when treated with total thyroidectomy, lymph node dissection, and postoperative iodine therapy.[96]

Other pediatric thyroid neoplasms include **lymphoma** and **teratoma.** In pediatric patients with Hashimoto's thyroiditis and a solitary or multiple hypoechoic lesions, lymphoma should be a primary consideration.[78]

Parathyroid Glands

The parathyroid glands are two paired endocrine glands arising from the third and fourth branchial pouches.[111] **Normal parathyroid tissue** is infrequently identified separate from the thyroid because their echotexture is similar. Sonographic imaging of the parathyroid may be helpful in the presence of primary or secondary **hyperparathyroidism.** Parathyroid **adenomas** are rare in children but the most common cause of primary hyperparathyroidism.[112-114] Children with chronic renal failure may develop a multinodular gland hyperplasia caused by secondary hyperparathyroidism.[115] Ultrasound

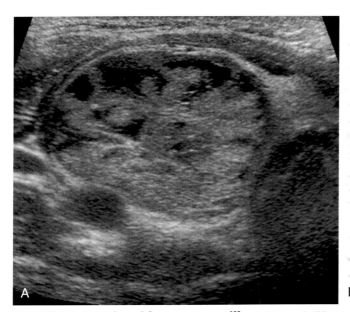

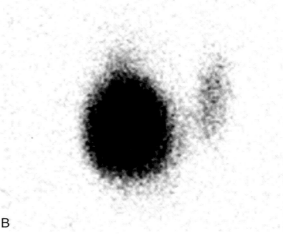

FIGURE 50-43. Thyroid cancer, papillary type. A, Heterogeneous, well-defined right thyroid lobe nodule with peripheral halo, favored to represent follicular adenoma. **B,** ^{99m}Tc-pertechnetate scan demonstrates increased uptake, suggesting hyperfunctioning adenoma. Pathology diagnosis was cancer.

is 80% to 90% sensitive in detecting parathyroid tumors and gland enlargement.[112] The typical sonographic imaging of an adenoma and hyperplasia are similar, appearing as an oblong, sharply demarcated, hypoechoic solid mass aligned craniocaudal and posterior to the thyroid[116] (Fig. 50-44). Less frequently, the mass may be cystic, calcified, multilobular, and giant.[43] Enlargement of the adjacent inferior thyroid artery may be identified as an **arc of vascularity,** providing clues to diagnosis of an adenoma.[117] Because 20% of the parathyroid tissue can be ectopic, MRI may be considered if ultrasound is unsuccessful in identifying the lesion.[118]

Other Lesions of the Visceral Space

Foregut cysts represent defective budding of the respiratory or intestinal tract. **Bronchogenic cysts** are usually mediastinal and rarely may present as a mass in the lower neck.[82,119] **Esophageal cysts** are typically centered close to the esophageal wall. Foregut lesions usually present as a palpable lump but can enlarge rapidly, causing airway obstruction and dysphasia.[120] With sonography, the lesions are typically unilocular but may be complicated by hemorrhage and infection, especially in the presence of persistent communication with the airway or esophagus.

   Laryngoceles are air/fluid-filled dilations of the laryngeal saccule, a small pouch arising from the roof of the laryngeal ventricle.[81] Internal laryngoceles remain within the larynx, whereas external masses project through the thyrohyoid membrane.[121] When the laryngeal saccule is totally obstructed, the outpouching will appear as a smooth-walled anechoic mass projecting into the endolaryngeal or preepiglottic space.[121] In 8% to 10% of cases, laryngoceles develop superimposed infection, and there

is a 15% association with neoplasm.[81] Children typically present with airway obstruction or feeding difficulties.

LACKING DEFINITION BY THE HYOID

The carotid space and deep cervical fascial layers extend above and below the hyoid bone.[13,14] The **carotid space,** enveloped by all three layers, extends from the skull base to aortic arch. Its contents include the internal carotid artery, jugular vein, cranial nerves IX to XII (vagus nerve, X), and deep cervical lymph node chain. The **retropharyngeal and prevertebral spaces** extend from the skull base to the level of the third thoracic (T3) vertebral body. The **danger space** is within the retropharyngeal space where a pathway exists for infection to spread inferiorly into the posterior mediastinum. The retropharyngeal space contains primarily lymph nodes, whereas the prevertebral space contains vertebral bodies, spinal cord, paraspinal and scalene muscles, and vertebral artery and vein. These spaces are not discussed separately because many diseases, especially nodal, involve multiple spaces simultaneously.

Congenital Abnormalities

Branchial Anomalies

The **branchial (pharyngeal) apparatus** develops between the fourth and sixth week of gestation. The structure consists of six pairs of mesodermal **branchial arches** separated by five paired internal endodermal **pharyngeal pouches** and five paired external ectodermal

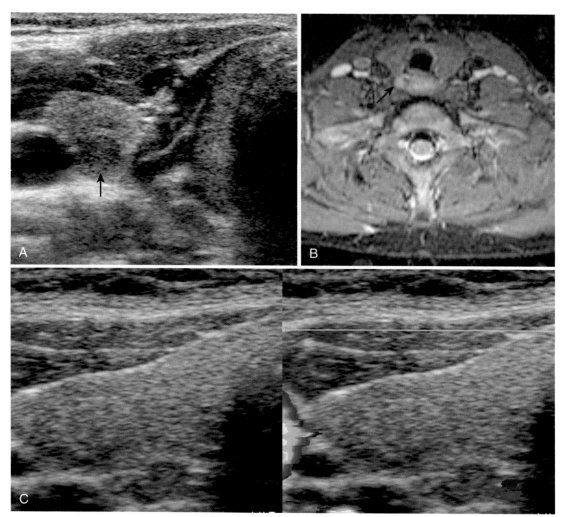

FIGURE 50-44. Parathyroid adenoma and hyperplasia. A, Patient with hyperparathyroidism demonstrates a hypoechoic nodule *(arrow)* posterior to the thyroid gland. **B,** Axial T1-weighted postgadolinium MR image shows enhancing nodule *(arrow)* posterior to right lobe of thyroid. **C,** Patient with renal failure shows hypoechoic lenticular lesions posterior to thyroid, consistent with parathyroid gland hyperplasia.

branchial clefts, or grooves. Table 50-3 lists the origin of structures from the branchial apparatus.[111,122,123] Abnormalities in development of this apparatus may result in the formation of a cyst, sinus tract, or fistula, although most present as cysts.[124,125] Branchial anomalies are the second most common congenital head and neck lesions in children, with the majority arising from the type II apparatus.[125] On sonography, branchial malformations typically appear as a simple or complex cyst with good through-transmission.[126] These lesions are susceptible to hemorrhage or superimposed infection, but predisposition to cancer remains controversial.[81] Treatment of choice is surgical resection.[122]

First branchial anomalies are 8% of all anomalies and present as a cyst or sinuses adjacent to the external auditory canal or parotid gland or along the pinnae, extending to the level of the mandible angle (Fig. 50-45). These lesions can be superficial or deep, even embedded into the parotid gland.[122,127] Some demonstrate a tract to the external auditory canal.

Second branchial anomalies represent 95% of all branchial apparatus malformations; 10% are bilateral.[127,128] Cysts of the type II branchial anomaly result from persistence of the cervical sinus.[122,123,127] During development of the branchial apparatus, the second arch expands downward to meet and merge with the fifth arch, thus covering the second, third, and fourth arches and forming a cervical sinus of His.[111,123] Because of this embryology, many anatomic type II cysts are possible. These cysts are differentiated (Bailey) into four types.[122] Type I is deep to the platysma muscle. Type II, the most common, is anterior to the sternocleidomastoid, posterior to the submandibular gland, and lateral to the carotid sheath (Fig. 50-46). Type III lies between the internal and external carotid arteries, posteromedial to the sternocleidomastoid and lateral to the pharynx. Type IV is adjacent to the pharyngeal wall.

Third and fourth branchial anomalies are rare. Third branchial apparatus cysts are typically located posterior to the carotid artery and jugular vein.[129] Third and fourth anomalies can present as a piriform sinus or fistula. The anatomy of the lesion is primarily a left-sided tract extending from the piriform sinus to the anterior lower neck adjacent to the thyroid.[89,130] Patients may present with recurrent neck infection or suppurative thyroiditis.[89] On sonography, the thyroid often appears heterogeneous because of inflammation from infection. In some cases, there is an air-containing intrathyroid or perithyroid cystic mass, representing a complicating abscess[57] (see Fig. 50-33). CT with oral barium or air is beneficial to define the tract usually inconspicuous on sonography.[89]

Ectopic Thymus

The thymus gland arises in the sixth week of gestation as outpouchings of primarily the third and a small portion of the fourth pharyngeal pouches.[81] Caudal elongation leads to the formation of tubular structures known as the **thymopharyngeal ducts.** By the ninth week, migration followed by obliteration of the duct occurs from the angle of the mandible, along the carotid sheath, to the level of the superior mediastinum because of attachment to the pericardium. The resulting solid masses fuse to form thymus tissue anatomically located below the thyroid gland.[131] Thymic lesions typically present between 2 and 13 years of age as asymptomatic masses. These lesions are more common on the left side and can be located anywhere along the course of descent.[123,131] The ectopic thymus can be differentiated from other masses with sonography because of isoechogenicity with normal thymus, sharp angulated margins, parallel septa, pliability, lack of mass effect, and absence of central hilum with color Doppler imaging[131] (Fig. 50-47). Occasionally, a bridge of tissue can be defined between normal thymus and a cervical mass.[43]

With persistence of the thymopharyngeal duct, a **thymic cyst** may occur.[87,111] Approximately 50% of cervical cysts are in continuity with a mediastinal mass.[43,132] On ultrasound, the lesions are typically large, unilocular or multilocular cysts intimately associated with the

---

TABLE 50-3. SIMPLIFIED CLASSIFICATION OF BRANCHIAL APPARATUS DERIVATIVES*: NORMAL ANATOMIC STRUCTURES FORMED

CLEFT	ARCH	POUCH
1st	EAC	Mandible, muscles of mastication, malleus, incus, auricle eustachian tube, mastoid of EAC, mandibular division cranial nerve V, tympanic cavity
2nd	Rudimentary	Muscles of facial expression, body and lesser horn of the palatine tonsil, hyoid, stapes, cranial nerves VII and VIII
3rd	Rudimentary	Superior constrictor muscles, internal carotid artery, inferior parathyroid, greater horn and body of hyoid, cranial nerve IX, piriform sinus, thymus
4th	Rudimentary	Thyroid and cuneiform cartilage, aortic arch, right superior parathyroid, apex, subclavian artery, laryngeal muscles, cranial nerve X, piriform sinus
5th	Rudimentary	Rudimentary parafollicular cells of thyroid gland
6th	—	Arytenoids and cricoid cartilages and cranial nerve X

EAC, External auditory canal.
Six pairs of branchial arches separated by five paired pharyngeal pouches internally and five paired branchial clefts externally.

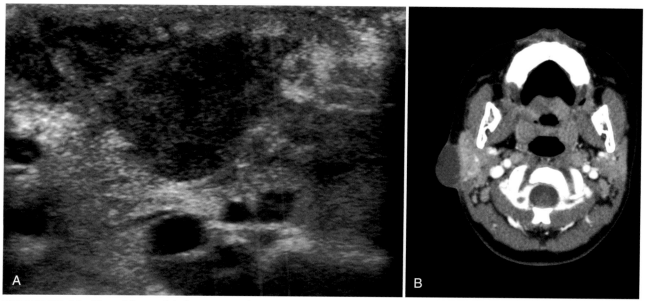

FIGURE 50-45. Type I branchial cyst. A, 7 year old presents with right ear swelling and pain. Longitudinal sonogram demonstrates poorly defined heterogeneous hypoechoic lesion superficial to the parotid gland. **B,** Axial CT scan obtained after 2 weeks of antibiotics confirms well-defined cystic lesion superficial to the parotid, which is enhancing asymmetrically due to resolving inflammation.

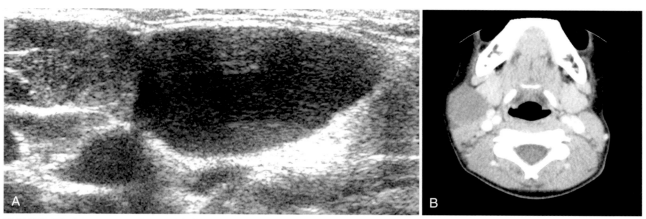

FIGURE 50-46. Type II branchial cyst. A, Unilocular, anechoic, thin-walled cystic lesion with through-transmission in the right neck adjacent to sternocleidomastoid muscle. **B,** Axial CT demonstrates the cyst in typical type II location, posterior to the submandibular gland and anterolateral to the sternocleidomastoid muscle.

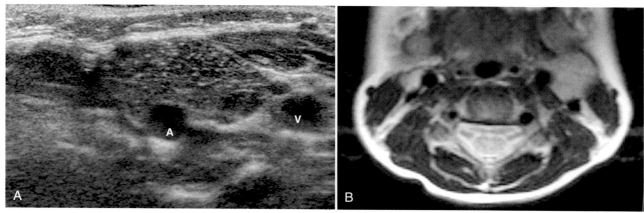

FIGURE 50-47. Ectopic thymus tissue. A, Angular soft tissue mass with thin septae in the carotid space splaying the carotid artery *(A)* and jugular vein *(V)*. **B,** Axial T2-weighted MR image shows soft tissue in the left carotid space, which was equal in signal to thymus in the superior mediastinum.

carotid space, often splaying the carotid artery and jugular vein[122,132] (Fig. 50-48). Intralesional debris can occur in the presence of hemorrhage or infection.[89] There are no reports of associated neoplasm.[81]

Dermoid/Epidermoid

Dermoid/epidermoid lesions represent 7% of head and neck lesions and 25% of midline cervical anomalies.[81,86] These lesions develop when there is inclusion of ectodermal tissue during the fusion of the branchial arches.[123,133] **Dermoid cysts** contain two germ layers, both ectoderm and mesoderm; whereas **epidermoid cysts** consist of only one germ layer, ectoderm.[87,124] Although the majority of these masses are found around the orbit or adjacent to the nose, approximately 11% of these cysts will present in the floor of the mouth in the submandibular space.[81] When imaging the neck, most present as painless midline neck masses in the floor of the mouth, or less often, thyroidal, suprasternal, or suboccipital.[43] Ultrasound of these lesions demonstrates a well-circumscribed, thin-

walled unilocular mass with internal echoes and minimal posterior echo enhancement[43,52] (Fig. 50-49). Surgical resection is recommended because these anomalies are at risk for rupture or infection, and 5% will undergo malignant degeneration to squamous cell neoplasms.[81,86]

Teratomas

Cervical teratomas are rare, occurring in 1 in 40,000 live births but representing 5% to 14% of all neonatal teratomas.[133-135] These lesions are believed to arise from pluripotential cells of two or three germ layers isolated at sites distant to the anatomic site of origin.[54,133] About 90% of childhood teratomas consist of all three germ layers with variable differentiation, and 75% to 85% of head and neck tumors contain neuroectodermal tissue.[133] Most cervical teratomas are benign, with rare malignant diagnosis.[54,135] These lesions typically present as a large, infiltrative cystic and solid mass in the anterior and lateral neck.[12,135] Airway impingement is the most common cause of morbidity; therefore prenatal

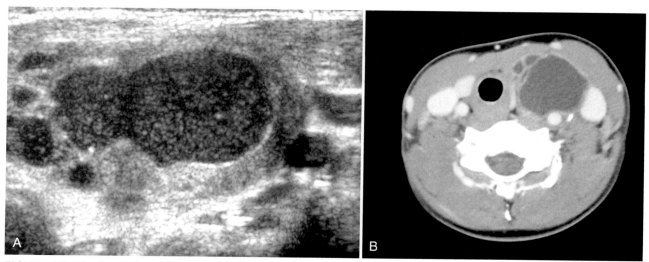

FIGURE 50-48. Complicated thymic cyst. A, Complex cystic mass with septation and thick peripheral wall splaying carotid artery and jugular vein. **B,** Axial CT scan shows complex mass at thoracic inlet displacing thyroid and airway.

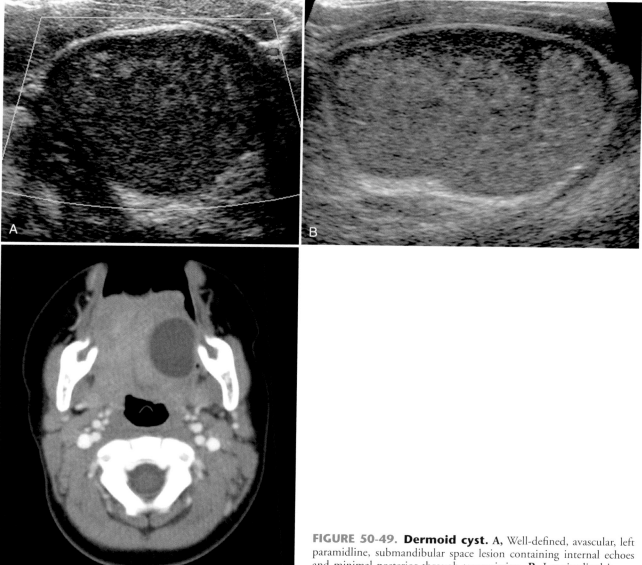

FIGURE 50-49. Dermoid cyst. A, Well-defined, avascular, left paramidline, submandibular space lesion containing internal echoes and minimal posterior through-transmission. **B,** Longitudinal image shows complex internal architecture. **C,** CT image suggests lesion is centered in the left tongue.

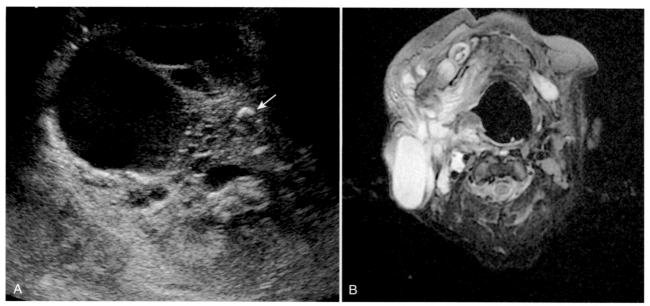

FIGURE 50-50. Cervical teratoma. A, Poor definition of soft tissue planes caused by a complex infiltrative mass containing cystic, solid, and calcified areas *(arrow)*. **B,** Axial T2-weighted MR image shows complex cystic and solid mass infiltrating the parotid, masseter, submandibular, parapharyngeal, and carotid space soft tissues.

identification of the lesion may help define management at delivery.[135,136] Sonography demonstrates a multilocular heterogeneous mass containing solid and cystic components, with calcifications in 50% of cases[135-137] (Fig. 50-50). Prognosis is almost 100% mortality if the lesions are not immediately managed and resected.[136,138]

Vascular Malformations or Tumors

In 1982, Mulliken and Glowacki[50] proposed a new classification, separating vascular anomalies into two groups, tumors versus malformations, based on lesion growth patterns. Vascular lesions that grow in proportion to the child and do not involute are considered **malformations.** Vascular masses that proliferate rapidly and can involute are regarded as **tumors.**[53] **Infantile hemangiomas,** described previously, are considered tumors. It is also significant to note that if one or multiple hemangiomas are present in a trigeminal dermatome distribution, the clinician should consider **PHACES syndrome** (**p**osterior fossa malformations, **h**emangiomas, **a**rterial anomalies, **c**oarctation of aorta and cardiac defects, **e**ye abnormalities, **s**ternal notching).[49]

Vascular malformations represent a spectrum of endothelial lesions ranging from purely vascular to lymphatic. Vascular malformations consist of combined, lymphatic, capillary, venous, and arterial elements.[50] These malformations can be further subdivided based on flow. **Fast-flow malformations** mainly contain arterial components. All other types are considered **slow–flow malformations.**[53] Gray-scale and color and duplex Doppler ultrasound can help determine whether the anomaly is cystic or solid and can identify the presence of high-flow

BINARY CLASSIFICATION OF VASCULAR ANOMALIES

TUMORS
Hemangioma
Hemangioendothelioma
Angiosarcoma
Miscellaneous

MALFORMATIONS
Slow Flow
Capillary
Lymphatic
Venous

Fast Flow
Arterial
Combined

From International Society for the Study of Vascular Anomalies.

vessels.[55] CT scans may be helpful when a patient cannot be sedated, to evaluate for intralesional calcification and bone changes. Because of soft tissue definition, multiplanar capabilities, and ability to define high-flow vessels, MRI is the preferred imaging modality for vascular malformations.[50,55]

Lymphatic malformations, originating from sequestered embryonic lymph sac, are composed of primitive lymphatic spaces of varying sizes separated by connective tissue stroma.[122] Formerly, microcystic lesions were termed "lymphangiomas" and macrocystic anomalies

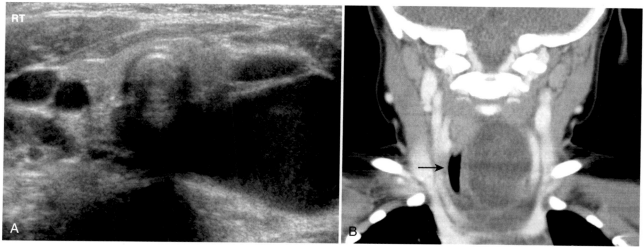

FIGURE 50-51. Lymphatic malformation. A, Multilocular cystic lesion extending posterior to the left lobe of the thyroid and distorting the airway. **B,** Coronal reformatted CT demonstrates a multilocular cystic mass in the left neck causing rightward compression and narrowing of the airway *(arrow).*

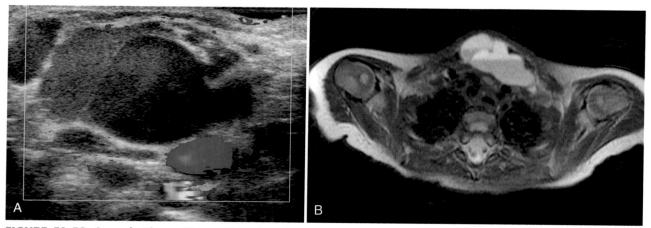

FIGURE 50-52. Lymphatic malformation. A, Infiltrative hypovascular multilocular cystic lesion with internal echoes. **B,** Axial T2-weighted MR image shows multiseptated cystic lesion containing fluid-fluid levels consistent with prior hemorrhage.

called "cystic hygromas." However, it is now believed that lesion cyst size is likely caused by the *stromal environment* rather than lesion behavior.[87] These terms are outdated and should be considered together under lymphatic malformations. Some lymphatic malformations are diagnosed prenatally, with 90% presenting by age 2 years.[49] Clinically, the skin is usually normal but may have a bluish hue, puckering, or tiny vesicles.[49,55] These lesions can be diffuse or focal, tend to invade multiple anatomic facial planes, and will rapidly enlarge if complicated by hemorrhage or infection. Hypertrophy and intraosseous invasion of adjacent bone, usually the mandible, can occur.

About 75% of lymphatic lesions occur in the neck, and most originate within the posterior triangle or oral cavity, with lesions occurring on the left side twice as often as on the right side.[43,53,69] Of infants with lymphatic malformations, 3% to 10% have airway compromise from respiratory obstruction or mediastinal extension.[49,52,54]

Although most children with lymphatic malformation have a normal karyotype, several syndromes are associated (e.g., Turner, Down, Noonan, Roberts), as well as trisomy 13 and 18.[124] On ultrasound, most lymphatic malformations are multiloculated cystic masses with septa of variable thickness and solid components[52] (Fig. 50-51). Fluid-fluid levels or echogenic debris can result from superimposed hemorrhage or infection (Fig. 50-52). MRI provides the optimum tissue characterization and anatomy of the lesion before surgical intervention.[139] Surgical resection is the treatment of choice but can be difficult if the lesion invades neural, vascular, and muscular structures; therefore sclerotherapy, radiofrequency ablation, and laser therapy are other options.[53,139]

Venous malformations are soft, compressible lesions that may distend with increased venous pressure (Valsalva maneuver). About 40% of these lesions present in the head and neck, and many invade multiple fascial planes and involve osseous structures.[55] These lesions,

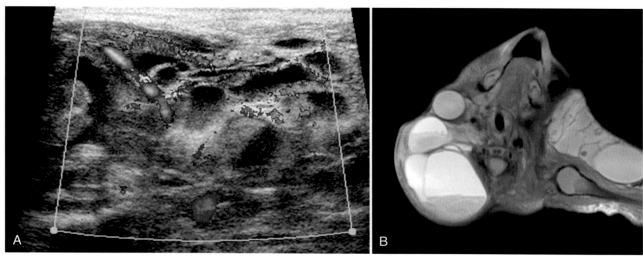

FIGURE 50-53. Venolymphatic malformation in patient with Klippel-Trénaunay syndrome. A, Multiple small, cystic areas and infiltrating soft tissue with anomalous vessels on color Doppler sonogram in neonate. **B,** Axial proton-density MRI 3 months later shows bilateral neck involvement and enlargement of the cystic spaces, now containing fluid-fluid levels related to prior hemorrhage.

appearing clinically as soft, bluish, compressible masses, consist of thin-walled, dilated, dysplastic, small and large venous channels deficient in smooth muscle.[43] Rapid enlargement may occur secondary to phlebothrombosis.[49] These malformations have been seen in conjunction with intracranial venous anomalies,[140] blue rubber bleb nevus, and Maffucci's syndrome. **Klippel-Trénaunay** and **Sturge-Weber** (Parkes Weber) syndromes have combined capillary and lymphatic components (Fig. 50-53). **Phleboliths** are present in 16% of cases and can help confirm the diagnosis. Ultrasound demonstrates hypoechoic lesions with heterogeneous architecture. Acoustic shadowing secondary to phleboliths and fluid-fluid levels may be identified[53] (Fig. 50-54). On Doppler sonography, venous low-velocity flow is identified. Treatment includes elastic compression, sclerotherapy, and surgical excision.[49]

Arteriovenous malformations (AVMs) represent collections of abnormal, thin-walled vessels connecting dilated feeding arteries to draining veins. These lesions may be centered in cutaneous, muscular, or intraosseous structures. Clinically, a blush hyperemia and thrill or bruit may be present. AVMs can enlarge acutely from increased blood flow, obstruction, or infection. An extensive lesion may cause congestive heart failure.[49] AVMs also are affected by hormones, often increasing in size at puberty and during pregnancy.[53] The most common sites of origin include the cheek, followed by the ear, nose, and forehead.[43] On gray-scale ultrasound, AVMs demonstrate heterogeneity, with multiple hypoechoic channels and absence of soft tissue mass. Doppler sonograms show a high-flow lesion with low-resistance arteries and arterialized venous waveforms[52] (Fig. 50-55). Transcatheter embolization, sclerotherapy, and surgical excision are the mainstays of management.[49,53]

Inflammatory Disease

Lymph Nodes

Lymph nodes consist of an outer cortex of lymphoid follicles and hilum containing lymphatic sinus, connective tissue, and blood vessels. Cervical lymph nodes, which number about 300, are located along the lymphatic vessels in the neck.[141] For ultrasound examinations, lymph node distribution can be classified according to eight regions[141,142] (Fig. 50-56). A normal infant lymph node measures less than 3 mm in diameter.[43] In children, lymph nodes larger than 1 cm in maximum dimension are considered enlarged.[142] On ultrasound, a normal node is ovoid in shape and hypoechoic, with an echogenic hilum containing central vascularity (Fig. 50-57). The normal length exceeds its width by 2:1.[64]

Lymph nodes can enlarge as a result of reactive hyperplasia, infection or inflammation, and malignancy.[143] Cervical lymphadenopathy is common and frequently a normal finding in children. From 47% to 55% of children at all ages and 80% to 90% of children between ages 4 and 8 years have palpable reactive hyperplastic lymph nodes not originating from infection or systemic illness. Palpable lymph nodes in infants, however, are not normal and should be evaluated further. **Supraclavicular lymphadenopathy** is highly significant, associated with malignancy in 60% of cases.[128,143]

Acute lymph node enlargement in children can be unilateral or bilateral. The anterior cervical nodes, which drain the mouth and pharynx, are most often affected.[128] In 80% of cases, acute unilateral pyogenic lymphadenitis is secondary to *Staphylococcus aureus* or group A beta-hemolytic streptococci.[64,128,144] Many patients present with respiratory tract infection, pharyngitis, tonsillitis, or

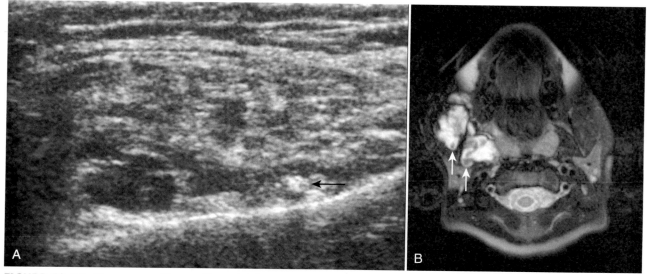

FIGURE 50-54. Venous malformation. A, Masseter muscle demonstrates round, hypoechoic areas and hyperechoic foci *(arrow)* with shadowing, consistent with phleboliths. **B,** Axial T2-weighted fat-saturated MR image demonstrates high signal lesion infiltrating the masseter muscle and parapharyngeal space. Dark foci are consistent with phleboliths *(arrows).*

otitis media in conjunction with tender, warm, and erythematous lymph nodes.

The etiology of **bilateral cervical lymphadenopathy** tends to be viral.[144] Viral infections, such as **Epstein-Barr virus** (EBV), however, can be difficult to differentiate from bacterial infections because the infection may be associated with exudative tonsillitis. In a patient with EBV, the presence of diffuse lymphadenopathy and hepatosplenomegaly may help confirm the diagnosis.[12] Noting the age of the child and the sites involved may provide other clues[145] (Tables 50-4 and 50-5).

The diagnosis of lymphadenitis is often clinical, and most cases are uncomplicated; therefore most patients are treated medically and require no additional imaging. If imaging is performed, key features include location, extent of cellulitis, myositis, presence of abscess, and vascular compromise.[124] With ultrasound imaging, **lymphadenitis** demonstrates multiple enlarged lymph nodes, normal in shape but with reduced echogenicity and increased central and peripheral vascularity[64,124,146] (Fig. 50-58). With progressive enlargement of the nodes and **cellulitis,** there is blurring of soft tissue planes, some septa may stand out, and Doppler imaging shows increased blood flow[45] (Fig. 50-59). When an **abscess** forms, the nodes coalesce, central vascularity disappears, and a hypoechoic center is noted, surrounded by a thick, hyperechoic, irregular capsule that is hypervascular[5] (Fig. 50-60). Pus fluid levels, fluid movement on Doppler ultrasound, and hyperechoic foci with comet-tail artifacts, signifying air, help confirm the diagnosis.[64] FNA and surgical incision may be necessary to resolve the infection.[128] In severe cases, sinus tracts and fistulas may develop.[45]

Subacute or chronic infection occurs when cervical lymph nodes enlarge slowly and are only minimally tender without significant associated cellulitis. Differential diagnosis includes viral, bacterial, atypical mycobacterial, or *Mycobacterium tuberculosis* infection; cat-scratch disease; and other, rare entities.[128] Most **mycobacterial infections** are caused by variant strains of *Mycobacterium avium-intracellulare scrofulaceum* (MAIS) complex.[128] Infection is typically unilateral and in children ages 1 to 5 years. *M. tuberculosis,* when it involves the cervical nodes, is thought to represent an extension of the primary pulmonary lesion or to be associated with acquired immunodeficiency syndrome (AIDS).[45] Nodes on sonography with low attenuation centers and small calcifications should suggest mycobacterial infection.[61,124] **Cat-scratch disease**, caused by the organism *Bartonella henselae,* presents typically with a dominant unilateral node 2 to 4 weeks after a minor cat scratch, usually a kitten[128] (Fig. 50-61). FNA for cytopathology and culture may help confirm the diagnosis.[45] Because malignancy may present similarly, persistence of a dominant lymph node for longer than 6 to 8 weeks despite appropriate antibiotic therapy indicates excisional biopsy.[128]

Other inflammatory causes of lymphadenopathy in children include collagen vascular disease, sarcoid, immunologic deficiencies (especially HIV), and postvaccination syndrome.[145] **Kawasaki's disease,** a multisystem vasculitis of unknown cause, causes cervical adenopathy in 50% to 70% of patients with the disease.[147] Children with Kawasaki's disease typically present before 5 years of age with enlarged nodes greater than 1.5 cm in diameter.[147]

Fibromatosis Coli

Fibromatosis coli occurs in 0.3% to 1.9% of children. The etiology is still unclear but may involve

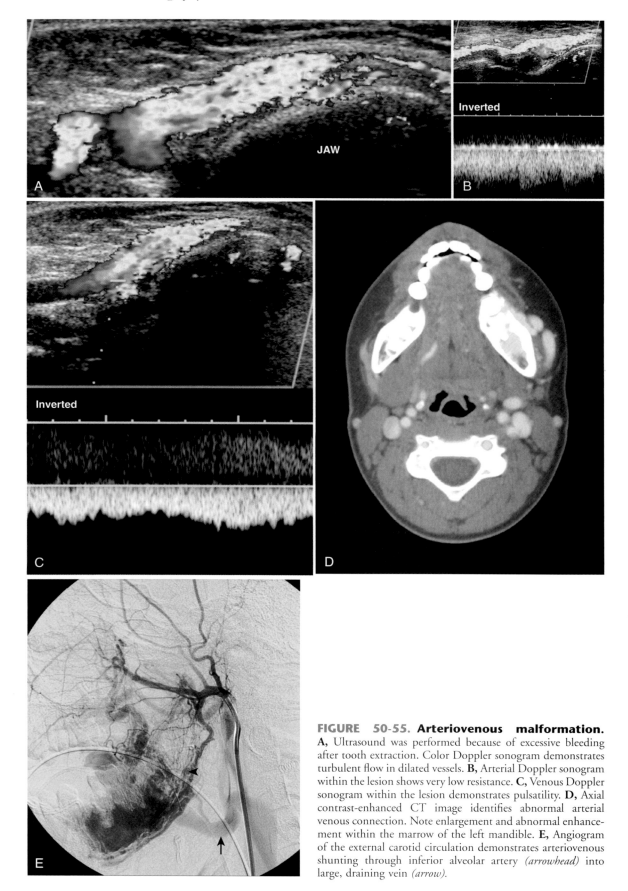

FIGURE 50-55. Arteriovenous malformation. **A,** Ultrasound was performed because of excessive bleeding after tooth extraction. Color Doppler sonogram demonstrates turbulent flow in dilated vessels. **B,** Arterial Doppler sonogram within the lesion shows very low resistance. **C,** Venous Doppler sonogram within the lesion demonstrates pulsatility. **D,** Axial contrast-enhanced CT image identifies abnormal arterial venous connection. Note enlargement and abnormal enhancement within the marrow of the left mandible. **E,** Angiogram of the external carotid circulation demonstrates arteriovenous shunting through inferior alveolar artery *(arrowhead)* into large, draining vein *(arrow).*

intramuscular hemorrhage, venous occlusion, birth trauma, or in utero torticollis.[69,124,128,148] Pathologically, fibromatosis coli results from fibrosis and shortening of the sternocleidomastoid muscle, producing a soft tissue mass.[149] Peak incidence of presentation is 2 to 8 weeks after birth. Fibromatosis coli typically affects the first-born boy with breech presentation or difficult delivery. Most infants present with ipsilateral head tilt, contralateral chin deviation, and a palpable soft tissue mass.[150,151]

From 6% to 20% of patients will have associated musculoskeletal anomalies, including hip dysplasia and facial asymmetry.[57]

Sonography is the best technique to image the fibromatosis coli lesion. A normal sternocleidomastoid muscle demonstrates decreased echogenicity and long, thin, echogenic lines denoting the muscle fascicles along the length of the muscle. In the presence of fibromatosis coli, there is a focal or diffuse enlargement of the

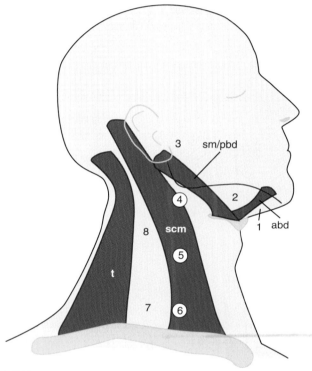

FIGURE 50-56. Cervical lymph node classification. *1,* Submental; *2,* submandibular; *3,* parotid; *4,* upper cervical, suprahyoid, along internal jugular chain; *5,* middle cervical; *6,* lower cervical; *7,* supraclavicular; *8,* posterior triangle; *t,* trapezius muscle; *scm,* sternocleidomastoid; *sm/pbd,* stylohyoid and posterior belly of digastric muscle; *abd,* anterior belly of digastric muscle.

TABLE 50-4. AGE AND CAUSES OF LYMPHADENOPATHY

PEDIATRIC CATEGORY	COMMON INFECTIOUS CAUSES
Newborn	*Staphylococcus aureus* most common Occasionally, late-onset group B streptococci
Infant and child <5 years	Group A streptococci and *S. aureus* Nontuberculous *Mycobacterium*
School-age child and adolescent	Epstein-Barr virus, cytomegalovirus, toxoplasmosis Tuberculosis or infectious mononucleosis

TABLE 50-5. SITE OF NODE AND CAUSES OF LYMPHADENOPATHY

NODE SITE	COMMON CAUSES
Occipital	Roseola, rubella, scalp infections
Periauricular	Eye infections, cat-scratch disease
Cervical	Streptococcal or staphylococcal adenitis or tonsillitis Mononucleosis, toxoplasmosis, malignancies, Kawasaki's disease
Submandibular	Hodgkin's or non-Hodgkin's lymphoma, tuberculosis, histoplasmosis

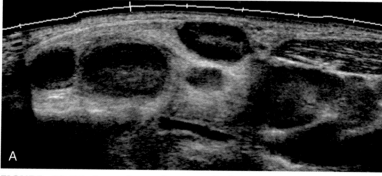
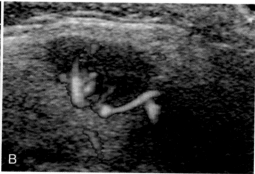

FIGURE 50-57. Lymph node morphology. A, Panoramic scan of multiple borderline lymph nodes, ovoid in shape and hypoechoic, with an echogenic hilum. **B,** Color Doppler sonogram demonstrates central hilar vessels.

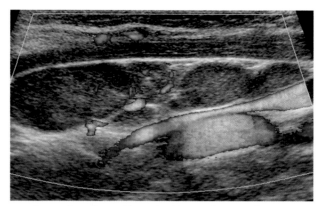

FIGURE 50-58. Lymphadenopathy related to Epstein-Barr virus. Left anterior cervical chain demonstrates multiple enlarged hypoechoic nodes with peripheral vascularity.

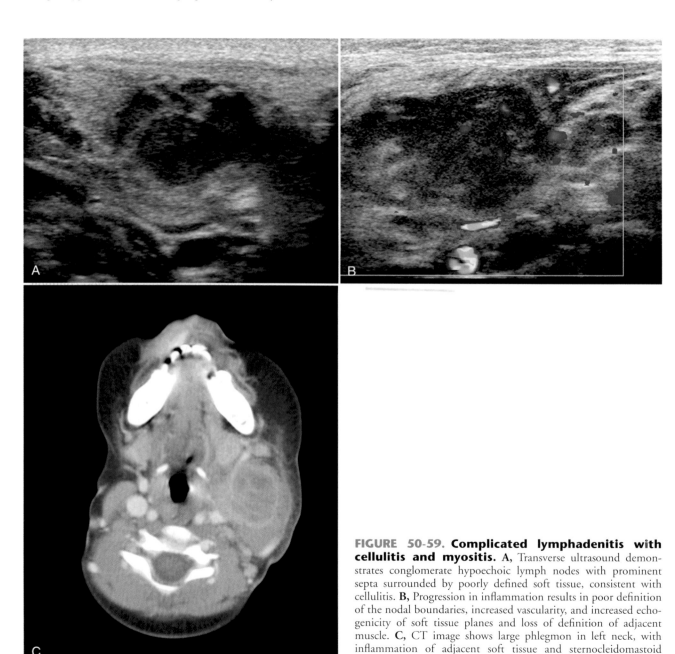

FIGURE 50-59. Complicated lymphadenitis with cellulitis and myositis. A, Transverse ultrasound demonstrates conglomerate hypoechoic lymph nodes with prominent septa surrounded by poorly defined soft tissue, consistent with cellulitis. **B,** Progression in inflammation results in poor definition of the nodal boundaries, increased vascularity, and increased echogenicity of soft tissue planes and loss of definition of adjacent muscle. **C,** CT image shows large phlegmon in left neck, with inflammation of adjacent soft tissue and sternocleidomastoid muscle.

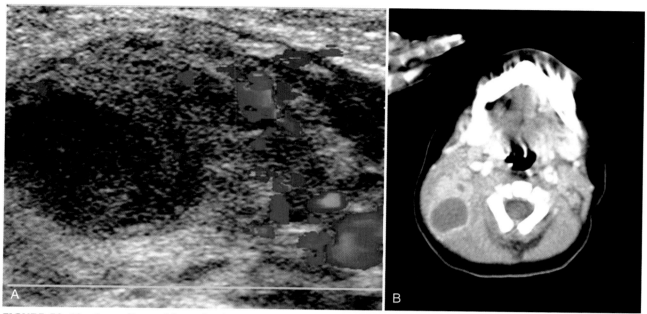

FIGURE 50-60. Complicated lymphadenitis with abscess. A, Color Doppler sonogram shows round, hypoechoic, avascular area with thick wall and peripheral vascularity. **B,** Axial contrast-enhanced CT image shows low-density lesion with peripheral wall enhancement, confirmed as abscess.

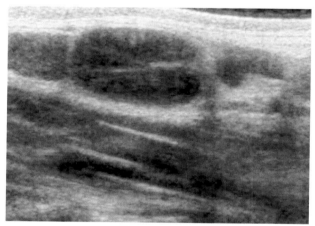

FIGURE 50-61. Cat-scratch lymphadenopathy. Imaging of the left anterior cervical neck in a child who was scratched by a kitten 2 weeks earlier. Multiple hypoechoic enlarged lymph nodes are identified.

sternocleidomastoid, which typically shows homogeneous or heterogeneous, increased echogenicity; however, mixed and hypoechoic lesions have been described[148,149] (Fig. 50-62). Focal lesions tend to involve the inferior third of the muscle.[148] In larger masses, there is distorted architecture with disruption of the normal muscle bundles.[149] Some cases may resolve spontaneously; however, physical therapy is the first line of therapy and effective in 95% of children.[57] If head tilt persists, muscle release or tenotomy is performed to prevent development of significant craniofacial asymmetry and scoliosis.[12]

Neoplasms

Cancers of the head and neck represent 5% of childhood cancers.[128] Lymphomas and sarcomas encompass 50% of these neoplasms. The most common cancers in children under 6 years are neuroblastoma, lymphoma, and rhabdomyosarcoma. Between ages 7 and 13 years, lymphoma, thyroid cancer, and rhabdomyosarcomas are prevalent. After puberty, lymphoma is the most common neoplasm.[128]

Imaging usually cannot differentiate reactive, inflammatory, or neoplastic disease.[124,130,142] Clinical concerns for neoplasm include onset in neonatal period, rapid growth, skin ulceration, fixation to skin, and large, hard masses.[144] With ultrasound, suspicious findings have been defined. Tumor invasion generally starts in the cortex, so changes in the normal nodal shape from ovoid to round or asymmetrical is a concern.[43] Other imaging clues to malignant diagnosis include large size (>3 cm), heterogeneous echotexture, lack of echogenic hilum, perinodal invasion, and lack of soft tissue edema and matted nodes.[135,136] Necrosis and calcification can be a sign of malignancy, but similar findings are noted in granulomatous lesions.[135]

Color Doppler sonography of lymph nodes can be helpful when classified into four categories: hilar, peripheral, mixed, and avascular.[123,134] Color Doppler sonograms of benign lesions are typically avascular or hilar; whereas malignant nodes demonstrate peripheral or mixed vascular flow[93,134,135] (Fig. 50-63). High Doppler resistive indices and pulsatility index have been noted in neoplastic adenopathy; however, other studies have not supported this finding. Therefore, the accuracy of this

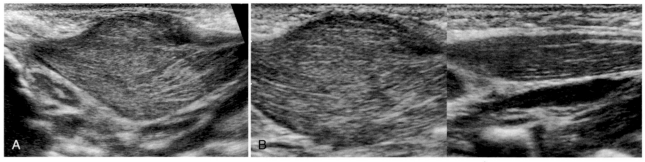

FIGURE 50-62. Fibromatosis coli. A, Longitudinal ultrasound shows sternocleidomastoid muscle with enlargement, attenuation of striations, and mild increase in echotexture. **B,** Longitudinal view shows comparison of abnormal left and normal right sternocleidomastoid muscle.

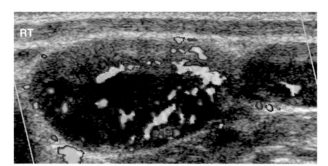

FIGURE 50-63. Hodgkin's lymphoma. Color Doppler ultrasound demonstrates mixed and peripheral arrangement of vessels.

technique is controversial.[123] Ultrasound is useful in guiding FNA biopsy.[135,138]

Lymphoma

Lymphoma is the most common head and neck malignancy, accounting for 50% in children. There is an equal 50% distribution of Hodgkin's lymphoma and non-Hodgkin's lymphoma.[124] **Hodgkin's lymphoma** typically presents in adolescence as upper cervical and less frequently supraclavicular masses.[130,152] **Non-Hodgkin's lymphoma** usually presents between ages 2 and 12 years with extranodal masses, diffuse nodal involvement, and rapid growth.[130,152] On gray-scale ultrasound, lymphoma often demonstrates a hypoechoic, pseudocystic appearance with sharp borders caused by reduced fat in lymph nodes, and absence of calcifications[153] (Fig. 50-64). Lymphomas do not necessarily follow malignant color vascular distribution, often with exaggerated hilar flow containing large, central branching vessels.[153] Extensive axillary and mediastinal adenopathy may be noted at presentation.[124] Imaging of these patients should include CT scans of the neck, chest, and abdomen and pelvis. Gallium-67 citrate scintigraphy and FDG-PET is also helpful in further depiction of disease extent.[152] Positron emission tomography (PET) and CT scans may also be considered in the future.

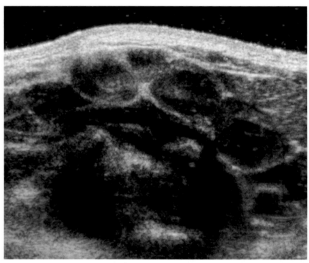

FIGURE   50-64. Hodgkin's   lymphoma. Multiple enlarged hypoechoic, pseudocystic lymph nodes demonstrate well-defined borders. The largest has a round configuration. No adjacent soft tissue edema noted.

Metastatic Nodal Disease

Metastatic nodal disease is uncommon in pediatrics.[124] Neuroblastoma, rhabdomyosarcoma, and thyroid cancer are the most likely etiologies. **Neuroblastoma,** a neoplasm derived from the sympathetic neural crest cells, typically metastasizes to the head and neck from a primary adrenal tumor.[69] Metastatic nodal disease is most common to the supraclavicular chain.[64] Primary cervical lesions are noted in 5% of cases and typically have a favorable prognosis.[146,154] Presenting symptoms include Horner syndrome and heterochromia (two different-colored eyes).[154] Ultrasound typically demonstrates an echogenic mass with or without calcification that displaces the great vessels of the neck and may extend into the mediastinum, spine, or skull base[154] (Fig. 50-65). Thyroid nodal metastases are typically identified in the low neck and supraclavicular area.[155] On sonography, thyroid nodal disease demonstrates the same neoplastic findings previously described, as well as

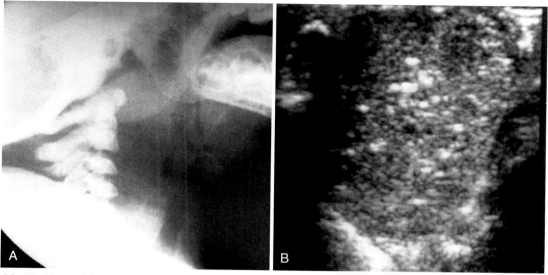

FIGURE 50-65. Neuroblastoma. A, Lateral neck with increased retropharyngeal soft tissues in 1-year-old child with difficulty breathing. **B,** Ultrasound shows mass with fine calcification, typical of neuroblastoma.

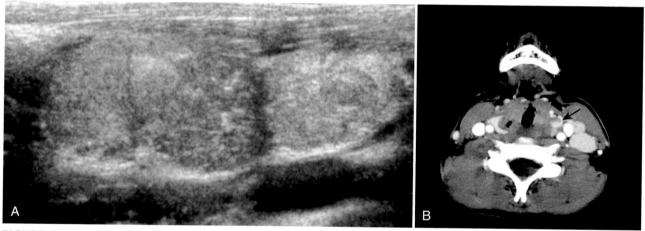

FIGURE 50-66. Lymph node metastasis from thyroid cancer. A, Enlarged conglomerate nodes with internal foci of increased echogenicity, consistent with microcalcification. **B,** Axial CT scan shows intensely enhancing lower cervical lymph nodes with subtle mass in the left lobe of the thyroid (arrow).

increased echogenicity and cystic degeneration, with greater than 50% containing internal calcifications[141,155] (Fig. 50-66).

Rhabdomyosarcoma

Rhabdomyosarcoma is a malignant tumor that arises from skeletal muscle cells. It is the most common soft tissue sarcoma of childhood, and 40% of cases originate in the head and neck.[124,156] About 85% of patients with rhabdomyosarcoma are under age 15 years.[157] A bimodal peak incidence occurs between 1 and 3 years and in early adolescence.[64] The two main histologic types are embryonal and alveolar.[156] **Embryonal rhabdomyosarcoma** represents 60% of cases, is most common in the young child, and frequently arises in the head and neck.[157,158] **Alveolar rhabdomyosarcoma,** 20% of tumors, are more common in the older child and have a poorer prognosis. The most common sites of origin include the orbit, nasopharynx, middle ear or mastoid, and sinonasal cavity. These tumors tend to be aggressive, metastasize to lymph nodes, and rapidly invade bone, often with intracranial extension. Because of this aggressive course, MRI and CT scans are typically the first line of imaging. If a lesion is detected with ultrasound, however, the tumors typically are poorly vascularized and heterogeneous, with ill-defined hypoechoic areas caused by necrosis.[64] If the mass is discovered on ultrasound, CT and MRI scans are necessary to define the full extent of the lesion and exclude intracranial extension.[69]

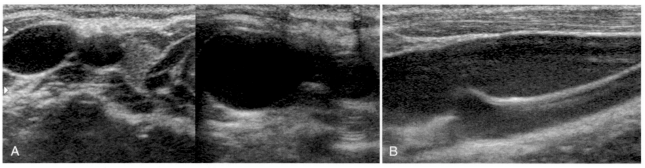

FIGURE 50-67. Internal jugular phlebectasia. A, Child was referred for bluish pulsation beneath the skin. Ultrasound through the carotid and jugular. On the left, imaging is without Valsalva, and on the right, with Valsalva. Note the dilation of the jugular vein with Valsalva. **B,** Longitudinal image shows aneurysmal dilation of the jugular vein.

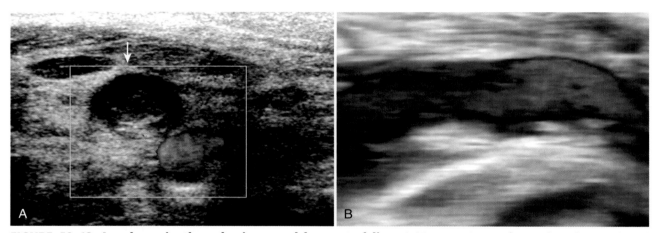

FIGURE 50-68. Jugular vein thrombosis caused by central line. A, Transverse image of internal jugular vein *(arrow)* with thrombus occlusion at tip of catheter. **B,** Three-dimensional ultrasound image shows complete occlusion of the vessel by clot.

Vascular Anomalies

Congenital Abnormalities

Cervical aortic arch is a rare congenital anomaly in which the arch is positioned high, usually in the right neck. These patients may present with a pulsatile anechoic mass, dysphasia, and respiratory symptoms.[43] **Internal jugular phlebectasia** is believed to represent a congenital fusiform dilation of the internal jugular vein.[43,159] The lesion typically presents with a swelling of the neck that increases with straining. Ultrasound demonstrates an echo-free, slow-flow vessel on color Doppler sonography that increases in size with Valsalva maneuver[159] (Fig. 50-67).

Iatrogenic Abnormalities

Color and duplex Doppler ultrasound are noninvasive techniques that provide information about blood vessel patency, size, and direction of blood flow.[160-162] Vascular lines are typically placed through the subclavian or jugular vein into the superior vena cava. Gray-scale and color Doppler sonograms well demonstrate **arterial** and **venous stenosis, thrombosis,** or **pseudoaneurysms,** which can result from central line placement or prior extracorporeal membrane oxygenation (ECMO) therapy[163] (Fig. 50-68). Ultrasound guidance has also proved useful for insertion of central venous and ECMO catheters to prevent morbidity related to malposition.[164-166]

Inflammatory Disease

Lemierre's syndrome is rare and typically occurs in an adolescence after a primary oropharyngeal infection. It is hypothesized that **thrombophlebitis** of tonsillar veins propagate into the internal jugular vein, resulting in *Fusobacterium* **septicemia** and **septic emboli,** primarily to the lungs.[167] Ultrasound demonstrates an engorged, noncompressible vein that may contain echogenic thrombus (Fig. 50-69). Color Doppler ultrasound can document absent flow, and duplex Doppler imaging may show a lack of pulsation with Valsalva maneuver. Blood cultures and chest radiography or CT scan secure the diagnosis so that appropriate antibiotic therapy may be instituted.[168]

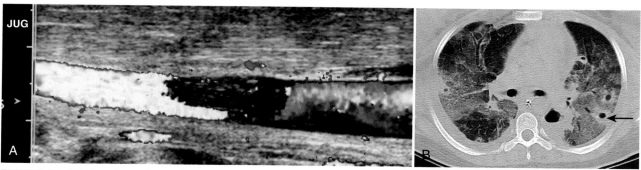

FIGURE 50-69. Lemierre's syndrome. A, Color Doppler sonogram of the internal jugular vein demonstrates occlusive clot within the lumen. **B,** Axial chest CT image shows bilateral parenchymal disease with multiple areas of nodular cavitation (largest denoted with *arrow*) caused by septic emboli.

References

Normal Cervical Anatomy

1. Koch BL. Avoiding sedation in pediatric radiology. Pediatr Radiol 2008;38(Suppl 2):225-226.
2. Pappas JN, Donnelly LF, Frush DP. Reduced frequency of sedation of young children with multisection helical CT. Radiology 2000;215:897-899.
3. Reed MH. Imaging utilization commentary: a radiology perspective. Pediatr Radiol 2008;38(Suppl 4):660-663.
4. Strauss KJ, Kaste SC. The ALARA (as low as reasonably achievable) concept in pediatric interventional and fluoroscopic imaging: striving to keep radiation doses as low as possible during fluoroscopy of pediatric patients—a white paper executive summary. Radiology 2006;240:621-622.
5. Glasier CM, Seibert JJ, Williamson SL, et al. High resolution ultrasound characterization of soft tissue masses in children. Pediatr Radiol 1987;17:233-237.
6. Oestreich AE. Ultrasound imaging of musculoskeletal and superficial tissues in infants and children. Appl Radiol 1984:83-93.
7. Chodosh PL, Silbey R, Oen KT. Diagnostic use of ultrasound in diseases of the head and neck. Laryngoscope 1980;90:814-821.
8. Friedman AP, Haller JO, Goodman JD, Nagar H. Sonographic evaluation of non-inflammatory neck masses in children. Radiology 1983;147:693-697.
9. Sherman NH, Rosenberg HK, Heyman S, Templeton J. Ultrasound evaluation of neck masses in children. J Ultrasound Med 1985;4:127-134.
10. Kraus R, Han BK, Babcock DS, Oestreich AE. Sonography of neck masses in children. AJR Am J Roentgenol 1986;146:609-613.
11. Reede DL, Whelan MA, Bergeron RT. CT of the soft tissue structures of the neck. Radiol Clin North Am 1984;22:239-250.
12. Malik A, Odita J, Rodriguez J, Hardjasudarma M. Pediatric neck masses: a pictorial review for practicing radiologists. Curr Probl Diagn Radiol 2002;31:146-157.
13. Harnsberger HR, Osborn AG. Differential diagnosis of head and neck lesions based on their space of origin. 1. The suprahyoid part of the neck. AJR Am J Roentgenol 1991;157:147-154.
14. Smoker WR, Harnsberger HR. Differential diagnosis of head and neck lesions based on their space of origin. 2. The infrahyoid portion of the neck. AJR Am J Roentgenol 1991;157:155-159.
15. Bergeron RT. Historical perspective: differential diagnosis of head and neck lesions. Parts I and II. AJNR Am J Neuroradiol 2001;22:1628-1629.

Suprahyoid Space

16. Currarino G, Votteler TP. Lesions of the accessory parotid gland in children. Pediatr Radiol 2006;36:1-7; quiz 84-85.
17. Lowe LH, Stokes LS, Johnson JE, et al. Swelling at the angle of the mandible: imaging of the pediatric parotid gland and periparotid region. Radiographics 2001;21:1211-1227.
18. Bialek EJ, Jakubowski W, Karpinska G. Role of ultrasonography in diagnosis and differentiation of pleomorphic adenomas. Work in progress. Arch Otolaryngol Head Neck Surg 2003;129:929-933.
19. Howlett DC. High resolution ultrasound assessment of the parotid gland. Br J Radiol 2003;76:271-277.
20. Weissman JL, Carrau RL. Anterior facial vein and submandibular gland together: predicting the histology of submandibular masses with CT or MR imaging. Radiology 1998;208:441-446.
21. Garcia CJ, Flores PA, Arce JD, et al. Ultrasonography in the study of salivary gland lesions in children. Pediatr Radiol 1998;28:418-425.
22. Ching AS, Ahuja AT. High-resolution sonography of the submandibular space: anatomy and abnormalities. AJR Am J Roentgenol 2002;179:703-708.
23. Yasumoto M, Inoue H, Ohashi I, et al. Simple new technique for sonographic measurement of the thyroid in neonates and small children. J Clin Ultrasound 2004;32:82-85.
24. McQuone SJ. Acute viral and bacterial infections of the salivary glands. Otolaryngol Clin North Am 1999;32:793-811.
25. Thoeny HC. Imaging of salivary gland tumours. Cancer Imaging 2007;7:52-62.
26. Mehta D, Willging JP. Pediatric salivary gland lesions. Semin Pediatr Surg 2006;15:76-84.
27. Saarinen RT, Kolho KL, Pitkaranta A. Cases presenting as parotid abscesses in children. Int J Pediatr Otorhinolaryngol 2007;71:897-901.
28. Myer C, Cotton RT. Salivary gland disease in children: a review. Part 1. Acquired non-neoplastic disease. Clin Pediatr (Phila) 1986;25:314-322.
29. Som PM, Shugar JM, Train JS, Biller HF. Manifestations of parotid gland enlargement: radiographic, pathologic, and clinical correlations. Part II. The diseases of Mikulicz syndrome. Radiology 1981;141:421-426.
30. Bianchi A, Cudmore RE. Salivary gland tumors in children. J Pediatr Surg 1978;13:519-521.
31. Gritzmann N. Sonography of the salivary glands. AJR Am J Roentgenol 1989;153:161-166.
32. Yousem DM, Kraut MA, Chalian AA. Major salivary gland imaging. Radiology 2000;216:19-29.
33. Martin X, Uffer S, Gailloud C. Ophthalmia nodosa and the oculoglandular syndrome of Parinaud. Br J Ophthalmol 1986;70:536-542.
34. Lewis GJS, Leithiser RE, Glasier CM, et al. Ultrasonography of pediatric neck masses. Ultrasound Q 1989;7:315-355.
35. Leerdam CM, Martin HC, Isaacs D. Recurrent parotitis of childhood. J Paediatr Child Health 2005;41:631-634.
36. Chitre VV, Premchandra DJ. Recurrent parotitis. Arch Dis Child 1997;77:359-363.
37. Sitheeque M, Sivachandran Y, Varathan V, et al. Juvenile recurrent parotitis: clinical, sialographic and ultrasonographic features. Int J Paediatr Dent 2007;17:98-104.
38. Nozaki H, Harasawa A, Hara H, et al. Ultrasonographic features of recurrent parotitis in childhood. Pediatr Radiol 1994;24:98-100.
39. Kawamura H, Taniguchi N, Itoh K, Kano S. Salivary gland echography in patients with Sjogren's syndrome. Arthritis Rheum 1990;33:505-510.
40. Martinoli C, Derchi LE, Solbiati L, et al. Color Doppler sonography of salivary glands. AJR Am J Roentgenol 1994;163:933-941.
41. Rosso R, Pretolesi F, del Bono V, et al. Benign lymphoepithelial parotid lesions in vertically HIV-infected patients. AIDS Patient Care STDS 2006;20:536-541.

42. Mandel L, Bijoor R. Imaging (computed tomography, magnetic resonance imaging, ultrasound, sialography) in a case of recurrent parotitis in children. J Oral Maxillofac Surg 2006;64:984-988.

43. Toma P, Rossi UG. Pediatric ultrasound. II. Other applications. Eur Radiol 2003;11:2369-2398.

44. Goddart D, Francois A, Ninane J, et al. Parotid gland abnormality found in children seropositive for the human immunodeficiency virus (HIV). Pediatr Radiol 1990;20:355-357.

45. Hudgins PA. Nodal and nonnodal inflammatory processes of the pediatric neck. Neuroimaging Clin North Am 2000;10:181-192, ix.

46. Hockstein NG, Samadi DS, Gendron K, et al. Pediatric submandibular triangle masses: a fifteen-year experience. Head Neck 2004; 26:675-680.

47. Soberman N, Leonidas JC, Berdon WE, et al. Parotid enlargement in children seropositive for human immunodeficiency virus: imaging findings. AJR Am J Roentgenol 1991;157:553-556.

48. Bentz BG, Hughes CA, Ludemann JP, Maddalozzo J. Masses of the salivary gland region in children. Arch Otolaryngol Head Neck Surg 2000;126:1435-1439.

49. Baker SR, Malone B. Salivary gland malignancies in children. Cancer 1985;55:1730-1736.

50. Mulliken JB, Glowacki J. Hemangiomas and vascular malformations in infants and children: a classification based on endothelial characteristics. Plast Reconstr Surg 1982;69:412-422.

51. Seibert RW, Seibert JJ. High resolution ultrasonography of the parotid gland in children. Pediatr Radiol 1986;16:374-379.

52. Petrovic S, Petrovic D, Pesic Z, Kovacevic P. Sonography of congenital neck masses in children. Med Biol 2005;12:164-169.

53. Fordham LA, Chung CJ, Donnelly LF. Imaging of congenital vascular and lymphatic anomalies of the head and neck. Neuroimaging Clin North Am 2000;10:117-136, viii.

54. Guarisco JL. Congenital head and neck masses in infants and children. Part II. Ear Nose Throat J 1991;70:75-82.

55. Robertson RL, Robson CD, Barnes PD, Burrows PE. Head and neck vascular anomalies of childhood. Neuroimaging Clin North Am 1999;9:115-132.

56. Hung W, August GP, Randolph JG, et al. Solitary thyroid nodules in children and adolescents. J Pediatr Surg 1982;17:225-229.

57. Turkyilmaz Z, Karabulut R, Bayazit YA, et al. Congenital neck masses in children and their embryologic and clinical features. B-ENT 2008;4:7-18.

58. Koral K, Sayre J, Bhuta S, et al. Recurrent pleomorphic adenoma of the parotid gland in pediatric and adult patients: value of multiple lesions as a diagnostic indicator. AJR Am J Roentgenol 2003;180: 1171-1174.

59. Kim J, Kim EK, Park CS, et al. Characteristic sonographic findings of Warthin's tumor in the parotid gland. J Clin Ultrasound 2004; 32:78-81.

60. Koch BL, Myer 3rd CM. Presentation and diagnosis of unilateral maxillary swelling in children. Am J Otolaryngol 1999;20:106-129.

61. Vazquez E, Enriquez G, Castellote A, et al. US, CT, and MR imaging of neck lesions in children. Radiographics 1995;15: 105-122.

62. Yasumoto M, Yoshimura R, Sunaba K, Shibuya H. Sonographic appearances of malignant lymphoma of the salivary glands. J Clin Ultrasound 2001;29:491-498.

63. Asai S, Okami K, Nakamura N, et al. Tortoiseshell appearance of bilateral submandibular glands by infiltration of mucosa-associated lymphoid tissue lymphoma. J Ultrasound Med 2008;27:969-973.

64. Dubois J, Patriquin H. Doppler sonography of head and neck masses in children. Neuroimaging Clin N Am 2000;10:215-252, ix.

65. Woodfield CA, Levine MS, Rubesin SE, et al. Pharyngeal retention cysts: radiographic findings in seven patients. AJR Am J Roentgenol 2005;184:793-796.

66. Gutierrez JP, Berkowitz RG, Robertson CF. Vallecular cysts in newborns and young infants. Pediatr Pulmonol 1999;27:282-285.

67. Leonardo GD, Federico M, Stefania N, et al. Endoscopic treatment of vallecular cyst in a newborn. Int J Pediatr Otorhinolaryngol 2009;4:10-13.

68. Cuillier F, Bidault J. Vallecular cyst. Reunion Island, France, 2001, Hospital Felix Guyon. www.thefetus.net.

69. Meuwly JY, Lepori D, Theumann N, et al. Multimodality imaging evaluation of the pediatric neck: techniques and spectrum of findings. Radiographics 2005;25:931-948.

70. Seibert RW, Seibert JJ. High resolution ultrasonography of the parotid gland in children. Part II. Pediatr Radiol 1988;19:13-18.

Suprahyoid Space

71. Schneider K. Sonographic imaging of the thyroid in children. Prog Pediatr Surg 1991;26:1-14.

72. Solomon JR, Rangecroft L. Thyroglossal-duct lesions in childhood. J Pediatr Surg 1984;19:555-561.

73. Babcock DS. Thyroid disease in the pediatric patient: emphasizing imaging with sonography. Pediatr Radiol 2006;36:299-308, quiz 372-373.

74. Tessler FN, Tublin ME. Thyroid sonography: current applications and future directions. AJR Am J Roentgenol 1999;173:437-443.

75. Ueda D. Normal volume of the thyroid gland in children. J Clin Ultrasound 1990;18:455-462.

76. Ueda D, Mitamura R, Suzuki N, et al. Sonographic imaging of the thyroid gland in congenital hypothyroidism. Pediatr Radiol 1992; 22:102-105.

77. Garel C, Leger J. Thyroid imaging in children. In: Van Vliet G, Polak M, editors. Thyroid gland development and function. Paris: S Karger, AG Basel; 2007. p. 43-61.

78. Toma P, Rossi UG, Magnaguagno F, Granata C. Imaging of the normal and affected thyroid in children with emphasis on sonography. Pediatr Endocrinol Rev 2003;1(Suppl 2):237-243; discussion 243.

79. Marinovic D, Garel C, Czernichow P, Leger J. Ultrasonographic assessment of the ectopic thyroid tissue in children with congenital hypothyroidism. Pediatr Radiol 2004;34:109-113.

80. De Bruyn R, Ng WK, Taylor J, et al. Neonatal hypothyroidism: comparison of radioisotope and ultrasound imaging in 54 cases. Acta Paediatr Scand 1990;79:1198-1199.

81. Masters F, Given CA. Cystic neck masses: a pictorial review of unusual presentations and complicating features. Appl Radiol 2008; 37:26-32.

82. Hsieh YY, Hsueh S, Hsueh C, et al. Pathological analysis of congenital cervical cysts in children: 20 years of experience at Chang Gung Memorial Hospital. Chang Gung Med J 2003;26:107-113.

83. Kutuya N, Kurosaki Y. Sonographic assessment of thyroglossal duct cysts in children. J Ultrasound Med 2008;27:1211-1219.

84. Wadsworth DT, Siegel MJ. Thyroglossal duct cysts: variability of sonographic findings. AJR Am J Roentgenol 1994;163: 1475-1477.

85. Ahuja AT, King AD, Metreweli C. Sonographic evaluation of thyroglossal duct cysts in children. Clin Radiol 2000;55:770-774.

86. Foley DS, Fallat ME. Thyroglossal duct and other congenital midline cervical anomalies. Semin Pediatr Surg 2006;15:70-75.

87. Lev S, Lev MH. Imaging of cystic lesions. Radiol Clin North Am 2000;38:1013-1027.

88. Judd ES. Thyroglossal duct cysts and sinuses. Surg Clin North Am 1963;43:1023-1032.

89. Wang HK, Tiu CM, Chou YH, Chang CY. Imaging studies of pyriform sinus fistula. Pediatr Radiol 2003;33:328-333.

90. Bar-Ziv J, Slasky BS, Sichel JY, et al. Branchial pouch sinus tract from the piriform fossa causing acute suppurative thyroiditis, neck abscess, or both: CT appearance and the use of air as a contrast agent. AJR Am J Roentgenol 1996;167:1569-1572.

91. Miller D, Hill JL, Sun CC, et al. The diagnosis and management of pyriform sinus fistulae in infants and young children. J Pediatr Surg 1983;18:377-381.

92. Rogers DG. Thyroid disease in children. Am Fam Physician 1994; 50:344-350.

93. Mahmutyazicioglu K, Turgut M. Doppler evaluation of the thyroid in pediatric goiter. J Clin Ultrasound 2004;32:24-28.

94. Niedziela M. Pathogenesis, diagnosis and management of thyroid nodules in children. Endocr Relat Cancer 2006;13:427-453.

95. Ardito G, Pintus C, Revelli L, et al. Thyroid tumors in children and adolescents: preoperative study. Eur J Pediatr Surg 2001;11: 154-157.

96. Reiners C, Demidchik YE. Differentiated thyroid cancer in childhood: pathology, diagnosis, therapy. Pediatr Endocrinol Rev 2003;1(Suppl 2):230-235; discussion 235-236.

97. Donohoo JH, Wallach MT. Cricoid cartilage on sonography in pediatric patients mimics a thyroid mass. J Ultrasound Med 2006;25:907-911.

98. Park CH, Oh KK, Kim EK, et al. Thyroid gland rupture after blunt cervical trauma. J Ultrasound Med 2006;25:943-946.

99. Cole-Beuglet C, Goldberg BB. New high-resolution ultrasound evaluation of diseases of the thyroid gland: a review article. JAMA 1983;249:2941-2944.

100. Bachrach LK, Daneman D, Daneman A, Martin DJ. Use of ultrasound in childhood thyroid disorders. J Pediatr 1983;103: 547-552.

101. Garcia CJ, Daneman A, Thorner P, Daneman D. Sonography of multinodular thyroid gland in children and adolescents. Am J Dis Child 1992;146:811-816.

102. Al-Fifi S, Rodd C. Multinodular goiter in children. J Pediatr Endocrinol Metab 2001;14:749-756.

103. Lyshchik A, Drozd V, Demidchik Y, Reiners C. Diagnosis of thyroid cancer in children: value of gray-scale and power Doppler US. Radiology 2005;235:604-613.

104. Crom DB, Kaste SC, Tubergen DG, et al. Ultrasonography for thyroid screening after head and neck irradiation in childhood cancer survivors. Med Pediatr Oncol 1997;28:15-21.

105. Segal K, Arad-Cohen A, Mechlis S, et al. Cancer of the thyroid in children and adolescents. Clin Otolaryngol Allied Sci 1997;22: 525-528.

106. Brkljacic B, Cuk V, Tomic-Brzac H, et al. Ultrasonic evaluation of benign and malignant nodules in echographically multinodular thyroids. J Clin Ultrasound 1994;22:71-76.

107. Shin JH, Han BK, Ko EY, Kang SS. Sonographic findings in the surgical bed after thyroidectomy: comparison of recurrent tumors and nonrecurrent lesions. J Ultrasound Med 2007;26:1359-1366.

108. Jun P, Chow LC, Jeffrey RB. The sonographic features of papillary thyroid carcinomas: pictorial essay. Ultrasound Q 2005;21:39-45.

109. Chammas MC, Gerhard R, de Oliveira IR, et al. Thyroid nodules: evaluation with power Doppler and duplex Doppler ultrasound. Otolaryngol Head Neck Surg 2005;132:874-882.

110. Frates MC, Benson CB, Charboneau JW, et al. Management of thyroid nodules detected at ultrasound. Society of Radiologists in Ultrasound consensus conference statement. Radiology 2005;237: 794-800.

111. Benson MT, Dalen K, Mancuso AA, et al. Congenital anomalies of the branchial apparatus: embryology and pathologic anatomy. Radiographics 1992;12:943-960.

112. Winzelberg GG, Hydovitz JD, O'Hara KR, et al. Parathyroid adenomas evaluated by Tl-201/Tc-99m pertechnetate subtraction scintigraphy and high-resolution ultrasonography. Radiology 1985; 155:231-235.

113. Rodriguez-Cueto G, Manzano-Sierra C, Villalpando-Hernandez S. Preoperative ultrasonographic diagnosis of a parathyroid adenoma in a child. Pediatr Radiol 1984;14:47-48.

114. Prasad TR, Bhatnagar V. Giant solitary parathyroid adenoma presenting with bone disease. Indian Pediatr 2002;39:1044-1047.

115. Scheible W. Recent advances in ultrasound: high-resolution imaging of superficial structures. Head Neck Surg 1981;4:58-63.

116. Simeone JF, Mueller PR, Ferrucci Jr JT, et al. High-resolution real-time sonography of the parathyroid. Radiology 1981;141:745-751.

117. Wolf RJ, Cronan JJ, Monchik JM. Color Doppler sonography: an adjunctive technique in assessment of parathyroid adenomas. J Ultrasound Med 1994;13:303-308.

118. Lee VS, Spritzer CE. MR imaging of abnormal parathyroid glands. AJR Am J Roentgenol 1998;170:1097-1103.

119. Sarin YK, Thambudorai R. Ectopic bronchogenic cyst. Indian Pediatr 1997;34:1035-1036.

120. Cohen SR, Thompson JW, Brennan LP. Foregut cysts presenting as neck masses: a report on three children. Ann Otol Rhinol Laryngol 1985;94:433-436.

Lacking Definition by the Hyoid

121. Da Cunha Pinho M, Viana PC, Omokawa M, et al. External laryngocele: sonographic appearance—a case report. Radiol Bras 2007;40: 279-282.

122. Koch BL. Cystic malformations of the neck in children. Pediatr Radiol 2005;35:463-477.

123. Nicollas R, Guelfucci B, Roman S, Triglia JM. Congenital cysts and fistulas of the neck. Int J Pediatr Otorhinolaryngol 2000;55: 117-124.

124. Koch BL. The child with a neck mass. Appl Radiol 2005;34:8-22.

125. Waldhausen JH. Branchial cleft and arch anomalies in children. Semin Pediatr Surg 2006;15:64-69.

126. Badami JP, Athey PA. Sonography in the diagnosis of branchial cysts. AJR Am J Roentgenol 1981;137:1245-1248.

127. Miller MB, Rao VM, Tom BM. Cystic masses of the head and neck: pitfalls in CT and MR interpretation. AJR Am J Roentgenol 1992; 159:601-607.

128. Brown RL, Azizkhan RG. Pediatric head and neck lesions. Pediatr Clin North Am 1998;45:889-905.

129. Mukherji SK, Fatterpekar G, Castillo M, et al. Imaging of congenital anomalies of the branchial apparatus. Neuroimaging Clin North Am 2000;10:75-93, viii.

130. Imhof H, Czerny C, Hormann M, Krestan C. Tumors and tumor-like lesions of the neck: from childhood to adult. Eur Radiol 2004; 14(Suppl 4):L155-L165.

131. Fitoz S, Atasoy C, Turkoz E, et al. Sonographic findings in ectopic cervical thymus in an infant. J Clin Ultrasound 2001;29:523-526.

132. Ballal HS, Mahale A, Hegde V, et al. Case report: cervical thymic cyst. Indian J Radiol Imaging 1999;9:187-189.

133. Smirniotopoulos JG, Chiechi MV. Teratomas, dermoids, and epidermoids of the head and neck. Radiographics 1995;15:1437-1455.

134. Al-Khateeb TH, Al-Zoubi F. Congenital neck masses: a descriptive retrospective study of 252 cases. J Oral Maxillofac Surg 2007;65: 2242-2247.

135. Kerner B, Flaum E, Mathews H, et al. Cervical teratoma: prenatal diagnosis and long-term follow-up. Prenat Diagn 1998;18:51-59.

136. Hasiotou M, Vakaki M, Pitsoulakis G, et al. Congenital cervical teratomas. Int J Pediatr Otorhinolaryngol 2004;68:1133-1139.

137. Kogutt MS, Cohen S. Cervical teratoma in infants and children. South Med J 1977;70:122-123.

138. Herman TE, Siegel MJ. Cervical teratoma. J Perinatol 2008; 28:649-651.

139. Edwards PD, Rahbar R, Ferraro NF, et al. Lymphatic malformation of the lingual base and oral floor. Plast Reconstr Surg 2005;115: 1906-1915.

140. Boukobza M, Enjolras O, Guichard JP, et al. Cerebral developmental venous anomalies associated with head and neck venous malformations. AJNR Am J Neuroradiol 1996;17:987-994.

141. Ying MTC, Ahuja AT. Ultrasonography of cervical lymph nodes. Hong Kong SAR, 2008. http://www.droid.cuhk.edu.hk/web/specials/lymph_nodes/lymph_nodes.htm.

142. Hajek PC, Salomonowitz E, Turk R, et al. Lymph nodes of the neck: evaluation with ultrasound. Radiology 1986;158:739-742.

143. Jordan N, Tyrrell J. Management of enlarged cervical lymph nodes. Curr Paediatr 2004;14:154-159.

144. Moore SW, Schneider JW, Schaaf HS. Diagnostic aspects of cervical lymphadenopathy in children in the developing world: a study of 1,877 surgical specimens. Pediatr Surg Int 2003;19:240-244.

145. Peters TR, Edwards KM. Cervical lymphadenopathy and adenitis. Pediatr Rev 2000;21:399-405.

146. Turkington JR, Paterson A, Sweeney LE, Thornbury GD. Neck masses in children. Br J Radiol 2005;78:75-85.

147. Kao HT, Huang YC, Lin TY. Kawasaki disease presenting as cervical lymphadenitis or deep neck infection. Otolaryngol Head Neck Surg 2001;124:468-470.

148. Bedi DG, John SD, Swischuk LE. Fibromatosis colli of infancy: variability of sonographic appearance. J Clin Ultrasound 1998; 26:345-348.

149. Cheng JC, Metreweli C, Chen TM, Tang S. Correlation of ultrasonographic imaging of congenital muscular torticollis with clinical assessment in infants. Ultrasound Med Biol 2000;26:1237-1241.

150. Hsu TC, Wang CL, Wong MK, et al. Correlation of clinical and ultrasonographic features in congenital muscular torticollis. Arch Phys Med Rehabil 1999;80:637-641.

151. Lin JN, Chou ML. Ultrasonographic study of the sternocleidomastoid muscle in the management of congenital muscular torticollis. J Pediatr Surg 1997;32:1648-1651.

152. Toma P, Granata C, Rossi A, Garaventa A. Multimodality imaging of Hodgkin disease and non-Hodgkin lymphomas in children. Radiographics 2007;27:1335-1354.

153. Evans RM. Ultrasound of cervical lymph nodes. Imaging 2003; 15:101-108.

154. Cardesa-Salzmann TM, Mora-Graupera J, Claret G, Agut T. Congenital cervical neuroblastoma. Pediatr Blood Cancer 2004;43: 785-787.

155. Kuna SK, Bracic I, Tesic V, et al. Ultrasonographic differentiation of benign from malignant neck lymphadenopathy in thyroid cancer. J Ultrasound Med 2006;25:1531-1537; quiz 1538-1540.

156. McCarville MB, Spunt SL, Pappo AS. Rhabdomyosarcoma in pediatric patients: the good, the bad, and the unusual. AJR Am J Roentgenol 2001;176:1563-1569.

157. Ng WK. Embryonal rhabdomyosarcoma in a young boy. Mcgill J Med 2007;10:16-19.
158. Bellah R. Ultrasound in pediatric musculoskeletal disease: techniques and applications. Radiol Clin North Am 2001;39:597-618, ix.
159. Hu X, Li J, Hu T, Jiang X. Congenital jugular vein phlebectasia. Am J Otolaryngol 2005;26:172-174.
160. Babcock DS. Sonographic evaluation of suspected pediatric vascular diseases. Pediatr Radiol 1991;21:486-489.
161. Taylor BJ, Seibert JJ, Glasier CM, et al. Evaluation of the reconstructed carotid artery following extracorporeal membrane oxygenation. Pediatrics 1992;90:568-572.
162. Simonetti G, Bozzao A, Floris R, Silvestrini M. Non-invasive assessment of neck-vessel pathology. Eur Radiol 1998;8:691-697.
163. Jacobs JP, Goldman AP, Cullen S, et al. Carotid artery pseudoaneurysm as a complication of ECMO. Ann Vasc Surg 1997;11:630-633.
164. Kuenzler KA, Arthur LG, Burchard AE, et al. Intraoperative ultrasound reduces ECMO catheter malposition requiring surgical correction. J Pediatr Surg 2002;37:691-694.
165. Liberman L, Hordof AJ, Hsu DT, Pass RH. Ultrasound-assisted cannulation of the right internal jugular vein during electrophysiologic studies in children. J Interv Card Electrophysiol 2001;5:177-179.
166. Lamperti M, Caldiroli D, Cortellazzi P, et al. Safety and efficacy of ultrasound assistance during internal jugular vein cannulation in neurosurgical infants. Intensive Care Med 2008;34:2100-2105.
167. De Sena S, Rosenfeld DL, Santos S, Keller I. Jugular thrombophlebitis complicating bacterial pharyngitis (Lemierre's syndrome). Pediatr Radiol 1996;26:141-144.
168. Castro-Marin F, Kendall JL. Diagnosis of Lemierre syndrome by bedside emergency department ultrasound. J Emerg Med 2007;10:44.

CHAPTER 51

The Pediatric Spinal Canal

Carol E. Barnewolt and Carol M. Rumack

Chapter Outline

*I*n normal infants, the spinal cord can be visualized because the nonossified state of the posteromedian intraneural synchondrosis provides an ample acoustic window (Fig. 51-1). The abnormal configuration of vertebral bodies in infants with certain dysraphic abnormalities opens the window even further. Although magnetic resonance imaging (MRI) is considered the examination of choice when evaluating the spine in children and adults, sonography of the spine in the newborn period can reveal details that are difficult to define with MRI.

EMBRYOLOGY

A detailed description of spinal column and spinal cord embryology is beyond the scope of this chapter, and the reader is referred to several excellent works covering this topic.[1-7] For a better understanding of spinal pathology, a general knowledge of the process of spinal cord and vertebral column formation is helpful. From the cervical through the second sacral segments, the spinal cord forms by the process of **primary neurulation.**[8] Distal to this level, the cord and the filum terminale are formed by a process termed **canalization and retrogressive differentiation** of the caudal cell mass, sometimes referred to as **secondary neurulation.**

Primary neurulation is the process by which **neural ectoderm** (neuroectoderm, neuroderm), the dorsal layer of the 18 to 28–day embryonic disc, becomes the **neural tube,** with the neural groove acting as a fulcrum. **Neural crest,** initially the lateral edge of the neural ectoderm,

moves to the top of the neural tube so that it is then dorsal to the neural tube, and gives rise to the sensory ganglia (dorsal root ganglia)[9] (Fig. 51-2). The process by which neuroectoderm separates from cutaneous ectoderm is termed **disjunction.**

The undifferentiated caudal cell mass coalesces caudal to the posterior neuropore and extends to the tail fold. This conglomerate of cells develops vacuoles that coalesce to form the most distal neural tube (canalization), which fuses with the rostral tube as it forms through primary neurulation. **Differentiation of the caudal cell mass** into the distal neural tube occurs between 28 to 48 days.

The spinal column develops in parallel with the spinal cord beginning at the future occipital region and sweeps caudally. Solid blocks of mesoderm form in a ventral position to the neural plate. This divides into paired blocks or **somites** by day 20. The dorsolateral portion of each somite will become skeletal muscle and dermis, whereas the ventromedial portion will become the cartilage, bone, and ligaments of the vertebral column. These latter cells migrate around the neural tube, forming a perichordal tube that will begin to segment into primitive precartilaginous vertebra at about day 24. One can readily see how failure of completion or error in organization at any of these levels might lead to open neural tube defects, tethered cord, caudal regression, and vertebral body anomalies.

Some spinal column and spinal cord anomalies are known to occur with other anomalies, such as cervical myelomeningoceles, split cord malformations, neurenteric cysts, certain complex intestinal malformations, and

Klippel-Feil syndrome. Several authors have theorized that these situations cannot be explained by the scenario previously described. Because these complex anomalies involve all three embryonic germ layers, a disorder of the earlier process of **gastrulation,** the conversion of a bilaminar embryonic disc to a trilaminar embryonic disc, has been proposed.[10]

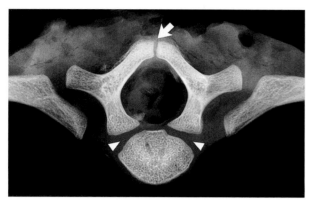

FIGURE 51-1. Cartilaginous gaps in vertebral ring allow penetration by scanning beam. Transverse radiograph through a thoracic vertebral body specimen from an infant demonstrates the cartilaginous posterior median intraneural synchondrosis *(arrow)* and the paired neurocentral synchondroses *(arrowheads). (Courtesy Dr. Paul Kleinman, Children's Hospital, Boston.)*

SONOGRAPHIC TECHNIQUE AND NORMAL ANATOMY

Infants are generally scanned in the prone position, although it is possible to scan in a decubitus position while the infant is fed with a bottle or even breast-fed. The decubitus position is much more challenging. A much better scan will be obtained if the caregiver is allowed to feed a struggling infant and return to the prone position in the postprandial state. If possible, the lumbar lordosis is accentuated by elevating the shoulders, to aid determination of vertebral body level by defining the lumbosacral junction.[11] An alternative approach is to place a rolled blanket under the lower abdomen in a prone position. Modern high-frequency linear transducers allow visualization of fine details of anatomy, with the additional aid of extended–field of view images (Fig. 51-3). Although different indications for imaging may require varying views, it is best to scan the entire back in both the longitudinal and the transverse plane. This allows a thorough search for contiguity of vertebral body rings, an assessment of contour and position of the spinal cord, and a survey of the paraspinous musculature and overlying skin.

The fine anatomic display possible with sonography has been shown in correlative studies between ultrasound and specimen anatomy.[12] Figure 51-4 demonstrates the

SONOGRAPHY OF NEONATAL SPINE

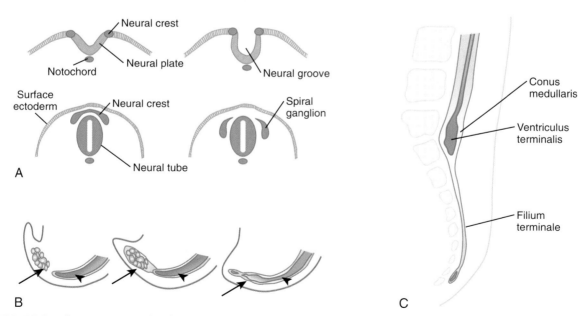

FIGURE 51-2. Three stages of spinal cord development. A, Neurulation (closure of neural tube) is the process of progression from neural plate to neural groove to neural tube. **B, Canalization** occurs when multiple microcysts form and coalesce in caudal cell mass *(arrows),* which fuses to distal neural tube *(arrowheads),* forming the primitive spinal cord. **C, Retrogressive differentiation** (programmed cell death) is the process by which the caudal cell mass and neural tube regress in size to form the **fetal conus medullaris, ventriculus terminalis,** and **filum terminale.** Note labeled structures. (*A from Sadler T.* Langman's medical embryology. *5th ed. Baltimore, 1985, Lippincott; B and C from Barkovich AJ.* Pediatric neuroimaging. *3rd ed. Philadelphia, 2000, Lippincott–Williams & Wilkins.)*

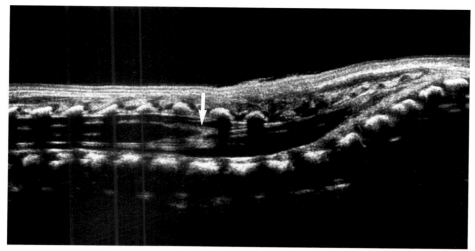

FIGURE 51-3. Lumbosacral spine in 2-week-old infant. Extended–field of view image reveals detailed anatomy of the course and contour of the lumbosacral spine. The tip of the conus medullaris is clearly visible *(arrow).*

basic landmarks that should be visible. In general, the cord is relatively hypoechoic, whereas the interfaces created by the fanning nerve rootlets are echogenic. In the past, controversy has surrounded the origin of the central echo complex in the hypoechoic cord. It is intuitively satisfying to presume that this represents the central canal of the spinal cord, but some authorities thought that the central echogenicity may actually indicate the interface between the myelinated ventral white commissure and central end of the anterior median fissure.[13,14] Images obtained with high-frequency transducers sometimes reveal a column of fluid within the center of the central echo complex. This implies that the structure represents a patent central spinal canal. This is seen so often in the neonate that it should probably be considered a normal finding (Fig. 51-5).

The normal **filum terminale** should be clearly visible and mobile with cerebrospinal fluid (CSF) pulsations. The center of the filum tends to be relatively hypoechoic compared to its bright outer margins (Fig. 51-6). Modern transducers may allow visualization of a cystic structure at the tip of the conus medullaris. A terminal ventricle or filar cyst should be considered a variant of normal development when there is no other suggestion of pathology[9,15] (Fig. 51-7). Some infants have more prominent epidural fat, which also should be considered a normal variant unless other signs suggest an abnormal fatty mass (Fig. 51-8). Color Doppler ultrasound can help localize the epidural venous plexus, anterior spinal arteries, and paired posterior spinal arteries. Malposition, compression, or distention of these vessels may help to distinguish an abnormal mass within the vertebral canal from normal nerve rootlets or epidural fat.

A careful determination of the **position of the tip of the conus medullaris** should always be included in a neonatal spine sonographic examination. This may be challenging in a squirming infant. Possible approaches

include (1) finding the 12th rib and counting down from this level, (2) defining the lumbosacral junction by accentuating the lumbar lordosis and using that as a reference, and (3) counting upward from the last ossified vertebral body. The third approach can be difficult because of the great variability in the ossification of the coccygeal vertebral bodies.[16] Generally, ossified coccygeal vertebral bodies have a rounded central nucleus, whereas sacral ossification centers take on a more squared contour (Fig. 51-9). If these methods prove problematic, the ultrasound transducer can be used to locate the tip of the conus, mark the skin at that level with a **radiopaque BB,** and obtain a radiograph of the entire spine to determine the corresponding vertebral level (Fig. 51-10). If this is done, a lateral film is most helpful because distortion from beam angulation is less problematic. The degree of ossification of the coccyx can also be addressed with this film. As the sonographer gains experience in scanning the neonatal spine, the tremendous variability in the shape of the cartilaginous coccyx also becomes evident (Fig. 51-11).

Opinion has varied over the years regarding the normal conus medullaris position and whether it changes in later fetal life and as a child grows. Studies of fetal and newborn spine anatomy in the historical literature suggest the vast majority of so-called cord ascent occurs before 25 weeks' gestation, and a **conus position at the third lumbar vertebra (L3) or above** by the beginning of the third trimester should be considered normal.[17-19] Current literature supports the view that the tip of the conus medullaris is normally located at the mid-L3 vertebral body level, or higher, at birth (even as early as 25 weeks' gestation), and that a conus tip at the L3-L4 disc space level is too low.[20-26] The trend is toward a higher conus position as the fetus approaches term[27,28] (Fig. 51-12). Some authorities consider a conus position of L3 proper in the term or preterm infant to be equivocal,

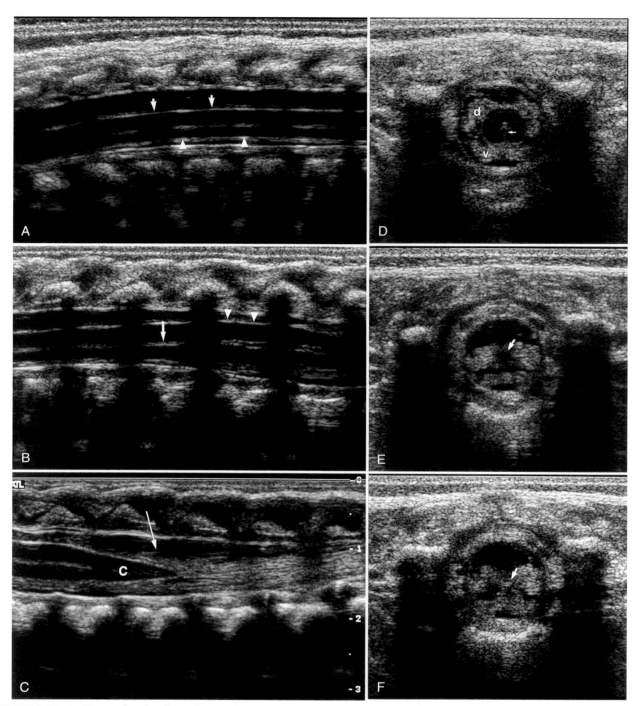

FIGURE 51-4. Normal spinal cord. A, Sagittal view shows posterior aspect *(arrows)* and anterior aspect of the thoracic spinal cord *(arrowheads)*. Normal thoracic spinal cord is more anteriorly positioned within the vertebral canal than the more distal spinal cord. **B,** Normal widening of the lumbar spinal cord *(arrowheads)*. The central spinal canal is visible as an echogenic line *(arrow)*. **C,** Tip of the conus medullaris *(C)* should taper gradually. Individual nerve rootlets are visible with modern equipment *(arrow)*. **D,** On transverse view of the lumbar spinal cord, dorsal *(d)* and ventral *(v)* nerve rootlets, as well as the anterior median fissure, are visible *(arrow)*. **E,** Transverse view near the tip of the conus medullaris demonstrates the relatively hypoechoic substance of the cord *(arrow)* in the center of the more echogenic nerve rootlets. **F,** The beginning of the filum terminale is seen as a central, slightly echogenic focus *(arrow)* in the transverse plane.

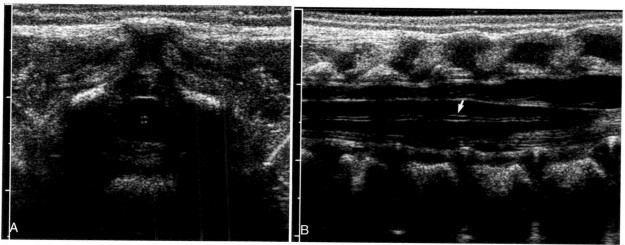

FIGURE 51-5. Fluid within central canal. A and **B,** Transverse and sagittal views of the lumbar spine. This is a common, normal variant *(arrow)* observed in many infants.

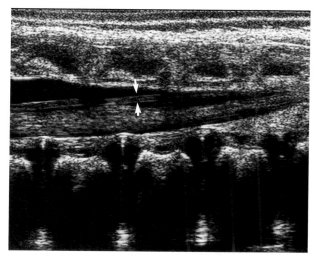

FIGURE 51-6. Normal filum terminale. This can be clearly distinguished from the nerve rootlets and should be less than 2 mm in diameter *(arrows)*. The external edges of the filum are relatively bright compared to the central portion of the filum.

requiring some form of follow-up.[3,24] The range of normal varies, and factors other than conus position alone need to be considered when determining the need, if any, for further evaluation with MRI. When an **experienced** spine sonographer finds that the tip of the conus medullaris is positioned over the upper third of the L3 vertebral body with normal nerve root pulsation, and if no other abnormalities are noted and the physical examination is not suspicious, we do not generally recommend further imaging at our hospital. A careful prospective study, beginning in fetal life, with high-resolution probes and long-term follow-up, including directed neurologic testing, will be necessary to put this question to rest.

If subsequent MRI is deemed prudent after an equivocal ultrasound examination, many pediatric neuroradiologists support waiting until the infant is at least 3 months old. Greater anatomic detail can be displayed with MRI in the larger infant using standard techniques.

THE CRANIOCERVICAL JUNCTION

In general, the linear transducer produces spine images of greatest quality. The one possible exception is the evaluation of the craniocervical junction. A smaller-footprint sector transducer allows scanning at the base of the skull and through the foramen magnum. This view allows visualization of the cisterna magna, brainstem, inferior cerebellum, and proximal cervical cord[29-31] (Fig. 51-13).

SPINAL DYSRAPHISM

The term *spinal dysraphism* stems from the Greek roots meaning "bad" *(dys)* "seam" or suture *(raphe)* and was first used in the literature by Tulpuis in 1641.[32] In 1886, von Recklinghausen first proposed the "non-closure theory," suggesting that failure of closure of the embryologic neural tube resulted in the overtly abnormal spectrum of open neural tube defects.[33] Currently, the term **dysraphism** is used to describe any abnormality that might be explained by an error in the embryologic processes of primary neurulation, disjunction, canalization, and retrogressive differentiation of the caudal cell mass. This includes infants with the grossly abnormal physical findings of open neural tube defects (**overt spinal**

Text continued on page 1742

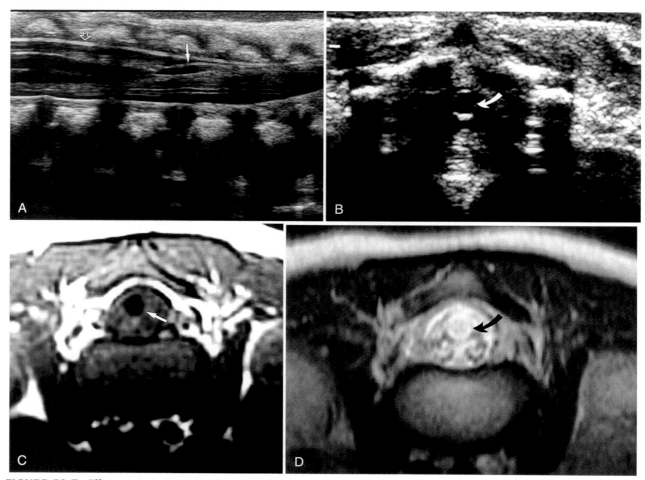

FIGURE 51-7. Filar cyst. A, Normal variant *(arrow)* on longitudinal view of the conus medullaris in a newborn. The dura is particularly bright and easy to visualize *(open arrow)*. **B** to **D,** Transverse views of a filar cyst in an older infant: **B,** ultrasound *(curved arrow)*; **C,** T1-weighted MRI *(arrow)*; **D,** T2-weighted MRI *(curved arrow)*.

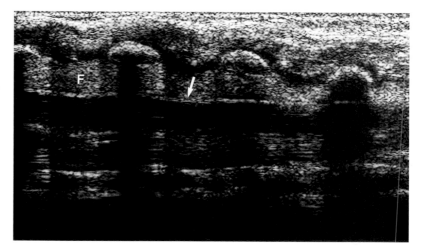

FIGURE 51-8. Epidural fatty layer. Unusually prominent epidural fatty layer *(F)* occurs in some infants; *arrow,* dura.

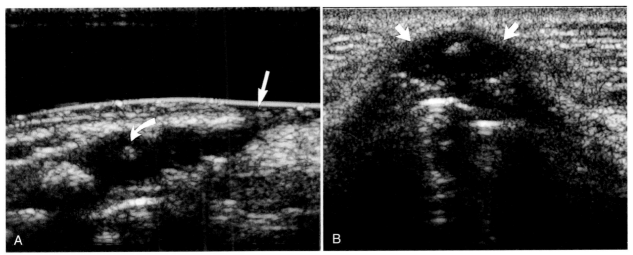

FIGURE 51-9. Almost entirely cartilaginous coccyx. A, Longitudinal view in a 4-week-old girl reveals the tiny, rounded beginnings of ossification of the first coccygeal segment *(curved arrow)* and the tip of the cartilaginous coccyx, which is positioned at the apex of an intergluteal dimple *(straight arrow)*. The cartilaginous coccyx should not be confused with a sinus tract. **B,** Early ossification is appropriately positioned in the center of the first segment on this transverse view *(outlined by arrows)*.

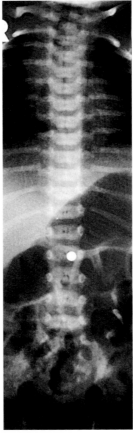

FIGURE 51-10. Determining level of conus medullaris. When it is difficult to determine the level of the conus medullaris by ultrasound alone, plain radiographs are often helpful. A BB is placed on the skin of the infant, corresponding to the position of the tip of conus medullaris during sonography, to help determine the associated vertebral body level.

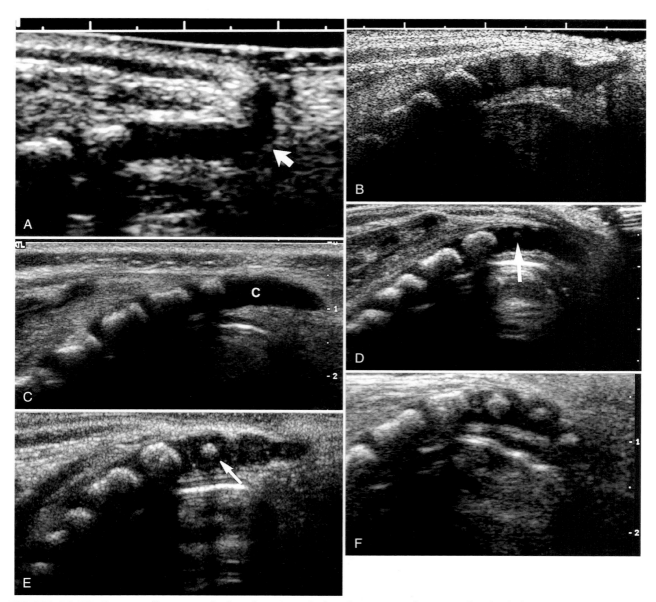

FIGURE 51-11. Extraordinary variation in normal development of coccyx in six infants. A, Unusually sharp curve of the distal coccyx *(arrow)*. **B,** The curve is less severe. **C,** Smooth, classic curve of the cartilaginous coccyx *(C)*. **D,** A tiny ossification nucleus is seen in the C1 segment *(arrow)*. **E,** Larger focus of ossification *(arrow),* and **F,** ossification nuclei are visible within all coccygeal segments.

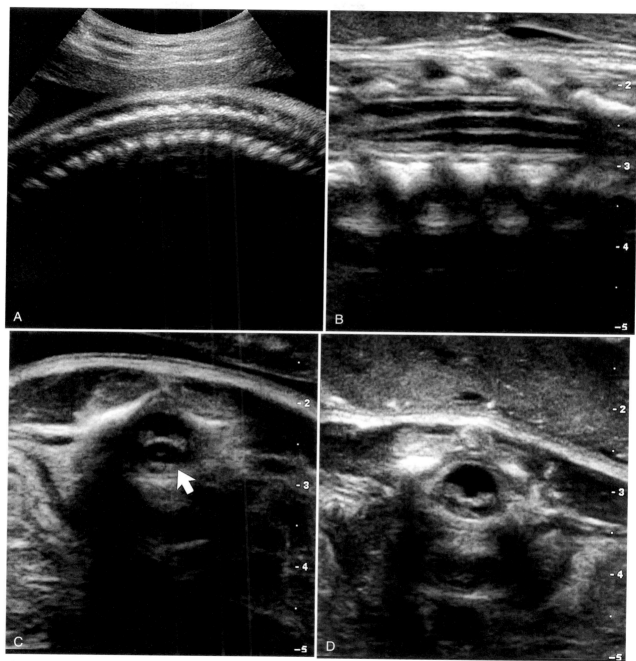

FIGURE 51-12. An amazing amount of detail of the normal fetal spine at 31 weeks with modern transducers. A and B, Sagittal views of the thoracolumbar spine (**A**) and lumbar spine (**B**) allow direct visualization of the spinal cord. **C** and **D,** Transverse views of the lumbar spine reveal a clearly defined cord (**C,** *arrow*) and more inferiorly, nerve rootlets (**D**). Visualization of the bony and cartilaginous vertebral rings is also possible.

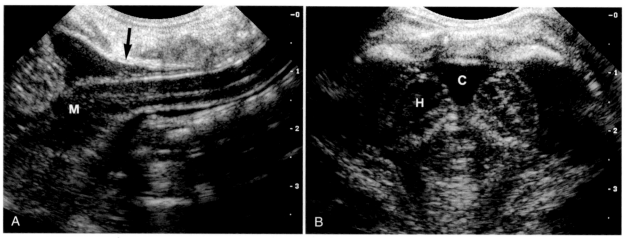

FIGURE 51-13. Brainstem, cisterna magna, and cerebellar hemispheres. A, Sagittal view of the craniocervical junction using the foramen magnum as a window. The arrow indicates the posterior margin of the foramen magnum. Visualization of the cerebellum and medulla *(M)* is also possible on this view. **B,** On transverse view, the cisterna magna *(C)* and cerebellar hemispheres *(H)* are well shown.

dysraphism) as well as the so-called occult or skin-covered lesions **(occult spinal dysraphism),** such as an intradural or filar lipoma.

OVERT SPINAL DYSRAPHISM

The terminology used to describe this spectrum of anomalies can be confusing because there is a tendency to use the terms imprecisely. **Spina bifida** simply refers to incomplete closure of the posterior bony elements of the spine.

NEURAL TUBE DEFECTS*

OVERT DYSRAPHISM
Myelocele
Meningomyelocele

OCCULT DYSRAPHISM
Spinal lipoma
  Intradural lipoma
  Lipomyelocele
  Lipomyelomeningocele
  Fibrolipoma of the filum terminale
Meningocele
Dorsal dermal sinus
Myelocystocele
Diastematomyelia
Split notochord syndrome

*Anomalies thought to result from errors in tubularization and disjunction.

Spina bifida aperta refers to the posterior protrusion of all or part of the contents of the vertebral canal through this posterior bony defect; *aperta* is Latin for "open" or "uncovered." The term **spina bifida cystica** introduces the additional requirement that the protrusion not only passes beyond the bony defect, but also passes beyond the expected demarcations of the skin of the back, such that a cystlike mass can be seen, most typically at the lumbosacral level. The classically uncovered lesions include **myelocele** and **myelomeningocele.** Infants with myelocele have a flat **neural placode** that is exposed to the environment (Fig. 51-14). In the more common myelomeningocele, this placode is further displaced posteriorly by expansion of the subarachnoid space. Newborns with myelocele or myelomeningocele generally are repaired on the first or second day of life without preoperative imaging because the defect is readily apparent. When lesion definition is deemed prudent, ultrasound can provide great anatomic detail by virtue of the deficiency in the involved posterior elements, which allows a clear acoustic window.

Myelomeningoceles are almost always associated with the **Chiari II malformation,** whereas meningoceles are rarely associated. The Chiari II malformation consists of a small posterior fossa with upward transincisural herniation of the superior cerebellum, as well as downward herniation through the foramen magnum with associated compression and distortion of the brainstem. This posterior fossa distortion can be seen readily by sonography of the brain through the anterior fontanelle and of the craniocervical junction through the foramen magnum.[34] Sonography also has a potential role in the evaluation of the spinal cord in patients with repaired myelomeningocele. Specifically, gray-scale two-dimensional (2-D) ultrasound and M-mode ultrasound,

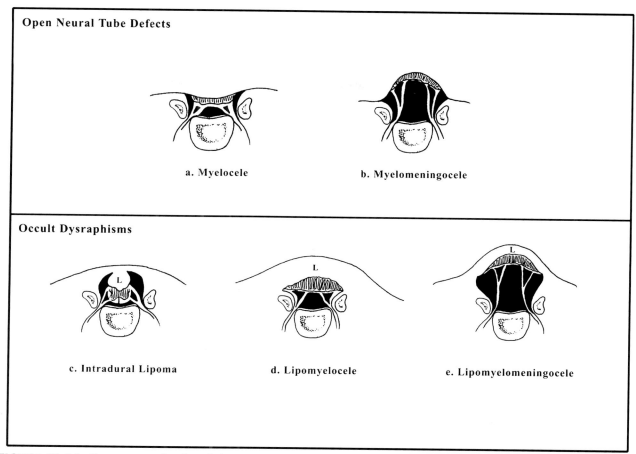

Open Neural Tube Defects

a. Myelocele   b. Myelomeningocele

Occult Dysraphisms

c. Intradural Lipoma   d. Lipomyelocele   e. Lipomyelomeningocele

FIGURE 51-14. Open neural tube defects and examples of occult dysraphisms. Each diagram is positioned with the dorsal side up as one would scan the spine of an infant; *L*, lipoma. *(Modified from Barkovich AJ. Pediatric neuroimaging. 3rd ed. Philadelphia, 2000, Lippincott–Williams & Wilkins.)*

in conjunction with MRI, have the potential to suggest the development of tethered cord syndrome, based on dampened nerve root pulsation, in this high-risk group.[35-38]

Although ultrasound of the newborn spine with unrepaired myelomeningocele is infrequently performed, sonography of the fetus being screened for this condition is well established.[39-41] This diagnosis is often first suspected on screening tests for elevated levels of alpha-fetoprotein (AFP) in amniotic fluid or maternal serum. Fetal cranial findings that support the diagnosis of the Chiari II malformation include the **lemon sign** (bitemporal narrowing of fetal skull) and **banana sign** (compression of fetal cerebellum). Both the level and the nature of the myelomeningocele, as well as associated findings (e.g., clubfoot), can be evaluated with fetal ultrasound (Fig. 51-15). In fact, three-dimensional (3-D) ultrasound of the fetal spine holds promise in increasing the precision with which the level of spinal involvement and thus extent of likely neurologic impairment are determined.[42,43] Fetal MRI may also play a role in defining spinal and brain anatomy in this situation,

particularly in the screening and follow-up of fetuses being considered for investigational in utero myelomeningocele repair.[44-49] Interestingly, the incidence of myelomeningocele seems to be decreasing, possibly the result of periconceptual folic acid or other vitamin supplementation, other environmental factors, or termination of affected pregnancies.[50]

OCCULT SPINAL DYSRAPHISM

Occult spinal dysraphisms are defined as the group of spinal dysraphisms that exist beneath an intact covering of dermis and epidermis and that are therefore not discovered with AFP screening. Many such patients are clearly identified by an abnormal physical examination. Frequently there is an obvious skin-covered mass or a hairy tuft, appendage, discolored skin, distorted spinal curvature, asymmetrical intergluteal cleft, or deep dimple.[51-54] These anomalies are occult only by virtue of a skin covering; they are not necessarily hidden from ready physical diagnosis. Infants with suspicious physical

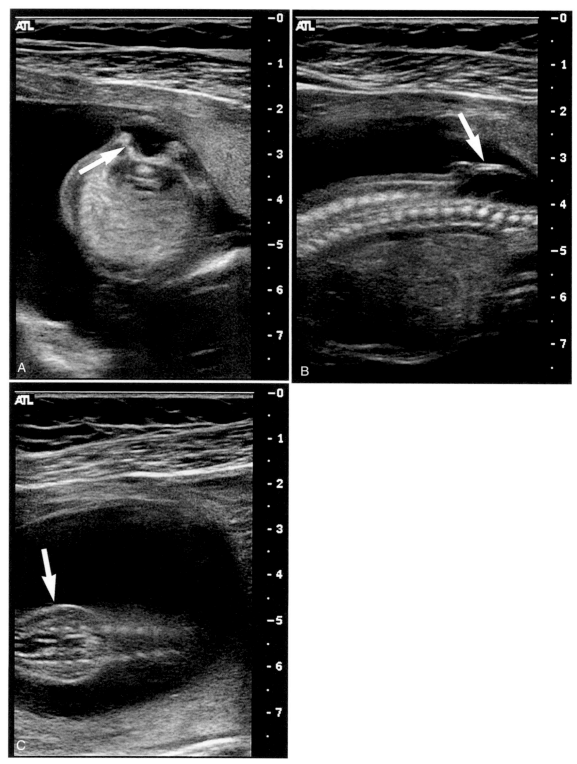

FIGURE 51-15. Lumbosacral myelomeningocele in 18-week fetus. A, Transverse view shows the open nature of the posterior elements of the affected vertebral ring *(arrow)*. **B,** Sagittal view shows the protuberance of the covering membrane and neural placode *(arrow)*. **C,** Coronal view shows the thin nature of the covering membrane *(arrow)*.

findings on the back or other abnormalities known to be associated with occult spinal dysraphism warrant radiologic evaluation. Beginning in the early 1980s, a series of excellent reviews of sonography of occult spinal dysraphisms began to appear.[55-60] At present, neonatal sonography plays a critical role in the diagnosis or exclusion of this category of dysraphism. Correlative studies with MRI suggest a high degree of accuracy.[61,62] Fatty masses, cord position, and relationship to any mass, as well as presence or absence of nerve root pulsations, can be seen clearly.

Spinal Lipoma

Spinal lipomas are fatty masses that have a connection with the leptomeninges or spinal cord.[63,64] These likely develop as a result of premature disjunction of neuroectoderm from cutaneous ectoderm. Sacral lipomas can be divided into four categories: intradural lipomas, lipomyelocele, lipomyelomeningocele, and fibrolipomas of the filum terminale (see Fig. 51-14). **Intradural lipomas** are situated in a subpial position in a dorsal cleft of the open spinal cord (Fig. 51-16). The **lipomyelocele** is analogous to the myelocele. Instead of an exposed neural placode, there is an overlying covering of attached lipoma and intact skin. The lipoma is in contiguity with the subcutaneous fatty layer. There is expansion of the subarachnoid space ventral to the placode in patients with **lipomyelomeningocele** (Fig. 51-17). This expansion and its associated lipoma can be asymmetrical, leading to large differences in the length of the paired dorsal roots and protrusion of the meningocele so that it extends posterior to the neural placode.[4]

It is also possible, but challenging, to make the fetal diagnosis of lipomyelomeningocele with sonography.[65,66] This can be difficult because the well-known signs of the Chiari II malformation almost universal in fetuses with myelomeningocele are generally not present in fetuses with a skin-covered lipomyelomeningocele. The clinician must depend on obtaining detailed views of the fetal back. Fetal position and maternal body habitus play a major role in the sensitivity of this sonographic approach.

Fibrolipomas of the filum terminale are a unique form of spinal lipoma that, in some situations, may represent a variant of normal development. This is a controversial issue.[63,64,67-69] In this entity, fatty tissue expands the filum terminale beyond its usual diameter of approximately 2 mm.[70] On ultrasound, this is seen as a thickened, echogenic filum terminale, sometimes with an undulating contour[71] (Fig. 51-18). If a fibrolipoma of the filum terminale is observed in the setting of an abnormally low position of the conus medullaris, it is termed a **tight filum terminale** or **tethered cord syndrome**[72] (Fig. 51-19). Some authorities believe that this term should apply whenever a fibrolipoma of the filum

terminale is observed, regardless of conus level.[63,64] A short, thickened filum terminale likely results from deficient retrogressive differentiation of the caudal cell mass. These patients may be asymptomatic initially, with onset of symptoms at any age (typically during an adolescent growth spurt). Symptoms include lower extremity weakness, abnormal lower extremity reflexes, bladder (and rarely bowel) dysfunction, scoliosis, foot deformities, painful or numb lower extremities, and back pain. Spinal cord injury is theorized to result from cord ischemia caused by excessive tension or stretching of nerve fibers.

Meningocele

The term *meningocele* requires further descriptors to be useful. Simple and complex **dorsal meningoceles** are composed of a dorsal herniation of dura, arachnoid, and CSF into the subcutaneous tissues of the back and are skin covered. A **simple** dorsal meningocele does not contain neural elements. A **complex** dorsal meningocele is associated with anomalies of the spinal cord and often the associated vertebral column. Dorsal meningoceles are easily observed with ultrasound as a cystic subcutaneous collection in contiguity with the vertebral canal. The spinal cord contained within the vertebral canal will appear normal when observing a so-called simple dorsal meningocele, but the cord may appear abnormal if the lesion is a complex dorsal meningocele.

For completeness, **lateral meningoceles** deserve mention. These CSF-filled protrusions of dura and arachnoid extend through enlarged neural foramina and are almost never observed in the newborn period. Most are found in patients with neurofibromatosis or with Marfan or Ehlers-Danlos syndrome.[4] Because lateral meningoceles tend to present in older children and adults, sonography is not the traditional method of evaluation.

Dorsal Dermal Sinuses

Dorsal dermal sinuses are thought to result from incomplete disjunction of cutaneous ectoderm from neuroectoderm and can also be seen by neonatal sonography and MRI. These sinuses may or may not penetrate the dura. If the dura is penetrated, the sinus may end in the subarachnoid space, the conus medullaris, filum terminale, a nerve root, or a dermoid or epidermoid cyst (Fig. 51-20). The lumbosacral region is the most common site of such sinuses, and if present, the skin opening tends to be positioned cephalad to the point of contact with the dura (Fig. 51-20, *D*). Occipital, cervical, and thoracic sinuses can all occur but are less common. Also, sinuses and other dysraphic lesions, such as myelomeningoceles, can coexist. The chief risks of undiagnosed dorsal dermal sinuses are infection and compression injury by any associated intradural mass.[73-78]

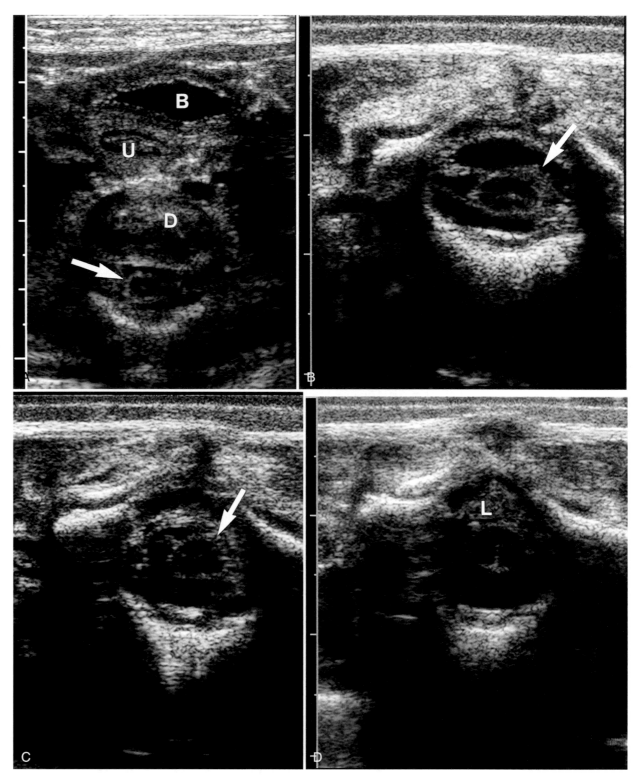

FIGURE 51-16. Intradural juxtamedullary lipoma in 2-week-old girl. A, Transverse view of the pelvis shows the partially full urinary bladder *(B)*, the newborn uterus *(U)*, and an intervertebral disc space of the sacrum *(D)*. The spinal cord is too low and is visible from an anterior approach *(arrow)*. **B** to **G,** Traditional views of the spine, scanning the neonatal back. **B, C,** and **D,** Progressively inferior transverse views reveal the rightward skew of the abnormally low spinal cord *(arrow)*, which is also pulled into an abnormally dorsal position by the lipoma *(L)*.

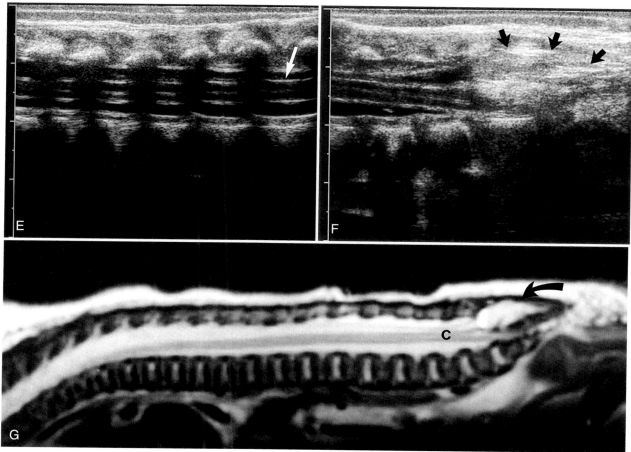

FIGURE 51-16, cont'd. E and **F,** Sagittal views of the low cord *(white arrow)* with the clearly visible tethering lipoma *(black arrows).* **G,** The correlative sagittal T2-weighted MR image, oriented to match the ultrasound, reveals the abnormally low cord *(C)* and the lipoma *(curved black arrow).*

Myelocystocele

A myelocystocele is a malformation in which the **dilated central canal** of the spinal cord protrudes dorsally through a bony spina bifida. Myelocystoceles can occur at the cervical, thoracic, or lumbosacral levels. They are quite distinct from myelomeningoceles and are skin covered.[4,61] When occurring at the lumbosacral level, they are designated **terminal myelocystoceles;** these are quite rare.[79] The diagnosis can be firmly established with ultrasound or MRI when the low-lying cord terminus ends in a cyst that is in communication with the central canal of the spinal cord. Expanded subarachnoid space tends to surround the distal cord and terminal cyst. Fluid within the terminal cyst does not communicate with the expanded subarachnoid space.[80-82] On fetal sonography, the terminal myelocystocele can mimic the diagnosis of myelomeningocele or even sacrococcygeal teratomas (Fig. 51-21). It is important to note that myelocystoceles are not usually associated with the Chiari II malformation, whereas myelomeningoceles almost always are associated. The precise antenatal diagnosis of terminal myelocystocele, versus myelomeningocele or

sacrococcygeal teratoma, is particularly important in the era of fetal surgery.[83,84]

Diastematomyelia

Diastematomyelia and **split cord malformation** are equivalent malformations in which there is sagittal division of the cord into two hemicords, each containing a central canal, a single ventral horn, and a single dorsal horn.[4] It is likely that this anomaly results from sagittal splitting of the embryonic notochord, perhaps resulting from an obstacle to cell migration from Henson's node.[85] The diagnosis of diastematomyelia can be made with ultrasound in the newborn period[61,80,86,87] (Fig. 51-22). About one half of patients with diastematomyelia have some surface stigmata of an underlying malformation, such as hypertrichosis, nevi, lipomas, dimples, or vascular lesions.[4] Despite this, it is not unusual for the diagnosis to be delayed until older childhood because scoliosis or other characteristic neurologic or orthopedic symptoms develop. MRI is necessary beyond the neonatal period to establish the diagnosis. Definition of any dividing cartilaginous or bony septum is an important part of

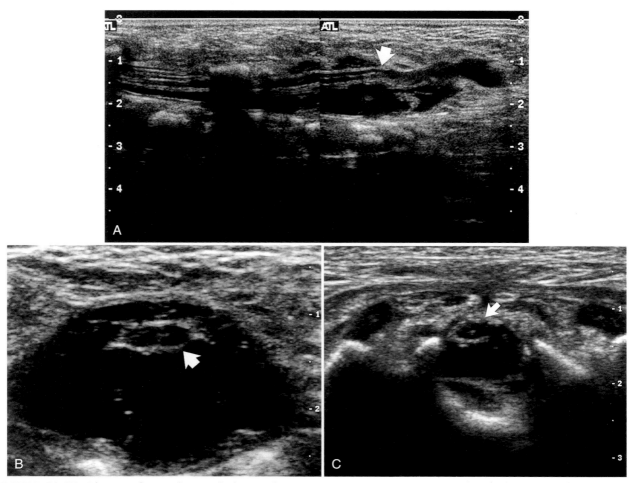

FIGURE 51-17. Lipomyelomeningocele in newborn. A, Sagittal split-screen collage of the low spinal cord *(arrow)*. **B,** Transverse view shows the neural placode posteriorly displaced *(arrow)* and the CSF-filled meningocele surrounding the placode. **C,** Distal end of the tethered cord is incorporated into the lipoma *(arrow)*.

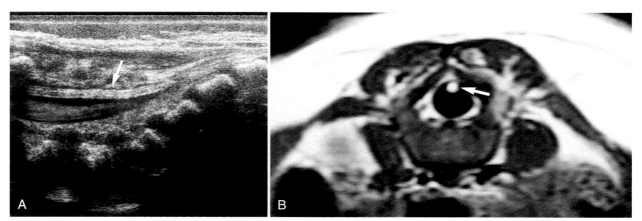

FIGURE 51-18. Fibrolipoma of filum terminale. A, Sagittal ultrasound, and **B,** transverse T1-weighted MR image, show that filum terminale is abnormally thickened and echogenic *(arrow)*, with high T1 signal in the filum *(arrow)* on MRI.

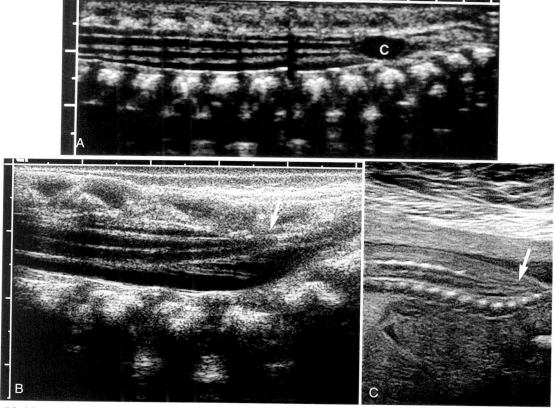

FIGURE 51-19. Tethered cord in two infants. A, Newborn with an interposed filar cyst *(C)*. **B,** Newborn, and **C,** fetus at 30 weeks, with a tethered cord in the setting of the VATER association (**v**ertebral defects, imperforate **a**nus, **t**racheo**e**sophageal fistula, and **r**adial and **r**enal anomalies. Arrow indicates the point of tethering.

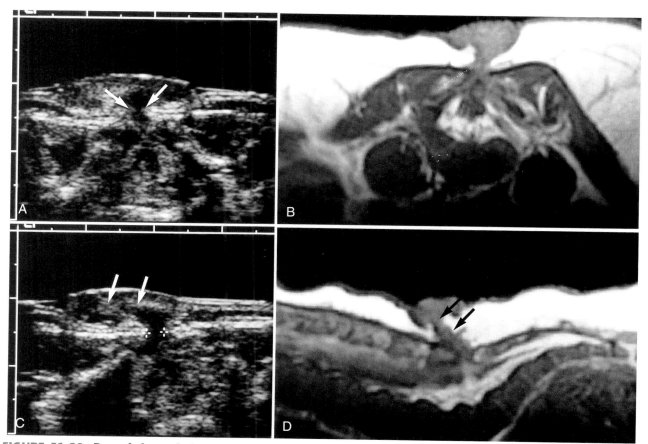

FIGURE 51-20. Dorsal dermal sinus. Transverse and sagittal views, pairing ultrasound and T1-weighted MRI. **A** and **B,** Transverse views reveal the open connection among the subcutaneous fatty layer, overlying muscles, and vertebral canal *(arrows)*. **C** and **D,** Sagittal views show the obliquity of the connecting sinus *(arrows)*. The skin-side opening is superior to the level of dural connection. This is a typical configuration.

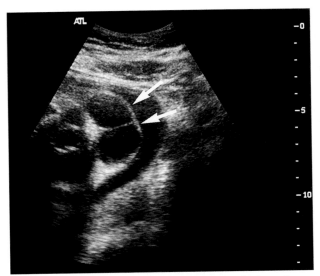

FIGURE 51-21. Terminal myelocystocele in a fetus at 31 weeks' gestation. Oblique coronal view shows the well-defined, echogenic skin covering characteristic of these lesions *(arrows).*

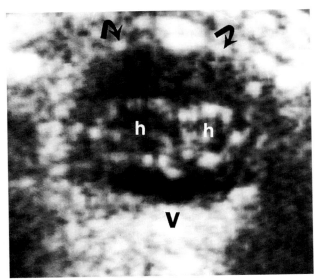

FIGURE 51-22. Diastematomyelia in 3-year-old girl. Transverse scan of lumbar canal shows two hemicords *(h),* confirmed on MRI and at surgery; *V,* vertebral body; *curved arrows,* dorsal dura.

surgical planning, sometimes necessitating the additional step of spinal CT.

The fetal diagnosis of diastematomyelia is heralded by the disorganized appearance of the vertebral column, with a fusiform segment of vertebral canal widening, and a visible dividing septum in the center of the area of widening.[88,89] Such early diagnosis should allow prompt surgical attention and may improve prognosis. Diastematomyelia may occur in isolation or in conjunction with other anomalies, such as myelomeningocele, lipomas, dermal sinuses, and dermoids.[4] There are rare reports of teratomas occurring in newborns in a position immediately dorsal to the site of diastematomyelia.[90]

Split Notochord Syndrome

The split notochord syndrome describes a complex group of anomalies thought to be caused by an abnormal, persistent connection between the dorsally located ectoderm and ventrally located endoderm of the early embryonic disc. This may occur during the process of gastrulation.[10] These malformations include dorsal enteric fistula, cyst, sinus, and diverticulum. The **dorsal enteric fistula** is an abnormal connection that runs from the intestinal cavity through the prevertebral soft tissues, vertebral bodies, vertebral canal, spinal cord, and posterior elements and ends on the dorsal skin surface in the midline.[4] The **dorsal enteric cyst, sinus,** and **diverticulum** occur at various positions along this course as portions of the dorsal enteric fistula are obliterated or persist. Included within this overall category are **neurenteric cysts,** which tend to be seen anterior to the vertebral column at a level well inferior to the associated vertebral anomaly.[91] More than one of these persistent anomalous

connections can occur in the same patient.[92] **Enteric cysts** can occur within the vertebral canal, typically ventral or ventrolateral to the spinal cord.[4] Lesions within the vertebral canal and large cysts immediately anterior or anterolateral to the vertebral body should be visible with spine sonography in the newborn period. The diagnosis of fetal neurenteric cyst has been reported in the setting of a cystic thoracic mass with associated vertebral anomalies.[93-95]

The long and complex list of anomalies termed **occult spinal dysraphism** includes both relatively common and extraordinarily rare diagnoses. As mentioned, there is often an abnormality in the contour or character of the overlying skin of the back. When this is the case, neonatal spine sonography is the ideal screening modality. The younger the infant, the better is the sonographic window and the more confident the diagnosis. As vertebral ossification progresses and the infant becomes more active, fewer details are visible with ultrasound (Fig. 51-23). Should an abnormality be detected, MRI is often requested. Because surgical correction is often not planned in the newborn period, MRI should be delayed until immediately before surgery so that as much information as possible can be gleaned from the study. Spine MRI in the newborn period can be technically challenging.

A well-established body of literature has shown an increased incidence of urogenital and anorectal anomalies in association with spinal dysraphism.[96-102] The following anomalies are listed in order of increasing incidence of associated dysraphism: **ectopic or low imperforate anus, high imperforate anus,** the **cloacal malformation,** and **cloacal exstrophy.**[97] About one third of infants with high imperforate anus, one half with the cloacal malformation, and essentially all with cloacal

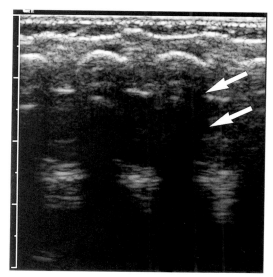

FIGURE 51-23. Sacral dimple in 4-month-old girl. On sagittal view of the lumbar spine, heavy posterior element calcification casts a shadow *(arrows)*, making it difficult to observe the spinal cord.

exstrophy have associated spinal cord anomalies. One could argue that the cloacal exstrophy group should forgo the ultrasound step and go straight to MRI. A large percentage of the other groups can avoid sedated MRI if they are shown on ultrasound to have a normal-appearing spine in the newborn period. Because patients with spinal dysraphism often have associated renal anomalies, the kidneys should always be examined as part of the routine newborn spine ultrasound examination (Fig. 51-24).

ANOMALIES AT RISK FOR SPINAL DYSRAPHISM

Cloacal exstrophy (100%)
Cloacal malformation (50%)
High imperforate anus (30%)
Ectopic or low imperforate anus

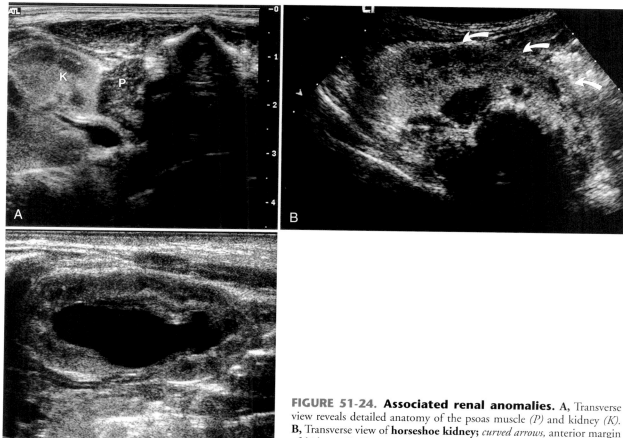

FIGURE 51-24. Associated renal anomalies. A, Transverse view reveals detailed anatomy of the psoas muscle *(P)* and kidney *(K)*. **B,** Transverse view of **horseshoe kidney;** *curved arrows,* anterior margin of kidney. **C,** Coronal view of moderate **hydronephrosis** in another patient.

CAUDAL REGRESSION

The syndrome of caudal regression traditionally encompasses a spectrum of anomalies from the extreme of **sirenomelia,** with fusion of the lower extremities, to varying degrees of **lumbosacral agenesis.**[103] The traditional embryologic explanation is an insult to the caudal mesoderm, including the cloaca and caudal cell mass, during secondary neurulation.[4] Because the caudal cell mass gives rise to the most distal spinal levels, beginning with the second sacral level, and because the spectrum of caudal regression can begin as high as the thoracic level, this lesion should begin during germ cell formation. Others have proposed that an interruption of the primitive streak results in an error of **both** primary and secondary neurulation to produce this spectrum of anomalies.[104]

About 15% of patients with caudal regression are **infants of diabetic mothers.**[105] These patients have varying degrees of absence of the caudal end of the spine. The spectrum includes isolated absence of the coccygeal vertebrae to absence of the distal thoracic, lumbar, sacral, and coccygeal vertebral bodies. Some patients with higher levels of vertebral agenesis have associated **imperforate anus, agenesis of the bladder,** and **absence of one or both kidneys.** The position of the **spinal cord terminus** tends to be unusually **high** and has an abnormally rounded or wedge shape (Fig. 51-25). An associated **cord tethering** by a fibrolipoma of the filum terminale is occasionally seen.[105,106] If the sacral vertebrae are absent, the iliac wings become closely opposed. There is often associated dislocation of the hips.

Detection of caudal regression is possible by fetal sonography.[107-109] The condition has been reported in one of a set of monozygotic twins of a diabetic mother. This suggests that some factor, other than isolated hyperglycemia, is implicated in its causation.[110] Genetic studies show a correlation between a terminal deletion of chromosome 7 and sacral agenesis with the additional anomaly of **holoprosencephaly.**[111-113] This implies that genes at this site are involved in the development of brain segmentation and the caudal region.

VERTEBRAL BODY ANOMALIES

Recall that the vertebral column arises from paired somites that organize around the developing spinal cord, differentiating in a cranial-to-caudal direction. Each pair gives rise to a single vertebral body and single set of posterior elements. During the sixth week, chondrification begins. Ossification begins at about week 9. The intervertebral disc develops from perinotochordal mesenchymal cells.[114] **Hemivertebrae** result from a disruption of the primary ossification center and pairing defects of the involved sclerotomes. Disorders of vertebral segmentation include **block vertebrae** and **unilateral unsegmented bars.** Fusion can occur at myriad sites, including the anterior and posterior spinal column, or at facet joints.[114]

Ultrasound of the newborn spine allows detailed visualization of both the cartilaginous and the bony elements of the vertebral column (Fig. 51-26). Therefore, both prenatal and postnatal ultrasound can visualize and characterize many of the formational vertebral anomalies and is probably an underutilized tool.[115-118] The suspicion of a subtle vertebral anomaly seen on radiographs in the newborn period when ossification is incomplete can often be proved or refuted with spine sonography (Figs. 51-27, 51-28, and 51-29).

Well-described syndromes in which hemivertebrae, fused vertebrae, and hypoplastic vertebrae are a major feature include the rare autosomal recessive **Jarcho-Levin syndrome,** also called **spondylothoracic dysostosis.** Vertebral body height is short, and the small size of the thorax often leads to severe respiratory compromise and early death.[119] Based on these striking vertebral anomalies and family history, diagnosis of Jarcho-Levin can be suggested on fetal sonography.[120,121] **Larsen syndrome** is another inherited disorder characterized by vertebral segmentation anomalies, particularly involving the upper thoracic and cervical levels. Multiple joint dislocations are also characteristic.[122,123] The fetal diagnosis of Larsen syndrome has been based on vertebral body segmentation anomalies and multiple joint dislocations.[124] **Klippel-Feil syndrome** also prominently involves cervical segmentation anomalies leading to limitations in neck motion.[125] The **MURCS association** (müllerian duct agenesis, renal agenesis or ectopia, and cervicothoracic somite dysplasia) has the additional characteristic of associated genitourinary anomalies.[126,127]

TUMORS

Tumors positioned in and around the vertebral canal are rare. In the neonatal period, **intraspinal neuroblastoma** is the most likely diagnosis when such a mass is discovered.[128] These lesions tend to calcify and extend into the vertebral canal from the retroperitoneum. Both the calcium and the course of extension can be observed with sonography (Fig. 51-30). These infants may present with a palpable abdominal mass or signs of spinal cord compression. Other differential possibilities in the situation of intraspinal tumor extension include **hemangioma** and **rhabdoid tumor.**[129] There are a few reports of primary intramedullary neoplasms, such as gliofibroma.[130]

Sacrococcygeal teratomas most often present in the fetal or newborn period as a sacral mass. These heterogeneous teratomas tend to recur and are generally described as **mature** or **immature.**[131-134] Altman's classification of sacrococcygeal teratomas describes the extent

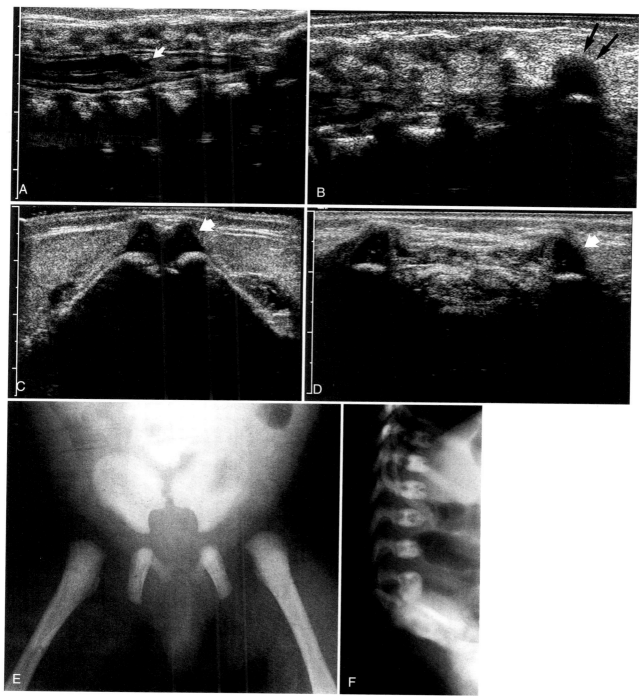

FIGURE 51-25. Caudal regression syndrome in 4-week-old girl. A, Sagittal view of the conus medullaris reveals its tip is abnormally rounded *(arrow)*. **B,** Sagittal view of the truncated, distal end of the vertebral column reveals an abnormally upturned and truncated cartilaginous tip *(black arrows)*. **C,** Transverse view of absent sacrum at the expected position of the sacral spine shows the cartilaginous posterior margin of the iliac wings to be directly apposed *(arrow)* with no separating sacrum. **D,** Normal comparison of the relationship of the posterior, cartilaginous iliac wings *(arrow)* in most infants. **E,** Frontal radiograph of the pelvis demonstrates the directly apposed medial aspects of the iliac wings, absent distal lumbar and sacral spine, and dislocated hips. **F,** Lateral radiograph demonstrates the truncated vertebral column.

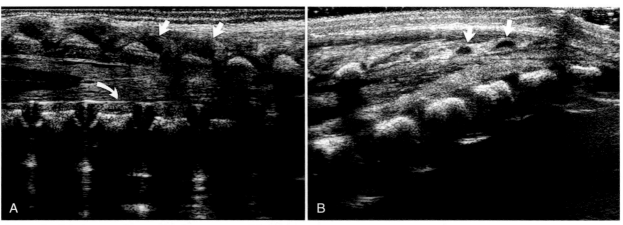

FIGURE 51-26. **Normal vertebral sonographic anatomy. A,** Sagittal view of the distal lumbar spine shows fine definition of vertebral body anatomy. The cartilaginous tips of the posterior spinous processes are seen *(arrows),* as well as the posterior margin of the cartilaginous portion of the L3 vertebral body *(curved arrow).* **B,** More distal sagittal view shows the cartilaginous posterior elements of the midsacral spine *(arrows).*

TABLE 51-1. ALTMAN'S CLASSIFICATION OF SACROCOCCYGEAL TERATOMAS	
TYPE	DESCRIPTION
I	The bulk of the mass is external, with only a minimal presacral component.
II	Both large external and large internal components are present.
III	A relatively small amount of tumor is external, but the bulk of the mass is internal.
IV	There is no external mass because the tumor is exclusively presacral.

of the mass and is helpful in presurgical planning[135] (Table 51-1). These masses tend to have a very heterogeneous appearance on ultrasound, including solid and cystic components (Figs. 51-31 and 51-32). Sacrococcygeal teratomas do not generally enter the vertebral canal, but there are rare reports of such extension.[136]

Modern fetal imaging, including ultrasound and MRI, makes the in utero diagnosis of sacrococcygeal teratoma possible[137-139] (Fig. 51-33). Occasionally, the distinction between the diagnosis of myelomeningocele and sacrococcygeal teratoma is challenging.[140] Demonstration of feeding vessels and relative hyperemia in teratomas with color Doppler sonography can aid in making this distinction[141] (Fig. 51-34). In fact, the extreme hyperemia of these tumors can sometimes lead to fetal demise from high-output cardiac failure or newborn death by exsanguination at delivery.[142-144] Therefore, in the situation of developing fetal hydrops, some centers are performing fetal excision of sacrococcygeal teratomas.[145]

An interesting hereditary association, the **Currarino triad,** includes **anorectal stenosis, sacral agenesis,** and a **presacral mass.**[146-150] The so-called sacral agenesis tends to occur in an asymmetrical pattern, and thus a partial crescent-shaped sacrum is observed. The presacral mass may consist of a teratoma, meningocele, or enteric cyst. Although a tendency exists to make the diagnosis of Currarino triad in childhood, screening with ultrasound in infancy might be warranted in patients with a provocative family history.

HEMORRHAGE AND INFECTION

Hemorrhage within the vertebral canal can occur in newborns in association with trauma, such as a birth injury, or with an invasive procedure, such as lumbar puncture. Hemorrhage from birth trauma can be centered at any vertebral level. Hemorrhage related to lumbar puncture is originally centered at the point of needle placement but can extend superiorly and inferiorly for some distance. These primarily epidural collections can be visualized acutely as echogenic fluid that quickly becomes heterogeneous and then anechoic in appearance[151,152] (Fig. 51-35). Injury to the spinal cord itself is also visible with ultrasound as a hyperechoic focus in the acute phase.[153] Echogenic debris within the subarachnoid space is sometimes visible with ultrasound after lumbar puncture (Fig. 51-36). This may represent hemorrhage from the trauma of the procedure or may be caused by redistribution of hemorrhage originally found in the cerebral ventricles of infants with known intraventricular hemorrhage.[154]

The importance of prompt recognition and treatment of epidural abscesses is well documented in the historical literature.[155] In the newborn period, and perhaps even later, ultrasound is useful in detecting such collections.[156,157] This is particularly true if the infant is

Text continued on page 1763

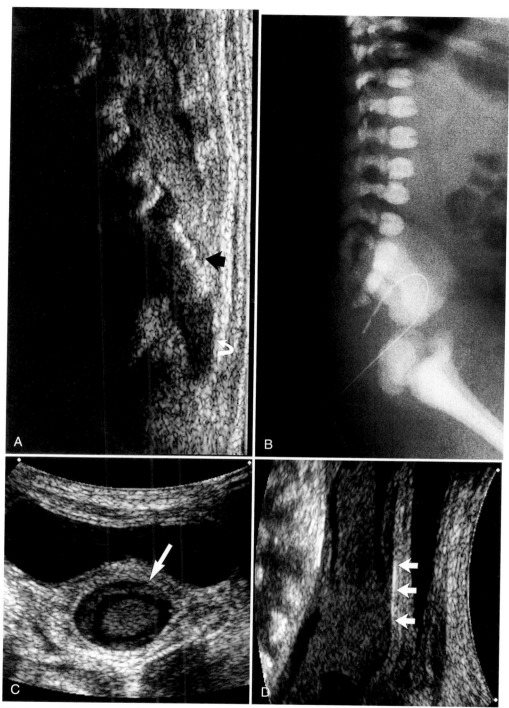

FIGURE 51-27. Imperforate anus in 2-month-old boy. A, Sagittal ultrasound view of the coccyx reveals an abnormally truncated sacrum. The very tip is cartilaginous *(curved arrow),* and there are block vertebral body anomalies *(black arrow).* **B,** The accompanying lateral radiograph of the spine reveals the same findings. **C** and **D,** Transverse and sagittal views of the pelvis show fecal material in the distended rectum *(arrows),* before surgical repair of the imperforate anus.

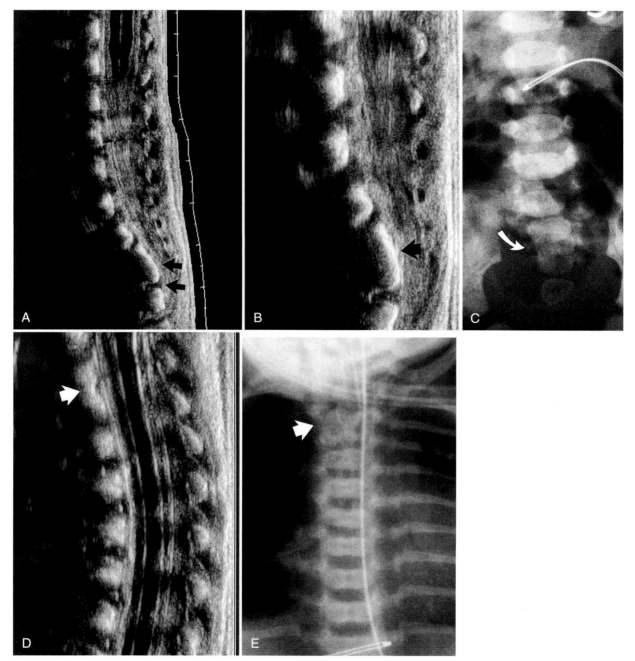

FIGURE 51-28. Imperforate anus. A, Extended–field of view image reveals the abnormal sacral truncation and block vertebrae *(arrows).* **B,** Enlarged view of the same region. **C,** Accompanying radiograph shows the area of vertebral fusion *(curved arrow).* **D,** Sagittal view of the thoracic spine, and **E,** frontal radiograph, reveal an additional block vertebrae *(arrows).*

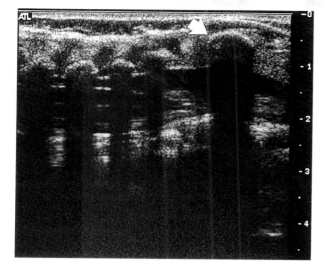

FIGURE 51-29. Abnormal fusion in 9-week-old boy. Abnormal fusion of the posterior elements *(arrow)* created a firm mass to palpation.

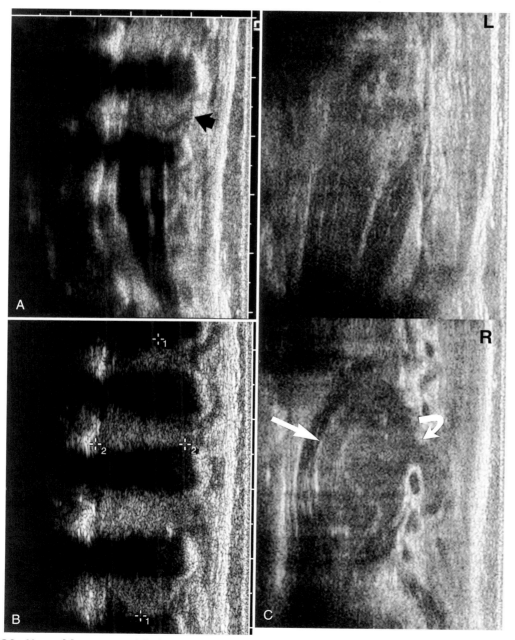

FIGURE 51-30. Neuroblastoma with intraspinal extension. This 4-week-old girl presented with rectal prolapse. Initial imaging included spinal sonography. **A** and **B,** On sagittal views (oriented to match MR images), a homogeneously echogenic mass was discovered within the lumbar vertebral canal *(arrow).* **C,** Paired sagittal left and right views of the psoas muscle demonstrate the clear asymmetry. On the right side, the mass can be seen to deviate the psoas muscle anteriorly *(straight arrow)* and to protrude through the neural foramen *(curved arrow).*

Continued

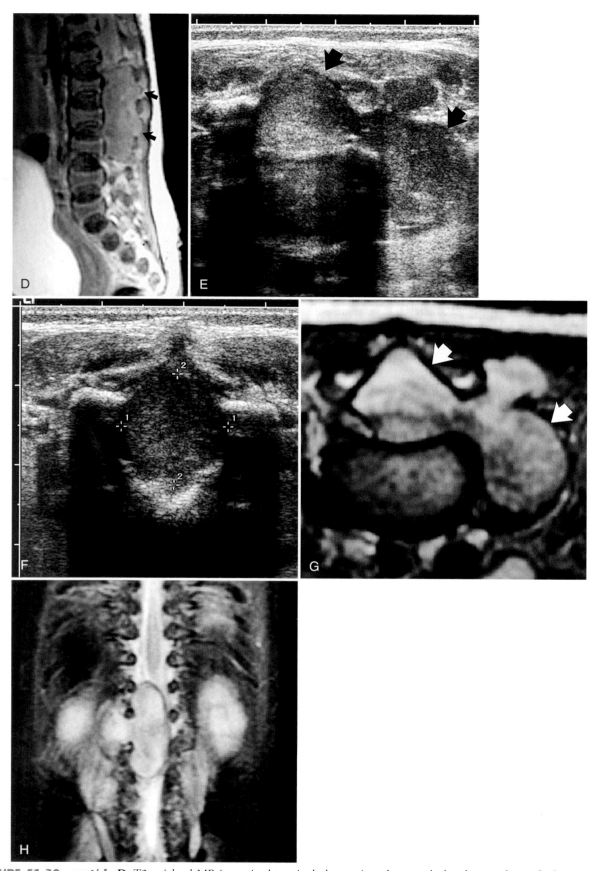

FIGURE 51-30, cont'd. D, T2-weighted MR image in the sagittal plane, oriented to match the ultrasound, reveals the same mass *(black arrows).* **E** and **F,** Transverse sonogram shows that the mass fills the canal, and there is also a clear connection with the retroperi- toneum on the right side *(black arrows).* **G,** T2-weighted MR image reveals the same unusual dumbbell-like configuration of an intraspinal mass with a visible connection to a paraspinal/retroperitoneal mass. **H,** Coronal T2-weighted MR image reveals the intraspinal mass compressing the conus medullaris and its contiguity with the retroperitoneal mass.

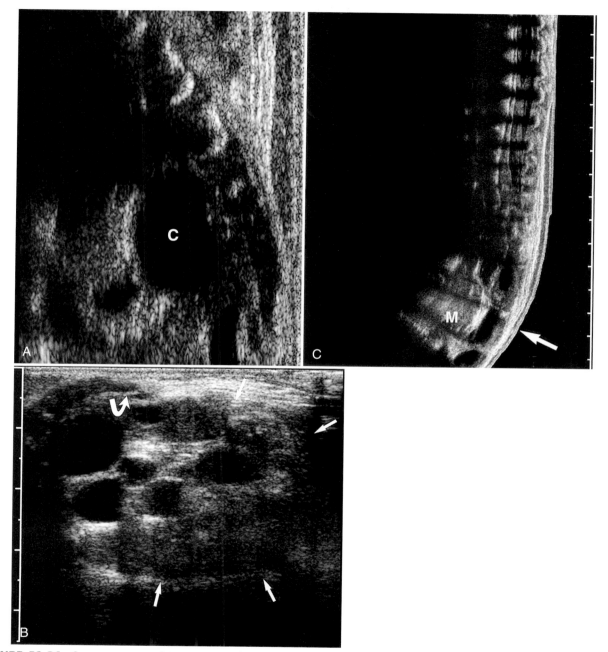

FIGURE 51-31. Sacrococcygeal teratoma. Three-day-old infant girl presented with "fullness" in the buttocks. **A,** Sagittal view shows a complex mass immediately anterior to the cartilaginous coccyx. Portions of the mass are cystic *(C)*. **B,** More distal view reveals the tip of the coccyx *(curved arrow)*. The large mass extended even below the end of coccyx *(straight arrows)*. **C,** Extended–field of view image gives another sense of the relative size of the mass *(M)* compared to the rest of the spine *(arrow,* end of coccyx), but the contour of the skin of the buttocks was not distorted.

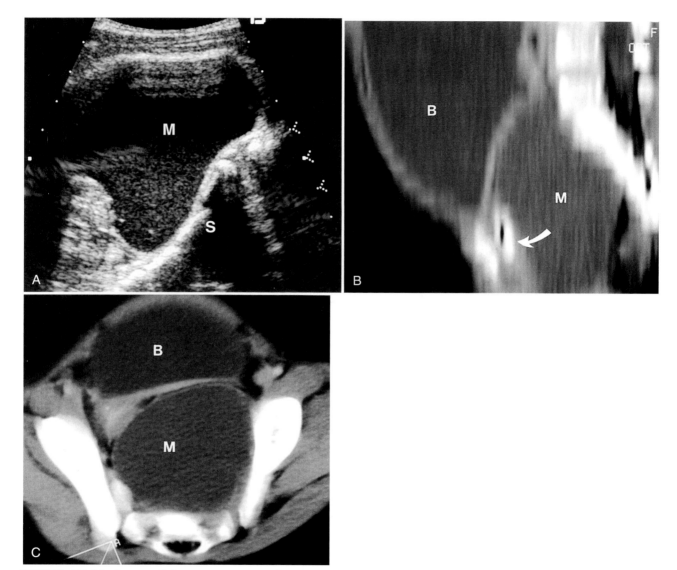

FIGURE 51-32. Intrapelvic sacrococcygeal teratoma. Three-year-old girl presented with bladder outlet obstruction. **A,** Sagittal ultrasound view of the pelvis shows a complex cystic mass *(M)* that might have been mistaken for the urinary bladder. The mass was compressed immediately against the anterior wall of the sacrum *(S)*. **B,** Reconstructed sagittal, and **C,** direct axial, CT views reveal the mass *(M)* and the distended urinary bladder *(B)*. High-intensity material is barium within the anteriorly displaced rectum *(curved arrow).*

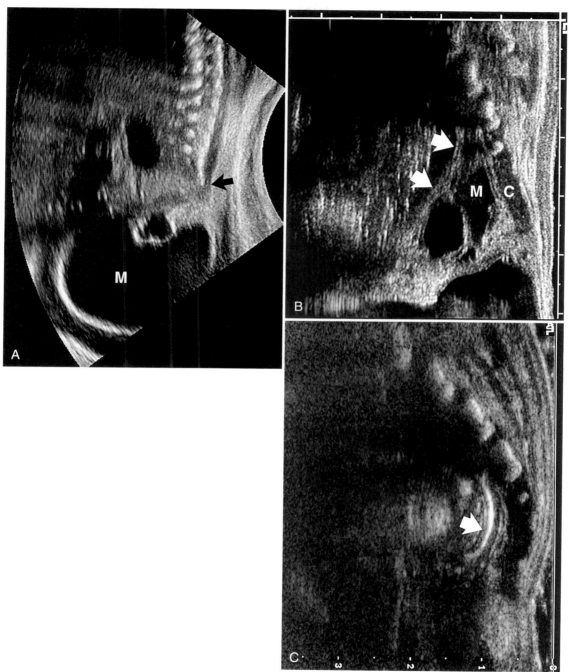

FIGURE 51-33. Cystic sacrococcygeal teratoma. A, Fetus at 25 weeks' gestation. The distal end of the calcified spine *(black arrow)* and the cystic portion of the mass *(M)* are demonstrated. **B,** Postnatal ultrasound. The mass *(M)* is positioned immediately anterior to the coccyx *(C)* and immediately posterior to the posterior wall of the rectum *(arrows)*. A large portion of the mass was external, and a small tongue of the tumor extended into a presacral, retrorectal position. **C, Normal infant,** sagittal view, shows air within the rectum *(arrow),* which hugs the anterior aspect of the coccyx.

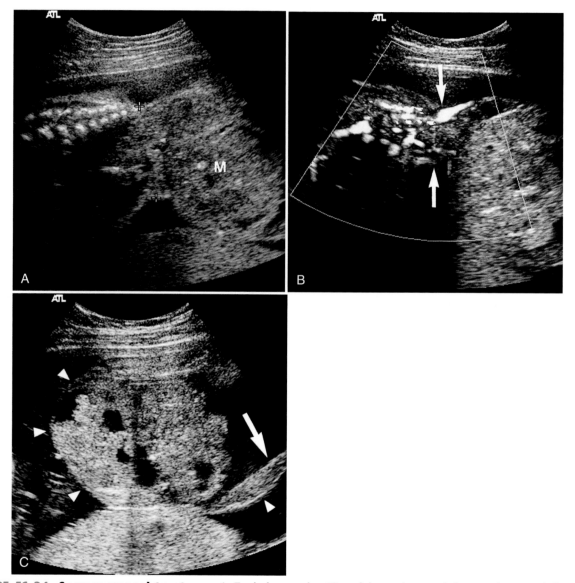

FIGURE 51-34. Sacrococcygeal teratoma. A, Fetal ultrasound at 30 weeks' gestation revealed a complex mass *(M)*. **B,** Color Doppler sonogram shows unusually prominent vessels feeding the mass *(arrows)*. **C,** Transverse view of mass *(arrowheads)* shows dependent fluid levels *(arrow)*, suggesting previous in utero hemorrhage.

medically unstable and transfer to the MRI suite is deemed too risky. It is important to scan the entire length of the vertebral column and to pay special attention to the integrity of the vertebral bodies in these patients.

OTHER POTENTIAL USES OF SPINAL SONOGRAPHY

Many authors have described the use of intraoperative spinal sonography in minimizing surgical invasion of the spinal cord and in analyzing normal and abnormal cord motion.[158-161] Once a **laminectomy** has been performed, the extended window into the vertebral canal makes highly detailed imaging possible, even in older patients.[162] Masses can be precisely localized, and optimal position of the neck and thus the cervical cord can be determined before cervical vertebral fusion. Ultrasound has successfully guided fine-needle aspiration biopsy of lytic vertebral body and paraspinal mass lesions.[163] Definition of postoperative collections is also possible (Fig. 51-37). In general, the superficial soft tissues of the back are well defined by ultrasound. Superficial **hemangiomas** of the back, frequently the impetus to perform spine sonography, are well delineated on ultrasound (Fig. 51-38).

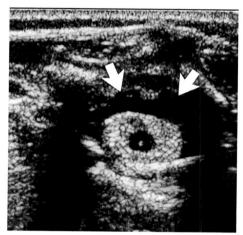

FIGURE 51-35. Epidural hemorrhage. Transverse view of the lumbar spine shows the hypoechoic spinal cord with closely positioned, echogenic nerve rootlets surrounded by a halo of anechoic fluid *(arrows),* caused by an epidural hemorrhage after a lumbar puncture. This hemorrhage became anechoic over time.

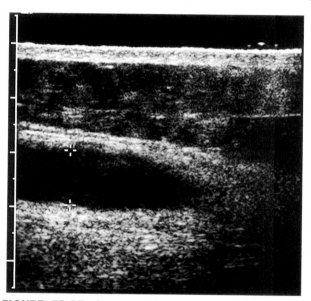

FIGURE 51-37. Seroma. Transverse view of the back in a 6-year-old child after posterior spinal fusion for scoliosis. Cursors indicate the presence of a seroma.

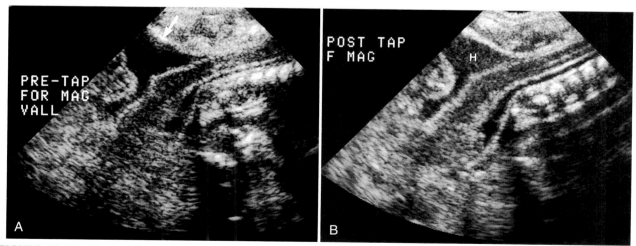

FIGURE 51-36. Hemorrhage in cisterna magna after lumbar tap. A, Sagittal view of the craniocervical junction before a lumbar tap using the foramen magnum as a window reveals anechoic fluid in the cisterna magna *(arrow).* **B,** The same region contains internal echoes, indicating the presence of hemorrhage *(H),* after lumbar tap.

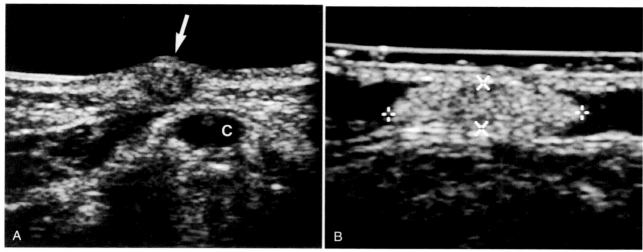

FIGURE 51-38. Subcutaneous hemangiomas. A, Transverse ultrasound of a palpable, red mass adjacent to the coccyx *(C)* in a newborn. There is no extension into the vertebral canal, and the underlying spinal cord *(arrow)* is normal. **B,** Sagittal ultrasound view of another infant shows an echogenic lesion that does not distort the skin surface. The standoff pad is helpful to demonstrate or exclude changes in skin contour.

References

Embryology

1. Jinkins JR. Embryology: embryology of the spine. In: John JR, editor. Atlas of neurologic embryology, anatomy, and variants. Philadelphia: Lippincott–Williams & Wilkins; 2000. p. 33-38.
2. Moore KL, Persaud TVN. The nervous system. In: The developing human: clinically oriented embryology. Philadelphia: Saunders; 2003. p. 427-463.
3. Barkovich AJ. The nervous system. In: Pediatric neuroimaging. Philadelphia: Lippincott–Williams & Wilkins; 2000. p. 13-69.
4. Barkovich AJ. Congenital anomalies of the spine. In: Pediatric neuroimaging. Philadelphia: Lippincott–Williams & Wilkins; 2000. p. 621-683.
5. O'Rahilly R, Gardner E. The timing and sequence of events in the development of the human nervous system during the embryonic period proper. Z Anat Entwicklungsgesch 1971;134:1-12.
6. Dias MS, Pang D. Human neural embryogenesis: a description of neural morphogenesis and a review of embryonic mechanisms. In: Pang D, editor. Disorders of the pediatric spine. New York: Raven Press; 1995. p. 1-26.
7. Dias MS, McLone DG. Normal and abnormal early development of the nervous system. In: McLone DG, editor. Pediatric neurosurgery: surgery of the developing nervous system. Philadelphia: Saunders; 2001. p. 31-71.
8. Muller F, O'Rahilly R. The development of the human brain, the closure of the caudal neuropore, and the beginning of secondary neurulation at stage 12. Anat Embryol (Berl) 1987;176:413-430.
9. Lowe LH, Johanek AJ, Moore CW. Sonography of the neonatal spine. Part 1. Normal anatomy, imaging pitfalls, and variations that may simulate disorders. AJR Am J Roentgenol 2007;188:733-738.
10. Dias MS, Walker ML. The embryogenesis of complex dysraphic malformations: a disorder of gastrulation? Pediatr Neurosurg 1992; 18:229-253.

Sonographic Technique and Normal Anatomy

11. Beek FJ, van Leeuwen MS, Bax NM, et al. A method for sonographic counting of the lower vertebral bodies in newborns and infants. AJNR Am J Neuroradiol 1994;15:445-449.
12. Gusnard DA, Naidich TP, Yousefzadeh DK, Haughton VM. Ultrasonic anatomy of the normal neonatal and infant spine: correlation with cryomicrotome sections and CT. Neuroradiology 1986;28:493-511.
13. St Amour TE, Rubin JM, Dohrmann GJ. The central canal of the spinal cord: ultrasonic identification. Radiology 1984;152:767-769.

14. Nelson Jr MD, Sedler JA, Gilles FH. Spinal cord central echo complex: histoanatomic correlation. Radiology 1989;170:479-481.
15. Lowe LH, Johanek AJ, Moore CW. Sonography of the neonatal spine. Part 2. Spinal disorders. AJR Am J Roentgenol 2007;188: 739-744.
16. Beek FJ, Bax KM, Mali WP. Sonography of the coccyx in newborns and infants. J Ultrasound Med 1994;13:629-634.
17. Ballantyne JW. The spinal column of the infant. Edinburgh Med J 1892;37:913-922.
18. Miller MM. Prenatal growth of the human spinal cord. J Comp Neurol 1913;23:39-70.
19. Streeter GL. Factors involved in the formation of the filum terminale. Am J Anat 1919;25:1-11.
20. Barson AJ. The vertebral level of termination of the spinal cord during normal and abnormal development. J Anat 1970;106: 489-497.
21. Wilson DA, Prince JR. John Caffey award. MR imaging determination of the location of the normal conus medullaris throughout childhood. AJR Am J Roentgenol 1989;152:1029-1032.
22. Hawass ND, el-Badawi MG, Fatani JA, et al. Myelographic study of the spinal cord ascent during fetal development. AJNR Am J Neuroradiol 1987;8:691-695.
23. DiPietro MA. The conus medullaris: normal US findings throughout childhood. Radiology 1993;188:149-153.
24. Robbin ML, Filly RA, Goldstein RB. The normal location of the fetal conus medullaris. J Ultrasound Med 1994;13:541-546.
25. Hill CA, Gibson PJ. Ultrasound determination of the normal location of the conus medullaris in neonates. AJNR Am J Neuroradiol 1995;16:469-472.
26. Sahin F, Selcuki M, Ecin N, et al. Level of conus medullaris in term and preterm neonates. Arch Dis Child Fetal Neonatal Ed 1997;77:F67-F69.
27. Beek FJ, de Vries LS, Gerards LJ, Mali WP. Sonographic determination of the position of the conus medullaris in premature and term infants. Neuroradiology 1996;38(Suppl 1):174-177.
28. Wolf S, Schneble F, Troger J. The conus medullaris: time of ascendance to normal level. Pediatr Radiol 1992;22:590-592.

The Craniocervical Junction

29. Goodwin L, Quisling RG. The neonatal cisterna magna: ultrasonic evaluation. Radiology 1983;149:691-695.
30. Cramer BC, Jequier S, O'Gorman AM. Sonography of the neonatal craniocervical junction. AJR Am J Roentgenol 1986;147:133-139.
31. Harlow CL, Drose JA. A special technique for cervical spine sonography. Illustrated by a patient with meningoencephalocele, Dandy-Walker variant, and syringomyelia. J Ultrasound Med 1992;11: 502-506.

Spinal Dysraphism

32. Leveuf J. Etudes sur le spina bifida. Paris: Masson & Cie; 1937.
33. Lichtenstein BW. Spinal dysraphism. Arch Neurol Psychiatry 1940;44:792-810.

Overt Spinal Dysraphism

34. De la Cruz R, Millan JM, Miralles M, Munoz MJ. Cranial sonographic evaluation in children with meningomyelocele. Childs Nerv Syst 1989;5:94-98.
35. Levy LM, Di Chiro G, McCullough DC, et al. Fixed spinal cord: diagnosis with MR imaging. Radiology 1988;169:773-778.
36. Schumacher R, Kroll B, Schwarz M, Ermert JA. M-mode sonography of the caudal spinal cord in patients with meningomyelocele. Work in progress. Radiology 1992;184:263-265.
37. Brunelle F, Sebag G, Baraton J, et al. Lumbar spinal cord motion measurement with phase-contrast MR imaging in normal children and in children with spinal lipomas. Pediatr Radiol 1996;26:265-270.
38. Gerscovich EO, Maslen L, Cronan MS, et al. Spinal sonography and magnetic resonance imaging in patients with repaired myelomeningocele: comparison of modalities. J Ultrasound Med 1999;18:655-664.
39. Fiske CE, Filly RA. Ultrasound evaluation of the normal and abnormal fetal neural axis. Radiol Clin North Am 1982;20:285-296.
40. Russ PD, Pretorius DH, Manco-Johnson ML, Rumack CM. The fetal spine. Neuroradiology 1986;28:398-407.
41. Dennis MA, Drose JA, Pretorius DH, Manco-Johnson ML. Normal fetal sacrum simulating spina bifida: "pseudodysraphism." Radiology 1985;155:751-754.
42. Johnson DD, Pretorius DH, Riccabona M, et al. Three-dimensional ultrasound of the fetal spine. Obstet Gynecol 1997;89:434-438.
43. Coniglio SJ, Anderson SM, Ferguson 2nd JE. Functional motor outcome in children with myelomeningocele: correlation with anatomic level on prenatal ultrasound. Dev Med Child Neurol 1996;38:675-680.
44. Whitby E, Paley MN, Davies N, et al. Ultrafast magnetic resonance imaging of central nervous system abnormalities in utero in the second and third trimester of pregnancy: comparison with ultrasound. BJOG 2001;108:519-526.
45. Meuli M, Meuli-Simmen C, Hutchins GM, et al. In utero surgery rescues neurological function at birth in sheep with spina bifida. Nat Med 1995;1:342-347.
46. Adzick NS, Sutton LN, Crombleholme TM, Flake AW. Successful fetal surgery for spina bifida. Lancet 1998;352:1675-1676.
47. Huisman TA, Wisser J, Martin E, et al. Fetal magnetic resonance imaging of the central nervous system: a pictorial essay. Eur Radiol 2002;12:1952-1961.
48. Kitano Y, Flake AW, Crombleholme TM, et al. Open fetal surgery for life-threatening fetal malformations. Semin Perinatol 1999;23:448-461.
49. Tulipan N, Hernanz-Schulman M, et al. Intrauterine myelomeningocele repair reverses preexisting hindbrain herniation. Pediatr Neurosurg 1999;31:137-142.
50. Smithells RW, Sheppard S, Schorah CJ, et al. Possible prevention of neural-tube defects by periconceptional vitamin supplementation. Lancet 1980;1:339-340.

Occult Spinal Dysraphism

51. Anderson FM. Occult spinal dysraphism: diagnosis and management. J Pediatr 1968;73:163-177.
52. Hall DE, Udvarhelyi GB, Altman J. Lumbosacral skin lesions as markers of occult spinal dysraphism. JAMA 1981;246:2606-2608.
53. Albright AL, Gartner JC, Wiener ES. Lumbar cutaneous hemangiomas as indicators of tethered spinal cords. Pediatrics 1989;83:977-980.
54. Kriss VM, Desai NS. Occult spinal dysraphism in neonates: assessment of high-risk cutaneous stigmata on sonography. AJR Am J Roentgenol 1998;171:1687-1692.
55. Miller JH, Reid BS, Kemberling CR. Utilization of ultrasound in the evaluation of spinal dysraphism in children. Radiology 1982;143:737-740.
56. Raghavendra BN, Epstein FJ, Pinto RS, et al. The tethered spinal cord: diagnosis by high-resolution real-time ultrasound. Radiology 1983;149:123-128.
57. Naidich TP, Fernbach SK, McLone DG, Shkolnik A. John Caffey Award. Sonography of the caudal spine and back: congenital anomalies in children. AJR Am J Roentgenol 1984;142:1229-1242.
58. Kangarloo H, Gold RH, Diament MJ, et al. High-resolution spinal sonography in infants. AJR Am J Roentgenol 1984;142:1243-1247.
59. Naidich TP, Radkowski MA, Britton J. Real-time sonographic display of caudal spinal anomalies. Neuroradiology 1986;28:512-527.
60. Zieger M, Dorr U, Schulz RD. Pediatric spinal sonography. Part II. Malformations and mass lesions. Pediatr Radiol 1988;18:105-111.
61. Korsvik HE, Keller MS. Sonography of occult dysraphism in neonates and infants with MR imaging correlation. Radiographics 1992;12:297-306; discussion 307-308.
62. Rohrschneider WK, Forsting M, Darge K, Troger J. Diagnostic value of spinal US: comparative study with MR imaging in pediatric patients. Radiology 1996;200:383-388.
63. Pierre-Kahn A, Zerah M, Renier D, et al. Congenital lumbosacral lipomas. Childs Nerv Syst 1997;13:298-334; discussion 335.
64. La Marca F, Grant JA, Tomita T, McLone DG. Spinal lipomas in children: outcome of 270 procedures. Pediatr Neurosurg 1997;26:8-16.
65. Seeds JW, Jones FD. Lipomyelomeningocele: prenatal diagnosis and management. Obstet Gynecol 1986;67:34S-37S.
66. Kim SY, McGahan JP, Boggan JE, McGrew W. Prenatal diagnosis of lipomyelomeningocele. J Ultrasound Med 2000;19:801-805.
67. McLendon RE, Oakes WJ, Heinz ER, et al. Adipose tissue in the filum terminale: a computed tomographic finding that may indicate tethering of the spinal cord. Neurosurgery 1988;22:873-876.
68. Uchino A, Mori T, Ohno M. Thickened fatty filum terminale: MR imaging. Neuroradiology 1991;33:331-333.
69. McLone DG, Thompson DNP. Lipomas of the spine. In: McLone DG, editor. Pediatric neurosurgery: surgery of the developing nervous system. Philadelphia: Saunders; 2001. p. 289-301.
70. Raghavan N, Barkovich AJ, Edwards M, Norman D. MR imaging in the tethered spinal cord syndrome. AJR Am J Roentgenol 1989;152:843-852.
71. Rypens F, Avni EF, Matos C, et al. Atypical and equivocal sonographic features of the spinal cord in neonates. Pediatr Radiol 1995;25:429-432.
72. Fitz CR, Harwood Nash DC. The tethered conus. Am J Roentgenol Radium Ther Nucl Med 1975;125:515-523.
73. Martinez-Lage JF, Esteban JA, Poza M, Casas C. Congenital dermal sinus associated with an abscessed intramedullary epidermoid cyst in a child: case report and review of the literature. Childs Nerv Syst 1995;11:301-305.
74. Walker AE, Bucy PC. Congenital dermal sinuses: a source of spinal meningeal infection and subdural abscesses. Brain 1934;57:401-421.
75. Mount LA. Congenital dermal sinuses as a cause of meningitis, intraspinal abscess and intracranial abscess. J Am Med Assoc 1949;139:1263-1268.
76. Haworth JC, Zachary RB. Congenital dermal sinuses in children: their relation to pilonidal sinuses. Lancet 1955;269:10-14.
77. Wright RL. Congenital dermal sinuses. Prog Neurol Surg 1971;4:175-191.
78. Barkovich AJ, Edwards M, Cogen PH. MR evaluation of spinal dermal sinus tracts in children. AJNR Am J Neuroradiol 1991;12:123-129.
79. McLone DG, Naidich TP. Terminal myelocystocele. Neurosurgery 1985;16:36-43.
80. Unsinn KM, Geley T, Freund MC, Gassner I. Ultrasound of the spinal cord in newborns: spectrum of normal findings, variants, congenital anomalies, and acquired diseases. Radiographics 2000;20:923-938.
81. Peacock WJ, Murovic JA. Magnetic resonance imaging in myelocystoceles: report of two cases. J Neurosurg 1989;70:804-807.
82. Nishino A, Shirane R, So K, et al. Cervical myelocystocele with Chiari II malformation: magnetic resonance imaging and surgical treatment. Surg Neurol 1998;49:269-273.
83. Meyer SH, Morris GF, Pretorius DH, James HE. Terminal myelocystocele: important differential diagnosis in the prenatal assessment of spina bifida. J Ultrasound Med 1998;17:193-197.
84. Midrio P, Silberstein HJ, Bilaniuk LT, et al. Prenatal diagnosis of terminal myelocystocele in the fetal surgery era: case report. Neurosurgery 2002;50:1152-1154; discussion 1154-1155.

85. Schijman E. Split spinal cord malformations: report of 22 cases and review of the literature. Childs Nerv Syst 2003;19:96-103.
86. Glasier CM, Chadduck WM, Burrows PE. Diagnosis of diastematomyelia with high-resolution spinal ultrasound. Childs Nerv Syst 1986;2:255-257.
87. Raghavendra BN, Epstein FJ, Pinto RS, et al. Sonographic diagnosis of diastematomyelia. J Ultrasound Med 1988;7:111-113.
88. Sepulveda W, Kyle PM, Hassan J, Weiner E. Prenatal diagnosis of diastematomyelia: case reports and review of the literature. Prenat Diagn 1997;17:161-165.
89. Allen LM, Silverman RK. Prenatal ultrasound evaluation of fetal diastematomyelia: two cases of type I split cord malformation. Ultrasound Obstet Gynecol 2000;15:78-82.
90. Ugarte N, Gonzalez-Crussi F, Sotelo-Avila C. Diastematomyelia associated with teratomas: report of two cases. J Neurosurg 1980;53:720-725.
91. Fernandes ET, Custer MD, Burton EM, et al. Neurenteric cyst: surgery and diagnostic imaging. J Pediatr Surg 1991;26:108-110.
92. Akgur FM, Ozdemir T, Olguner M, et al. A case of split notochord syndrome: presence of dorsal enteric diverticulum adjacent to the dorsal enteric fistula. J Pediatr Surg 1998;33:1317-1319.
93. Macaulay KE, Winter 3rd TC, Shields LE. Neurenteric cyst shown by prenatal sonography. AJR Am J Roentgenol 1997;169:563-565.
94. Uludag S, Madazli R, Erdogan E, et al. A case of prenatally diagnosed fetal neurenteric cyst. Ultrasound Obstet Gynecol 2001;18:277-279.
95. Almog B, Leibovitch L, Achiron R. Split notochord syndrome: prenatal ultrasonographic diagnosis. Prenat Diagn 2001;21:1159-1162.
96. Long FR, Hunter JV, Mahboubi S, et al. Tethered cord and associated vertebral anomalies in children and infants with imperforate anus: evaluation with MR imaging and plain radiography. Radiology 1996;200:377-382.
97. Appignani BA, Jaramillo D, Barnes PD, Poussaint TY. Dysraphic myelodysplasias associated with urogenital and anorectal anomalies: prevalence and types seen with MR imaging. AJR Am J Roentgenol 1994;163:1199-1203.
98. Carson JA, Barnes PD, Tunell WP, et al. Imperforate anus: the neurologic implication of sacral abnormalities. J Pediatr Surg 1984;19:838-842.
99. Warf BC, Scott RM, Barnes PD, Hendren 3rd WH. Tethered spinal cord in patients with anorectal and urogenital malformations. Pediatr Neurosurg 1993;19:25-30.
100. Chestnut R, James HE, Jones KL. The Vater association and spinal dysraphia. Pediatr Neurosurg 1992;18:144-148.
101. Karrer FM, Flannery AM, Nelson Jr MD, et al. Anorectal malformations: evaluation of associated spinal dysraphic syndromes. J Pediatr Surg 1988;23:45-48.
102. Beek FJ, Boemers TM, Witkamp TD, et al. Spine evaluation in children with anorectal malformations. Pediatr Radiol 1995;25(Suppl 1):28-32.

Caudal Regression
103. Duhamel B. From the mermaid to anal imperforation: the syndrome of caudal regression. Arch Dis Child 1961;36:152-155.
104. Harlow CL, Partington MD, Thieme GA. Lumbosacral agenesis: clinical characteristics, imaging, and embryogenesis. Pediatr Neurosurg 1995;23:140-147.
105. Barkovich AJ, Raghavan N, Chuang S, Peck WW. The wedge-shaped cord terminus: a radiographic sign of caudal regression. AJNR Am J Neuroradiol 1989;10:1223-1231.
106. Muthukumar N. Surgical treatment of nonprogressive neurological deficits in children with sacral agenesis. Neurosurgery 1996;38:1133-1137; discussion 1137-1138.
107. Baxi L, Warren W, Collins MH, Timor-Tritsch IE. Early detection of caudal regression syndrome with transvaginal scanning. Obstet Gynecol 1990;75:486-489.
108. Twickler D, Budorick N, Pretorius D, et al. Caudal regression versus sirenomelia: sonographic clues. J Ultrasound Med 1993;12:323-330.
109. Adra A, Cordero D, Mejides A, et al. Caudal regression syndrome: etiopathogenesis, prenatal diagnosis, and perinatal management. Obstet Gynecol Surv 1994;49:508-516.
110. Zaw W, Stone DG. Caudal regression syndrome in twin pregnancy with type II diabetes. J Perinatol 2002;22:171-174.
111. Morichon-Delvallez N, Delezoide AL, Vekemans M. Holoprosencephaly and sacral agenesis in a fetus with a terminal deletion 7q36→7qter. J Med Genet 1993;30:521-524.
112. Schrander-Stumpel C, Schrander J, Fryns JP, Hamers G. Caudal deficiency sequence in 7q terminal deletion. Am J Med Genet 1988;30:757-761.
113. Nowaczyk MJ, Huggins MJ, Tomkins DJ, et al. Holoprosencephaly, sacral anomalies, and situs ambiguus in an infant with partial monosomy 7q/trisomy 2p and SHH and HLXB9 haploinsufficiency. Clin Genet 2000;57:388-393.

Vertebral Body Anomalies
114. Brockmeyer DL, Smith JT. Congenital vertebral anomalies. In: McLone DG, editor. Pediatric neurosurgery: surgery of the developing nervous system. Philadelphia: Saunders; 2001. p. 428-441.
115. Abrams SL, Filly RA. Congenital vertebral malformations: prenatal diagnosis using ultrasonography. Radiology 1985;155:762.
116. Benacerraf BR, Greene MF, Barss VA. Prenatal sonographic diagnosis of congenital hemivertebra. J Ultrasound Med 1986;5:257-259.
117. Rouse GA, Filly RA, Toomey F, Grube GL. Short-limb skeletal dysplasias: evaluation of the fetal spine with sonography and radiography. Radiology 1990;174:177-180.
118. Zelop CM, Pretorius DH, Benacerraf BR. Fetal hemivertebrae: associated anomalies, significance, and outcome. Obstet Gynecol 1993;81:412-416.
119. Jarcho S, Levin PM. Hereditary malformation of the vertebral bodies. Bull Johns Hopkins Hosp 1938;62:216.
120. Tolmie JL, Whittle MJ, McNay MB, et al. Second trimester prenatal diagnosis of the Jarcho-Levin syndrome. Prenat Diagn 1987;7:129-134.
121. Lawson ME, Share J, Benacerraf B, Krauss CM. Jarcho-Levin syndrome: prenatal diagnosis, perinatal care, and follow-up of siblings. J Perinatol 1997;17:407-409.
122. Larsen LJ, Schottstaedt ER, Bost FC. Multiple congenital dislocations associated with characteristic facial abnormality. J Pediatr 1950;37:574-581.
123. Latta RJ, Graham CB, Aase J, et al. Larsen's syndrome: a skeletal dysplasia with multiple joint dislocations and unusual facies. J Pediatr 1971;78:291-298.
124. Tongsong T, Wanapirak C, Pongsatha S, Sudasana J. Prenatal sonographic diagnosis of Larsen syndrome. J Ultrasound Med 2000;19:419-421.
125. Ulmer JL, Elster AD, Ginsberg LE, Williams 3rd DW. Klippel-Feil syndrome: CT and MR of acquired and congenital abnormalities of cervical spine and cord. J Comput Assist Tomogr 1993;17:215-224.
126. Duncan PA, Shapiro LR, Stangel JJ, et al. The MURCS association: müllerian duct aplasia, renal aplasia, and cervicothoracic somite dysplasia. J Pediatr 1979;95:399-402.
127. Fernandez CO, McFarland RD, Timmons C, et al. MURCS association: ultrasonographic findings and pathologic correlation. J Ultrasound Med 1996;15:867-870.

Tumors
128. Patel RB. Sonographic diagnosis of intraspinal neuroblastoma. J Clin Ultrasound 1985;13:565-569.
129. Garcia CJ, Keller MS. Intraspinal extension of paraspinal masses in infants: detection by sonography. Pediatr Radiol 1990;20:437-439.
130. Windisch TR, Naul LG, Bauserman SC. Intramedullary gliofibroma: MR, ultrasound, and pathologic correlation. J Comput Assist Tomogr 1995;19:646-648.
131. Gonzalez-Crussi F, Winkler RF, Mirkin DL. Sacrococcygeal teratomas in infants and children: relationship of histology and prognosis in 40 cases. Arch Pathol Lab Med 1978;102:420-425.
132. Ein SH, Adeyemi SD, Mancer K. Benign sacrococcygeal teratomas in infants and children: a 25-year review. Ann Surg 1980;191:382-384.
133. Lahdenne P, Heikinheimo M, Nikkanen V, et al. Neonatal benign sacrococcygeal teratoma may recur in adulthood and give rise to malignancy. Cancer 1993;72:3727-3731.
134. Altman RP, Randolph JG, Lilly JR. Sacrococcygeal teratoma: American Academy of Pediatrics Surgical Section Survey—1973. J Pediatr Surg 1974;9:389-398.

135. Noseworthy J, Lack EE, Kozakewich HP, et al. Sacrococcygeal germ cell tumors in childhood: an updated experience with 118 patients. J Pediatr Surg 1981;16:358-364.
136. Ribeiro PR, Guys JM, Lena G. Sacrococcygeal teratoma with an intradural and extramedullary extension in a neonate: case report. Neurosurgery 1999;44:398-400.
137. Teal LN, Angtuaco TL, Jimenez JF, Quirk Jr JG. Fetal teratomas: antenatal diagnosis and clinical management. J Clin Ultrasound 1988;16:329-336.
138. Chisholm CA, Heider AL, Kuller JA, et al. Prenatal diagnosis and perinatal management of fetal sacrococcygeal teratoma. Am J Perinatol 1999;16:89-92.
139. Avni FE, Guibaud L, Robert Y, et al. MR imaging of fetal sacrococcygeal teratoma: diagnosis and assessment. AJR Am J Roentgenol 2002;178:179-183.
140. Yu JA, Sohaey R, Kennedy AM, Selden NR. Terminal myelocystocele and sacrococcygeal teratoma: a comparison of fetal ultrasound presentation and perinatal risk. AJNR Am J Neuroradiol 2007;28:1058-1060.
141. Sherer DM, Fromberg RA, Rindfusz DW, et al. Color Doppler aided prenatal diagnosis of a type 1 cystic sacrococcygeal teratoma simulating a meningomyelocele. Am J Perinatol 1997;14:13-15.
142. Bond SJ, Harrison MR, Schmidt KG, et al. Death due to high-output cardiac failure in fetal sacrococcygeal teratoma. J Pediatr Surg 1990;25:1287-1291.
143. Langer JC, Harrison MR, Schmidt KG, et al. Fetal hydrops and death from sacrococcygeal teratoma: rationale for fetal surgery. Am J Obstet Gynecol 1989;160:1145-1150.
144. Hoehn T, Krause MF, Wilhelm C, et al. Fatal rupture of a sacrococcygeal teratoma during delivery. J Perinatol 1999;19:596-598.
145. Currarino G, Coln D, Votteler T. Triad of anorectal, sacral, and presacral anomalies. AJR Am J Roentgenol 1981;137:395-398.
146. Deprest JA, Lerut TE, Vandenberghe K. Operative fetoscopy: new perspective in fetal therapy? Prenat Diagn 1997;17:1247-1260.
147. O'Riordain DS, O'Connell PR, Kirwan WO. Hereditary sacral agenesis with presacral mass and anorectal stenosis: the Currarino triad. Br J Surg 1991;78:536-538.
148. Gaskill SJ, Marlin AE. The Currarino triad: its importance in pediatric neurosurgery. Pediatr Neurosurg 1996;25:143-146.
149. Ashcraft KW, Holder TM. Hereditary presacral teratoma. J Pediatr Surg 1974;9:691-697.
150. Cohn J, Bay-Nielsen E. Hereditary defect of the sacrum and coccyx with anterior sacral meningocele. Acta Paediatr Scand 1969;58:268-274.

Hemorrhage and Infection
151. Leadman M, Seigel S, Hollenberg R, Caco C. Ultrasound diagnosis of neonatal spinal epidural hemorrhage. J Clin Ultrasound 1988;16:440-442.
152. Coley BD, Shiels 2nd WE, Hogan MJ. Diagnostic and interventional ultrasonography in neonatal and infant lumbar puncture. Pediatr Radiol 2001;31:399-402.
153. Filippigh P, Clapuyt P, Debauche C, Claus D. Sonographic evaluation of traumatic spinal cord lesions in the newborn infant. Pediatr Radiol 1994;24:245-247.
154. Rudas G, Almassy Z, Papp B, et al. Echodense spinal subarachnoid space in neonates with progressive ventricular dilatation: a marker of noncommunicating hydrocephalus. AJR Am J Roentgenol 1998;171:1119-1121.
155. Stammers FAR. Spinal epidural suppuration, with special reference to osteomyelitis of the vertebrae. Br J Surg 1938;26:366-374.
156. Gudinchet F, Chapuis L, Berger D. Diagnosis of anterior cervical spinal epidural abscess by US and MRI in a newborn. Pediatr Radiol 1991;21:515-517.
157. Rubaltelli L, De Gerone E, Caterino G. Echographic evaluation of tubercular abscesses in lumbar spondylitis. J Ultrasound Med 1990;9:67-70.

Other Potential Uses of Spinal Sonography
158. Rubin JM, DiPietro MA, Chandler WF, Venes JL. Spinal ultrasonography: intraoperative and pediatric applications. Radiol Clin North Am 1988;26:1-27.
159. Jokich PM, Rubin JM, Dohrmann GJ. Intraoperative ultrasonic evaluation of spinal cord motion. J Neurosurg 1984;60:707-711.
160. Maiuri F, Iaconetta G, de Divitiis O. The role of intraoperative sonography in reducing invasiveness during surgery for spinal tumors. Minim Invasive Neurosurg 1997;40:8-12.
161. Theodotou BC, Powers SK. Use of intraoperative ultrasound in decision making during spinal operations. Neurosurgery 1986;19:205-211.
162. Braun IF, Raghavendra BN, Kricheff, II. Spinal cord imaging using real-time high-resolution ultrasound. Radiology 1983;147:459-465.
163. Gupta S, Takhtani D, Gulati M, et al. Sonographically guided fine-needle aspiration biopsy of lytic lesions of the spine: technique and indications. J Clin Ultrasound 1999;27:123-129.

CHAPTER 52

The Pediatric Chest

Chetan Chandulal Shah and S. Bruce Greenberg

Chapter Outline

INDICATIONS FOR CHEST SONOGRAPHY

Extracardiac chest sonography is limited by air in the lungs and bone in the rib cage. However, ultrasound is valuable for evaluating the abnormal chest in which fluid and solid densities interpose between the chest wall and lung. Sonography is particularly well suited for the evaluation of **pleural effusions.** The thymus, liver, and spleen provide windows for chest sonography. Any radiographically opaque chest can be further evaluated by sonography to determine whether there is pleural fluid, a chest mass, atelectasis, consolidation, or lung hypoplasia. Ultrasound can be used to guide thoracentesis, chest tube placement, or biopsy of the pleura, the lung, or a mediastinal mass.

ULTRASOUND TECHNIQUE

Linear transducers with frequencies ranging from 5 to 15 MHz are used for chest ultrasound.[1] Diaphragmatic motion can be assessed using M-mode ultrasound and real-time video comparison of right-to-left motion. Color flow Doppler imaging is useful to demonstrate vascular supply, which is important in the diagnosis of sequestration. The selection of the frequency of the transducer is inversely dependent on patient size. Higher frequencies are used for infants and lower frequencies for adolescents.[2]

Sector or vector transducers are used for intercostal and suprasternal approaches. Linear transducers with the long axis of the transducer aligned with the intercostal space can also be used. We have found that the smaller footprint of newer linear transducers provide improved resolution compared to vector transducers using the intercostal window (Fig. 52-1).

Acoustic windows are better in infants because of the unossified sternum and larger thymus. Transabdominal ultrasound of the lower chest, including the diaphragm, can be performed using the liver, spleen, or fluid-filled stomach as acoustic windows. Sector, vector, or linear array transducers can be used for this purpose.

Free pleural fluid is dependent in position and will shift with patient repositioning. Ultrasound of the dependent areas will identify free pleural fluid and will show loculated fluid, which is not dependent.

SONOGRAPHIC SIGNS OF PLEURAL FLUID

The most frequent use of chest sonography is for the evaluation of a completely radiopaque hemithorax (Fig. 52-2) or a partially radiopaque hemithorax (Fig. 52-3). Ultrasound distinguishes pleural from pulmonary causes of opacification. Chest ultrasound is more sensitive than decubitus radiographs for detecting small amounts of pleural fluid (Fig. 52-4). Pleural fluid collections less than 4 mm in thickness can be physiologic and detected in normal children placed into the elbow position after lying for 5 minutes in a left lateral decubitus position.[3] Pleural effusions transmit sound waves, allowing visualization of structures deep to the pleura that are not normally identifiable, including the posterior wall. The

INDICATIONS FOR CHEST SONOGRAPHY

Fluid Detection and Treatment
Pleural effusions
Pericardial effusion
Thoracentesis and chest tube placement

Masses
Mediastinal masses
Thymus relationship to masses
Extension of neck masses into chest
Peripheral lung mass
Chest wall mass
Needle biopsy of masses
Sclerotherapy of lymphatic malformation

Differentiation
Subpulmonic vs. subphrenic fluid
Tumor vs. large or persistent pleural effusion
Chest wall mass vs. pleural fluid
Cystic vs. solid masses
Consolidation vs. atelectasis
Round pneumonia vs. mediastinal mass
Thymus vs. mediastinal mass

Diaphragm Disorders
Diaphragmatic paralysis
Diaphragmatic hernia
Diaphragm defect
Rupture of diaphragm

Vascular Indications
Vascular access
Catheter position in vessels
Vascular thrombi

Uncommon Indications
Pneumothorax
Rib fracture
Rib osteomyelitis

SONOGRAPHIC SIGNS OF PLEURAL FLUID

Hypoechoic fluid collection under chest wall
Moving septations are loculated.
Posterior chest wall is visualized behind the fluid.
Hypoechoic fluid is above diaphragm.
Free fluid moves with respiration.
Septations move if loculated fluid.
Color Doppler signal between visceral and parietal pleura
Color Doppler signal at costophrenic angle
Diaphragm sign (fluid outside or peripheral to diaphragm)
Displaced-crus sign
Bare-area sign

posterior chest wall is normally obscured when the liver is used as an acoustic window because intervening aerated lung reflects the sound beam.

Intercostal and subdiaphragmatic windows are used to access the pleural space. The **spleen** and **liver** are good windows to the pleural space because they are relatively homogeneous, solid organs that provide good through-transmission (Figs. 52-5 and 52-6). The classic appearance of transudative pleural effusion is an echo-free or hypoechoic collection without septations immediately deep to the chest wall, but exudates can also be anechoic.[4] In a recent report, transudative pleural effusions were anechoic in only 45% of patients, with a complex non-septated pattern present in 55% of transudates.[4] The improved resolution of modern ultrasound equipment allows for better resolution of small particles in transudates. Therefore, echogenicity in pleural collections does not exclude the diagnosis of a transudate.

Exudates can be anechoic but are more likely than **transudates** to be complex collections with associated fibrin septations. The collections may be multiloculated with a honeycomb appearance.[5] Exudates are associated with pleural thickening and underlying parenchymal abnormality.[6] Complex collections such as a **hemothorax** (Fig. 52-7) or **empyema** (Fig. 52-8) have thicker fluid with **septations** (Fig. 52-9). Underlying consolidated or atelectatic lung is more echogenic than an effusion. Complicated effusions are characterized by an irregular or indistinct interface between pleura and the adjacent lung. A **fibrothorax** has a thick pleural rind that is echogenic. Multiple hyperechoic foci in the lung are caused by residual air within bronchi and alveoli and are called **sonographic air bronchograms** (Fig. 52-10).

Free fluid changes position with changes in the patient's position. Fluid will move posterior to the liver and lungs when the patient is in a supine position (Fig. 52-11). When the patient is upright, the fluid will move between the lung and diaphragm. Free fluid is indicated by change in the shape of pleural fluid with inspiration and expiration and the presence of **moving septations** within the pleural fluid[7] **(Video 52-1).** These septations are fibrin strands. To-and-fro motion is unequivocal evidence that the fluid has a relatively low viscosity.

Fluid Color Flow Doppler Signal

Color flow Doppler ultrasound aids in distinguishing pleural effusion from pleural thickening or complex collections.[7] Color Doppler signal is identified during respiratory motion between the visceral and parietal pleura in the presence of pleural effusion. Cell movement, debris, and fibrin scatter sound waves, producing the color flow Doppler signal in the pleural fluid collection (Fig. 52-12). Organized pleural thickening will appear as a colorless pleural lesion with no Doppler signal. The color flow Doppler signal has high sensitivity and specificity in determining if a fluid collection can be aspirated.[2]

Text continued on page 1776

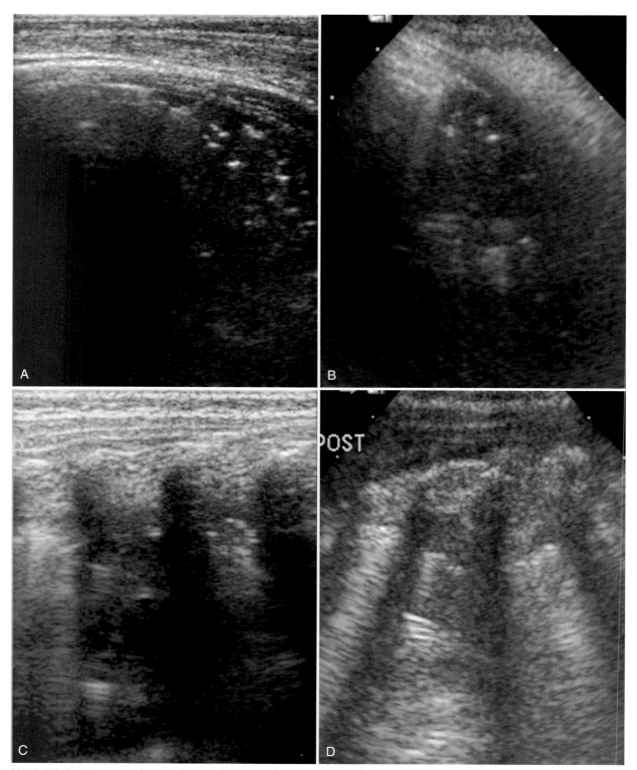

FIGURE 52-1. Pneumonia on chest ultrasound. A, Linear transducer. **B,** Vector transducer. **Air bronchograms** from pneumonia are seen better with linear transducers than vector transducers, especially when the air bronchograms are closer to the chest wall and there is no intervening pleural fluid. **C** and **D,** Air bronchograms within a round pneumonia in another child are better visualized with a linear transducer (**C**) than with a vector transducer (**D**), despite the intervening rib shadows.

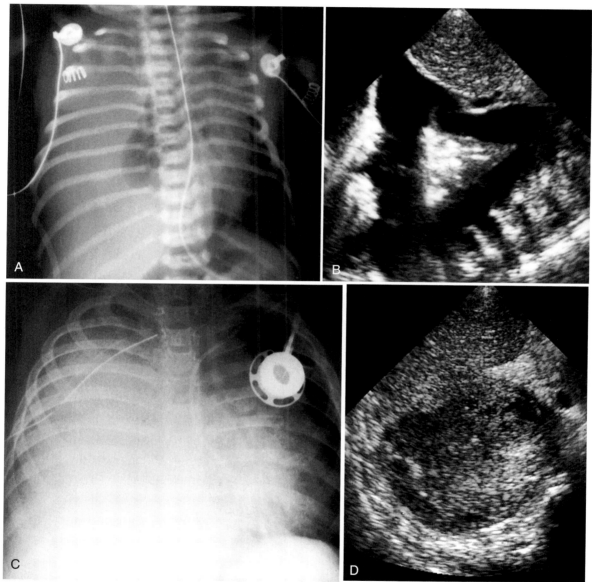

FIGURE 52-2. Radiopaque hemithorax: neonatal chylothorax. A, Anteroposterior chest radiograph in 2-week-old infant shows opacified right chest and shift of heart and mediastinum to left. **B,** Sonogram through liver shows that the opacity is a large accumulation of fluid around a collapsed lung. **C,** Right chest opacification with shift of the heart to the left side, suggesting fluid in the right pleural space. No drainage was obtained from a chest tube. **D,** Sonogram through liver shows that the right chest is filled with solid tissue, which at surgery was infected with **aspergillosis** extending from the liver. *(From Seibert RW, Seibert JJ, Williams SL: The opaque chest: when to suspect a bronchia foreign body. Pediatric Radiol 1986;16:193-196.)*

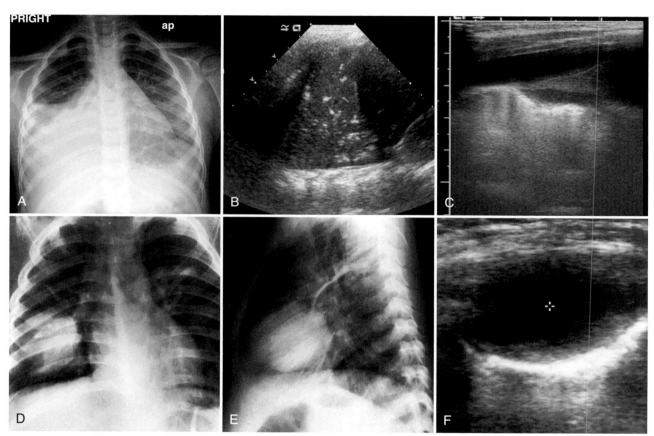

FIGURE 52-3. Partially radiopaque hemithorax. A, Radiograph. **B** and **C,** Sonograms show left upper lobe pneumonia with left pleural fluid. **D** to **F,** Another patient with partially opaque right hemithorax. **D** and **E,** Posteroanterior and lateral chest radiographs. **F,** Sonogram shows that the radiopacity is hypoechoic, loculated fluid collection in the minor fissure.

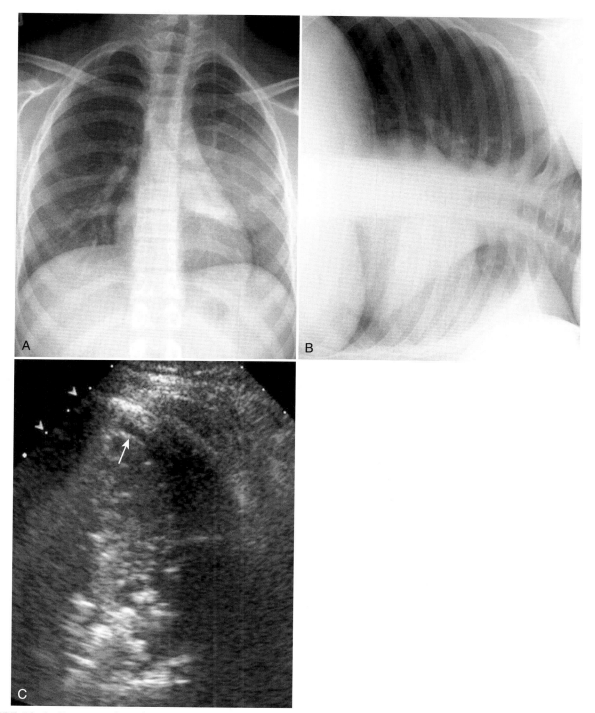

FIGURE 52-4. Pneumonia with small amount of pleural fluid. A and **B,** Posteroanterior and left lateral decubitus chest radiographs did not show pleural fluid. **C,** Sonography performed in upright position shows small amount of pleural fluid in the dependent region *(arrow)*. Echogenic air bronchograms within the consolidated lung confirm presence of underlying pneumonia.

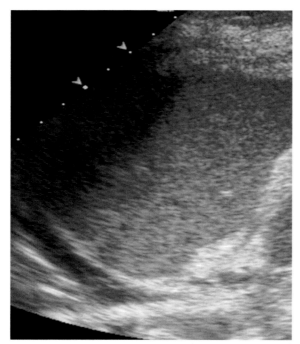

FIGURE 52-5. Pleural fluid seen through splenic window. Longitudinal sonogram shows a small amount of fluid in the left pleural space.

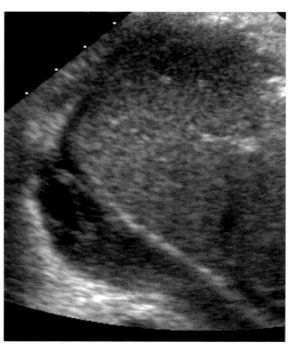

FIGURE 52-6. Empyema seen through hepatic window. Sonography of pleural space through the hepatic window shows presence of echogenic fluid in the right pleural space.

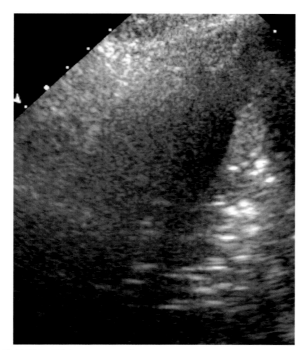

FIGURE 52-7. Hemothorax. Moderately echogenic right effusion is present after trauma from four-wheeler crash. Atelectasis of the right lower lung is present, with some hyperechoic air bronchograms visible.

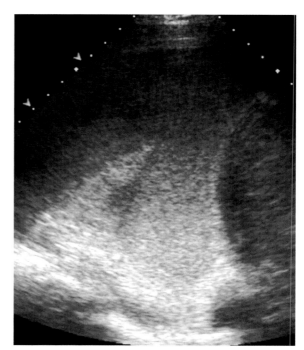

FIGURE 52-8. Empyema caused by pneumonia. Longitudinal sonogram shows echogenic fluid in the right pleural space above the diaphragm. Purulent drainage contained gram-positive and gram-negative rods and gram-positive cocci.

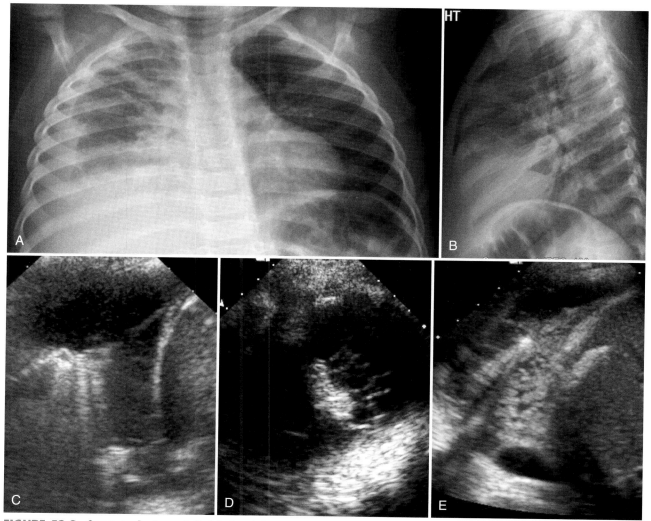

FIGURE 52-9. Septated pleural fluid. A and **B,** Posteroanterior and lateral radiographs show right pleural fluid with obliterated right hemidiaphragm. **C,** Longitudinal sonogram shows septated pleural fluid. **D** and **E,** Transverse and longitudinal sonograms of two other patients with septated pleural fluid.

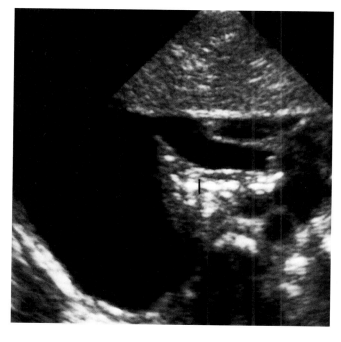

FIGURE 52-10. Sonographic air bronchograms within pneumonia. Multiple echogenic linear air shadows called sonographic air bronchograms are seen within the consolidated lung *(L)* in this child with pneumonia.

The fluid color flow Doppler signal is particularly useful in distinguishing if small, loculated collections can be aspirated.

Diaphragm Sign

When the liver or spleen is used as an acoustic window and fluid is seen adjacent to them, the location of the fluid is determined in reference to the diaphragm's

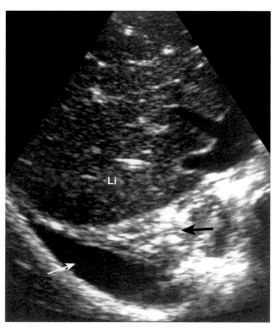

FIGURE 52-11. Posterior pleural fluid over bare area of liver. Transverse scan through liver with patient in supine position shows triangular consolidated lung (air bronchograms) behind the liver *(black arrow)* and fluid *(white arrow)* posterior to lung and liver *(Li).*

position. If the fluid is inside the diaphragm and more centrally located, it is **ascites.** If the fluid is outside the diaphragm and more peripherally located, it is in the pleural space (see Fig. 52-5).

Displaced-Crus Sign

There is fluid in the pleural space if the fluid is interposed between the crus and the vertebral column, displacing the crus away from the spine.

Bare-Area Sign

The posterior aspect of the right lobe of the liver is directly attached to the posterior diaphragm without peritoneum. Thus, ascitic fluid in the subhepatic or subphrenic space cannot extend behind the liver at the level of the bare area. Pleural fluid will extend behind the liver at the level of the bare area (see Fig. 52-11).

Advantages and Disadvantages of Sonography

Ultrasound, unlike computed tomography (CT), is a portable, bedside technique, making it ideal for evaluating chest opacification detected by conventional radiographs in the critically ill infant or child, to distinguish pulmonary from pleural disease (Fig. 52-13). Septations are better visualized by ultrasound than CT (Fig. 52-14). CT is better at identifying pulmonary parenchymal abnormalities, but this does not improve the outcome in managing empyema.[8]

A limitation of chest sonography is that very homogeneous, solid, hypoechoic lesions may appear fluid filled (Fig. 52-15). The criteria for fluid-filled structures in the abdomen are (1) lack of internal echoes, (2) a sharp

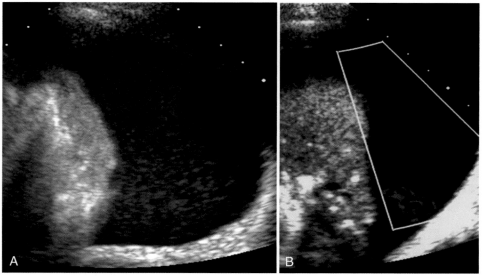

FIGURE 52-12. Color flow Doppler signal in pleural fluid with debris. A, Gray-scale sonogram shows left pleural fluid with much debris. **B,** Color flow Doppler signal.

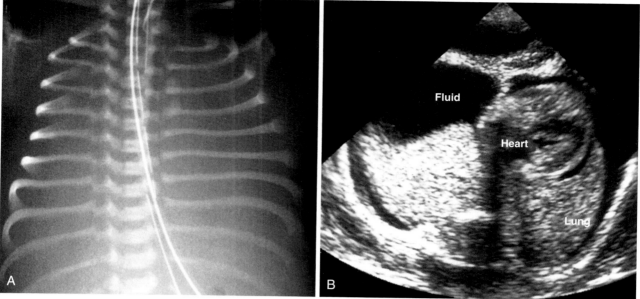

FIGURE 52-13. Bilateral pleural fluid and pericardial fluid in critically ill patient. A, Chest radiograph of infant receiving extracorporeal membrane oxygenation (ECMO) shows complete lung opacification. **B,** Transverse sonogram shows pleural fluid around both collapsed lungs and a small amount of pericardial fluid.

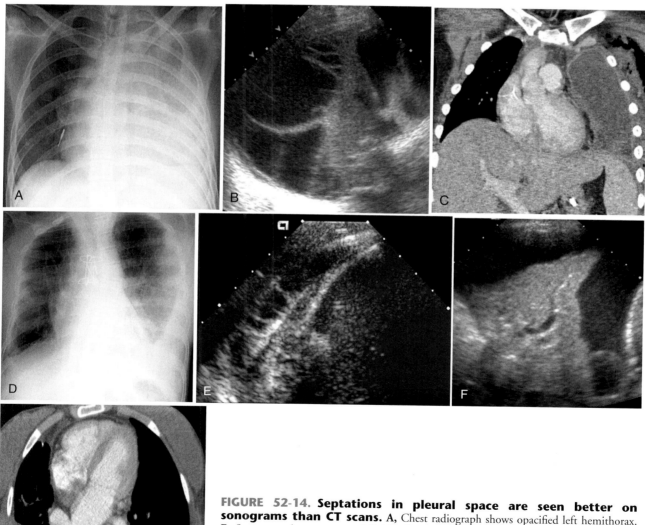

FIGURE 52-14. Septations in pleural space are seen better on sonograms than CT scans. A, Chest radiograph shows opacified left hemithorax. **B,** Sonogram shows a septated fluid collection. **C,** CT scan shows pleural fluid, but the septa are not well visualized. **D,** In another child with cystic fibrosis, radiograph shows left-sided pleural fluid with an obliterated right costophrenic angle. Postoperative changes of lung transplant and cholecystectomy are noted. **E,** Sonogram shows septated pleural fluid on the right side, in addition to **F,** echogenic pleural fluid with few septations on the left side. **G,** CT scan shows bilateral pleural fluid, but septations at the right base are not well visualized.

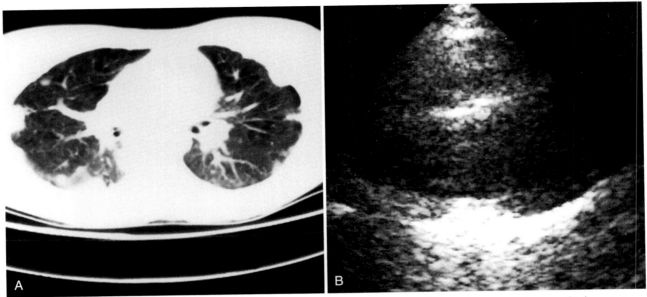

FIGURE 52-15. Hypoechoic metastases from renal cell carcinoma. A, CT scan in teenager shows multiple metastases. **B,** Sonogram shows large pleural mass that is relatively hypoechoic.

posterior wall, and (3) increased through-transmission of sound deep to the collection of fluid. The lack of echogenicity is a relative phenomenon that is judged by the echogenicity of the surrounding structures. The air-filled lung deep to a pleural collection will have a strong echogenic interface regardless of the nature of the pleural collection. Fluid in the pleural space produces **acoustic enhancement.** The lack of referenced solid or cystic structures in the chest makes detection of increased through-transmission difficult to judge within the chest. Observing a change in shape of the pleural fluid during respiration, the movement of echogenic particles, and the fluid color flow Doppler signal is helpful in distinguishing thick pleural fluid from solid masses. Consolidated lung superficial to aerated lung will have increased through-transmission compared with the aerated lung and can be identified as lung parenchyma by the presence of **air or fluid bronchograms.** Collapsed or consolidated lung tissue often has the appearance of the liver or spleen.

Another pitfall in the sonographic evaluation of the chest is the acoustic shadow cast by a rib **(rib shadowing),** which may confuse the inexperienced sonographer into misinterpreting that a mass is anechoic. The transducer should be placed between the ribs to avoid this pitfall. The echogenicity of the mass or pleural lesion can be compared with that of the liver.

PARAPNEUMONIC COLLECTIONS AND LUNG ABSCESS

Parapneumonic collections occur in up to 40% of children with bacterial pneumonia and are especially common in those younger than 4 years.[9] Most collections are not infected, but many evolve into **empyemas** with frank pus. Parapneumonic effusions detected by ultrasound can be prognostic in children with pneumonia. Children with complicated collections characterized by septations have longer hospital stays and benefit from intrapleural fibrinolytic therapy or surgical procedures.[10]

An **empyema** or **lung abscess** adjacent to the chest wall or to acoustic windows such as the liver or spleen usually appears as a complex collection with fluid-debris levels and septations. Abscesses and empyemas usually exhibit different types of motion when visualized by ultrasound. An abscess demonstrates expansion of the entire circumference with inspiration, whereas with an empyema, only the internal wall adjacent to the lung shows slight motion. Lung abscesses may be difficult to differentiate from empyema when the empyema contains multiple, loculated air collections caused by thoracentesis. Air-fluid collections move with patient repositioning, which can aid in distinguishing empyema from abscess (Figs. 52-16 and 52-17).

LUNG PARENCHYMA

Consolidated lung is hypoechoic relative to the highly reflective, air-filled, normal surrounding lung. Consolidated lung echogenicity is similar to the liver (Fig. 52-18), but sonographic air bronchograms differentiate it from liver. Strong, nonpulsatile, branching, linear echoes produced by air-filled bronchi converge toward the root of the lung. The linear pattern of bright echoes is observed when scanning parallel to the long axis of the

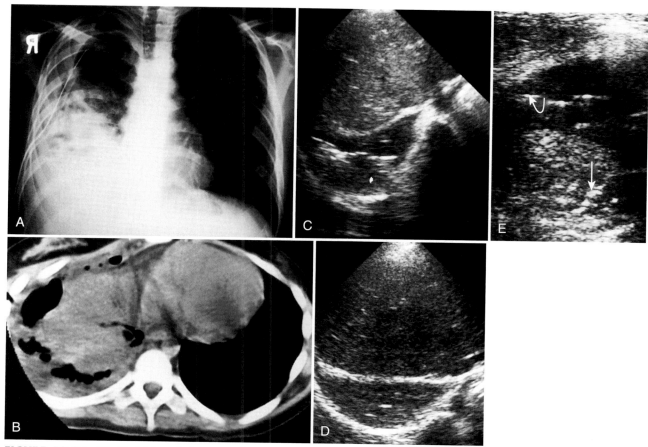

FIGURE 52-16. Air-fluid levels in complex empyema. A, Chest radiograph; **B,** CT scan; and **C,** sonogram through liver. **D,** Upright sonogram. Air-fluid levels change when patient is erect (air moved up and out of this transverse scan through lower chest). **E,** Transverse intercostal scan through anterior chest wall shows both the linear lines of bronchi *(arrow)* at random pattern and the linear lines of air *(curved arrow)* in the pleural fluid, all at one level in a supine view.

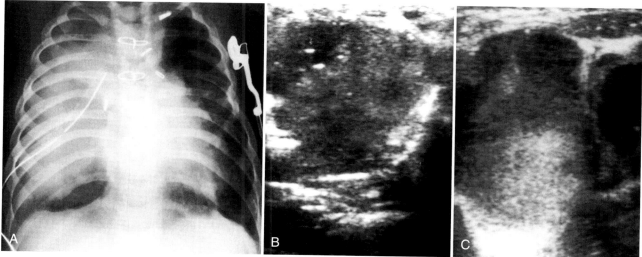

FIGURE 52-17. Thick pleural fluid with changing appearance in empyema. A, Chest radiograph shows pleural fluid that is not draining by chest tube. **B,** Transverse sonogram shows very thick fluid with no air bronchograms. **C,** Differential thick fluid-fluid level caused by change in position.

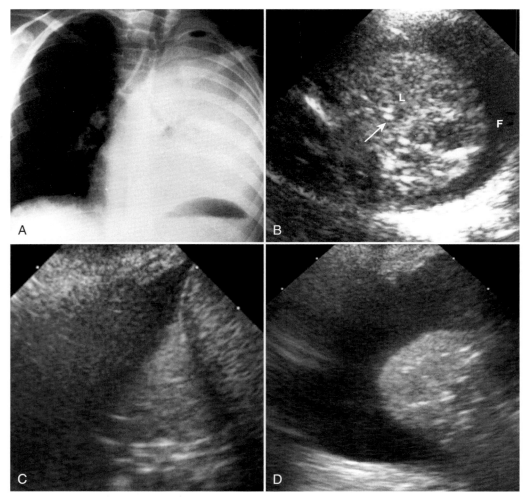

FIGURE 52-18. Echogenicity of air bronchograms in consolidated lung. A, Chest radiograph shows an opacified left chest with some air bronchograms. **B,** Transverse scan shows fluid *(F)* around consolidated lung *(L)*, which has echogenicity similar to the liver. Air bronchograms within the consolidated lung *(arrow)*. **C** and **D,** Sonograms of another patient show consolidated lung with air bronchograms and surrounded by fluid.

bronchi (Fig. 52-19). When the scanning is done at more acute angles, scattered echoes of variable lengths produced by the sonographic air bronchograms are observed (Fig. 52-20). Posterior reverberation and acoustic shadowing can be seen and are related to the large, proximal, air-filled bronchi. If there is adjacent pleural fluid, the hypoechoic consolidated lung can be differentiated from the hypoechoic-to-anechoic pleural effusion by identification of these sonographic air bronchograms.

Round Pneumonia

Round pneumonia is more common in children under 8 years of age, but 15% occur between 8 and 12 years.[11] Poor development of the pores of Kohn and channels of Lambert in children lead to centrifugal spread of pneumonia.[12] The advancing front is sharply demarcated from unaffected lung, causing the characteristic focal round mass that mimics a posterior mediastinal mass. Most round pneumonias are posterior within the lower lobes. Ultrasound shows air bronchograms in the mass, confirming that it is a round pneumonia (Fig. 52-21).

Atelectasis

Atelectatic lung is similar in echogenicity to liver (Fig. 52-22). Sonographic air bronchograms may be present in atelectatic lung, but the air bronchograms are more crowded than in pneumonia because the lung volume is decreased. Bronchi can be filled with fluid rather than air, creating fluid bronchograms. The echogenic, parallel, branching walls are filled with hypoechoic fluid, without the acoustic shadowing and reverberation artifacts normally seen with air. Color flow Doppler sonography differentiates fluid-filled bronchi from vessels.

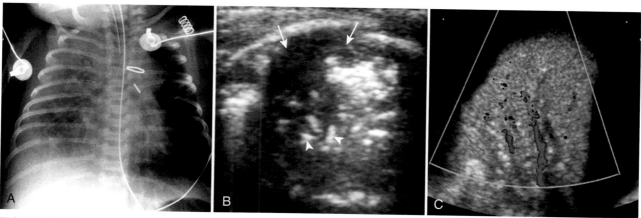

FIGURE 52-19. Pneumonia showing branching, tubular air bronchograms. This 2-week-old girl had persistent fever and purulent endotracheal drainage after coarctation repair. **A,** Chest radiograph shows right parenchymal infiltrates and possible pleural fluid. **B,** Transverse sonogram shows consolidated lung parenchyma *(arrows)* with echogenic, branching, tubular *(arrowheads)* air-filled bronchi. No pleural fluid was seen. At autopsy, necrotizing pneumonia was found throughout right lung without evidence of empyema. **C,** Color flow Doppler sonogram in another patient shows echogenic branching air bronchograms with intervening branching vessels.

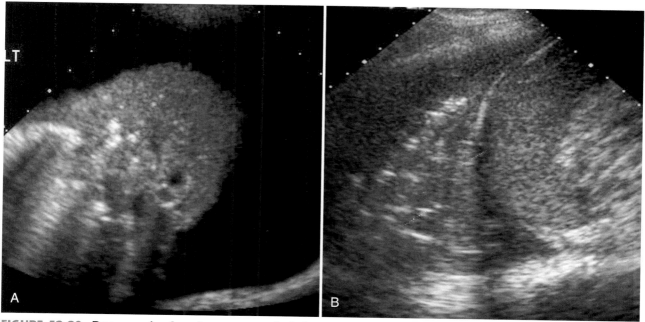

FIGURE 52-20. Pneumonia showing scattered air bronchograms. A and **B,** Transverse and longitudinal sonograms of two patients in a plane that is not parallel to the long axis of the bronchi show scattered echoes of variable lengths from scattered air bronchograms. Fluid surrounds the consolidated lung.

MEDIASTINUM

Chest Vessels

The normal thymus is an excellent acoustic window to view normal mediastinal structures and mediastinal masses. The thymus is anterior to the great vessels and extends inferiorly to the upper portion of the heart. The great vessels, including the superior vena cava (SVC),

aorta, and pulmonary artery, are well imaged through the thymus. These vessels are more conspicuous with color Doppler ultrasound (Fig. 52-23). The left brachiocephalic vein courses transversely from left to right, posterior to the thymus, to enter the SVC. This is useful to determine catheter position (Fig. 52-24) and the presence of a thrombus in children with central venous catheters.

Doppler examination is useful in identifying **thrombus** within the subclavian vein, SVC, and pulmonary

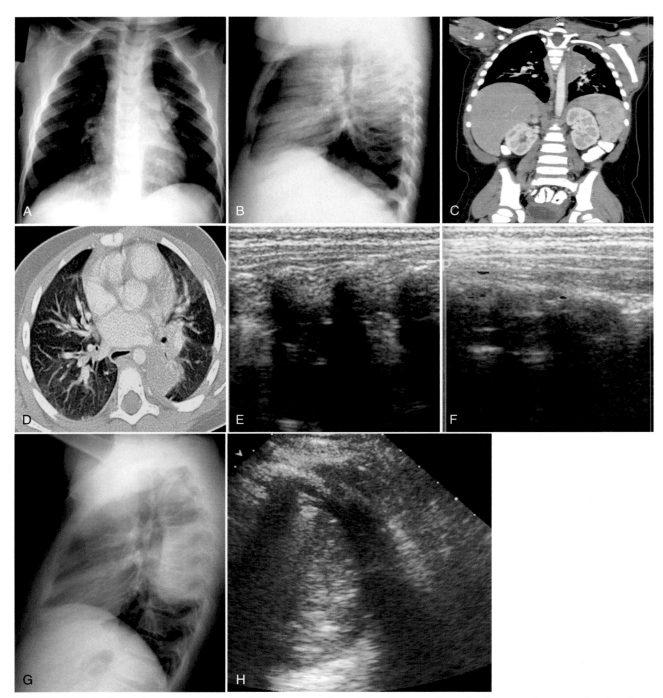

FIGURE 52-21. Round pneumonia. A and **B,** Posteroanterior and lateral chest radiographs show round pneumonia referred as a posterior mediastinal mass in this 2-year-old child. **C** and **D,** CT scans of chest, abdomen and pelvis show pneumonia. **E** and **F,** Sonograms done through posterior chest wall shows presence of air bronchograms within the lesion, confirming round pneumonia. Ionizing radiation from CT scan of chest, abdomen, and pelvis could have been avoided. **G,** Lateral chest radiograph shows a rounded opacity posteriorly in this 12-year-old child. **H,** Transverse sonogram shows air bronchograms within the lesion, confirming it as round pneumonia, with a small amount of pleural fluid surrounding the consolidated lung. Ultrasound diagnosis helped avoid ionizing radiation from a CT scan.

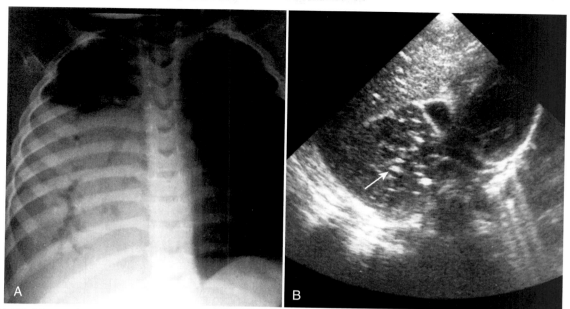

FIGURE 52-22. Atelectasis from foreign body. A, Chest radiograph shows air bronchograms in opacified right side of chest with shift of the heart to the right, indicating volume loss. **B,** Transverse sonogram through liver shows no fluid in chest. Multiple air bronchograms *(arrow)* are seen within collapsed lung. At endoscopy, foreign body was found in right main stem bronchus. *(From Seibert RW, Seibert JJ, Williamson SL: The opaque chest: when to suspect a bronchial foreign body. Pediatr Radiol 1986;16:193-196.)*

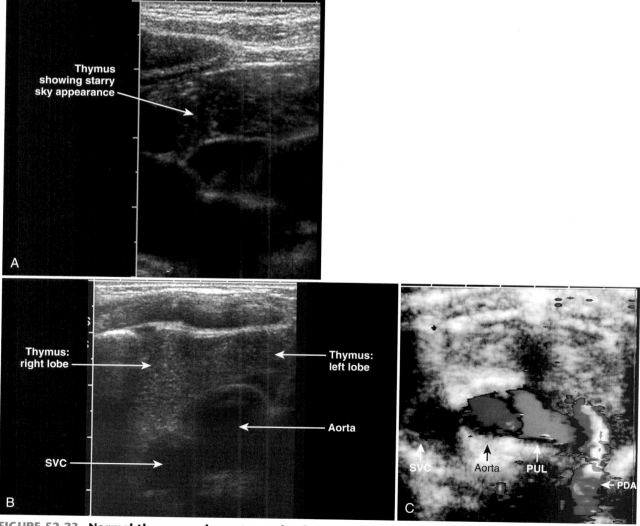

FIGURE 52-23. Normal thymus and great vessels of chest. A and **B,** Longitudinal and transverse sonograms show normal thymus echotexture in a 31-month-old boy. Superior vena cava and aorta are seen through the thymic window. **C,** Color flow Doppler image shows normal great vessels in the chest in transverse scan through the thymus in another child. *SVC,* Superior vena cava; *PUL,* pulmonary artery; *PDA,* posterior descending artery.

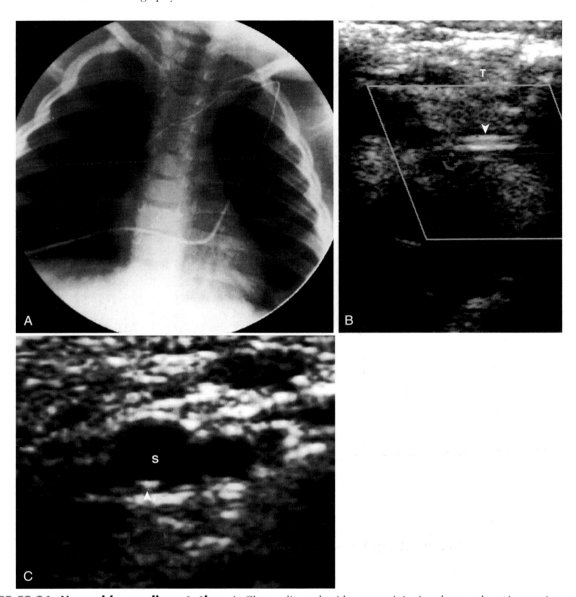

FIGURE 52-24. Normal hyperalimentation. A, Chest radiograph with contrast injection shows catheter in superior vena cava. **B,** Longitudinal sonogram. **C,** Transverse sonogram shows no clot on catheter *(arrowhead).* Thymus *(T)* was used as window. *S,* Superior vena cava.

artery (Fig. 52-25). Thrombosis of the axillary or sub-clavian vein secondary to thoracic outlet syndrome[13] is seen on ultrasound Doppler study in **Paget-Schroetter syndrome**[14,15] (Fig. 52-26). It results from an abnormal insertion of the costoclavicular ligament laterally on the first rib, along with hypertrophy of the scalenus anticus muscle.

The Doppler waveform is abnormal when **thrombosis** or **obstruction** of the SVC is present. Doppler ultrasound findings include (1) loss of biphasic SVC waveform, (2) continuous forward flow rather than distinct systolic and diastolic peaks, (3) a turbulent flow profile, (4) increased velocity downstream, and (5) decreased velocity upstream.[16] Venous thrombosis is reported in 20% of children receiving extracorporeal

membrane oxygenation (ECMO).[17] Doppler waveforms may be different in patients receiving ECMO because their resistive indices are low. Recurrent SVC thrombosis has been reported in a child with activated protein C resistance.[18]

SUPERIOR VENA CAVA THROMBOSIS: DOPPLER SONOGRAPHIC FINDINGS

Loss of biphasic waveform
Continuous forward flow (no systolic or diastolic peaks)
Turbulent flow
Increased downstream velocity
Decreased velocity upstream

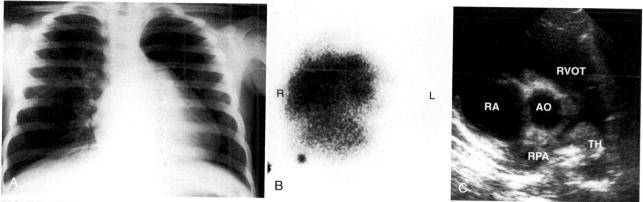

FIGURE 52-25. Pulmonary embolus. A, Chest radiograph shows hyperlucent left lung in 4-year-old child. **B,** Pulmonary perfusion scan shows no perfusion to left lung. **C,** Transverse sonogram through heart shows saddle embolus in main pulmonary artery. *TH,* Thrombus; *RVOT,* right ventricular outflow tract; *AO,* aorta; *RA,* right atrium; *RPA,* right pulmonary artery.

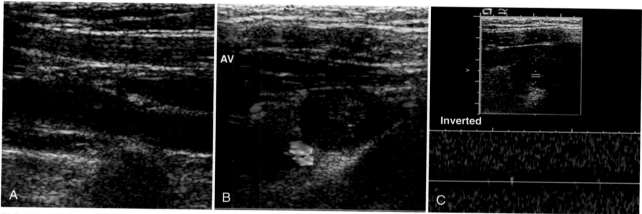

FIGURE 52-26. Paget-Schroetter syndrome. A, Gray-scale; **B,** color flow; and **C,** spectral Doppler waveform *(C)* images show subclavian vein thrombosis with absence of color flow and absence of Doppler signal secondary to a thoracic outlet syndrome in a 17-year-old female equestrian. *(Courtesy Dr. Charles A. James, Arkansas Children's Hospital, Little Rock.)*

Mediastinal Masses

A CT scan and magnetic resonance imaging (MRI) are the primary modalities for evaluation of mediastinal masses detected by chest radiography. A widened superior mediastinum detected on chest radiography can be evaluated initially by sonography. Detection of normal, but prominent thymus rather than a mediastinal mass precludes the need for CT. **Lymphatic malformations** (Fig. 52-27) are composed of dilated lymphatic sacs of variable size, which may appear unilocular or multilocular. Lymphatic malformations may undergo hemorrhage, in which case the lesion appears as a uniformly echogenic mass or multiple cysts containing echogenic debris. Septations in cystic masses are better identified by ultrasound than by CT or MRI. Mediastinal ultrasound can also determine whether chest masses extend into the neck. **Retrosternal thyroid** mass extension detection by ultrasound is helpful for surgical planning. In children less than 1 year old, sternal ossification centers are unfused, the mineral content of the bones and cartilage

is lower than in older children, and the thymus is much larger relative to other structures. Acoustic windows through the sternum, costal cartilages, and thymus allow ultrasound evaluation of mediastinal structures.

Three longitudinal planes can be identified in the mediastinum (Fig. 52-28): right parasagittal through the SVC, sagittal through the aortic root, and left parasagittal through the pulmonary outflow tract. **Two distinct transverse planes** through the mediastinum can be identified (Fig. 52-29): the superior plane at the confluence of the brachiocephalic veins and SVC and a lower transverse plane where the SVC, aorta, and pulmonary outflow tract are visualized.

Ultrasound-guided percutaneous biopsy of anterior and superior mediastinal masses abutting chest wall is safe and can provide a tissue diagnosis.[19] Color Doppler ultrasound before biopsy can rule out vascular lesions that would preclude biopsy.

Suprasternal sonography can also be useful for detecting small and large mediastinal masses, particularly lymphoma. Mediastinal sonography for masses should

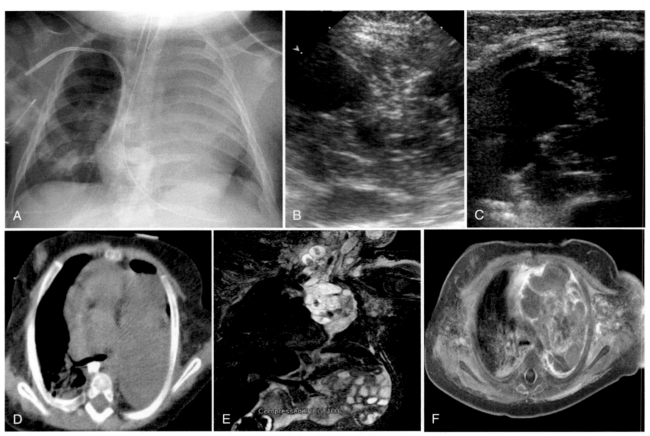

FIGURE 52-27. Macrocystic lymphatic malformation in 7-month-old girl. A, Chest radiograph shows opacity in left upper chest and neck. **B** and **C,** Sonograms show multiple cystic spaces. **D,** CT scan. **E,** T2-weighted coronal, and **F,** T1-weighted post-contrast, axial MR images are better at defining the extent of the lesion. CT scan fails to show multicystic architecture of the lesion.

include major vessels or cardiac chambers in the field of view so that mass and vessel echogenicity can be compared directly. This prevents the pitfall created by reducing the gain setting in response to the hyperechoic appearance of adjacent lung. The reduced gain setting gives a false hypoechoic appearance to a solid mass. **Juxtaphrenic paravertebral masses** may be detected with a subxiphoid or transdiaphragmatic approach. Ultrasound allows characterization of masses as solid or cystic and detection of calcifications.

Posterior mediastinal masses, including neurogenic tumors, make up the majority of mediastinal masses in young infants. The most common mediastinal mass in older children is lymphadenopathy resulting from leukemia or lymphoma.

Lymphadenopathy appears as hypoechoic nodules. Lymph nodes in lymphoma are more hypoechoic and more hypovascular than inflammatory lymph nodes.[20] Germ cell tumors can have variable appearance. **Teratomas** are heterogenous masses that contain fat, bone, and cystic elements.

Neurogenic tumors appear as a lobulated or well-defined hypoechoic mass with granular or flecklike calcifications. Neurenteric cysts are well-defined, anechoic lesions with thin walls. When inflammation and hemor-

rhage occur, the cyst may contain echogenic debris from proteinaceous fluid, mucus, or blood.

Thymus

The thymus is located in the superior mediastinum anterior to the great vessels in the superior mediastinum, from superior edge of the manubrium to the fourth costal cartilage. The thymus is mildly hypoechoic relative to liver, spleen, and thyroid. It shows some echogenic strands. A fine granular echotexture gives the thymus a "starry sky" appearance (see Fig. 52-23). A fibrous capsule gives the thymus a smooth, well-defined margin.

Thymic index is the product of thymic width measured on transverse images and the area of the largest lobe measured on a longitudinal image[21-23] (Table 52-1). The thymic index has acceptable correlation with actual thymus weight and volume. The measurement is performed during expiration to obtain a standardized size. Thymic index is greater in children with active atopic dermatitis than in healthy controls[24] (Fig. 52-30). Larger thymic index at birth is associated with lower infant mortality rate.[25] Thymic size varies with age, and normal thymic index values have been established[21-23] (Table 52-2).

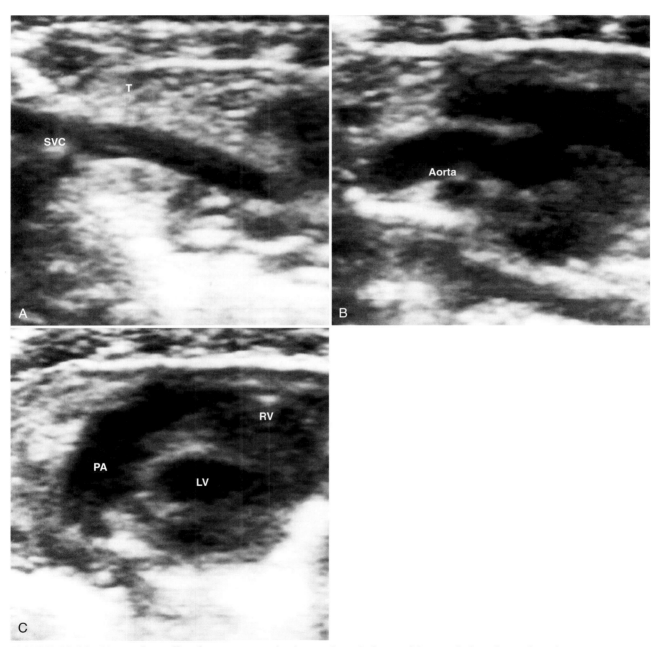

FIGURE 52-28. Normal mediastinum. Longitudinal views through thymus *(T)*. **A,** Right lateral view through superior vena cava *(SVC)*. **B,** Midline view through aorta. **C,** Left lateral view through pulmonary outflow tract. *LV,* Left ventricle; *PA,* pulmonary artery; *RV,* right ventricle.

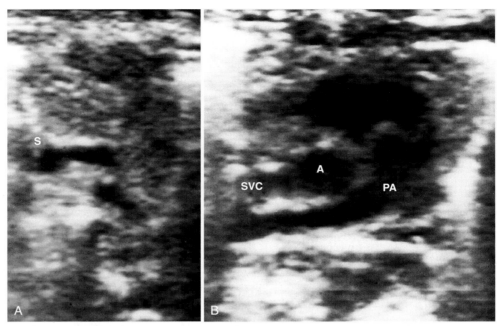

FIGURE 52-29. Normal mediastinum, transverse view. A, Superior plane with innominate vein catheter running through thymus to superior vena cava *(S)*. **B,** Inferior plane through superior vena cava *(SVC)*, aorta *(A)*, and pulmonary artery *(PA)*.

TABLE 52-1. FORMULA FOR CALCULATION OF THYMIC INDEX

Thymic index (cm³)	=	Area of the largest lobe (cm²)	× Transverse dimension of thymus from right lateral edge to left lateral edge (cm)
Area of the lobe of thymus (cm²)	=	Craniocaudad dimension (cm)	× Anteroposterior dimension (cm)

Superior herniation of thymus into the neck is a rare entity in which there is intermittent migration of the broadest part of the normal thymus out of the thorax into the suprasternal region. Real-time ultrasound shows that the mass moves into the neck during Valsalva maneuver, with an increase in the intrathoracic pressure, and has typical echotexture of thymus, thereby avoiding unnecessary biopsy and surgery.[26]

Cervical ectopic thymus is an uncommon variant. A hypoechoic mass with characteristic thymic ultrasound echotexture is identified along the track of the thymopharyngeal duct.[27,28] The thymus can protrude into the chest wall as a bulging mass because of a congenital sternal defect. Real-time ultrasound can demonstrate movement of herniated thymus during respiratory cycles.

Benign abnormalities of thymus in children include thymic cyst, intrathymic hemorrhage, thymolipoma, and thymoma. Thymus may also be involved by hemangioma, lymphatic malformation, or Langerhans cell histiocytosis. Malignant infiltration of thymus is also seen in lymphoma and leukemia. **Thymic cysts** are anechoic. The other abnormalities of thymus may show irregular or lobular margin, heterogeneous echogenicity, coarse echotexture, and calcifications.

EXTRACARDIAC CHEST MASSES

Chest sonography can be used to evaluate chest masses outside of the mediastinum if they are adjacent to the pleura or to an acoustic window such as the liver or spleen. A patient with persistent pleural fluid not responding to drainage can be evaluated by ultrasound for a possible underlying tumor (Fig. 52-31). It is important to compare the echogenicity of the mass with adjacent structures such as the liver, spleen, or heart. Doppler imaging may be helpful in evaluating whether a chest mass is vascular in origin. Malignant chest masses demonstrate a low-impedance, high-diastolic-flow Doppler signal.[29]

Sonography is particularly valuable in evaluating a paradiaphragmatic mass, which may be a **diaphragm eventration**, a **diaphragmatic hernia** (Fig. 52-32), or an **intrathoracic kidney.**[30] These abnormalities

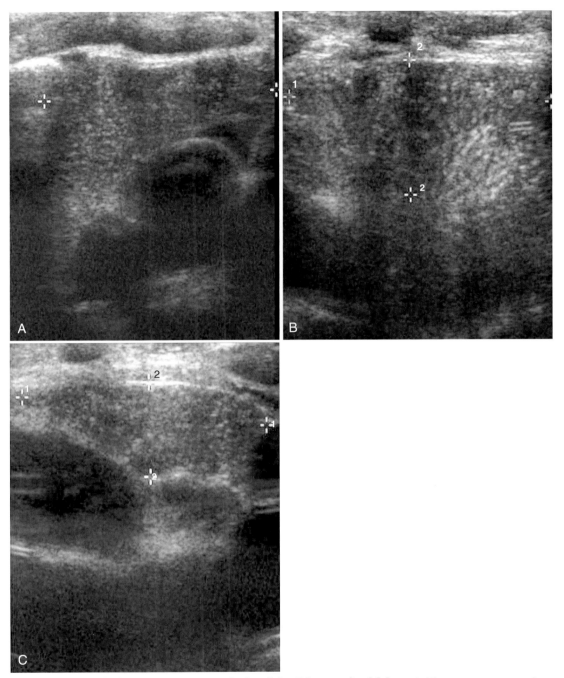

FIGURE 52-30. Thymic index measurement in healthy 31-month-old boy. A, Transverse sonogram shows measurement of transverse dimension of the thymus from right lateral edge to the left lateral edge. **B** and **C,** Longitudinal images of right lobe and left lobe of thymus, respectively. Area of each lobe is measured by multiplying the craniocaudad and anteroposterior dimensions. Images were obtained during expiratory phase. Area of the right lobe (5.9 cm²) is larger than the left lobe (3.5 cm²). Thymic index (19.5 cm³) is the product of area of the larger lobe (5.9 cm²) and transverse dimension (3.3 cm) of the thymus.

frequently are associated with respiratory compromise, making bedside, portable sonography the study of choice. Less common diaphragmatic masses detected by sonography include hemangioma,[31] primitive neuroectodermal tumor,[32] and primary embryonal rhabdomyosarcoma.[33]

Pulmonary sequestrations may be extralobar or intralobar.[34,35] Extralobar sequestration is congenital and has pulmonary tissue with separate pleura. Children with extralobar sequestration typically present in infancy. Intralobar sequestration is acquired following pneumonia and is associated with bronchial obstruction and compromised pulmonary artery supply. Hypertrophy of parasitized systemic arteries, such as the phrenic and inferior pulmonary ligament arteries, supply the

TABLE 52-2. NORMAL THYMIC INDEX FOR CHILDREN UNDER 2 YEARS OF AGE

| AGE (MONTHS) | Thymic Index (cm³) | |
	AVERAGE	STANDARD DEVIATION (SD)
Premature	11.9	3.9
0-1	18.1	6.7
1-2	25.4	9.4
2-3	22.3	6.9
3-4	26.8	10.3
4-5	29.7	17.6
5-6	24.2	9.3
6-8	22.2	8.9
8-10	21.5	6.8
10-12	23.2	7.2
12-18	17.2	6.4
18-24	15.4	5.6

Modified from Yekeler E, Tambag A, Tunaci A, et al. Analysis of the thymus in 151 healthy infants from 0 to 2 years of age. J Ultrasound Med 2004;23:1321-1326.

sequestered lung. The intralobar sequestered lung is typically present in the lower lobes and is enclosed by the visceral pleura of the parent lung. Ultrasound may show a hypoechoic mass in the lower lobe (Fig. 52-33). Color Doppler can demonstrate a systemic vessel supplying the hypoechoic mass in both extralobar and intralobar sequestration.

Congenital pulmonary airway malformation (CPAM),[36] previously known as **congenital cystic adenomatoid malformation** (CCAM), is of three types. Type I has one or more large cysts measuring more than 2 cm in size. Type II has multiple small cysts. Type III has microcysts but appears solid on ultrasound and on gross examination.[1] Unlike pulmonary sequestration, no systemic vascular supply can be demonstrated in CPAM. The type I variety shows anechoic rounded areas that measure more than 2 cm in size. Type II shows multiple small anechoic areas that are smaller than 2 cm. Type III appears echogenic and solid. The cysts are too small to be delineated.

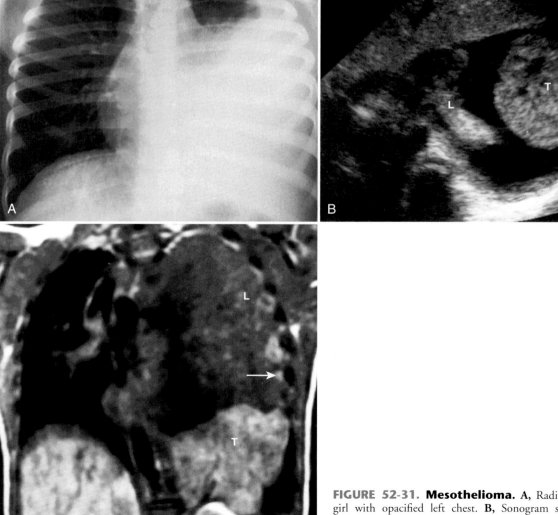

FIGURE 52-31. Mesothelioma. A, Radiograph of young girl with opacified left chest. **B,** Sonogram shows fluid with multiple echogenic pleural nodules *(arrow). T,* Tumor; *L,* lung. **C,** MRI shows the pleural *(arrow)* and parenchymal tumors.

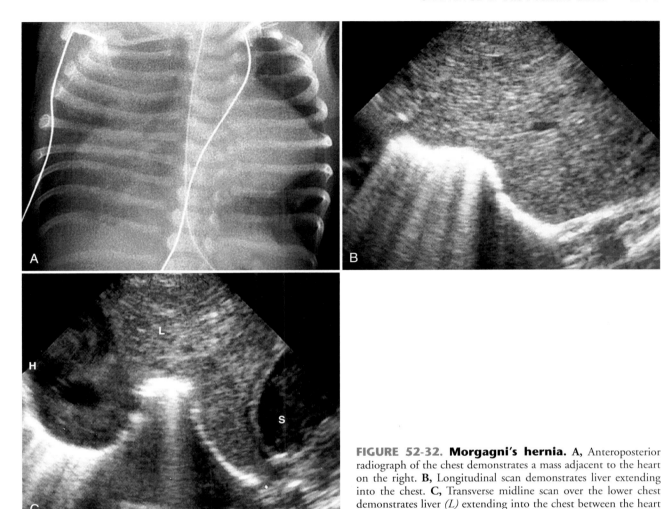

FIGURE 52-32. **Morgagni's hernia. A,** Anteroposterior radiograph of the chest demonstrates a mass adjacent to the heart on the right. **B,** Longitudinal scan demonstrates liver extending into the chest. **C,** Transverse midline scan over the lower chest demonstrates liver *(L)* extending into the chest between the heart *(H)* and stomach *(S)*.

Pulmonary masses except for **metastasis** are rare in children. Ultrasound may show the pulmonary mass but may not be able to provide a specific diagnosis. CT is required for evaluation of extent of mass. Biopsy might be required to arrive at a specific diagnosis. **Pulmonary blastoma** is a rare mass that starts at the lung periphery and can be viewed on ultrasound.[37]

Bronchogenic cysts or **bronchopulmonary foregut malformations** may be identified by chest ultrasound if they are adjacent to the chest wall (Fig. 52-34). Subphrenic abscesses, pericardial cysts, and pericardial fat pads are visualized adjacent to the diaphragm using the liver or spleen as a window. Chest wall masses may be evaluated by sonography.

DIAPHRAGM

Ultrasound is the bedside examination of choice for evaluation of suspected diaphragmatic motion abnormalities. Real-time sonography is the only imaging procedure that simultaneously evaluates the paradiaphragmatic spaces, the hemidiaphragms, and their motion.

Bilateral comparison of hemidiaphragm motion can be observed by placing the transducer in the subxiphoid position in a transverse orientation, angled upward toward the posterior leaflets of the hemidiaphragms (Fig. 52-35). Such comparison can be done with transverse sonographic scanning in infants **(Video 52-2),** but in older children **(Video 52-3),** unilateral sagittal scanning of each diaphragm is necessary. A comparison of the maximal excursion of the diaphragm for each side using B-mode or B/M-mode is more accurate than fluoroscopy in demonstrating diaphragmatic movement abnormality.[38] In the artificially ventilated patient, the respirator must be disconnected for approximately 5 to 10 seconds to observe unassisted respiration. With paralysis, there is absent or **paradoxical motion** on one side and exaggerated excursions on the opposite side. **Diaphragm paralysis** show right hemidiaphragm paralysis is a frequent concern after cardiac surgery[39,40] **(Video 52-4).** Severe eventration and a diaphragmatic hernia may also show

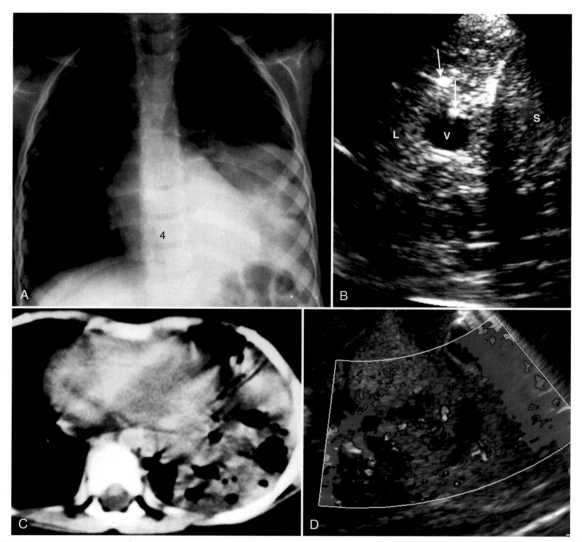

FIGURE 52-33. Sequestration. A, Chest radiograph of 4-year-old child shows large mass in left lower chest. **B,** Left longitudinal sonogram shows solid mass with air bronchograms *(arrows)* and appearance of lung *(L)* above spleen *(S); V,* blood vessel in mass. **C,** CT scan shows diffuse areas of bronchiectasis throughout mass. **D,** Color Doppler ultrasound shows arterial feeding vessel from aorta to sequestration in another patient. *(Courtesy Carol M. Rumack, MD.)*

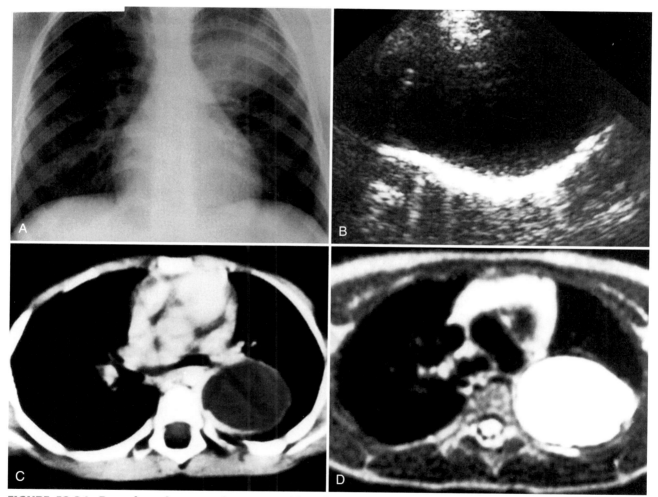

FIGURE 52-34. Bronchopulmonary foregut malformation (duplication cyst). A, Posteroanterior radiograph shows round mass in left upper lung. **B,** Posterior sonogram shows fluid-filled cyst with "back-wall enhancement due to increased through transmission." **C,** CT scan, and **D,** MR image, show fluid-filled chest mass.

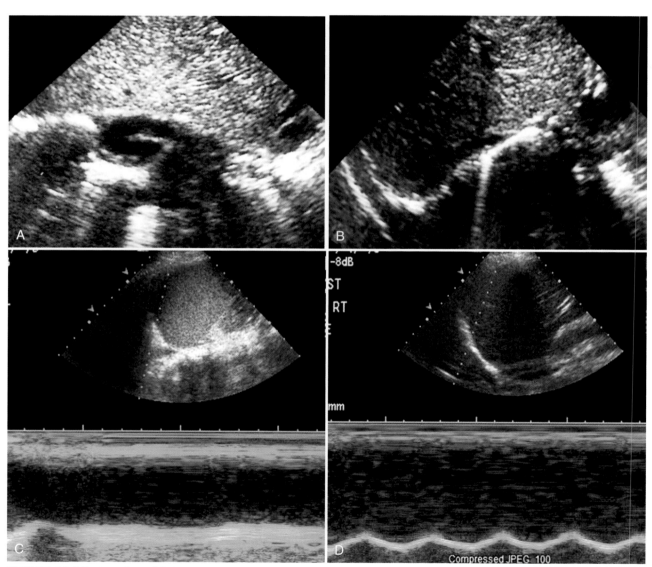

FIGURE 52-35. Paralyzed left hemidiaphragm compared to normal right hemidiaphragm. Bilateral diaphragmatic motion comparison using gray-scale ultrasound shows change in position and shape of right hemidiaphragm *(R)* on **A** and **B**, but no change on left. **C,** M-mode sonogram in another patient shows left hemidiaphragmatic paralysis. **D,** Normal excursions of right side.

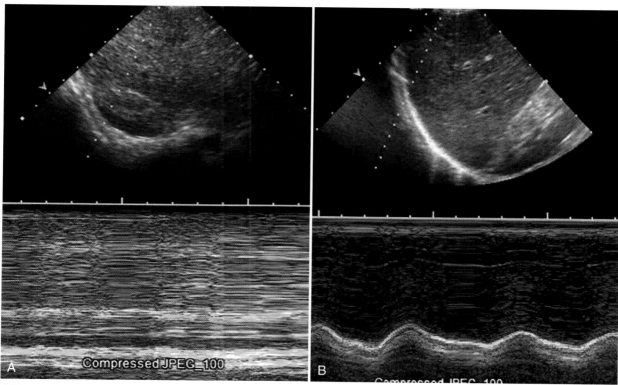

FIGURE 52-36. Follow-up of diaphragmatic paralysis. Gray-scale real-time and M-mode ultrasound. **A,** Child with complex congenital heart disease shows left hemidiaphragmatic paralysis. **B,** Spontaneous recovery of left hemidiaphragmatic motion was observed on follow-up sonogram.

paradoxical motion. During real-time evaluation of diaphragm motion, M-mode sonography can also be used in follow-up to monitor changes in diaphragm function[41] (Fig. 52-36). Sonography can demonstrate **rupture of the diaphragm**[42] (Fig. 52-37).

ULTRASOUND-GUIDED PROCEDURES

Sonography is an excellent method for guiding **pleural fluid aspiration** and chest wall **lesion biopsy.** Ultrasound can be used either for marking the skin overlying a fluid collection or for directly visualizing a needle during insertion into a collection (Fig. 52-38). Skin marking for fluid aspiration is usually performed at the bedside with the patient in the upright position. Ultrasound is particularly helpful in determining whether the pleural effusion will respond to **simple drainage** or will require **surgical decortication.**[43] If the fluid is relatively anechoic or clear, simple drainage with thoracentesis or chest tube drainage is an adequate treatment. If the fluid is thick with multiple septations, and if the patient does not respond promptly to antibiotic therapy, decortication or video-assisted thoracic surgery may be recommended.[10,44] More recently, complicated parapneumonic

effusions and empyemas have been successfully treated in up to 93% of children using tissue plasminogen activator administered through a small-bore chest tube.[45]

Empyema surrounded by lung may appear to be a pulmonary abscess on sonography. Changing the patient position and the viewing planes can help distinguish an empyema from a lung abscess (Fig. 52-39). An **abscess** should be visualized in two planes.

Ultrasound is useful in the evaluation of pulmonary consolidation. It can be used to guide needle aspiration for etiologic diagnosis in patients with complicated pneumonia, as well as aspiration of microabscesses in necrotizing pneumonia.

Sonography can detect **pneumothoraces** after thoracentesis.[46] Before and after thoracentesis, the ipsilateral pulmonary apex and adjacent lung should be examined in the upright position for normal pleural respiratory movement. If the pleural respiratory motion is absent, a pneumothorax should be suspected.

Sclerotherapy for macrocystic lymphatic malformation under ultrasound guidance has the advantage of dynamically visualizing the procedure reaction that causes obliteration of the macrocysts[47] (Fig. 52-40). Unlike fluoroscopy guidance, the residual cysts are easily seen under ultrasound guidance and can be targeted for further sclerotherapy.

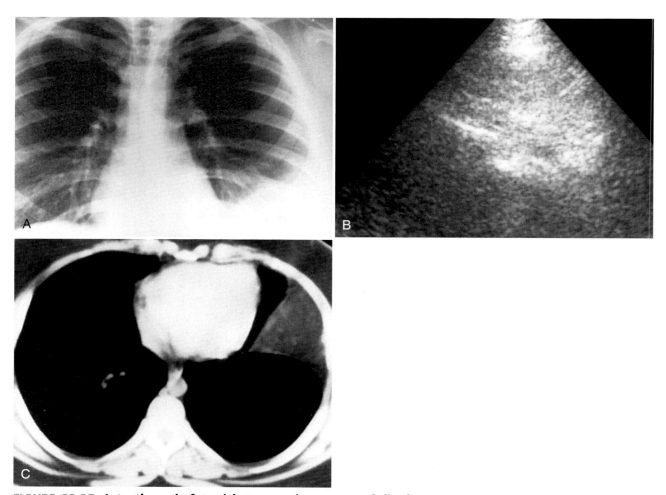

FIGURE 52-37. Intrathoracic fat with traumatic rupture of diaphragm. A, Chest radiograph shows round mass in left lower lung adjacent to left cardiophrenic border. **B,** Transverse sonogram shows echogenic mass. **C,** CT shows mass with fat density. During drainage of empyema 4 years earlier, chest tube had ruptured through diaphragm and omental fat-filled defect at surgery.

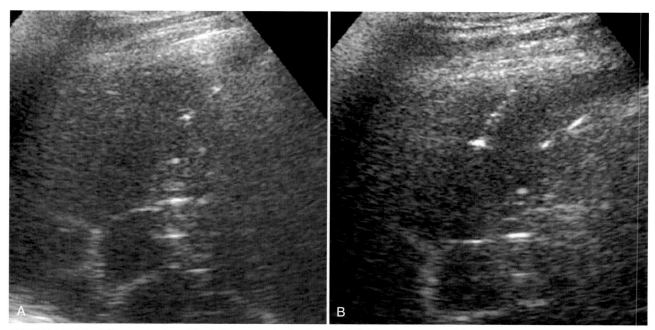

FIGURE 52-38. Ultrasound-guided thoracentesis. A, Pleural fluid with septa and debris. **B,** Sonogram shows position of the needle tip within the pleural fluid.

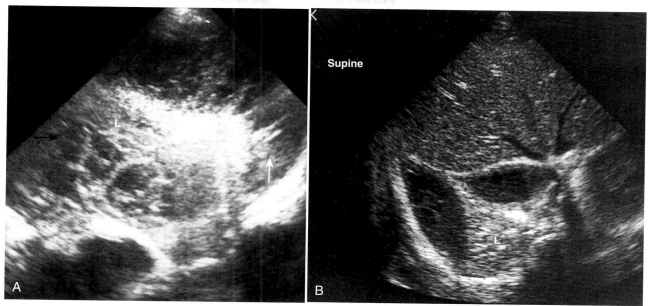

FIGURE 52-39. Empyema requiring surgical decortications in patient with sickle cell anemia. A, Thick fluid *(black arrow)* around lung *(L)* with multiple loculations. Thick, putty rind was found at surgery. Possible intraparenchymal abscesses *(white arrow)* on upright transverse scan. **B,** On supine scan through the liver, only empyema surrounds the lung *(L);* no abscess is present.

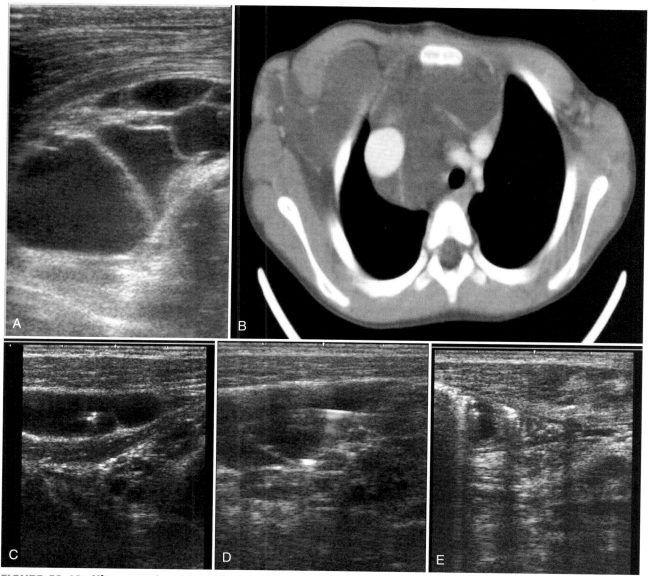

FIGURE 52-40. Ultrasound-guided sclerotherapy of macrocystic lymphatic malformation. A, Sonogram shows multiple cysts within the right chest wall and axilla extending into the mediastinum. **B,** CT scan shows extent of the lesion. **C** and **D,** Sonograms show needle and dilator, respectively, within the lesion. **E,** Sonogram immediately after sclerotherapy injection shows excellent response.

OSTEOMYELITIS AND RIB FRACTURES

Ultrasound may be used to demonstrate the soft tissue swelling associated with **osteomyelitis** of the ribs. The ultrasound demonstration of thickening around the ribs may be the first sign of periosteal edema associated with early osteomyelitis before the radiographic changes of bone destruction are present. **Rib fractures** in infants that might be difficult to identify on radiography can be detected by ultrasound.[48]

References

Ultrasound Technique

1. Coley BD. Pediatric chest ultrasound. Radiol Clin North Am 2005;43:405-418.
2. Riccabona M. Ultrasound of the chest in children (mediastinum excluded). Eur Radiol 2008;18:390-399.

Sonographic Signs of Pleural Fluid

3. Kocijancic K. Ultrasonographic forms of pleural space in healthy children. Coll Antropol 2007;31:999-1002.
4. Chen HJ, Tu CY, Ling SJ, et al. Sonographic appearances in transudative pleural effusions: not always an anechoic pattern. Ultrasound Med Biol 2008;34:362-369.
5. Kim OH, Kim WS, Kim MJ, et al. Ultrasound in the diagnosis of pediatric chest diseases. Radiographics 2000;20:653-671.
6. Feller-Kopman D. Ultrasound-guided thoracentesis. Chest 2006;129:1709-1714.
7. Wu RG, Yang PC, Kuo SH, Luh KT. "Fluid color" sign: a useful indicator for discrimination between pleural thickening and pleural effusion. J Ultrasound Med 1995;14:767-769.
8. Jaffe A, Calder AD, Owens CM, et al. Role of routine computed tomography in paediatric pleural empyema. Thorax 2008;63:897-902.

Parapneumonic Collections and Lung Abscess

9. Pinotti KF, Ribeiro SM, Cataneo AJ. Thorax ultrasound in the management of pediatric pneumonias complicated with empyema. Pediatr Surg Int 2006;22:775-778.
10. Chen KY, Liaw YS, Wang HC, et al. Sonographic septation: a useful prognostic indicator of acute thoracic empyema. J Ultrasound Med 2000;19:837-843.

Lung Parenchyma

11. Kim YW, Donnelly LF. Round pneumonia: imaging findings in a large series of children. Pediatr Radiol 2007;37:1235-1240.
12. Gaston B. Pneumonia. Pediatr Rev 2002;23:132-140.

Mediastinum

13. Arthur LG, Teich S, Hogan M, et al. Pediatric thoracic outlet syndrome: a disorder with serious vascular complications. J Pediatr Surg 2008;43:1089-1094.
14. Urschel Jr HC, Patel AN. Surgery remains the most effective treatment for Paget-Schroetter syndrome: 50 years' experience. Ann Thorac Surg 2008;86:254-260; discussion 260.
15. Serial quantitative coronary analyses for the evaluation of one-year change in saphenous vein grafts (retraction). Ann Thorac Surg 2008;86:1726.
16. Lv FQ, Duan YY, Yuan LJ, et al. Doppler superior vena cava flow evolution and respiratory variation in superior vena cava syndrome. Echocardiography 2008;25:360-365.
17. Riccabona M, Kuttnig-Haim M, Dacar D, et al. Venous thrombosis in and after extracorporeal membrane oxygenation: detection and follow-up by color Doppler sonography. Eur Radiol 1997;7:1383-1386.
18. Provenzale JM, Frush DP, Ortel TL. Recurrent thrombosis of the superior vena cava associated with activated protein C resistance: imaging findings. Pediatr Radiol 1998;28:597-598.

19. Sheth S, Hamper UM, Stanley DB, et al. Ultrasound guidance for thoracic biopsy: a valuable alternative to CT. Radiology 1999;210:721-726.
20. Na DG, Lim HK, Byun HS, et al. Differential diagnosis of cervical lymphadenopathy: usefulness of color Doppler sonography. AJR Am J Roentgenol 1997;168:1311-1316.
21. Hasselbalch H, Ersboll AK, Jeppesen DL, Nielsen MB. Thymus size in infants from birth until 24 months of age evaluated by ultrasound: a longitudinal prediction model for the thymic index. Acta Radiol 1999;40:41-44.
22. Jeppesen DL, Hasselbalch H, Nielsen SD, et al. Thymic size in preterm neonates: a sonographic study. Acta Paediatr 2003;92:817-822.
23. Yekeler E, Tambag A, Tunaci A, et al. Analysis of the thymus in 151 healthy infants from 0 to 2 years of age. J Ultrasound Med 2004;23:1321-1326.
24. Olesen AB, Andersen G, Jeppesen DL, et al. Thymus is enlarged in children with current atopic dermatitis: a cross-sectional study. Acta Derm Venereol 2005;85:240-243.
25. Aaby P, Marx C, Trautner S, et al. Thymus size at birth is associated with infant mortality: a community study from Guinea-Bissau. Acta Paediatr 2002;91:698-703.
26. Senel S, Erkek N, Otgun I, et al. Superior herniation of the thymus into the neck: a familial pattern. J Thorac Imaging 2008;23:131-134.
27. De Foer B, Vercruysse JP, Marien P, et al. Cervical ectopic thymus presenting as a painless neck mass in a child. JBR-BTR 2007;90:281-283.
28. Chu WC, Metreweli C. Ectopic thymic tissue in the paediatric age group. Acta Radiol 2002;43:144-146.

Extracardiac Chest Masses

29. Hsu WH, Yu YH, Tu CY, et al. Color Doppler US pulmonary artery vessel signal: a sign for predicting the benign lesions. Ultrasound Med Biol 2007;33:379-388.
30. Chu IW, Yeh SJ, Lin YC. Intrathoracic kidney in a case of trisomy 18. Turk J Pediatr 2008;50:176-178.
31. Cacciaguerra S, Vasta G, Benedetto AG, et al. Neonatal diaphragmatic hemangioma. J Pediatr Surg 2001;36:E21.
32. Smerdely MS, Raymond G, Fisher KL, Bhargava R. Primitive neuroectodermal tumor of the diaphragm: a case report. Pediatr Radiol 2000;30:702-704.
33. Gupta AK, Mitra DK, Berry M. Primary embryonal rhabdomyosarcoma of the diaphragm in a child: case report. Pediatr Radiol 1999;29:823-825.
34. Frazier AA, Rosado de Christenson ML, Stocker JT, Templeton PA. Intralobar sequestration: radiologic-pathologic correlation. Radiographics 1997;17:725-745.
35. Gosselin MV. Intralobar sequestration. In: Gurney JW, Winer-Muram HT, editors. Diagnostic imaging: chest. Salt Lake City, 2006, Amirsys, II-2-14-17.
36. Stocker JT. Non-neoplastic lung disease. Histopathology 2002;41(Suppl 2):424-458.
37. Ucar B, Akgun N, Bor O, et al. Biphasic pulmonary blastoma in a child. Turk J Pediatr 2000;42:258-263.

Diaphragm

38. Houston JG, Fleet M, Cowan MD, McMillan NC. Comparison of ultrasound with fluoroscopy in the assessment of suspected hemidiaphragmatic movement abnormality. Clin Radiol 1995;50:95-98.
39. Lemmer J, Stiller B, Heise G, et al. Postoperative phrenic nerve palsy: early clinical implications and management. Intensive Care Med 2006;32:1227-1233.
40. Lerolle N, Guerot E, Dimassi S, et al. Ultrasonographic diagnostic criterion for severe diaphragmatic dysfunction after cardiac surgery. Chest 2009;135:401-407.
41. Gerscovich EO, Cronan M, McGahan JP, et al. Ultrasonographic evaluation of diaphragmatic motion. J Ultrasound Med 2001;20:597-604.
42. Eren S, Kantarci M, Okur A. Imaging of diaphragmatic rupture after trauma. Clin Radiol 2006;61:467-477.

Ultrasound-Guided Procedures

43. McBride SC. Management of parapneumonic effusions in pediatrics: current practice. J Hosp Med 2008;3:263-270.

44. Chiu CY, Wong KS, Huang YC, et al. Echo-guided management of complicated parapneumonic effusion in children. Pediatr Pulmonol 2006;41:1226-1232.
45. Feola GP, Shaw LC, Coburn L. Management of complicated parapneumonic effusions in children. Tech Vasc Interv Radiol 2003;6:197-204.
46. Pihlajamaa K, Bode MK, Puumalainen T, et al. Pneumothorax and the value of chest radiography after ultrasound-guided thoracocentesis. Acta Radiol 2004;45:828-832.

47. Duman L, Karnak I, Akinci D, Tanyel FC. Extensive cervical-mediastinal cystic lymphatic malformation treated with sclerotherapy in a child with Klippel-Trenaunay syndrome. J Pediatr Surg 2006;41:e21-e24.

Osteomyelitis and Rib Fractures
48. Kelloff J, Hulett R, Spivey M. Acute rib fracture diagnosis in an infant by ultrasound: a matter of child protection. Pediatr Radiol 2009;39:70-72.

CHAPTER 53

The Pediatric Liver and Spleen

Sara M. O'Hara

Chapter Outline

ANATOMY

The anatomy of the liver can be explored in many planes with sonography. The usual course of intrahepatic vessels and their normal variants can be traced.[1] There is a simple sonographic approach to the segmental anatomy of the liver based on the nomenclature of the French surgeon Couinaud,[2] who described the segments according to the distribution of the portal and hepatic veins. Each segment has a branch (or a group of branches) of the **portal vein** at its center and a **hepatic vein** at its periphery. Each lobe of the liver contains **four segments.** The segments are numbered counterclockwise: 1 through 4 make up the **left lobe,** and 5 through 8, the **right lobe.** Segment 1 is the **caudate lobe** or Spiegel lobe. The right and left lobes are separated by the **main hepatic fissure,** a line connecting the neck of the gallbladder and the left side of the inferior vena cava (IVC) (Fig. 53-1).

The segmental branches of the portal vein (each one of which leads into a segment) can be outlined in the form of two Hs turned sideways, one for the left lobe (segments 1-4) and one for the right lobe (segments 5-8) (Fig. 53-2).

Portal Vein Anatomy

Left Lobe of Liver

The H of the left lobe is visualized with an oblique, upwardly tilted subxiphoid view. The H is formed by the left portal vein, the branch entering segment 2, the umbilical portion of the left portal vein, and the branches to segments 3 and 4 (see Fig. 53-2). To this recumbent H are attached two ligaments, the **ligamentum venosum,** also called the lesser omentum or the hepatogastric ligament, and the **falciform ligament.** The ligamentum

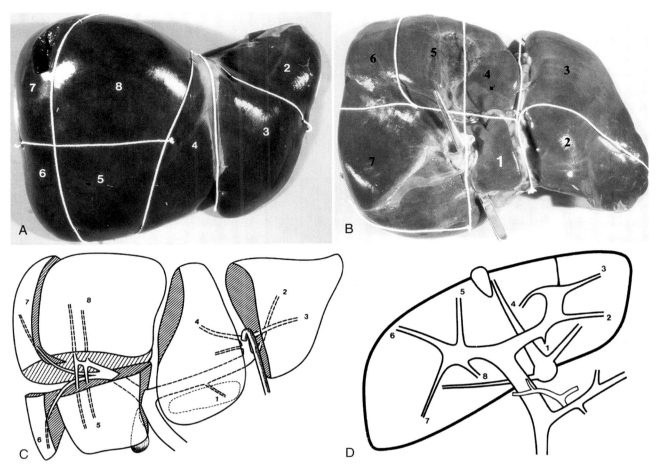

FIGURE 53-1. External segmental anatomy of the liver. Segments are numbered in a counterclockwise direction. Their borders are marked with string. **A,** Upper and anterior surface. Note the whitish falciform ligament that separates segments 3 and 4. **B,** Lower surface: the forceps are in the main portal vein. The gallbladder has been removed from its bed, which separates segments 4 and 5. The vertical string between segments 4 and 5 and between 1 and 7 follows the gallbladder/middle hepatic vein axis and marks the main hepatic fissure, the division between right and left lobes. Segment 1, the caudate lobe, is to the right of the forceps. Segments 3 and 4 are separated by the falciform ligament; 1 and 2 by the ligamentum venosum. **C,** Schema of the hepatic segments with their portal venous branches (upper anterior, viewed as in **A**). **D,** Diagram of the portal and hepatic veins and their relationship to the segments (lower liver surface, viewed as in **B**). *(From Ikeda S, Sera Y, Yamamoto H, et al. Effect of phenobarbital on serial ultrasonic examination in the evaluation of neonatal jaundice. Clin Imaging 1994;18:146-148.)*

venosum separates segment 1 from segment 2 (Figs. 53-1, *B,* and 53-2, *A*). The falciform ligament is seen between the umbilical portion of the left portal vein[2] and the outer surface of the liver (Figs. 53-1, *A* and *B,* and 53-2, *A* and *C*). It separates segment 3 from segment 4.

Segment 1, the caudate lobe, is bordered posteriorly by the IVC, laterally by the ligamentum venosum, and anteriorly by the left portal vein (Fig. 53-1, *B*). Unlike the other segments of the liver, segment 1 may receive branches of the left and right portal veins. The portal veins to segment 1 are usually small and are rarely seen sonographically. The caudate lobe has one or more hepatic veins that drain directly into the IVC, separately from the three main hepatic veins.[3] This special vascularization is a distinctive characteristic of segment 1.

The portal vein leading to **segment 2** is a linear continuation of the left portal vein, completing the lower horizontal limb of the H. Segmental branches to segments 3 and 4 form the other horizontal limb (Fig. 53-2). Segments 2 and 3 are thus located to the left of the umbilical portion of the left portal vein, the ligamentum venosum, and the falciform ligament. **Segment 4, the quadrate lobe,** is situated around the right anterior limb of the portal venous H, to the right of the umbilical portion of the left portal vein and the falciform ligament (Fig. 53-2). Segment 4 is separated from segment 5 by the main hepatic fissure (Fig. 53-1, *B*) and from segments 5 and 8 by the middle hepatic vein. The quadrate lobe is separated from segment 1 by the left portal vein.

Right Lobe of Liver

The right portal vein and its branches are best seen with a sagittal or oblique midaxillary intercostal approach. In

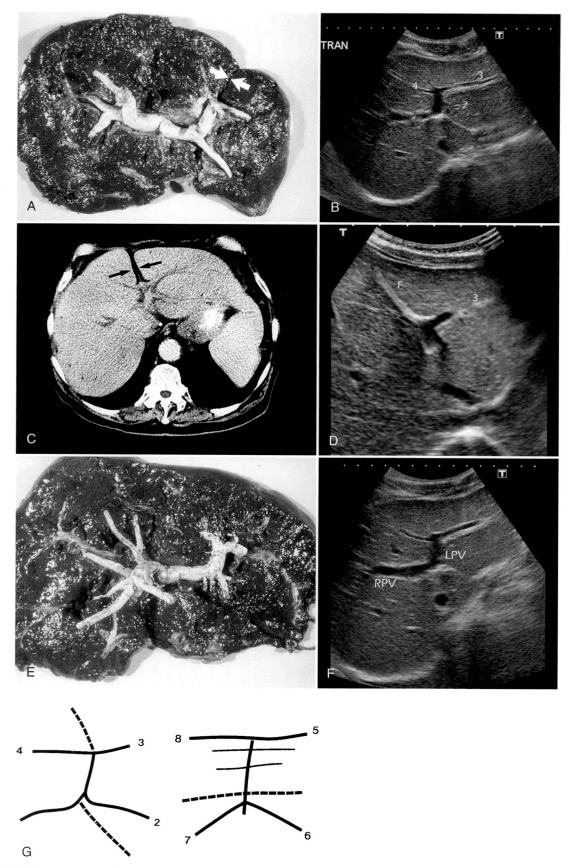

FIGURE 53-2. Anatomy of segmental portal veins. A, Left hepatic lobe, shown on a dissected specimen (with pale-blue dye in portal vein); **B,** on a subxiphoid transverse sonogram; **C,** on CT; and **D,** on more cephalad transverse sonogram. The left portal vein, with branches to segments 2, 3, and 4, forms a horizontally placed H. The umbilical portion of the left portal vein forms the crossbar of the H. Falciform ligament, indicated by arrows in **A** and **C** and "F" in **D,** is an extension of the umbilical part of the left portal vein. **E,** Right hepatic lobe of a dissected specimen, and **F,** on a transverse sonogram obtained at the branch point of the main portal vein into right and left branches. **G,** *Left* and *right,* Diagrams of the portal vein branches to the left and right lobes. Portal vein branches to segments 5 through 8 and 6 and 7 form the main limbs of the H, and the right portal vein forms its crossbar. Once again, the H is turned horizontally. *(From Bismuth H. Surgical anatomy and anatomical surgery of the liver. World J Surg 1982;6:3-9.)*

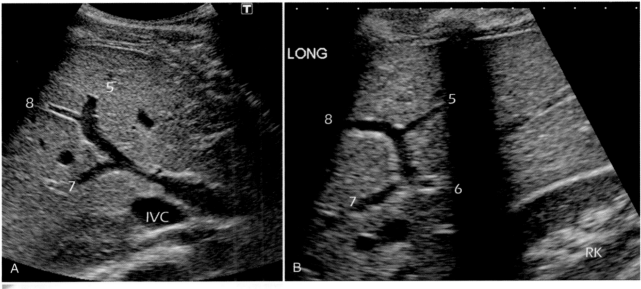

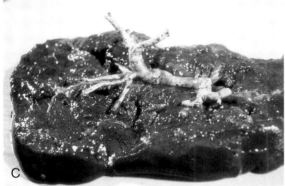

FIGURE 53-3. Right portal vein and branches. Intercostal midaxillary sonograms with varying obliquity show the right portal vein forming the crossbar of the right H. **A,** Transverse view of the right portal vein branching into segments 5 to 8; *IVC,* inferior vena cava. **B,** Intercostal view angled more posteriorly and longitudinally shows the portal vein branch to segment 7 to better advantage. Segmental branch 6 is directed toward the right kidney *(RK)*. **C,** Right portal vein and its branches. Dissected specimen shows the segmental branches and their oblique course. *(From Bismuth H. Surgical anatomy and anatomical surgery of the liver. World J Surg 1982;6:3-9.)*

some subjects, a subcostal approach is also useful. The right portal vein follows an oblique or vertical course, directed anteriorly.

The branches leading to the segments of the right lobe of the liver are also distributed in the shape of a sideways H. The right portal vein forms the crossbar of the H. The branches to segments 5 and 8 form the upper limb of the H (Fig. 53-2), whereas the branches to segments 6 and 7 form its lower portion. The branches of segments 6 and 7 are more obliquely oriented, and the transducer should be rotated slightly upward for segment 7 and downward in the direction of the right kidney for segment 6.

The middle hepatic vein separates segments 5 and 8 from segment 4. The right hepatic vein separates segments 5 and 8 from the segments 6 and 7 (Fig. 53-3).

Segment 5 is bordered medially by the gallbladder and the middle hepatic vein and laterally by the right hepatic vein. The right portal vein serves as a landmark for the separation of segment 5 from segment 8. Segment 8 is separated from segment 7 by the right hepatic vein and from segment 4 by the middle hepatic vein (Fig. 53-3).

Segments 6 and 7 are separated from segments 5 and 8 by the right hepatic vein. **Segment 6** is the part of the liver closest to the kidney; its lateral border is the rib cage. **Segment 7** is separated from segment 8 by the right hepatic vein and is bordered laterally by the rib cage and cephalically by the dome of the diaphragm.

Hepatic Vein Anatomy

When seen with an oblique coronal subxiphoid view, the three hepatic veins form a W, with its base on the IVC. The left and middle hepatic veins join the left anterior part of the IVC (Fig. 53-4). The hepatic veins separate the following segments: the **left hepatic vein** separates segment 2 from segment 3; the **middle hepatic vein** separates segment 4 from segments 5 and 8; and the **right hepatic vein** separates segments 5 and 8 from segments 6 and 7 (see Fig. 53-1, *D*). With the oblique subxiphoid view, the right portal vein is seen en face, which helps separate the superficial segment 5 from the more deeply situated segment 8.

The sonographic examination of the child's liver should include visualization of the **right and left portal**

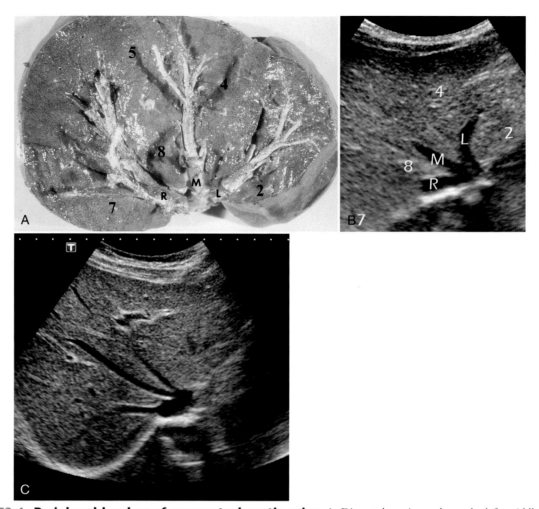

FIGURE 53-4. Peripheral borders of segments: hepatic veins. A, Dissected specimen shows the left, middle, and right hepatic veins *(L, M, R).* The position of the segments is indicated by numbers. **B** and **C,** Subxiphoid, oblique sonogram at a similar plane as **A** shows the three hepatic veins. *(From Bismuth H: Surgical anatomy and anatomical surgery of the liver. World J Surg 1982;6:3-9.)*

veins and their segmental branches, as well as the hepatic veins. Not only can focal lesions be identified and accurately localized, but thrombosis, compression, or tumor invasion of vessels can be outlined. Doppler sonography is added when the presence and direction of blood flow within these veins need to be assessed. Exploring the liver through its vessels is an excellent way to ensure that the sonographic examination is complete and not just an arbitrary glance at this otherwise homogeneous organ with variable contours and few landmarks except for its veins. Because the branches of the hepatic artery and the bile ducts are neighbors of the portal veins, the examination of the lobar and segmental portal veins ensures a complete look at these structures as well.

NEONATAL JAUNDICE

The cause of persistent jaundice in the newborn is often difficult to define because clinical and laboratory features may be similar in hepatocellular and obstructive jaundice. If bile obstruction, biliary atresia, or metabolic diseases such as galactosemia and tyrosinemia are to be treated effectively with surgery or specific diet and medication, the diagnosis must be made early, in the first 2 to 3 months, before irreversible cirrhosis has occurred.

Sonography plays an important role in defining causes of **extrahepatic obstruction to bile flow** that may be effectively treated with early surgery, including choledochal cyst, biliary atresia, and spontaneous perforation of the bile ducts. (Other causes of bile duct obstruction, such as cholelithiasis, tumors of the bile ducts or pancreas, and congenital stenosis of the common bile duct, usually appear later in childhood.) Intrahepatic causes of neonatal jaundice include **hepatitis** (bacterial, viral, or parasitic) and **metabolic diseases** (e.g., galactosemia, tyrosinemia, fructose intolerance, α_1-antitrypsin deficiency, cystic fibrosis, paucity of interlobular bile ducts, North American Indian cirrhosis). **Systemic diseases** that cause cholestasis include heart failure, shock, sepsis, neonatal lupus, histiocytosis, and severe hemolytic disease.

CAUSES OF NEONATAL JAUNDICE

OBSTRUCTION OF BILE DUCTS
Choledochal cyst
Biliary atresia
Spontaneous perforation of the bile ducts
Paucity of interlobular bile ducts (Alagille
  syndrome)

HEPATOCELLULAR DAMAGE (CHOLESTASIS)
Hepatitis
Bacterial
  Syphilis
  Listeria
  Staphylococcus
Viral
  Hepatitis B
  Hepatitis C
  Cytomegalovirus
  Human immunodeficiency virus
  Rubella
  Herpesvirus
  Epstein-Barr virus
Parasitic
  Toxoplasma

Systemic Diseases
Shock
Sepsis
Heart failure
Neonatal lupus
Histiocytosis
Hemolytic diseases

METABOLIC LIVER DISEASES
Galactosemia
Tyrosinemia
Fructose intolerance
α_1-Antitrypsin deficiency
  Cystic fibrosis

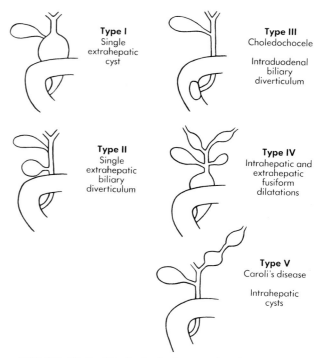

FIGURE 53-5. Choledochal cyst classification.

Choledochal Cyst

Dilation of varying lengths and severity of the common bile duct, termed choledochal cyst, has been detected in utero and usually presents as jaundice in infancy, clinically mimicking neonatal hepatitis and biliary atresia (Fig. 53-5). Todani's classification,[6] a modification of that proposed by Alonson-Lej, describes five types. Type I, **cylindrical or saccular dilation of the common bile duct** (CBD), is most common (80%-90%) and is thought to be caused by an abnormal insertion of the CBD into the pancreatic duct, forming a common channel and facilitating reflux of enzymes into the CBD, with consequent inflammation. Because choledochal cysts have been detected in 15-week-old fetuses, when amylase is not yet present, and because surgically treated cysts in the newborn period show minimal inflammation, there must be causative factors (as yet unknown) other than the common-channel theory. Two rare but well-documented causes of bile duct dilation (choledochal cyst) in the newborn are localized atresia of the CBD and multiple intestinal atresias in which the CBD empties into a blind pouch of bowel.[7] A choledochal cyst presenting later in childhood may have a different pathogenesis. It is usually complicated by cholangitis and classically causes abdominal pain, obstructive jaundice, and fever. In some cases the cyst is palpable as a mass.

Choledochal cyst type II consists of one or more **diverticula** of the CBD (2% of cysts). **Choledochocele** (type III) is a dilation of the intraduodenal part of the CBD (1%-5%). **Multiple intrahepatic and**

The infant with jaundice is usually screened with sonography. When dilation of the bile ducts is found, percutaneous cholangiography or cholecystography may be performed if the cause and anatomy of the obstruction are unclear. If sonography fails to outline an anatomic abnormality, hepatobiliary scintigraphy may define patency of the common bile duct, unless hepatocyte damage is extensive. If no radionuclide reaches the gut, liver biopsy is generally performed. Both scintigraphy and the sonographic search for the gallbladder seem to be enhanced by the bile-stimulating effect of phenobarbital administered for 3 to 5 days before the test.[4] The **triangular cord sign,** an echogenic cone-shaped density just cranial to the portal vein bifurcation on longitudinal or transverse scans, is highly predictive of biliary atresia. An **absent or small gallbladder** (<1.5 cm in length) coupled with the triangular cord sign is even more specific for the diagnosis.[5]

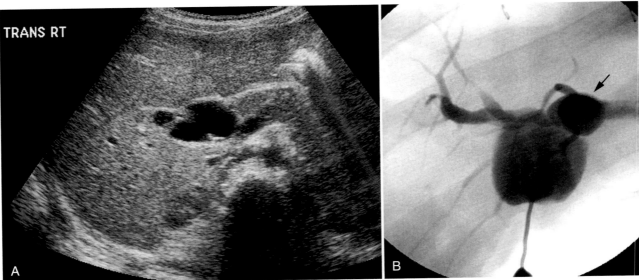

FIGURE 53-6. Choledochal cyst type I in infant with jaundice. A, Transverse sonogram. A large cyst that is the greatly dilated common bile duct is visible entering the pancreatic head. **B,** Intraoperative cholangiogram shows injection of the gallbladder and filling of the choledochal cyst *(arrow).*

extrahepatic cysts make up type IV (10%). **Caroli's disease** (type V) affects intrahepatic bile ducts.

Sonographic screening of the jaundiced infant shows one or several thin-walled cysts at the liver hilum or within the liver (choledochal cyst type I; Fig. 53-6). The gallbladder is identified separately. Dilation of intrahepatic ducts, as well as stones, may occur later as a result of bile stasis and cholangitis. Scintigraphy is used to document bile flow into the cyst, and percutaneous cholecystography/cholangiography or endoscopic retrograde cholangiopancreatography is performed if detailed mapping of the bile system is deemed necessary before surgery.

Caroli's disease (type V choledochal cyst) consists of nonobstructive dilation of intrahepatic bile ducts[8,9] and is often associated with congenital hepatic fibrosis and infantile polycystic disease.[10] The disease is caused by the arrest or derangement in embryologic remodeling of ducts, resulting in segmental dilation. Patients tend to seek medical attention later than with other types of choledochal cysts, usually after cholangitis and stones have formed in childhood (Fig. 53-7). At sonography, Caroli's disease has dilated ducts surrounding branches of the portal vein.[9] Sludge and stones are often visible within the dilated ducts. Abscesses complicating cholangitis are seen as cavities with walls thicker than those of the ducts and filled with heterogeneous material. Polycystic kidneys, when present, are another clue to the diagnosis of Caroli's disease.

Spontaneous Rupture of Bile Duct

Rupture of the bile duct is rare. Rupture in newborns leads to jaundice, abdominal distention, and death unless it is repaired. The cause is unknown. Because the site of rupture is usually the junction of the cystic and common bile ducts, it is believed that a developmental weakness at this site leads to the rupture. The biliary system is undilated, but there are ascites and loculated fluid collections around the gallbladder.[11]

Paucity of Interlobular Bile Ducts and Alagille Syndrome

Presenting with chronic cholestasis, usually within the first 3 months of life, ductal paucity and **arteriohepatic dysplasia** (Alagille syndrome) are diagnosed histologically by noting a reduced number of interlobular bile ducts compared to the total number of portal areas. Because of cholestasis, the gallbladder may be very small (disuse). The liver is usually enlarged, especially the left lobe. Portal hypertension ensues, with splenomegaly and esophageal varices. In children with Alagille syndrome, paucity of bile ducts is associated with a particular facies, pulmonary stenosis, butterfly vertebrae, and, infrequently, renal abnormalities (renal tubular acidosis).[12] Alagille syndrome appears to be inherited as an autosomal dominant disease with variable penetrance.

Biliary Atresia

The incidence of biliary atresia varies from 1 in 8000 to 10,000 births. Boys and girls are equally affected and are usually born at term. Biliary cirrhosis occurs early, often present in the first weeks after birth.

Biliary atresia is characterized by absence or obliteration of the lumen of the extrahepatic and intrahepatic bile ducts (Fig. 53-8). This disease was once thought to

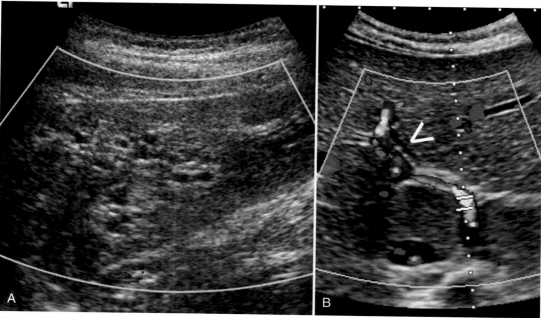

FIGURE 53-7. Biliary ductal dilation. A, Caroli's disease, type V choledochal cyst. Longitudinal color Doppler image of the left lobe of the liver shows saccular dilation of bile ducts with thickened echogenic walls and few vessels in the deeper aspect of the liver. Cholangitis, caused by obstruction of the bile ducts or by ascending infection, leads to dilation of the intrahepatic and common bile ducts. **B,** Central bile duct dilation on transverse sonogram in a different patient, with concentric smooth dilation of main intrahepatic duct *(arrowhead)* caused by distal common bile obstruction.

be caused by faulty development of the bile system. It is associated with the **polysplenia syndrome** (biliary atresia, situs inversus, polysplenia, symmetrical liver, interrupted IVC, preduodenal portal vein) in about 20% of patients,[13] as well as with **trisomy 17 or 18.** Because the disease is extremely rare in fetuses and stillborn or newborn infants, and because the pancreatic duct, which develops with the bile ducts, is normal in affected children, biliary atresia likely develops after the bile ducts have formed. An in utero insult to the hepatobiliary system, either infectious, immunologic, toxic, or vascular, results in a progressive sclerosis of the extrahepatic and intrahepatic bile ducts. Certain drugs (e.g., carbamazepine) have been associated with biliary atresia, conclusive serologic evidence of in utero infection in affected children has not been found.[14]

Jaundice classically develops gradually, 2 to 3 weeks after birth. The diagnosis is readily made if there are radiologic or sonographic signs of the polysplenia syndrome (Fig. 53-8, *C-G*). Because the flow of bile is interrupted, the gallbladder is very small (20%) or absent (80%) in the majority of patients.[13] After having the infant fast for 4 to 6 hours, a specific search with a high-frequency transducer will demonstrate a very small gallbladder (**microgallbladder**) in about 20% of cases. When the gallbladder is visible, the "ghost triad" appearance has been reported to help in making the correct diagnosis of biliary atresia.[15] The **ghost triad** consists of gallbladder length less than 1.9 cm, irregular or incomplete mucosal lining, and irregular or lobular contour.

The echogenic fibrotic remnant of the CBD seen adjacent to the portal vein has been called the **triangular cord sign.** The combination of a small gallbladder, less than 1.5 cm in length, and the triangular cord sign are very specific for the diagnosis of biliary atresia.[5] Any intrahepatic bile duct remnants may dilate and be visible at sonography as bile duct dilation or small cysts. In addition, the cholangitis that complicates biliary atresia may result in cystic areas within the liver.[16]

Surgical treatment creates contact between a loop of jejunum (transposed to the liver after a Roux-en-Y anastomosis) and any patent bile "ductules" at the liver hilum. This is the classic hepatoportoenterostomy described by Kasai in 1959. Even if there is no mucosal contact between intestine and the bile ducts, the procedure permits bile drainage, with complete clinical remission in 30% and partial drainage in 30% of affected children. The prognosis becomes much more guarded when the Kasai procedure is delayed to more than 60 days after birth.[17] Despite successful Kasai procedures, 75% of patients require liver transplantation before age 20 years.[18]

Neonatal Hepatitis

Defined as an infection of the liver occurring before the age of 3 months, neonatal hepatitis is now considered an entity distinct from toxic or metabolic diseases affecting the neonate. The causative agent (bacterium, virus, or parasite) reaches the liver through the placenta, the

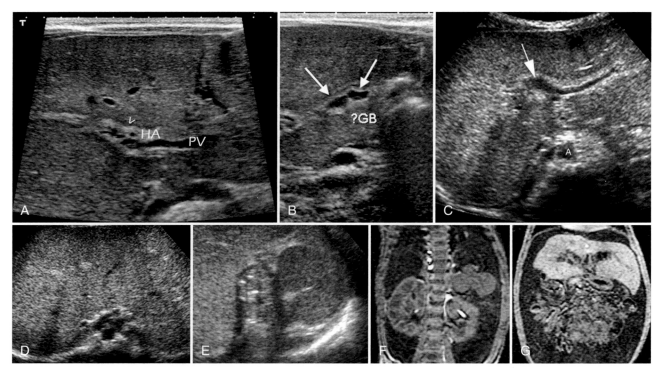

FIGURE 53-8. Biliary atresia spectrum. A, Transverse sonogram near the porta hepatis. **Triangular cord sign** is linear, echogenic fibrous tissue *(arrowhead)* anterior to a normal portal vein and hepatic artery. Failure to visualize the common bile duct in a newborn with jaundice is strongly suggestive of biliary atresia. **B, Gallbladder ghost triad:** small gallbladder *(arrows)*, irregular/incomplete echogenic lining, and indistinct/lobular wall. Highly specific finding for biliary atresia. **C to G, Polysplenia syndrome** in a different patient, with preduodenal portal vein and interruption of inferior vena cava (IVC). **C,** Transverse liver sonogram shows aorta *(A)* anterior and left of the spine in newborn girl. The bifurcation of the portal vein *(arrow)* is more anterior than usual. **D, "Transverse liver."** Right transverse sonogram shows liver extending across the entire upper abdomen. IVC is missing on both views. **E,** In left upper quadrant, several small spleens are present. No gallbladder was found in this patient with biliary atresia. **F, Polysplenia.** Coronal MR SPGR images performed for ascites and elevated liver enzymes. **G,** Transverse liver with anteriorly positioned portal vein several months after Kasai procedure.

vagina from infected maternal secretions, or through catheters or blood transfusions. Transplacental infection occurs most readily during the third trimester, and syphilis, *Toxoplasma,* rubella, and cytomegalovirus (CMV) are the most common agents.[14]

Neonatal bacterial hepatitis is usually secondary to upward spread of organisms from the vagina, infecting endometrium, placenta, and amniotic fluid. (In twin pregnancies, the fetus nearest the cervix is more frequently affected.) *Listeria* and *Escherichia coli* are the usual organisms. During vaginal delivery, direct contact with herpesvirus, CMV, human immunodeficiency virus (HIV), and *Listeria* may lead to hepatitis. Blood transfusions may contain the hepatitis viruses B or C, CMV, Epstein-Barr virus (EBV), and HIV. Infected umbilical vein catheterization usually results in bacterial hepatitis or abscesses.[14]

With the exception of diffuse hepatomegaly, there are no specific sonographic signs of hepatitis, unless abscesses (usually bacterial in origin) occur[19,20] (Fig. 53-9). The gallbladder wall may be thickened, probably from hypoalbuminemia.

Neonatal Jaundice and Urinary Tract Infection/Sepsis

The association of jaundice with urinary tract infection or sepsis occurs more often in male than female newborns. Jaundice, hepatomegaly, and vomiting are common clinical signs. Urinary tract symptoms are uncommon, as are shock and fever. A thorough examination of the kidneys, ureters, and bladder should therefore accompany sonography of the liver in the infant with jaundice. Similarly, the diaphragm and lung bases should be examined to look for pleural effusions and pneumonia, which may be accompanied by sepsis and jaundice in the newborn.

Inborn Errors of Metabolism

Because these disorders cause liver damage in the newborn, some rapidly destroying the liver if untreated, and because several can be treated effectively with diet or drugs once diagnosed, pediatricians and radiologists should be well acquainted with inborn errors of

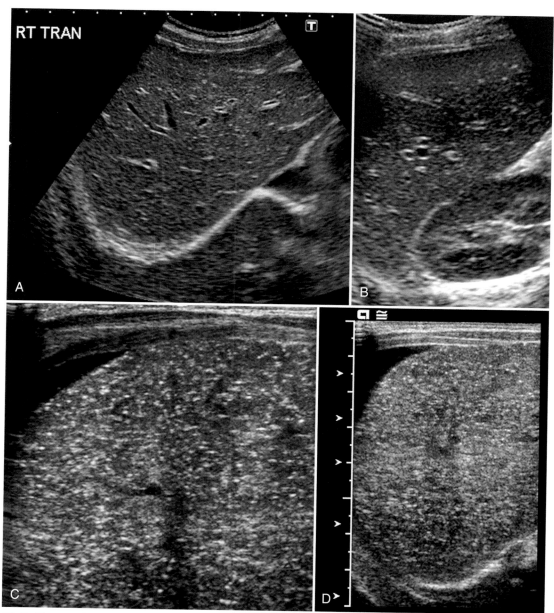

FIGURE 53-9. Hepatitis. A, Transverse sonogram in a teenage boy with acute hepatitis shows echogenic portal triads and hypoechoic parenchyma. **B,** Longitudinal image in same patient showing hepatic hypoechoic echotexture similar to adjacent right kidney. **C,** Transverse magnified sonogram, and **D,** conventional linear array image, show **congenital herpes infection** in an infant with dystrophic calcification throughout the liver. No similar calcifications were seen in the spleen.

metabolism. Liver damage is caused by storage of a hepatotoxic metabolite or by absence of an essential enzyme that impairs the detoxification process of the liver.

Steatosis is especially prominent in the glycogen storage diseases, galactosemia, tyrosinemia, and cystic fibrosis. **Cirrhosis** eventually develops in all the diseases that cause liver damage, and portal hypertension then follows. The risk of **hepatocellular carcinoma** is significantly increased in α_1-antitrypsin deficiency, in tyrosinemia, and in glycogen storage disease type I. **Liver adenomas** also develop in the latter two entities, as does

renal tubular disease, which is usually characterized by acidosis and nephrocalcinosis.[14]

Tyrosinemia is now best treated by transplantation. Until drug therapy became available for the treatment of the acute neurologic crises in infants with acute tyrosinemia, transplantation was performed as a lifesaving procedure as soon as surgically feasible. Currently, transplantation is done once liver nodules appear because hepatocarcinoma develops in about 30% of children with tyrosinemia who survive the neonatal period. A review of livers dissected at liver transplantation found

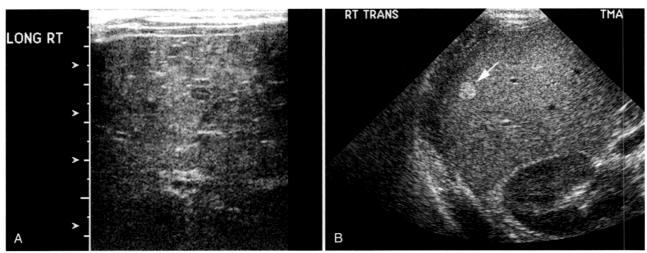

FIGURE 53-10. Tyrosinemia and glycogen storage disease (type I, von Gierke's disease). A, Longitudinal sonogram shows heterogeneous echotexture, likely a combination of regenerating nodules and adenomas of the liver, in a patient with tyrosinemia awaiting liver transplant. B, **Echogenic adenoma** *(arrow)* in the liver of another child with glycogen storage disease type I. Follow-up was done because of this patient's increased risk of hepatocellular carcinoma.

INBORN ERRORS OF METABOLISM

HEPATOCYTE INJURY CONSISTENTLY
Glycogen storage disease type IV
Galactosemia
Fructose intolerance
Tyrosinemia
Wolman disease
Zellweger syndrome
Neonatal iron storage disease
Wilson's disease

HEPATOCYTE INJURY SOMETIMES
α_1-Antitrypsin deficiency
Cystic fibrosis
Glycogen storage disease (I and III)

NO HEPATOCYTE DAMAGE (STORE METABOLITES)
Mucopolysaccharidoses
Gaucher's disease

that preoperative sonograms and CT scans were not accurate in distinguishing regeneration nodules, adenomas, and carcinomas, nor was alpha-fetoprotein (AFP) analysis[21] (Fig. 53-10).

The sonographic examination of children with possible metabolic disease includes a careful analysis of liver size and architecture, searching for steatosis, cirrhosis, and nodules; an analysis of renal architecture, searching for increased size and nephrocalcinosis; and a Doppler examination of the abdomen searching for signs of portal hypertension.

STEATOSIS (FATTY DEGENERATION OR INFILTRATION)

Fat accumulates in hepatocytes after cellular damage (fatty degeneration), through the overloading of previously healthy cells with excess fat (fatty infiltration), or in certain enzyme deficiency syndromes, through the inability of fat to be mobilized out of the liver. Drugs (acetylsalicylic acid, tetracycline, valproate, warfarin [Coumadin]) and toxins (aflatoxin, hypoglycine) as well as alcohol abuse lead to fatty degeneration of liver cells. Steatosis is also seen in metabolic liver disorders such as galactosemia, fructose intolerance, and Reye's syndrome. Obesity, corticosteroid therapy, hyperlipidemia, and diabetes are examples of increased fat mobilization and its entry into the liver. In malnutrition, nephrotic syndrome, and cystic fibrosis, not only does excess fat enter the liver, but mobilization of fat out of the hepatocyte is deficient as well. When parenteral nutrition does not include lipids, steatosis results from a deficiency of essential fatty acids. Most inherited disorders of the liver mentioned previously involve an enzyme deficiency and result in steatosis.

Fatty changes are reversible, may be diffuse or focal, and are often detected by ultrasonography before clinically suspected.[22] On sonography, areas of steatosis are highly echogenic, blurring vessel walls. The nearby kidney cortex appears much less echogenic. When focal, steatosis usually has smooth, geometric, or fingerlike borders[23] (Fig. 53-11). Intervening normal liver may appear hypoechogenic and masquerade as mass lesions (metastases or abscesses), especially if the ultrasound gain

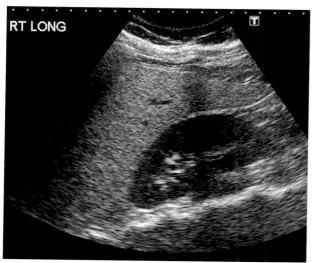

FIGURE 53-11. Fatty infiltration of liver (steatosis) in patient with cystic fibrosis. Sagittal view shows increased hepatic echotexture, with some sparing posteriorly. The cortex of the right kidney is much less echogenic than the fatty liver.

CAUSES OF STEATOSIS

Drugs
    Acetylsalicylic acid
    Tetracycline
    Valproate
    Warfarin (Coumadin)
Toxins
    Aflatoxin
    Hypoglycine
Alcohol abuse
Metabolic liver disease
    Galactosemia
    Fructose intolerance
    Reye's syndrome
Obesity
Corticosteroid therapy
Hyperlipidemia
Diabetes
Malnutrition
Nephrotic syndrome
Cystic fibrosis

is adjusted by using the fatty areas as a normal reference. Segments 4 and 5 are often spared in steatosis, perhaps because of favorable blood supply by the gallbladder and its vessels.[24] Nodules of steatosis may mimic metastases on CT. Areas of abnormal echotexture on ultrasonographic studies can be further evaluated with CT; the two modalities are complementary in this situation.

Despite sophisticated imaging, ultrasound- or CT-guided biopsy may be necessary.

CIRRHOSIS

The usual forms of cirrhosis in childhood are **biliary** and **postnecrotic.** Morphologically, the cirrhotic liver consists of regenerating nodules devoid of central veins and surrounded by variable amounts of connective tissue. Hepatic architecture is sufficiently distorted to disturb hepatic circulation and hepatocellular function. Increased resistance to blood flow through the liver leads to portal hypertension.

The sonographic appearance of the liver depends on the severity of the cirrhosis. With progressive replacement of hepatocytes by fibrous tissue, the liver attenuates sound increasingly, and sound penetration of the liver, even with low-frequency (2 or 3 MHz) transducers, becomes difficult. The macronodules of advanced cirrhosis become visible sonographically at the surface of the liver (contrasted to the neighboring lesser omentum, peritoneum, or ascites, if present) or within its substance (nodular architecture, increased hyperechogenic fibrous tissue around portal vein branches and the ligamentum teres).[23] The caudate lobe is often prominent[25] (Fig. 53-12). Parts of segment 4 of the right lobe of the liver may atrophy in advanced disease.

CHOLELITHIASIS

Gallstones are less common in children than in adults and are usually related to an associated disease. Their composition can be mixed or of calcium bilirubinate. The "adult" cholesterol stone is rare except in children with cystic fibrosis.[26] Gallstones are mobile and hyperechogenic, and they cast acoustic shadows only if they are of appropriate size and composition.

In some children, especially those receiving total parenteral nutrition (TPN), thick bile can be observed to form **sludge,** loosely formed "sludge balls" or "tumefactive sludge," and finally **stones,** when serial sonograms are performed over several weeks (Fig. 53-13). **Stasis of bile flow** is the probable cause of sludge and stone formation, also seen in utero and in premature infants and usually regressing spontaneously.[27]

Gallbladder wall thickening occurs in children with acute hepatitis, hypoalbuminemia, obstructed hepatic venous return, and ascites.[19,20] The classic signs of impacted gallstone, thick gallbladder wall, and fluid around the gallbladder seen in adults with **acute cholecystitis** are rare in children. The gallbladder becomes dilated and rounded (rather than the normal oval shape) in fasting children (especially infants receiving TPN),

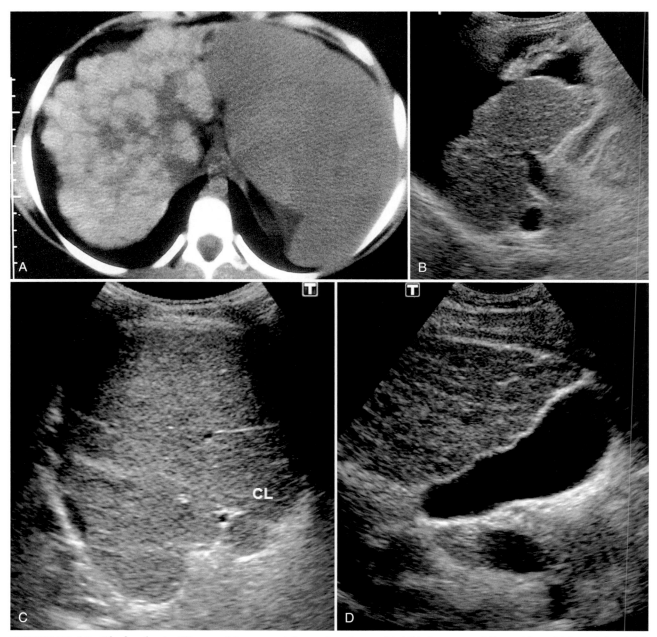

FIGURE 53-12. Cirrhosis. A, CT scan of the upper abdomen in a 6-year-old child shows a small liver with multiple nodules visible both along the cortex and within the liver. Microscopy of the native liver after transplantation showed regenerating nodules and severe cirrhosis (portal hypertension). **B,** Sonogram of another child shows macronodules of cirrhosis at the surface of the liver outlined by ascitic fluid. **C,** Sonogram in a teenager with cystic fibrosis and cirrhosis shows diffusely increased echotexture of the liver. Note the nodular lateral surface of the liver and the larger caudate lobe *(CL)*. **D,** Nodular contour may also be appreciated against a fluid-filled gallbladder margin in patients without ascites. This 17-year-old patient had autoimmune hepatitis and developing cirrhosis.

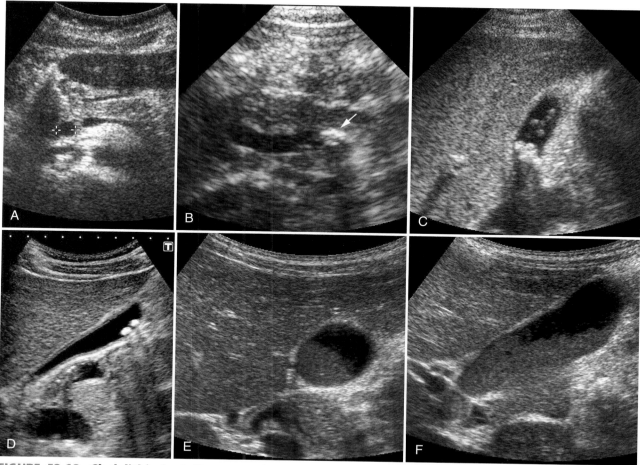

FIGURE 53-13. Cholelithiasis. A, Transverse, and **B,** longitudinal, views of a dilated common bile duct (between cursors in **A**) containing an echogenic shadowing stone (stone seen only on **B,** *arrow*) in a teenager with acute right upper quadrant pain. **C** and **D,** Multiple echogenic, shadowing gallstones in two other patients, with hemolytic anemia. Note that the stones show variable degrees of shadowing, likely related to their mineral composition. **E** and **F,** Gallbladder sludge without stones or gallbladder wall thickening in a patient receiving total parenteral nutrition.

DISEASES ASSOCIATED WITH GALLSTONES IN CHILDREN

HEMATOPOIETIC
Hemolytic anemias or hemolysis (artificial heart valve)
Rh incompatibility
Blood transfusions
Sickle cell anemia

GASTROINTESTINAL
Cystic fibrosis
Bile duct anomalies
Ileal dysfunction (Crohn's disease, short bowel)
Total parenteral nutrition (TPN)
Metabolic liver diseases

OTHER
Immobilization (scoliosis surgery)
Dehydration
Obesity
Sepsis
Oral contraceptives

children with sepsis (especially streptococcal), and those in the acute phase of Kawasaki disease. When distended, the gallbladder may become tender and painful. It heals with the underlying disease. **Acalculous cholecystitis** in children is rare and should be diagnosed only if no disease causing gallbladder distention or wall edema is found.[28] The distinction between gallbladder atony and obstruction cannot always be made with scintigraphic gallbladder ejection fractions.

LIVER TUMORS

Identification

It is sometimes difficult to define the origin of an abdominal mass, especially when it is large. The following questions are helpful in tracing a mass to hepatic origin:

• **Vascular anatomy:** Can a feeding hepatic vessel be identified by means of Doppler sonography? Are segmental portal veins displaced or invaded by the tumor?[29] What liver segments are involved? Is the main hepatic artery enlarged? (This usually signals the presence of a highly vascular hemangioendothelioma.)

- **Biliary anatomy:** Are the bile ducts normal? Has the gallbladder been identified?
- **Anatomy of the abdomen:** Does the mass move with the liver during respiration? Is the liver parenchyma normal or cirrhotic? Is there ascitic fluid available for cytology? Is there another abdominal, retroperitoneal, para-aortic, or pelvic mass that could be a primary tumor?

Benign Liver Tumors

About 40% of primary liver tumors in children are benign. Hemangiomas are by far the most common. Mesenchymal hamartomas, adenomas, and focal nodular hyperplasia together constitute about one half of benign liver tumors in the child.[30]

LIVER MASSES IN CHILDREN

SOLID
Hemangioendothelioma (single or multiple)
Adenoma, hamartoma
Focal nodular hyperplasia
Regeneration nodules in cirrhosis
Hepatoblastoma
Hepatocellular carcinoma
Biliary rhabdomyosarcoma (can be cystic)
Lymphoma
Metastasis

CYSTS IN OR NEAR THE LIVER
Congenital cysts
Congenital hepatic fibrosis
Choledochal cysts
Duodenal duplication cyst
Hydatid cyst ("sand," daughter cysts)
Caroli's disease
   Hamartoma

Hemangiomas

Hemangiomas are vascular, mesenchymal masses characterized initially by active endothelial growth (angiogenesis). At this stage, the tumor is highly vascular and may cause sufficient arteriovenous (AV) shunting to result in high-output heart failure. When associated with hydrops or congestive heart failure and thrombocytopenia, this lesion may be called **neonatal hemangiomatosis.** Hemangiomas in the liver may be solitary or multiple and are sometimes associated with cutaneous hemangiomas as well (Fig. 53-14). When numerous with complications

of hemorrhage, cardiac compromise, hepatic failure, or coagulopathy, hemangiomas may be treated with corticosteroids or rarely chemotherapy.[31] As a typical solitary hemangioma matures, vessel growth slows. Existing vessels may enlarge and form "lakes" with minimal blood flow. This is the cavernous hemangioma typically seen in adults and rarely in children.[32]

Infantile Hemangioendotheliomas

Infantile hemangioendotheliomas are single or multiple solid masses of varying echogenicity, often containing fine, linear foci of calcium.[33] Doppler sonography shows blood flow in multiple tortuous vessels both within and at the periphery of the mass (Fig. 53-15). Doppler shifts exceed those seen in normal intrahepatic arteries. When AV shunting is severe, the celiac axis, hepatic artery, and veins are dilated, and the infraceliac aorta is small. Doppler shifts from hemangioendothelioma vessels may resemble those from malignant tumors.[34] The vascular nature of these lesions is confirmed by bolus injection CT and the search for rapid filling and rapid washout in these masses. Angiography is usually reserved for patients considered for embolization.

Mesenchymal Hamartomas

Mesenchymal hamartomas are rare, usually multiseptate, cystic masses derived from periportal mesenchyma. Calcifications occur rarely. Hamartoma typically presents as an asymptomatic mass in the right lobe of the liver in children younger than 2 years.[35]

Adenomas

Adenomas are rare except in association with metabolic liver disease, especially **glycogen storage disease type I;**[36] **oral contraceptive therapy;** and **anabolic steroid therapy** for Fanconi's anemia. The latter may develop hepatocellular carcinoma. Serum AFP levels are normal. Sonographic appearance varies from hyperechogenic to hypoechogenic and is nonspecific. Malignant degeneration is rare. The distinction between adenoma and a malignant mass is difficult with sonography, CT, and MRI because imaging findings vary and are nonspecific. In patients with Fanconi's anemia after bone marrow transplant, adenomas may mimic abscess during sepsis evaluation.

Focal Nodular Hyperplasia

Focal nodular hyperplasia typically shows a central scar, which may be visible sonographically or at CT. The normal or increased uptake of technetium-99m sulfur colloid by the mass helps to distinguish it from malignant masses, which typically fail to take up the radiolabeled material.[37]

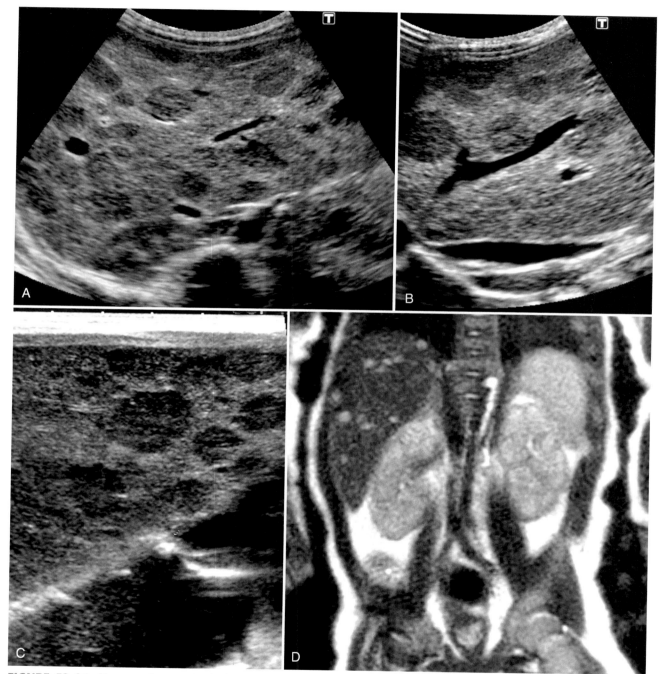

FIGURE 53-14. Hemangiomas. Multiple visceral and cutaneous hemangiomas were found in this newborn with enlarged liver at birth. **A,** Transverse sonogram showing innumerable hypoechoic lesions enlarging the liver. **B,** Longitudinal sonogram of the liver showing one hemangioma deforming the adjacent hepatic vein. **C,** Transverse linear array image showing the lesions in greater detail. **D,** Coronal MRI SSFSE image shows only a few remaining liver lesions several months after a course of steroids.

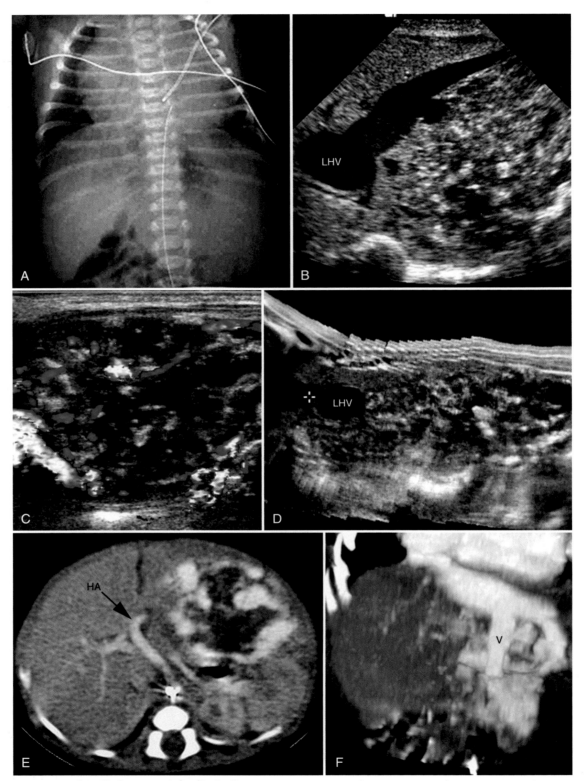

FIGURE 53-15. Infantile hemangioendothelioma. A, Chest and abdominal radiograph of newborn shows left upper quadrant soft tissue mass and congestive heart failure. **B,** Longitudinal gray-scale ultrasound; *LHV,* left hepatic vein. **C,** Color Doppler ultrasound. **D,** Extended-view longitudinal ultrasound. **E,** Contrast medium–enhanced axial CT. **F,** Images of the mass show an enlarged hepatic artery (*HA* in **E**) feeding the lesion and large veins (*V* in **F**) draining into the right atrium and creating a left-to-right shunt and heart failure.

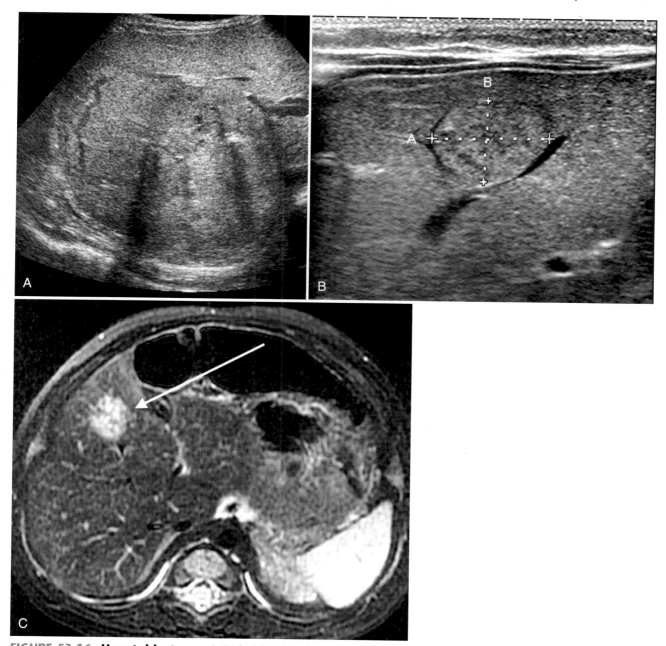

FIGURE 53-16. Hepatoblastoma. A, Right lobe of the liver contains a large heterogeneous mass with scattered, shadowing calcifications in a 1-month-old girl with palpable abdominal mass. **B** and **C,** Images from a different newborn infant, with prenatally diagnosed hepatic mass. **B,** Longitudinal linear array image shows a relatively small mass (between cursors) deforming adjacent vessels. **C,** Axial MR fast spin-echo T2-weighted image of high-signal-intensity lesion *(arrow)* found to be hepatoblastoma on surgical resection.

Malignant Liver Tumors

Most solid liver tumors are malignant and are derived from epithelium.

Hepatoblastoma

Hepatoblastoma, the most common primary liver tumor in childhood, presents in children younger than 3 years and may be considered the infantile form of hepatocellular carcinoma. There is an association with **Beckwith-Wiedemann syndrome, hemihypertrophy,** and the **11p13 chromosome.**[38] Serum AFP levels are almost always elevated. Some tumors secrete gonadotropins and lead to precocious puberty.

The tumor is usually single, solid, large, of mixed echogenicity, and poorly marginated, with small cysts and rounded or irregularly shaped deposits of calcium (Fig. 53-16). These calcifications are quite different from the fine, linear calcifications seen in hemangioendotheliomas.[39] The remaining liver is usually normal, although metastases may be found at diagnosis. Intrahepatic vessels are displaced and amputated by the mass. Tumor thrombi are less common than in hepatocellular carcinoma. Doppler sonography is helpful in diagnosing vessel invasion and detecting flow in malignant neovasculature.[40,41] Complete resection of the tumors results in a 50% to 60% cure rate. Resectability depends on the number of segments and vessels involved and is best determined with MRI.[42]

Hepatocellular Carcinoma

The incidence of hepatocellular carcinoma, the second most common malignant tumor, has two peaks, at 4 to 5 years and at 12 to 14 years. About one half of affected children have preexisting liver disease, especially tyrosinemia, glycogen storage type I, α_1-antitrypsin deficiency, post–hepatitis B or C cirrhosis or biliary cirrhosis following biliary atresia, Byler's disease, and Alagille syndrome. Serum AFP levels are usually elevated. The tumor is often multicentric; masses are solid, rarely calcify, and have variable echogenicity. Portal venous invasion is common and easily detected with Doppler sonography, as is the high-velocity flow in peripheral neovasculature.[40,41,43]

Undifferentiated Embryonal Sarcoma

Undifferentiated embryonal sarcoma (malignant mesenchymoma) is considered the malignant counterpart of the hamartoma. It is rare; occurs in children 6 to 10 years of age, which is older than those with hamartomas; grows rapidly; and develops central necrosis and cysts. Serum AFP levels are normal. Masses are typically large and appear heterogeneous.

Biliary Rhabdomyosarcoma

An unusual site for primary rhabdomyosarcoma, tumors of the biliary tree tend to occur in young children, with a mean age of $3\frac{1}{2}$ years. Rhabdomyosarcoma may originate in the intrahepatic and extrahepatic ducts, gallbladder, cystic duct, or ampulla of Vater. Children typically present with intermittent obstructive jaundice, hepatomegaly, abdominal distention and pain, weight loss, dark urine, and acholic stools. Intraductal location is the best imaging clue to the diagnosis of this otherwise heterogeneous, occasionally cystic mass (Fig. 53-17). Tumors spread locally and metastasize to lung and bone.

Metastases

Metastases to the liver usually arise from **neuroblastoma** (Fig. 53-18), **Wilms' tumor, leukemia,** or **lymphoma.** Diffuse infiltration of the liver (or multiple nodules) in stage 4S neonatal neuroblastoma is remarkable for its good prognosis.

Detection of Tumor Angiogenesis

Hepatoblastoma and hepatocellular carcinoma frequently produce a network of microscopic, parasitic tumor vessels at their periphery. Flow in these vessels, which lack a normal muscularis, produces Doppler shifts (low-resistance, high-velocity flow) greater than those seen in the aorta.[41,43]

LIVER ABSCESS AND GRANULOMAS

Pyogenic Abscess

Pyogenic liver abscesses are rare in the normal child. Abscesses generally occur in association with sepsis, in children with depressed immunity (leukemia, drugs), in those with primary immune defects (chronic granulomatous disease, dysgammaglobulinemia), and with contiguous infection (appendicitis, cholangitis). At sonography, abscesses are generally well-defined masses, with or without heterogeneous fluid content and small air bubbles producing ringdown artifacts (Fig. 53-19). Abscesses displace but do not invade neighboring vessels. A Doppler examination may be used to confirm the patency of nearby portal venous branches. Fluid in the pleural space or in Morison's pouch should be sought in the supine position. **Aspiration,** with or without drainage of abscesses, under sonographic or CT guidance is becoming the preferred treatment in many centers. Some abscesses, especially those accompanying chronic granulomatous disease, gradually calcify during medical treatment.[44] Multiple small abscesses, usually seen in the immunosuppressed child, may result in an enlarged, painful liver. Distinguishing these tiny hypoechogenic lesions from normal liver parenchyma is a challenge to the resolution of the equipment and the skill of the examiner. Scanning the anterior surface of the liver with a high-frequency linear transducer often outlines some of the multiple lesions that are otherwise missed. We routinely complement the ultrasound examination with high-resolution CT in these children because small abscesses are often better seen with CT.

Parasitic Abscesses

Amebiasis

The incidence of parasitic abscesses in children, although low, is increasing because of expanding travel and immigration. Amebiasis is endemic in the tropics and spreads through person-to-person contact. The protozoan *Entamoeba histolytica* is ingested, invades the colonic mucosa, enters intestinal veins, and spreads into portal venous branches. The organism secretes proteolytic enzymes, and hepatic abscess formation occurs rapidly. It is the

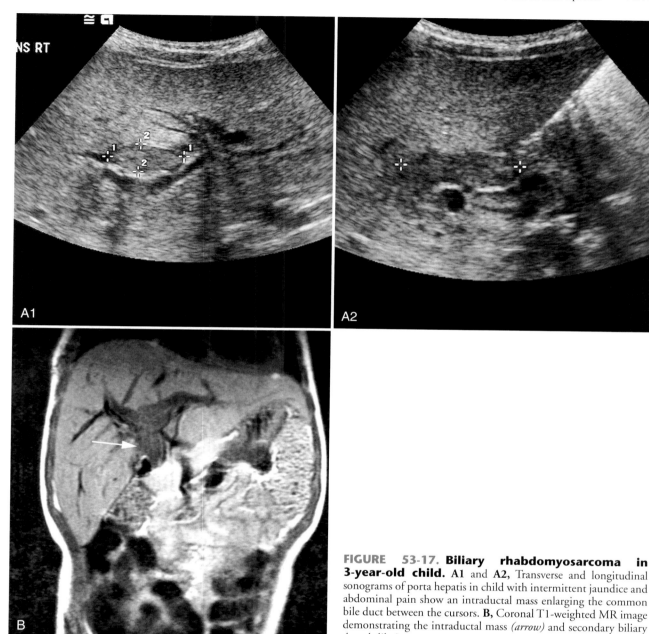

FIGURE 53-17. Biliary rhabdomyosarcoma in 3-year-old child. A1 and **A2,** Transverse and longitudinal sonograms of porta hepatis in child with intermittent jaundice and abdominal pain show an intraductal mass enlarging the common bile duct between the cursors. **B,** Coronal T1-weighted MR image demonstrating the intraductal mass *(arrow)* and secondary biliary ductal dilation.

most frequent extraintestinal complication of **amebic infection.** In children, abscesses are usually multiple and occur most often in infants younger than 1 year and are life threatening. Fever spikes and hepatomegaly without jaundice are the usual forms of presentation. Diagnosis is made by serologic testing, although this is not always positive in infants.

Both sonographic and CT imaging are highly sensitive but fail to differentiate amebic from pyogenic abscesses. The sonographic pattern of hypoechoic, homogeneous, or heterogeneous target masses may mimic that of hematoma or neoplasm. Abscess rupture into the thorax, although rare in childhood, is pathognomonic for amebic abscess. Extension into subphrenic or perihepatic spaces, peritoneum, and nearby abdominal organs is more fre-

quent. Diagnostic puncture is disappointing because of the low yield of organisms. Because pyogenic abscesses usually occur in the immunodeficient child, an abscess occurring in an otherwise healthy infant should be considered amebic until proven otherwise. In the past, high mortality rates (60% in infants) have been caused by late diagnosis. They have been reduced to near-zero with early detection through the use of refined imaging techniques (scintigraphy, sonography, and CT).[45]

Echinococcosis

The adult tapeworm, *Echinococcus,* lives in the jejunum of the dog, where it lays its eggs, which are spread through feces and then swallowed by the intermediate

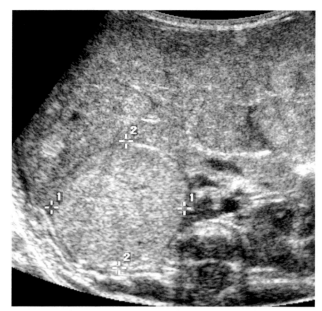

FIGURE 53-18. Metastatic liver disease in 4-year-old child. Transverse sonogram in right upper quadrant shows well-defined right adrenal neuroblastoma *(cursors)* and multiple echogenic hepatic metastases.

host (usually sheep but sometimes humans). Endemic areas include the Middle East, the southern United States, and northern Canada. Embryos, freed in the duodenum, invade the mucosa to enter a mesenteric vein, which flows to the liver, where a slowly growing cyst composed of an acellular outer layer and an endothelialized inner layer may develop. Compressed surrounding liver tissue forms a third layer. The inner layer forms freely floating embryos (scolices), or "hydatid sand," which is visible with sonography. **Daughter cysts** form within the main cyst under certain circumstances and, when seen sonographically, suggest the diagnosis of **hydatid cyst** (Fig. 53-19, *C*). Ruptured daughter cysts form floating membranes. A dead cyst decreases in size and gradually calcifies.[46,47]

Schistosomiasis

Invasion of the portal vein by the ova of *Schistosoma* leads to portal hypertension without cirrhosis. Liver disease progresses so slowly that portal hypertension is rarely seen in a child.

Granulomas of the Liver

Granulomas are circumscribed, focal, inflammatory lesions that may be of bacterial (*Mycobacterium tuberculosis,* other mycobacteria, *Listeria,* spirochetes), fungal *(Candida, Histoplasma, Aspergillus),* parasitic *(Toxocara, Ascaris),* or malignant (lymphoma) origin. Clinical features are those of the underlying disease, and the liver is

usually enlarged. Confluent granulomas or abscesses may be recognized as distinct masses at sonography.

DOPPLER ASSESSMENT OF LIVER DISEASE AND PORTAL HYPERTENSION

Basic Principles

The physics of Doppler ultrasound and the details of instrumentation have been well described.[48-50] The principles essential to the performance of a successful clinical examination with real-time ultrasound coupled to a spectral or color Doppler display are discussed in Chapter 1.

The main factors that affect the Doppler shift in the clinical situation are the **velocity** (v) and the **vessel-transducer angle** (Θ). Commercial machines express the Doppler shift in kilohertz (kHz) or centimeters per second (cm/sec). It must be remembered that true velocity calculations require a vessel beam-angle measurement. When the Doppler beam is perpendicular to the vessel axis, flow will not be registered. At that angle, there is no motion toward or away from the transducer. Therefore the vessel beam angle to detect blood flow should be small, ideally less than 60 degrees. The ultrasound image is best when the transducer is perpendicular to a structure, whereas the Doppler angle is best at up to 60 degrees. The art of performing abdominal Doppler ultrasound consists of placing the transducer at a location where the angle between the Doppler beam and the axis of the vessel is optimal.

The basic technique of the **duplex Doppler ultrasound** consists of visualizing the vessel with real-time or color Doppler and then placing a Doppler beam with a small "aperture," the sample volume, within the vessel, which should be slightly less than the diameter of the vessel. The transducer alternately sends and receives sound waves from the aperture. If there are cells moving within the vessel, a Doppler shift will result.

Most of the abdominal vessels studied in children have a low flow velocity. Therefore the wall filter should be as low as possible, preferably at 50 Hz or less. The pulse repetition frequency should be as low as possible for the same reason, unless there is **aliasing,** the projection of a "cutoff" spectral image on the opposite side of the reference line, or a light, reverse-color image. Thus, flow approaching the transducer is seen above the reference line, and flow receding from the transducer is seen below the reference line. In this way the presence or absence of flow in a vessel can be determined, as can the direction of that flow. If the vessel to beam angle can be measured, velocity of flow can be estimated. When the diameter of the vessel can be determined accurately, an estimate of flow volume can be made (with some limitations of accuracy).[50]

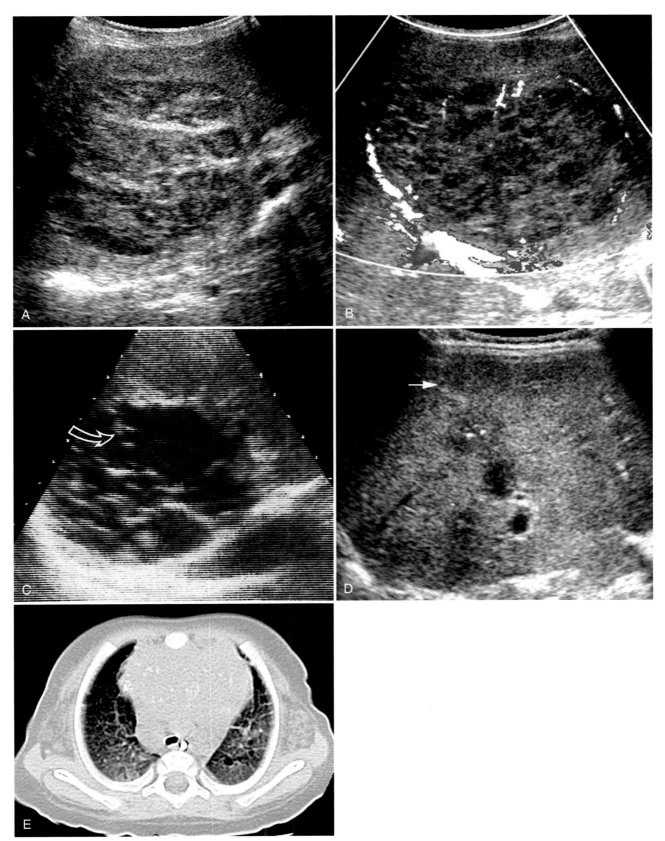

FIGURE 53-19. Hepatic infections. A and **B, Intrahepatic abscess.** Longitudinal gray-scale and transverse color Doppler images in a patient with severe combined immunodeficiency. Note the peripheral hyperemia and decreased vascularity centrally. **C, Hydatid cyst.** Sagittal sonogram of the liver shows a cyst with multiple septa. There are several small (daughter) cysts in the center *(arrow)*. **D** and **E, Langerhans cell histiocytosis. D,** Longitudinal sonogram shows multiple hypoechoic areas in the liver mimicking tiny abscesses *(arrow)* in this infant with failure to thrive. **E,** Axial CT of chest shows mediastinal calcifications and lung cysts.

Color Doppler ultrasound is another method of displaying the Doppler shift arising from moving blood cells within a vessel.[51] Instead of interrogating a small volume within a vessel, the Doppler receiver detects signals from many scan lines. The resultant numerous Doppler signals are displayed as color signals; high-frequency shifts are light-colored (yellow or white), and by convention, flow toward the transducer is red and flow away from it is blue. Turbulent flow is displayed as a mosaic of shades of red and blue. There are great advantages to color mapping because entire segments of vessels are seen at a glance (e.g., portosystemic collateral veins in portal hypertension or stenoses of vessels). The limitations of the vessel/beam angle remain, and no flow may be detected in the part of the vessel perpendicular to the transducer. Flow in tortuous vessels may be difficult to understand because it will have both red and blue segments. When examining small vessels in children, motion may produce flashes or dots of color artifact. Pulsed Doppler sampling of such doubtful signals distinguishes these artifacts from flow signals.

Power Doppler sonography measures the force (power) of the Doppler signal but gives no indication of direction or velocity. It is much less angle dependent than color or pulsed Doppler and is more sensitive to slowly flowing blood. It is most useful in detecting slow flow in small vessels or in vessels perpendicular to the ultrasound beam. Arterial and venous flow cannot be distinguished, but a pulsed Doppler examination can be made at any point in the vessel identified with power Doppler. Because of their small body size and ready access to the Doppler beam, children are particularly suited to color, power, and pulsed Doppler abdominal examinations.

Normal Flow Patterns in Splanchnic Vessels

Arteries to the liver and spleen supply a low-resistance vascular bed and normally show forward flow throughout the cardiac cycle (systole and entire duration of diastole). Blood flow in the mesenteric arteries shows few or no diastolic Doppler shifts. The superior mesenteric artery in the fasting person has very little forward flow during diastole. Shortly after a meal, its diastolic flow increases considerably.[52] The Doppler profile of the abdominal aorta changes throughout its course. Continuous forward diastolic flow in the upper abdominal aorta is no longer seen beyond the origins of the low-resistance branches to the liver, spleen, intestine, and kidneys. In the distal abdominal aorta, flow reverses during diastole. Figure 53-20 shows curves of some arteries and veins pertinent to this discussion.[53]

The **systemic veins of the abdomen** (IVC and hepatic and renal veins) show a pulsatile flow pattern that reflects cardiac contractions; two flow peaks toward the heart occur during atrial and ventricular diastole (filling). A short spurt of reversed flow occurs in the hepatic veins and proximal IVC. This reversed flow accompanies atrial systole (P wave of electrocardiogram). In addition, the phase of respiration will influence the flow pattern of the systemic intra-abdominal veins (with increasing velocity in expiration). Consequently, the Doppler sonographic characteristics of these veins are variable in the breathing child.

Flow in splanchnic veins is more steady, with only gentle undulations that mirror cardiac motion[53] (Fig. 53-20). Blood is constantly directed toward the portal vein and into the liver. Flow velocity in the portal vein increases greatly after a meal and decreases with exercise.[54,55] **Hepatofugal** portal venous flow (away from liver) can be reversed to **hepatopetal** (into liver) flow after a meal.[55]

Possibilities and Pitfalls

An excellent complement to splanchnic angiography and MRI, Doppler sonography answers the queries from an injection contrast examination with or without pharmaceutical manipulation. Doubts may remain about direction of flow or whether a vessel is obstructed or simply inaccessible to the contrast medium, such as reversed flow in the portal vein. The Doppler examination is a reliable indicator of direction of flow and assesses the splanchnic system in its physiologic state.

The hepatic veins, difficult to outline with angiography, are easily identified with sonography and their flow pattern outlined. The major splanchnic vessels, such as the splenic, mesenteric, and portal veins, are readily opacified with arterioportography, but small vessels are difficult to explore. This is particularly true of the branches of the **left portal vein,** which often are not opacified. The intrahepatic portal circulation can be readily studied with Doppler sonography, both in health and in disease. Each segmental branch of the portal vein is usually accessible to the Doppler beam. Regional flow patterns and the result of compression, obstruction of flow, reversal of flow, or AV fistulas can be assessed. With angiography and MRI, to-and-fro flow in a splanchnic vein is difficult to perceive. The Doppler examination yields clear signals of to-fro flow motions both on spectral display signal above, then below reference line) and with color (alternating red and blue signals). If questions remain about examination details or changes in the patient's condition, the Doppler examination can be repeated without risk.

These advantages are counterbalanced by certain limitations, most of which are identical to those of real-time sonography. The examination is operator dependent and requires some training not only in sonography but also in the physics of Doppler and in the normal anatomy and physiology of the liver and splanchnic circulation. Doppler sonography is subject to the same physical laws as is real-time ultrasound. One cannot expect a good

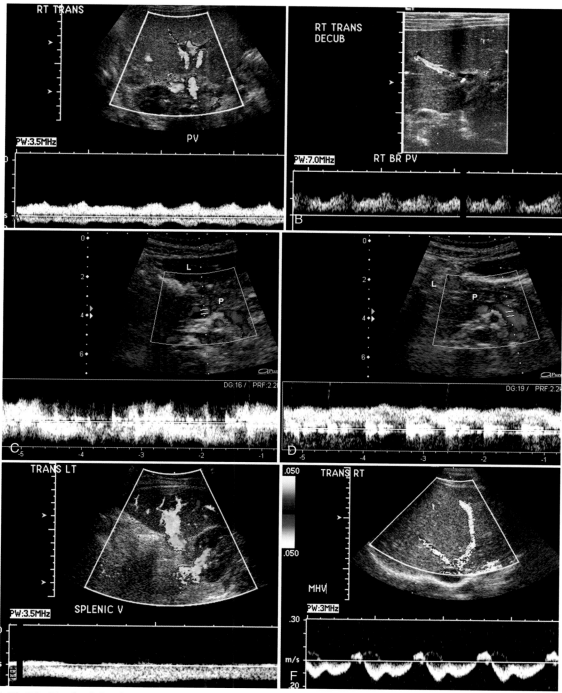

FIGURE 53-20. Typical duplex Doppler images of splanchnic vessels of various patients. A, Normal portal vein examined through a transverse, paramedian, subcostal approach. Flow fluctuates slightly with cardiac systole. Note aliasing artifact from low pulse repetition frequency. **B,** Normal right branch of portal vein seen from an oblique right subcostal approach. **C,** Normal splenic vein. Doppler sample volume is in vein near splenomesenteric confluence and in its middle third; *P,* pancreas; *L,* liver. **D,** Normal splenic vein with cardiac-related modulation of flow. **E,** Normal splenic vein at hilum, seen from a left intercostal approach. Note the lack of transmitted pulsations from the heart in the splenic vein. Normal left renal artery and vein are also seen. **F,** Normal hepatic vein, transverse subcostal view, with flow away from transducer and modulated by pulsations of nearby right atrium.

Doppler examination in a patient who just had a poor real-time sonogram. The child's cirrhotic liver may be enlarged with increased sound attenuation. Penetrating all this tissue with a real-time or Doppler beam can be a challenge to the sonographer and instrumentation.

Quantitative analysis of splanchnic blood flow with Doppler instrumentation could allow more intensive study of physiologic flow as well as portal hypertension and response to various drugs. However, because the technique depends on exact vessel beam angle and vessel diameter measurements, it is currently fraught with inaccuracies.[50,56]

In the present state of the art, despite the limitations just cited, the Doppler examination of the splanchnic circulation is valuable. If a noninvasive test can determine whether the patient has portal hypertension, the location of the level of obstruction to blood flow, and whether esophageal varices exist, it is indeed a useful clinical tool. For this reason, the Doppler examination has become the screening method of choice for children with liver disease and potential portal hypertension.

Sonographic Technique

Children older than 5 years are usually examined after a 4- to 6-hour fast. Normally, their cooperation can be obtained if the procedure is explained to them. Sedation is seldom necessary. Whenever possible, respiration is stopped during the Doppler examination of a vessel so as to minimize its movement. The usual Doppler frequency is 3.0 or 5.0 MHz, even though the appropriate real-time frequency for the examination may vary from 3.0 to 7.5 MHz. Because a small or upset child tends to breathe rapidly, the examiner must be familiar with the Doppler equipment to manipulate it quickly. All technical settings should be preadjusted. The vessel to be examined is identified with real-time sonography. Color Doppler ultrasound can be used to guide the placement of the sample volume. A spectral display of the Doppler shift is then usually readily obtained, even though it may disappear during part of the respiratory cycle.

Child with Liver Disease: Doppler Examination for Portal Hypertension

The aim of the Doppler examination is to assess the presence and direction of flow in splanchnic veins, the main portal vein and its segmental intrahepatic branches, the hepatic veins, and the IVC[57-60] (Fig. 53-21). In addition, the presence of flow in the main hepatic artery and its intrahepatic branches should be determined. When the clinical or basic Doppler examination raises the suspicion of **portal hypertension,** a systematic search for portosystemic collateral veins follows. Figure 53-22 outlines the usual sites for spontaneous portosystemic shunts.[59,61] The lesser omentum[62] (from splanchnomesen-

teric junction to esophagus) and the renal, splenic, and hepatic hila as well as the pelvis are screened for the presence of dilated, tortuous veins. If hepatofugal (reversed) flow is found in a splanchnic vein, this vein is traced to the recipient systemic vessel. In cases of portal hypertension, the **left gastric vein** drains blood into the inferior esophageal vein; the **splenic vein** drains into the renal (or pararenal) veins; the **superior and inferior mesenteric veins** drain into gonadal, retroperitoneal, or hemorrhoidal veins; and the **paraumbilical veins** follow the round and falciform ligaments to drain into the anterior abdominal and iliac veins to form the classic **caput medusae** or into veins of the anterior chest wall and the internal mammary vein.

Direction of flow in one or several veins of the portal venous system may change in portal hypertension, and it is essential to record the flow direction accurately. The clinician must carefully check that the orientation of the spectral or color Doppler sonographic display is normal and not inverted before starting the examination. The Doppler sample volume should be placed in the center of the vessel lumen. If the direction of flow within a vessel is difficult to ascertain, a nearby vessel with known flow direction can be used as a reference (e.g., splenic or hepatic artery or adjacent vein).

The **main portal vein** and its right hepatic branches are best studied through a right intercostal approach. Sometimes the superior mesenteric vein is also clearly seen from this position. The **left portal vein** and three of its four branches (portal branch to caudate lobe is rarely seen) and the **hepatic veins** are best seen through an oblique subcostal approach. The **splenic vein** is explored through a transverse approach over the spleen. The **superior mesenteric vein** and **main portal vein** are best visualized through a sagittal right paramedian approach (see Fig. 53-20). The **left gastric vein** usually ends near the splenoportal junction and, when enlarged, is easily observed through a sagittal left paramedian view. The **inferior mesenteric vein,** when normal, can rarely be outlined. When enlarged, it may be traced through a left lateral approach to its junction with the splenic or superior mesenteric vein.

The various possible origins of the **hepatic artery** may be difficult to recognize. We first look for the artery at its usual origin from the celiac axis and also as it passes between the portal vein and the common bile duct. When the left hepatic artery arises from the superior mesenteric artery, it passes through the ligamentum venosum. The intrahepatic arterial branches accompany branches of the portal vein and can be detected with a slightly enlarged Doppler sample volume placed over a portal venous branch, even when the arterial branch cannot be seen with real-time ultrasound. Flow in the arteries to the right lobe of the liver (especially segments 5, 7, and 8) is usually easy to identify in this manner. The hepatic arterial branch accompanying the umbilical portion of the left portal vein (to segment 4) is especially

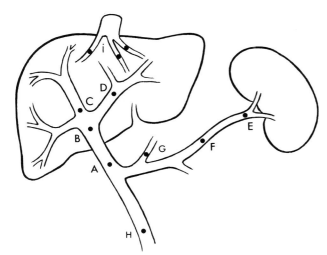

FIGURE 53-21. Essential splanchnic vein reference points in Doppler sampling for possible portal hypertension in children with liver disease. *A,* Main portal vein; *B,* intrahepatic portal vein; *C,* right portal vein; *D,* left portal vein; *E,* splenic vein at hilum; *F,* splenic vein; *G,* left coronary vein; *H,* superior mesenteric vein; *I,* hepatic veins. Evaluation of the hepatic artery and inferior vena cava should be done as well. *(From Patriquin HB, Lafortune M, Burns PH, et al. Duplex Doppler examination in portal hypertension: technique and anatomy. AJR Am J Roentgenol 1987;149:71-76.)*

easy to examine with Doppler imaging because of the almost ideal vessel beam angle, which can be obtained through an anterior abdominal approach (Fig. 53-23). For this reason, we routinely look for arterial Doppler signals at this site in children who have undergone liver transplantation (see Fig. 53-2).

Abnormal Flow Patterns within Portal System

Absent Doppler Signal

Proof of absence of a Doppler signal is much more difficult to establish than is its presence. The examiner who fails to obtain a Doppler signal from a given vessel usually questions the sensitivity of the machine and tests other nearby vessels. Failure to obtain a pulsed, color, or power Doppler signal from a splanchnic vein examined at an angle of less than 60 degrees, full Doppler gain, and low pulse repetition frequency, with 50-Hz wall filter and restricted Doppler window, means that blood is flowing at a velocity of less than 4 cm/sec (extremely slow). Thus, absence of a Doppler signal in this situation generally means absence of flow or a prethrombotic state.

Arterialized Flow Patterns

The normal, gently undulating flow within a portal vein is replaced by systolic peaks and high diastolic Doppler shifts. The arterialized flow pattern may signal the presence of an arterioportal fistula.[63]

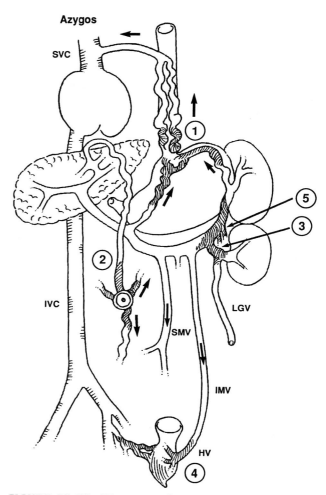

FIGURE 53-22. Diagram of common spontaneous portosystemic collateral routes. *SVC,* Superior vena cava; *IVC,* inferior vena cava; *SMV, IMV,* superior, inferior mesenteric veins; *LGV,* left gonadal vein; *HV,* hemorrhoidal vein; *1,* left gastric-azygos route (esophageal varices); *2,* paraumbilical-hypogastric/internal mammary route (caput medusa); *3,* splenorenal route; *4,* IMV-hemorrhoidal route; *5,* spleno-retroperitoneal-gonadal route. *(From Patriquin HB, Lafortune M. Syllabus in pediatric radiology. 1994, Society for Pediatric Radiology.)*

CAUSES OF ABSENT DOPPLER SIGNAL

Doppler angle greater than 60 degrees
Low Doppler gain
Low pulse repetition frequency
High filter (best is 50 Hz)
Small sample volume
Portal vein flow decreases when fasting.
Hepatic artery flow decreases after a meal.

Reversed or To-and-Fro Flow

Reversed flow in a splanchnic or intrahepatic portal vein is the most reliable Doppler sign of portal hypertension. However, hepatofugal flow in the portal vein occurs late and relatively rarely in patients with liver disease.

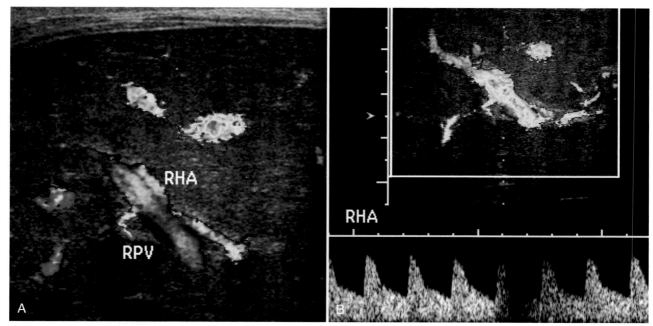

FIGURE 53-23. Normal liver and right hepatic artery (RHA) in an infant. Oblique subcostal color Doppler sonograms. **A,** Right portal vein *(RPV).* **B,** Cursor in RHA shows normal arterial flow waveform. Doppler shifts from normal hepatic artery and portal vein have identical directions of flow.

To-and-fro flow in the portal vein also suggests the presence of portal hypertension. Highly pulsatile or to-fro flow in the portal vein may also be seen in right-sided heart failure (Fig. 53-24) or tricuspid insufficiency, resulting from transmitted pressure across the hepatic sinusoids.

Abnormal Hepatic Arterial Doppler Patterns

Absence of a hepatic artery Doppler signal suggests arterial thrombosis or reduced flow in prethrombotic states.[63] Locally increased systolic Doppler shifts or peripheral tardus-parvus curves may be the result of stenosis of the hepatic artery, as at any other arterial site.

The portal vein and hepatic artery act in concert to nourish the liver. Changes in flow volumes in one affect the other. After a meal, portal venous flow increases and hepatic arterial flow diminishes, probably by vasoconstriction. Postprandially, hepatic arterial diastolic flow is decreased and systolic peaks are lower when measured at the same sites in the same person.[64] Arterial signals within the liver may be difficult to find after a meal. This is particularly disturbing in the patient who has received a liver transplant, in whom a false diagnosis of thrombosis may be considered.

Portal Venous Hypertension

Portal venous hypertension is a pathologic condition characterized by increased pressure in the portal vein or one of its tributaries. The normal pressure in the portal vein is between 5 and 10 mm Hg. When the pressure in the portal vein is more than 5 mm Hg above IVC pressure, portal hypertension is present.

The many sequelae of portal hypertension include splenomegaly, collateral vein formation, and a thickened lesser omentum. In children the lesser omentum is observed between the left lobe of the liver and the aorta on sagittal images. Lesser omentum thickness should not exceed the diameter of the aorta[64,65] (Fig. 53-25). In portal hypertension it is thickened by lymphatic stasis and an engorged left gastric vein. Morphologic changes of the liver architecture are usually present as well.

An increased caliber of the portal vein and a lack of variation in the caliber of the splenic and mesenteric veins have been described in portal hypertension in adults. The accuracy of these findings in the assessment of portal hypertension in children has not been established. Anecdotally, in children with biliary cirrhosis, portal venous caliber has decreased as cirrhosis progressed.

The hemodynamic information gleaned from the Doppler examination usually answers the following questions: Is portal hypertension present? What is the level of obstruction? What is the direction of flow within the system? Are there portosystemic collaterals?

Hepatofugal flow in a portosystemic collateral vein establishes the diagnosis of portal hypertension. Clinically, the most significant route is through the left gastric vein, which supplies esophageal varices. The **left gastric vein** is rarely visible sonographically in the normal child. When it dilates to a diameter of greater than 2 to 3 mm,

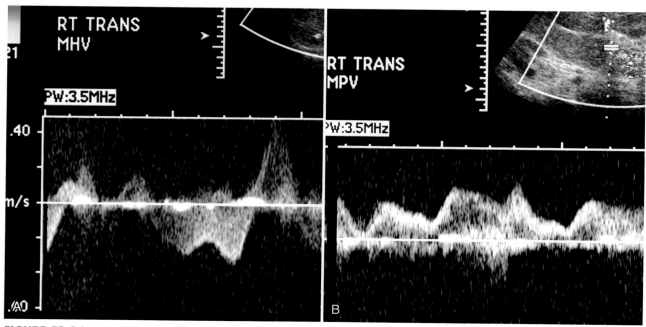

FIGURE 53-24. A, Highly pulsatile hepatic venous flow, and **B,** portal venous flow, in a child with congenital heart disease after Fontan procedure. Right atrial pressure is transmitted through the hepatic veins, across the hepatic sinusoids to the portal vein. Compare with the gently undulating flow in Figure 53-20, *F.*

it can be traced from the splenic vein near the spleno-mesenteric junction through the lesser omentum (behind left lobe of liver and anterior to aorta) to the esophagus (see Figs. 53-20, *E,* and 53-25). A venous Doppler flow pattern makes it possible to distinguish the vein from the nearby left gastric or hepatic arteries. Flow direction is determined at the same time. The caliber of the left gastric vein is usually related to the size of esophageal varices and probably to the likelihood of bleeding.[66]

The **paraumbilical vein** classically shunts blood from the left portal vein to the periumbilical venous network. It follows a vertical, right paramedian course to enter the falciform ligament through the left lobe of the liver[67,68] (Fig. 53-26). With a high-frequency transducer (7.5-10 MHz), its subcutaneous course is easily seen on sonography from the lower tip of the left lobe of the liver to the umbilicus. Other spontaneous portosystemic collateral veins should be sought near the spleen, left kidney, and flanks, where splenorenal shunts (Fig. 53-27) or dilated perirenal, retroperitoneal, or gonadal veins receive blood from the splenic or mesenteric veins; in the pelvis (Fig. 53-28), around the right kidney; and near the porta hepatis and gallbladder (Figs. 53-29 and 53-30), where portocaval, paraduodenorenal, or veins of Sappey may shunt the blood between portal and hepatic veins. The variety of spontaneous portosystemic collaterals is almost limitless.

All portosystemic collaterals should be traced to their recipient systemic vein, which is usually dilated where the shunt enters. The "donor" splanchnic vein is also dilated. When portal hypertension decreases after shunt surgery or transplantation, portosystemic collaterals decrease in size (as do the enlarged spleen and lesser omentum).

If a spontaneous or surgical portosystemic shunt is large, hepatic encephalopathy may ensue. The Doppler examination, being "physiologic," may reveal unusual portosystemic collateral routes difficult to demonstrate with arterioportographic studies (locally inverted flow in intrahepatic portal venous branches, "neo" veins leading from portal veins to abdominal wall, or hepatofugal flow in splenic vein).

Prehepatic Portal Hypertension

Prehepatic portal hypertension results from obstruction of the splenic, mesenteric, or portal vein. As with other venous thromboses, predisposing factors involve the vessel wall (trauma, catheters), stagnant blood flow, and abnormal clotting factors. Principal causes of **thrombosis of the portal vein** include (1) trauma such as umbilical venous catheterization; (2) dehydration or shock; (3) pyophlebitis following appendicitis or abdominal sepsis; (4) coagulopathy, with protein C deficiency increasingly recognized; (5) portal vein invasion by adjacent tumors; (6) compression of the vein by pancreatitis, lymph nodes, or tumor; and (7) increased resistance to portal venous flow into the liver in cirrhosis or the Budd-Chiari syndrome.

Recanalization of portal venous thrombi usually occurs rapidly in children. In addition, paraportal venous channels and the cystic veins draining the gallbladder

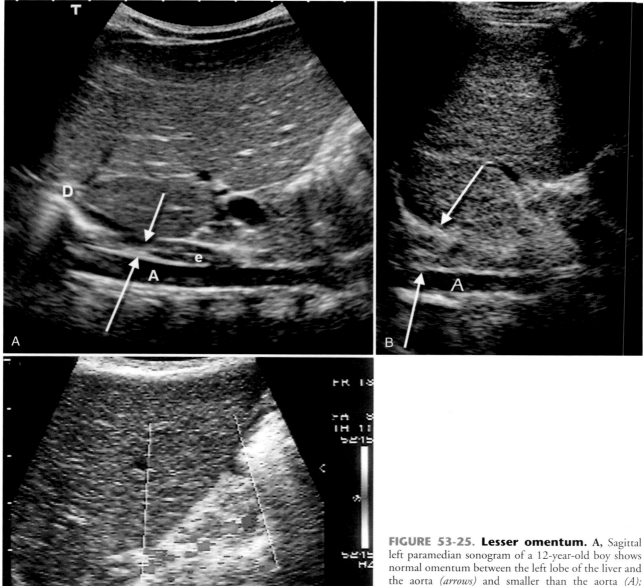

FIGURE 53-25. Lesser omentum. A, Sagittal left paramedian sonogram of a 12-year-old boy shows normal omentum between the left lobe of the liver and the aorta *(arrows)* and smaller than the aorta *(A); e,* esophagus; *D,* diaphragm. **B,** Thickened lesser omentum *(arrows)* by a tortuous, dilated left gastric vein in cirrhosis. **C,** Abnormal left gastric vein. Color Doppler image shows flow signals toward the esophagus *(blue).*

CAUSES OF PORTAL VEIN THROMBOSIS

Trauma
Catheters
Dehydration
Shock
Pyelophlebitis
Coagulopathy, especially protein C deficiency
Portal vein invasion
Portal vein compression
Cirrhosis
Budd-Chiari syndrome

dilate and channel blood into the liver if there is no obstruction at this site (in cirrhosis or hepatic vein thrombosis). The resultant collection of tortuous veins is called a **cavernoma** (see Fig. 53-29). Hepatopetal flow in these vessels is easily detected with Doppler sonography. Despite these collateral channels, portal hypertension follows, often with esophageal varices.[69]

After thrombosis of the portal vein, the peripheral intrahepatic portal veins become small and threadlike. The lumen may not be visible. Careful examination of these vessels with Doppler sonography usually shows hepatopetal venous flow, likely the result of shunting through the vessels at the porta hepatis, which constitute

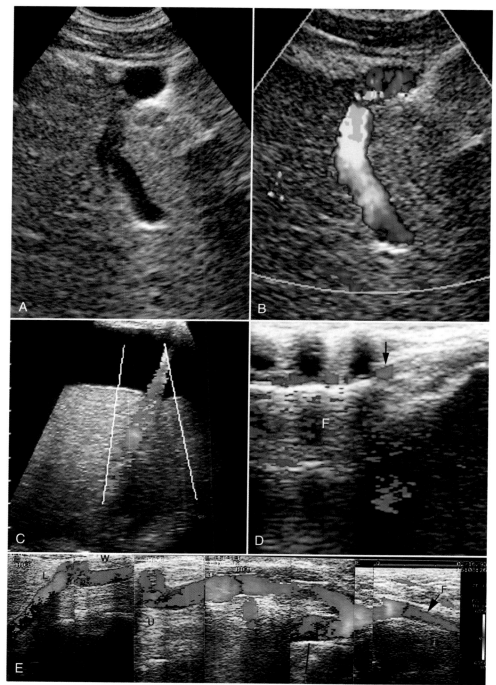

FIGURE 53-26. Paraumbilical collateral route. A and **B,** Transverse paramedian gray-scale and color Doppler sonograms show left lobe of liver in a 14-year-old boy with cirrhosis and portal hypertension from cystic fibrosis (CF). **Recanalized umbilical vein,** with venous flow signals directed toward the transducer, anteriorly out of the liver. **C** thru **E,** Sagittal color Doppler images of a 10-year-old boy with cystic fibrosis and ascites. Blood flow leaves the liver through a patent paraumbilical vein that enters the falciform ligament, which is surrounded by fluid. **D,** Cirrhosis and portal hypertension. In the parasternal region of another child, color Doppler images show cephalad pulsatile flow in the internal mammary veins, originating from a paraumbilical vein *(arrow).* Flash color artifacts *(F)* are from the moving lungs. **E,** Composite sagittal sonogram (7.5-MHz transducer) of the abdominal wall *(W)* shows the paraumbilical vein leaving the liver *(L),* surrounding the umbilicus *(U),* and entering the iliac vein *(I). (From Taylor KJW, Burns PH, Wells PNT, editors.* Clinical applications of Doppler ultrasound. *Philadelphia, 1996, Lippincott-Raven; and Patriquin HB.* Pediatric diseases test and syllabus. *Vol 35. Reston, Va, 1993, American College of Radiology.)*

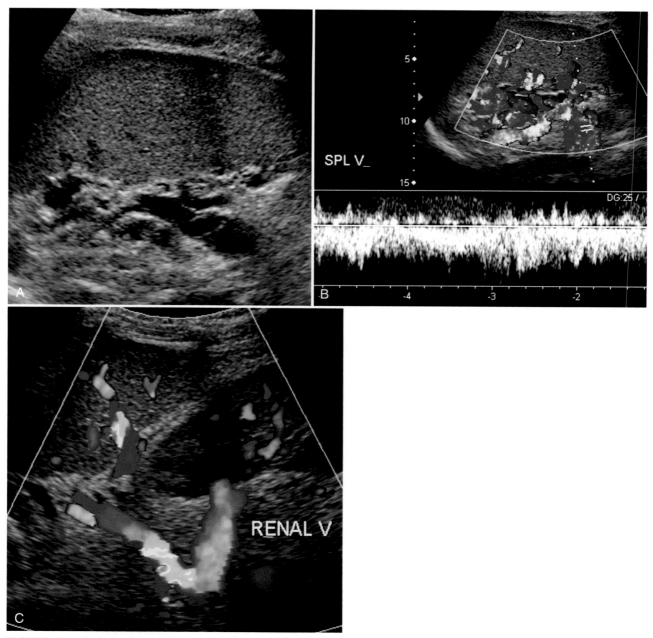

FIGURE 53-27. Splenic varices and splenorenal shunt. A, Splenic varices in a patient with cirrhosis shown on longitudinal gray-scale image of the left upper quadrant. **B,** Color and pulsed Doppler sonogram shows tortuous veins leaving the spleen, with largest vessel (*blue* with Doppler gate) demonstrating venous flow toward the left kidney. **C,** Color Doppler image of this spontaneous splenorenal shunt shows flow away from the spleen toward the kidney.

the "cavernoma." Because the obstruction to venous flow occurs at the porta hepatis, it is not surprising that children with portal venous thrombosis do not have enlarged paraumbilical veins and a caput medusa; this portosystemic route relies on abundant flow in the left portal vein.[69]

Another cause of prehepatic (or intrahepatic "presinusoidal") portal hypertension in children is **congenital hepatic fibrosis.** This inherited, autosomal recessive disease is characterized by fibrosis at the portal triad,

where terminal branches of the portal vein and small bile ducts are compressed. Hepatocytes are found to be normal, as is liver function.[10] Liver architecture is disturbed by linear or cystlike structures representing variable bile duct ectasia, as well as paraportal collaterals (cavernoma)[70,71] (Fig. 53-30). These children usually present with bleeding esophageal varices. Sonography shows hallmarks of portal hypertension: splenomegaly and a thick lesser omentum in which a dilated tortuous left gastric vein may be visible, with hepatofugal flow

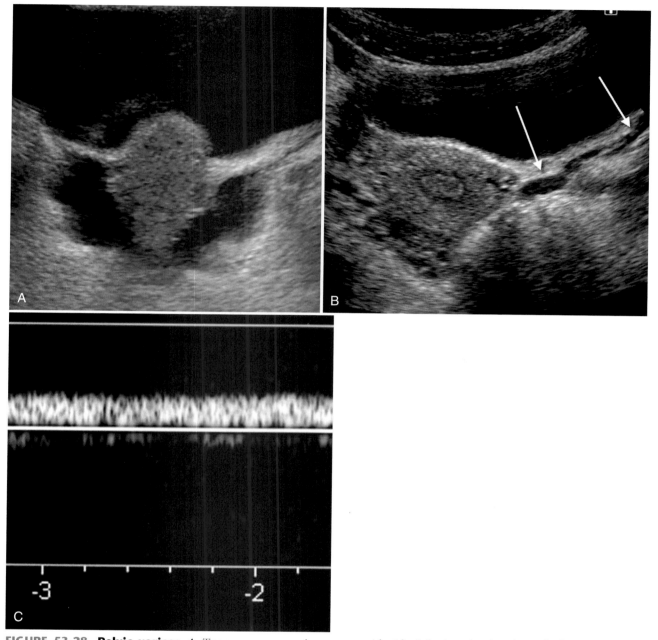

FIGURE 53-28. Pelvic varices. A, Transverse sonogram in a teenage girl with cirrhosis and ascites shows fluid surrounding the uterus and adnexal structures. **B,** In a different patient with cirrhosis and pelvic varices, a prominent vein *(arrows)* is seen in the left adnexal region on transverse view. **C,** Pulsed Doppler waveform of paraovarian varix shunting blood toward the renal veins or inferior vena cava.

detected with Doppler sonography (see Fig. 53-25). Congenital hepatic fibrosis is usually associated with **recessive polycystic kidney disease**[72] (Fig. 53-30). The dilation of renal collecting ducts in these children is variable and less severe than in the neonatal form, and renal impairment is less marked. However, renal architecture is greatly disturbed. The pyramids are hyperechogenic and may contain calcium; small cysts may be seen; and the kidneys are usually enlarged. These features enable informed sonographers to find the cause of upper intestinal bleeding in these children during their first abdominal sonogram.

Intrahepatic Portal Hypertension

Serious insult to the hepatocyte results in **necrosis.** Unless necrosis is overwhelming, scarring and the formation of multiple regenerating nodules follow. The process of **cirrhosis** results in scarred and obstructed sinusoids and abnormal portal venous blood flow through the regenerated nodules. In children, cirrhosis results from the following:

• Hepatitis
• Destruction of the hepatocyte by toxins accumulated in inherited metabolic diseases, such as tyrosinemia,

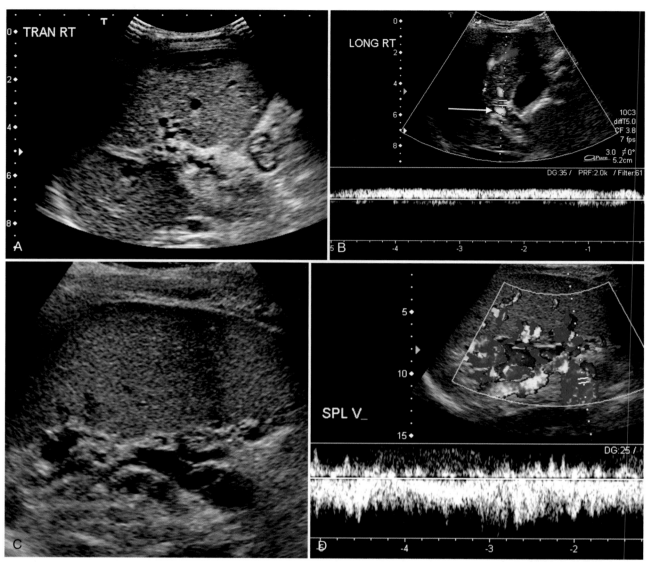

FIGURE 53-29. Cavernous transformation of portal vein in child after umbilical vein catheterization in infancy. A, Transverse sonogram of the liver shows several tortuous tubular veins, but no large main portal vein at the porta hepatis. **B,** Color and pulsed Doppler waveform within one of these veins shows slow hepatopetal flow. The **main hepatic artery** is large *(arrow)* just deep to the vein being interrogated, a typical finding in cavernous transformation of the portal vein. **C,** Despite the venous collaterals transporting blood into the liver around the thrombosed main portal vein, the child had **splenic varices** seen on longitudinal sonogram. **D,** Color and pulsed Doppler waveform of the splenic varices shows more brisk venous flow than that seen in the porta.

some forms of glycogen storage disease, and Wilson's disease
• Bile stasis, as in biliary atresia and cystic fibrosis
Although different types of cirrhosis cause initial obstruction at presinusoidal (schistosomiasis, biliary

CAUSES OF CIRRHOSIS IN CHILDREN

Hepatitis
Toxins accumulated in inherited metabolic diseases
Biliary atresia
Cystic fibrosis

cirrhosis), sinusoidal (Laennec's cirrhosis), and postsinusoidal levels, progressive scarring usually spreads to the entire sinusoid. As intrahepatic portal venous flow stagnates, portosystemic collaterals open. Portal blood flow decreases. Total hepatic blood supply is usually maintained by an increase of blood flow in the hepatic artery.

Sonographically, these changes in hemodynamics are signaled by decreasing diameter of the portal vein and its segmental branches, to the point they are reduced to threadlike structures. Flow velocity, when measurable, is reduced. Conversely, branches of the hepatic artery (normally difficult to see in children) may become visible with gray-scale sonography. Doppler sonography mirrors the increased hepatic arterial caliber and flow

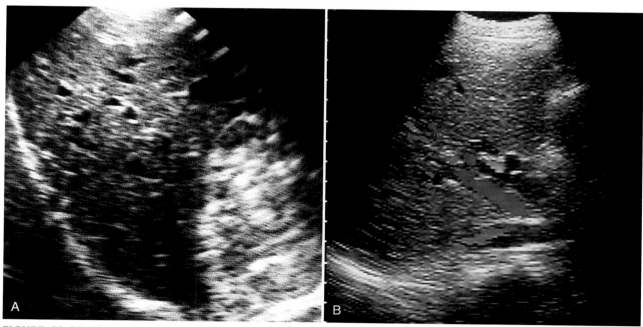

FIGURE 53-30. Congenital hepatic fibrosis causes portal vein and biliary obstruction: portal cavernoma and bile duct ectasia. A, Sagittal view shows multiple small cystic structures in the right lobe of the liver. The adjacent kidney is large and contains multiple hyperechoic foci throughout the cortex and medulla caused by recessive polycystic kidney disease. **B,** The liver hilum in a 12-year-old girl contains three tubular structures: two "portal veins" and a dilated bile duct (devoid of color flow signals). *(From Patriquin HB. Pediatric diseases test and syllabus. Vol 35. Reston, Va, 1993, American College of Radiology.)*

seen angiographically. Doppler shifts from segmental arteries are increased compared to their portal venous neighbors.

Two hemodynamic mechanisms appear to operate in patients with portal hypertension, especially in those with cirrhosis. The **backward-flow theory** explains portal hypertension by the increased resistance to portal venous flow caused by the intrahepatic block described earlier. In response to stagnating intrahepatic flow, portosystemic collaterals form and drain blood away from the liver, finally resulting in hepatofugal flow in some or all segmental branches and in the main portal vein, which is easily demonstrated with Doppler sonography. Why does the portal pressure remain elevated despite the presence of such a decompression mechanism? This question may be answered by the **forward-flow theory.** In the backward-flow theory, portal blood flow is unchanged or even diminished. The forward-flow theory proposes that splanchnic arterioles dilate in patients with cirrhosis. The resultant decreased splanchnic resistance leads to increased flow in the intestinal arteries and veins, with subsequently increased portal venous blood flow. This would explain why portal hypertension is maintained despite extensive portosystemic shunting.

Because the obstruction to portal blood flow in cirrhosis is within the liver, periportal and cystic venous collaterals rarely develop. However, blood is often shunted from the left portal vein through one or several tortuous **paraumbilical veins** to veins of the anterior

wall of the abdomen and thorax. Documenting hepatofugal flow in such a vein situated within the falciform ligament is an easy way to establish the diagnosis of portal hypertension in children. The superficial abdominal (thoracic) wall collaterals are readily traced with color Doppler sonography if a high-frequency transducer is used (see Fig. 53-26, *E*).

The **left gastric vein,** shunting blood from the liver to esophageal varices, although dilated, becomes increasingly difficult to detect sonographically in children with advanced cirrhosis. Atrophy of the left lobe of the liver abolishes the acoustic window through which the lesser omentum is normally explored.

All the other portosystemic shunts described in Figure 53-22 are possible in children with cirrhosis; thus the entire abdomen and pelvis should be explored with sonography. The principle of **shunting** is constant in all portosystemic collaterals; a dilated, often tortuous splanchnic vein with reversed (hepatofugal) flow shunts blood into a systemic vein that is equally dilated at the site of the shunt. Rapid venous blood flow produces high, steady Doppler shifts. Turbulence and bidirectional flow often occur at the shunt site. A diagram that summarizes the Doppler findings is extremely helpful in visualizing the entire shunt route as well as the intrahepatic circulation (see Fig. 53-22). A few patients with severe portal hypertension develop reversal of flow in the main portal vein, sometimes because of the proximity of a large shunt near the porta hepatis (see Fig. 53-28). *If* *one were to depend on reversed portal venous flow to make the diagnosis of portal hypertension, one would miss the diagnosis in the majority of such patients.[73]*

Suprahepatic (Posthepatic) Portal Hypertension

The clinical quartet of ascites, abdominal pain, jaundice, and hepatomegaly that follows obstruction of the hepatic veins is called the **Budd-Chiari syndrome** (Fig. 53-31). It is rare in children. Doppler sonography is particularly useful in excluding the diagnosis, because the four clinical signs that make up the syndrome are quite common in children with other forms of portal hypertension. The first patients with thrombosis of the hepatic veins described by Budd (1846), Fredrichs, Lange, and Chiari (1899) were thought to have hepatic phlebitis secondary to sepsis or syphilis, with primary involvement of small branches of the hepatic veins. Since then, other causes have been recognized, now classified as obstruction of the central and sublobular veins, the major hepatic veins, or the IVC near the hepatic vein ostia.[74] **Small-vessel hepatic venous occlusive disease** (VOD) is caused by toxins, especially pyrrolizidine alkaloids contained in ragwort or Jamaican bush tea; chemotherapy; bone marrow transplantation; lupus erythematosus; hepatic irradiation; and oral contraceptives. This VOD involves primarily small hepatic venous radicles, although the major branches may be secondarily involved.

Sonographic findings of VOD include splenomegaly, ascites, small-caliber hepatic veins, and flow in paraumbilical veins. The sonographic diagnosis of VOD remains difficult; clinical and laboratory criteria are better indicators of the severity of VOD and its response to medical therapy.[75] **Thrombosis of the main hepatic veins** is usually caused by coagulation abnormalities or congenital malformations of the hepatic vein ostia. Obstruction of the hepatic portion of the IVC may result in thrombosis of the hepatic veins. Congenital membranes of the IVC resulting from faulty embryologic fenestration of its lumen can also lead to obstruction of hepatic veins.[76,77] The most common position for such a membrane is below an obstructed left hepatic vein and above a patent right hepatic vein, probably a result of an obstructing fibrous remnant of the left umbilical vein and ductus venosus.

CAUSES OF HEPATIC VENOUS OCCLUSIVE DISEASE

Toxins
    Ragwort or Jamaican bush tea
Chemotherapy
Bone marrow transplantation
Lupus erythematosus
Hepatic irradiation
Oral contraceptives
Coagulation abnormalities
Congenital malformations of hepatic vein ostia
Obstruction of hepatic portion of inferior vena cava
Congenital membranes of inferior vena cava

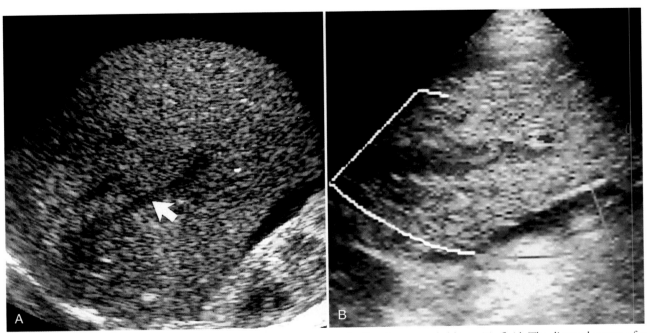

FIGURE 53-31. Budd-Chiari syndrome. A, Acute appearance: the liver is surrounded by ascitic fluid. The diagonal course of a hepatic vein is filled with echogenic clot *(arrow).* **B,** Several days later, color Doppler image shows almost complete absence of flow within the hepatic vein *(blue). (Courtesy M. Lafortune, MD, Montreal.)*

After any obstruction of the hepatic veins, the liver becomes enlarged and congested. Because the caudate lobe has its own hepatic vein that drains into the IVC below the others, it is often spared and serves as the only initial venous drainage route for the entire liver. The caudate lobe enlarges quickly and often compresses the IVC. This is followed by ascites, often pleural effusions, splenomegaly, and the formation of portosystemic collaterals. Doppler sonography shows absence or reversal of flow in the hepatic veins (Fig. 53-31). Areas of high-velocity flow near stenoses of hepatic veins are easily detected with color-guided, pulsed Doppler sonography. In the absence of hepatic venous drainage, arterial blood may be shunted into the portal vein through microscopic shunts at the portal triad or through larger intrahepatic shunts. Portal venous flow may reverse. Alternately, the portal vein may thrombose when liver congestion is severe. All these changes can be detected with Doppler sonography. **Wedge hepatic venography,** which shows a spider web network of intrahepatic veins instead of the usual hepatic venous lumens, is now rarely performed.

The patient with acute Budd-Chiari syndrome rarely has time to form portosystemic collateral routes. If present, shunt routes are similar to those seen in cirrhosis. (Periportal and cystic veins do not usually serve as shunt routes because they drain into the segmental branches of the right portal vein, which are highly congested in response to hepatic vein obstruction.) Extensive intrahepatic shunts may form and can be demonstrated with color Doppler sonography.

The treatment of hepatic vein occlusion is anticoagulant therapy, ablation of obstructive webs, or emergency portocaval shunting. The recanalization of hepatic veins, the regression of portal hypertension (decreased caliber and flow velocity in portosystemic shunts, smaller spleen, absorption of ascites), and the patency of therapeutic shunts can be assessed with Doppler sonography.

Surgical Portosystemic Shunts

Previously, definitive treatment of children with bleeding esophageal varices was surgical portosystemic shunts. These shunts are now created only when sclerotherapy of varices has failed or liver transplantation is not feasible. Children with healthy livers and prehepatic portal hypertension are still candidates for shunt procedures. **Transjugular intrahepatic portosystemic shunts** (TIPS) are being performed as an alternate to classic surgical shunts in adults, with increasing use in children. The patency of transjugular shunts is being monitored with Doppler sonography, which shows blood flowing from the "donor" right portal vein through the intrahepatic stent and into the right (or another) hepatic vein. Shunt stenoses, thrombosis, and flow around the stent are readily visible with Doppler sonography.

Surgical portosystemic shunts can be total or partial. **Total shunts** direct the entire venous blood flow from the congested splanchnic system into a systemic vein, as in the end-to-side portocaval shunt, in which the main portal vein is redirected. The hepatic end is ligated and the splanchnic end is connected to the IVC. In this situation, portal venous perfusion of the liver is minimal. **Partial shunts** divert only some of the splanchnic blood into a systemic vein, thereby yielding better liver perfusion and reducing the incidence of hepatic encephalopathy. The distal splenorenal (Warren) shunt connects the splenic vein to the left renal vein. The side-to-side, H-type, portocaval shunt connects the portal vein to the IVC at the porta hepatis. The REX shunt connects the left portal vein to the IVC using a donor vein. Many variants of these surgical procedures exist.

Doppler study of the intrahepatic portal veins is invaluable in the assessment of **portocaval shunt patency.** In the majority of patent shunts, flow in the intrahepatic portal veins is hepatofugal.[78] It is easy to understand why this should be so in side-to-side portocaval shunts, where high-pressure intrahepatic venous blood flows through the shunt into the low-pressure vena cava. It is more difficult to explain hepatofugal flow in the intrahepatic portal veins in patients with an end-to-side portocaval shunt, in whom the hepatic end of the portal vein has been ligated and cut. Blood may leave the liver through a system of collateral veins between intrahepatic branches of the portal vein and low-pressure systemic veins. This phenomenon has been demonstrated on angiography.[79]

Signs of shunt obstruction include the following:
- The shunt site is difficult or impossible to detect, and no Doppler signals can be obtained.
- Blood in the splanchnic vein feeding the shunt no longer flows toward the shunt.
- The direction of intrahepatic portal venous flow returns to normal.
- Spontaneous portosystemic shunts and other signs of portal hypertension reappear.

DOPPLER SONOGRAPHY IN CHILDREN RECEIVING LIVER TRANSPLANT

Pretransplantation Evaluation

Before liver transplantation can be considered, the caliber and patency of the main portal vein and IVC must be assessed. This is usually done with Doppler sonography and supplemented with MRI.[80,81] If the portal vein diameter is less than 4 mm (as in advanced cirrhosis) or if Doppler flow studies are equivocal, MRI or angiography may be performed. Children with biliary atresia may have an associated **polysplenia syndrome** (see Fig. 53-8, C-G), which includes intestinal malrotation, bilaterally symmetrical patterns of the major bronchi, abnormal location of the portal vein anterior to the duodenum, and interruption of the IVC.[13,80] Liver transplantation may be more difficult in these children. It is essential that the surgeon be aware of this anatomic abnormality before transplantation.

In addition, portocaval or mesenteric-caval shunts, whether created surgically or occurring naturally, change both the flow pattern and the caliber of the main portal vein and may alter the surgical approach to transplantation. The anatomic variants of the hepatic artery are not always demonstrated on sonography, but angiography is rarely performed for the purpose of outlining the anatomy of the hepatic artery. The examination of the child before transplantation should also include several organs: the kidneys, lungs, heart, and intestinal tract.[80]

During liver transplantation in the child, the donor hepatic artery is sometimes removed with a cuff of aorta and anastomosed to the recipient's abdominal aorta or iliac artery. An adult liver is usually divided before being transplanted into a small child. Although the left lobe (segments 2 and 3) is preferred, an adult liver may be divided and used for two recipients. A **transient fluid collection** often forms around the cut surface of the transplanted lobe or segments, even though the cut is packed with hemostatic material such as Gelfoam or fibrin glue. Because the anatomy involved in segmental or lobar liver transplantation differs considerably from the normal anatomy and from the anatomy involved in whole-organ transplantation, a diagram of the procedure is a useful guide for the sonographer assessing patency of anastomosed vessels.

Posttransplantation Evaluation

The most common complication in the immediate postoperative period is **hepatic artery stenosis** and thrombosis. Although collateral vessels may form in the child and shunt arterial blood into the liver, bile duct injury frequently occurs, followed by the formation of bile lakes and recurrent infection. Retransplantation is almost invariably necessary.

Immediate Doppler examination either in the surgical suite or at the child's bedside soon after surgery and then daily for 5 to 7 days is typically performed to confirm patency of the anastomosed vessels, before clinical or biochemical liver examinations become abnormal. The hepatic arterial anastomosis can be difficult to see adjacent to the Roux loop, so it is important to examine the intrahepatic arterial branches adjacent to intrahepatic portal veins, with both gray-scale and Doppler techniques. Optimal sites for the detection of hepatic arterial Doppler signals in whole-liver transplants are adjacent to the umbilical branch of the left portal vein and adjacent to the branch to segments 3 and 4, and alongside the right portal vein and the branches to segments 6 and 7 (see Fig. 53-23). The presence of arterial signals at these sites usually establishes patency of the hepatic artery. In segmental liver transplants, the "porta hepatis" is located eccentrically along the right lateral costal margin.[82] Given the variability of graft size and orientation in the right upper quadrant, the sonographer must find optimal imaging windows by trial and error. In the immediate postoperative period, hepatic arterial flow (both systolic and diastolic) is generally brisk. However, in the next 2 to 3 days, graft edema may result in transiently decreased diastolic flow. As long as systolic upstroke remains sharp and there are other signs of graft swelling (i.e., periportal edema), patients are watched expectantly. If the patient's liver enzyme levels rise, further Doppler evaluation or surgical reexploration is generally performed.

Children with clinically undetected, chronic obstruction of the main hepatic artery have been reported in whom dampened intrahepatic arterial flow was detected with Doppler sonography. Angiography in these patients shows obstruction of the hepatic artery and liver perfusion through extensive arterial collaterals around the site of a portoenterostomy at the porta hepatis.

In patients well enough to eat or receive gastric tube feedings, remember that hepatic arterial Doppler shifts are difficult to detect after a meal.[64] A repeat examination after a fast may show much stronger signals. Failure to detect intrahepatic arterial Doppler shifts indicates thrombosis or a prethrombotic state. Given the risk of graft injury, arteriography is generally performed in this situation, with the intent to treat with thrombolytics or angioplasty.

Although hepatic artery interrogation is the most important part of the posttransplant examination, the Doppler study is also helpful in assessing the patency of the venous anastomoses—the portal and hepatic veins and the IVC. The sites of venous anastomosis are clearly visible with gray-scale sonography and should be demonstrated (Fig. 53-32). **Portal venous thrombosis** at the anastomosis may occur but is less frequent than arterial occlusion. Turbulence may be expected at the anastomotic site of the portal vein (Fig. 53-33). **Stenosis** or compression of the portal vein is accompanied by locally increased Doppler shifts. Portal hypertension may follow. Poststenotic dilation of the portal vein may occur without serious sequelae. In some patients with a small portal vein from a segmental transplant, prolonged fasting may increase hepatic arterial flow and make visualization of the portal vein difficult. A limited follow-up scan, after feeding the patient, can vastly improve visualization of portal venous flow.

Inferior vena cava thrombosis is usually asymptomatic in the child because collateral flow through the paravertebral venous system is quickly established. The sonographic diagnosis of an IVC thrombus in a child with lobar transplantation can be difficult. The IVC lumen is obliterated by thrombus, and the vessel becomes very difficult to find (Fig. 53-34, *A* and *B*). However,

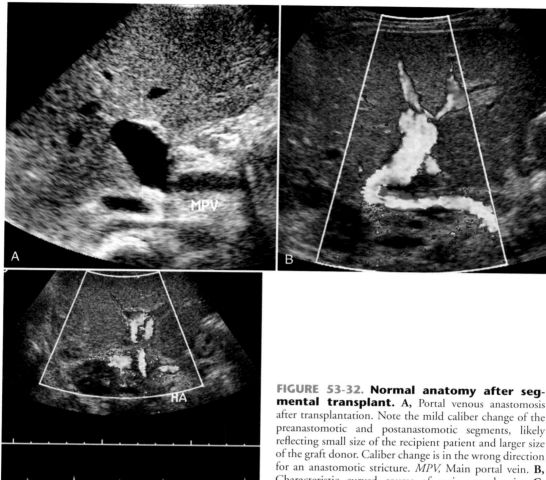

FIGURE 53-32. Normal anatomy after segmental transplant. A, Portal venous anastomosis after transplantation. Note the mild caliber change of the preanastomotic and postanastomotic segments, likely reflecting small size of the recipient patient and larger size of the graft donor. Caliber change is in the wrong direction for an anastomotic stricture. *MPV,* Main portal vein. **B,** Characteristic curved course of main portal vein. **C,** Normal pulsed Doppler tracing of hepatic artery *(HA).* Note the sharp systolic upstroke and good forward flow throughout diastole.

even a patent IVC can be difficult to find because anatomic relationships are greatly altered in these children. At Doppler sonography, flow in a hemiazygos vein is easily mistaken for flow in the IVC. The IVC is frequently compressed by a large donor graft, so careful examination of the draining hepatic veins is important in these patients.

During segmental transplantation, the recipient's IVC is left intact and the hepatic vein(s) directly anastomosed to the IVC or right atrium. Both the hepatic veins and the IVC may thrombose, starting at the anastomosis. The immediate postoperative examination outlines the surgical anatomy in these children and serves as a useful standard for comparison in assessing the continued patency of the anastomosed vessels. Stumps of oversewn graft IVC are also frequently encountered, lying between the liver parenchyma and native IVC. Thrombus in the remnant of donor IVC seldom propagates but can be seen as intraluminal echoes perioperatively. With time, these donor IVC remnants become less visible,

collapsing and blending into the medium-level echoes of the retroperitoneum.

Graft rejection does not result in predictable flow alterations of the hepatic artery, unlike the increased intrarenal resistance to flow noted in acute renal allograft rejection. However, changes in the normal phasicity of hepatic venous blood flow have been linked to graft rejection. Specifically, when normal triphasic hepatic venous blood flow becomes monophasic, biopsy specimens show evidence of acute rejection (sensitivity 92%, specificity 48%) or other hepatic disease (cholangitis, fibrosis, centrilobular congestion/necrosis, lymphoproliferative disease, cholestasis, hepatitis).[83] Some liver transplant recipients never demonstrate triphasic flow, presumably because of poor elasticity in the donor graft, and thus these criteria are not useful.

Biliary air or **pneumobilia** is another common finding in patients after liver transplant (Fig. 53-34, *I*). Anecdotally, it is less frequent in the immediate postoperative period (despite routine stenting of the duct) and

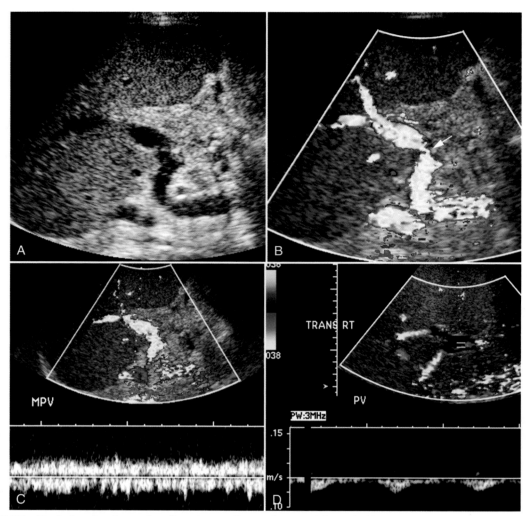

FIGURE 53-33. Portal vein stenosis after transplantation. A, Subcostal oblique sonogram, and **B,** color Doppler image, show a narrowed segment of the portal vein at the anastomotic site *(arrow).* **C,** Pulsed Doppler tracing just beyond the site of stenosis shows turbulent, high-velocity, bidirectional flow; *MPV,* main portal vein. **D,** Color and pulsed Doppler images in a different transplant patient show impending thrombosis of the portal vein *(PV),* with absent color signal and minimal flow on low scale settings.

is more likely to be noted on routine follow-up scans several months later. The source of air is retrograde passage from the gastrointestinal tract, through the Roux loop and choledochoenterostomy and into the bile ducts. Careful examination of the liver parenchyma on routine follow-up sonography is important to exclude biliary tree abnormalities, abscess, focal areas of ischemia, and complications of percutaneous biopsy (e.g., bile lake, AV shunts, hemorrhage). Biliary ductal dilation may be caused by stenosis of the choledochoenterostomy, bile duct ischemia with secondary stricture, stone disease, and compression of ducts by external masses, fluid collections, or adenopathy. Perioperative **fluid collections** are common and typically resolve in weeks to months. Persistent collections may represent lymphocele or persistent bile leak. New collections are most often related to infection, iatrogenic injury, trauma, or graft failure.

Long-term survival of pediatric liver transplant patients continues to improve, bringing a new set of long-term complications to search out during imaging examina-

tions. **Aneurysms** may develop in the portal vein or hepatic arteries (Fig. 53-34, *E-H*), particularly at anastomoses or where segments of donor vessel were used. A careful search of the entire length of donor portal vein and hepatic artery to the point of connection to native vasculature is recommended. In the case of infrarenal aortic anastomoses, the entire length of the hepatic artery conduit may be difficult to identify. Intervening bowel gas may be compressed out of the way, or a far lateral, midaxillary line of scanning through the flank may show the graft site along the anterior surface of the aorta just below the renal arteries. Cross-sectional imaging with CT angiogram, MRI, and occasionally angiography are occasionally needed. Hepatic vein stenosis can also be a cause of cryptic graft failure. Careful examination of the hepatic venous outflow may still show only indirect evidence of stenosis: loss of phasicity in the hepatic veins, with change in phasicity in only one of the three hepatic veins. Given the location of the upper hepatic venous or caval anastomosis, sonographic evaluation is challenging.

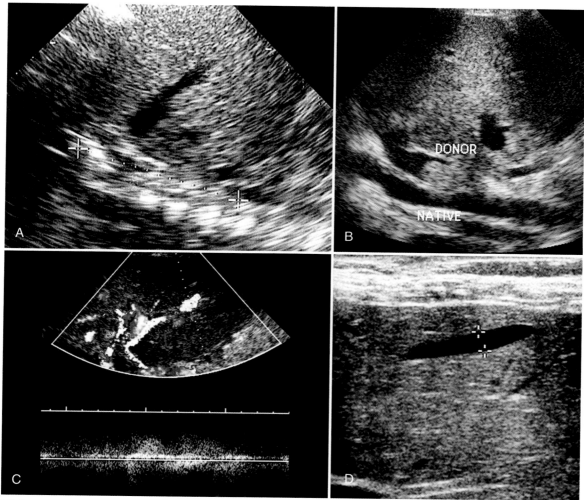

FIGURE 53-34. Transplant complications. A, Thrombosis (*cursors*) of inferior vena cava (IVC) after bisegmental liver transplantation in a 2-year-old child contrasts with the hypoechoic lumen of a nearby patent hepatic vein. **B, Partial thrombosis** of oversewn donor IVC interposed between native inferior vena cava and hepatic parenchyma. This is not usually problematic unless the clot propagates. **C,** Color and pulsed Doppler image shows **arteriovenous fistula** with turbulent flow in a transplant liver after biopsy. **D,** Focal dilation (*cursors*) of a bile duct in the left lobe of the transplant liver. This may be caused by hepatic arterial compromise and duct stenosis or ductal injury from previous percutaneous biopsy.

Occasionally, venography will clearly show a tight stenosis where one was only suspected sonographically. Fortunately, venous access in these cases can also be used to treat the lesion with angioplasty.

Additional complications in the long-term liver transplant survivors include renal cystic disease,[84] chronic renal failure, graft-versus-host disease, lymphoproliferative disorders, and other complications of immune suppression.

Multiorgan Transplants

A growing new subset of liver transplant recipients involves those receiving combined liver–small intestine transplants. Sonographic evaluation of the whole-liver transplant is unchanged, although the addition of a second donor pancreas and donor aorta with celiac and superior mesenteric arteries can create Doppler imaging challenges.[85] Evaluation of the small bowel is limited when there is postoperative ileus. Color Doppler evaluation of donor small bowel wall perfusion is useful in the immediate perioperative period. As bowel function returns, other clinical parameters replace Doppler evaluation of bowel viability. When complications arise, sonographic evaluation of the small bowel is similar to the approach used for necrotizing enterocolitis, looking for pneumatosis, poor perfusion, complicated ascites, and signs suggesting perforation. Sonographic imaging experience with these patients continues to expand.

THE SPLEEN

Examination of the spleen is an integral part of the sonographic assessment of the child with liver or pancreatic disease or with infection or trauma.

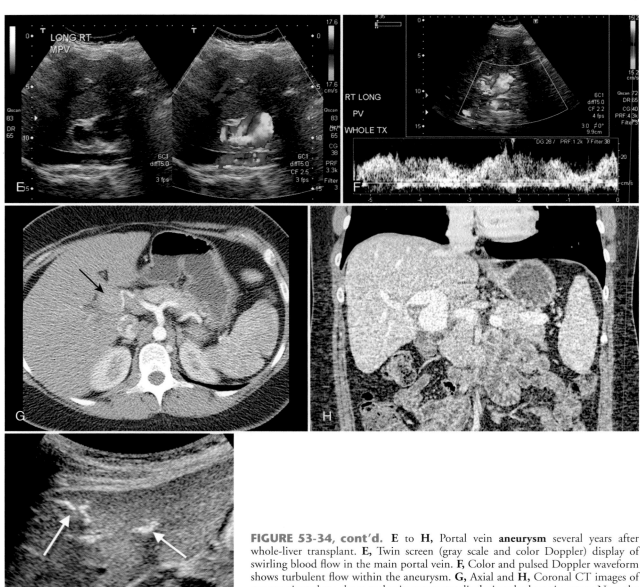

FIGURE 53-34, cont'd. E to **H,** Portal vein **aneurysm** several years after whole-liver transplant. **E,** Twin screen (gray scale and color Doppler) display of swirling blood flow in the main portal vein. **F,** Color and pulsed Doppler waveform shows turbulent flow within the aneurysm. **G,** Axial and **H,** Coronal CT images of same patient show the portal vein aneurysm displacing the hepatic artery. Note the perisplenic and perigastric varices, best seen on the coronal reformatted CT image. **I, Pneumobilia.** Transverse sonogram shows branching echogenic lines of air with "dirty" shadowing. Air within the biliary tree is common after choledochoenterostomy and is not itself a complication, although it can impair sonographic evaluation of the transplant liver.

Cysts of the spleen are congenital (epithelial lined),[86] posttraumatic (pseudocyst without lining),[87] or hydatid (unilocular and later daughter cysts).[46] Splenic cysts associated with polycystic kidney disease are rare in childhood. Splenic **abscesses** are found most frequently in immunosuppressed or leukemic children with candidiasis. The abscesses within the enlarged spleen usually become visible long after the diagnosis of candidal sepsis has been made. Cat-scratch disease is another cause of multiple splenic abscesses. Splenic **calcifications** may be the result of granulomatous infections (histoplasmosis, tuberculosis) or chronic granulomatous disease of childhood.

Splenic enlargement accompanies many systemic infections, including infectious mononucleosis (EBV) and other viral infections, typhoid fever, malaria, and fungal infections. Both the length and the width of the spleen increase (Fig. 53-35). The lower tip of the spleen becomes rounded. Other causes of enlargement include congestion in portal hypertension and infiltration with leukemic or lymphomatous tissue, which is usually impossible to distinguish from normal splenic parenchyma sonographically. These conditions underline the importance of examining the spleen in the context of the entire abdomen (e.g., for liver disease and portosystemic collaterals or for lymphadenopathy).[28]

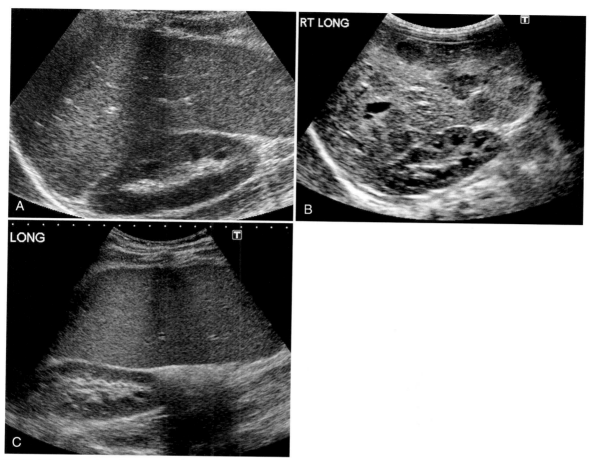

FIGURE 53-35. Hepatosplenomegaly. When the liver or spleen extends below the inferior pole of the ipsilateral kidney, enlargement is always present. **A,** Coronal sonogram of an enlarged liver in a teenager with elevated liver function tests. **B,** Hepatomegaly in a newborn with multiple hemangiomas. Note the fetal lobation and newborn echotexture of the right kidney. **C,** Longitudinal sonogram of splenomegaly in a teenager with mononucleosis.

CAUSES OF SPLENIC ENLARGEMENT

Infection (bacterial, viral, protozoal, fungal)
Lymphoma, leukemia
Lymphoproliferative disorders
  Chronic granulomatous disease
Cirrhosis, portal hypertension
Sequestration
  Sickle cell disease
Hemolytic anemia, extramedullary hematopoiesis
Langerhans cell histiocytosis
Storage diseases
  Gaucher's disease
  Niemann-Pick disease
  Mucopolysaccharidoses
Collagen vascular disease
Congestive heart failure
Sarcoidosis

The spleen is one of the most frequently injured organs when abdominal trauma has occurred. **Splenic hematomas** are usually hypoechoic lesions, often located under the capsule (Fig. 53-36, *C*). Fresh hematomas may be isoechoic or hyperechoic, and some linear lacerations are difficult to see on sonography. Hemoperitoneum is almost always present. Sonography is being used as the initial screening examination in children with abdominal trauma with variable results.[88,89] Not all studies routinely compare **focused abdominal sonography for trauma** (FAST) scanning with CT, the "gold standard." CT may be used only in doubtful cases or when there is concomitant spinal or head trauma. Proponents of sonography state that despite underdiagnosing some pancreatic and exceptional splenic hematomas as well as some mesenteric tears, the surgical management of their children was not affected, and no child died because lesions were missed at the initial examination.[89] In their cases, CT was performed if sonography was difficult because of rib fractures, or if there was doubt or increasing unexplained hemoperitoneum. CT remains the standard of care for pediatric abdominal trauma in the United States, whereas ultrasound is favored in Canada and some European countries.

Spontaneous rupture of the spleen occurs in the enlarged fragile organ in infectious mononucleosis[90] and is heralded by hemoperitoneum.

Splenic infarcts occur frequently in children with sickle cell anemia and also in children with various forms

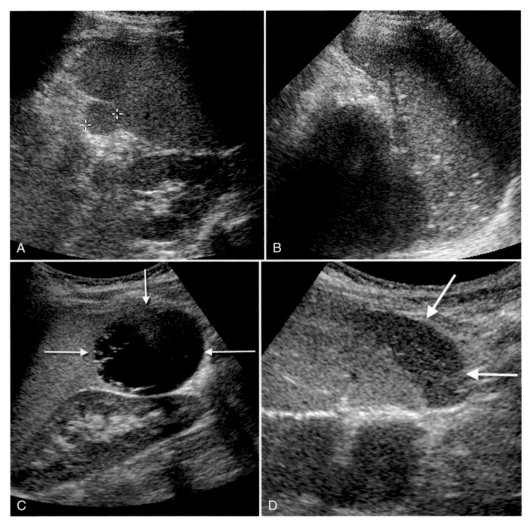

FIGURE 53-36. Splenic abnormalities. A, Transverse sonogram shows small **accessory spleen** near the splenic hilum *(cursors).* **B, Granulomas.** Multiple echogenic, faintly shadowing foci. **C,** Subacute **hematoma/contusion,** which is evolving into a posttraumatic cyst *(arrows).* A well-defined hypoechoic area in the splenic tip after sports trauma in a teenager. **D,** Splenic infarct *(arrows)* in a patient after bone marrow transplant with sepsis.

of vasculitis (Fig. 53-36, *D*). Lesions are usually triangular and hypoechoic. If the ligamentous attachments of the spleen are lax or absent, the spleen may move about in the abdomen (**wandering spleen**) and occasionally may undergo torsion on its pedicle. Torsion and splenic infarction can present as acute abdominal pain or a palpable mass.

Acknowledgment

This chapter is an update and revision of the previous excellent work by Heidi Patriquin, MD, who passed away in November 2000. Dr. Patriquin was a pioneer in pediatric ultrasound and particularly in abdominal visceral Doppler. She developed novel techniques for evaluating blood flow, described important differences in pediatric and adult sonography, and was well published and world renowned in the field. I had the pleasure of knowing her briefly and found her enthusiasm for pediatric ultrasound

contagious. I think she would enjoy the advances described and new images included in the chapter.

References

Anatomy
1. Bismuth H. Surgical anatomy and anatomical surgery of the liver. World J Surg 1982;6:3-9.
2. Couinaud CLF. Etudes anatomiques et chirurgicales. Paris: Masson; 1957.
3. Dodds WJ, Erickson SJ, Taylor AJ, et al. Caudate lobe of the liver: anatomy, embryology, and pathology. AJR Am J Roentgenol 1990; 154:87-93.

Neonatal Jaundice
4. Ikeda S, Sera Y, Yamamoto H, et al. Effect of phenobarbital on serial ultrasonic examination in the evaluation of neonatal jaundice. Clin Imaging 1994;18:146-148.
5. Tan Kendrick AP, Phua KB, Ooi BC, et al. Making the diagnosis of biliary atresia using the triangular cord sign and gallbladder length. Pediatr Radiol 2000;30:69-73.
6. Todani T, Watanabe Y, Narusue M, et al. Congenital bile duct cysts: classification, operative procedures, and review of thirty-seven cases

including cancer arising from choledochal cyst. Am J Surg 1977;134: 263-269.

7. McHugh K, Daneman A. Multiple gastrointestinal atresias: sonography of associated biliary abnormalities. Pediatr Radiol 1991;21: 355-357.
8. Caroli J, Soupault R, Kossakowski J, et al. La dilatation polykystique congenitale des foies biliaires intrahepatiques: essai de classifcation [Congenital polycystic dilation of the intrahepatic bile ducts: attempt at classification]. Sem Hop 1958;34:488-495.
9. Levy AD, Rohrmann Jr CA, Murakata LA, Lonergan GJ. Caroli's disease: radiologic spectrum with pathologic correlation. AJR Am J Roentgenol 2002;179:1053-1057.
10. Davies CH, Stringer DA, Whyte H, et al. Congenital hepatic fibrosis with saccular dilatation of intrahepatic bile ducts and infantile polycystic kidneys. Pediatr Radiol 1986;16:302-305.
11. Haller JO, Condon VR, Berdon WE, et al. Spontaneous perforation of the common bile duct in children. Radiology 1989;172: 621-624.
12. Alagille D, Estrada A, Hadchouel M, et al. Syndromic paucity of interlobular bile ducts (Alagille syndrome or arteriohepatic dysplasia): review of 80 cases. J Pediatr 1987;110:195-200.
13. Abramson SJ, Berdon WE, Altman RP, et al. Biliary atresia and noncardiac polysplenic syndrome: US and surgical considerations. Radiology 1987;163:377-379.
14. Roy CC, Silverman A, Alagille D. Pediatric clinical gastroenterology. 4th ed. St Louis: Mosby; 1994.
15. Tan Kendrick AP, Phua KB, Ooi BC, Tan CE. Biliary atresia: making the diagnosis by the gallbladder ghost triad. Pediatr Radiol 2003;33: 311-315.
16. Betz BW, Bisset 3rd GS, Johnson ND, et al. MR imaging of biliary cysts in children with biliary atresia: clinical associations and pathologic correlation. AJR Am J Roentgenol 1994;162:167-171.
17. Kasai M, Suzuki H, Ohashi E, et al. Technique and results of operative management of biliary atresia. World J Surg 1978;2:571-579.
18. Bezerra JA, Balistreri WF. Cholestatic syndromes of infancy and childhood. Semin Gastrointest Dis 2001;12:54-65.
19. Maresca G, De Gaetano AM, Mirk P, et al. Sonographic patterns of the gallbladder in acute viral hepatitis. J Clin Ultrasound 1984;12: 141-146.
20. Patriquin HB, DiPietro M, Barber FE, Teele RL. Sonography of thickened gallbladder wall: causes in children. AJR Am J Roentgenol 1983;141:57-60.
21. Dubois J, Garel L, Patriquin H, et al. Imaging features of type 1 hereditary tyrosinemia: a review of 30 patients. Pediatr Radiol 1996; 26:845-851.

Steatosis (Fatty Degeneration or Infiltration)
22. Henschke CI, Goldman H, Teele RL. The hyperechogenic liver in children: cause and sonographic appearance. AJR Am J Roentgenol 1982;138:841-846.
23. Tchelepi H, Ralls PW, Radin R, Grant E. Sonography of diffuse liver disease. J Ultrasound Med 2002;21:1023-1032; quiz 33-34.
24. Aubin B, Denys A, Lafortune M, et al. Focal sparing of liver parenchyma in steatosis: role of the gallbladder and its vessels. J Ultrasound Med 1995;14:77-80.

Cirrhosis
25. Patriquin HB, Roy CC, Weber AM, Filiatrault D. Liver diseases and portal hypertension. Clin Diagn Ultrasound 1989;24:103-127.

Cholelithiasis
26. Lobe TE. Cholelithiasis and cholecystitis in children. Semin Pediatr Surg 2000;9:170-176.
27. Keller MS, Markle BM, Laffey PA, et al. Spontaneous resolution of cholelithiasis in infants. Radiology 1985;157:345-348.
28. Littlewood Teele R Chrestman Share J. Ultrasonography of infants and children. Philadelphia, 1991, Saunders.

Liver Tumors
29. Brunelle F, Chaumont P. Hepatic tumors in children: ultrasonic differentiation of malignant from benign lesions. Radiology 1984; 150:695-699.
30. Isaacs Jr H. Fetal and neonatal hepatic tumors. J Pediatr Surg 2007;42:1797-1803.
31. Gottschling S, Schneider G, Meyer S, et al. Two infants with life-threatening diffuse neonatal hemangiomatosis treated with cyclophosphamide. Pediatr Blood Cancer 2006;46:239-242.

32. Mulliken JB, Glowacki J. Hemangiomas and vascular malformations in infants and children: a classification based on endothelial characteristics. Plast Reconstr Surg 1982;69:412-422.
33. Dachman AH, Lichtenstein JE, Friedman AC, Hartman DS. Infantile hemangioendothelioma of the liver: a radiologic-pathologic-clinical correlation. AJR Am J Roentgenol 1983;140:1091-1096.
34. Paltiel HJ, Patriquin HB, Keller MS, et al. Infantile hepatic hemangioma: Doppler US. Radiology 1992;182:735-742.
35. Ros PR, Goodman ZD, Ishak KG, et al. Mesenchymal hamartoma of the liver: radiologic-pathologic correlation. Radiology 1986;158: 619-624.
36. Brunelle F, Tammam S, Odievre M, Chaumont P. Liver adenomas in glycogen storage disease in children: ultrasound and angiographic study. Pediatr Radiol 1984;14:94-101.
37. D'Souza VJ, Sumner TE, Watson NE, Formanek AG. Focal nodular hyperplasia of the liver imaging by differing modalities. Pediatr Radiol 1983;13:77-81.
38. Koufos A, Hansen MF, Copeland NG, et al. Loss of heterozygosity in three embryonal tumours suggests a common pathogenetic mechanism. Nature 1985;316:330-334.
39. Dachman AH, Pakter RL, Ros PR, et al. Hepatoblastoma: radiologic-pathologic correlation in 50 cases. Radiology 1987;164:15-19.
40. Bates SM, Keller MS, Ramos IM, et al. Hepatoblastoma: detection of tumor vascularity with duplex Doppler US. Radiology 1990;176: 505-507.
41. Van Campenhout I, Patriquin H. Malignant microvasculature in abdominal tumors in children: detection with Doppler sonography. Radiology 1992;183:445-448.
42. Boechat MI, Kangarloo H, Ortega J, et al. Primary liver tumors in children: comparison of CT and MR imaging. Radiology 1988;169: 727-732.
43. Taylor KJ, Ramos I, Morse SS, et al. Focal liver masses: differential diagnosis with pulsed Doppler US. Radiology 1987;164:643-647.

Liver Abscess and Granulomas
44. Garel LA, Pariente DM, Nezelof C, et al. Liver involvement in chronic granulomatous disease: the role of ultrasound in diagnosis and treatment. Radiology 1984;153:117-121.
45. Merten DF, Kirks DR. Amebic liver abscess in children: the role of diagnostic imaging. AJR Am J Roentgenol 1984;143:1325-1329.
46. Andronikou S, Welman CJ, Kader E. Classic and unusual appearances of hydatid disease in children. Pediatr Radiol 2002;32: 817-828.
47. Lewall DB, McCorkell SJ. Hepatic echinococcal cysts: sonographic appearance and classification. Radiology 1985;155:773-775.

Doppler Assessment of Liver Disease and Portal Hypertension
48. Taylor KJ, Burns PN. Duplex Doppler scanning in the pelvis and abdomen. Ultrasound Med Biol 1985;11:643-658.
49. Taylor KJ, Burns PN, Woodcock JP, Wells PN. Blood flow in deep abdominal and pelvic vessels: ultrasonic pulsed-Doppler analysis. Radiology 1985;154:487-493.
50. Burns PN, Jaffe CC. Quantitative flow measurements with Doppler ultrasound: techniques, accuracy, and limitations. Radiol Clin North Am 1985;23:641-657.
51. Nelson TR, Pretorius DH. The Doppler signal: where does it come from and what does it mean? AJR Am J Roentgenol 1988;151: 439-447.
52. Sato S, Ohnishi K, Sugita S, Okuda K. Splenic artery and superior mesenteric artery blood flow: nonsurgical Doppler ultrasound measurement in healthy subjects and patients with chronic liver disease. Radiology 1987;164:347-352.
53. Patriquin HB, Paltiel H. Abdominal Doppler ultrasound in children: clinical applications. In Pediatric radiology categorical course syllabus. Chicago: Radiological Society of North America; 1989. p. 185-196.
54. Ohnishi K, Saito M, Nakayama T, et al. Portal venous hemodynamics in chronic liver disease: effects of posture change and exercise. Radiology 1985;155:757-761.
55. Tochio H, Kudo M, Nishiuma S, Okabe Y. Intrahepatic spontaneous retrograde portal flow in patients with cirrhosis of the liver: reversal by food intake. AJR Am J Roentgenol 2001;177:1109-1112.
56. Burns P, Taylor K, Blei AT. Doppler flowmetry and portal hypertension. Gastroenterology 1987;92:824-826.
57. Lafortune M, Madore F, Patriquin H, Breton G. Segmental anatomy of the liver: a sonographic approach to the Couinaud nomenclature. Radiology 1991;181:443-448.

58. Patriquin H, Lafortune M, Burns PN, Dauzat M. Duplex Doppler examination in portal hypertension: technique and anatomy. AJR Am J Roentgenol 1987;149:71-76.
59. Subramanyam BR, Balthazar EJ, Madamba MR, et al. Sonography of portosystemic venous collaterals in portal hypertension. Radiology 1983;146:161-166.
60. Van Leeuwen MS. Doppler ultrasound in the evaluation of portal hypertension. Clin Diagn Ultrasound 1990;26:53-76.
61. Patriquin HB, LaFortune M. Syllabus in pediatric radiology. Society for Pediatric Radiology; 1994.
62. Patriquin HB, Tessier G, Grignon A, Boisvert J. Lesser omental thickness in normal children: baseline for detection of portal hypertension. AJR Am J Roentgenol 1985;145:693-696.
63. Segel MC, Zajko AB, Bowen A, et al. Hepatic artery thrombosis after liver transplantation: radiologic evaluation. AJR Am J Roentgenol 1986;146:137-141.
64. Lafortune M, Dauzat M, Pomier-Layrargues G, et al. Hepatic artery: effect of a meal in healthy persons and transplant recipients. Radiology 1993;187:391-394.
65. Brunelle F, Alagille D, Pariente D, Chaumont P. An ultrasound study of portal hypertension in children. Ann Radiol (Paris) 1981;24:121-130.
66. Lebrec D, De Fleury P, Rueff B, et al. Portal hypertension, size of esophageal varices, and risk of gastrointestinal bleeding in alcoholic cirrhosis. Gastroenterology 1980;79:1139-1144.
67. Patriquin H. Current concepts in pediatric radiology. Chicago: Radiological Society of North America; 1994.
68. Taylor KJW, Burns PN, Wells PNT, editors. Clinical applications of Doppler ultrasound. Philadelphia: Lippincott-Raven; 1996.
69. De Gaetano AM, Lafortune M, Patriquin H, et al. Cavernous transformation of the portal vein: patterns of intrahepatic and splanchnic collateral circulation detected with Doppler sonography. AJR Am J Roentgenol 1995;165:1151-1155.
70. Besnard M, Pariente D, Hadchouel M, et al. Portal cavernoma in congenital hepatic fibrosis. angiographic reports of 10 pediatric cases. Pediatr Radiol 1994;24:61-65.
71. Odievre M, Chaumont P, Montagne JP, Alagille D. Anomalies of the intrahepatic portal venous system in congenital hepatic fibrosis. Radiology 1977;122:427-430.
72. Patriquin HB. Pediatric diseases test and syllabus. Vol 35. Reston, Va: American College of Radiology; 1993.
73. Bolondi L, Gandolfi L, Arienti V, et al. Ultrasonography in the diagnosis of portal hypertension: diminished response of portal vessels to respiration. Radiology 1982;142:167-172.
74. Stanley P. Budd-Chiari syndrome. Radiology 1989;170:625-627.
75. Lassau N, Auperin A, Leclere J, et al. Prognostic value of Doppler ultrasonography in hepatic veno-occlusive disease. Transplantation 2002;74:60-66.
76. Hosoki T, Kuroda C, Tokunaga K, et al. Hepatic venous outflow obstruction: evaluation with pulsed duplex sonography. Radiology 1989;170:733-737.
77. Rodgers BM, Kaude JV. Real-time ultrasound in determination of portasystemic shunt patency in children. J Pediatr Surg 1981;16:968-971.
78. Novak D, Butzow GH, Becker K. Hepatic occlusion venography with a balloon catheter in patients with end-to-side portacaval shunts. AJR Am J Roentgenol 1976;127:949-953.
79. Ledesma-Medina J, Dominguez R, Bowen A, et al. Pediatric liver transplantation. Part I. Standardization of preoperative diagnostic imaging. Radiology 1985;157:335-338.

Doppler Sonography in Children Receiving Liver Transplant

80. Hernanz-Schulman M, Ambrosino MM, Genieser NB, et al. Current evaluation of the patient with abnormal visceroatrial situs (pictorial essay). AJR Am J Roentgenol 1990;154:797-802.
81. Longley DG, Skolnick ML, Zajko AB, Bron KM. Duplex Doppler sonography in the evaluation of adult patients before and after liver transplantation. AJR Am J Roentgenol 1988;151:687-696.
82. Caron KH, Strife JL, Babcock DS, Ryckman FC. Left-lobe hepatic transplants: spectrum of normal imaging findings. AJR Am J Roentgenol 1992;159:497-501.
83. Jequier S, Jequier JC, Hanquinet S, et al. Orthotopic liver transplants in children: change in hepatic venous Doppler wave pattern as an indicator of acute rejection. Radiology 2003;226:105-112.
84. Calvo-Garcia MA, Campbell KM, O'Hara SM, et al. Acquired renal cysts after pediatric liver transplantation: association with cyclosporine and renal dysfunction. Pediatr Transplant 2008;12:666-671.
85. Sudan DL, Iyer KR, Deroover A, et al. A new technique for combined liver/small intestinal transplantation. Transplantation 2001;72:1846-1848.

The Spleen

86. Daneman A, Martin DJ. Congenital epithelial splenic cysts in children: emphasis on sonographic appearances and some unusual features. Pediatr Radiol 1982;12:119-125.
87. Paterson A, Frush DP, Donnelly LF, et al. A pattern-oriented approach to splenic imaging in infants and children. Radiographics 1999;19:1465-1485.
88. Emery KH, McAneney CM, Racadio JM, et al. Absent peritoneal fluid on screening trauma ultrasonography in children: a prospective comparison with computed tomography. J Pediatr Surg 2001;36:565-569.
89. Filiatrault D, Longpre D, Patriquin H, et al. Investigation of childhood blunt abdominal trauma: a practical approach using ultrasound as the initial diagnostic modality. Pediatr Radiol 1987;17:373-379.
90. Johnson MA, Cooperberg PL, Boisvert J, et al. Spontaneous splenic rupture in infectious mononucleosis: sonographic diagnosis and follow-up. AJR Am J Roentgenol 1981;136:111-114.

CHAPTER 54

The Pediatric Kidney and Adrenal Glands

*Diane S. Babcock and Heidi B. Patriquin**

Chapter Outline

PEDIATRIC RENAL SONOGRAPHY

Improvement in resolution of ultrasound equipment and the development of higher-frequency transducers have resulted in the widespread use of sonography for diagnosing and studying diseases of the kidney and adrenal gland in the pediatric patient. Sonography has the advantages of requiring no contrast material and of using nonionizing radiation. It is the primary imaging modality of the pediatric urinary tract.

Technique

The examination of the urinary tract in the pediatric patient should include images of the kidneys, ureters if visualized, and urinary bladder. The child's parents are asked to bring the patient for the study with a full urinary bladder. The child may be given fluid to drink

and asked not to void for [½] hour before the examination. For a young child who is not yet toilet-trained, the examination may be timed to bladder filling, with the patient being given fluids to drink while in the ultrasound department. The bladder must be checked first and frequently; the patient may fill and void suddenly.

Although children vary in their ability to hold still for a sufficient period, sedation is rarely needed. Infants under 1 year of age can be fed or given a pacifier during the examination. The patient older than 1 year can be distracted or entertained during the examination by watching movies, playing with toys, or reading a book. The addition of cine loop with clips often compensates for the movement of the child.

We use the services of child life specialists available through our hospital. Child life specialists are professionally trained and certified members of the health care team. They are experts in child development who promote effective coping through play, preparation, education, and self-expression activities. By providing

*In her memory, for all she did for pediatric radiology.

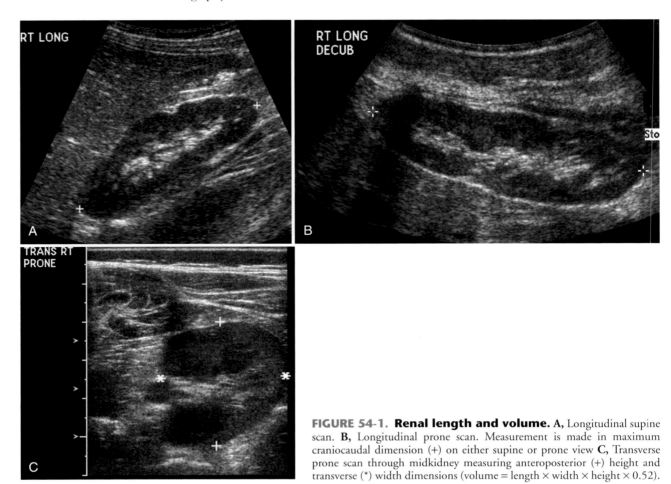

FIGURE 54-1. Renal length and volume. A, Longitudinal supine scan. **B,** Longitudinal prone scan. Measurement is made in maximum craniocaudal dimension (+) on either supine or prone view **C,** Transverse prone scan through midkidney measuring anteroposterior (+) height and transverse (*) width dimensions (volume = length × width × height × 0.52).

developmentally appropriate preparation and support before and during medical procedures, child life specialists help to lower levels of fear, stress, and anxiety. A child life specialist who is present with a parent during a procedure can also enhance the parent's ability to support the child. This psychosocial approach in collaboration with the health care team can contribute to a patient's ability to cope more effectively, with greater cooperation and success during medical procedures.

A variety of ultrasound equipment can be used. The highest-frequency transducer that will penetrate the area being examined is optimal. In an infant, this is usually a 14-6 MHz transducer, and in a child, a 6.0-MHz transducer. Harmonic imaging may aid in visualization of the difficult-to-scan patient. Different types of transducers are used for different parts of the body. Scans of the kidneys from the back are best performed with a linear or curved linear transducer, whereas frontal scans of the kidney are best performed with a curved linear or sector transducer that penetrates between the ribs. Views of the bladder are performed with a curved linear transducer. The ureters are evaluated as they leave the renal pelvis and enter the bladder. The images are recorded on digital storage.

Routine examination includes longitudinal and transverse views of both kidneys (Fig. 54-1). In the pediatric patient the kidneys are imaged in the supine and prone positions. The supine sagittal or coronal image allows optimal visualization of the upper pole, which may be obscured by ribs in the prone position. The echogenicity of the kidney can also be compared to the adjacent liver and spleen. Decubitus positioning is helpful to visualize the upper pole for measurement when the upper kidney is obscured by the ribs. The prone image allows optimal visualization of the lower pole of the kidney, but the upper pole may be obscured by overlying ribs or aerated lung in the costophrenic angle.

The maximum **renal length** obtained on the supine or prone images is utilized and is plotted against age[1] (Fig. 54-2, *A*). In cases where the patient is unusually tall or short or obese for age, the renal length may be plotted against patient height or weight (Fig. 54-2, *B* and *C*). **Kidney volumes** may be determined by obtaining a transverse image through the midkidney and measuring anteroposterior (AP) and transverse dimensions. (Fig. 54-1, *C*) The following volume formula for an ellipsoid kidney shape is used:

$$\text{Kidney volume} = \text{Length} \times \text{Width} \times \text{Height} \times 0.523$$

Several references are available for normal renal size, including length and volume[1-4] (Fig. 54-3 and Table 54-1). Data for length of a single functioning kidney in

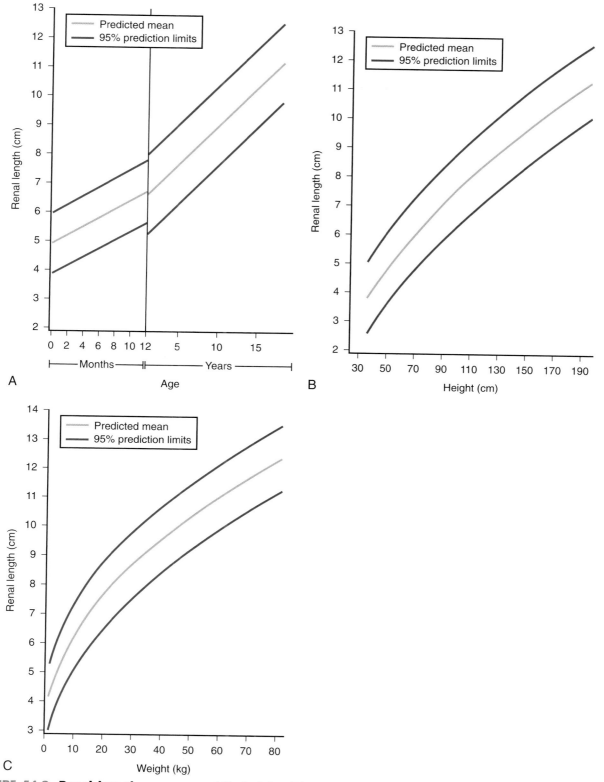

FIGURE 54-2. Renal length versus age (A), height (B), and weight (C). *(From Han BK, Babcock DS. Sonographic measurements and appearance of normal kidneys in children. AJR Am J Roentgenol 1985;145:611-616.)*

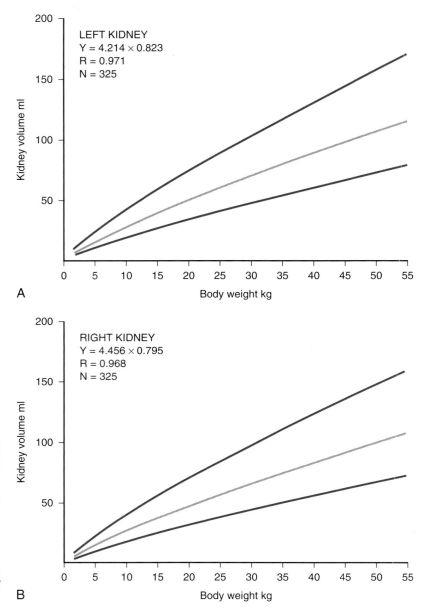

LEFT KIDNEY
Y = 4.214 × 0.823
R = 0.971
N = 325

RIGHT KIDNEY
Y = 4.456 × 0.795
R = 0.968
N = 325

FIGURE 54-3. Volume of left kidney (A) and right kidney (B) correlated to body weight. Median values and the 95% regions of tolerance are determined by statistical analysis of 325 children. Regression line and tolerance limits were computed after logarithmic transformation of volume and weight and then retransformed. There is only a slight difference between the left and right kidneys. *(From Dinkel E, Ertel M, Dittrich M, et al. Kidney size in childhood: sonographical growth charts for kidney length and volume. Pediatr Radiol 1985;15:38-43.)*

children has also been reported.[5] Compensatory renal growth of a single functional kidney occurs in utero, and its relative size difference continues throughout infancy and childhood (Table 54-2). Renal size in premature infants has also been compared to gestational age or birth weight[3,4] (Fig. 54-4). Renal size should be measured and compared to charts[1-5] (see Figs. 54-2 and 54-3). In patients with chronic problems, such as recurrent urinary tract infections, reflux, or neurogenic bladder, renal growth should be plotted on follow-up examinations.

Longitudinal and transverse views are obtained of the urinary bladder in both distended and postvoid states (Fig. 54-5). Images are obtained with a convex linear transducer using the highest frequency that will penetrate the patient. Harmonic imaging may be useful to minimize artifacts. **Bladder volume** may be determined on longitudinal and transverse views of the urinary bladder when maximally but comfortably distended.

Because the bladder varies in shape, various formulas have been suggested to calculate its volume. A correction coefficient, k, has been calculated on the basis of bladder shape using the following formula[6] (Table 54-3):

$$Volume = Height \times Weight \times Depth \times k$$

Bladder capacity may also be compared with normal data obtained during radionuclide cystography[7] (Table 54-4). Bladder volume is also determined by age, as follows:

$$Volume = Age(yr) + 2 \times 30\ mL$$

Bladder wall thickness is determined on the maximally distended bladder in a sagittal plane. The posteroinferior wall is measured (Fig. 54-5). Wall thickness can also be measured in the transverse plane lateral to the trigone. Normal measurements are reported for both a full and an empty bladder[8] (see Normal Bladder Anatomy).

Both the bladder volume and bladder wall thickness are affected by the degree of bladder distention. Spurious measurements can be obtained with a less than fully distended bladder.

TABLE 54-1. NORMAL STANDARDS FOR BODY WEIGHT VS. KIDNEY LENGTH IN NEWBORNS

	Kidney Length (mm)*	
BODY WEIGHT (g)	LOWER LIMIT	UPPER LIMIT
600	26.4	35.7
700	27.2	36.5
800	27.9	37.2
900	28.7	38.0
1000	29.4	38.7
1100	30.1	39.5
1200	30.9	40.2
1300	31.6	41.0
1400	32.4	41.7
1500	33.1	42.5
1600	33.9	43.2
1700	34.6	43.9
1800	35.1	44.7
1900	36.1	45.4
2000	36.9	46.2
2100	37.6	46.9
2200	38.4	47.7
2300	39.1	48.4
2400	39.9	49.2
2500	40.6	49.9
2600	41.3	50.7
2700	42.1	51.4
2800	42.8	52.2
2900	43.6	52.9
3000	44.3	53.7

*Upper and lower limits are determined from 95% confidence limits.
From Schlesinger AE, Hedlund GL, Pierson WP, Null DM. Normal standards for kidney length in premature infants: determination with US. Work in progress. Radiology 1987;164:127-129.

Scans of the bladder are performed with the bladder comfortably full so that abnormalities, including wall thickening and trabeculation, can be seen. Dilation of the distal ureters and ureteroceles are also sought. The thickness of the bladder wall may be increased with inflammation or muscular hypertrophy. Postvoid views of the bladder and kidneys may be helpful in patients with a neurogenic bladder or dilated upper collecting system, because a distended bladder may cause increased dilatation.

Doppler sonography is used in selected clinical situations to evaluate the **ureteric jets** (Fig. 54-5, C). Doppler ultrasound of the kidneys is performed in select patients when renal vein or arterial disease is suspected, using similar technique as in adults. Three-dimensional (3-D) Doppler technique has been recently added, with applications yet to be explored (Fig. 54-6). Surface-rendered views of the bladder and distal ureters have been helpful in select patients.[9] Volume measurement of the kidney parenchyma may be useful, especially with hydronephrosis.[10]

Normal Renal Anatomy

Throughout the second trimester, the fetal kidney consists of a collection of **renunculi** (small kidneys), each composed of a central large pyramid with a thin peripheral rim of cortex. As the renunculi fuse progressively, their adjoining cortices form a **column of Bertin.** The former renunculi are then called **lobes.** Remnants of these lobes with somewhat incomplete fusion are recognized by a lobulated surface of the kidney. This **"renal lobulation"** (sometimes called fetal lobulation) should not be confused with renal scars[11] and may persist into adulthood[12] (Fig. 54-7). The **renal junctional defect** (junctional parenchymal defect, interrenicular septum or fissure) is the most prominent of these grooves, extending from the hilum to the cortex and caused by perirenal

TABLE 54-2. MEAN AND STANDARD DEVIATION (SD) OF RENAL LENGTH OVER FIXED AGE RANGES IN PATIENTS WITH SINGLE FUNCTIONING KIDNEY AND A GROUP OF CONTROL SUBJECTS

AGE RANGE (wk)	Single Kidney				Control Kidney				
	MEAN AGE (wk)	MEAN LENGTH (mm)	SD	n	MEAN AGE (wk)	MEAN LENGTH (mm)	SD	n	p
0-4	2	51.0	5.8	13	0	44.8	3.1	10	<0.002
5-15	9	56.8	6.3	40	9	52.8	6.6	54	<0.01
17-34	23	62.8	5.6	25	26	61.5	6.7	20	<0.5
34-52	46	69.6	6.8	18	41	62.3	6.3	8	<0.01
53-94	63	71.7	7.9	33	78	66.5	5.4	28	<0.01
103-153	112	78.0	8.0	32	130	73.8	5.4	12	<0.046
156-207	172	79.6	8.2	17	182	73.6	6.4	30	<0.046
208-258	225	86.7	9.5	14	234	78.7	5.0	26	<0.01
260-312	279	91.0	7.9	12	286	80.9	5.4	10	<0.01

From Rottenberg GT, De Bruyn R, Gordon I: Sonographic standards for a single functioning kidney in children. AJR Am J Roentgenol 1996;167:1255-1259.

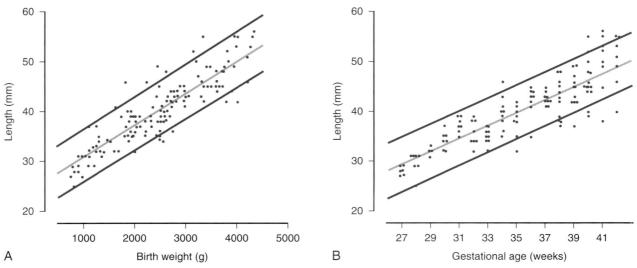

FIGURE 54-4. Kidney length versus birth weight (A) and gestational age (B). *(From Chiara A, Chirico G, Barbarini M, et al. Ultrasonic evaluation of kidney length in term and preterm infants. Eur J Pediatr 1989;149:94-95.)*

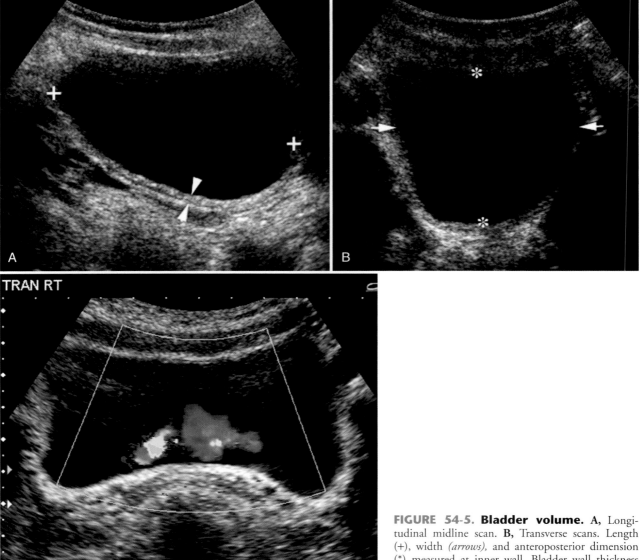

FIGURE 54-5. Bladder volume. A, Longitudinal midline scan. **B,** Transverse scans. Length (+), width *(arrows),* and anteroposterior dimension (*) measured at inner wall. Bladder wall thickness *(arrowheads)* measured at posterior wall. **C,** Ureteric jets.

TABLE 54-3. SHAPE AND CORRECTION COEFFICIENT (k) FOR BLADDER VOLUME

BLADDER SHAPE	k (SE)	PEARSON'S r	p	MEAN PERCENTAGE ERROR ±SD
Whole sample*	0.66 (0.011)	0.927	<0.01	19.19 ± 9.59
Round	0.561 (0.013)	0.940	<0.01	5.10 ± 8.30
Cuboid	0.923 (0.012)	0.982	<0.01	5.53 ± 6.86
Ellipsoid	0.802 (0.006)	0.992	<0.01	3.09 ± 3.52
Triangular	0.623 (0.007)	0.988	<0.01	7.71 ± 8.66
Undefined	0.749 (0.048)	0.976	<0.01	15.18 ± 17.21

SE, Standard error; SD, standard deviation.
  *Regardless of shape.
  Modified from Kuzmic AC, Brkljacic B, Ivankovic D. The impact of bladder shape on the ultrasonographic measurement of bladder volume in children. Pediatr Radiol 2003;33:530-534.

TABLE 54-4. PEDIATRIC BLADDER VOLUMES (mL): FUNCTIONAL BLADDER CAPACITY VS. AGE

AGE (yr)	MEAN −2 SD	MEAN −1.68 SD	MEAN +2 SD	MEAN	SD
<1	21	34	189	105	42
1-2	54	72	274	164	55
2-3	85	104	321	203	59
3-4	99	121	379	239	70
4-5	114	136	390	252	69
5-6	121	145	417	269	74
6-7	126	150	430	278	76
7-8	125	152	457	291	83
8-9	145	172	481	313	84
9-10	171	197	499	335	82
10-11	168	198	540	354	93
11-12	180	212	576	378	99
12-13	203	233	579	391	94
13-14	181	219	661	421	120
Girls 13-14	194	232	666	430	118
Boys 13-14	122	162	622	371	125

n = 5165; SD, standard deviation.
  Modified from Treves ST, Zurakowski D, Bauer SB, et al. Functional bladder capacity measured during radionuclide cystography in children. Radiology 1996;198:269-272.

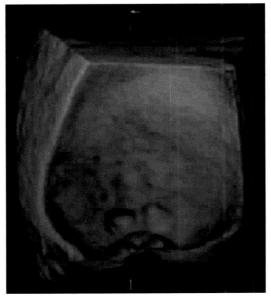

FIGURE 54-6. Three-dimensional sonogram of bladder. Surface-rendered three-dimensionally acquired image of bladder base.

fat adherent to the renal capsule along a cleft on the renal surface. It is frequently seen in the anterosuperior aspect of the kidney.[12] At birth, the pyramids are still large and hypoechoic compared with the thin rim of echogenic cortex that surrounds them. Glomerular filtration rate shortly after birth is low and increases rapidly after the first week postpartum. Throughout childhood, there is significant growth of the cortex, and the pyramids gradually become proportionately smaller.

The renal sonographic appearance and anatomy of the pediatric patient depends on age. The anatomy in the **teenager and older child** is similar to that in the adult[13,14] (Fig. 54-8). The renal parenchyma consists of the cortex, which is peripheral, contains the glomeruli, and has several extensions to the edge of the renal sinus (the septa of Bertin), and the medulla (containing the renal pyramids), which is more central and adjacent to the calices. The normal cortex produces low-level, back-scattered echoes. The medullary pyramids are relatively hypoechoic and arranged around the central, echo-producing renal sinus. The arcuate vessels can be

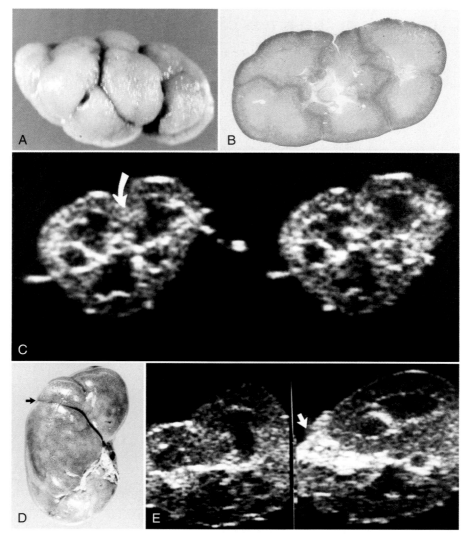

FIGURE 54-7. Renal lobulation changes with maturation. A, Fetal kidney of 16 weeks' gestation. The external surface shows individual lobes, or renunculi, separated by deep grooves. **B,** Microscopic section of a whole kidney at 23 weeks' gestation (hematoxylin and eosin stain). Individual renunculi, each composed of a central pyramid and a thin peripheral eosinophilic cortex, are visible. **C,** In vitro sonogram shows kidney at 1 month after birth. The lobes are well seen, each with a central pyramid and a thin rim of cortex. A line of fusion *(arrow)* is faintly seen in the center of a column of Bertin. **D,** Renal lobes are fused, and the external surface of a cadaver kidney is smooth except for three grooves; the most prominent is the interrenicular junction or junctional parenchymal defect, which extends from the hilum to the cortex *(arrow).* **E,** In vitro longitudinal and transverse sonographic cuts of the same kidney as in **D** shows the junctional parenchymal defect extending from the hilum to the cortex *(arrow).*

demonstrated as intense specular echoes at the corticomedullary junction.[13] This **corticomedullary differentiation** can be identified in most children but occasionally cannot be visualized in those with increased overlying soft tissues. The **central echo complex** consists of strong specular echoes from the renal sinus, including the renal collecting system, calices and infundibula, arteries, veins, lymphatics, peripelvic fat, and part of the renal pelvis. With distention of the renal collecting system, these echoes become separated and small degrees of hydronephrosis can be demonstrated. Mild degrees of distention can be seen in normal children, particularly after recent high intake of fluids or diuretics. A normally distended urinary bladder can also cause functional

ureteral obstruction and mild distention of the renal collecting systems. Rescanning when the bladder is empty will resolve this question.

In the **infant** the normal kidney has several features that differ from the normal adult patient[14] (Fig. 54-8). The central echo complex is much less prominent compared to the renal parenchyma because there is less peripelvic fat in the infant than in the adult. The echogenicity of the renal cortex in the normal term infant is often the same echogenicity as the adjacent normal liver, whereas in the older child and adult, the renal cortex is less echogenic than the liver. The renal cortex echogenicity is typically increased in the **very premature infant** compared to the liver and spleen. The medullary

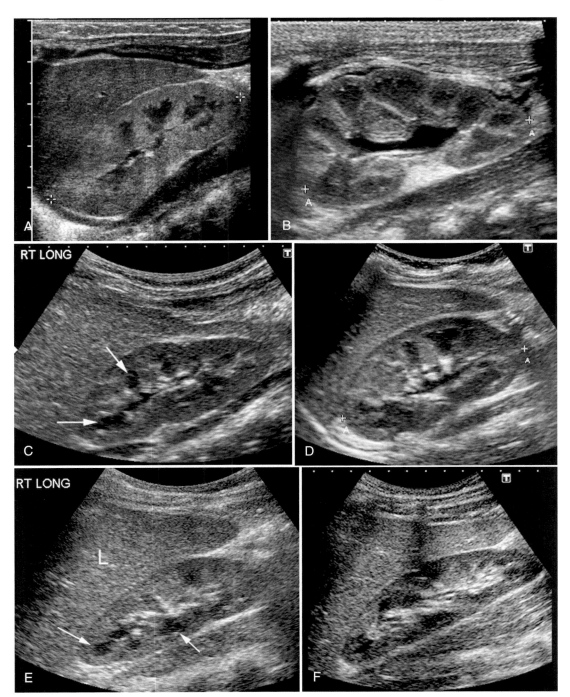

FIGURE 54-8. Normal renal appearances at different ages. A, Premature infant. Cortex is prominent and more echogenic than the liver. **B, Term infant.** Normal fetal lobulations of renal cortex are isoechoic or slightly hyperechoic to liver and spleen. Prominent renal pyramids are hypoechoic. **C, Infant.** Central echo complex is not prominent because of less peripelvic fat; the renal cortex equals the liver in echogenicity; and the medullary pyramids *(arrows)* are relatively larger and appear more prominent. **D, 2-year-old child.** Renal cortex is slightly less echogenic than liver. Renal sinus fat begins to develop central echogenicity around vessels. **E, 10-year-old child.** Normal cortex produces low-level echoes, whereas the medullary pyramids *(arrows)* are relatively hypoechoic and are arranged around the central echo complex consisting of strong specular echoes. The renal cortex is equally or less echogenic than the adjacent liver *(L)*. **F, 14-year-old child.** Renal cortex is less echogenic than liver or spleen. Pyramids are much less prominent. Renal sinus fat is increased.

pyramids in the infant are relatively larger and tend to appear more prominent. The corticomedullary differentiation is greater in the infant and child's kidney than in the adult, possibly because of increased resolution from higher-frequency transducers and less overlying body fat

tissue. It may also result from differences in the cellular composition of the renal parenchyma in the infant. These prominent pyramids in the pediatric kidney can easily be mistaken for multiple cysts or dilated calices by those not familiar with the differences; normal pyramids

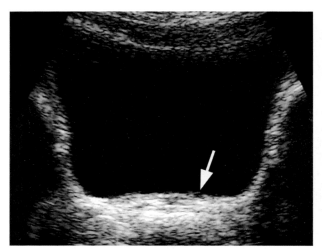

FIGURE 54-9. Normal urinary bladder and ureter.
Transverse sonogram of distended bladder with thin wall (<3 mm).
Distal ureteric insertion visible at trigone *(arrow)*.

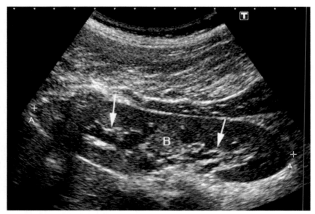

FIGURE 54-10. Renal duplication. The central echo complex *(arrows)* is separated into two parts with an interposed column of normal renal parenchyma (column of Bertin).

line up around the central echo complex in a characteristic pattern and can therefore be differentiated from cysts. Also, the position of the arcuate artery at the corticomedullary junction can help to identify a structure as a pyramid.

Indentations between lobes are between pyramids, whereas scars are indentations within pyramids and not on the edge.

Normal Bladder Anatomy

The normal urinary bladder is thin walled in the distended state (<3 mm). When empty, the wall thickness increases but is still less than 5 mm.[8] The distal ureters may be visible at the bladder base, especially if the child is well hydrated[9] (Fig. 54-9).

Both the bladder volume and the bladder wall thickness are affected by the degree of bladder distention. Spurious measurements can be obtained with a less than fully distended bladder. The thickness of the bladder wall may be increased with inflammation or muscular hypertrophy.

CONGENITAL ANOMALIES OF THE URINARY TRACT

Renal Duplication

A common congenital anomaly of the urinary tract is duplication of the collecting system, which may be partial or complete. In **complete duplication,** two pelves and two separate ureters drain the kidney. The lower-pole collecting system usually inserts into the bladder at the normal site; however, the intramural portion may be shorter than usual, and vesicoureteral reflux frequently results. The upper-pole system often inserts ectopically, inferior and medial to the site of the

normal ureteral insertion **(Weigert-Meyer rule).** Its orifice may be stenotic and obstructed. Ballooning of the submucosal portion of this upper-pole ureter causes a ureterocele. The upper-pole ureter may have an insertion entirely outside the bladder; in the urethra; above, at, or below the external urinary sphincter; into the uterus or vagina; or into the ejaculatory duct, seminal vesicle, or vas deferens.[15]

Patients with unobstructed duplications have no more clinical problems than their normal counterparts. Patients with complicated renal duplications may present with urinary tract infections, failure to thrive, abdominal mass, hematuria, or symptoms of bladder outlet obstruction from a ureterocele. Female patients with urethral insertions of the upper-pole ureter below the external urinary sphincter or with vaginal or uterine insertions may present with chronic, constant urinary incontinence or dribbling.

Duplication of the renal collecting system is diagnosed on sonography when the central echo complex separates into two parts with an interposed column of normal renal parenchyma (column of Bertin)[16] (Fig. 54-10). It is usually impossible to distinguish a partial, uncomplicated duplication from a complete one because the normal ureter is difficult to visualize sonographically.[17]

With **obstruction of an upper-pole moiety**, dilation of the upper-pole collecting system and its entire ureter is seen (Fig. 54-11). The renal parenchyma may be thinned over this upper-pole collecting system. If the obstruction is associated with a simple ureterocele, views of the bladder may demonstrate the ureterocele as a curvilinear structure within the bladder, in addition to the dilated distal ureter adjacent to the bladder. A large ureterocele may cross the midline and obstruct the contralateral ureter or bladder outlet and cause bilateral hydronephrosis. Ureteroceles can be difficult to diagnose if they are so large as to mimic the bladder. If this is a question, a postvoid scan will be diagnostic.

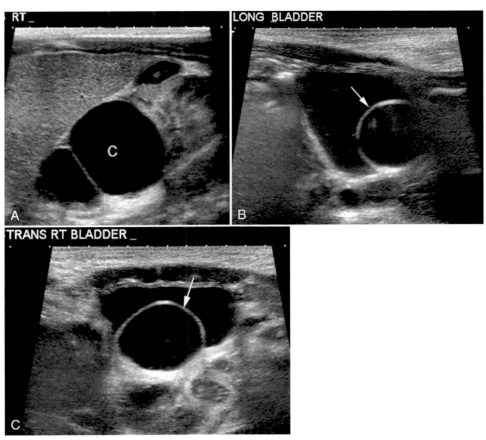

FIGURE 54-11. Renal duplication with obstructing ureterocele. A, Longitudinal scan of the right kidney shows upper-pole cyst *(C)* caused by dilated upper-pole collecting system. **B** and **C,** Longitudinal and transverse scans of the bladder demonstrate ureterocele *(arrow)* projecting into the bladder.

With **reflux into the lower-pole moiety,** the lower-pole collecting system and its ureter will be dilated to varying degrees. If reflux is mild, there may be no lower-pole dilation.

Other Renal Anomalies

Other renal anomalies include congenital absence of the kidney, abnormal position of the kidney (e.g., pelvic kidney, cross-fused ectopia), and horseshoe kidney with fusion of the lower poles in the midline.[18] **Absence of the kidney** is suspected when no renal tissue can be identified on sonography. At birth, the adrenal gland will take on a flat shape instead of the usual inverted V above the kidney (a lying-down adrenal). Care must be taken to search for the kidney not only in its usual position in the renal fossa, but also in the lower abdomen or pelvis. The contralateral kidney, when healthy, shows compensatory hypertrophy when one kidney is absent or severely damaged. Nuclear renal scan may be helpful in identifying a small, functioning kidney not visualized by ultrasound.

With a **horseshoe kidney** the longitudinal axis of the kidneys is abnormal, with the lower poles located more medially than usual and fusing in the midline anterior to the spine (Fig. 54-12). The fusion may be a fibrous band or actual fusion of the renal parenchyma. The

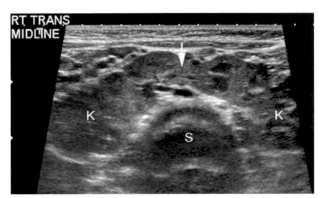

FIGURE 54-12. Horseshoe kidney. Transverse supine scan demonstrates lower poles of kidneys *(K)* more medial than usual in the midline anterior to the spine *(S)*. Fusion is by band of renal parenchyma *(arrow)*.

lower poles of the kidneys are rotated medially and may be positioned somewhat lower than usual. In **cross-fused ectopy,** both kidneys are located on the same side of the abdomen and are fused inferior to the ipsilateral kidney. They can also be fused in an L-shaped configuration. The ureters normally insert into each side of the bladder.[18] A horseshoe kidney may be missed easily if the abnormal axis of the kidney is not recognized. The central renal tissue may also be thin and easy to miss, particularly if it is only fibrous tissue.

HYDRONEPHROSIS

Dilation of the renal collecting system—hydronephrosis—is a fairly common problem in the pediatric patient. It is frequently, but not always, associated with obstruction; ultrasound is particularly sensitive for its detection. Hydronephrosis may be detected on fetal sonography and the infant referred for evaluation after birth. Small amounts of fluid may be detected in the normal renal pelvis. Dilation of the renal calices is abnormal and suggests significant pathology. To make a more precise diagnosis and to estimate severity, information on degree of dilation, unilateral or bilateral, ureters and bladders dilated, and status of the renal parenchyma should be obtained with sonography. Dilation may be caused by obstruction, reflux, or abnormal muscle development. A cystogram and nuclear renogram with furosemide (Lasix) are often performed for complete evaluation.

Ureteropelvic Junction Obstruction

The most common neonatal abdominal mass is hydronephrosis,[19] and obstruction is most common at the level of the ureteropelvic junction (UPJ), secondary to a functional stricture. Stricture results in a functional disturbance in either the initiation or the propagation of the normal peristaltic activity within the ureter. The obstruction produces proximal dilation of the collecting system, whereas the ureter is normal in caliber. There is an increased incidence of abnormalities of the contralateral kidney.[18]

The investigation of a child with suspected hydronephrosis usually begins with sonography to evaluate the anatomy of the kidneys, ureters, and bladder. The degree of functional obstruction is evaluated by nuclear renogram with furosemide. If mild, the patient is followed; the obstruction and dilation often resolve as the patient grows older.[20] The typical appearance of a hydronephrotic kidney is a cystic mass in the renal fossa, which maintains its reniform shape (Fig. 54-13). With a UPJ obstruction, a larger cyst medially represents a dilated medial pelvis, whereas smaller cysts arranged around the periphery of the pelvis represent the dilated renal calices. A variable amount of renal parenchymal tissue can be visualized. With obstruction at the ureteropelvic junction, the ureter is normal in size and usually is not visualized by ultrasound.

Ureteral Obstruction

The ureter can be obstructed anywhere along its course by extrinsic compression by a mass, such as a lymphoma or abscess. The exact site of obstruction may be difficult to visualize by ultrasound because of overlying bowel gas. The ureter is more often obstructed by intrinsic abnormalities, such as stones, blood clot, and fungus balls.

Obstruction can occur at the ureterovesical junction because of primary megaureter, **atresia,** or an ectopically inserted ureter. With **primary megaureter,** the juxtavesicular segment of the ureter near the bladder is narrowed by an increase in fibrous tissue or by circumferential tissue that is devoid of muscle. There is a variable degree of dilation of the intrarenal collecting system and the ureter proximal to the narrowing. Sonography typically shows hydronephrosis and hydroureter with a narrow segment of the distal ureter behind the bladder[21] (Fig. 54-14). Increased peristalsis in the ureter proximal to the obstruction may be detected with real-time sonography. Doppler sonography often shows a diminished or abnormal ureteric jet on the side of obstruction.[22,23] **Ectopic insertion of a ureter** can occur with or without a ureterocele and results in dilation of the more proximal collecting system and ureter. As discussed previously, this is usually associated with a duplication.

Bladder Outlet Obstruction

Bilateral hydronephrosis is frequently caused by obstruction at the level of the bladder or bladder outlet. A **neurogenic bladder** (e.g., with meningomyelocele) can result in a thickened and dilated bladder and bilateral dilation of the collecting systems and ureters. The bladder and bladder outlet may be obstructed by congenital anomalies, such as **posterior urethral valves** or **polyps,** or it may be obstructed by a pelvic mass, such as a **tumor** distorting the bladder base. In either case, the bladder will be enlarged and have a thickened, irregular wall.[24] Congenital anomalies of the spine should be sought with radiographs and spinal ultrasound in neonates, if not obvious clinically. Posterior urethral valves can sometimes be diagnosed by ultrasound, with demonstration of a dilated posterior urethra[18,24](Fig. 54-15). Voiding cystography should be performed for optimal visualization of the posterior urethral valves.

Dilation of the renal collecting system is not always caused by obstruction, and other abnormalities, such as **vesicoureteral reflux,** should be considered. In a patient with hydronephrosis detected by ultrasound, the bladder and urethra should be further evaluated with a voiding cystourethrogram. Bladder size, contractility, and the urethra can be evaluated. In addition, vesicoureteral reflux can be assessed and even may be the cause of the urinary tract dilation.

Prune-Belly Syndrome

Abdominal muscle deficiency (Eagle-Barrett, prune-belly) syndrome includes congenital absence or deficiency of the abdominal musculature, large hypotonic dilated tortuous

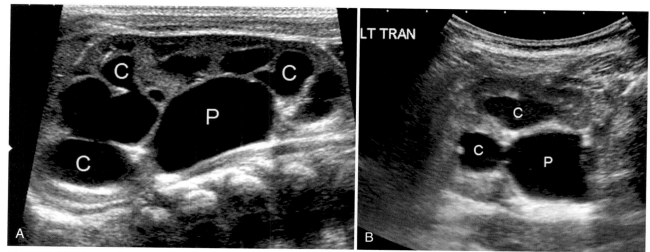

FIGURE 54-13. Hydronephrosis with ureteropelvic junction obstruction. A and **B,** Longitudinal and transverse scans show marked dilation of the collecting system with a larger cyst *(P)* medially, which is a dilated renal pelvis, and smaller connecting cysts from dilated renal calices *(C).* The ureter is normal in size and not visualized.

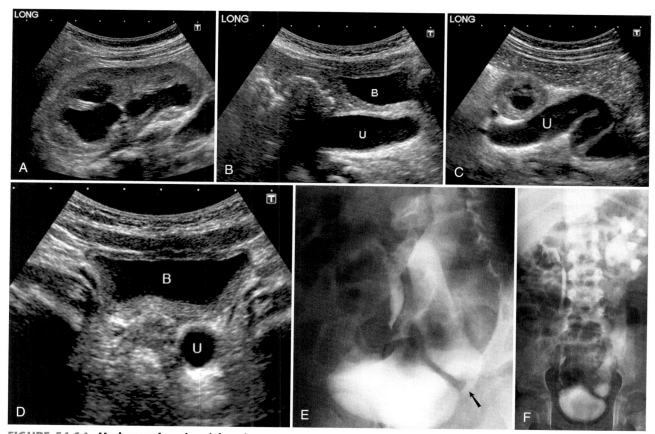

FIGURE 54-14. Hydronephrosis with primary megaureter. A, Longitudinal scan demonstrates moderate hydronephrosis. **B,** Medial longitudinal scan shows dilated ureter *(U)* extending toward the bladder *(B).* **C,** Longitudinal scan through right pelvis, and **D,** transverse scan, show dilated distal ureter *(U)* near the insertion into the bladder *(B).* **E** and **F,** Excretory urogram in another patient demonstrates hydronephrosis and hydroureter with narrowed segment of distal ureter *(arrow)* behind the bladder.

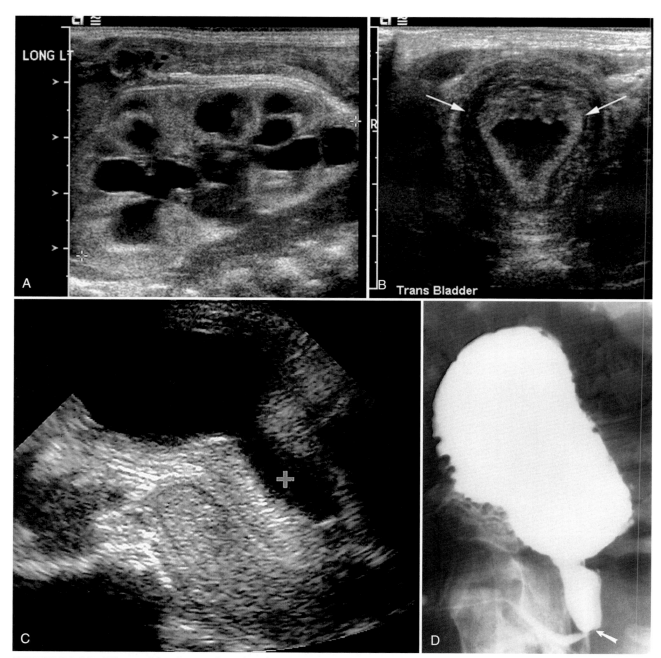

FIGURE 54-15. Bilateral hydronephrosis with posterior urethral valves. A, Longitudinal scan of kidney shows hydronephrosis, which was present bilaterally. **B,** Scan of the pelvis shows trabeculated bladder *(B)* with thick walls *(arrows),* indicating bladder outlet obstruction. **C,** Longitudinal scan of midbladder base in another patient shows dilated posterior urethra (+). **D,** Voiding cystourethrogram shows dilated prostatic urethra and obstructing valves *(arrow).*

ureters, a large bladder, a patent urachus (see Urachal Anomalies), bilateral cryptorchidism, and dilated prostatic urethra. There are decreased muscular fibers throughout the urinary tract and prostate, resulting in dilation and hypoperistalsis. Renal dysplasia and hydronephrosis can occur to varying degrees. Associated pulmonary hypoplasia may lead to Potter's syndrome and death.[18]

Megacystis-Microcolon-Malrotation–Intestinal Hypoperistalsis Syndrome

This rare syndrome occurs in girls who are born with a grossly distended abdomen. An enlarged bladder, hydronephrosis, and hydroureter are demonstrated sonographically. Microcolon, malrotation, and diminished-to-absent

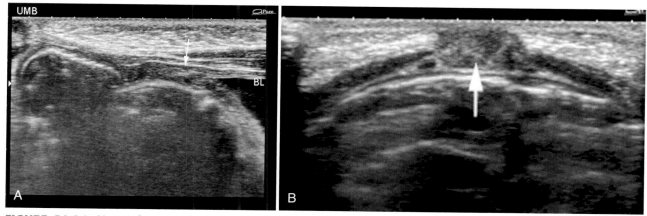

FIGURE 54-16. Normal urachal remnant. A and **B,** Longitudinal and transverse scans demonstrate an elliptical, hypoechoic structure on middle of anterosuperior surface of urinary bladder *(BL),* often visible using high-frequency transducer.

peristalsis of the bowel are seen with contrast examination of the gastrointestinal tract. The condition is fatal unless the patient can be maintained with total parenteral hyperalimentation.[18]

Bladder Exstrophy

Exstrophy of the bladder is a rare anomaly in which the pubic bones are far apart and the bladder and urethral mucosa are exposed. The kidneys and ureters are usually normal. After surgical repair, the bladder is small and irregularly shaped.[25] There may be hydronephrosis secondary to poor bladder emptying. A bladder augmentation procedure using bowel may then be performed. The bladder is then more normal in size but still irregular, and there may be peristalsis and echogenic debris (e.g., mucus).

Urachal Anomalies

The fetal **urachus** is a tubular structure extending from the umbilicus to the bladder. It normally closes by birth, and a **urachal remnant** may be visible as a hypoechoic elliptical–shaped mass on the anterosuperior aspect of the bladder[26] (Fig. 54-16). If it remains patent, urine may leak from the umbilicus. If part of the urachus closes, patent parts may form **urachal cysts,** which may become infected. The proximal portion of the urachus may remain open, producing a diverticulum-like structure from the dome of the bladder.[25] These anomalies may be associated with prune-belly syndrome. Urachal abnormalities are evaluated with cystography in the lateral projection and with sonography. Ultrasound is particularly useful in demonstrating urachal cysts and masses near the abdominal wall, along the site of the urachal tract[26,27] (Fig. 54-17).

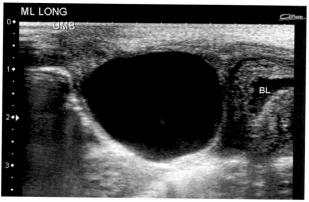

FIGURE 54-17. Urachal cyst. Midline longitudinal scan of the pelvis shows compression of the bladder dome *(BL)* by a cystic mass containing low-level echoes.

RENAL CYSTIC DISEASE

Autosomal Recessive Polycystic Kidney Disease

Renal cystic disease is a complex subject, with overlapping classifications; this discussion summarizes the most common forms. Autosomal recessive polycystic kidney disease (ARPKD; Potter type 1) is a phenotypically variable disorder with varying degrees of nonobstructing renal collecting duct ectasia, hepatic biliary duct ectasia, and fibrosis of the liver and kidneys. ARPKD in the kidney is characterized by dilated collecting ducts, seen as radially arranged, fusiform cysts that are most prominent in the medullary portions of the kidney.[28] This disease has a spectrum of severity and a reciprocal relationship with liver involvement (e.g., periportal fibrosis, often with proliferation and variable dilation of bile ducts).[29,30] Severe renal involvement can be diagnosed in the second trimester by enlarged hyperechogenic kidneys,

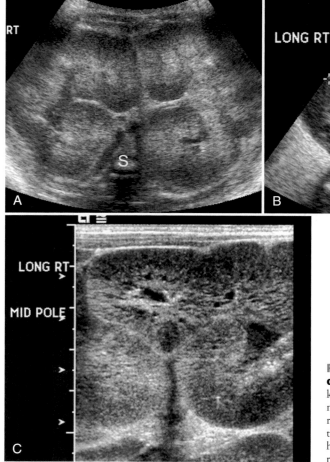

FIGURE 54-18. Autosomal recessive polycystic kidney disease (ARPKD). Newborn with symmetrically enlarged kidneys almost filling the entire abdomen. **A,** Transverse scan of midabdomen. **B,** Longitudinal scan of right kidney. **C,** High-resolution scan shows hyperechoic medullary region with dilated tubuli and hyperechoic foci. The subcapsular region is relatively hypoechoic, reflecting compressed cortex. Pyramids are no longer recognizable. *S,* Spine.

followed by oligohydramnios. In the third trimester the kidneys occupy almost the entire abdomen and cause it to enlarge. On antenatal and newborn sonography, the kidneys are hyperechogenic and greatly enlarged, often with a hypoechogenic outer rim, which probably represents the cortex compressed by the greatly expanded pyramids[31] (Fig. 54-18). High-resolution sonography shows a spectrum of abnormalities, including dilated tubules, cysts, and hyperechoic foci.[32] Intravenous urography (IVU) outlines a little of the stagnation of urine that occurs within the tubules; the enlarged kidneys show a striated, increasingly dense nephrogram and poor visualization of the collecting system.[33] Children with ARPKD generally succumb to their renal failure, and no clinical liver disease is noted. If they survive, the appearance of the kidneys may evolve, with increasing echogenicity and larger cysts.[34]

Autosomal Recessive Polycystic Kidney Disease with Severe Hepatic Fibrosis

At the other end of the ARPKD spectrum is the teenager who presents with bleeding esophageal varices caused by portal hypertension secondary to congenital hepatic fibrosis. In these children, approximately 10% of kidney tubules are cystic, and renal failure presents much later in life. The kidneys in these children are often slightly or moderately enlarged with echogenic pyramids that often contain calcium (Fig. 54-18). At IVU, the pattern resembles that of adult medullary sponge kidney, with pooling of contrast medium in the dilated collecting ducts. In more advanced cases the entire kidney may be replaced by tiny cysts.

Autosomal Dominant Polycystic Kidney Disease

Although more than 90% of patients with autosomal dominant polycystic kidney disease (ADPKD; Potter type 3) have a gene locus on the short arm of chromosome 16, and although penetrance is complete, disease severity varies greatly. ADPKD has been diagnosed in utero and in early childhood, but the typical presentation is between ages 30 and 40 years, at which time hypertension or azotemia is present. At the extreme end of the spectrum, the disease has been discovered incidentally in otherwise healthy persons in the seventh or eighth

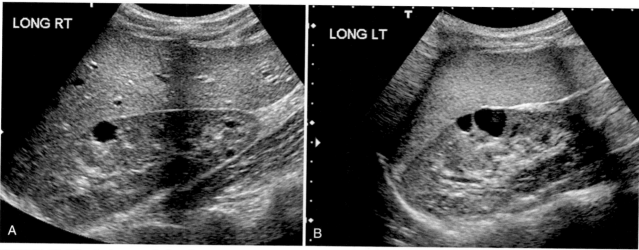

FIGURE 54-19. Autosomal dominant polycystic kidney disease (ADPKD) in 18-year-old. Longitudinal scans of right kidney **(A)** and left kidney **(B)** demonstrate cysts of varying size. The kidneys are mildly enlarged.

decade. About 25% of patients have a negative family history. ADPKD is characterized by a weakness in basement membranes, likely because of a generalized defect in collagen formation. All parts of the nephron are affected, although only 5% to 10% of the nephrons are involved. Cysts therefore can occur anywhere and are usually macroscopic and of varying size[35-37] (Fig. 54-19). The incidence of cysts in other organs depends on the stage and severity of the disease. About 10% of patients with ADPKD have hepatic cysts, and there is a much lower incidence of splenic, pancreatic, and pulmonary cysts. These patients may also have cerebral aneurysms, colonic diverticulosis, and cysts in the ovaries, seminal vesicles, and brain. Extrarenal cysts are rare in children.

Multicystic Renal Dysplasia

Multicystic dysplastic kidney (MCDK; Potter type 2) is the most common form of cystic disease in infants and is associated with an increased incidence of abnormalities in the contralateral kidney, including UPJ stenosis, multicystic dysplastic kidney (in which case the disease is fatal), primary megaureter, and vesicoureteral reflux. Multicystic renal dysplasia is now usually detected sonographically in utero; large cysts of varying sizes are arranged like a bunch of grapes, and there is no recognizable renal pelvis (Fig. 54-20). Ureteral obliteration causes renal function to diminish and then cease. When MCDK cysts resemble the dilated calices of severe UPJ stenosis, scintigraphy is useful to detect any remaining renal function. The calices in severe hydronephrosis from UPJ stenosis communicate, whereas MCDK cysts do not.[38] Surgery for multicystic renal dysplasia is usually not necessary unless the kidney is massively enlarged.[25,39] Periodic follow-up sonography shows a decrease in the size of the cysts as urine production stops, to the point that the kidney may no longer be visible.[40]

Medullary Cystic Disease and Juvenile Nephronophthisis

Medullary cystic disease and juvenile nephronophthisis are morphologically indistinguishable. Both cause chronic renal failure in adolescents or young adults. At sonography, the kidneys are small, echogenic, and contain cysts of variable sizes at the corticomedullary junction and elsewhere[18] (Fig. 54-21). Medullary cystic disease is inherited as autosomal dominant, whereas juvenile nephronophthisis as autosomal recessive.

Cysts

Tuberous Sclerosis and Von Hippel–Lindau Disease

Cysts of various sizes and location occur in a variety of syndromes. Tuberous sclerosis is an autosomal dominant disease consisting of mental retardation, epilepsy, adenoma sebaceum, multiple ectodermal lesions, and mesodermal hamartomas. Renal lesions are present in more than 40% of patients and include cysts, which can be multiple and resemble adult-type polycystic kidney disease with renal enlargement. **Angiomyolipomas** can occur and vary in their echogenicity depending on the type of tissue, being extremely echogenic when containing considerable fat[41] (Fig. 54-22).

In von Hippel–Lindau disease, there are cysts and an increased incidence of renal cell carcinoma, which is often bilateral.

Acquired Cysts

Patients with chronic renal failure, especially those receiving dialysis, often develop multiple small renal cysts. The kidneys usually remain small, and large cysts

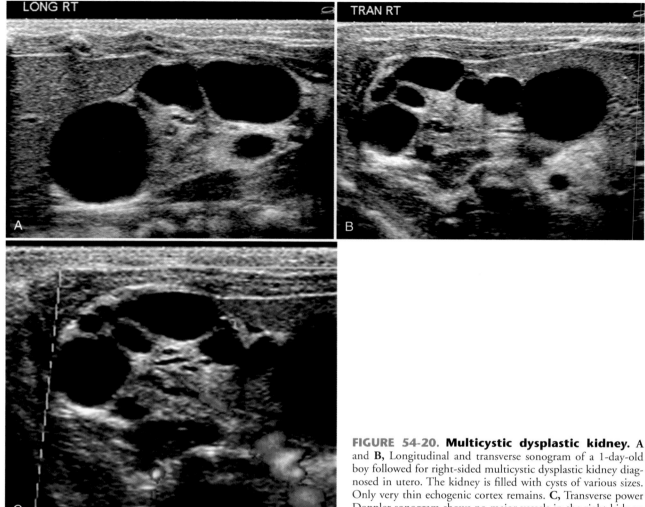

FIGURE 54-20. Multicystic dysplastic kidney. A and **B,** Longitudinal and transverse sonogram of a 1-day-old boy followed for right-sided multicystic dysplastic kidney diagnosed in utero. The kidney is filled with cysts of various sizes. Only very thin echogenic cortex remains. **C,** Transverse power Doppler sonogram shows no major vessels in the right kidney. No right kidney function was seen on DTPA scan.

are rare. There is an increased incidence of formation of adenomas and a slightly increased incidence of adenocarcinoma in patients receiving long-term dialysis. Spontaneous hemorrhage may occur.

Renal cysts have also been reported in patients with **liver transplant.** Those at risk are at least 10 years after transplant and have been treated with cyclosporine and have impaired renal function.[42]

Simple cysts are much less common in children than adults and typically appear as a single mass arising from the kidney. Simple cysts are clinically important only because they can be associated with hematuria or infection.[18]

URINARY TRACT INFECTION

Urinary tract infection (UTI) is a common clinical problem in children and a common indication for renal sonography. The imaging workup of the child with a UTI is usually performed after the first culture has documented infection in a male or female infant or child. The purpose of the workup is to identify congenital anomalies, obstructions, and other abnormalities that may predispose the patient to infections. Sonography of the urinary tract, including the kidneys and bladder, is used for initial screening. The lower urinary tract, the bladder, and the urethra are evaluated by radiographic voiding cystography. Cystography is performed in younger patients, but not routinely in older patients.[18] Nuclear radiographic cystography or ultrasound contrast cystography[43] can be used to evaluate vesicoureteral reflux. Our approach is to perform a radiographic cystogram in males, in whom it is important to visualize the urethral anatomy, and in girls if abnormalities are seen at sonography. The nuclear cystogram is associated with a lower radiation dose to the gonads in males. It is used in females with normal renal and bladder sonograms, in whom urethral abnormalities are rare, and for follow-up examinations for reflux in both males and females. If

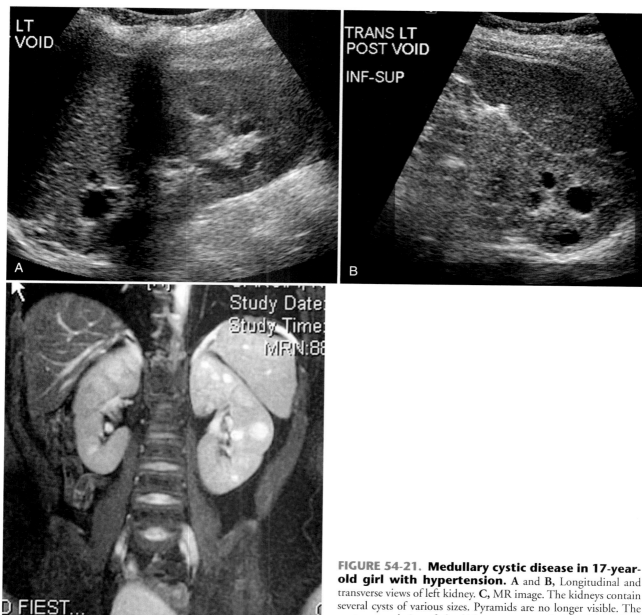

FIGURE 54-21. Medullary cystic disease in 17-year-old girl with hypertension. A and **B,** Longitudinal and transverse views of left kidney. **C,** MR image. The kidneys contain several cysts of various sizes. Pyramids are no longer visible. The contours and size of the kidneys are normal. Juvenile nephronophthisis (autosomal recessive form) will have the same sonographic appearance.

abnormalities that require further investigation are detected on the renal sonogram or the cystogram, renal nuclear scintigraphy with pertechnetate (DTPA) or mertiatide (MAG3) can be performed. Renal nuclear scintigraphy with technetium-99m glucoheptonate or succimer (DMSA) is extremely sensitive for demonstrating focal areas of inflammation and parenchymal scars. Mild scars may be missed with sonography. Sonography with power Doppler increases the sensitivity.[44] It is thought that mild scars are of little practical importance and do not alter the course of therapy; therefore the radiation dose of a renal cortical scan is not warranted.[45-48] The increased time and expense of Doppler sonography may also be unnecessary.

Patients with reflux are often treated with a **deflux procedure,** and follow-up sonography of the bladder shows the **deflux mounds** (Fig. 54-23).

Acute Pyelonephritis

Acute pyelonephritis, or **infectious interstitial nephritis,** is usually diagnosed by the clinical features of sudden fever, flank pain, and costovertebral angle tenderness, with microscopic evidence of urinary infection. The infection usually occurs as an ascending infection from the bladder through reflux but can occur by hematogenous spread.[49] The findings on sonography or excretory urography are usually few but include swelling of the

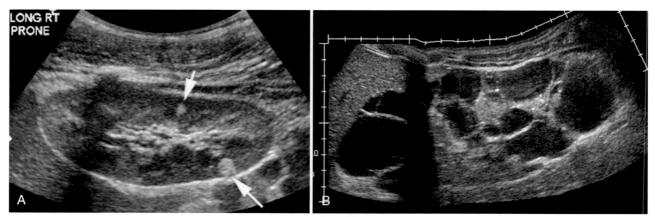

FIGURE 54-22. Tuberous sclerosis. A, Teenager with multiple hyperechoic masses consistent with angiomyolipoma *(arrows).* **B,** Infant with bilaterally enlarged kidneys and multiple cysts.

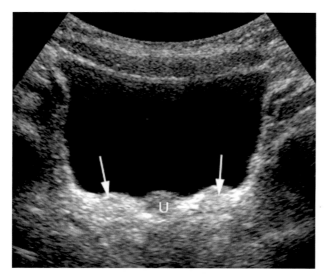

FIGURE 54-23. Deflux mounds. Transverse view of bladder demonstrates bilateral echogenic masses in posterior bladder wall at region of ureter insertion *(arrows); U,* uterus.

infected kidney, altered renal parenchymal echogenicity from edema,[18] or triangular areas of increased echogenicity (Fig. 54-24). There may be thickening of the wall of the renal pelvis and ureter, also caused by edema and inflammation[50] (Fig. 54-25).

Scintigraphy, computed tomography (CT), magnetic resonance imaging (MRI), and Doppler sonography may show absent or decreased perfusion in a diffuse or lobar distribution, especially at the upper or lower poles.[18,51,52] Pyelonephritis may involve one portion of the kidney more than other parts.[49] Sonography may demonstrate a localized renal mass with altered echogenicity compared to the remainder of the kidney and low-level echoes that disrupt the corticomedullary definition of the kidney in that area.[18] Sequential examinations will demonstrate a rapid change, with resolution of the mass in response to antibiotic therapy. If response to antibiotic therapy is inadequate, the mass may liquefy centrally and become

a **renal abscess** that requires drainage. Sonography of an abscess shows a focal mass with a hypoechoic central area representing liquefied pus (Fig. 54-26). On long-term follow-up, **focal scarring** and clubbed calices may result from the focal infection (Figs. 54-27 and 54-28). Another complication that requires drainage is **pyonephrosis,** identified on sonography as echogenic material filling a dilated collecting system (Fig. 54-29). When patients with UTIs do not respond rapidly to antibiotic therapy, repeat sonographic and/or CT examinations are indicated to search for these complications that require drainage.

Chronic Pyelonephritis

Chronic pyelonephritis is caused by repeated episodes of acute pyelonephritis and results in a small, scarred kidney, indicative of end-stage renal disease. The kidney is usually irregular in outline because of focal parenchymal loss. The renal cortex becomes more echogenic than the liver parenchyma. The pyramids are difficult to outline on sonography (Fig. 54-30). These findings are not specific and can also be seen in chronic glomerulonephritis, dysplastic kidneys, and hypertensive or ischemic disease.

Neonatal Candidiasis

Candida albicans is a saprophytic fungus that usually infects immunocompromised patients, particularly neonates with indwelling catheters receiving broad-spectrum antibiotics. Systemic candidiasis leads to infection of multiple organs, including the kidneys, and neonates may present with anuria, oliguria, a flank mass, or hypertension. Sonography may show diffuse enlargement of the kidney, with loss of normal architecture and presence of abnormal parenchymal echogenicity. Mycelial clumping **(fungus ball formation)** may occur in the collecting system, causing hydronephrosis and echogenic filling defects (Fig. 54-31). The filling defects may obstruct the

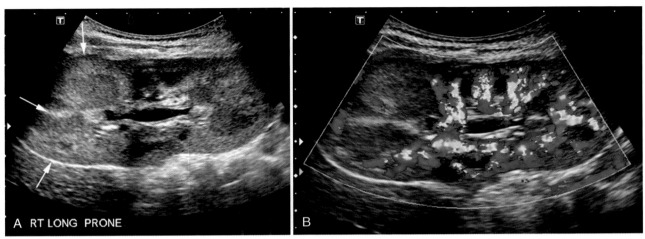

FIGURE 54-24. Acute pyelonephritis in 1-year-old boy. A, Sagittal sonogram of the right kidney shows a swollen upper pole *(arrows).* **B,** On power Doppler sonography, this area is devoid of flow signals.

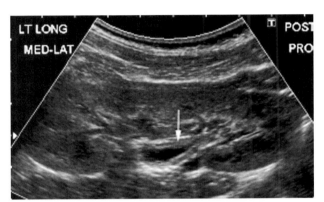

FIGURE 54-25. Thickening of renal pelvis wall. Edema of the wall of the renal pelvis and ureter can occur with inflammation or reflux. The wall *(arrow)* is thickened with medium-level echoes less than the adjacent sinus fat.

collecting system and require drainage procedures (e.g., nephrostomy).[53]

Cystitis

Inflammation of the urinary bladder may occur in children as a result of infection or drug therapy, as with cyclophosphamide (Cytoxan). The bladder wall becomes thickened (>3 mm) and irregular. Echogenic debris or blood clot may be seen in the urine[27] (Fig. 54-32). Rarely an inflammatory pseudotumor may result, with visualization of a bladder mass.

MEDICAL RENAL DISEASE

Glomerulonephritis

The glomerulonephritides include lesions resulting from glomerular reaction to immunologic injury. In **acute**

poststreptococcal glomerulonephritis the kidneys are moderately swollen and have cellular infiltrate in the glomerular tufts. There may be interstitial edema, followed by atrophy. Sonographic findings include normal or bilaterally enlarged kidneys, with diffuse increase in the echogenicity of the renal cortex (Fig. 54-33). The renal cortical echogenicity may be greater than that of the adjacent liver, and the medullary pyramids appear prominent, in contrast to the hyperechoic cortex. The echogenicity of the renal cortex decreases with regression of acute disease, as sonography can demonstrate, obviating the need for serial renal biopsies. The findings in acute glomerulonephritis are those of type I medical renal disease, as described by Rosenfield and Siegel,[54] and are nonspecific, also seen in amyloidosis, nephrosclerosis, **acute tubular necrosis** (ATN), leukemia, Goodpasture's syndrome, Henoch-Schönlein purpura, sepsis, malakoplakia, and the nephrotic syndrome.

In **chronic glomerulonephritis** the kidneys are small, diffusely hyperechogenic, and show loss of corticomedullary differentiation. These findings are also nonspecific and identical to those of end-stage renal disease of any cause.[18]

Elevated Renal Rind

Bilateral perirenal hyperechoic bands several millimeters thick, surrounding a thin hypoechoic rim of fluid, have been described during the acute phase of illness (Fig. 54-34). It is believed that the changes are likely secondary to systemic inflammatory mediators with fluid leakage into the perirenal tissues. The patients were in shock, and the finding resolved in those who survived.[55]

Nephrocalcinosis

Causes of the deposition of calcium within the kidney in childhood include hypervitaminosis D, milk alkali

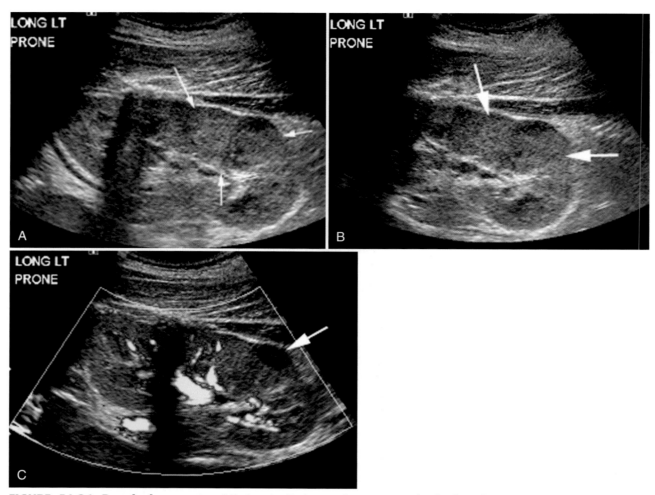

FIGURE 54-26. Renal abscess. A and **B,** Longitudinal scans demonstrates a localized renal mass *(arrows)* and destruction of the cortical medullary definition by an area of focal bacterial nephritis. **C,** Power Doppler image shows decreased flow and anechoic fluid area *(arrow).*

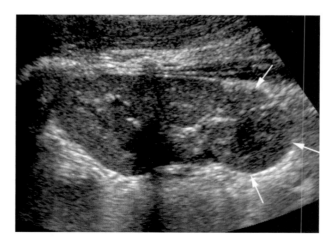

FIGURE 54-27. Focal renal scar. Longitudinal image shows focal thinning of renal parenchyma *(arrows)* of the lower pole.

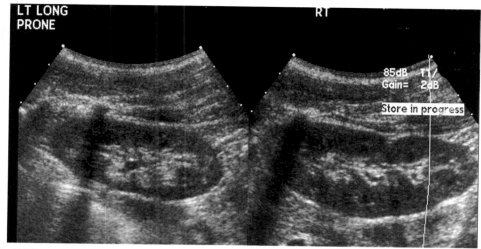

FIGURE 54-28. Diffuse parenchymal loss. Patient with prior infection. Left kidney is small (7.1 cm) compared with normal right kidney (9.2 cm).

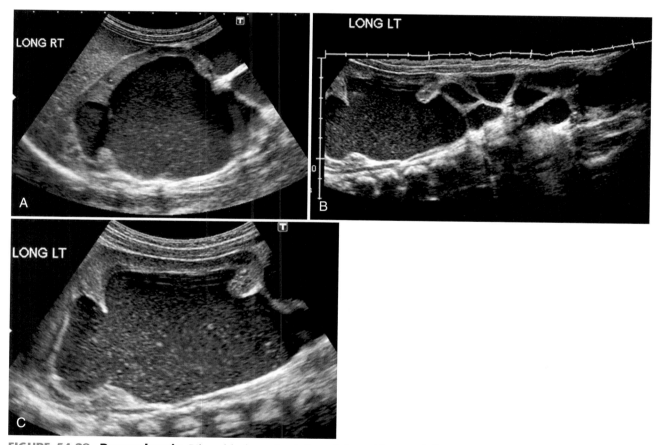

FIGURE 54-29. Pyonephrosis. Bilateral hydronephrosis in an infant with prune-belly syndrome. Sagittal sonograms of the right kidney (**A**) and the left kidney (**B** and **C**) show bilateral hydronephrosis and hydroureter. Urine contains low-level echoes.

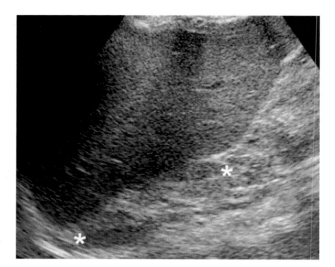

FIGURE 54-30. **Chronic pyelonephritis.** Longitudinal scan of right kidney and liver shows small hyperechoic kidney with poor corticomedullary differentiation *(between cursors).*

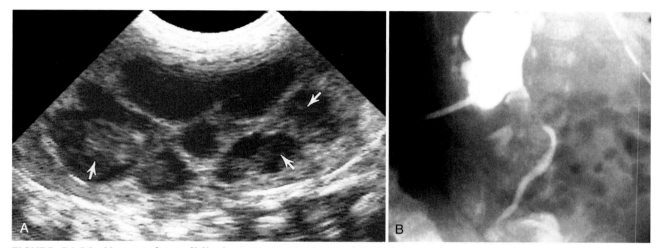

FIGURE 54-31. **Neonatal candidiasis.** **A,** Longitudinal scan of the right kidney shows hydronephrosis with echogenic filling defects *(arrows)* representing fungus ball formation. **B,** Nephrostomy was performed under ultrasound guidance to drain obstructed system.

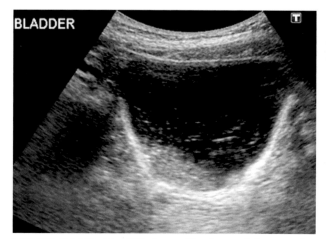

FIGURE 54-32. **Cystitis in patient receiving cyclophosphamide.** Longitudinal scan of pelvis shows thick-walled bladder and echogenic debris and blood clot in urine.

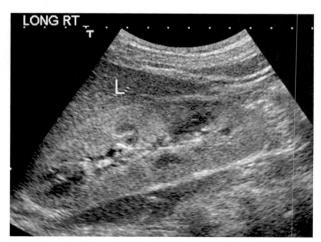

FIGURE 54-33. **Acute glomerulonephritis.** Longitudinal scan of right kidney demonstrates renal enlargement with diffuse increase in renal cortical echogenicity greater than adjacent liver *(L).*

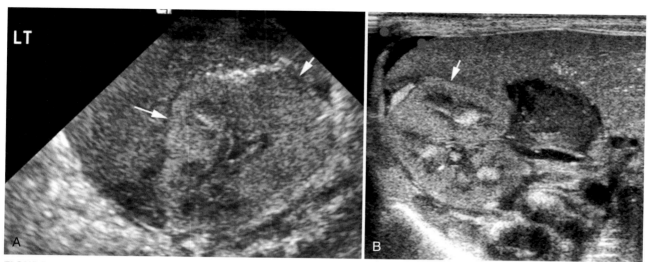

FIGURE 54-34. Renal rind. A, Longitudinal scan of left kidney. **B,** Transverse scan of right kidney. Hypoechoic rim of fluid is seen surrounding the kidney. Changes are likely secondary to systemic inflammation, with fluid leaking into the perirenal tissues.

syndrome, renal tubular acidosis, hyperparathyroidism, hyperoxaluria, sarcoidosis, Cushing's syndrome, Williams' syndrome, and chronic treatment with furosemide (in premature infants). In these conditions an increased load of calcium is presented to the kidney. The mineral content within the kidney increases progressively from the glomerulus to the collecting ducts, and thus the greatest concentration of calcium is found in the pyramids, especially at their tips. Randall, Anderson, and Carr described calcareous deposits at the tips or sides of pyramids at microscopy in normal pediatric and adult cadaver kidneys. Bruwer[56] outlined identical deposits in cadaver kidney slices using high-resolution radiography. These authors postulate that the concentration of calcium is high in fluids about the renal tubules, and that calcium is normally removed from this area by lymphatic flow. If the calcium load exceeds the lymphatic capacity, microscopic calcium aggregates occur in the medulla, mainly at the tips of the fornix and at the margins. They may fuse to form plaque (e.g., Randall's) and migrate toward the caliceal epithelium, finally perforating it. A nidus for urinary stones is provided. Bruwer termed this process the "Anderson-Carr-Randall progression" of calculus formation.

CAUSES OF NEPHROCALCINOSIS

Hypervitaminosis D
Milk alkali syndrome
Renal tubular acidosis
Hyperparathyroidism
Hyperoxaluria
Sarcoidosis
Cushing's syndrome
Williams' syndrome
Chronic treatment with furosemide (Lasix)

Sonography is more sensitive than radiography in detecting calcium deposits within the kidney. Four patterns of calcium deposition within the kidney show the progression from nephrocalcinosis to formation of macroscopic plaques of calcium near the calyx[57] (Fig. 54-35). These later perforate into the calyx and form a ureteral stone. Any form of urinary stasis predisposes not only to infection, but also to calcium formation.[18] Thus the tubular ectasia encountered in **medullary sponge kidney** and also in autosomal recessive polycystic kidney disease associated with congenital hepatic fibrosis often shows deposits of calcium, once again in the pyramids, at the site of the dilated tubules. Similarly, milk of calcium may deposit in **caliceal diverticula** or in UPJ obstruction[58] (Fig. 54-36). **Staghorn calculi** occur occasionally in children with obstruction and infection (Fig. 54-37).

The finely branching calcifications within the cortex and medulla of the kidney found after **renal vein thrombosis** are actually calcified microthrombi in the intrarenal veins.[59] **Chronic infections,** such as mycoses and tuberculosis, **tumors,** and tubular or papillary **necrosis** or infection cause dystrophic calcification at the renal site affected.[60]

RENAL TRAUMA

Because the child's kidneys are relatively larger and less protected than the adult's, the kidneys are frequently affected when the abdomen is injured. Preexisting and often clinically silent renal abnormalities such as hydronephrosis may make the kidney more susceptible to injury by minor trauma. Renal trauma is often associated with other organ injury, particularly of the liver and spleen. CT has become the primary imaging modality for suspected multiorgan blunt abdominal trauma in the

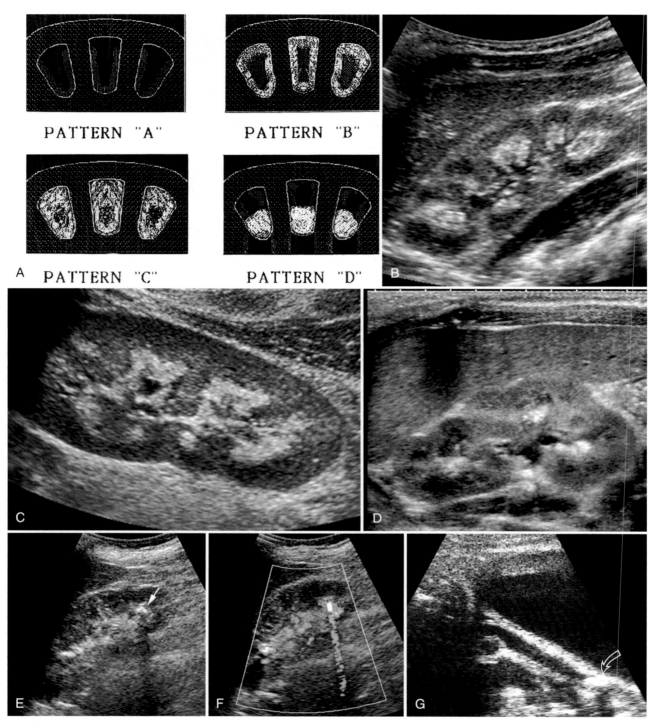

FIGURE 54-35. Nephrocalcinosis. A, Diagram of four sonographic patterns of renal medullary **calcium deposition.** Patterns A, B, and C represent increasing stages of calcium deposition beginning in the periphery of the renal pyramids. Pattern D shows stone formation at fornices. **B,** Nephrocalcinosis (type B) in a boy with **renal tubular acidosis.** Calcium deposits are at the periphery of the pyramids. **C,** Type C pattern in a 7-month-old boy with **glycogenosis.** Sonogram of the right kidney shows pyramids virtually completely filled with calcium deposits. **D,** Pattern D. Sonogram of right kidney shows hyperechoic foci with acoustic shadows in the tips of the pyramids (fornices), suggesting presence of calcium. **E,** A small renal stone at edge of calyx *(arrow).* **F,** Color Doppler shows "twinkle" phenomenon. **G,** Longitudinal sonogram shows a stone impacted in dilated distal right ureter *(arrow). (A from Patriquin H, Robitaille P. Renal calcium deposition in children: sonographic demonstration of the Anderson-Carr progression. AJR Am J Roentgenol 1986;146: 1253-1256.)*

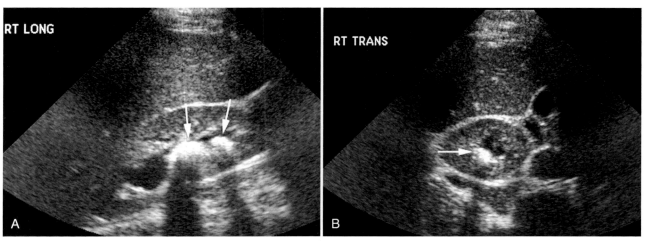

FIGURE 54-36. Urinary calculi. A, Supine longitudinal scan, and **B,** transverse sonogram, show urine–milk of calcium levels in dependent part of dilated calices. The milk of calcium moved with change in patient position.

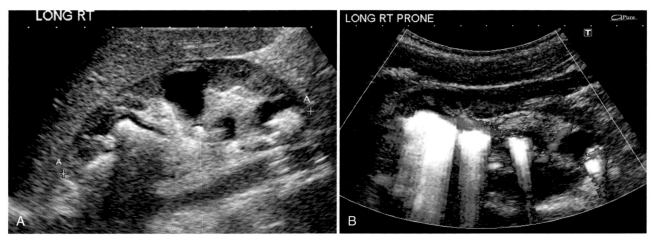

FIGURE 54-37. Staghorn calculi. A, Teenager with chronic hydronephrosis and multiple echogenic foci in dilated calices. **B,** Color Doppler demonstrates ringdown artifact.

pediatric patient.[61] Ultrasound is used primarily in the follow-up of the injuries found on CT.[62] Sonography in renal trauma shows distortion of the normal renal architecture (Fig. 54-38). Renal hematoma can vary but is usually echogenic at first and becomes hypoechoic as it liquefies. Extravasation of urine may occur around the kidney, which can be difficult to distinguish from hypoechoic blood. Injuries to the vascular renal pedicle are uncommon but constitute a surgical emergency. Doppler sonography can demonstrate both arterial and venous patency. Absent flow signals in part of or all the kidney—when signals are detected elsewhere in the abdomen—herald arterial obstruction. The sonographic gray-scale appearance of the kidney acutely deprived of its arterial blood supply is normal. Power Doppler ultrasound can increase sensitivity in detecting areas of decreased perfusion and hemorrhage.

RENAL AND ADRENAL TUMORS

The most common abdominal masses in the child are of renal origin: hydronephrosis and multicystic renal dysplasia (MCDK).[19] Solid tumors are less common. Initial imaging includes sonography and often a plain film of the abdomen. The site of origin of the mass, its architecture (cystic or solid), and vascularization can usually be outlined with sonography. Metastases and tumoral invasion of the renal vein or inferior vena cava are sought during the sonographic survey of the abdomen. If the mass is cystic and arises from the kidney, the most likely differential diagnosis is between a hydronephrotic kidney and MCDK. The configuration of the cysts on sonography and presence of function on nuclear renogram help distinguish these two entities. If the mass is solid and

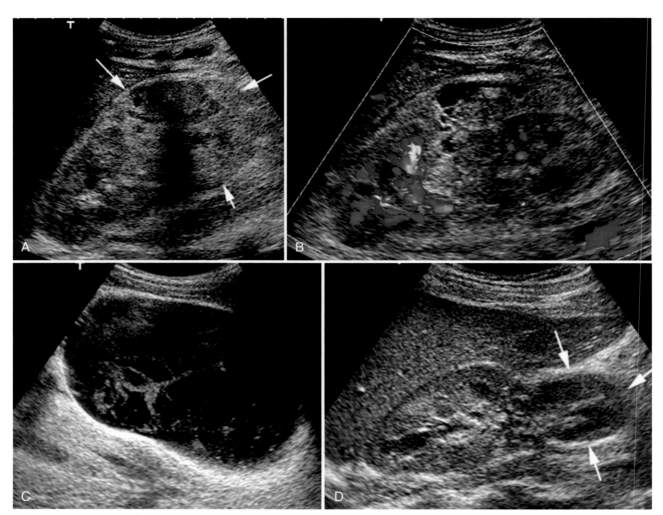

FIGURE 54-38. Renal trauma. A, Longitudinal scan shows heterogeneous echogenicity in the lower pole area of injury *(arrows).* **B,** Power Doppler image shows decreased flow in the area of injury *(arrow).* **C,** Bladder contains echogenic clot. **D,** Lower pole has parenchymal atrophy 2 months later.

related to the kidney, Wilms' tumor is the most likely diagnosis. Staging of the tumor is usually done with CT or MRI. If the kidney is normal and the mass is related to another organ, the work-up continues with imaging that is optimal for that organ. Several types of renal tumors occur in the pediatric patient.[18,63]

MALFORMATIONS ASSOCIATED WITH WILMS' TUMOR

Congenital hemihypertrophy
Beckwith-Wiedemann syndrome
Sporadic aniridia
Neurofibromatosis
Cerebral gigantism

Wilms' Tumor

Wilms' tumor, or **nephroblastoma,** is the most common intra-abdominal malignant tumor to occur in the child. Its incidence peaks between 2 and 5 years of age.[64] When large, it may be difficult to differentiate from neuroblastoma, which frequently arises from the adrenal gland and occurs in a similar age group. Wilms' tumor is usually bulky and expands within the renal parenchyma, resulting in distortion and displacement of the collecting system and capsule. It is usually sharply marginated.[18] Typically, a large solid mass distorting the sinus, pyramids, cortex, and contour of the kidney is outlined with sonography (Fig. 54-39). Although usually quite hyperechoic and homogeneous, there may be hypoechoic areas that represent hemorrhage and necrosis.[65,66] Power Doppler and contrast ultrasound will show decreased perfusion. From 5% to 10% of patients have bilateral

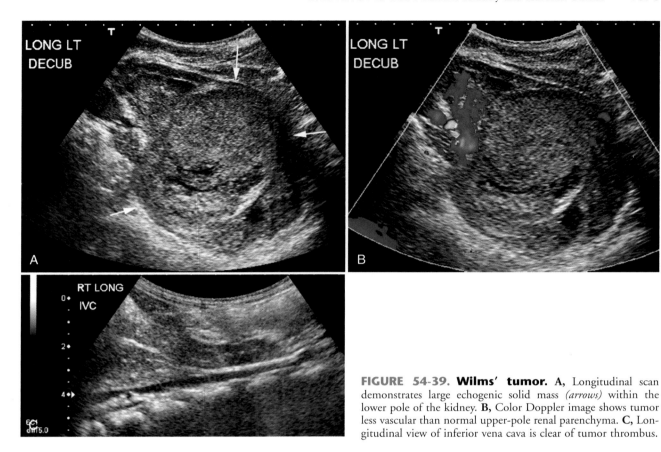

FIGURE 54-39. Wilms' tumor. A, Longitudinal scan demonstrates large echogenic solid mass *(arrows)* within the lower pole of the kidney. **B,** Color Doppler image shows tumor less vascular than normal upper-pole renal parenchyma. **C,** Longitudinal view of inferior vena cava is clear of tumor thrombus.

tumors, and nephroblastomatosis may be present in both kidneys in children with unilateral Wilms' tumors.[67] Specific malformations associated with Wilms' tumors and nephrogenic rests include congenital hemihypertrophy, Beckwith-Wiedemann syndrome, sporadic aniridia, neurofibromatosis, and cerebral gigantism.[64]

Wilms' tumor spreads through direct extension into the renal sinus and peripelvic soft tissues, the lymph nodes in the renal hilum, and the para-aortic areas. Because extension is possible into the renal vein, inferior vena cava, right atrium, and liver, these areas should also be examined for the presence of tumor (Fig. 54-39, *C*). Color and spectral Doppler sonography is useful in detecting residual flow around a tumor clot, as well as tumor arterial signals both from the periphery of the tumor[68] and from within the tumor thrombus. The opposite kidney should be carefully examined for the presence of bilateral tumor. CT and MRI are usually performed for further work-up and staging. CT is often favored because the chest can also be evaluated for metastases,[69] which most frequently involve the lungs.

Neuroblastoma

The second most common abdominal tumor of childhood, occurring mainly between ages 2 months and 2 years, is neuroblastoma. It arises from the adrenal gland or the sympathetic nervous chain. Its extrarenal origin displaces and compresses the kidney without otherwise distorting the internal renal architecture. Neuroblastoma spreads early and widely, so the majority of patients have metastases at presentation. Its spread around the aorta and celiac and superior mesenteric arteries occurs early and helps to distinguish neuroblastoma from Wilms' tumor at sonography. Wilms' tumor is usually well defined and relatively homogeneous, whereas neuroblastoma is poorly defined and heterogeneous, with irregular hyperechogenic areas caused by calcifications[70,71] (Fig. 54-40). Syndromes associated with neuroblastoma include Beckwith-Wiedemann syndrome, Klippel-Feil syndrome, fetal alcohol and phenylhydantoin syndromes, and Hirschsprung's disease. Sonography is followed by CT or MRI for staging of the disease. MRI is particularly useful because the tumor can extend into the spinal canal and cause neurologic symptoms. It is critical to know if this extension has occurred before the tumor is surgically removed because the child may develop neurologic symptoms postoperatively if the tumor is not carefully resected.

Mesoblastic Nephroma

Mesoblastic nephroma or **fetal renal hamartoma** (congenital Wilms' tumor) is the most common neonatal

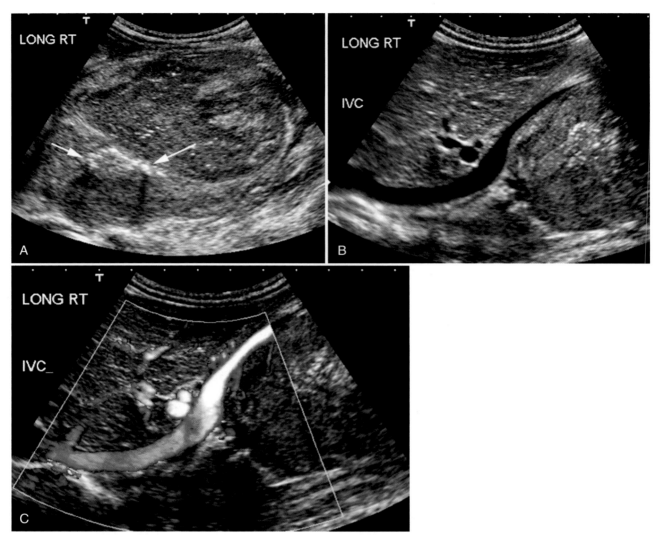

FIGURE 54-40. Neuroblastoma. A and **B,** Longitudinal scans of the right upper abdomen demonstrate inhomogeneously solid mass with focal areas of calcification *(arrows)* and shadowing. **C,** Color Doppler ultrasound. The aorta is displaced arteriorly by the mass.

renal neoplasm in the first few months of life and is sometimes detected in the fetus. It is a benign tumor but can spread by local invasion and is usually treated by simple nephrectomy. Sonography demonstrates a mass arising within the kidney, appearing similar to a Wilms' tumor. The tumor is solid but may have cystic-appearing areas of hemorrhage and necrosis (Fig. 54-41). The young age of the patient, the tumor's benign biologic behavior, and its more favorable outcome help to differentiate mesoblastic nephroma from the classic Wilms' tumor.[72]

Renal Cell Carcinoma

Renal cell carcinoma, rare in childhood, occurs later (mean age 12 years) than Wilms' tumor. Its presentation and sonographic appearance are similar to those in adults.

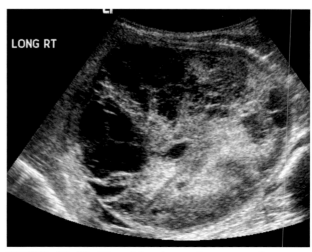

FIGURE 54-41. Mesoblastic nephroma. Infant with a large abdominal mass. Tumor is mixed in echogenicity without calcifications.

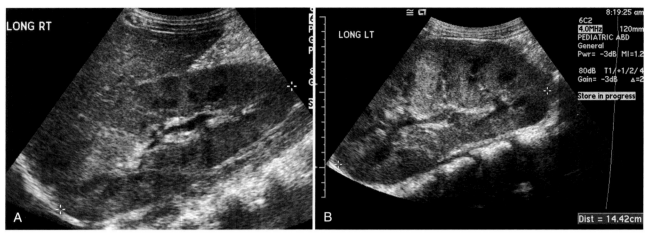

FIGURE 54-42. Renal lymphoma. Longitudinal scans of right kidney (**A**) and left kidneys (**B**) demonstrate bilateral renal enlargement with thickened cortex and increased echogenicity.

Angiomyolipoma

Angiomyolipoma is a form of hamartoma that can cause symptoms related to hemorrhage and rupture. In children, these tumors are usually multiple and are associated with **tuberous sclerosis.**[41] Sonography typically shows multiple masses of varying echogenicity and, because of the fat content, some masses may be hyperechogenic (see Fig. 54-22, *A*). There may be associated cysts within the kidney, and the kidneys may be enlarged.

Multilocular Renal Cyst

Also called a **cystic nephroma,** the multilocular renal cyst is a rare lesion that is generally considered benign. It can occur at any age but is uncommon in children younger than 2 years. The mass is composed of multiple cysts of varying size joined by connective tissue septa. It may be difficult to distinguish from cystic, well-differentiated Wilms' tumor, with nephroblastoma components in the walls of the cysts. Sonography demonstrates a well-circumscribed, multiloculated cystic mass with septations. Some suggest a malignant potential for these lesions and recommend nephrectomy.[63,73]

Renal Lymphoma

Lymphomatous involvement of the kidney is usually a secondary process and can be seen on sonography as single or multiple, relatively hypoechoic or weakly echogenic masses within the kidney. The kidney may be enlarged and lobulated in outline. Diffuse infiltration of the kidney can also occur[74,75] (Fig. 54-42).

Bladder Tumors

Primary tumors of the lower urinary tract are uncommon in children. **Sarcoma botryoides** is a rhabdomyosarcoma arising in the bladder base in males, presenting with bladder outlet obstruction (Fig. 54-43). In girls, this rare tumor typically occurs in the uterus or vagina. Polyps can occur in the urethra.[27]

DOPPLER OPTIMIZATION FOR SLOW FLOW

Highest transducer frequency
Restriction of color area of interest
Low pulse repetition frequency (PRF)
Aliasing corrected by increasing PRF
Small sample volume
Lowest vessel/beam angle

DOPPLER ASSESSMENT OF RENAL VASCULAR DISEASE IN CHILDREN

Kidney Examination Technique

Infants and small children are examined without special preparation, but they may be given juice or milk to drink during the examination to calm them, to increase hydration, and to provide an acoustic window through the fluid-filled stomach. Sedation is rarely necessary. The older child is examined after a 4- to 6-hour fast (to reduce intestinal gas) only if a detailed examination of the main renal artery is planned. Color and pulsed Doppler examinations are performed. Power Doppler may also be useful to evaluate the presence of vascular flow. Doppler settings are adjusted for maximal detection of slow flow: highest possible transducer frequency, relatively small color area of interest, low pulse repetition frequency, and low wall filter. Pulse repetition frequency is augmented if aliasing occurs. A small sample volume and the lowest possible vessel/beam angle are used.

The aorta and main renal arteries are examined by means of an anterior left paramedian as well as a left axillary approach, with longitudinal and transverse views. The color Doppler mode is used to trace the renal arteries, which are then examined with serial pulsed Doppler samples, especially in areas of high-velocity

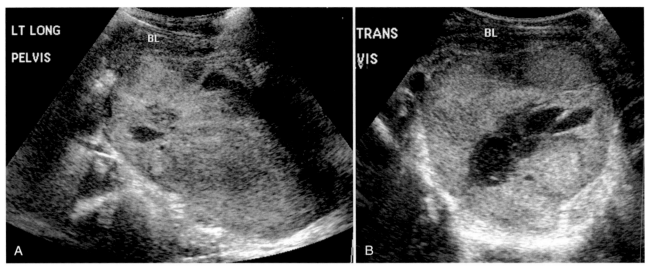

FIGURE 54-43. Bladder rhabdomyosarcoma. A and **B,** Longitudinal and transverse scans of the pelvis demonstrate large, heterogeneous mass filling the pelvis. Bladder *(BL)* is compressed anteriorly.

flow. Even if the entire renal artery cannot be outlined because of overlying intestinal gas, the retrocaval portion of the right renal artery and the hilar arteries can usually be analyzed. A segmental or interlobar artery in each third of the kidney (upper, middle, and lower) is then studied with pulsed Doppler, and the resistive index (Pourcelot) or pulsatility index is calculated.

Normal Vascular Anatomy and Flow Patterns

The intrarenal arteries and veins and their relationship to the renal cortex, pyramids, and calices are exceptionally well outlined with color Doppler technology.[76] The main renal artery(ies) divides in the renal hilum to form several pairs (anterior and posterior) of segmental arteries. These course toward the pyramids and there divide into interlobar branches, which follow the periphery of the pyramids. At the outer edge of the pyramids, interlobar arteries give rise to arcuate arteries, which follow the outer contour of the pyramids. Cortical arteries arise from the arcuate arteries and radiate into the cortex, following a direction similar to that of interlobar vessels. The venous circulation follows that of the arteries, and simultaneous adjacent signals are often visible both with color Doppler sonography and on spectral analysis (Fig. 54-44).

The renal arterial bed normally has low resistance, and there is a constant flow into the kidney throughout the cardiac cycle. The normal **adult resistive index** (RI) is estimated at 0.65 ± 0.10. In the **neonatal** period, probably concurrent with the physiologic low glomerular filtration rate, the resistance of the renal arterial bed is somewhat higher: RI = 0.7 to 0.8. Because there is a range of normal RI values, the diagnosis of abnormal intrarenal resistance is much more reliably made by comparing waveforms from the pathologic kidney to those of the normal kidney, or tracings one day to the next of the pathologic kidney.

Pulsed Doppler tracings from the normal intrarenal and main renal veins are somewhat variable: in some children the pulsations from right atrial diastole and systole are clearly visible, whereas in others the flow is steadier (Fig. 54-44). To-and-fro venous flow throughout the cardiac cycle may be seen in right-sided heart failure or in the absence of arterial perfusion of end-stage renal disease.

Causes of Increased Resistance to Intrarenal Arterial Flow

Any increase in intrarenal arterial pressure results in decreased flow. Diastolic flow occurs at the lowest pressure during the cardiac cycle, so it will decrease or disappear before systolic Doppler flow curves are affected appreciably. The causes of increased intrarenal resistance to flow can be classified as **intravascular, perivascular,** and **perirenal** (Fig. 54-45). Any decrease in the size of the lumen of small intrarenal arteries or arterioles (spasm, as in shock; endothelial inflammation, as in hemolytic uremic syndrome) leads to increased resistance to arterial inflow. However, compression of small vessels by intrarenal edema (e.g., renal vein thrombosis) may result in identical arterial Doppler tracings. Back pressure from an acutely obstructed ureter has the same result. Finally, significant compression from hematomas, lymphangiomas, or the tight abdominal wall around an adult kidney transplanted into a small child may have the same effect.

The successful Doppler examination of intrarenal arteries therefore comprises the following two steps:
1. Comparing the RI either to the other side or to a previous examination.
2. Reviewing the pertinent pathophysiologic factors involved in a patient with high RI.

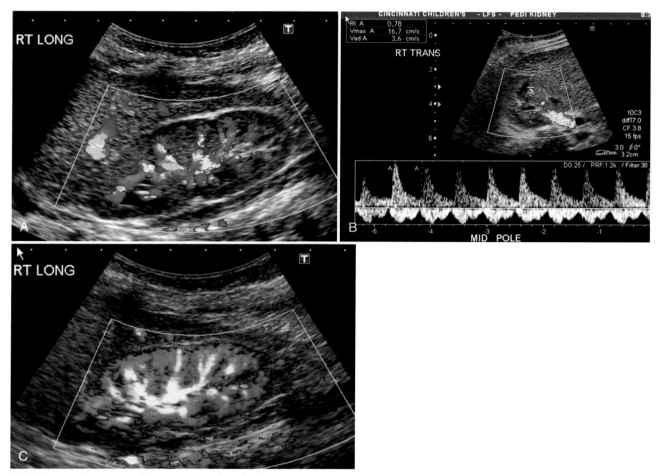

FIGURE 54-44. Normal intrarenal circulation. A, Color Doppler sonogram of an infant shows the position of intrarenal vessels at the hilum (segmental) alongside the pyramids (interlobar) and at the inner edge of the cortex (arcuate). **B,** Spectral display from a normal segmented artery (parabolic, low resistance, allowing high diastolic flow) and vein (triphasic flow reflecting right atrial pulsations). **C,** Power Doppler ultrasound with increased sensitivity demonstrates flow in the renal cortex to the periphery.

CAUSES OF INCREASED RESISTIVE INDEX IN RENAL ARTERIES

INTRAVASCULAR
Vascular spasm in shock
Endothelial inflammation in hemolytic uremic
  syndrome

PERIVASCULAR
Intrarenal edema
Renal vein thrombosis
Acutely obstructed ureter

PERIRENAL COMPRESSION
Hematoma
Lymphangioma
Tight abdominal wall

Clinical Applications

Vessel Patency

The Doppler examination is a reliable indicator of the patency of the renal arteries, of the veins, and of the presence of intrarenal perfusion. Therefore the examination is particularly useful in the evaluation of allograft perfusion immediately after surgery. It is also useful in the exclusion of arterial injury after trauma, especially when the renal architecture is sonographically normal and other, more invasive examinations are not indicated. Color Doppler sonography is especially valuable in the search for postbiopsy arteriovenous (AV) fistulas and aneurysms.[77]

Acute Renal Vein Thrombosis

Acute renal vein thrombosis may follow shock or occur after the nephrotic syndrome, in abnormal coagulation,

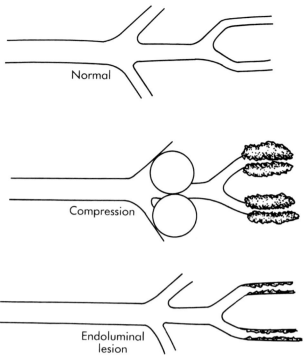

FIGURE 54-45. Causes of increased resistance to intrarenal arterial flow. Diagram of intrarenal circulation.

CAUSES OF ACUTE RENAL VEIN THROMBOSIS

Shock
Nephrotic syndrome
Coagulopathy
Adjacent tumors (e.g., Wilms' tumor)
Neonatal dehydration, especially infants of diabetic
  mothers

---

or in the presence of a nearby malignant mass, such as Wilms' tumor. In the neonate, thrombosis is usually associated with dehydration, decreased renal perfusion and oxygenation, and polycythemia. It is more prevalent in infants of diabetic mothers. The clinical presentation includes hematuria, palpable flank mass, proteinuria, and decreased renal function. Sonography typically shows an enlarged kidney with altered parenchymal echogenicity (Figs. 54-46 and 54-47). The normal corticomedullary differentiation is obliterated. Patchy areas of decreased and increased echogenicity are secondary to edema and parenchymal hemorrhage.[78] Sonography may demonstrate echogenic thrombus within the renal vein and inferior vena cava. Thrombi start in small venules and propagate toward the hilum, so renal parenchymal abnormalities are often present without clear visualization of a thrombus. (In the renal allograft, thrombosis usually starts at the anastomosis.)

Doppler sonography has shown decreased or absent flow in the renal veins, as well as a significantly increased RI in the involved renal arteries. This decreased renal arterial diastolic flow is caused by edema and obstruction to outflow of arterial blood entering the kidney. In babies these signs are much less reliable because flow is rapidly reestablished in the main renal vein, as well as within intrarenal veins. Diastolic flow, although affected in the early stages of the process, is rapidly reestablished to 80% or 90% of that of the opposite kidney. There appears to be an increased number of collateral veins around the hilum of the kidney and around the vertebral column (see Fig. 54-46). This reestablishment of venous flow occurs not only in native kidneys but also in renal transplants, although the process takes much longer, up to 3 weeks in the transplanted kidney.[78,79]

CAUSES OF RENAL ARTERY STENOSIS

Fibromuscular hyperplasia
Neurofibromatosis
Radiation arteritis
Coarctation of the aorta
Takayasu's disease

SIGNS OF RENAL ARTERY STENOSIS

Increased resistance to flow proximally
Decreased or absent diastolic or even systolic flow
High velocity at the site of narrowing (>180 cm/
  sec)
Turbulence immediately distally
Downstream circulation showing parvus-tardus
  curve

Renal Artery Stenosis

Renovascular disease accounts for up to 10% of cases of hypertension in children. Many cases are associated with established disorders including vasculitides (Takayasu's disease, moyamoya), syndromes (Turner, Marfan, Williams, Klippel-Trenaunay-Weber, midaortic), neurofibromatosis and previous renal artery surgery. Hypertensive children without these comorbid conditions often have single, focal branch artery stenoses.[80]

Sonography of the abdominal aorta and of renal size and architecture is useful to exclude global nephropathy, mass, or focal scarring. Doppler ultrasound is not routinely performed because the small renal arteries are not seen sonographically, and Doppler is not highly sensitive for detecting renal vascular disease in these children with small branch vessel stenosis. Detailed examination of the renal arteries with angiography may be performed to detect renovascular disease.

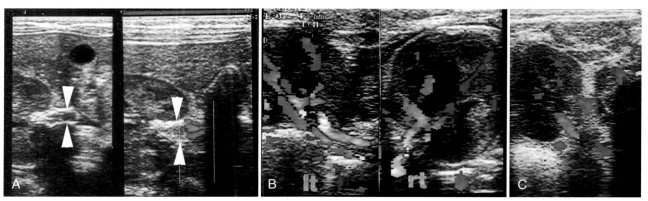

FIGURE 54-46. Renal vein thrombosis. A, Coronal sonograms of the right renal hilum in a 12-day-old infant show a calcified thrombus dilating the renal vein, with color Doppler signals around the clot. **B,** Prone coronal sonograms of the normal left *(lt)* and thrombosed right *(rt)* kidneys showing arterial and venous flow signals in both kidneys. There is venous flow around the renal vein clot at the right hilum. **C,** Left renal vein thrombosis in a 1-year-old infant on prone sonogram. Note tiny calcifications, mainly in the medulla, and numerous collateral renal veins at the hilum and near the spine.

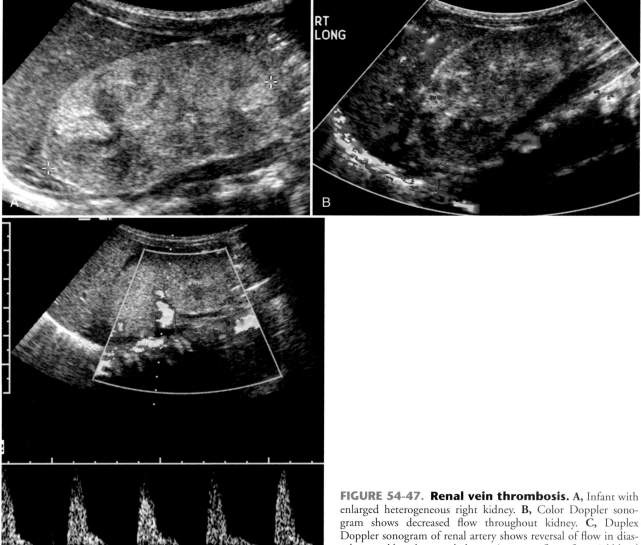

FIGURE 54-47. Renal vein thrombosis. A, Infant with enlarged heterogeneous right kidney. **B,** Color Doppler sonogram shows decreased flow throughout kidney. **C,** Duplex Doppler sonogram of renal artery shows reversal of flow in diastole caused by edema and obstruction to outflow of arterial blood entering the kidney.

The **classic signs of stenosis** include increased resistance to flow proximally (decreased or absent diastolic or even systolic flow), high velocity at the site of narrowing (>180 cm/sec), turbulence immediately distally, and flow possibly returning to normal at some distance from the stenosis. The following renal arterial Doppler criteria have been found to suggest significant stenosis[81]:

1. Flow velocity measurements exceeding 180 cm/sec
2. Velocity ratio between renal artery and abdominal aorta greater than 3.5:1.

In addition, the effects of severe arterial stenosis on the downstream circulation can be used to diagnose stenosis. These **downstream effects**, caused by a loss of kinetic energy and the normal high elastic recoil of renal arteries, include the following[81,82]:

• Decreased flow velocity
• Dampened systolic wave
• Slowed acceleration of systolic upstroke

Because the intrarenal arteries are almost always accessible to Doppler interrogation, the secondary effects of severe (>75%) renal arterial stenosis may well be reflected here[81,82] (Fig. 54-48). Doppler curves return to normal immediately after repair of stenosis. It must be remembered that the **parvus-tardus curve** (described in the downstream circulation) reflects any stenosis occurring upstream, including Takayasu's disease or coarctation of the aorta.

Intrarenal Arterial Disease

The **hemolytic uremic syndrome** (HUS), consisting of anemia, thrombocytopenia, and acute renal failure (ARF), usually follows gastroenteritis, especially *Escherichia coli* 0157:H7 infection and its resultant toxins. HUS is a major cause of ARF in children and leads to multiple glomerular thrombi and vasculitis affecting arterioles in the kidney. These lesions cause increased resistance to arterial flow into the kidney. At sonography, the renal cortex is uniformly hyperechogenic, and the pyramids are sharply demarcated (Fig. 54-49). The kidneys may greatly enlarge. During a study of 20 children with HUS, we found that during the phase of anuria, there was no diastolic flow.[83] As the acute vascular lesions healed, diastolic flow returned, followed by diuresis within 24 to 48 hours. Because the Doppler examinations predicted the onset of diuresis, the duration of peritoneal dialysis was kept to a minimum, thus reducing the risk of complications.

Hydronephrosis

Not all dilated renal collecting systems in children are obstructed, and an acutely obstructed ureter can go into spasm and not dilate at all. DTPA-furosemide scintigraphy and the Whitaker test are being used to distinguish dilated from truly obstructed ureters, with incomplete success.

No reliable distinguishing test exists, so the Doppler examinations in this field are being watched with interest, especially in pediatric urology. Acute ureteral obstruction causes immediate intrarenal vasodilation, followed several hours later by vasoconstriction. During days or weeks, this vasoconstriction lessens because pressure is relieved by forniceal rupture or because of hormone-mediated adaptation.[84] The effect of acute vasoconstriction has been shown on angiography in animals in which ureteral ligation was followed by absence of arteriolar filling after injection of contrast material into the renal artery.[85] Platt et al.[86] showed decreased diastolic flow, reflecting increased arterial resistance, on Doppler sonography in adults with acute ureteral obstruction. The RI measurements are best compared to the patient's own norm: the normal kidney in unilateral disease (see Fig. 54-45) or a preoperative baseline examination in the case of a single kidney or a renal allograft. Garcia-Pena et al.[87] showed that the RI in the obstructed kidney of children exceeds that from the healthy kidney by 0.08 or more. Increased resistance appears to be detectable only in the acutely obstructed kidney. In an ongoing study of 110 children with unilateral urinary obstruction, we have found no significant alterations in RI from chronically obstructed kidneys, such as in utero–detected UPJ stenosis.

Ureteral Jets

Visible at both urography and vesical sonography, ureteric jets are easily perceptible with Doppler imaging.[88] The jet is measured within the bladder, near the ureterovesical junction, in transverse section. It has a near-vertical upsweep, a short peak, and a rapid downsweep. In partial ureteral obstruction, the normal jet is replaced by a slow, almost constant dribble of urine entering the bladder (Fig. 54-50). However, abnormally located ureteral orifices can be outlined with this method, because the more lateral the orifice, the greater the probability of vesicoureteral reflux. Doppler sonography of ureteric jets is reportedly sensitive enough to use for monitoring treatment of reflux.[88]

Renal Transplantation

Common causes of malfunction of a renal allograft soon after surgery include dehydration; obstruction of the renal artery, vein, or ureter; ATN; acute rejection; cyclosporine toxicity; and infection (pyelonephritis). Sonography is the screening examination of choice in the search for anatomic abnormalities. The hemodynamic information obtained with Doppler is useful in several ways. The Doppler examination is a reliable indicator of the patency of the newly anastomosed renal artery and vein and the flow in the intrarenal (segmental, interlobar, arcuate) arteries and veins,[89] as well as into postbiopsy AV shunts.[90] The renal artery and its anastomosis to the

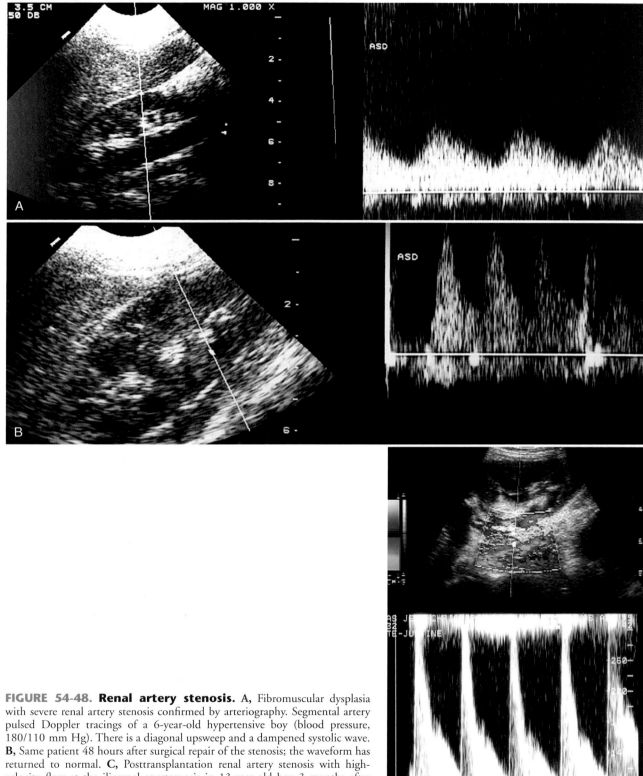

FIGURE 54-48. Renal artery stenosis. A, Fibromuscular dysplasia with severe renal artery stenosis confirmed by arteriography. Segmental artery pulsed Doppler tracings of a 6-year-old hypertensive boy (blood pressure, 180/110 mm Hg). There is a diagonal upsweep and a dampened systolic wave. **B,** Same patient 48 hours after surgical repair of the stenosis; the waveform has returned to normal. **C,** Posttransplantation renal artery stenosis with high-velocity flow at the iliorenal anastomosis in 13-year-old boy 3 months after renal transplantation. Sagittal color Doppler image of the graft shows high-velocity *(yellow)* turbulent flow (Doppler *cursor*). The spectral display shows velocity of 280 cm/sec (angle 60 degrees). *(From Patriquin HB, Lafortune M, Jequier JC, et al. Stenosis of the renal artery: assessment of slowed systole in the downstream circulation with Doppler sonography. Radiology 1992;184:479-485.)*

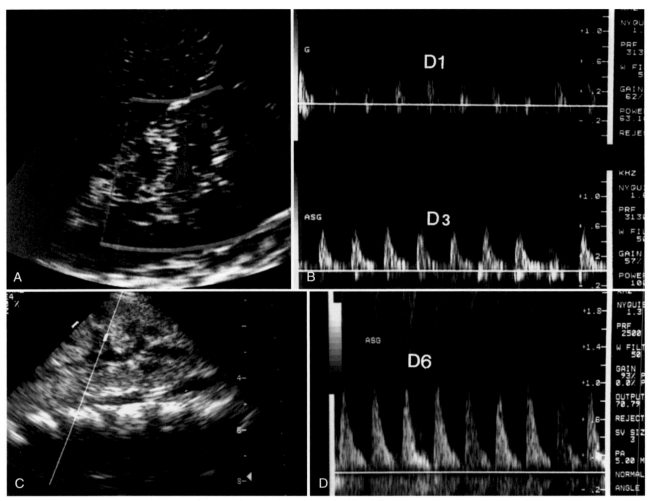

FIGURE 54-49. Hemolytic uremic syndrome in 2-year-old girl. A, Color Doppler ultrasound shows patent segmental and interlobar artery *(red)* outlined against the side of a pyramid, well seen because of the intensely hyperechoic cortex. **B,** Spectral Doppler display from a segmental artery during the anuric phase. Day 1 *(top):* systole is very short; there is no diastolic flow; the resistive index is therefore 1.0. Day 3 *(bottom):* systole has lengthened and there is some diastolic flow. **C** and **D,** Spectral Doppler ultrasound, day 6: diastolic flow is much improved even though end diastolic flow is not yet normal.

iliac artery are usually seen with real-time and Doppler ultrasound; the detection of renal artery stenosis in a **graft** is much easier than in the native kidney (Fig. 54-51). The renal artery is traced from the hilum to the iliac artery. The Doppler pattern changes from pan-diastolic flow in the renal artery to the typical high-resistance pattern with reversed early diastolic flow in the iliac artery distal to the graft. Stenosis is signaled by a zone of high-frequency Doppler shift. The flow pattern beyond the stenosis and within the kidney may be normal or may show a pulsus parvus-tardus waveform.

Rejection of the Renal Allograft

Histocompatibility difference between donor and recipient (unless they are monozygotic twins) leads to rejection of the renal allograft. The two types of rejection are interstitial or **cellular,** mediated by T cells, and vascular or **humoral,** mediated by B cells. In the **interstitial** type of rejection, T cells activated by graft antigens stimulate

the production of inflammatory cells that in turn cause cellular infiltration of the cortex, edema of the interstitium, and ATN. Inflammatory cells are found within interlobular capillaries, venules, and lymphatics, but arterioles and glomeruli are usually spared. Interstitial rejection resembles **tubulointerstitial nephritis** histologically. Vessel lumina are not reduced in caliber, and thus renal impedance and diastolic flow are not primarily affected. In the **vascular** type of rejection, activated B cells produce antigraft antibodies directed against the endothelium of arterioles and capillaries. The result is swelling and inflammation of the endothelium, which leads to vessel wall damage. Stasis of blood flow is greatly increased, which leads to decreased, absent, or reversed diastolic flow.[91]

Posttransplant Resistance

Timing of Rejection Acute rejection occurs mainly between posttransplantation weeks 3 and 12 but may

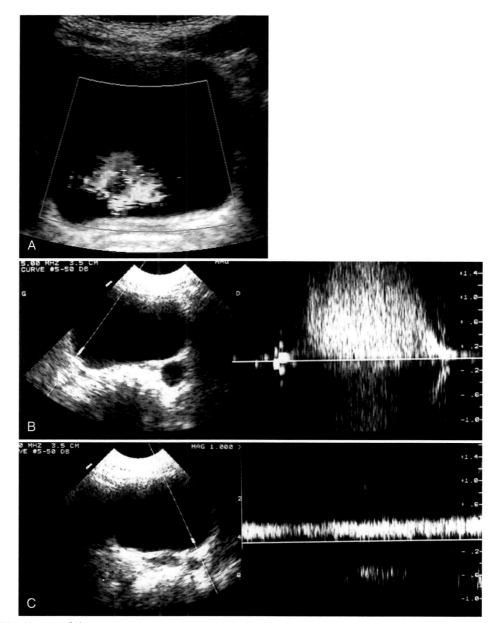

FIGURE 54-50. Ureteral jets. Transverse sonograms of the bladder base in 8-year-old boy. **A,** Color Doppler sonogram aids in locating jet. **B,** Normal bell-curve jet from the normal right ureter. **C,** *Bottom:* Constant Doppler signal from the dilated obstructed left ureter. Urine appears to be reaching the bladder in a more or less constant dribble. *(From Patriquin HB, Paltiel H: Pediatric radiology categorical course syllabus. 1989, Radiological Society of North America.)*

CAUSES OF RENAL TRANSPLANT DYSFUNCTION

Hyperacute rejection: hours after transplant, caused by antibodies from presensitization
Accelerated rejection: 1 to 7 days after transplant, from poorly matched donors; presensitization
Acute rejection: 3 to 12 weeks after transplant, caused by antibodies newly formed
Graft dysfunction: 1 to 7 days
Acute tubular necrosis (ATN)
Obstruction of collecting system
Large perirenal fluid collection
Cyclosporine toxicity
Acute renal vein thrombosis
Pyelonephritis
Chronic rejection: months to years, from repeated acute rejection

recur later. Because T or B cells must be stimulated, the rejection response usually takes a week or more to occur. Hyperacute rejection occurs during or within hours of transplantation from antibodies against the graft tissue already present in the host. Hyperacute rejections are rare with modern assays for presensitization. Accelerated rejection occurs on days 1 through 7 in poorly matched living donor grafts and also results from presensitization. Other causes of graft dysfunction in the first days or week after transplantation include ATN, obstructive uropathy, large perirenal fluid collections, cyclosporine toxicity, acute renal vein thrombosis, and pyelonephritis. Clinical findings in all are similar: decreasing urine output, rising serum creatinine, abdominal pain, fever, and leukocytosis. Hydronephrosis and perirenal fluid collections are easily detected with gray-scale sonography.

Doppler sonography is a sensitive indicator of the increasing intrarenal impedance that accompanies **acute vascular rejection.** If serial measurements can be obtained by performing a baseline study shortly after surgery, the RI can be compared to the patient's own values rather than population norms (Fig. 54-51). Single measurements have been disappointing in distinguishing ATN and cyclosporine toxicity from acute rejection. Sonography is used for an initial investigation of a failing graft. The diagnosis of rejection is established by biopsy.

To assess alterations in intrarenal arterial resistance in conditions often encountered in the transplanted kidney, Pozniak et al.[91] studied four groups of dog allografts with pulsed Doppler: normal, ATN, cyclosporine-toxicity, and rejection (Table 54-5). In the normal and ATN groups, the RI rose immediately after surgery and returned to baseline levels after 10 days. Renal length also increased slightly. No significant change in RI or renal length was noted in the cyclosporine toxicity group. The acute rejection group showed an initial slight decrease in the RI and then a rapid and progressive rise in the RI after day 5. Renal length also increased

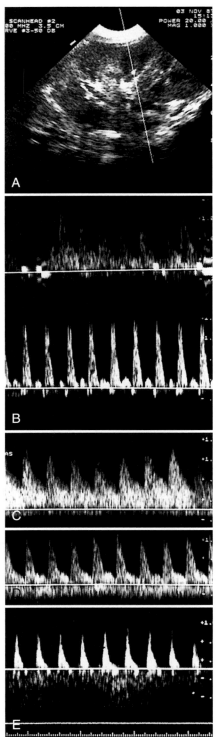

FIGURE 54-51. Renal allograft rejection and treatment. A, Doppler cursor adjacent to a pyramid (within an interlobar artery) records a normal flow pattern 2 days after transplantation. **B,** One week later, normal diastolic flow has disappeared; flow reverses at the end of diastole. The serum creatinine level had risen, and there was oliguria. **C,** At 12 hours after completion of a course of antirejection therapy with monoclonal antibodies, normal intrarenal flow has resumed (urine flow and creatinine level had returned almost to normal levels). **D,** Within 1 week, creatinine level rose again. Diastolic flow diminished. **E,** Two days later, during oliguria, reversal of diastolic flow heralded another severe episode of rejection. *(From Patriquin HB, Paltiel H: Pediatric radiology categorical course syllabus. 1989, Radiological Society of North America.)*

TABLE 54-5. POSTTRANSPLANT INTRARENAL ARTERIAL RESISTANCE

	RI EARLY	RI LATE	RENAL LENGTH
Normal	↑	Baseline after 10 days	↑Slightly
Acute tubular necrosis	↑	Baseline after 10 days	↑Slightly
Cyclosporine toxicity	No change	No change	No change
Acute rejection	↑RI	↑RI after 5 days	↑

RI, Resistive index.

From Pozniak MA, Kelcz F, D'Alessandro A, et al. Sonography of renal transplants in dogs: the effect of acute tubular necrosis, cyclosporine nephrotoxicity, and acute rejection on resistive index and renal length. AJR Am J Roentgenol 1992;158:791-797.

steadily. This study is an elegant demonstration of the temporal changes in renal impedance in three of the most common diseases affecting the recent renal allograft. It also illustrates the difficulty in attempting to diagnose a specific disease process from a single RI or renal length measurement and emphasizes the importance of serial examinations and their correlation with clinical findings.

When acute vascular rejection is effectively treated (with cyclosporine, which prevents proliferation of T cells, or with polyclonal or monoclonal antibodies, which "blind" T cells to graft antigens), the decrease in intrarenal resistance is dramatic and is well demonstrated with pulsed Doppler sonography[91] (Fig. 54-51). Chronic rejection occurs months to years after transplantation and is the result of many episodes of unsuccessfully treated acute rejection. Chronic rejection may start as early as the first few months after transplantation and is characterized by **sclerosing arteritis** and **tubular atrophy.** The glomeruli are small or hyalinized, and there is vascular intimal proliferation, especially of interlobar and arcuate arteries. The resultant decreased diameter of small intrarenal vessels leads to increased vascular impedance and low or absent diastolic flow.[18]

PEDIATRIC ADRENAL SONOGRAPHY

The adrenal gland is relatively prominent in the neonate and is easily visualized with ultrasound. In the older child the adrenal gland is usually not visible.

The adrenal glands are superior to the kidneys; longitudinal and transverse images are obtained with a high-frequency convex or sector transducer. From the transverse images of the gland, AP and transverse dimensions are measured. From the longitudinal images, the cephalocaudal length is measured from the apex to the midpoint of the base of the gland (Fig. 54-52). Table

54-6 lists the results, including change (decrease) over time expressed as percentage size at the time in question compared with the size at birth.[92]

At birth, the adrenal gland is relatively large, representing 0.2% to 0.3% of total body weight, compared with 0.001% in adults. There is a linear relationship between body weight and gland lengths in healthy neonates. In premature neonates there is a linear relationship between gestational age and gland size. The linear dimensions continually decrease during the first 6 months of life. In addition, the appearance changes as the cortex decreases in size and the echogenicity changes.[92]

Normal Anatomy

The success of sonographic visualization of the normal adrenal gland varies with the child's age and size. In the neonatal period the normal adrenal gland can be readily visualized because it is relatively large, there is relatively little perirenal fat to obscure the gland, and high-frequency transducers can be used. Normal adrenal glands are readily identified in the suprarenal location and have a V-, Y-, or Z-shaped configuration (Fig. 54-52). The gland has a thin echogenic core that represents the adrenal medulla. This is surrounded by a less echogenic rim that represents the adrenal cortex.[93] In the neonate, there is a thick fetal zone that occupies about 80% of the cortex of the gland. After birth, the fetal zone of the adrenal cortex undergoes involution.

At birth, vascular congestion is present throughout the fetal zone; involution occurs by hemorrhagic necrosis; and the fetal zone gradually shrinks and is replaced by connective tissue by 1 year of age. Values for the normal size of the adrenal gland in the infant are available (Table 54-6). Adrenal length ranges between 3.6 and 0.9 cm (mean 1.5 cm); width ranges between 0.5 and 0.2 cm (mean 0.3 cm).[92] The mean adrenal length increases with gestational age. The adrenal gland in the older child and teenager is not easily seen by ultrasound, and other imaging modalities are preferable for its evaluation. If there is **renal agenesis,** the neonatal adrenal will be seen as a long linear structure (lying flat) still recognizable by the normal cortex and medulla (Fig. 54-53).

Congenital Adrenal Hyperplasia

Infants with deficiency of 21-hydroxylase, which is necessary for adrenal production of cortisol, have an excessive accumulation of androgenic precursors, with enlarged adrenal glands[94] and virilization of the genitalia in female infants. Sivit et al.[95] reported enlarged width of the adrenal gland (>0.5 cm) in four of six patients, with preservation of the normal architecture. Hernanz-Schulman et al.[96] described enlarged adrenal glands in 8 of 16 patients. However, a normal-sized gland does not exclude the diagnosis. A typical cerebriform appearance has been described[97] (Fig. 54-54).

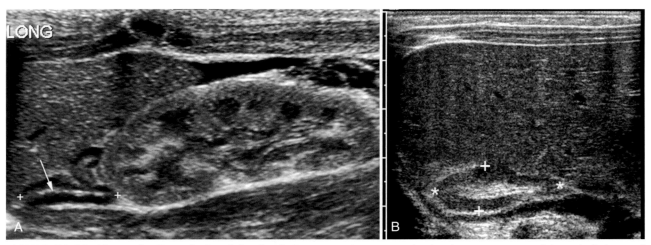

FIGURE 54-52. Normal adrenal gland in the infant. A and B, Longitudinal and transverse scans of the right kidney and adrenal gland shows a Y-shaped gland with an echogenic central area *(arrow)* representing the adrenal medulla and a less echogenic peripheral rim representing the fetal adrenal cortex. Length (+) and width (*) and AP (+) measurement are made.

TABLE 54-6. ADRENAL MEASUREMENTS IN NEONATES: MEAN ±SD (MEAN PERCENTAGE CHANGE ±SD)

DAY	TRANSVERSE	ANTEROPOSTERIOR	CIRCUMFERENCE	AREA (cm²)	LENGTH
1	17.0 ± 2.7	9.6 ± 2.1	44.5 ± 5.3	1.3 ± 0.3	17.3 ± 1.8
3	14.8 ± 3.3	7.5 ± 2.2	36.7 ± 8.4	0.95 ± 0.5	12.8 ± 3.2
	(84.0 ± 19.9)	(78.6 ± 16.9)	(82.4 ± 16.3)	(68.3 ± 24.5)	(73.9 ± 18.7)
5	13.7 ± 2.1	6.9 ± 1.6	33.4 ± 5.1	0.75 ± 0.2	11.4 ± 2.7
	(77.5 ± 11.3)	(62.0 ± 20.6)	(65.2 ± 19.4)	(44.5 ± 29.2)	(51.9 ± 12.6)
11	11.8 ± 2.5	5.9 ± 1.4	28.6 ± 6.1	0.57 ± 0.3	8.9 ± 2.0
	(67.4 ± 17.2)	(62.0 ± 20.6)	(65.2 ± 19.4)	(44.5 ± 19.4)	(51.9 ± 12.6)
21	10.8 ± 1.9	5.6 ± 0.5	25.3 ± 3.9	0.45 ± 0.1	8.2 ± 1.2
	(61.5 ± 13.4)	(61.1 ± 16.3)	(57.8 ± 11.3)	(35.7 ± 13.7)	(47.9 ± 8.0)
42	9.5 ± 1.5	5.7 ± 1.0	23.8 ± 2.8	0.4 ± 0.1	7.7 ± 0.9
	(53.9 ± 11.6)	(61.3 ± 14.8)	(54.4 ± 10.4)	(32.5 ± 11.5)	(45.0 ± 6.4)

From Scott EM, Thomas A, McGarrigle HH, Lachelin GC. Serial adrenal ultrasonography in normal neonates. J Ultrasound Med 1990;9:279-283.

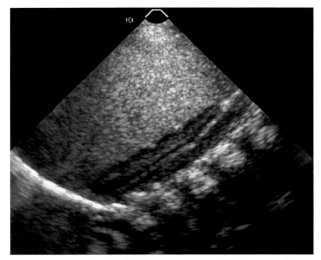

FIGURE 54-53. "Lying-flat adrenal" in newborn with renal agenesis. Longitudinal sonogram with only an adrenal in the right renal fossa, typical hypoechoic cortex, echogenic medulla, and a flat shape to the adrenal.

Neonatal Adrenal Hemorrhage

Hemorrhage into the adrenal gland occurs in the neonate and is associated with stress, trauma at birth, anoxia, sepsis, bleeding disorders, and diabetes in the mother. It occurs most frequently between the second and seventh day of life, and patients present with an abdominal mass, hyperbilirubinemia, and occasionally, hypovolemic shock. In some cases the hemorrhage is asymptomatic. If a palpable abdominal mass is found, an adrenal hemorrhage must be differentiated from a tumor of the adrenal gland or kidney. Sonography demonstrates a suprarenal mass with variable echogenicity.[98,99] In the acute phase the hemorrhage is usually echogenic, representing clot formation. Over several weeks, the hemorrhage becomes echo free as the clot lyses and becomes liquefied (Fig. 54-55). The hemorrhage gradually decreases in size and may result in adrenal calcification. Differentiation from a neonatal neuroblastoma is important. Follow-up that demonstrates the mass decreasing

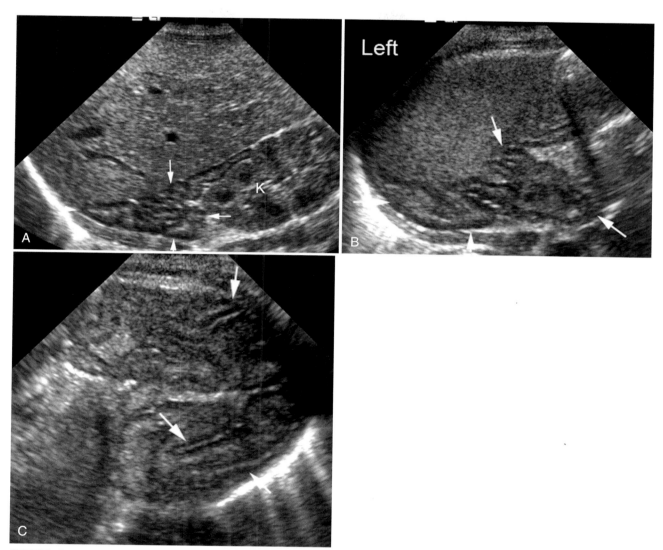

FIGURE 54-54. Cerebriform adrenal gland in neonate with congenital adrenal hyperplasia. A, Longitudinal image with redundant adrenal coils *(arrows)* crowning the right kidney apex *(K).* **B** and **C,** Longitudinal and transverse left images show coils with echogenic central gland and hypoechoic cortex *(arrows).*

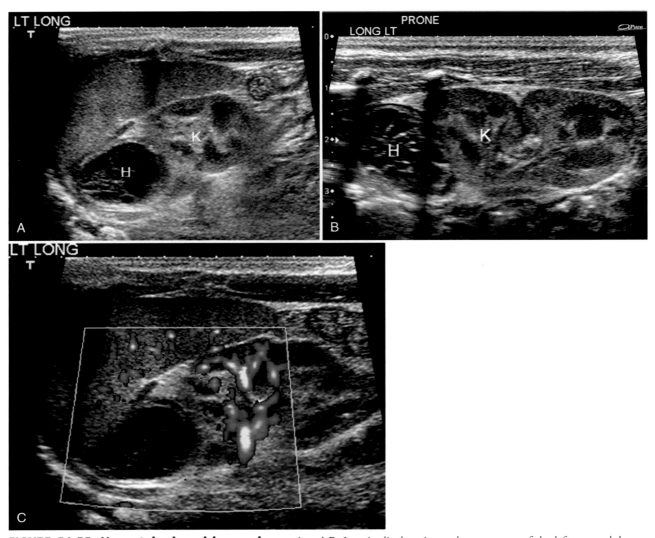

FIGURE 54-55. Neonatal adrenal hemorrhage. A and **B,** Longitudinal supine and prone scans of the left upper abdomen show inferior displacement of the left kidney *(K)* by a suprarenal mass. The adrenal gland is enlarged secondary to hemorrhage with hypoechoic hematoma *(H).* **C,** Power Doppler ultrasound shows that hematoma has no flow.

in size and eventually resolving confirms the diagnosis of an adrenal hemorrhage.

References

Pediatric Renal Sonography

1. Han BK, Babcock DS. Sonographic measurements and appearance of normal kidneys in children. AJR Am J Roentgenol 1985;145: 611-616.
2. Dinkel E, Ertel M, Dittrich M, et al. Kidney size in childhood: sonographical growth charts for kidney length and volume. Pediatr Radiol 1985;15:38-43.
3. Chiara A, Chirico G, Barbarini M, et al. Ultrasonic evaluation of kidney length in term and preterm infants. Eur J Pediatr 1989;149: 94-95.
4. Schlesinger AE, Hedlund GL, Pierson WP, Null DM. Normal standards for kidney length in premature infants: determination with US. Work in progress. Radiology 1987;164:127-129.
5. Rottenberg GT, De Bruyn R, Gordon I. Sonographic standards for a single functioning kidney in children. AJR Am J Roentgenol 1996; 167:1255-1259.
6. Kuzmic AC, Brkljacic B, Ivankovic D. The impact of bladder shape on the ultrasonographic measurement of bladder volume in children. Pediatr Radiol 2003;33:530-534.
7. Treves ST, Zurakowski D, Bauer SB, et al. Functional bladder capacity measured during radionuclide cystography in children. Radiology 1996;198:269-272.
8. Jequier S, Rousseau O. Sonographic measurements of the normal bladder wall in children. AJR Am J Roentgenol 1987;149:563-566.
9. Riccabona M, Pilhatsch A, Haberlik A, Ring E. Three-dimensional ultrasonography–based virtual cystoscopy of the pediatric urinary bladder: a preliminary report on feasibility and potential value. J Ultrasound Med 2008;27:1453-1459.
10. Riccabona M, Fritz GA, Schollnast H, et al. Hydronephrotic kidney: pediatric three-dimensional US for relative renal size assessment: initial experience. Radiology 2005;236:276-283.
11. Patriquin H, Lefaivre JF, Lafortune M, et al. Fetal lobation: an anatomo-ultrasonographic correlation. J Ultrasound Med 1990;9: 191-197.
12. Currarino G, Lowichik A. The Oddono's sulcus and its relation to the renal "junctional parenchymal defect" and the "interrenicular septum." Pediatr Radiol 1997;27:6-10.
13. Rosenfield AT, Taylor KJ, Crade M, DeGraaf CS. Anatomy and pathology of the kidney by gray scale ultrasound. Radiology 1978;128: 737-744.

14. Hricak H, Slovis TL, Callen CW, et al. Neonatal kidneys: sonographic-anatomic correlation. Radiology 1983;147:699-702.

Congenital Anomalies of the Urinary Tract
15. Mackie GG, Awang H, Stephens FD. The ureteric orifice: the embryologic key to radiologic status of duplex kidneys. J Pediatr Surg 1975;10:473-481.
16. Hayden Jr CK, Swischuk LE. Pediatric ultrasonography. Baltimore: Williams & Wilkins; 1987. p. 263-345.
17. Schaffer RM, Shih YH, Becker JA. Sonographic identification of collecting system duplications. J Clin Ultrasound 1983;11:309-312.
18. Slovis TL. Caffey's pediatric diagnostic imaging. 11th ed. Philadelphia: Mosby-Elsevier; 2007.

Hydronephrosis
19. Brown T, Mandell J, Lebowitz RL. Neonatal hydronephrosis in the era of sonography. AJR Am J Roentgenol 1987;148:959-963.
20. Zerin JM. Hydronephrosis in the neonate and young infant: current concepts. Semin US CT MR 1994;15:306-316.
21. Wood BP, Ben-Ami T, Teele RL, Rabinowitz R. Ureterovesical obstruction and megaloureter: diagnosis by real-time ultrasound. Radiology 1985;156:79-81.
22. Jequier S, Paltiel H, Lafortune M. Ureterovesical jets in infants and children: duplex and color Doppler US studies. Radiology 1990;175:349-353.
23. De Bessa Jr J, Denes FT, Chammas MC, et al. Diagnostic accuracy of color Doppler sonographic study of the ureteric jets in evaluation of hydronephrosis. J Pediatr Urol 2008;4:113-117.
24. Gilsanz V, Miller JH, Reid BS. Ultrasonic characteristics of posterior urethral valves. Radiology 1982;145:143-145.
25. Docimo SG, Canning D, Khoury A. The Kelalis-King-Belman textbook of clinical pediatric urology. Philadelphia: Saunders-Elsevier; 2007.
26. Cacciarelli AA, Kass EJ, Yang SS. Urachal remnants: sonographic demonstration in children. Radiology 1990;174:473-475.
27. Fernbach SK, Feinstein KA. Abnormalities of the bladder in children: imaging findings. AJR Am J Roentgenol 1994;162:1143-1150.

Renal Cystic Disease
28. Osathanondh V, Potter E. Pathogenesis of polycystic kidneys. Arch Pathol 1964;77:458-512.
29. Blyth H, Ockenden BG. Polycystic disease of kidney and liver presenting in childhood. J Med Genet 1971;8:257-284.
30. Premkumar A, Berdon WE, Levy J, et al. The emergence of hepatic fibrosis and portal hypertension in infants and children with autosomal recessive polycystic kidney disease: initial and follow-up sonographic and radiographic findings. Pediatr Radiol 1988;18:123-129.
31. Melson GL, Shackelford GD, Cole BR, McClennan BL. The spectrum of sonographic findings in infantile polycystic kidney disease with urographic and clinical correlations. J Clin Ultrasound 1985;13:113-119.
32. Traubici J, Daneman A. High-resolution renal sonography in children with autosomal recessive polycystic kidney disease. AJR Am J Roentgenol 2005;184:1630-1633.
33. Lonergan GJ, Rice RR, Suarez ES. Autosomal recessive polycystic kidney disease: radiologic-pathologic correlation. Radiographics 2000;20:837-855.
34. Avni FE, Guissard G, Hall M, et al. Hereditary polycystic kidney diseases in children: changing sonographic patterns through childhood. Pediatr Radiol 2002;32:169-174.
35. Rosenfield AT, Lipson MH, Wolf B, et al. Ultrasonography and nephrotomography in the presymptomatic diagnosis of dominantly inherited (adult-onset) polycystic kidney disease. Radiology 1980;135:423-427.
36. Kaariainen H, Koskimies O, Norio R. Dominant and recessive polycystic kidney disease in children: evaluation of clinical features and laboratory data. Pediatr Nephrol (Berl) 1988;2:296-302.
37. Jain M, LeQuesne GW, Bourne AJ, Henning P. High-resolution ultrasonography in the differential diagnosis of cystic diseases of the kidney in infancy and childhood: preliminary experience. J Ultrasound Med 1997;16:235-240.
38. Stuck KJ, Koff SA, Silver TM. Ultrasonic features of multicystic dysplastic kidney: expanded diagnostic criteria. Radiology 1982;143:217-221.

39. Gordon AC, Thomas DF, Arthur RJ, Irving HC. Multicystic dysplastic kidney: is nephrectomy still appropriate? J Urol 1988;140:1231-1234.
40. Strife JL, Souza AS, Kirks DR, et al. Multicystic dysplastic kidney in children: US follow-up. Radiology 1993;186:785-788.
41. Narla LD, Slovis TL, Watts FB, Nigro M. The renal lesions of tuberosclerosis (cysts and angiomyolipoma): screening with sonography and computerized tomography. Pediatr Radiol 1988;18:205-209.
42. Calvo-Garcia MA, Campbell KM, O'Hara SM, et al. Acquired renal cysts after pediatric liver transplantation: association with cyclosporine and renal dysfunction. Pediatr Transplant 2008;12:666-671

Urinary Tract Infection
43. Darge K, Trusen A, Gordjani N, Riedmiller H. Intrarenal reflux: diagnosis with contrast-enhanced harmonic ultrasound. Pediatr Radiol 2003;33:729-731.
44. Stogianni A, Nikolopoulos P, Oikonomou I, et al. Childhood acute pyelonephritis: comparison of power Doppler sonography and Tc-DMSA scintigraphy. Pediatr Radiol 2007;37:685-690.
45. Lebowitz RL, Mandell J. Urinary tract infection in children: putting radiology in its place. Radiology 1987;165:1-9.
46. Jequier S, Forbes PA, Nogrady MB. The value of ultrasonography as a screening procedure in a first-documented urinary tract infection in children. J Ultrasound Med 1985;4:393-400.
47. Mason Jr WG. Urinary tract infections in children: renal ultrasound evaluation. Radiology 1984;153:109-111.
48. Gelfand MJ, Parker BR, Kushner DC, et al. Urinary tract infection: American College of Radiology appropriateness criteria. Radiology 2000;215(Suppl):847-854.
49. Talner LB, Davidson AJ, Lebowitz RL, et al. Acute pyelonephritis: can we agree on terminology? Radiology 1994;192:297-305.
50. Babcock DS. Sonography of wall thickening of the renal collecting system: a nonspecific finding. J Ultrasound Med 1987;6:29-32.
51. Majd M, Rushton HG. Renal cortical scintigraphy in the diagnosis of acute pyelonephritis. Semin Nucl Med 1992;22:98-111.
52. Dacher JN, Pfister C, Monroc M, et al. Power Doppler sonographic pattern of acute pyelonephritis in children: comparison with CT. AJR Am J Roentgenol 1996;166:1451-1455.
53. Robinson PJ, Pocock RD, Frank JD. The management of obstructive renal candidiasis in the neonate. Br J Urol 1987;59:380-382.

Medical Renal Disease
54. Rosenfield AT, Siegel NJ. Renal parenchymal disease: histopathologic-sonographic correlation. AJR Am J Roentgenol 1981;137:793-798.
55. Paterson A, Frush DP, Sweeney LE, Thomas PS. Elevated renal rind. J Ultrasound Med 2000;19:459-463.
56. Bruwer A. Primary renal calculi: Anderson-Carr-Randall progression? AJR Am J Roentgenol 1979;132:751-758.
57. Patriquin H, Robitaille P. Renal calcium deposition in children: sonographic demonstration of the Anderson-Carr progression. AJR Am J Roentgenol 1986;146:1253-1256.
58. Patriquin H, Lafortune M, Filiatrault D. Urinary milk of calcium in children and adults: use of gravity-dependent sonography. AJR Am J Roentgenol 1985;144:407-413.
59. Jayogapal S, Cohen HL, Brill PW, et al. Calcified neonatal renal vein thrombosis demonstration by CT and US. Pediatr Radiol 1990;20:160-162.
60. Gilsanz V, Fernal W, Reid BS, et al. Nephrolithiasis in premature infants. Radiology 1985;154:107-110.

Renal Trauma
61. Stalker HP, Kaufman RA, Stedje K. The significance of hematuria in children after blunt abdominal trauma. AJR Am J Roentgenol 1990;154:569-571.
62. Furtschegger A, Egender G, Jakse G. The value of sonography in the diagnosis and follow-up of patients with blunt renal trauma. Br J Urology 1988;62:110-116.

Renal and Adrenal Tumors
63. Lowe LH, Isuani BH, Heller RM, et al. Pediatric renal masses: Wilms tumor and beyond. Radiographics 2000;20:1585-1603.
64. Bryd R. Wilms' tumor: medical aspects. In Broecher BH, Klein FA, editors. Pediatric tumor of the genitourinary tract. New York: Alan R Liss; 1988. p. 61-73.

65. Jaffe MH, White SJ, Silver TM, Heidelberger KP. Wilms tumor: ultrasonic features, pathologic correlation, and diagnostic pitfalls. Radiology 1981;140:147-152.

66. De Campo JF. Ultrasound of Wilms' tumor. Pediatr Radiol 1986; 16:21-24.

67. Lonergan GJ, Martinez-Leon MI, Agrons GA, et al. Nephrogenic rests, nephroblastomatosis, and associated lesions of the kidney. Radiographics 1998;18:947-968.

68. Van Campenhout I, Patriquin H. Malignant microvasculature in abdominal tumors in children: detection with Doppler US. Radiology 1992;183:445-448.

69. White KS. Helical/spiral CT scanning: a pediatric radiology perspective (invited article). Pediatr Radiol 1996;26:5-14.

70. Bousvaros A, Kirks DR, Grossman H. Imaging of neuroblastoma: an overview. Pediatr Radiol 1986;16:89-106.

71. Hartman DS, Sanders RC. Wilms' tumor versus neuroblastoma: usefulness of ultrasound in differentiation. J Ultrasound Med 1982;1: 117-122.

72. Hartman DS, Lesar MS, Madewell JE, et al. Mesoblastic nephroma: radiologic-pathologic correlation of 20 cases. AJR Am J Roentgenol 1981;136:69-74.

73. Agrons GA, Wagner BJ, Davidson AJ, Suarez ES. Multilocular cystic renal tumor in children: radiologic-pathologic correlation. Radiographics 1995;15:653-669.

74. Hartman DS, David Jr CJ, Goldman SM, et al. Renal lymphoma: radiologic-pathologic correlation of 21 cases. Radiology 1982;144: 759-766.

75. Heiken J, McClennan B, Gold R. Renal lymphoma. Semin US CT MR 1986;7:58-66.

Doppler Assessment of Renal Vascular Disease in Children

76. Chavhan GB, Parra DA, Mann A, Navarro OM. Normal Doppler spectral waveforms of major pediatric vessels: specific patterns. Radiographics 2008;28:691-706.

77. Hubsch PJ, Mostbeck G, Barton PP, et al. Evaluation of arteriovenous fistulas and pseudoaneurysms in renal allografts following percutaneous needle biopsy: color-coded Doppler sonography versus duplex Doppler sonography. J Ultrasound Med 1990;9:95-100.

78. Rosenfield AT, Zeman RK, Cronan JJ, Taylor KJ. Ultrasound in experimental and clinical renal vein thrombosis. Radiology 1980; 137:735-741.

79. Laplante S, Patriquin HB, Robitaille P, et al. Renal vein thrombosis in children: evidence of early flow recovery with Doppler US. Radiology 1993;189:37-42.

80. Vo NJ, Hammelman BD, Racadio JM, et al. Anatomic distribution of renal artery stenosis in children: implications for imaging. Pediatr Radiol 2006;36:1032-1036.

81. Stavros AT, Parker SH, Yakes WF, et al. Segmental stenosis of the renal artery: pattern recognition of tardus and parvus abnormalities with duplex sonography. Radiology 1992;184:487-492.

82. Patriquin HB, Lafortune M, Jequier JC, et al. Stenosis of the renal artery: assessment of slowed systole in the downstream circulation with Doppler sonography. Radiology 1992;184:479-485.

83. Patriquin HB, O'Regan S, Robitaille P, Paltiel H. Hemolytic-uremic syndrome: intrarenal arterial Doppler patterns as a useful guide to therapy. Radiology 1989;172:625-628.

84. Tublin ME, Dodd 3rd GD, Verdile VP. Acute renal colic: diagnosis with duplex Doppler US. Radiology 1994;193:697-701.

85. Ryan PC, Maher KP, Murphy B, et al. Experimental partial ureteric obstruction: pathophysiological changes in upper tract pressures and renal blood flow. J Urol 1987;138:674-678.

86. Platt JF, Rubin JM, Ellis JH, DiPietro MA. Duplex Doppler ultrasound of the kidney: differentiation of obstructive from nonobstructive dilatation. Radiology 1989;171:515-517.

87. Garcia-Pena BM, Keller MS, Schwartz DS, et al. The ultrasonographic differentiation of obstructive versus nonobstructive hydronephrosis in children: a multivariate scoring system. J Urol 1997;158: 560-565.

88. Leung VY, Chu WC, Yeung CK, Metreweli C. Doppler waveforms of the ureteric jet: an overview and implications for the presence of a functional sphincter at the vesicoureteric junction. Pediatr Radiol 2007;37:417-425.

89. Mutze S, Turk I, Schonberger B, et al. Colour-coded duplex sonography in the diagnostic assessment of vascular complications after kidney transplantation in children. Pediatr Radiol 1997;27:898-902.

90. Taylor KJ, Morse SS, Rigsby CM, et al. Vascular complications in renal allografts: detection with duplex Doppler US. Radiology 1987;162:31-38.

91. Pozniak MA, Kelcz F, D'Alessandro A, et al. Sonography of renal transplants in dogs: the effect of acute tubular necrosis, cyclosporine nephrotoxicity, and acute rejection on resistive index and renal length. AJR Am J Roentgenol 1992;158:791-797.

Pediatric Adrenal Sonography

92. Scott EM, Thomas A, McGarrigle HH, Lachelin GC. Serial adrenal ultrasonography in normal neonates. J Ultrasound Med 1990;9:279-283.

93. Oppenheimer DA, Carroll BA, Yousem S. Sonography of the normal neonatal adrenal gland. Radiology 1983;146:157-160.

94. Bryan PJ, Caldamone AA, Morrison SC, et al. Ultrasound findings in the adreno-genital syndrome (congenital adrenal hyperplasia). J Ultrasound Med 1988;7:675-679.

95. Sivit CJ, Hung W, Taylor GA, et al. Sonography in neonatal congenital adrenal hyperplasia. Ajr 1991;156:141-143.

96. Hernanz-Schulman M, Brock 3rd JW, Russell W. Sonographic findings in infants with congenital adrenal hyperplasia. Pediatr Radiol 2002;32:130-137.

97. Avni EF, Rypens F, Smet MH, Galetty E. Sonographic demonstration of congenital adrenal hyperplasia in the neonate: the cerebriform pattern. Pediatr Radiol 1993;23:88-90.

98. Mittelstaedt CA, Volberg FM, Merten DF, Brill PW. The sonographic diagnosis of neonatal adrenal hemorrhage. Radiology 1979; 131:453-457.

99. Heij HA, Taets van Amerongen AH, Ekkelkamp S, Vos A. Diagnosis and management of neonatal adrenal haemorrhage. Pediatr Radiol 1989;19:391-394.

CHAPTER 55

The Pediatric Gastrointestinal Tract

Susan D. John and Caroline Hollingsworth

Chapter Outline

ESOPHAGUS AND STOMACH

Normal Anatomy and Technique

Sonography has become an important diagnostic imaging modality in the evaluation of the gastrointestinal (GI) tract of children. Ultrasound permits direct visualization of the various mural layers of the GI tract, adding a new dimension to the imaging of this body system. The ability to observe gastrointestinal dynamics without exposure to ionizing radiation is an added asset of sonography. Video clips done during scanning can be a valuable resource to view peristalsis. Ultrasound is most suitable for portions of the GI tract that are not surrounded by or filled with large amounts of gas. The stomach is best evaluated after allowing the patient to ingest clear fluids. Sugar water works well for infants.

STOMACH: OPTIMAL MEASUREMENTS

Normal pyloric muscle thickness ≤2 mm
Normal gastric mucosa thickness ≤2-3 mm
Peristalsis through pylorus

Esophagus

Most of the esophagus is inaccessible by sonography because of surrounding aerated lung. Only the subdiaphragmatic portion of the esophagus is usually visible. The gastroesophageal junction can be seen by examining the patient with sagittal images in the supine or right-side-down decubitus position.[1-3] This technique permits observation of the function of the gastroesophageal junction and can be used to detect gastroesophageal reflux. Reflux is noted when fluid is regurgitated into the retrocardiac portion of the esophagus (Fig. 55-1). Color Doppler sonography may facilitate the detection of gastroesophageal reflux.[4] **Hiatal hernias** can also be detected with sonography, which may be more sensitive than barium studies for detecting small degrees of herniation, especially if color Doppler ultrasound is also used.[5,6] However, the sonographic techniques required are operator dependent and have not gained much popularity. Therefore, esophageal abnormalities are usually assessed with other imaging modalities, such as fluoroscopy or endoscopy.

Stomach

Most abnormalities of the stomach in infants and children involve the gastric antrum and distal third of the stomach. This portion of the stomach is easily evaluated using the liver as an acoustic window. Distending the stomach with clear fluid facilitates evaluation of the mucosal, submucosal, and muscular layers of the stomach (Fig. 55-2). Furthermore, gastric peristalsis and emptying can be evaluated.

Normal gastric mucosa, including the muscularis mucosae and submucosal layers, measures 2 to 3 mm, whereas the outer circular muscle layer measures between 1 and 2 mm in thickness.[7,8] These measurements should

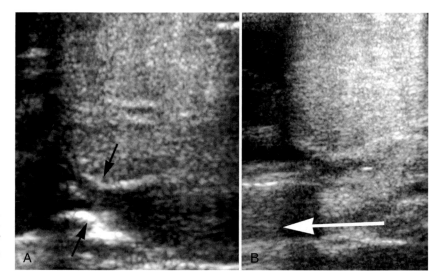

FIGURE 55-1. Gastroesophageal reflux. A, Normal contracted gastroesophageal junction *(arrows)*. **B,** Later, the lower esophageal sphincter opens, and reflux of fluid and formula into the esophagus is visible *(arrow)*.

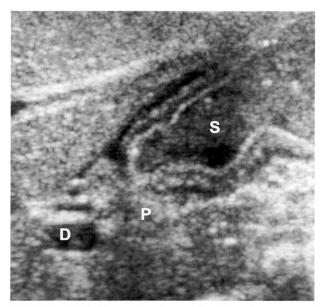

FIGURE 55-2. Normal stomach. Normal antrum of stomach *(S)*, pyloric canal *(P)*, and proximal duodenum *(D)*. Four gastric wall layers are visible (from inside out): echogenic mucosa, hypoechoic muscularis mucosae, echogenic submucosa, and hypoechoic outer circular muscle.

be obtained with the stomach fully distended with fluid, and the scan should be performed in the midlongitudinal plane of the stomach or, on cross section, proximal to the pyloric canal. On cross-sectional imaging, if the image obtained is too close to the contracted pyloric canal, thickening of the pyloric muscle can be suggested erroneously. Similarly, if tangential images are obtained on the longitudinal plane, the muscle may erroneously appear thickened (Fig. 55-3). This same phenomenon is also seen with the echogenic mucosal layer.

HYPERTROPHIC PYLORIC STENOSIS

Muscle width ≥3 mm
Pyloric canal length ≥1.2 cm
No peristalsis through pylorus

Hypertrophic Pyloric Stenosis

During the past decade, sonography has almost completely replaced the radiographic upper GI series for the diagnosis of infantile hypertrophic pyloric stenosis (HPS). Unlike the upper GI series that demonstrates only the indirect effects of pyloric muscle hypertrophy on the gastric lumen, ultrasound allows direct visualization of the gastric muscle thickening that is the hallmark of the disease. Although a few pitfalls in the sonographic diagnosis of HPS exist, the technique is relatively easily mastered and results in greatly improved accuracy of diagnosis and patient outcome. Indeed, the accuracy approaches 100%, and ultrasound is now the procedure of choice for the detection of pyloric stenosis.[9-12]

After the initial documentation of the sonographic detection of the hypertrophied pyloric muscle in pyloric stenosis by Teele and Smith,[13] many studies described the characteristic findings of HPS.[14-18] Increased pyloric muscle thickness and canal length, increased transverse diameter of the pylorus, estimation of degree of gastric outlet obstruction, and calculation of pyloric muscle volume have all been used to diagnose pyloric stenosis. However, of all the criteria, thickening of the pyloric muscle and elongation of the pyloric canal have emerged as the most consistently useful. The thickness at which the muscle is considered **hypertrophied is 3 mm or greater.**[7] Pyloric canal length of 1.5 cm is considered

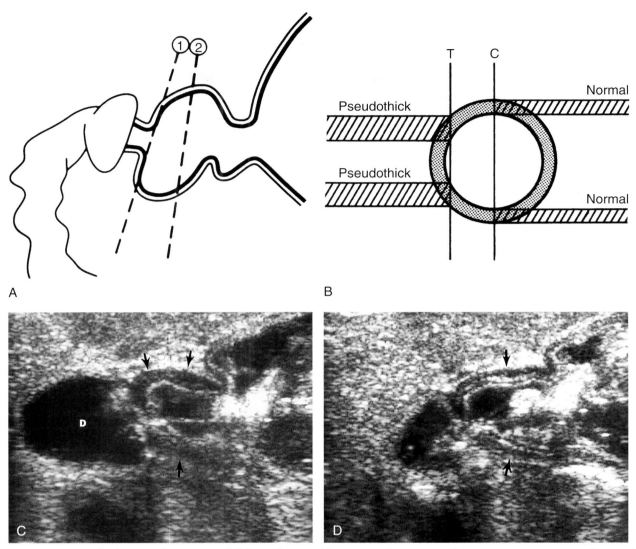

FIGURE 55-3. Pyloric muscle tangential imaging artifacts. A, When imaging the antrum in cross section, the muscle will appear thickened if obtained through plane 1, but will show normal thickness if obtained through plane 2. **B,** Longitudinal scan, tangential plane *(T),* shows pseudothickening. Imaging in center *(C)* shows true normal muscle thickness. **C,** Tangential scan shows muscle pseudothickening *(arrows); D,* duodenum. **D,** Antrum distended with fluid shows normal muscle *(arrows).*

diagnostic of pyloric stenosis when seen in conjunction with thickened pyloric muscle. In practice, however, normal canal length is much shorter than this and is often impossible to measure. Measurement of canal length is more problematic than measurement of muscle thickness and therefore a less reliable criterion.

In the classic case of HPS, the thickened muscle mass is seen as a hypoechoic layer just superficial to the more echogenic mucosal layer of the pyloric canal (Fig. 55-4, *A*). In cross section, this "**olive,**" on clinical palpation, resembles a sonolucent "**doughnut**" medial to the gall-bladder and anterior to the right kidney (Fig. 55-4, *B*). Often, small amounts of fluid are visible trapped between the echogenic mucosal folds, corresponding to the "**string**" (elongated canal) and "**double tract**" (folded mucosa) signs seen on radiographic upper GI series.[19] In longitudinal section, sonography also permits evaluation

of functional alterations at the pylorus. Active gastric peristalsis that ends abruptly at the margin of the hypertrophied muscle, absence of a normal opening of the pylorus, and diminished passage of fluid from the stomach into the duodenum are useful adjunctive findings in pyloric stenosis. Thickened mucosa within the pylorus often accompanies the muscle hypertrophy[20] (Fig. 55-4, *C*). Although most often an isolated abnormality, HPS occasionally accompanies other obstructive antropyloric lesions, such as duodenal feeding tubes (Fig. 55-5, *A*), eosinophilic gastroenteritis, antral polyps,[21] and idiopathic or prostaglandin-induced foveolar hyperplasia.[22]

Ultrasound also is very useful for the evaluation of persistent vomiting in the postpyloromyotomy patient. The fluoroscopic upper GI series is of limited value in such cases because it tends to show persistent deformity

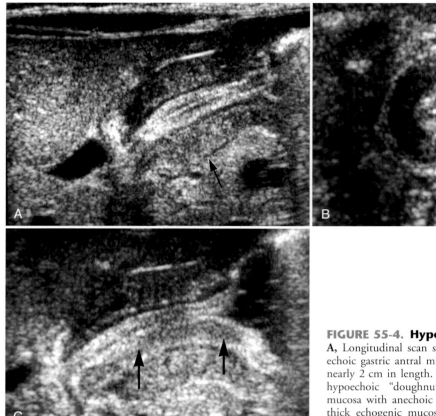

FIGURE 55-4. Hypertrophic pyloric stenosis. **A,** Longitudinal scan shows markedly thickened, hypoechoic gastric antral muscle *(arrows)*. Elongated canal is nearly 2 cm in length. **B,** Transverse scan shows typical, hypoechoic "doughnut" *(arrows)*. Central echogenic mucosa with anechoic fluid-filled crevices. **C,** Note the thick echogenic mucosa *(arrows)* within the thickened muscle mass.

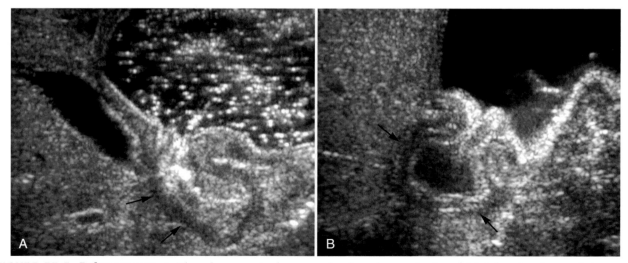

FIGURE 55-5. Pylorospasm. A, The pylorus remained contracted early in the examination of this infant, but the muscle is normal in thickness *(arrows)*. **B,** After slightly extended period of viewing, the pylorus relaxed and appeared normal *(arrows)*.

and narrowing of the canal even in asymptomatic patients. However, sonography can definitively identify persistently thickened muscle, although cautious interpretation in postpyloromyotomy patients is recommended because the pyloric muscle may not return to normal thickness for up to 5 months.[23]

Pylorospasm and Minimal Muscular Hypertrophy

In some vomiting infants, sonography shows a persistently contracted and elongated canal, but the degree of muscular thickening is less than the criterion of 3 mm

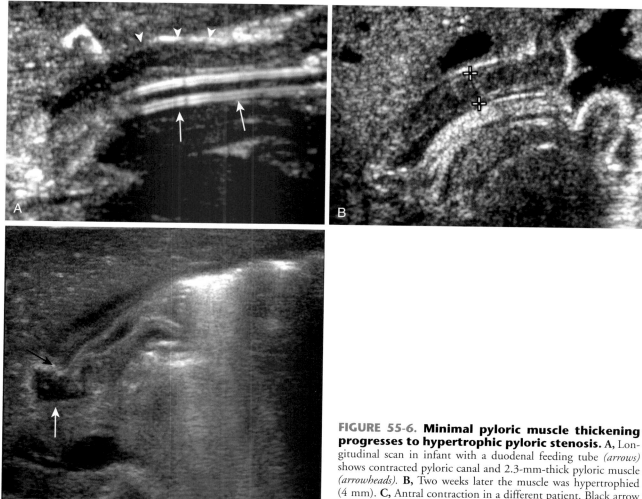

FIGURE 55-6. Minimal pyloric muscle thickening progresses to hypertrophic pyloric stenosis. A, Longitudinal scan in infant with a duodenal feeding tube *(arrows)* shows contracted pyloric canal and 2.3-mm-thick pyloric muscle *(arrowheads).* **B,** Two weeks later the muscle was hypertrophied (4 mm). **C,** Antral contraction in a different patient. Black arrow indicates position of the normal pylorus. White arrow depicts the normal, fluid-filled duodenal bulb.

for surgically correctible HPS. With extended observation, eventually the canal opens and fluid is seen to pass into the duodenum,[24] but the periods of spasm predominate (Fig. 55-6, *A* and *B*). In the vast majority of cases, there is no thickening of the pyloric muscle or mucosa, and the problem is primarily nonspecific **pylorospasm** (antral dyskinesia) (Fig. 55-6, *C*). This condition can accompany milk allergy or other forms of gastritis.

In some cases the pyloric muscle is mildly thickened, measuring 2 to 3 mm.[7] Such patients should be distinguished from those with normal muscle thickness (<2 mm) because some patients with minimal muscle hypertrophy can eventually progress to classic pyloric stenosis (see Fig. 55-5). Many of these infants will respond to medical therapy and require no surgery (Fig. 55-7). In other infants, minimal muscle thickening will resolve spontaneously, but such patients should be followed closely with ultrasound until the muscle regresses to a normal thickness.

Pitfalls in Sonographic Diagnosis

The echogenicity of the pyloric muscle varies according to the angle at which the ultrasound beam crosses the muscle fibers. During sonography of HPS, the hypertrophied muscle appears echogenic rather than hypoechoic when imaged in the midlongitudinal plane. This alteration of echogenicity is caused by an artifact called the **anisotropic effect,** which occurs at about the 6- and 12-o'clock positions of the muscle, where the ultrasound beam is perpendicular to the muscle fibers.[25] With current high-resolution linear array transducers, the echogenic appearance of the muscle does not significantly decrease its visibility (Fig. 55-8, *A*). The position of the antropyloric canal can change during the examination, especially if the stomach becomes overdistended with fluid. The distended antrum causes the pylorus to become more posteriorly directed, making it more difficult to follow with ultrasound. In such cases the gastric

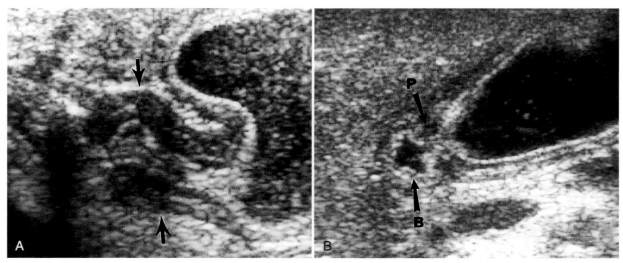

FIGURE 55-7. Minimal pyloric muscle thickening responds to medical therapy. A, Infant with a contracted canal and 2-mm-thick gastric muscle *(arrows).* **B,** After medical therapy, the pyloric muscle returned to a normal thickness; *B,* duodenal bulb; *P,* pylorus.

antrum may have a **squared-off configuration** (Fig. 55-8, *B*). When this occurs, the pylorus may be located by cephalad angulation of the transducer or by imaging from a more lateral position on the abdomen.

PITFALLS IN DIAGNOSIS OF HYPERTROPHIC PYLORIC STENOSIS (HPS)

Echogenic muscle at 90 degrees to beam (anisotropic effect)
Posteriorly oriented antropyloric canal (overdistended stomach)
Prostaglandin-induced HPS (mucosal, not muscular thickening)
Minimal pyloric muscle thickening; may progress to HPS.

Perhaps the most common pitfall in the sonographic diagnosis of pyloric muscle hypertrophy is inadequate distention of the gastric antrum with fluid. When the antrum is relatively empty, it remains contracted, and the muscle layer can appear falsely thickened (Fig. 55-9). When administering oral fluids for this study, keeping the infant in a right posterior oblique position helps to ensure that the fluid will fully distend the antrum. Despite these occasional pitfalls, the sonographic diagnosis of pyloric stenosis is generally straightforward.

Gastric Diaphragm

The gastric diaphragm, or antral web, consists of a congenital membrane that extends across the gastric antrum. These diaphragms most often lie less than 2 cm from the pylorus and are therefore usually visible on ultrasound examination. Complete diaphragms are considered one form of gastric atresia, but many diaphragms are incomplete and cause variable degrees of obstruction. On sonography, the web appears as an echogenic band across the distal gastric antrum (Fig. 55-10). Care must be taken to image such webs in the true midlongitudinal plane because if an incomplete diaphragm is imaged at its periphery, a complete diaphragm may be erroneously suggested.

Gastritis and Ulcer Disease

Peptic ulcer disease in pediatric patients is probably more common than generally is appreciated.[26] **Gastric ulcers** are more common in younger children (median age of 6.5 years) and *Helicobacter pylori* infection is less prevalent with gastric ulcers than with duodenal ulcers.[26] Sonography is not particularly helpful with duodenal ulcers, but gastric inflammatory disease may be visible sonographically. Barium radiographic studies often reveal nothing more than persistent deformity or spasm of the antropyloric region. Ultrasound of the fluid-filled stomach permits direct visualization of the thickened gastric mucosa and submucosa,[27] which often is accompanied by loss of definition of the individual layers of the gastric wall (Fig. 55-11). The ulcer crater itself usually is not visualized sonographically. Ultrasound can also be used to follow therapy, showing a return of the normal gastric wall layers as the ulcer heals. Thickening of the gastric mucosa is not a specific finding and can be seen with other conditions, such as **eosinophilic gastritis, inflammatory pseudotumor,**[28] **chronic granulomatous disease, Ménétrier's disease,**[29] **milk allergy,** and **prostaglandin-induced antral foveolar hyperplasia.**[30,31] The latter condition is self-limiting and can be seen in asymptomatic infants.[32]

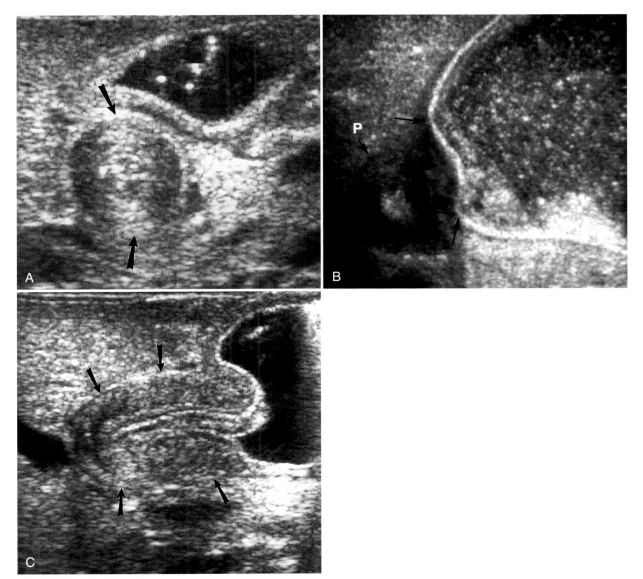

FIGURE 55-8. Hypertrophic pyloric stenosis. A, Echogenicity artifact at 6- and 12-o'clock positions (anisotropic effect). Cross-sectional image through the pylorus shows the thickened muscle with increased echogenicity at 6- and 12-o'clock positions *(arrows).* **B,** Posteriorly directed canal artifact. Note the squared-off appearance of the gastric antrum *(arrows).* The thickened pylorus *(P)* is only partially visible in this imaging plane. **C,** Longitudinal scan shows elongated canal. Anisotropic effect causes muscle to be more echogenic *(arrows).*

Bezoar

Lactobezoars are the most common form of bezoar in children, occurring predominantly in infants who are fed improperly reconstituted powdered formula. In older children, **trichobezoars,** caused by the ingestion of hair, are more common. Both types of bezoar can be easily identified with ultrasound, especially if the patient is given clear fluid to help outline the mass. Lactobezoars appear as a solid, heterogeneous, echogenic intraluminal mass[33] (Fig. 55-12). With trichobezoars, air tends to be trapped in and around the hair fibers, which causes a characteristic arc of echogenicity that obscures the mass but conforms to the shape of the distended stomach.[34]

DUODENUM AND SMALL BOWEL

Normal Anatomy and Technique

Normally, intestinal gas prevents complete visualization of the duodenum and small bowel with ultrasound. However, if the stomach is filled with fluid, it is often possible to identify the duodenal bulb and descending duodenum (see Figs. 55-2 and 55-3). In addition, gradual compression of the abdomen with the transducer during scanning often encourages the gas to move to other areas, allowing previously obscured small bowel loops to be examined. The mucosa, submucosa, and muscular layers can be delineated,[24] especially in those loops that contain fluid (Fig. 55-13).

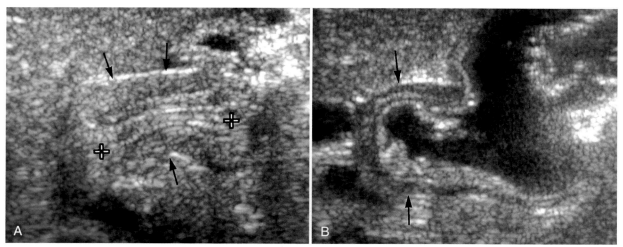

FIGURE 55-9. Empty stomach artifact. A, Before fluid is administered, the antrum is contracted and the pyloric muscle appears thickened *(arrows).* **B,** When fluid distends the antrum, the true normal thickness of the muscle is seen *(arrows).*

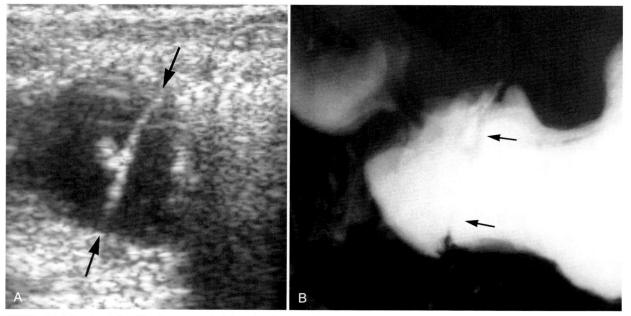

FIGURE 55-10. Gastric diaphragm. A, Note the thin membrane *(arrows)* crossing the fluid-filled gastric antrum. **B,** The same diaphragm seen during a contrast upper GI series *(arrows).*

Congenital Duodenal Obstruction

Sonography can readily identify an obstructed, fluid-filled, distended duodenum, and frequently the level of obstruction can be determined. Complete duodenal obstruction in the newborn is often readily apparent on radiographs, and ultrasound generally provides little additional useful information. However, in patients in whom the stomach and duodenum are filled with fluid rather than air, ultrasound can be quite useful.

Proximal duodenal obstruction resulting in the **classic double-bubble sign** occurs with **duodenal atresia,** with or without associated annular pancreas (Fig. 55-14). Plain radiograph findings usually are diagnostic, showing two air-filled bubbles representing the dilated stomach and proximal duodenum. Similar findings can be seen with **severe duodenal stenosis** and **duodenal diaphragms or webs.** Usually, sonography is not needed to identify obstructions in this portion of the duodenum. However, when duodenal atresia is associated with esophageal atresia, air cannot reach the stomach and duodenum, making radiographic diagnosis more difficult. Sonography is diagnostic in such infants by demonstrating the grossly distended, fluid-filled duodenal bulb, stomach, and distal esophagus.[35,36]

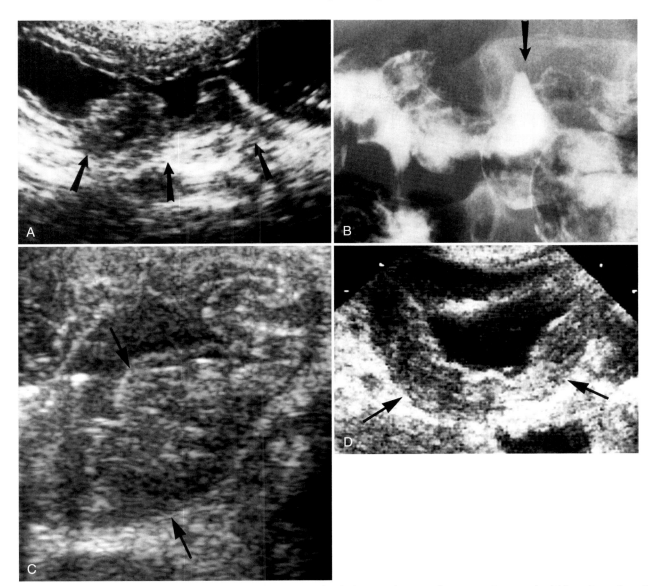

FIGURE 55-11. Gastritis. A, Gastric ulcer disease. Longitudinal ultrasound image of antrum. Note greatly thickened gastric wall with poorly defined mural layers *(arrows)*. An ulcer crater is suggested. **B,** Contrast study shows a large gastric ulcer *(arrow)*. **C, Immunosuppressed transplant patient.** Marked thickening of the gastric mucosa *(arrows)*. **D, Chronic granulomatous disease.** Marked thickening of the gastric wall *(arrows)* in a child. *(Courtesy W. McAlister, MD.)*

Sonography has been used for diagnosis of **intestinal malrotation with midgut volvulus** in an infant with bilious vomiting, although fluoroscopic upper GI series remains the "gold standard." If an ultrasound is performed in a patient with volvulus, vigorous peristalsis of the obstructed duodenal C-loop is seen, and characteristic tapering of the distal, twisted end often can be visualized[37] (Fig. 55-15). Above all, it is the location of the obstruction (i.e., third or fourth portion of duodenum) that most strongly suggests the diagnosis of midgut volvulus. Obstruction from **peritoneal** (Ladd's) **bands,** which also accompanies rotational anomalies of the intestine, can have an identical appearance. In addition to these findings, an abnormal position of the superior mesenteric vein and artery can be seen in patients with intestinal malrotation, with or without volvulus (Fig. 55-16, *B*). Failure of normal embryologic bowel rotation leaves the superior mesenteric vein anterior to or to the left of the superior mesenteric artery[38,39] as opposed to its normal position to the right of the artery. Although this finding is not always present in volvulus,[40] it is probably worthwhile to observe the relationship of these vessels in any child who is undergoing sonography for the evaluation of vomiting. When color Doppler ultrasound is used, the twisted mesenteric vessels are seen swirling in a clockwise direction **(whirlpool sign),** and this finding is highly suggestive of midgut volvulus[41] (Fig. 55-16, *C*). Although these findings are valuable for

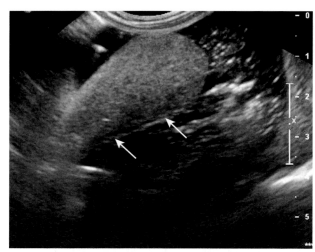

FIGURE 55-12. Lactobezoar. Longitudinal ultrasound of the stomach. Note large filling defect caused by the lactobezoar in an otherwise fluid-filled stomach. The child had been NPO for 6 hours.

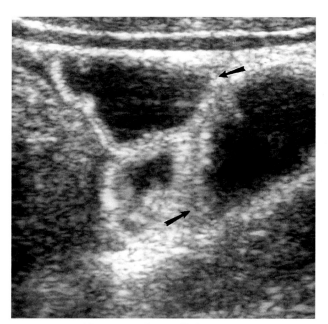

FIGURE 55-13. Normal small bowel. Note the thin-walled, fluid-distended loops *(arrows)*.

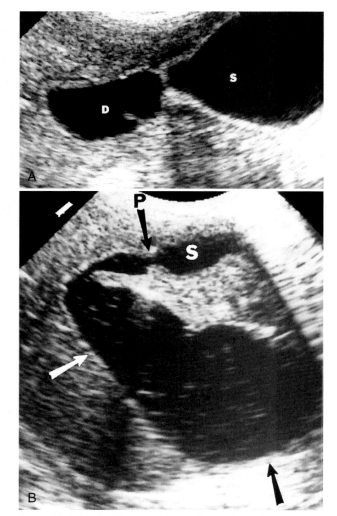

FIGURE 55-14. Duodenal obstruction. A, Duodenal **atresia.** Grossly distended duodenal bulb *(D)* and stomach *(S)*. **B, Duodenal diaphragm.** Grossly distended, obstructed descending duodenum *(arrows); P,* pyloric canal; *S,* stomach.

suggesting the diagnosis, absence of these findings does not exclude malrotation or volvulus.[42]

A final cause of distal duodenal obstruction is a **duodenal diaphragm** that has stretched into a windsock configuration (Fig. 55-14, *B*). The distal end of the obstructed duodenum will have a rounded shape in this condition,[43] as opposed to the tapered end, which is seen more often with midgut volvulus (Fig. 55-15).

Duodenal Hematoma

Duodenal hematoma is a common complication of blunt abdominal trauma in children, including those

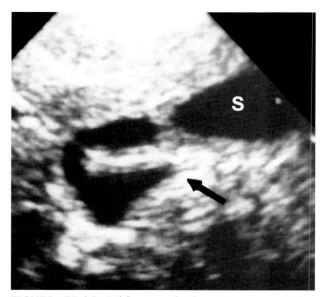

FIGURE 55-15. Midgut volvulus. Vigorous peristaltic activity fails to empty the duodenum, and the third portion of the duodenum has **beak deformity** *(arrow); S,* stomach.

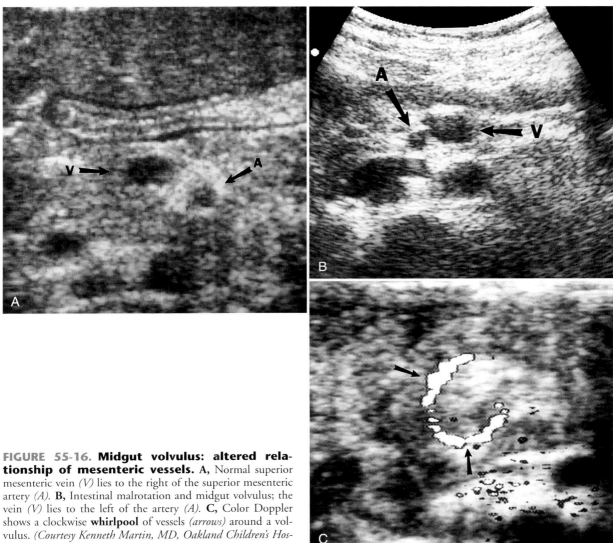

FIGURE 55-16. Midgut volvulus: altered relationship of mesenteric vessels. A, Normal superior mesenteric vein *(V)* lies to the right of the superior mesenteric artery *(A)*. **B,** Intestinal malrotation and midgut volvulus; the vein *(V)* lies to the left of the artery *(A)*. **C,** Color Doppler shows a clockwise **whirlpool** of vessels *(arrows)* around a volvulus. *(Courtesy Kenneth Martin, MD, Oakland Children's Hospital, Oakland, Calif.)*

with battered child syndrome. Sonography can demonstrate the dilated, obstructed duodenum and more specifically can show evidence of an intramural hematoma[44-46] (Fig. 55-17). The intramural hemorrhage initially causes echogenic thickening of the wall of the duodenum, but as time passes, the hematoma undergoes liquefaction and the thickened wall becomes hypoechoic. Similar hematomas can occur with Henoch-Schönlein purpura[47] (see later discussion).

Small Bowel Obstruction

The diagnosis of small bowel obstruction is usually accomplished with plain radiographs. At times, however, ultrasound can be used to help determine the site or cause of the obstruction. In cases of mechanical small bowel obstruction, the fluid-filled, dilated, hyperperistaltic loops of small bowel proximal to the obstruction are usually clearly visible with ultrasound (Fig. 55-18).

In neonates with congenital causes of small bowel obstruction (e.g., ileal atresia, meconium ileus), prenatal intestinal perforation can occur, releasing variable amounts of meconium into the peritoneal cavity. In some of these fetuses, the perforation heals in utero, and the only clues that remain after birth are scattered calcifications in the peritoneal cavity. In patients in whom larger amounts of meconium have leaked, or in whom an active leak remains after birth, cystic masses can be found in the peritoneal cavity, giving rise to the term **cystic meconium peritonitis**. Sonographically, these cysts appear as variably sized, fairly well-defined cystic collections, often with very heterogeneous cystic fluid.[48,49] The highly echogenic calcifications can also be found with ultrasound (Fig. 55-19). Echogenic ascitic fluid may also be present after perforation, whether in utero or neonatal. It may be missed if only still images are recorded, so video clips may be useful for later review (if saved on PACS).

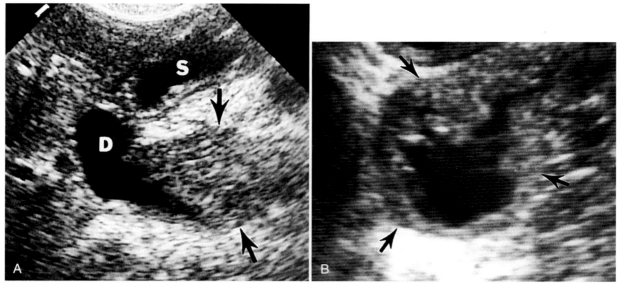

FIGURE 55-17. Duodenal hematoma. A, Large echogenic hematoma *(arrows),* compressing and obstructing duodenum *(D),* caused by blunt abdominal trauma; *S,* stomach. **B,** Asymmetrical thickening of the duodenal wall *(arrows)* caused by intramural hemorrhage in a patient with Henoch-Schönlein purpura. Note central cystic area as hematoma liquefies. *(Courtesy C. K. Hayden, Jr, MD, Fort Worth, Texas.)*

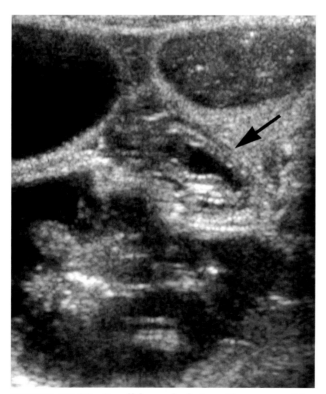

FIGURE 55-18. Small bowel obstruction caused by Meckel's diverticulum and fibrous bands. Dilated, fluid-filled, obstructed small bowel loops surround the small tubular diverticulum *(arrow).*

Small bowel obstruction from **intestinal hematomas** usually occurs as a result of Henoch-Schönlein purpura, blunt abdominal trauma, or coagulopathies. In any of these conditions, the mural hemorrhage can be detected sonographically as asymmetrical or circumferential areas of intestinal wall thickening that can vary from echogenic to hypoechoic in texture.[47]

Intussusception

Intussusception is the most common cause of small bowel obstruction in children between the ages of 6 months and 4 years. Clinical findings of crampy, intermittent abdominal pain, vomiting, palpable abdominal mass, and "currant jelly" stools are classic. Patients with these characteristic symptoms probably do not require ultrasound diagnosis before attempted enema reduction. Many of these clinical features are present in young children with abdominal pain for other reasons, and some children with intussusception do not exhibit all the classic features. In such children, sonography can help confirm or exclude intussusception. Sensitivity and specificity for the diagnosis of intussusception with ultrasound is virtually 100%.[50-54] If an intussusception is not demonstrated sonographically, an enema need not be performed unless clinical suspicion is high.

SONOGRAPHIC SIGNS OF INTUSSUSCEPTION

Oval hypoechoic mass
   Pseudokidney or doughnut sign
Hypoechoic rim with central echogenicity
Multiple layers and concentric rings
Small amount of peritoneal fluid
Large amount of peritoneal fluid
   Suggests perforation, especially echogenic ascites

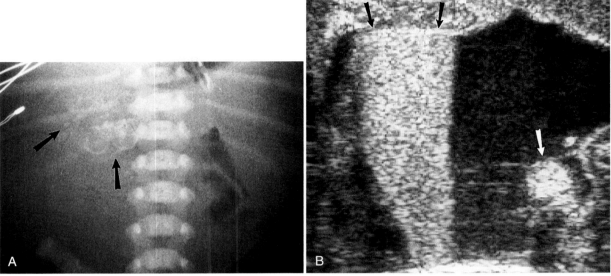

FIGURE 55-19. Cystic meconium peritonitis with calcification. A, Curvilinear calcifications in the right upper quadrant *(arrows)* of the distended abdomen in a newborn. **B,** Sonography revealed large, loculated areas of fluid with echogenic debris *(black arrows).* Echogenic calcifications were also noted *(white arrow).*

The sonographic appearance of intussusception can vary slightly depending on the type of ultrasound transducer that is used for the examination. When a 5-MHz sector scanner is used, the intussusception appears as an oval, hypoechoic mass with bright, central echoes on longitudinal imaging (i.e., **pseudokidney**) and a **hypoechoic doughnut,** or **target configuration,** on cross-sectional imaging.[55-57] The hypoechoic rim represents the edematous wall of the intussusceptum, and the central echogenicity represents compressed mesentery, mucosa, and intestinal contents. Linear array transducers, however, display the intussusceptum with greater clarity, showing multiple layers and concentric rings (Fig. 55-20), representing the bowel wall, mesentery, and even lymph nodes that have been drawn into the intussusception[58,59] (Fig. 55-21). In some cases, anechoic fluid is also seen trapped within the incompletely compressed head of the intussusception.

Once an intussusception has been documented by sonography, the patient usually proceeds to nonsurgical reduction, unless clinical or radiographic evidence of perforation is found. Currently, air reduction is the most popular method of treatment, although hydrostatic reduction using water-soluble contrast remains a viable alternative. **Ultrasound-guided hydrostatic reduction** has been suggested as a method to avoid the ionizing radiation of standard fluoroscopic examinations. The procedure has been used successfully in several centers,[60-62] but this technique has not achieved universal acceptance. Consequently, the primary role of ultrasound continues to be the diagnosis of intussusception. Sonography can also be used to identify the ileo-ileal intussusception that sometimes remains after the successful hydrostatic reduction of the ileocolic portion of

an intussusception. **Recurrent intussusception** occurs in approximately 4% to 10% of cases, and thus ultrasound is worthwhile in children with recurrent symptoms after successful enema reduction. Small bowel intussusception is less common in children, but it can occur when lead points such as **polyps** or **Meckel's diverticulum** are present or may occur as a postoperative complication of major abdominal surgeries.[63] Enema examinations are not helpful for diagnosis or treatment of intussusceptions restricted to small bowel, but ultrasound can provide prompt identification of the abnormality in most cases.[64]

Spontaneous reduction of intussusception is a well-known phenomenon that has been documented sonographically. In such patients, when symptoms subside between the time the diagnosis is made and the time a reduction procedure is begun, ultrasound can verify resolution of the intussusception and spare the patient an unnecessary enema procedure.[65] **Transient small bowel intussusception** is a common occurrence, especially in patients with hyperperistalsis. These intussusceptions are not associated with significant edema in the intussuscepted loops, and therefore the peripheral rim of the intussusception appears thinner and more echogenic than firmly impacted intussusceptions[66,67] (Fig. 55-20, *E* and *F*). The patient is usually asymptomatic, and spontaneous resolution of the intussusception usually can be observed at ultrasound with a little patience. Intussusception of the small bowel associated with gastrojejunal feeding tubes can also be identified sonographically.[68]

The only absolute contraindication to nonsurgical reduction of an intussusception is radiographic evidence of free intraperitoneal air or clinical signs of peritonitis. A small amount of free peritoneal fluid is typically seen

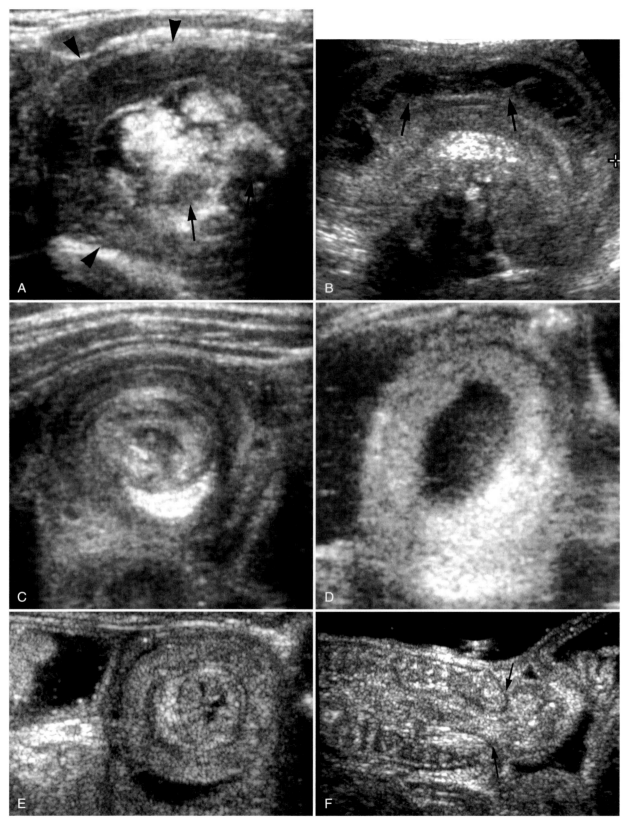

FIGURE 55-20. Intussusception. A, Linear transducers clearly show the concentric rings of the edematous intussusceptum *(arrowheads)* with echogenic fat, mesenteric lymph nodes *(arrows),* and hypoechoic fluid trapped in the center. **B,** Another intussusception, demonstrating a large amount of trapped fluid *(arrows).* **C,** Intussusception, showing concentric rings of bowel within bowel. **D,** Same intussusception as in **C,** showing only trapped fluid at different level. **E,** Transient intussusception with echogenic texture of the rim. **F,** Same intussusception as in **E.** Longitudinal image in real time shows in-and-out movement of the intussusception *(arrows)* and multiple transient intussusceptions, but patient remained asymptomatic.

during ultrasound in patients with intussusception, even in the absence of perforation.[69,70] Therefore, a small amount of ascites is not a contraindication to nonsurgical reduction. However, if a large amount of ascites is found or the fluid appears complex, perforation should be considered.

Investigators have attempted to correlate certain ultrasound features of intussusception with the subsequent ability to reduce them nonsurgically. Findings such as peripheral rim thickness of greater than 1 cm, large amounts of internal trapped fluid, and lymph nodes larger than 1 cm within the intussusception have shown some correlation with decreased success of enema reduction.[59,71] Color Doppler assessment of blood flow to the intussusceptum has been used to identify patients who have significant bowel ischemia and who may be at greater risk of perforation during attempted nonsurgical reduction[72,73] (Fig. 55-22). The true reliability of these findings has yet to be determined.

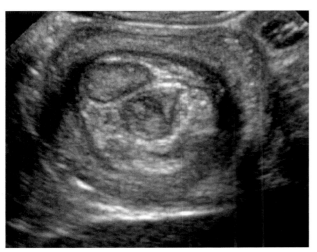

FIGURE 55-21. Intussusception. Transverse ultrasound of the right lower quadrant demonstrates an ileocolic intussusception with multiple lymph nodes that have been drawn into the intussusception.

COLON

Normal Anatomy and Technique

Sonographic evaluation of the colon can be compromised by the gas and fecal material that are frequently present. When sufficient fluid is present within the colon, the characteristic haustral markings in the multilayered wall can be identified. When pathologic wall thickening occurs, it tends to displace the gas and intestinal contents. These abnormal areas of colon are often more easily visible than is the normal colon. Ultrasound may be a useful adjunct in the evaluation of colitis in children. Patterns of inflammation and mural stratification have been described to assist in the diagnosis of colitis. However, sonography in the colon mainly focuses on imaging inflammatory disease and imperforate or ectopic anus. Some authors advocate graded compression for sonographic evaluation of colonic polyps.[74]

Ectopic or Imperforate Anus

In patients with ectopic or imperforate anus, it is important to determine where the distal end of the hindgut terminates. Well-known pitfalls in attempting this with plain radiographs include those taken in the cross-table prone position. Radiographically, the colon can erroneously appear to end in a high position if the air column fails to progress to the end of the colon because of impacted meconium. Sonography can directly visualize the end of the hindgut pouch, and the corresponding sacral level can be determined (Fig. 55-23). Thereafter, the level can be transferred to the plain radiographs, and the M-line of Cremin can be drawn.[75] The M-line corresponds to the level of the puborectalis sling, and if the hindgut ends above the line, a **high fistula** is presumed. If the hindgut ends below this line, **a low fistula** should be present.

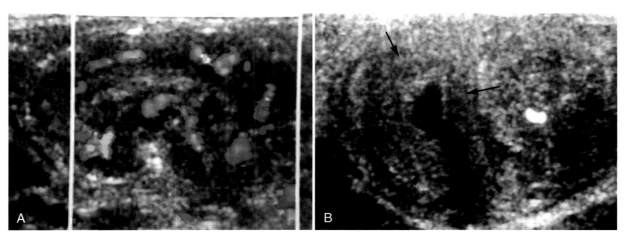

FIGURE 55-22. Intussusception: Doppler imaging. A, Color Doppler ultrasound demonstrates substantial blood flow within the wall of the intussusceptum. Hydrostatic reduction was successful in this patient without complication. **B,** Power Doppler ultrasound in another patient shows minimal flow within the wall of the intussusceptum *(arrows)*. At surgery, the bowel was necrotic.

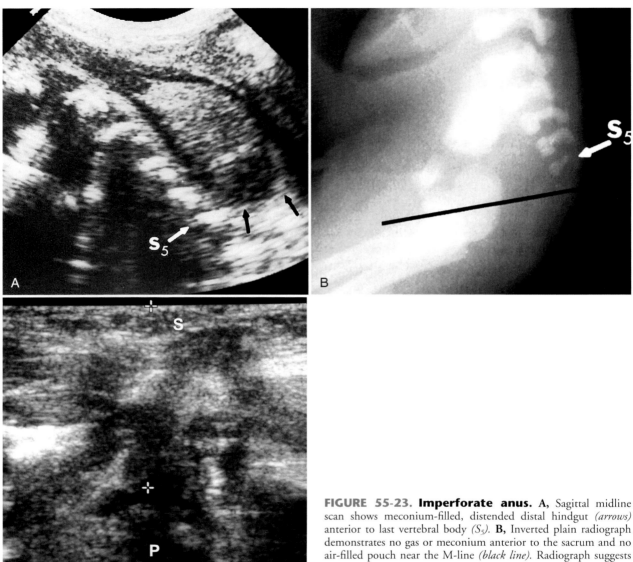

FIGURE 55-23. Imperforate anus. A, Sagittal midline scan shows meconium-filled, distended distal hindgut *(arrows)* anterior to last vertebral body *(S₅).* **B,** Inverted plain radiograph demonstrates no gas or meconium anterior to the sacrum and no air-filled pouch near the M-line *(black line).* Radiograph suggests that the hindgut ends quite high, but ultrasound clearly demonstrates a low pouch filled with meconium. **C,** Transverse perineal approach shows the pouch *(P)* less than 1.5 cm from the skin surface *(S).*

Sonographic images can also be obtained from a perineal approach at the site of the anal dimple. In this way, the distance between the skin surface and the blind-ending hindgut can be measured, and a distance of less than 1.5 mm suggests a **low pouch.**[76-78] In some cases, this procedure can be tricky to perform and lacks precision.

INTESTINAL INFLAMMATORY DISEASE

Although computed tomography (CT) and radiographic contrast studies are often used for evaluating inflammatory conditions of the intestines, ultrasound can provide similar information and avoids the ionizing radiation associated with CT. High-resolution linear array transducers allow direct and detailed evaluation of the intestinal wall, and areas of intestinal wall thickening can often be identified. Such thickening is nonspecific[79] and can be seen in a variety of inflammatory conditions, including regional enteritis,[80,81] ulcerative colitis,[81] pseudomembranous colitis,[82,83] neutropenic colitis (typhlitis),[84] bacterial ileocolitis,[85-87] allergic colitis,[88] Kawasaki disease,[89] necrotizing enterocolitis,[90] hemolytic-uremic syndrome,[91] graft-versus-host disease,[92,93] glycogen storage disease type 1B,[94] and chronic granulomatous disease of childhood. Even viral gastroenteritis can produce mild mucosal thickening in fluid-filled loops with diminished peristalsis.

CAUSES OF INTESTINAL WALL THICKENING

Inflammatory bowel disease (Crohn's or regional
  enteritis, ulcerative colitis)
Yersinia, Campylobacter ileocolitis
Colitis
Perforated appendicitis
Rotavirus
Cytomegalovirus (CMV) infection (AIDS)
Typhlitis
Chronic granulomatous disease
Eosinophilic enteritis
Hematoma (Henoch-Schönlein purpura, trauma)
Hemolytic uremic syndrome
Graft-versus-host disease
Intussusception
Lymphoma
Benign tumors
Tuberculosis (rare)
Celiac disease

Sonography can sometimes differentiate **mucosal** from **transmural** inflammation. If the inflammatory process involves primarily the mucosa (e.g., ulcerative colitis, pseudomembranous colitis, typhlitis), the inner echogenic mucosal layer becomes thickened and sometimes nodular or irregular, but the outer muscular layer of the wall remains thin (Fig. 55-24). When the inflammation involves the entire intestinal wall (e.g., regional enteritis), thickening of the entire wall is seen (Fig. 55-25). Color Doppler sonography demonstrates increased blood flow to the thickened intestinal loops with most inflammatory bowel conditions,[95] but hypovascularity is more typical in hemolytic uremic syndrome.[91] Doppler measurement of the resistive index (RI) in the superior mesenteric artery has been used to assess progression of disease in patients with active Crohn's disease.[96] Sonography is indicated in most of these children with regional enteritis to identify distal right ureteral involvement by the inflammatory mass that can result in hydronephrosis. Although the fistulas and sinus tracts that develop in regional enteritis are usually not discernible sonographically, ultrasound can be used to identify associated intra-abdominal abscesses. Recent advances in contrast-enhanced ultrasound and development of high-frequency probes may allow evaluation of disease activity and treatment efficacy in Crohn's disease.[97]

Henoch-Schönlein purpura, a condition probably caused by an allergic vasculitis of small vessels in a variety of body systems, frequently involves the GI tract. Of these patients, 50% to 60% develop abdominal pain from intramural hemorrhage in the intestines, and this symptom may precede the development of the more characteristic purpuric skin rash. In such patients, sonography may detect the involved intestinal loops, which usually show circumferential, echogenic wall thickening, sometimes associated with small amounts of free abdominal fluid[47] (Fig. 55-26). Sonography also can be used to follow the resolution of the intestinal hemorrhage. **Intussusception** is a major complication of Henoch-Schönlein purpura, and sonography is highly useful to identify such an intussusception,[98] which usually involves only the small bowel and does not extend into the colon. Intestinal hemorrhage may also complicate bleeding diatheses or blunt abdominal trauma (Fig. 55-27).

A variety of other conditions can result in thickening of the wall of the small bowel or colon, but few show distinguishing characteristics at imaging. **Hemolytic uremic syndrome** (HUS) is associated with *Escherichia coli* 0157:H7 infection, characterized by hemolytic anemia, thrombocytopenia, and renal failure. HUS is usually preceded by a severe hemorrhagic colitis. Color Doppler imaging reveals that the thickened bowel segments are hypovascular,[91] probably secondary to fibrin microthrombi that develop from factors released by the damaged endothelium (see Fig. 55-24, *E,* and Chapter 54). **Graft-versus-host disease** in bone marrow transplant patients occurs when the transplanted tissue mounts an attack on host tissues. Skin, liver, and GI involvement is common. Diffuse, circumferential, small bowel wall thickening and hyperemia are the predominant findings on ultrasound, with relatively less involvement of the colon. Intestinal injury results in abdominal pain, vomiting, and diarrhea. The thickened, featureless intestinal loops are visible with ultrasound. A thin rim of echogenic material lining the mucosal surface of the affected loops has been described[92] (Fig. 55-28). This membrane is thought to represent the fibrinous exudate often seen covering the ulcerated mucosa at endoscopy in this condition.

Necrotizing enterocolitis (NEC) in newborns is usually detected radiographically, but early in the disease, the classic findings of bowel dilation and pneumatosis intestinalis may not be apparent. In such cases, sonography may detect early thickening of the intestinal loops (Fig. 55-29, *A* and *D*). **Pneumatosis intestinalis** may be visible on sonography before it is seen on radiographs, appearing as small, punctate, echogenic foci in the nondependent wall or as a continuous echogenic ring[99] within the wall of affected bowel loops (Fig. 55-29, *B*). In addition, sonography can detect small amounts of gas within the portal venous system, which appear as small echogenic foci within the liver[100,101] (Fig. 55-29, *C*). **Pericholecystic hyperechogenicity** has also been described in infants with NEC.[102] The most serious complication is **bowel necrosis with perforation.** Increased flow velocity in the splanchnic arteries, most likely caused by vasoconstriction, has been suggested as a reliable early finding on Doppler sonography in NEC infants.[103] Free intra-abdominal air may not be detectable in infants who have minimal intestinal gas to escape

Text continued on p. 1912

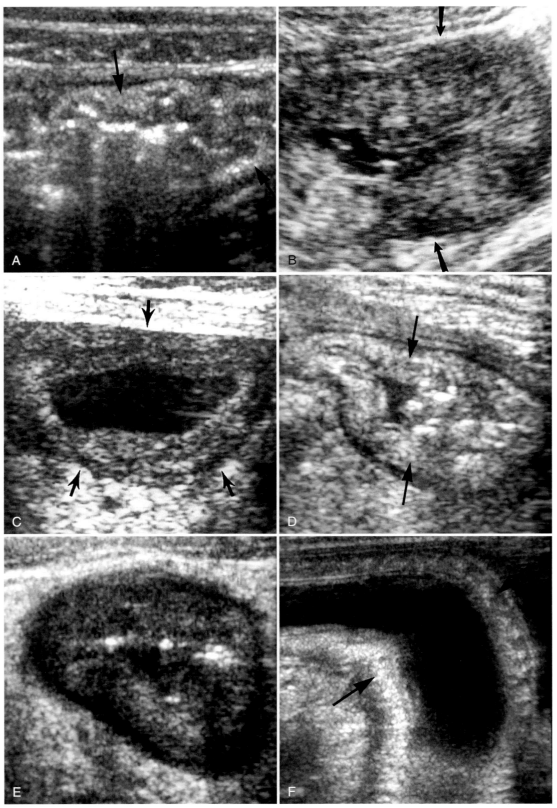

FIGURE 55-24. Inflammatory disease: mucosal thickening. A, Pseudomembranous colitis. Mild mucosal thickening *(arrow).* **B, Leukemia,** complicated by typhlitis. Echogenic thickening of the cecum *(arrows).* **C, Chronic granulomatous disease.** Echogenic thickening of small bowel mucosa *(arrows).* **D, Immunosuppressed transplant patient.** Thick colonic mucosa *(arrows).* **E, Hemolytic uremic syndrome.** Greatly thickened colonic mucosa. **F, Rotavirus infection.** Echogenic mucosal thickening *(arrows).*

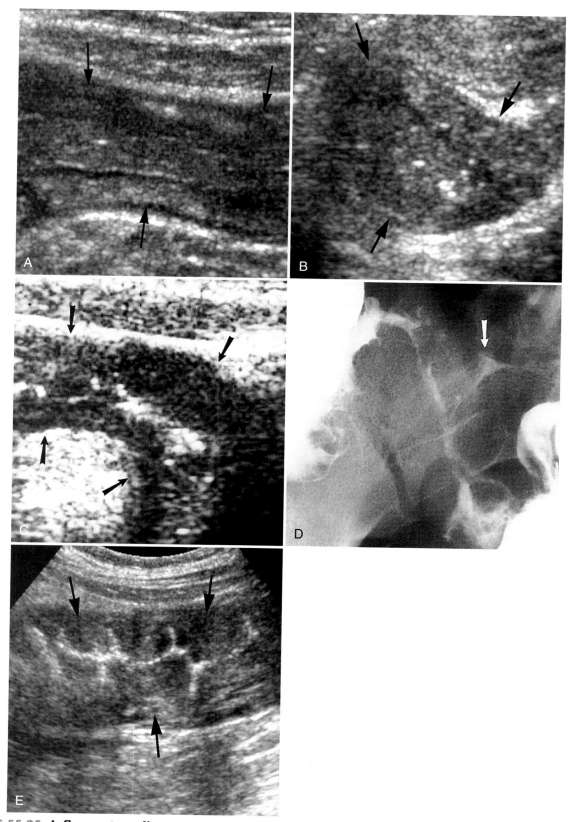

FIGURE 55-25. Inflammatory disease: transmural thickening. A, Regional enteritis. Hypoechoic thickening of the wall of the ileum *(arrows)* in a 13-year-old child. **B,** Same patient as **A.** An abscess was found nearby in the left lower quadrant *(arrows).* **C, Regional enteritis.** Hypoechoic thickening of the entire wall of the terminal ileum *(arrows).* **D,** Same patient as **C.** Narrowed lumen and a small fistula *(arrow)* on a contrast study. **E, Colitis and severe pyelonephritis.** Greatly thickened colonic wall *(arrows).*

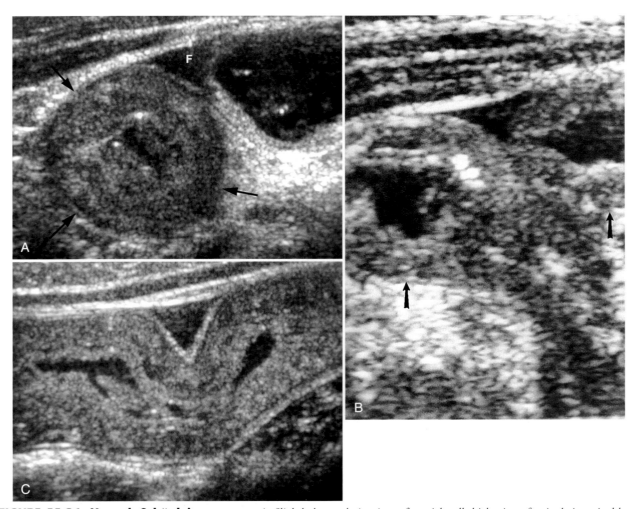

FIGURE 55-26. Henoch-Schönlein purpura. A, Slightly hypoechoic, circumferential wall thickening of a single intestinal loop *(arrows),* with a small amount of adjacent anechoic free fluid *(F).* Note the normal thin wall of the adjacent bowel loop. **B, Intramural hemorrhage** in a different patient, showing adjacent loops with echogenic wall thickening *(arrows).* **C,** Another child with echogenic, small bowel thickening caused by Henoch Schönlein purpura.

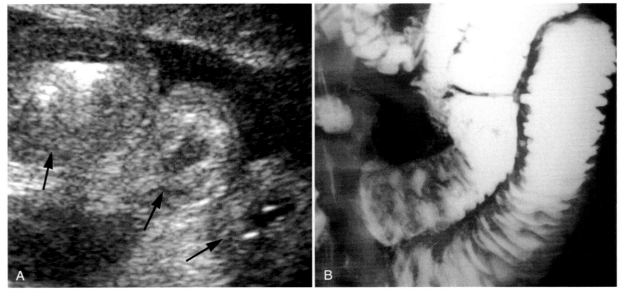

FIGURE 55-27. Hemophilia. A, Intramural hemorrhage in an adolescent. Multiple loops of small bowel with echogenic wall thickening *(arrows).* **B,** Upper GI series shows partial bowel obstruction and thick mucosal folds.

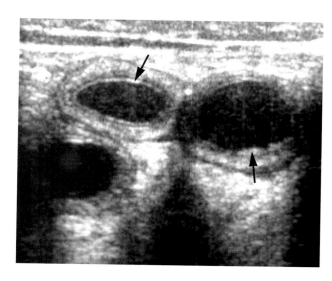

FIGURE 55-28. Graft-versus-host disease. Multiple thick-walled small bowel loops. A thin echogenic layer on the superficial surface of the mucosa *(arrows)* represents characteristic fibrinous deposit.

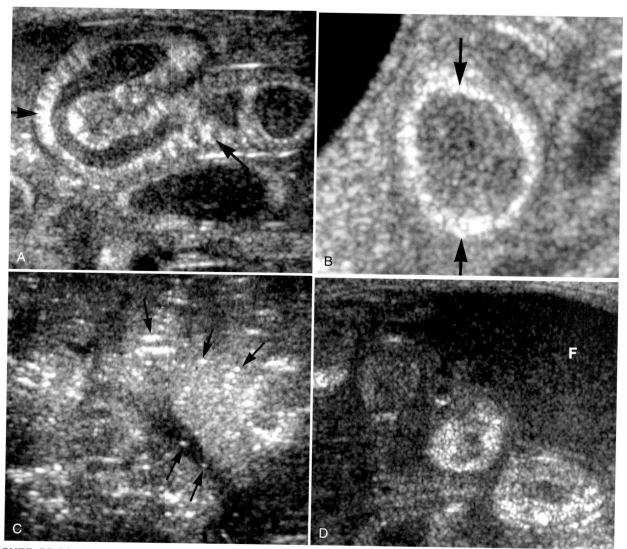

FIGURE 55-29. Necrotizing enterocolitis. A, Mucosal and submucosal thickening *(arrows).* **B,** Intramural gas (pneumatosis intestinalis) creates an echogenic ring *(arrows).* **C,** Widespread echogenic bubbles of gas in the portal veins *(arrows).* **D,** Fluid with echogenic debris *(F)* lies adjacent to thick loops.

through the perforation, but the sonographic demonstration of **ascites with fluid-debris levels** can suggest perforation in such patients[104] (Fig. 55-29, D).

SONOGRAPHIC SIGNS OF NECROTIZING ENTEROCOLITIS

Thickened bowel loops
Echogenic foci caused by portal venous air
Echogenic ring of intramural pneumatosis
Pericholecystic hyperechogenicity
Increased flow in superior mesenteric artery and celiac artery
Ascites with fluid-debris levels if perforation occurred

Appendicitis

Sonography is now accepted as a highly accurate modality for the detection of appendicitis in children.[105-108] Sonography is especially useful in children with ambiguous clinical findings,[109,110] and when appendicitis is not found, ultrasound often can help to suggest or confirm an alternative diagnosis.[111] In the end, the diagnostic approach to the acute abdomen remains a surgical management decision, but sonography is increasingly used to help diagnose appendicitis and to help manage postoperative complications.

SONOGRAPHIC SIGNS OF APPENDICITIS

Noncompressible, blind-ended, tubular structure
Diameter of tube ≥6 mm
Fluid trapped within nonperforated appendix
Target appearance of echogenic mucosa around fluid center surrounded by hypoechoic muscle
Fecalith: echogenic foci with pronounced posterior acoustic shadowing
Lymphadenopathy: nonspecific
Hypervascular appendix on color Doppler ultrasound
Gangrenous appendix: lack of flow on color Doppler ultrasound

---

Sonography of a child with acute abdominal pain is a procedure that requires patience and experience. The examination is facilitated by clinically localizing the pain, and even young children can help to guide the examination if asked to point with one finger to the site of maximal tenderness. Posterior manual compression may help to identify the appendix in patients whose appendix is not seen with graded-compression technique.[112] The normal appendix can be visualized in a variable percentage of cases, depending on operator experience and amount of intestinal gas. The normal appendix is easily compressible and smaller than the inflamed appendix, usually measuring less than 6 mm in diameter (Fig. 55-30). When the appendix cannot be found sonographically, the study is generally considered indeterminate. However, the absence of other secondary findings of appendicitis proves to be useful information when clinical suspicion is low. Confidence in sonographic interpretation is a major limiting factor in the use of ultrasound for appendicitis that improves as one gains greater experience.

Sonographically, the acute, inflamed appendix appears as a blind-ending tubular structure that is noncompressible and measures 6 mm or greater in diameter.[113] Size of the appendix can vary significantly in patients with both normal and abnormal appendices, and the 6-mm criterion is more useful for excluding appendicitis than for confirming it.[114] Demonstration of other, associated sonographic abnormalities improves confidence in the diagnosis. **Fluid** is often seen trapped within a nonperforated appendix, and the surrounding echogenic mucosal layer and hypoechoic muscular layer of the appendiceal wall, combined with the central anechoic fluid, give the appendix a target appearance in cross section (Fig. 55-31). **Fecaliths,** even those not calcified, can often be identified, appearing as echogenic foci with pronounced posterior acoustic shadowing (Fig. 55-31, D). A small amount of fluid may be seen adjacent to the appendix, even in the absence of perforation. Mesenteric lymphadenopathy frequently accompanies appendicitis, but alone is a nonspecific finding seen with other types of abdominal inflammation[115] (Fig. 55-32).

An advantage of sonography over other imaging modalities is the ability to correlate the pain of appendicitis with the imaging findings. Pinpoint tenderness with compression over the appendix is diagnostic in many children.[113] In cases of **perforated** appendicitis, the appendix itself is often more difficult to identify than in acute nonperforated appendicitis.[116] With perforation, the appendix becomes decompressed, and increasing intestinal gas from adynamic ileus and functional obstruction can interfere with the ultrasound examination (Fig. 55-33). Nevertheless, a careful, graded-compression technique may allow detection of focal loops of paralyzed bowel in the right lower quadrant, or a complex fluid collection representing an **abscess**[117] (Fig. 55-33, C). Loss of the normal echogenic submucosal layer suggests a **gangrenous appendix** (Fig. 55-33, D), often associated with perforation.

The use of color Doppler sonography for appendicitis can be helpful in some cases. Studies suggest that color Doppler imaging not only facilitates the identification of the inflamed appendix and increases confidence in the diagnosis,[117-119] but also provides clues to the presence of perforation. In acute nonperforated appendicitis the appendix itself is hypervascular (see Fig. 55-31, C), but as necrosis progresses, the amount of flow within the appendix decreases. After perforation, increasing flow may be seen in the soft tissues surrounding the appendix, and an abdominal fluid collection with peripheral hyper-

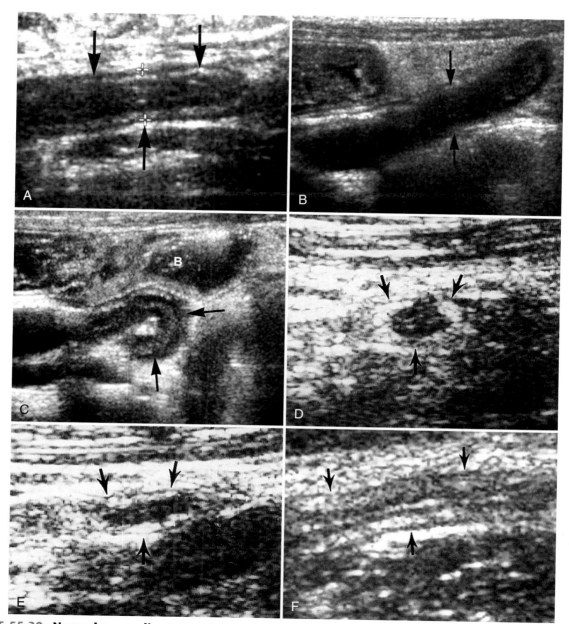

FIGURE 55-30. Normal appendix. Compression is critical to diagnosis. **A,** Fluid-filled but normal appendix *(arrows)*. **B,** Another patient, with a nontender but slightly large appendix *(arrows)*. **C,** Same patient as **B.** Appendix moves freely with peristalsis of adjacent bowel loops. **D,** In transverse section, this appendix measures 4.5 mm in diameter *(arrows)*. **E,** With compression, the appendix in **D** decreases to 3 mm *(arrows)*. **F,** Another normal appendix, with no intraluminal fluid, measuring 4 mm *(arrows)*.

emia is a fairly reliable indicator of abscess formation.[118,119] It is important to remember that many inflammatory conditions of the intestine other than appendicitis may be associated with small amounts of **free fluid surrounding the bowel loops.** Therefore, small collections of fluid without other definitive evidence of appendicitis should not necessarily suggest an appendiceal abscess.

Other inflammatory conditions in the right lower quadrant may resemble appendicitis clinically but may be identified sonographically. **Mesenteric adenitis** refers

SONOGRAPHIC SIGNS OF APPENDICEAL PERFORATION

Appendix difficult to find
Appendix decompressed
Focal loops of paralyzed bowel
Complex fluid collection in an abscess
Loss of normal, echogenic submucosal layer, suggesting gangrene
Decreased vascular flow with necrosis starts in center of appendix

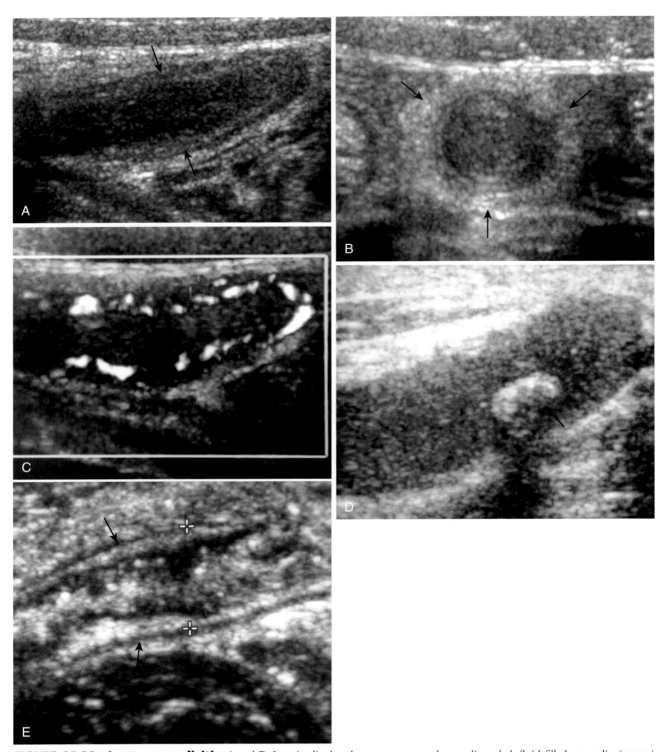

FIGURE 55-31. Acute appendicitis. A and **B,** Longitudinal and transverse scans show a distended, fluid-filled appendix *(arrows)* that measured 7 mm in diameter. **C,** Power Doppler imaging reveals hyperemia of the appendiceal wall. **D,** Echogenic fecalith with posterior shadowing *(arrow)* within a fluid-filled dilated appendix. **E,** Another dilated appendix *(arrows),* containing a large amount of fecal sludge.

to inflammation confined to the mesenteric lymph nodes in patients with a normal appendix. The condition is often associated with viral infection and usually is self-limited. Clusters of enlarged mesenteric lymph nodes that number more than five and are tender with com-

pression suggest the diagnosis,[95] especially when a normal appendix is also seen. Mild mucosal thickening in the distal ileum is a common associated finding (Fig. 55-32). Isolated mesenteric lymph nodes are common and should not be considered abnormal. **Omental infarc-**

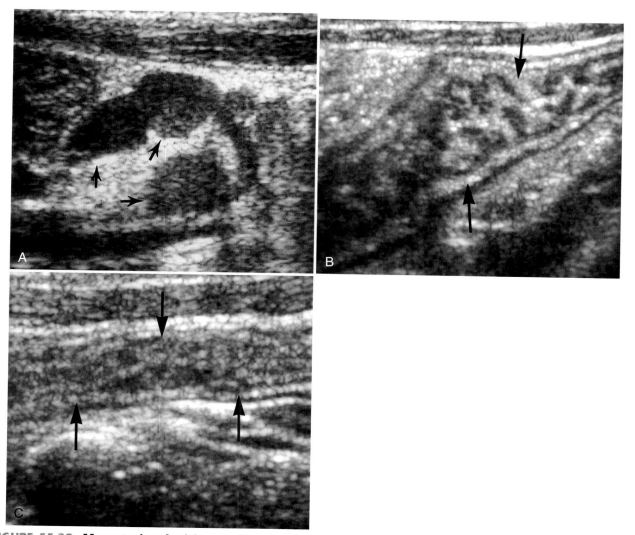

FIGURE 55-32. Mesenteric adenitis. A, Enlarged lymph nodes in ileocecal region *(arrows)*. **B,** Mild mucosal thickening in the terminal ileum *(arrows)*. **C,** More proximal small bowel loop *(arrows)* shows normal-thickness mucosa and peristalsis.

tion is a less common cause of acute abdominal pain in children. Ultrasound may reveal a heterogeneous mass or a localized focus of increased echogenicity in the omentum, characteristically located between the anterior abdominal wall and the colon.[120,121] **Meckel's diverticulum** may become torsed or inflamed and may resemble an inflamed appendix or a complex pelvic mass sonographically[122,123] (Fig. 55-34).

Gastrointestinal Neoplasms and Cysts

The superior ability of sonography to distinguish solid from cystic masses makes this examination an excellent choice for the diagnosis of the various types of cysts that can occur in the abdomen. The most common cysts associated with the GI tract are mesenteric cysts and GI duplication cysts. Characteristically, **gastrointestinal duplication cysts** are filled with anechoic fluid and have a well-defined, double-layered wall that consists of an inner echogenic mucosal layer and a thin, outer hypoechoic muscular layer (Fig. 55-35). These two layers are usually continuous throughout the cyst wall,[124,125] helping to distinguish GI duplication cysts from other simple-walled cysts, such as **mesenteric cysts** or **pseudocysts** (Figs. 55-36, *D,* and 55-35, *E*). Occasionally, single-walled cysts appear to have a double-layered wall because of a fibrinous layer that can be deposited along the inner cyst wall after intracystic bleeding, but this is a relatively uncommon occurrence. Duplication cysts frequently contain foci of ectopic gastric mucosa, which can become inflamed and ulcerated. In such cases, intracystic hemorrhage may occur, and the resulting debris within the cystic fluid can cause the cyst to appear solid[126] (Fig. 55-35, *D*). Some GI duplication cysts are pedunculated and therefore may be located at a site remote from the actual point of origin (Fig. 55-35, *C*). Occasionally, active peristalsis of the cyst wall can be seen at real-time ultrasound.

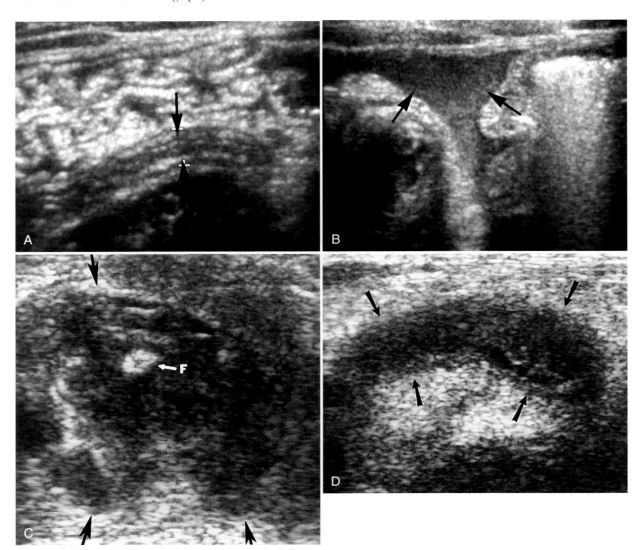

FIGURE 55-33. Perforated appendicitis. Fluid collections are a key finding. **A,** Decompressed appendix *(arrows)* that measures 5.9 mm in diameter. **B,** Same patient as **A.** Free fluid with debris in the right lower quadrant *(arrows).* **C,** In a different patient, the appendix was not found, but a heterogeneous, hypoechoic collection *(arrows)* was found in the right lower quadrant, representing an abscess. Note the echogenic fecalith *(F).* **D,** Enlarged, hypoechoic appendix with near-complete loss of the normal echogenic mucosal stripe *(arrows),* indicating a gangrenous appendix and likely perforation.

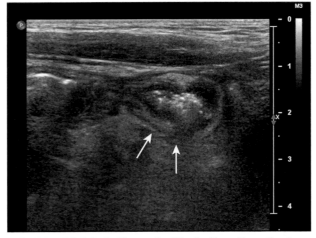

FIGURE 55-34. Inflamed Meckel's diverticulum *(arrows).* Transverse ultrasound of the right lower quadrant in a child with clinically suspected acute appendicitis.

Sonography does not play a major role in the evaluation of GI neoplasms, but masses or polyps may be identified in some cases when the bowel is filled with fluid.[74,127] More often, intraluminal GI masses in children present with obstruction caused by intussusception. The mass that acts as a lead point for the intussusception may not always be sonographically discernible. Most solid tumors appear with a variably echogenic pattern and cannot be reliably distinguished by their sonographic characteristics.[40,128-130] **Lymphoma** tends to be hypoechoic and may be associated with ulceration. The tumors most likely to appear predominantly cystic are teratomas and lymphangiomas.[131-135] **Abdominal lymphangiomas** most frequently occur in the mesentery and can appear as solitary cysts or as multiloculated cystic masses[135] (Fig. 55-36, *A*). **Gastrointestinal teratomas** usually have large cystic components, but echogenic fat and calcifications

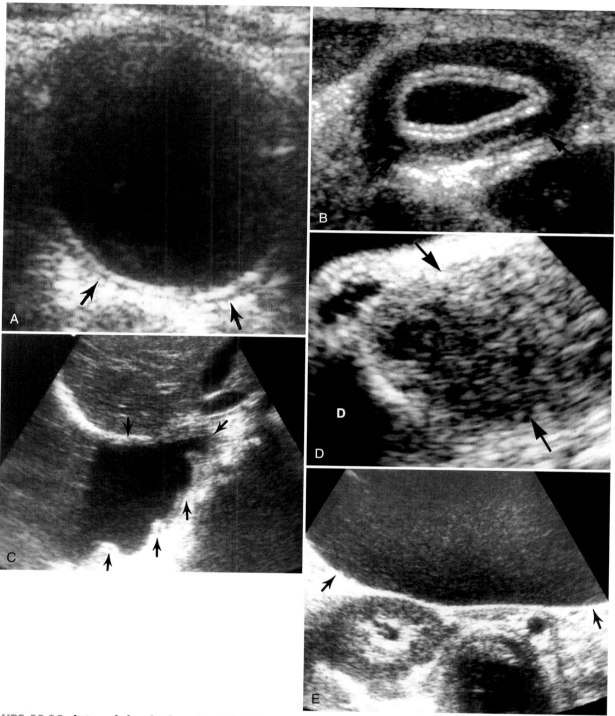

FIGURE 55-35. Intra-abdominal cysts. A, Ileal duplication cyst had a typical double-layered wall consisting of an inner echogenic mucosal layer and an outer hypoechoic muscular layer *(arrows)*. **B, Gastric duplication cyst** with a thick, double-layered wall *(arrows)*. **C, Duodenal duplication cyst** had an undulating, double-layered wall and extended above the diaphragm *(arrows)*. Active peristalsis of the cyst wall was seen. **D, Duodenal duplication cyst** *(arrows)* filled with thick, proteinaceous fluid, giving a more solid appearance. Adjacent obstructed duodenum *(D)*. **E, Mesenteric cyst** had only a single-layered wall *(arrows)*.

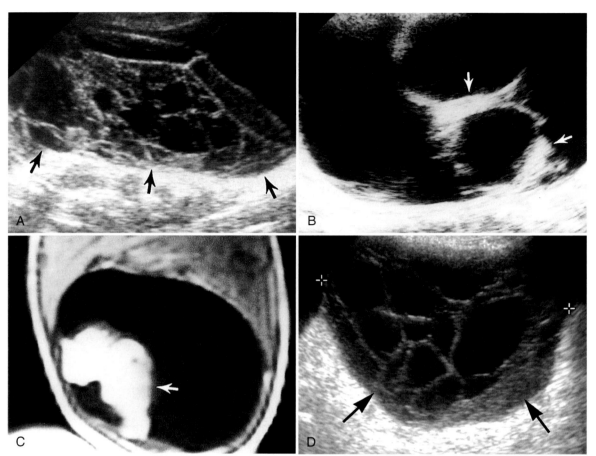

FIGURE 55-36. Cystic masses. A, Mesenteric lymphangioma with a multiloculated appearance *(arrows).* **B, Teratoma**. Large, multiloculated abdominal cyst also contained echogenic areas representing fat *(arrows).* **C,** MR image of teratoma shows fat within the cyst *(arrow).* **D,** Multiloculated cerebrospinal fluid **pseudocyst** *(arrows)* obstructing the peritoneal end of a VP shunt.

are also often visible[131,133,134] (Fig. 55-36, *B* and *C*). **Hemangiomas** may involve the mesentery and are usually associated with hypervascularity and large feeding vessels (Fig. 55-37).

PANCREAS

Normal Anatomy and Technique

The pancreas is easily imaged in children and normally appears relatively generous in size compared to the pancreas of an adult. The normal echotexture of the pancreas in childhood is homogeneous and most often isoechoic or hyperechoic compared to the liver. The normal pancreatic duct is usually not visible sonographically, unless a high-resolution linear transducer is used.

Pancreatitis

Pancreatitis is less common in children than in adults and is more likely to be acute rather than chronic. The most

common causes of acute pancreatitis in children include blunt abdominal trauma (including the battered child syndrome), viral infection, and drug toxicity. Regardless of the cause, sonographic findings are usually sparse unless a complicating pseudocyst arises. The most common abnormal sonographic finding is pancreatic enlargement, but a normal-sized pancreas does not exclude the diagnosis (Fig. 55-38). Decreased echogenicity of the pancreas can occur with pancreatitis,[136,137] but this is a difficult finding to substantiate because of the variable echogenicity of the normal pancreas in children.[137] Occasionally, increased echogenicity of the pararenal space may be encountered, the result of lipolysis of normal fat by pancreatic enzymes that have leaked into the hepatorenal space.[138] Peripancreatic fluid collections often accompany acute pancreatitis, but such collections are not considered **pseudocysts** until they become persistent and are surrounded by a well-defined echogenic wall (Fig. 55-39). Many pancreatic pseudocysts are now treated conservatively, and sonography is useful for following such patients to verify the spontaneous resolution of the fluid collection.[139] When the pseudocyst does not adequately resolve,

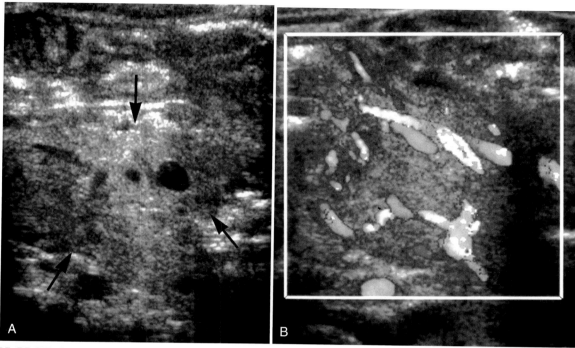

FIGURE 55-37. **Mesenteric hemangioma. A,** Large echogenic mass involving the mesentery *(arrows)* in an infant with chronic GI bleeding. **B,** Color Doppler ultrasound shows numerous internal vessels.

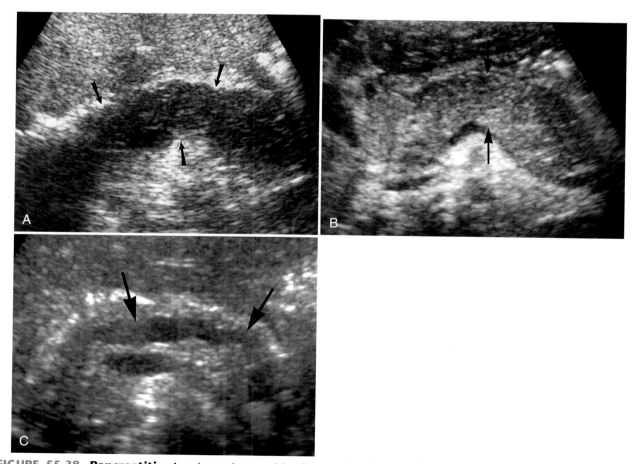

FIGURE 55-38. **Pancreatitis. A,** L-Asparaginase toxicity. Pancreas is enlarged and hypoechoic *(arrows).* **B,** Another child with pancreatic enlargement and pancreatitis *(arrows).* **C,** Chronic pancreatitis in a 7-year-old child with **pancreas divisum** shows atrophic pancreas and a dilated pancreatic duct *(arrows).*

sonography can be used to suggest suitability for percutaneous or endoscopic drainage.[140,141]

Chronic or recurrent pancreatitis in children is most likely caused by congenital abnormalities affecting the biliary tract (e.g., choledochal cysts, pancreas divisum anomaly, cystic fibrosis). With **cystic fibrosis,** precipitation or coagulation of secretions in the small pancreatic ducts leads to ductal concretions and obstruction. Distention of the ducts and acini leads to degeneration and replacement by small cysts. This ductal obstruction, along with atrophy of glandular elements and ensuing fibrosis, creates increased echogenicity of the pancreas[142-144] (Fig. 55-38, *C*). The gland is often small, and calcifications may be seen as punctate, echogenic foci within the hyperechoic pancreas. A similar appearance may be found in patients with hereditary autosomal dominant pancreatitis.[145]

Pancreatic Masses

Tumors of the pancreas are extremely uncommon in children. The most common primary neoplasms are the benign insulinoma and adenocarcinoma.[146] **Insulinomas** are often difficult to detect sonographically, but intraoperative sonography has been used with more success. **Carcinoma** of the pancreas usually appears as an echogenic or complex pancreatic mass. **Pancreatoblastoma** is a rare invasive tumor that is heterogeneous in texture, can encase vessels, and may metastasize widely.[147-149] Cystic masses of the pancreas include **lymphangioma, papillary-cystic neoplasm** of the pancreas (Fig. 55-40), and the rare **congenital pancreatic cyst.**[150,151]

Diffuse echogenic enlargement of the pancreas can be seen with **nesidioblastosis** (Fig. 55-41, *A*). This is a tumorlike condition of the pancreas characterized by diffuse proliferation and persistence of primitive ductal epithelial cells. Nesidioblastosis is often associated with hypoglycemia and the Beckwith-Wiedemann syndrome. Diffusely increased echogenicity of the pancreas can also occur with fatty infiltration in the **Shwachman-Diamond syndrome** (Fig. 55-41, *B*), but in this condition the pancreas usually remains normal in size. Rarely, other types of tumors, such as in **leukemia,**[152] can infiltrate and enlarge the pancreas.

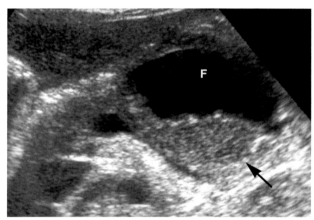

FIGURE 55-39. Pancreatic pseudocyst in battered child. Fluid collection *(F)* between the stomach and the focally enlarged pancreas *(arrow).*

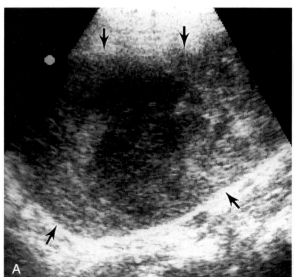
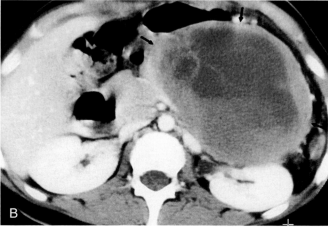

FIGURE 55-40. Pancreatic masses. A, Papillary-cystic neoplasm of the pancreas. Large, heterogeneous but predominantly cystic mass in the tail of the pancreas *(arrows).* **B,** CT also shows the predominantly cystic nature of this large, well-defined tumor *(arrows).*

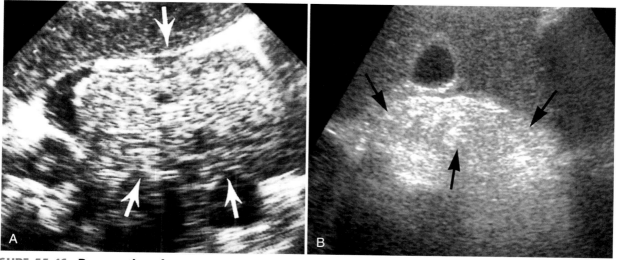

FIGURE 55-41. Pancreatic enlargement. A, Beckwith-Wiedemann syndrome and nesidioblastosis. Pancreas is greatly enlarged *(arrows).* **B,** Lipomatosis associated with Shwachman-Diamond syndrome. Echogenic enlargement of the pancreas *(arrows).*

References

Esophagus and Stomach

1. Wright LL, Baker KR, Meny RG. Ultrasound demonstration of gastroesophageal reflux. J Ultrasound Med 1988;7:471-475.
2. Gomes H, Lallemand A, Lallemand P. Ultrasound of the gastroesophageal junction. Pediatr Radiol 1993;23:94-99.
3. Esposito F, Lombardi R, Grasso AC, et al. Transabdominal sonography of the normal gastroesophageal junction in children. J Clin Ultrasound 2001;29:326-331.
4. Farina R, Pennisi F, La Rosa M, et al. Contrast-enhanced colour-Doppler sonography versus pH-metry in the diagnosis of gastro-oesophageal reflux in children. Radiol Med 2008;113:591-598.
5. Hirsch W, Kedar R, Preiss U. Color Doppler in the diagnosis of the gastroesophageal reflux in children: comparison with pH measurements and B-mode ultrasound. Pediatr Radiol 1996;26:232-235.
6. Jang HS, Lee JS, Lim GY, et al. Correlation of color Doppler sonographic findings with pH measurements in gastroesophageal reflux in children. J Clin Ultrasound 2001;29:212-217.
7. O'Keeffe FN, Stansberry SD, Swischuk LE, Hayden Jr CK. Antropyloric muscle thickness at US in infants: what is normal? Radiology 1991;178:827-830.
8. Hulka F, Campbell JR, Harrison MW, Campbell TJ. Cost-effectiveness in diagnosing infantile hypertrophic pyloric stenosis. J Pediatr Surg 1997;32:1604-1608.
9. Swischuk LE, Hayden Jr CK, Stansberry SD. Sonographic pitfalls in imaging of the antropyloric region in infants. Radiographics 1989;9:437-447.
10. Hernanz-Schulman M, Sells LL, Ambrosino MM, et al. Hypertrophic pyloric stenosis in the infant without a palpable olive: accuracy of sonographic diagnosis. Radiology 1994;193:771-776.
11. Hernanz-Schulman M, Zhu Y, Stein SM, et al. Hypertrophic pyloric stenosis in infants: US evaluation of vascularity of the pyloric canal. Radiology 2003;229:389-393.
12. Rohrschneider WK, Mittnacht H, Darge K, Troger J. Pyloric muscle in asymptomatic infants: sonographic evaluation and discrimination from idiopathic hypertrophic pyloric stenosis. Pediatr Radiol 1998;28:429-434.
13. Teele RL, Smith EH. Ultrasound in the diagnosis of idiopathic hypertrophic pyloric stenosis. N Engl J Med 1977;296:1149-1150.
14. Blumhagen JD, Maclin L, Krauter D, et al. Sonographic diagnosis of hypertrophic pyloric stenosis. AJR Am J Roentgenol 1988;150:1367-1370.
15. Cohen HL, Blumer SL, Zucconi WB. The sonographic double-track sign: not pathognomonic for hypertrophic pyloric stenosis; can be seen in pylorospasm. J Ultrasound Med 2004;23:641-646.
16. Haller JO, Cohen HL. Hypertrophic pyloric stenosis: diagnosis using ultrasound. Radiology 1986;161:335-339.
17. Lund Kofoed PE, Host A, Elle B, Larsen C. Hypertrophic pyloric stenosis: determination of muscle dimensions by ultrasound. Br J Radiol 1988;61:19-20.
18. Stunden RJ, LeQuesne GW, Little KE. The improved ultrasound diagnosis of hypertrophic pyloric stenosis. Pediatr Radiol 1986;16:200-205.
19. Cohen HL, Schechter S, Mestel AL, et al. Ultrasonic "double track" sign in hypertrophic pyloric stenosis. J Ultrasound Med 1987;6:139-143.
20. Hernanz-Schulman M, Neblett 3rd WW, Polk DB, Johnson JE. Hypertrophied pyloric mucosa in patients with hypertrophic pyloric stenosis. Pediatr Radiol 1998;28:901.
21. Kim S, Chung CJ, Fordham LA, Specter BB. Coexisting hyperplastic antral polyp and hypertrophic pyloric stenosis. Pediatr Radiol 1997;27:912-914.
22. Callahan MJ, McCauley RG, Patel H, Hijazi ZM. The development of hypertrophic pyloric stenosis in a patient with prostaglandin-induced foveolar hyperplasia. Pediatr Radiol 1999;29:748-751.
23. Yoshizawa J, Eto T, Higashimoto Y, et al. Ultrasonographic features of normalization of the pylorus after pyloromyotomy for hypertrophic pyloric stenosis. J Pediatr Surg 2001;36:582-586.
24. Cohen HL, Zinn HL, Haller JO, et al. Ultrasonography of pylorospasm: findings may simulate hypertrophic pyloric stenosis. J Ultrasound Med 1998;17:705-711.
25. Spevak MR, Ahmadjian JM, Kleinman PK, et al. Sonography of hypertrophic pyloric stenosis: frequency and cause of nonuniform echogenicity of the thickened pyloric muscle. AJR Am J Roentgenol 1992;158:129-132.
26. Roma E, Kafritsa Y, Panayiotou J, et al. Is peptic ulcer a common cause of upper gastrointestinal symptoms? Eur J Pediatr 2001;1 60:497-500.
27. Hayden Jr CK, Swischuk LE, Rytting JE. Gastric ulcer disease in infants: ultrasound findings. Radiology 1987;164:131-134.
28. Maves CK, Johnson JF, Bove K, Malott RL. Gastric inflammatory pseudotumor in children. Radiology 1989;173:381-383.
29. Goldwag SS, Bellah RD, Ward KJ, Kogutt MS. Sonographic detection of Menetrier's disease in children. J Clin Ultrasound 1994;22:567-570.
30. Mercado-Deane MG, Burton EM, et al. Prostaglandin-induced foveolar hyperplasia simulating pyloric stenosis in an infant with cyanotic heart disease. Pediatr Radiol 1994;24:45-46.
31. McAlister WH, Katz ME, Perlman JM, Tack ED. Sonography of focal foveolar hyperplasia causing gastric obstruction in an infant. Pediatr Radiol 1988;18:79-81.
32. Joshi A, Berdon WE, Brudnicki A, et al. Gastric thumbprinting: diffuse gastric wall mucosal and submucosal thickening in infants with ductal-dependent cyanotic congenital heart disease maintained on long-term prostaglandin therapy. Pediatr Radiol 2002;32:405-408.

33. Naik DR, Bolia A, Boon AW. Demonstration of a lactobezoar by ultrasound. Br J Radiol 1987;60:506-508.
34. Malpani A, Ramani SK, Wolverson MK. Role of sonography in trichobezoars. J Ultrasound Med 1988;7:661-663.

Duodenum and Small Bowel

35. Crowe JE, Sumner TE. Combined esophageal and duodenal atresia without tracheoesophageal fistula: characteristic radiographic changes. AJR Am J Roentgenol 1978;130:167-168.
36. Hayden Jr CK, Schwartz MZ, Davis M, Swischuk LE. Combined esophageal and duodenal atresia: sonographic findings. AJR Am J Roentgenol 1983;140:225-226.
37. Hayden Jr CK, Boulden TF, Swischuk LE, Lobe TE. Sonographic demonstration of duodenal obstruction with midgut volvulus. AJR Am J Roentgenol 1984;143:9-10.
38. Loyer E, Eggli KD. Sonographic evaluation of superior mesenteric vascular relationship in malrotation. Pediatr Radiol 1989;19:173-175.
39. Zerin JM, DiPietro MA. Superior mesenteric vascular anatomy at US in patients with surgically proved malrotation of the midgut. Radiology 1992;183:693-694.
40. Weinberger E, Winters WD, Liddell RM, et al. Sonographic diagnosis of intestinal malrotation in infants: importance of the relative positions of the superior mesenteric vein and artery. AJR Am J Roentgenol 1992;159:825-828.
41. Shimanuki Y, Aihara T, Takano H, et al. Clockwise whirlpool sign at color Doppler US: an objective and definite sign of midgut volvulus. Radiology 1996;199:261-264.
42. Ashley LM, Allen S, Teele RL. A normal sonogram does not exclude malrotation. Pediatr Radiol 2001;31:354-356.
43. Cremin BJ, Solomon DJ. Ultrasonic diagnosis of duodenal diaphragm. Pediatr Radiol 1987;17:489-490.
44. Hayashi K, Futagawa S, Kozaki S, et al. Ultrasound and CT diagnosis of intramural duodenal hematoma. Pediatr Radiol 1988;18:167-168.
45. Hernanz-Schulman M, Genieser NB, Ambrosino M. Sonographic diagnosis of intramural duodenal hematoma. J Ultrasound Med 1989;8:273-276.
46. Orel SG, Nussbaum AR, Sheth S, et al. Duodenal hematoma in child abuse: sonographic detection. AJR Am J Roentgenol 1988;151:147-149.
47. Couture A, Veyrac C, Baud C, et al. Evaluation of abdominal pain in Henoch-Schönlein syndrome by high-frequency ultrasound. Pediatr Radiol 1992;22:12-17.
48. Carroll BA, Moskowitz PS. Sonographic diagnosis of neonatal meconium cyst. AJR Am J Roentgenol 1981;137:1262-1264.
49. Bowen A, Mazer J, Zarabi M, Fujioka M. Cystic meconium peritonitis: ultrasonographic features. Pediatr Radiol 1984;14:18-22.
50. Applegate KE. Clinically suspected intussusception in children: evidence-based review and self-assessment module. Am J Roentgenol 2005;185:S175-S183.
51. Bhisitkul DM, Listernick R, Shkolnik A, et al. Clinical application of ultrasonography in the diagnosis of intussusception. J Pediatr 1992;121:182-186.
52. Verschelden P, Filiatrault D, Garel L, et al. Intussusception in children: reliability of US in diagnosis—a prospective study. Radiology 1992;184:741-744.
53. Shanbhogue RL, Hussain SM, Meradji M, et al. Ultrasonography is accurate enough for the diagnosis of intussusception. J Pediatr Surg 1994;29:324-327; discussion 327-328.
54. Pracros JP, Tran-Minh VA, Morin de Finfe CH, et al. Acute intestinal intussusception in children: contribution of ultrasonography (145 cases). Ann Radiol (Paris) 1987;30:525-530.
55. Parienty RA, Lepreux JF, Gruson B. Sonographic and CT features of ileocolic intussusception. AJR Am J Roentgenol 1981;136:608-610.
56. Morin ME, Blumenthal DH, Tan A, Li YP. The ultrasonic appearance of ileocolic intussusception. J Clin Ultrasound 1981;9:516-518.
57. Swischuk LE, Hayden CK, Boulden T. Intussusception: indications for ultrasonography and an explanation of the doughnut and pseudokidney signs. Pediatr Radiol 1985;15:388-391.
58. Del-Pozo G, Albillos JC, Tejedor D. Intussusception: ultrasound findings with pathologic correlation—the crescent-in-doughnut sign. Radiology 1996;199:688-692.
59. Del-Pozo G, Gonzalez-Spinola J, Gomez-Anson B, et al. Intussusception: trapped peritoneal fluid detected with ultrasound—relationship to reducibility and ischemia. Radiology 1996;201:379-383.
60. Riebel TW, Nasir R, Weber K. Ultrasound-guided hydrostatic reduction of intussusception in children. Radiology 1993;188:513-516.
61. Rohrschneider WK, Troger J. Hydrostatic reduction of intussusception under ultrasound guidance. Pediatr Radiol 1995;25:530-534.
62. Wood SK, Kim JS, Suh SJ, et al. Childhood intussusception: ultrasound-guided hydrostatic reduction. Radiology 1992;182:77-80.
63. Carnevale E, Graziani M, Fasanelli S. Post-operative ileo-ileal intussusception: sonographic approach. Pediatr Radiol 1994;24:161-163.
64. Ko SF, Lee TY, Ng SH, et al. Small bowel intussusception in symptomatic pediatric patients: experiences with 19 surgically proven cases. World J Surg 2002;26:438-443.
65. Swischuk LE, John SD, Swischuk PN. Spontaneous reduction of intussusception: verification with US. Radiology 1994;192:269-271.
66. Munden MM, Bruzzi JF, Coley BD, Munden RF. Sonography of pediatric small-bowel intussusception: differentiating surgical from nonsurgical cases. AJR Am J Roentgenol 2007;188:275-279.
67. Park NH, Park SI, Park CS, et al. Ultrasonographic findings of small bowel intussusception, focusing on differentiation from ileocolic intussusception. Br J Radiol 2007;80:798-802.
68. Hughes UM, Connolly BL, Chait PG, Muraca S. Further report of small-bowel intussusceptions related to gastrojejunostomy tubes. Pediatr Radiol 2000;30:614-617.
69. Feinstein KA, Myers M, Fernbach SK, Bhisitkul DM. Peritoneal fluid in children with intussusception: its sonographic detection and relationship to successful reduction. Abdom Imaging 1993;18:277-279.
70. Swischuk LE, Stansberry SD. Ultrasonographic detection of free peritoneal fluid in uncomplicated intussusception. Pediatr Radiol 1991;21:350-351.
71. Koumanidou C, Vakaki M, Pitsoulakis G, et al. Sonographic detection of lymph nodes in the intussusception of infants and young children: clinical evaluation and hydrostatic reduction. AJR Am J Roentgenol 2002;178:445-450.
72. Lam AH, Firman K. Value of sonography including color Doppler in the diagnosis and management of long-standing intussusception. Pediatr Radiol 1992;22:112-114.
73. Lim HK, Bae SH, Lee KH, et al. Assessment of reducibility of ileocolic intussusception in children: usefulness of color Doppler sonography. Radiology 1994;191:781-785.

Colon

74. Baldisserotto M, Spolidoro JV, Bahu Mda G. Graded compression sonography of the colon in the diagnosis of polyps in pediatric patients. AJR Am J Roentgenol 2002;179:201-205.
75. Cremin BJ. The radiological assessment of anorectal anomalies. Clin Radiol 1971;22:239-250.
76. Haber HP, Seitz G, Warmann SW, Fuchs J. Transperineal sonography for determination of the type of imperforate anus. AJR Am J Roentgenol 2007;189:1525-1529.
77. Donaldson JS, Black CT, Reynolds M, et al. Ultrasound of the distal pouch in infants with imperforate anus. J Pediatr Surg 1989;24:465-468.
78. Oppenheimer DA, Carroll BA, Shochat SJ. Sonography of imperforate anus. Radiology 1983;148:127-128.

Intestinal Inflammatory Disease

79. Lim JH, Ko YT, Lee DH, et al. Sonography of inflammatory bowel disease: findings and value in differential diagnosis. AJR Am J Roentgenol 1994;163:343-347.
80. Dinkel E, Dittrich M, Peters H, Baumann W. Real-time ultrasound in Crohn's disease: characteristic features and clinical implications. Pediatr Radiol 1986;16:8-12.
81. Worlicek H, Lutz H, Heyder N, Matek W. Ultrasound findings in Crohn's disease and ulcerative colitis: a prospective study. J Clin Ultrasound 1987;15:153-163.
82. Ros PR, Buetow PC, Pantograg-Brown L, et al. Pseudomembranous colitis. Radiology 1996;198:1-9.

83. Downey DB, Wilson SR. Pseudomembranous colitis: sonographic features. Radiology 1991;180:61-64.

84. Alexander JE, Williamson SL, Seibert JJ, et al. The ultrasonographic diagnosis of typhlitis (neutropenic colitis). Pediatr Radiol 1988;18:200-204.

85. Puylaert JB, Lalisang RI, van der Werf SD, Doornbos L. *Campylobacter* ileocolitis mimicking acute appendicitis: differentiation with graded-compression ultrasound. Radiology 1988;166:737-740.

86. Ueda D, Sato T, Yoshida M. Ultrasonographic assessment of *Salmonella* enterocolitis in children. Pediatr Radiol 1999;29:469-471.

87. Matsumoto T, Iida M, Sakai T, et al. *Yersinia* terminal ileitis: sonographic findings in eight patients. AJR Am J Roentgenol 1991;156:965-967.

88. Patenaude Y, Bernard C, Schreiber R, Sinsky AB. Cow's-milk-induced allergic colitis in an exclusively breast-fed infant: diagnosed with ultrasound. Pediatr Radiol 2000;30:379-382.

89. Chung CJ, Rayder S, Meyers W, Long J. Kawasaki disease presenting as focal colitis. Pediatr Radiol 1996;26:455-457.

90. Kodroff MB, Hartenberg MA, Goldschmidt RA. Ultrasonographic diagnosis of gangrenous bowel in neonatal necrotizing enterocolitis. Pediatr Radiol 1984;14:168-170.

91. Friedland JA, Herman TE, Siegel MJ. *Escherichia coli* O157:H7–associated hemolytic-uremic syndrome: value of colonic color Doppler sonography. Pediatr Radiol 1995;25(Suppl 1):65-67.

92. Haber HP, Schlegel PG, Dette S, et al. Intestinal acute graft-versus-host disease: findings on sonography. AJR Am J Roentgenol 2000;174:118-120.

93. Klein SA, Martin H, Schreiber-Dietrich D, et al. A new approach to evaluating intestinal acute graft-versus-host disease by transabdominal sonography and colour Doppler imaging. Br J Haematol 2001;115:929-934.

94. Schulman H, Weizman Z, Barki Y, et al. Inflammatory bowel disease in glycogen storage disease type 1 B. Pediatr Radiol 1995;25 (Suppl 1):160-162.

95. Quillin SP, Siegel MJ. Gastrointestinal inflammation in children: color Doppler ultrasonography. J Ultrasound Med 1994;13:751-756.

96. Giovagnorio F, Diacinti D, Vernia P. Doppler sonography of the superior mesenteric artery in Crohn's disease. AJR Am J Roentgenol 1998;170:123-126.

97. Migaleddu V, Quaia E, Scano D, Virgilio G. Inflammatory activity in Crohn disease: ultrasound findings. Abdom Imaging 2008;33:589-597.

98. Hu SC, Feeney MS, McNicholas M, et al. Ultrasonography to diagnose and exclude intussusception in Henoch-Schönlein purpura. Arch Dis Child 1991;66:1065-1067.

99. Goske MJ, Goldblum JR, Applegate KE, et al. The "circle sign": a new sonographic sign of pneumatosis intestinalis—clinical, pathologic and experimental findings. Pediatr Radiol 1999;29:530-535.

100. Merritt CR, Goldsmith JP, Sharp MJ. Sonographic detection of portal venous gas in infants with necrotizing enterocolitis. AJR Am J Roentgenol 1984;143:1059-1062.

101. Malin SW, Bhutani VK, Ritchie WW, et al. Echogenic intravascular and hepatic microbubbles associated with necrotizing enterocolitis. J Pediatr 1983;103:637-640.

102. Avni EF, Rypens F, Cohen E, Pardou A. Peri-cholecystic hyper-echogenicities in necrotizing enterocolitis: a specific sonographic sign? Pediatr Radiol 1991;21:179-181.

103. Deeg KH, Rupprecht T, Schmid E. Doppler sonographic detection of increased flow velocities in the celiac trunk and superior mesenteric artery in infants with necrotizing enterocolitis. Pediatr Radiol 1993;23:578-582.

104. Miller SF, Seibert JJ, Kinder DL, Wilson AR. Use of ultrasound in the detection of occult bowel perforation in neonates. J Ultrasound Med 1993;12:531-535.

105. Vignault F, Filiatrault D, Brandt ML, et al. Acute appendicitis in children: evaluation with US. Radiology 1990;176:501-504.

106. Rioux M. Sonographic detection of the normal and abnormal appendix. AJR Am J Roentgenol 1992;158:773-778.

107. Dilley A, Wesson D, Munden M, et al. The impact of ultrasound examinations on the management of children with suspected appendicitis: a 3-year analysis. J Pediatr Surg 2001;36:303-308.

108. Wan MJ, Krahn M, Ungar WJ, et al. Acute appendicitis in young children: cost-effectiveness of US versus CT in diagnosis—a Markov decision analytic model. Radiology 2009;250:378-386.

109. Sivit CJ, Newman KD, Boenning DA, et al. Appendicitis: usefulness of US in diagnosis in a pediatric population. Radiology 1992;185:549-552.

110. Axelrod DA, Sonnad SS, Hirschl RB. An economic evaluation of sonographic examination of children with suspected appendicitis. J Pediatr Surg 2000;35:1236-1241.

111. Siegel MJ, Carel C, Surratt S. Ultrasonography of acute abdominal pain in children. JAMA 1991;266:1987-1989.

112. Lee JH, Jeong YK, Hwang JC, et al. Graded compression sonography with adjuvant use of a posterior manual compression technique in the sonographic diagnosis of acute appendicitis. AJR Am J Roentgenol 2002;178:863-868.

113. Kao SC, Smith WL, Abu-Yousef MM, et al. Acute appendicitis in children: sonographic findings. AJR Am J Roentgenol 1989;153:375-379.

114. Rettenbacher T, Hollerweger A, Macheiner P, et al. Outer diameter of the vermiform appendix as a sign of acute appendicitis: evaluation at US. Radiology 2001;218:757-762.

115. Puylaert JB. Mesenteric adenitis and acute terminal ileitis: ultrasound evaluation using graded compression. Radiology 1986;161:691-695.

116. Hayden Jr CK, Kuchelmeister J, Lipscomb TS. Sonography of acute appendicitis in childhood: perforation versus nonperforation. J Ultrasound Med 1992;11:209-216.

117. Quillin SP, Siegel MJ, Coffin CM. Acute appendicitis in children: value of sonography in detecting perforation. AJR Am J Roentgenol 1992;159:1265-1268.

118. Patriquin HB, Garcier JM, Lafortune M, et al. Appendicitis in children and young adults: Doppler sonographic-pathologic correlation. AJR Am J Roentgenol 1996;166:629-633.

119. Quillin SP, Siegel MJ. Diagnosis of appendiceal abscess in children with acute appendicitis: value of color Doppler sonography. AJR Am J Roentgenol 1995;164:1251-1254.

120. Schlesinger AE, Dorfman SR, Braverman RM. Sonographic appearance of omental infarction in children. Pediatr Radiol 1999;29:598-601.

121. Grattan-Smith JD, Blews DE, Brand T. Omental infarction in pediatric patients: sonographic and CT findings. AJR Am J Roentgenol 2002;178:1537-1539.

122. Daneman A, Lobo E, Alton DJ, Shuckett B. The value of sonography, CT and air enema for detection of complicated Meckel diverticulum in children with nonspecific clinical presentation. Pediatr Radiol 1998;28:928-932.

123. Farris SL, Fernbach SK. Axial torsion of Meckel's diverticulum presenting as a pelvic mass. Pediatr Radiol 2001;31:886-888.

124. Barr LL, Hayden Jr CK, Stansberry SD, Swischuk LE. Enteric duplication cysts in children: are their ultrasonographic wall characteristics diagnostic? Pediatr Radiol 1990;20:326-328.

125. Hur J, Yoon CS, Kim MJ, Kim OH. Imaging features of gastrointestinal tract duplications in infants and children: from oesophagus to rectum. Pediatr Radiol 2007;37:691-699.

126. Segal SR, Sherman NH, Rosenberg HK, et al. Ultrasonographic features of gastrointestinal duplications. J Ultrasound Med 1994;13:863-870.

127. Walter DF, Govil S, Korula A, et al. Pedunculated colonic polyp diagnosed by colonic sonography. Pediatr Radiol 1992;22:148-149.

128. Park JM, Yeon KM, Han MC, et al. Diffuse intestinal arteriovenous malformation in a child. Pediatr Radiol 1991;21:314-315.

129. Schneider K, Dickerhoff R, Bertele RM. Malignant gastric sarcoma: diagnosis by ultrasound and endoscopy. Pediatr Radiol 1986;16:69-70.

130. Cremin BJ, Brown RA. Carcinoma of the colon: diagnosis by ultrasound and enema. Pediatr Radiol 1987;17:319-320.

131. Bowen B, Ros PR, McCarthy MJ, et al. Gastrointestinal teratomas: CT and US appearance with pathologic correlation. Radiology 1987;162:431-433.

132. McCullagh M, Keen C, Dykes E. Cystic mesothelioma of the peritoneum: a rare cause of "ascites" in children. J Pediatr Surg 1994;29:1205-1207.

133. Prieto ML, Casanova A, Delgado J, Zabalza R. Cystic teratoma of the mesentery. Pediatr Radiol 1989;19:439.

134. Shah RS, Kaddu SJ, Kirtane JM. Benign mature teratoma of the large bowel: a case report. J Pediatr Surg 1996;31:701-702.

135. Steyaert H, Guitard J, Moscovici J, et al. Abdominal cystic lymphangioma in children: benign lesions that can have a proliferative course. J Pediatr Surg 1996;31:677-680.

Pancreas

136. Coleman BG, Arger PH, Rosenberg HK, et al. Gray-scale sonographic assessment of pancreatitis in children. Radiology 1983;146:145-150.

137. Fleischer AC, Parker P, Kirchner SG, James Jr AE. Sonographic findings of pancreatitis in children. Radiology 1983;146:151-155.

138. Siegel MJ, Martin KW, Worthington JL. Normal and abnormal pancreas in children: US studies. Radiology 1987;165:15-18.

139. Swischuk LE, Hayden Jr CK. Pararenal space hyperechogenicity in childhood pancreatitis. AJR Am J Roentgenol 1985;145:1085-1086.

140. Shilyansky J, Sena LM, Kreller M, et al. Nonoperative management of pancreatic injuries in children. J Pediatr Surg 1998;33:343-349.

141. Slovis TL, VonBerg VJ, Mikelic V. Sonography in the diagnosis and management of pancreatic pseudocysts and effusions in childhood. Radiology 1980;135:153-155.

142. Daneman A, Gaskin K, Martin DJ, Cutz E. Pancreatic changes in cystic fibrosis: CT and sonographic appearances. AJR Am J Roentgenol 1983;141:653-655.

143. Patty I, Kalaoui M, Al-Shamali M, et al. Endoscopic drainage for pancreatic pseudocyst in children. J Pediatr Surg 2001;36:503-505.

144. Phillips HE, Cox KL, Reid MH, McGahan JP. Pancreatic sonography in cystic fibrosis. AJR Am J Roentgenol 1981;137:69-72.

145. Willi UV, Reddish JM, Teele RL. Cystic fibrosis: its characteristic appearance on abdominal sonography. AJR Am J Roentgenol 1980;134:1005-1010.

146. Khanna G, O'Dorisio SM, Menda Y, et al. Gastroenteropancreatic neuroendocrine tumors in children and young adults. Pediatr Radiol 2008;38:251-259, quiz 358-359.

147. Berrocal T, Prieto C, Pastor I, et al. Sonography of pancreatic disease in infants and children. Radiographics 1995;15:301-313.

148. Gupta AK, Mitra DK, Berry M, et al. Sonography and CT of pancreatoblastoma in children. AJR Am J Roentgenol 2000;174:1639-1641.

149. Montemarano H, Lonergan GJ, Bulas DI, Selby DM. Pancreatoblastoma: imaging findings in 10 patients and review of the literature. Radiology 2000;214:476-482.

150. Auringer ST, Ulmer JL, Sumner TE, Turner CS. Congenital cyst of the pancreas. J Pediatr Surg 1993;28:1570-1571.

151. Crowley JJ, McAlister WH. Congenital pancreatic pseudocyst: a rare cause of abdominal mass in a neonate. Pediatr Radiol 1996;26:210-211.

152. Rausch DR, Norton KI, Glass RB, Kogan D. Infantile leukemia presenting with cholestasis secondary to massive pancreatic infiltration. Pediatr Radiol 2002;32:360-361.

CHAPTER 56

Pediatric Pelvic Sonography

Henrietta Kotlus Rosenberg and Humaira Chaudhry

Chapter Outline

SONOGRAPHIC TECHNIQUE

High-resolution, real-time, duplex color Doppler sonography has emerged as the modality of choice for the evaluation of the pelvis in infants, children, and adolescents. Using the distended bladder as an acoustic window, the lower urinary tract, uterus, adnexa, prostate gland, seminal vesicles, and pelvic musculature and vessels can be easily evaluated.[1-6]

Depending on the size of the child, a 5-2, 9-4, or 8-5 MHz real-time curvilinear broad-bandwidth or sector scanhead is used to obtain scans, usually in the transverse and sagittal planes. Linear probe technology is useful for evaluation of the bowel, peritoneum, perineum, and superficial lesions using a 12-5 MHz, a 17-5 MHz, or the 15-7io ("hockey stick") broad-bandwidth probes. Patients should be well hydrated before pelvic sonography so that the bladder will be optimally filled. In infants and young children who are unable to maintain a full bladder despite drinking clear liquids, it may be necessary to catheterize and fill the bladder with sterile water through a 5- or 8-French feeding tube, although this is rarely necessary. The use of sterile water as a contrast agent to outline the vagina (**hydrosonovaginography**) (Fig. 56-1), rectum (water enema)[7,8] (Fig. 56-2), or urogenital sinus may be very helpful in the evaluation of

the pediatric patient with a pelvic mass or complex congenital anomalies of the genitourinary tract. Meticulous real-time scanning is essential because these structures are filled in a retrograde manner. When transabdominal sonography provides suboptimal images in mature, sexually active teenage girls, **endovaginal ultrasound** can provide higher resolution with more detailed sonograms, thus aiding in the elucidation of the origin and characteristics of pelvic masses and complex adnexal lesions.[9]

The wall of the urinary bladder should be smooth in a distended state, with the wall thickness not greater than 3 mm during bladder distention, with a mean of 1.5 mm.[10] The wall should not be greater than 5 mm thick with the bladder empty or partially distended. In the nondistended state the internal aspect of the bladder wall generally appears slightly irregular sonographically. A **urachal remnant** may be visualized on sonography, as a structure of variable form and size, lying ventral to the peritoneum and situated between the umbilicus and the apex of the urinary bladder.[11] The distal ureters, with the exception of the submucosal intravesical portion, are not usually visualized unless abnormally dilated.[12] The **trigone,** however, is easily demonstrated (Fig. 56-3). The bladder neck and urethra can be demonstrated in both males and females by angling the transducer inferiorly[13] (Fig. 56-4). If a urethral abnormality is noted on

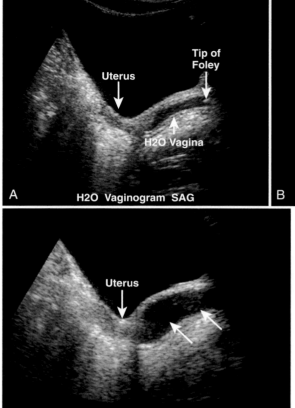

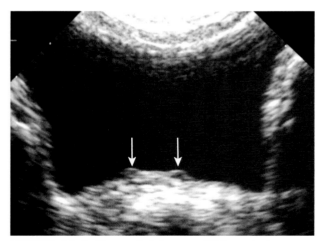

FIGURE 56-1. Normal hydrosono-vaginography in prepubertal female with prior vaginal rhabdomyosarcoma. A, Sagittal sonogram obtained during early filling of the vagina with sterile water. The water was hand-injected through a Foley catheter with the balloon inflated outside the vaginal introitus to prevent leakage. **B** and **C,** Transverse and sagittal sonograms, when the vaginal vault is well distended, show that the uterus is normal in size, echotexture, and configuration for a prepubertal female. The bright speckles within the water are caused by air.

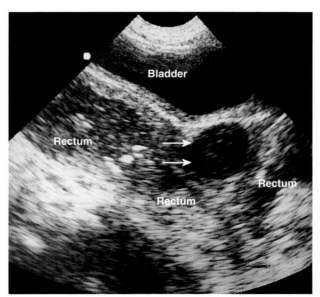

FIGURE 56-2. Water enema technique in 5-year-old boy with appendiceal abscess. Sagittal sonogram shows a small, hypoechoic fluid collection *(arrows)* located posterior to the bladder and anterior to the water-filled rectum.

FIGURE 56-3. Normal trigone. With meticulous scanning, it is possible to identify the trigone *(arrows)* in pediatric patients.

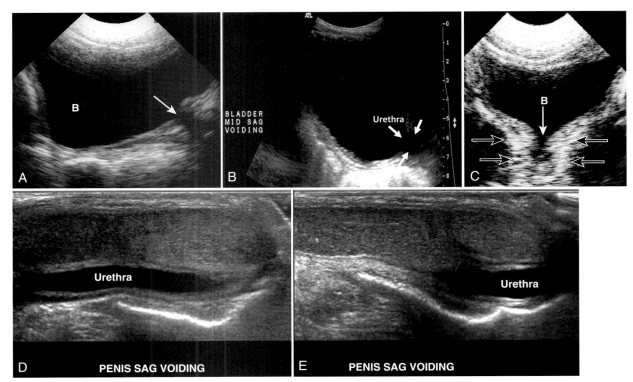

FIGURE 56-4. Normal urethras. A, Normal female urethra. Using bladder *(B)* as an acoustic window, urethra *(arrow)* may be seen. **B,** Voiding sonourethrography in a female. Using a sagittal suprapubic approach during voiding, the female urethra can be seen as a fluid-distended structure. **C,** Normal posterior urethra in young male child. Transverse scan through moderately distended bladder *(B)* shows posterior urethra *(white arrow)* and prostate gland *(black arrowheads)* surrounding the urethra. **D** and **E,** Voiding sonourethrography in a male. Sagittal scan demonstrating normal-appearing penile urethra in **D,** and the normal-appearing, most distal urethra at the fossa navicularis in the glans of the penis. *(**C** from Rosenberg HK. Sonography of the pediatric urinary tract. In Bush WH, editor:* urologic imaging and interventional techniques. *Baltimore, 1989, Urban & Schwarzenberg, pp 164-179.)*

suprapubic imaging, scans through the perineum or transrectally can confirm these findings using a different imaging plane.[14]

Hydrosonourethrography may be used to detect anterior urethral abnormalities (strictures, calculi, anterior or posterior urethral valves, foreign bodies, bladder neck dyssynergia, diverticula, trauma) by scanning the penis with a linear array transducer during real-time observation during voiding or during a retrograde hand injection of saline into the urethra.[15] **Postvoid scanning** of the bladder can provide information about bladder function, differentiate the bladder from cystic masses or fluid collections in the pelvis, and evaluate the degree of drainage from dilated upper urinary tracts. When children cannot void, films taken after a Credé maneuver or catheterization indicate the effectiveness of these bladder-emptying procedures. We measure the postvoid residual of the bladder using the following formula:

$$\text{Length} \times \text{Width} \times \text{Depth (in cm)} \div 2 = \text{Volume (in mL)}$$

NORMAL FEMALE ANATOMY

The Uterus

The uterus and ovaries undergo a series of changes in size and configuration during normal growth and development.[13] The **newborn female uterus** is prominent and thickened with a brightly echogenic endometrial lining caused by in utero hormonal stimulation[16] (Fig. 56-5). The uterine configuration is spade shaped, and the length is approximately 3.5 cm, with a fundus-to-cervix ratio of 1:2. At 2 to 3 months of age, the prepubertal uterus regresses to a smaller size and flat configuration (Fig. 56-6), with the length measuring 2.5 to 3 cm, the fundus/cervix ratio 1:1, and the endometrial stripe (when seen) appears as thin as a pencil line. This tubular uterine configuration is maintained until puberty. The **postpubertal uterine length** gradually increases to 5 to 7 cm, and the fundus/cervix ratio becomes 3:1 (Table 56-1).[13,16] The echogenicity and thickness of the endometrial lining then varies according to the phase of the menstrual cycle, as in adult women. The uterus is supplied by bilateral uterine arteries, which are branches of the internal iliac arteries. Color flow Doppler imaging generally demonstrates flow in the myometrium, with little or no flow in the endometrium.[15]

The Vagina

In children, digital and visual examination of the vagina is difficult. Often, physical examination of the vagina is performed under general anesthesia. High-resolution, real-time sonography can now obviate this need in many

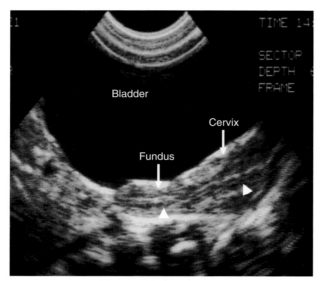

FIGURE 56-5. Normal newborn uterus. Sagittal view shows that ratio of fundus to cervix is 1:2 for length, and the somewhat thick endometrial lining is prominently echogenic as a result of in utero hormonal stimulation *(arrowheads)*.

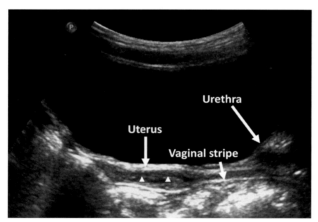

FIGURE 56-6. Normal prepubertal uterus in 2-year-old girl. Sagittal sonogram through the bladder demonstrates a fundus/cervix ratio of 1:1 and shows a pencil-line thin, unstimulated endometrial stripe *(arrowheads)*.

TABLE 56-1. PEDIATRIC UTERINE MEASUREMENTS

AGE	UTERINE LENGTH	FUNDUS-TO-CERVIX RATIO
Newborn	3.5 cm	1:2
Prepubertal*	2.5-3 cm	1:1
Postpubertal	5-8 cm	3:1

From Comstock CH, Boal DK. Pelvic sonography of the pediatric patient. Semin Ultrasound 1984;5:54-67; Rosenberg HK. Sonography of the pediatric urinary tract. In Bush WH, editor. *Urologic imaging and interventional techniques.* Baltimore, 1989, Urban & Schwarzenberg, pp 164-179.
*Beginning at age 2 to 3 months.

cases. In the infant or young girl presenting with an interlabial mass, sonography in conjunction with other imaging modalities can usually determine the cause. The vagina is best visualized on midline longitudinal scans through the distended bladder. It appears as a long, tubular structure in continuity with the uterine cervix. The apposed mucosal surfaces cause a long, bright, slender, central linear echo. Hydrosonovaginography under real-time sonography guidance can provide additional information about vaginal patency or confirm the presence or absence of a vaginal mass.

The Ovary

Sonographic visualization of the ovaries in children can vary, depending on their location, size, and the age of the patient (Fig. 56-7). Because of a generally long pedicle and a small pelvis, the neonatal ovaries may be found anywhere between the lower pole of the kidneys and the true pelvis (Fig. 56-8). Ovarian size is most reproducible and best described by measurement of the ovarian volume, which is calculated by a simplified prolate ellipse formula, as follows[17]:

$$\text{Length} \times \text{Depth} \times \text{Width (in cm)} \times 0.523 = \text{Volume (in mL)}$$

The **mean ovarian volume** in neonates and girls less than 6 years of age is usually 1 mL or less.[18] Ovarian volume gradually begins to increase at about age 6 years. The mean ovarian volume measurement in **premenarchal girls** between ages 6 and 11 years ranges between 1.2 and 2.5 mL (Table 56-2). There is marked enlargement in ovarian size after puberty; thus ovarian sizes in **menstruating females** in late childhood will be larger than their premenarchal counterparts. Cohen et al.[19] reported a mean ovarian volume of 9.8 mL, with a 95% confidence interval between 2.5 and 21.9 mL, in menstruating females.

Beginning in the neonatal period, the appearance of the typical ovary is heterogeneous secondary to small cysts. Cohen et al.[18] reported observing **ovarian cysts** in 84% of children 1 day to 2 years of age and 68% of children 2 to 12 years of age. **Macrocysts** (>9 mm) were more frequently seen in the ovaries of girls in their first year of life compared with those in their second year. This probably accounts for the larger mean and top-normal ovarian volume measurements obtained in girls up to 3 months of age (mean ovarian volume, 1.06 mL; range, 0.7-3.6 mL) versus those 13 to 24 months of age (mean ovarian volume, 0.67 mL; range, 0.1-1.7 mL). These findings probably result from the higher residual maternal hormone level in younger infants. Orbak et al.[20] concluded that ovarian volume was reduced in newborns with relatively low birth weight and intrauterine growth restriction, and that functional cysts were more prevalent among low-birth-weight girls. We suggest that small ovaries and ovarian dysfunction may have a

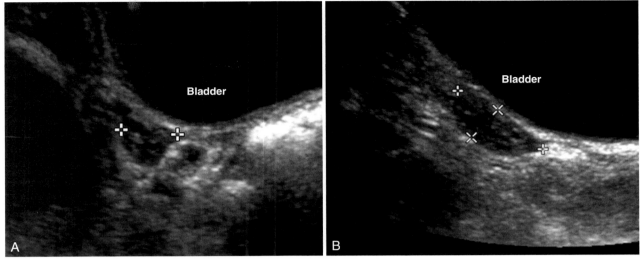

FIGURE 56-7. Normal ovary in 2-year-old child. A and **B,** Transverse and sagittal views of the ovary. Note that small follicles are normal in the prepubertal ovary and can be easily visualized with high-resolution technology.

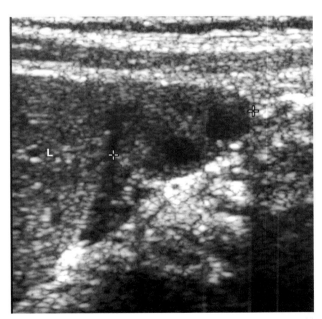

FIGURE 56-8. Ectopic ovary. Ectopic ovary in 18-year-old female with cyclic right upper quadrant pain thought to be caused by recurrent "gallbladder attacks." The liver and gallbladder were normal (not shown). The ectopic right ovary *(cursors)* is just below the inferior edge of the right lobe of the liver *(L).*

TABLE 56-2. PEDIATRIC OVARIAN VOLUME MEASUREMENTS

AGE	MEAN OVARIAN VOLUME mL (±SD)	
	Premenarchal	
0-5 yr	≤1 mL	
1 day to 3 mo		1.06 (±0.96)
4-12 mo		1.05 (±0.67)
13-24 mo		0.67 (±0.35)
3 yr		0.7 (±0.4)
4 yr		0.8 (±0.4)
5 yr		0.9 (±0.02)
6-8 yr	1.2 mL	
6 yr		1.2 (±0.4)
7 yr		1.3 (±0.6)
8 yr		1.1 (±0.5)
9-10 yr*	2.1 mL	
9 yr		2.0 (±0.8)
10 yr		2.2 (±0.7)
11 yr*	2.5 mL (±1.3)	
12 yr*		3.8 mL (±1.4)
13 yr*		4.2 mL (±2.3)
	Menstrual	
		9.8 mL (±5.8)

From Rosenberg HK. Sonography of the pediatric urinary tract. In Bush WH, editor. *Urologic imaging and interventional techniques.* Baltimore, 1989, Urban & Schwarzenberg, pp 164-179; and Cohen HL, Shapiro MA, Mandel FS, Shapiro ML. Normal ovaries in neonates and infants: a sonographic study of 77 patients 1 day to 24 months old. AJR Am J Roentgenol 1993;160:583-586.

*Note that these measurements may differ, depending on degree of maturation and presence of menarche.

prenatal origin, and further studies on normal and growth-restricted newborns are needed.

The blood supply of the ovary is dual, arising from the **ovarian artery,** which originates directly from the aorta, and from the **uterine artery,** which supplies an adnexal branch to each ovary. Blood flow can be seen in 90% of the adolescent ovary, but Doppler imaging cannot distinguish between the two blood supplies. Typically, on color flow Doppler imaging, the intraovarian arteries appear as short, straight branches located centrally within the normal ovary.[21]

OVARIAN ABNORMALITIES

Ovarian Cysts

Since the advent of sonography, simple ovarian cysts in children have been found to be more common than previously reported.[22] Small cysts (1-7 mm) have been detected

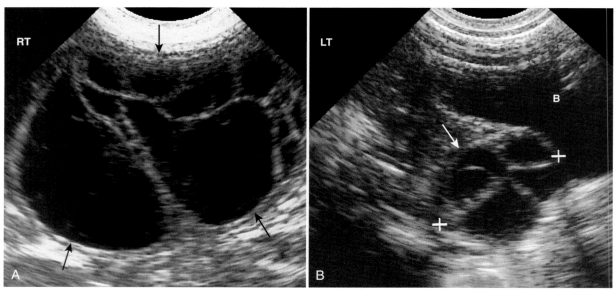

FIGURE 56-9. Ovarian cysts in newborn girl. A, Right ovary. **B,** Left ovary. Cysts presented as a lower abdominopelvic mass. Multiple anechoic cystic areas with septations are noted in ovaries bilaterally *(arrows)*. Ovarian cysts were believed to be secondary to in utero hormonal stimulation. Follow-up studies showed complete regression. *B,* Bladder.

on sonograms in the third-trimester fetus and the neonate and are secondary to maternal and placental chorionic gonadotropin. There is a higher incidence of larger ovarian cysts in infants of mothers with toxemia, diabetes, and Rh isoimmunization, all of which are associated with a greater-than-normal release of placental chorionic gonadotropin.[23] Large ovarian cysts in the fetus can cause mechanical complications during vaginal delivery. As a result of the small size of the true pelvis in infants and young children, ovarian cysts are often intra-abdominal in location and must be differentiated from **mesenteric** or **omental cysts, gastrointestinal duplication cysts,**[24] and **urachal cysts.** Ovarian cysts are associated with **cystic fibrosis, congenital juvenile hypothyroidism,**[25] **McCune-Albright syndrome** (fibrous dysplasia and patchy cutaneous pigmentation), and **peripheral sexual precocity.** Autonomously functioning ovarian cysts can cause **precocious pseudopuberty.**

Although neonatal ovarian cysts were surgically removed in the past, spontaneous resolution of some cysts has been demonstrated on sonography[23] (Fig. 56-9). When a follicle continues to grow after failed ovulation or when it does not collapse after ovulation, follicular and corpus luteal cysts may result. Most **follicular cysts** are unilocular, contain clear serous fluid, and range in size between 3 and 20 cm. **Corpus luteal cysts** can contain serous or hemorrhagic fluid and generally range in size from 5 to 11 cm. **Theca lutein cysts** are thought to represent hyperstimulated follicles caused by gestational trophoblastic disease or a complication of drug therapy to stimulate ovulation. Rarely, **parovarian cysts** are diagnosed in childhood (Fig. 56-10). They are of mesothelial or paramesonephric origin and arise in the broad ligament or fallopian tubes.

Complications: Torsion, Hemorrhage, Rupture

Most ovarian cysts are asymptomatic. Symptoms of pain, tenderness, nausea, vomiting, and low-grade fever usually indicate complications of torsion, hemorrhage, or rupture. **Torsion** can occur in normal ovaries but it is more often caused by an ovarian cyst or tumor. In children, torsion of the normal ovary can occur because the fallopian tube is relatively long and the ovary is more mobile. The typical presentation is acute onset of acute lower abdominal pain, often associated with nausea, vomiting, and leukocytosis. Torsion of **normal adnexa** usually occurs in prepubertal girls and is thought to be related to excessive mobility of the adnexa, allowing torsion at the mesosalpinx with changes in intra-abdominal pressure or body position. Torsion of the **ovary and fallopian tube** results from partial or complete rotation of the ovary on its vascular pedicle. This results in compromise of arterial and venous flow, congestion of the ovarian parenchyma, and, ultimately, hemorrhagic infarction.[26] The sonographic findings in **acute ovarian torsion** are often nonspecific and include ovarian enlargement, fluid in the cul-de-sac, and other adnexal pathologic findings, such as cyst or tumor (Fig. 56-11). A predominantly cystic or complex adnexal mass with a fluid-debris level or septa correlates with pathologic evidence of ovarian hemorrhage or infarction. In 28 of 32 patients, Lee et al.[27] showed that ultrasound could demonstrate preoperatively the twisted vascular pedicle in surgically proven torsion, giving a diagnostic accuracy of 87%. This appeared as a round, hyperechoic structure with multiple concentric hypoechoic stripes (target appearance), as a beaked

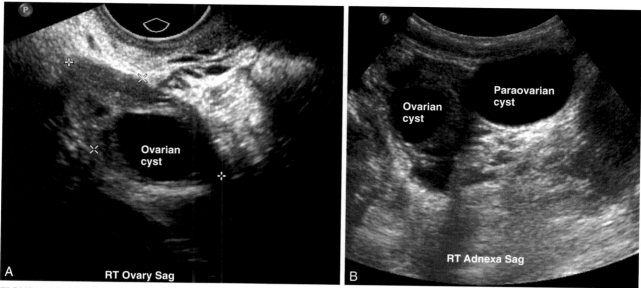

FIGURE 56-10. Ovarian cysts in teenager. A and **B,** Sonograms demonstrate a simple cyst within the right ovary. In addition, a simple paraovarian cyst is demonstrated in **B.**

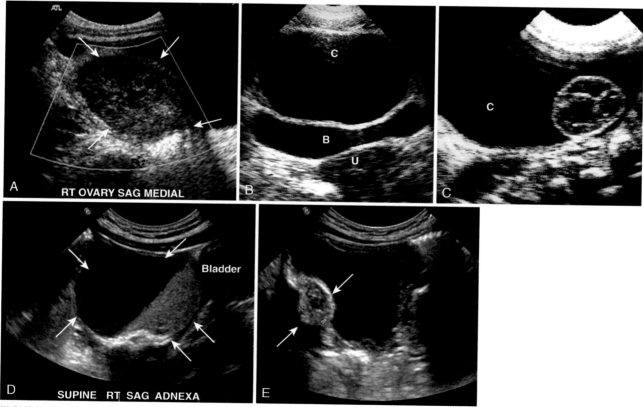

FIGURE 56-11. Ovarian torsion. A, Sagittal sonogram in 9-year-old girl with right lower quadrant pain demonstrates a greatly enlarged avascular right ovary that contains multiple, variably sized cysts. The ovary was easily untwisted at surgery and immediately regained normal color. **B,** Ovarian torsion complicating an ovarian cyst in a 16-year-old girl with pelvic pain. Transverse view of the pelvis shows the large anterior ovarian cyst *(C)* compressing the bladder *(B)* (surgical proof of torsion). No ovarian parenchymal tissue was seen sonographically; *U,* Uterus. **C,** Infarcted, encysted, ovarian torsion in a 6-day-old girl with an abdominal mass. Sonogram of the right lower abdomen and pelvis demonstrates an oval-shaped, complex structure within a larger cystic mass *(C).* **D,** Sagittal view shows infarcted, encysted, torsed right ovary in newborn with cystic mass noted on prenatal sonogram. A fluid-debris level is noted within the cyst *(arrows).* **E,** Transverse left decubitus scan shows encysted right ovary *(arrows)* embedded in the wall of the cyst.

structure with concentric hypoechoic stripes, or as an ellipsoid or tubular structure with internal heterogeneous echoes. Concentric hypoechoic intrapedicular structures could be identified as vascular structures by color Doppler sonography ("whirlpool sign"). The absence of flow at color Doppler ultrasound is not a reliable diagnostic criterion because peripheral (or even central) arterial flow can be seen in surgically proven twisted ovaries. This may be explained by the duality of the ovarian arterial perfusion.[28] The demonstration of **multiple follicles** (8-12 mm in size) **in the cortical or peripheral portion of a unilaterally enlarged ovary** has been reported as a specific sonographic sign of torsion.[29-31] These cystic changes occur in up to 74% of twisted ovaries and are attributed to transudation of fluid into follicles secondary to vascular congestion. At times, isolated fallopian tube torsion occurs in perimenarcheal girls who present with acute pelvic pain and demonstrate a cystic mass in a midline position (either in the cul-de-sac or superior to the uterus) associated with a normal ipsilateral ovary.[32]

Hemorrhagic ovarian cysts occur in adolescents and have a variety of sonographic patterns caused by internal blood clot formation and lysis (Fig. 56-12). The most common appearance is a heterogeneous mass, which is predominantly anechoic, containing hypoechoic material. Less often, hemorrhagic ovarian cysts are homogeneous, either hypoechoic or hyperechoic. Almost all hemorrhagic cysts (92%) have increased sound through-transmission, indicating the cystic nature of the lesion. Additional sonographic features include a thick wall (e.g., 4 mm), septations, and fluid in the cul-de-sac. Although the sonographic findings are nonspecific, the changing appearance of hemorrhagic ovarian cysts over time, as a result of clot lysis, can help establish the diagnosis.[33] In some cases the diagnosis can be confused with **appendiceal abscess, dermoid cyst,** or **teratoma.** Rarely, **pelvic varices** can masquerade as a multiseptated cystic mass (Fig. 56-13).

Polycystic Ovarian Disease (Stein-Leventhal)

The primary clinical manifestations of polycystic ovarian disease (polycystic ovary syndrome, Stein-Leventhal syndrome) are hirsutism and irregular menstrual bleeding caused by excess ovarian androgens and chronic anovulation.[34] These features emerge late in puberty or shortly thereafter. In patients with obesity or insulin resistance, the severity of the presentation is amplified. The evolution of this condition during early adolescence is not well understood, but it appears that abnormal activation of the hypothalamic-pituitary-ovarian-adrenal axis occurs, accompanied by specific morphologic changes in the ovaries.[34] The ovaries are bilaterally rounded and enlarged in 70% of affected patients, with mean ovarian volume of 14 mL. Follicle-stimulating hormone (FSH) levels are decreased, whereas luteinizing hormone (LH) levels are elevated. Sonography shows increased numbers of developing follicles, seen as multiple small cysts (0.5-0.8 cm in diameter) throughout the ovaries, in about 40% of patients, although maturing follicles are rare (Fig. 56-14). Long-term follow-up is important in these patients because of the increased incidence of **endometrial carcinoma** from long-term unopposed estrogen.[35] Dolz et al.[36] conducted a three-dimensional (3-D) sonographic evaluation of the size and structure of the ovaries of women who had clinical and biochemical findings suggestive of polycystic ovary syndrome and a comparative color Doppler flow (frequency) and power Doppler (amplitude) study of the vascular patterns of these ovaries. Compared to controls, these women had larger ovaries and thicker stroma, increased impedance in the uterine arteries, increased stromal vascularity with decreased impedance that persisted throughout the menstrual cycle, and a lack of luteal conversion.

Massive Ovarian Edema

Massive edema of the ovary is manifested by marked enlargement of the affected ovary caused by accumulation of edema fluid in the stroma, separating normal follicular structures (Fig. 56-15). It is thought to result from partial or intermittent torsion that interferes with venous and lymphatic drainage. It affects patients during their second to third decade of life and presents with acute abdominal pain, palpable adnexal mass, menstrual disturbances at times, masculinization, and Meigs' syndrome. Two thirds of patients have right-sided ovarian

---

ACUTE OVARIAN TORSION: SONOGRAPHIC FINDINGS

Ovarian enlargement
Fluid in cul-de-sac
Adnexal mass (ovarian hemorrhage or infarction)
Cystic or complex
Fluid-debris level
Septated
Peripheral, multiple follicles

OVARIAN MASSES IN CHILDREN

Benign ovarian teratomas (almost 60%)
Dysgerminoma
Embryonal carcinoma
Endodermal sinus tumor
Epithelial tumors of ovary (postpuberty)
Granulosa theca cell tumor (precocious puberty)
Arrhenoblastoma (rare, virilizing)
Gonadoblastoma (in dysplastic gonads, e.g., Turner's syndrome)
Acute leukemia

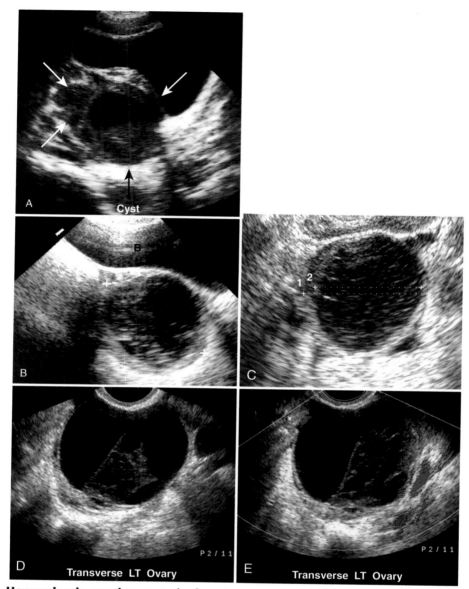

FIGURE 56-12. Hemorrhagic ovarian cysts in four teenagers with left pelvic pain: spectrum of appearances. A, Transverse view of the pelvis reveals a large, round cystic mass within the ovary (*arrows,* ovary) that contains a fluid-debris level representing a hemorrhagic cyst. **B,** Transabdominal sagittal sonogram shows enlargement of the left ovary with a rim of ovary surrounding a cyst that contains multiple, echogenic, streaky densities; *B,* bladder. **C,** Endovaginal sonography of the cyst confirms the presence of surrounding ovarian tissue and the heterogeneous appearance of the contained fluid. **D** and **E,** Transvaginal sonograms of the left ovary demonstrate jagged pseudosolid material within the clearly defined cyst.

edema, thought to be related to high pressure in the right ovarian vein caused by direct drainage into the inferior vena cava (IVC) or increased pressure secondary to uterine dextroposition. The ovaries may be massively enlarged, with diameter up to 35 cm. Grossly, the external surface is soft and pearly white and appears similar to **fibromatosis,** a condition likely to occur in young women (up to 25 years of age) in which primary proliferation of the ovarian stroma may result in torsion and

ultimately edema. The sonographic features of ovarian edema include a solid, hypoechoic mass, enhanced through-transmission, and cystic follicles within the lesion.[37,38] The masculinization is thought to be caused by stromal luteinization that results from mechanical stretching of the stromal cells by the edema fluid. In addition, human chorionic gonadotropin–like substance may accumulate in edema fluid and promote luteinization, and level of 17-ketosteroids may be increased.

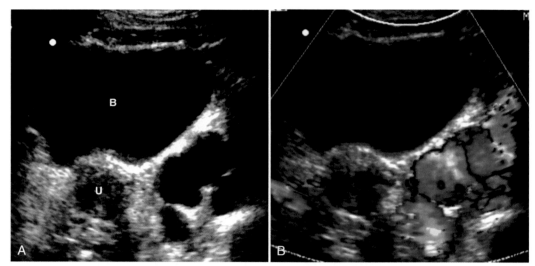

FIGURE 56-13. Pelvic varices mimicking a multiseptated ovarian cyst. Young woman with chronic liver disease and portal hypertension. **A,** Transverse sonogram of pelvis shows a multiseptated left adnexal mass; *B,* bladder; *U,* uterus. **B,** Transverse color Doppler sonography of pelvis clearly demonstrates the vascular nature of the lesion. Pulsed Doppler showed venous waveforms (not shown).

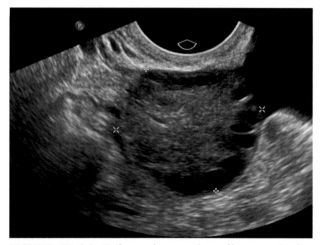

FIGURE 56-14. Polycystic ovarian disease: Stein-Leventhal syndrome. Sagittal sonogram of the left ovary in 21-year-old woman with secondary amenorrhea, obesity, and hirsutism. The ovary is round and contains multiple peripheral cysts ("string of pearls"), each of which measures greater than 5 mm.

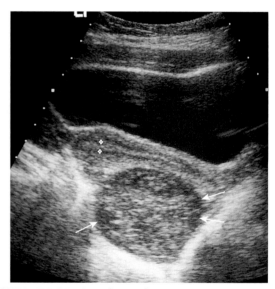

FIGURE 56-15. Ovarian edema. Massive ovarian edema in a 13-year-old girl with masculinization and intermittent pelvic and abdominal pain. Sagittal sonographic image demonstrates a large, heterogeneous, primarily hypoechoic mass posterior and separate from the uterus. This mass contains marked sound through-transmission and multiple tiny follicles *(arrows). Calipers,* Endometrial stripe. *(Case courtesy Marilyn Goske, MD.)*

Ovarian Neoplasms

Ovarian neoplasms account for 1% of all childhood tumors, and 10% to 30% of these are malignant. These neoplasms may develop at any age but most frequently occur at puberty. Abdominal pain or a palpable abdominal or pelvic mass is the usual presenting symptom. Symptoms may develop as a result of torsion or hemorrhage into the tumor. Ovarian torsion is more common in adolescents than in adults; however, ascites is less common in girls.[39]

Primary ovarian tumors can be classified into three types of cell origins: **germ cells**, **epithelial cells,** and **stromal cells.** In children, 60% of primary ovarian tumors are of germ cell origin, in contrast to adults, in whom 90% are epithelial in origin. About 75% to 95%

of germ cell tumors in childhood are benign teratomas. However, there is a higher incidence of malignancy in younger patients. In girls younger than 10 years, 84% of ovarian germ cell tumors are malignant. The presence of ascites suggests malignancy.

Benign teratomas have a wide spectrum of sonographic characteristics (Fig. 56-16). Teratomas may be predominantly cystic, with or without a mural nodule. Solid masses and complex lesions with fat-fluid levels, hair-fluid levels, and calcification have been described.[40] Cystic teratomas are usually freely mobile on a pedicle;

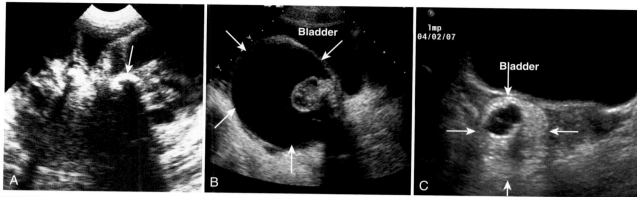

FIGURE 56-16. Benign ovarian teratomas. A, Transverse sonogram of pelvis in 6-year-old girl with constipation and large abdominal mass revealed very large, complex mass filling pelvis and lower two thirds of abdomen, containing multiple shadowing, echogenic foci *(arrows)* consistent with calcifications. **B,** Midline sonogram in a 12-year-old girl with right lower quadrant pelvic pain demonstrates a complex, primarily cystic mass that contains a small area of shadowing calcification in the dermal plug. **C,** Young girl presented with a history of urinary tract infection. A mass effect was noted effacing her bladder during an outside voiding cystourethrography. Sonography at our institution demonstrated a complex, round, primarily brightly echoic mass with smaller, hypoechoic cystic areas. A large fatty component was noted at surgery.

10% are bilateral, and 90% are less than 15 cm in diameter.[41]

Dysgerminoma is the most common malignant germ cell tumor of the ovary in childhood. This tumor frequently occurs before puberty, and 10% are bilateral. The tumor is usually a large, solid, encapsulated, rapidly growing mass containing hypoechoic areas as a result of hemorrhage, necrosis, and cystic degeneration. Retroperitoneal lymph node metastases may occur. Dysgerminoma is more radiosensitive than the other malignant ovarian tumors.

Embryonal carcinoma and **endodermal sinus tumors** are less common malignant germ cell tumors. **Choriocarcinoma** is rare in children. All these are rapidly growing, highly malignant, solid neoplasms. Embryonal carcinoma is often associated with abnormal hormonal stimulation. All these tumors tend to spread by direct extension to the opposite adnexa and retroperitoneal lymph nodes. Peritoneal seeding and hematogenous metastases to liver, lung, bone, and mediastinum are common. Molar pregnancy may occur in teenage patients (Fig. 56-17).

Epithelial tumors of the ovary, which include serous and mucinous **cystadenoma** or **cystadenocarcinoma,** represent 20% of ovarian tumors in children.[42] Epithelial lesions are rare before puberty. On sonography, they are predominantly cystic masses with septa of variable thickness. It is often difficult to differentiate benign from malignant and serous from mucinous cystadenomas or cystadenocarcinomas based only on sonographic criteria.

Granulosa theca cell tumor is the most common stromal tumor in children. It is often associated with feminizing effects and precocious puberty as a result of estrogen production. Of these tumors, 10% are bilateral; only 3% are malignant. Sonographic appearance is non-specific, and these tend to be predominantly solid tumors.[43] **Arrhenoblastoma** (Sertoli-Leydig cell tumor)

is rare but may result in virilization. **Gonadoblastoma** is composed of germ cells admixed with sex cell and stromal elements and usually arises in dysplastic gonads. Bilateral involvement occurs in one third of cases, and 50% contain dysgerminoma elements.

In **leukemic infiltration,** the ovaries, as well as the testes and central nervous system, are sanctuary sites for acute leukemia. Ovarian involvement in autopsy series ranges from 11% to 50%. In leukemia with ovarian relapse, most patients present with large, hypoechoic, pelvic masses with smooth, lobulated margins. The tumor can infiltrate the pelvic organs and bowel loops to such a degree that the uterus and ovaries cannot be separately identified. Secondary hydronephrosis may develop. Bickers et al.[44] suggest that pelvic sonography should be used to monitor and detect early leukemic relapse in the ovaries of children in clinical remission. The ovaries may also be a site for metastatic spread from **neuroblastoma, lymphoma,** and **colon carcinoma.** The tumors rarely grow large enough to produce a mass and are usually asymptomatic. Typically, the secondary neoplasms appear on sonography as enlargement of one or both ovaries, which are hypoechoic or hyperechoic to the uterus. Less often, a discrete solid or complex mass is seen.

It was originally thought that Doppler sonography would serve to differentiate between benign and malignant ovarian masses. In adolescents and adult women, malignant ovarian tumors generally have central, low-resistance arterial Doppler waveforms (RI [resistive index] <0.4, or PI [pulsatility index] <1.0), thought to be caused by a relative paucity of a muscular layer in the neoplastic vessels,[45] thereby limiting the specificity of Doppler imaging.[46] Benign ovarian masses tend to have peripheral, high-resistance flow (RI or PI >1.0). However, nonneoplastic lesions (e.g., tubo-ovarian abscess, ectopic pregnancy, functioning corpus luteum) also have low-resistance flow, and some malignant tumors show high-resistance flow.

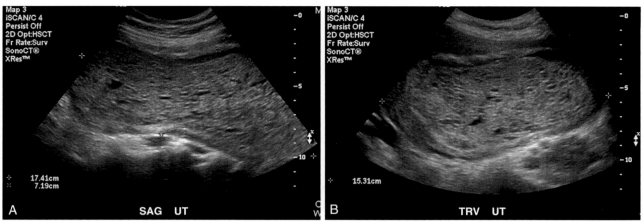

FIGURE 56-17. Molar pregnancy in 20-year-old patient with vaginal bleeding and abdominal pain. A and **B,** Sagittal and transverse sonograms of the uterus demonstrate a 17.4 × 15.3 × 7.2–cm complex, mainly solid mass, throughout the uterus with the exception of the distal end of the cervix, which is characterized by diffuse heterogeneity from a myriad of tiny cystic spaces. The mass is hypovascular and does not contain calcifications.

UTERINE AND VAGINAL ABNORMALITIES

Congenital Anomalies

Congenital anomalies of the uterus and vagina in children are uncommon and usually present as an abdominal or pelvic mass secondary to obstruction (Fig. 56-18). There is a high incidence of associated renal anomalies (50%) and an increased incidence of skeletal anomalies (12%).[47] The uterus, cervix, and upper two thirds of the vagina are formed by the fused caudal ends of the müllerian (paramesonephric) duct. The paired fallopian tubes are formed by the unfused upper ends. The lower third of the vagina is derived from the urogenital sinus. Müllerian duct development into the uterus is dependent on the formation of the wolffian (mesonephric) duct. Therefore, abnormal development of the müllerian duct, resulting in uterine and vaginal anomalies, is often associated with renal anomalies.[48,49]

The **bicornuate uterus** is the most common congenital uterine anomaly. It results when the two müllerian ducts fuse only inferiorly[50] (Fig. 56-19). The two separate uterine horns, which are joined at a variable level above the cervix, are best demonstrated on transverse sonograms through the superior portion of the uterus. Only one cervix and vagina are identified. With **complete duplication of the müllerian ducts**, there is a septated vagina and duplicated cervix and uterus. In either anomaly, obstruction of one uterine horn can result in a pelvic mass from unilateral hydrometra or hematometra. Other septation anomalies of the uterus cán result from incomplete involution of the midline septum between the paired müllerian ducts. A **unicornuate uterus** is formed from the agenesis of one müllerian duct.[51] In utero exposure to **diethylstilbestrol**

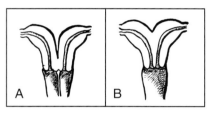

A, Uterus didelphys bicollis (septate vagina).
B, Uterus bicornis bicollis (vagina simplex).

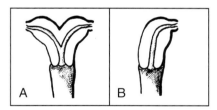

A, Uterus bicornis unicollis (vagina simplex). B, Uterus unicornis.

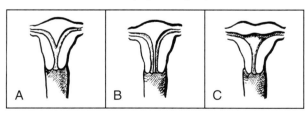

A, Uterus subseptus. B, Uterus septus. C, Uterus arcuatus.

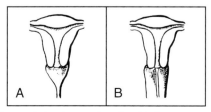

A, Congenital stricture of vagina. B, Septate vagina.

FIGURE 56-18. Uterine anomalies. *(From Wilson SR, Beecham CT, Carrington ER, editors: Obstetrics and gynecology, 8th ed. St Louis, 1987, Mosby.)*

(DES) has been associated with development of a **T-shaped uterus.** Sonography shows a narrow uterus caused by absence of the normal, superior, bulbous expansion of the uterine fundus. Three-dimensional sonography is an excellent modality for obtaining planar reformatted sections through the uterus, which allows for precise evaluation of the anatomy.[49]

Hydrocolpos or **hydrometrocolpos,** caused by obstruction of the vagina, accounts for 15% of abdominal masses in newborn girls (Fig. 56-20). The obstruction is secondary to an **imperforate hymen,** a **transverse vaginal septum,** or a **stenotic or atretic vagina.** There is an accumulation of mucous secretions proximal to the obstruction. The secretions are secondary to intrauterine and postnatal stimulation of uterine and cervical glands by maternal estrogens. A simple imperforate hymen is not usually associated with other congenital anomalies. However, there is a high incidence of genitourinary, gastrointestinal, and skeletal anomalies associated with **vaginal atresia** or a **midtransverse or high-transverse vaginal septum.** Combined perineal-abdominal sonography is an excellent method for accurate assessment of these anomalies.[52] Although transabdominal scanning is useful to determine if hydrocolpos or hydrometrocolpos is present, this method does not allow measurement of the thickness of a caudally placed obstructive septum. On sonographic examination, hydrocolpos appears as a large, tubular, cystic mass posterior to the bladder and extending inferior to the symphysis pubis.[53] Low-level echoes within the fluid represent mucous secretions in neonates and blood in postpubertal girls[54] (Fig. 56-21). There may be secondary urinary retention and hydronephrosis. Imperforate anus, cloacal exstrophy, and persistent urogenital sinus often have associated hydrometrocolpos.[55-57] Rarely, one may see peritoneal calcifications complicating hydrometrocolpos because of a sterile inflammatory reaction to spillage into the peritoneal cavity of accumulated secretions.[58]

The **Mayer-Rokitansky-Küster-Hauser syndrome,** the second most common cause of primary amenorrhea, comprises vaginal atresia, rudimentary bicornuate uterus, normal fallopian tubes and ovaries, and broad and round ligaments.[47] The spectrum of uterine anomalies (hypoplasia or duplication) range from a partial lumen to a septate or bicornuate uterus with unilateral or bilateral obstruction. These girls have a normal female karyotype, secondary sexual development, and external genitalia. There is a high incidence of unilateral renal (50%) and skeletal (12%) anomalies. Unilateral renal agenesis or ectopia is the most common renal anomaly. The most

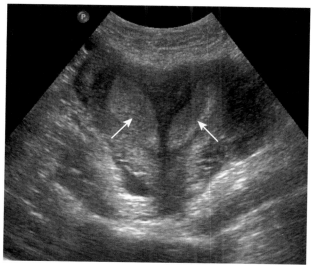

FIGURE 56-19. Bicornuate uterus. Transverse image of the uterus in a 20-year-old woman with acute lower abdominal and pelvic pain reveals two separate endometrial cavities *(arrows)* in the middle to fundal region of the uterus.

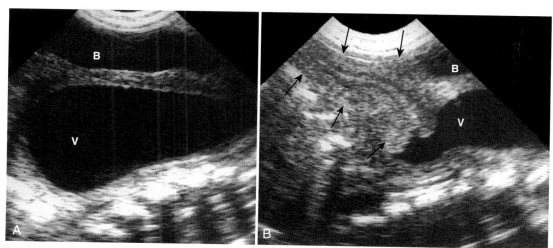

FIGURE 56-20. Hydrocolpos. A, Sagittal scan of pelvis in newborn showing large, conical, fluid-filled mass representing obstructed vagina *(V)* behind bladder *(B).* **B,** Sagittal scan, angled higher than in **A,** shows uterus *(arrows)* with cervix projecting into dilated vagina *(V); B,* bladder. *(From Rosenberg HK: Sonography of pediatric urinary tract abnormalities. Part I. Am Urol Assoc Weekly Update Series 1986;35:1-8.)*

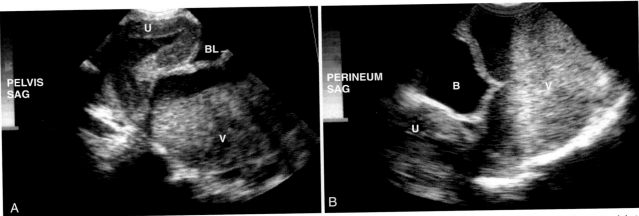

FIGURE 56-21. Hematometrocolpos. A, Sagittal scan of pelvis shows dilated uterine cavity *(U)* filled with echogenic debris (blood). Fluid-debris level is seen in dilated, obstructed vagina *(V)*. **B,** Perineal scan confirming the massively dilated vagina with the distal end immediately below the skin surface; *U,* uterus, *V,* vagina; *B,* bladder. *(From Fisher MR, Kricun ME, editors:* Imaging of the pelvis. *Gaithersburg, Md, 1989, Aspen.)*

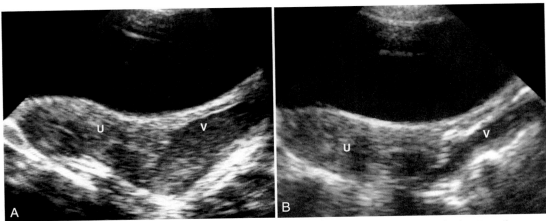

FIGURE 56-22. Mayer-Rokitansky-Kuster-Hauser syndrome. This 13-year-old girl had duplication of uterus and vagina, obstructed right-sided vagina, and fenestrated vaginal septum with cyclic pelvic pain and normal menstrual periods. **A,** Sagittal scan of pelvis demonstrates a normal right uterus *(U)* and a distended vagina *(V)* filled with echogenic material that moved at real time. **B,** Left-sided uterus *(U)* is clearly seen in the sagittal plane, and following hand injection of sterile water into the single introitus, the left-sided vagina *(V)* was demonstrated. During real-time observation, tiny amounts of water could be seen intermittently in the right-sided vagina, suggesting the presence of a fenestrated vaginal septum.

common sonographic findings are uterine didelphys with unilateral hydrometrocolpos and ipsilateral renal agenesis. Water vaginography can help identify the septated vagina with unilateral vaginal obstruction[47] (Fig. 56-22). The analogous genitourinary defects in the male result in duplicated müllerian duct remnants (müllerian cyst and dilated prostatic utricle) with unilateral renal agenesis.

Neoplasm

Tumors of the uterus and vagina are uncommon in the pediatric patient. Malignant tumors are more common than are benign tumors, and the vagina is a more common site than is the uterus. **Rhabdomyosarcoma** is the most common primary malignant neoplasm.[59] It can arise from the uterus or vagina, although uterine involvement is more frequent by direct extension from a vaginal tumor. These children usually present at 6 to 18 months of age with vaginal bleeding or protrusion of a polypoid

cluster of masses (**sarcoma botryoides**) through the introitus. Rhabdomyosarcoma most often arises from the anterior wall of the vagina near the cervix. It may also arise in the distal vagina or labia. Direct extension of the tumor into the bladder neck is common, but posterior invasion of the rectum is infrequent. Lymphadenopathy and distant metastases are uncommon at presentation. On sonographic examination, these tumors are solid, homogeneous masses that fill the vaginal cavity or cause enlargement of the uterus with an irregular contour. Tumors of the endometrium are rare in the pediatric age range. When the sonographic findings demonstrate a fairly well-defined, heterogeneous endometrial mass—in the appropriate clinical setting—one should consider the possibility of retained products of conception (Fig. 56-23).

Endodermal sinus tumor, a less common genital neoplasm, is a highly malignant germ cell tumor that can arise in the vagina. It has a similar clinical and

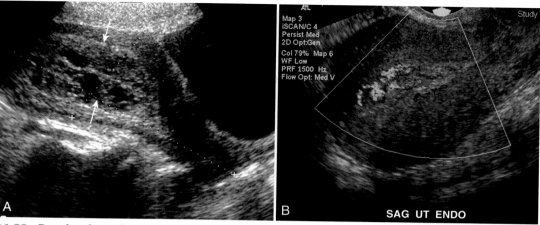

FIGURE 56-23. Retained products of conception. A, This 15-year-old girl presented with ongoing cramps and vaginal bleeding after a spontaneous abortion. Sagittal sonography shows elongation of the uterus (12.9 cm) with a heterogeneous, fairly well-defined, oval-shaped masslike area *(arrows)* occupying the fundus. **B,** Another teenager presented with vaginal bleeding a few days after a therapeutic abortion. Sagittal color Doppler sonogram of the uterus demonstrates hypervascularity throughout the insonated portion of the endometrium, consistent with retained products of conception.

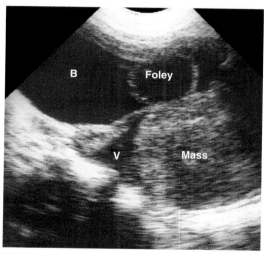

FIGURE 56-24. Endodermal sinus tumor of vagina. Sagittal scan of pelvis shows solid, homogeneous mass filling vagina *(V)*. Foley catheter balloon is seen in bladder *(B)*. *(From Fisher MR, Kricun ME, editors:* Imaging of the pelvis. *Gaithersburg, Md, 1989, Aspen.)*

sonographic presentation as rhabdomyosarcoma (Fig. 56-24). Other malignant tumors of the uterus and vagina are rare. Adenocarcinoma of the cervix in adults arises from the endocervix, whereas in children it is a polypoid lesion that originates from the ectocervix and upper vagina. **Carcinoma of the vagina** (usually clear cell adenocarcinoma) usually occurs in teenagers with a history of in utero DES exposure. Leukemic infiltration of the uterus can occur secondary to contiguous extension from an ovarian relapse. Sonography shows a large, homogeneous, hypoechoic, pelvic mass incorporating the uterus and ovaries, which cannot be separately identified. There may be associated hydronephrosis caused by distal ureteral obstruction.

Benign, solid neoplasms of the uterus and vagina are rare in children. However, benign cystic vaginal masses

can occur. The most common cystic lesion of the vagina is **Gartner's cyst.** A remnant of the distal wolffian (mesonephric) duct, Gartner's cysts may be single or multiple and typically arise from the anterolateral vaginal wall. They appear as fluid-filled cysts within the vagina on ultrasound. Other cystic vaginal masses include **paraurethral cysts, inclusion cysts,** and **paramesonephric (müllerian) duct cysts.**

Pregnancy

Intrauterine pregnancy must always be considered in the differential diagnosis of a pelvic mass in girls 9 years of age or older. There is an increased incidence of complications in pediatric pregnancy. These include **toxemia, preeclampsia, placental abruption, lacerations,** and **cesarean section.** Prematurity and perinatal mortality are also increased in infants of teenage mothers. Although **ectopic pregnancy** accounts for approximately 2% of all pregnancies and is less common in young adolescents, the diagnosis should be considered in the presence of pelvic pain, an abnormal **beta human chorionic gonadotropin** (β-hCG) level, irregular vaginal bleeding, and missed menstrual period. An ectopic pregnancy is most likely located in a fallopian tube (ampulla 70%, isthmus 12%, fimbria 11.1%). The two most common sonographic signs of ectopic pregnancy include an **adnexal mass** that is separate from the ovary and the **tubal ring sign** (Fig. 56-25). The diagnosis is more certain when a yolk sac or a living embryo is demonstrated within the adnexal mass.[60] The tubal ring sign consists of a hyperechoic ring surrounding an extrauterine gestational sac. The additional demonstration of the **"ring of fire" sign,** which consists of high-velocity, low-impedance flow within the hyperechoic ring, may be another useful finding.[61] However, this sign is nonspecific and may be seen surrounding a normal maturing follicle or a corpus luteal cyst. About 10% of patients with an ectopic

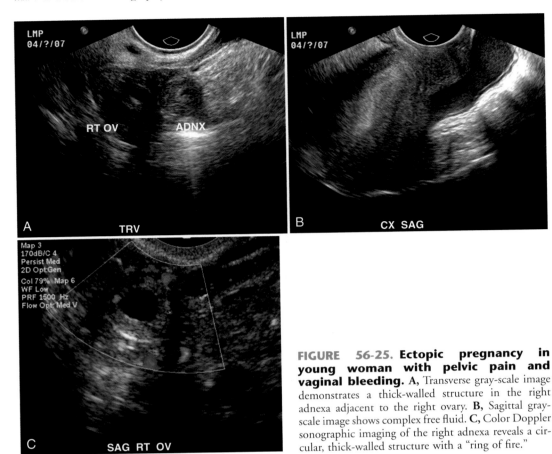

FIGURE 56-25. Ectopic pregnancy in young woman with pelvic pain and vaginal bleeding. A, Transverse gray-scale image demonstrates a thick-walled structure in the right adnexa adjacent to the right ovary. **B,** Sagittal gray-scale image shows complex free fluid. **C,** Color Doppler sonographic imaging of the right adnexa reveals a circular, thick-walled structure with a "ring of fire."

pregnancy demonstrate a pseudogestational sac, which in the absence of a double–decidual sac sign, is more likely an indication of an ectopic pregnancy in the right setting.[62] Hypotension or overt shock suggests ruptured ectopic pregnancy. Although endovaginal sonography has greatly improved the diagnostic evaluation of suspected ectopic pregnancy, transabdominal scanning plays a complementary role by providing a global view of the pelvis and abdominal contents.[63] β-hCG measurements are essential for establishing the diagnosis. This glycoprotein hormone begins to increase in a curvilinear fashion early in pregnancy and continues to increase until approximately 9 to 11 weeks, when it normally reaches a plateau. The plateau lasts for a few days and declines at 20 weeks. β-hCG doubles on an average of approximately 48 hours when the pregnancy is normal and viable. In the presence of an ectopic pregnancy, however, serum β-hCG levels often rise much more slowly, and a plateau is reached early in the pregnancy. A less than 50% increase in β-hCG level in a 48-hour period is almost always associated with a nonviable pregnancy, whether intrauterine or extrauterine.[64] Wherry et al.[65] showed that color Doppler RI of the endometrium could help differentiate an early intrauterine pregnancy from an ectopic pregnancy. Trophoblastic flow was defined as an RI of less than 0.6 within the endometrium. The negative predictive value for the presence of endometrial low-resistance flow for excluding ectopic pregnancy was 97%.

Infection

Pelvic Inflammatory Disease

Pelvic inflammatory disease (PID) is an infection of the upper genital tract, usually related to *Neisseria gonorrhoeae* or *Chlamydia trachomatis* infection. The serious sequelae of this disease include ectopic pregnancy, infertility, and chronic pelvic pain. Adolescent females are in a higher-risk group, and thus PID should be considered in sexually active females presenting with pelvic pain. The ascending infection may affect uterus, fallopian tubes, and ovaries, causing endometritis, salpingitis, oophoritis, pelvic peritonitis, and tubo-ovarian abscess.

In a study by Bulas et al.,[66] anatomic detail was improved with endovaginal scanning compared with transabdominal scanning. Endovaginal scans showed new abnormalities in 71% of patients, and the level of disease severity was changed in 33% of patients, which affected treatment decisions in many of these patients.

Acutely, the pelvic sonogram may be normal.[63,65] In the **endometritis** stage of PID, the uterus may be enlarged and more hyperechoic, may contain a small amount of fluid in the endometrial canal, and may have indistinct margins. The normal fallopian tube is usually not visualized on sonography. As the infection ascends, however, the fallopian tubes become thick walled and fill with purulent material[66] (Fig. 56-26). A **pyosalpinx** is a

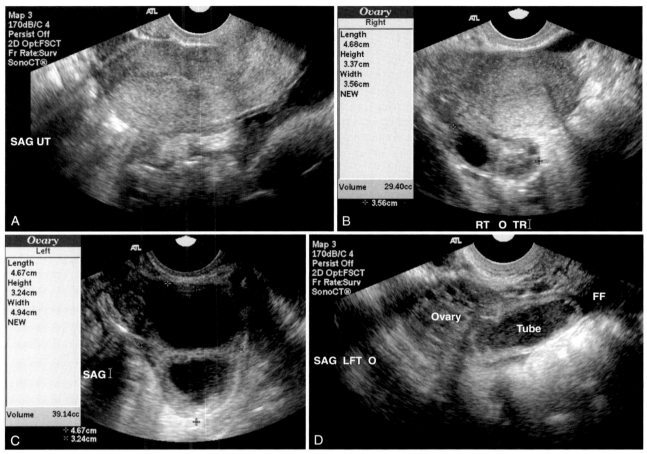

FIGURE 56-26. Pelvic inflammatory disease with tubo-ovarian complex. Endovaginal sonography in 16-year-old girl with pelvic pain. **A,** Sagittal image of the uterus shows free fluid in the cul de sac. **B,** The right ovary is normal size, although there is an anechoic dominant cyst. **C,** Sagittal image of greatly enlarged left adnexa demonstrates a tubo-ovarian complex (one cyst within ovary and one anterior to ovarian border). **D,** Fluid-distended fallopian tube is noted with surrounding free fluid (FF). The fluid within the tube is hypoechoic, implying purulent material.

PELVIC INFLAMMATORY DISEASE: SONOGRAPHIC FINDINGS

Enlarged, hyperechoic uterus
Indistinct uterine margins
Fluid in endometrial canal
Hydrosalpinx with echogenic fluid
Ovarian enlargement with tiny cysts
Tubo-ovarian abscess (heterogeneous adnexal mass)

dilated, occluded fallopian tube that contains echogenic purulent fluid. A residual **hydrosalpinx** is a tubular or round structure with anechoic fluid. Ovarian changes from PID may include enlargement secondary to the production of inflammatory exudate and edema and development of many tiny cysts, which may represent small follicles or abscesses (Fig. 56-27).

Periovarian adhesions may form, resulting in fusion of the ovary and thickened tube, forming a tubo-ovarian complex. Further progression leads to tissue breakdown

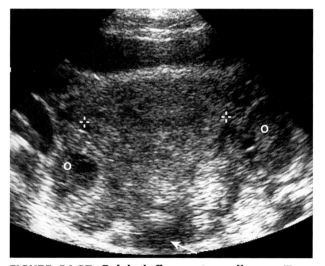

FIGURE 56-27. Pelvic inflammatory disease. Transverse transabdominal image of the pelvis reveals increased, poorly defined, soft tissue echogenicity representing inflammatory material causing indistinct uterine and ovarian margins and haziness in the parametrial area. A small amount of echogenic fluid is seen posteriorly (arrow). Calipers, Uterus; O, ovary.

and formation of a **tubo-ovarian abscess,** which usually appears as a well-defined, heterogeneous, adnexal mass with enhanced through-transmission. Most contain internal debris and septations. Color flow Doppler evaluation of pelvic masses in patients with PID is not specific and overlaps with other entities. Flow in an abscess may be seen along its periphery; however, this pattern may also be seen in other cystic lesions.[21,66] In **extensive cases of PID** the pelvis is diffusely filled with a heterogeneous echo pattern containing cystic and solid components that obscure tissue planes and uterine margins.

A complication of PID is **gonococcal or chlamydial perihepatitis** (Fitz-Hugh–Curtis syndrome). The patient presents with right upper quadrant pain caused by localized peritonitis of the anterior liver surface and parietal peritoneum of the anterior abdominal wall. Sonographic findings include the presence of ascitic fluid and thickening of the right anterior extrarenal tissue between the liver and right kidney.[67,68]

Foreign Bodies

A vaginal discharge may be a sign of vaginal infection or trauma. Foreign bodies in the vagina are a cause of 4% of cases of **vaginitis.** A wad of toilet paper is the most common foreign body in the vagina. Vaginal foreign bodies are seen in 18% of children with vaginal bleeding and discharge and in 50% of children with vaginal bleeding and no discharge. Sonography, either transabdominal or transperineal, with or without water vaginography, can identify both radiopaque and nonradiopaque foreign bodies within the vagina as echogenic material with distal acoustic shadowing. A retained vaginal foreign body can be demonstrated on sonography as a slight indentation on the posterior bladder wall. Acoustic shadowing is characteristic, but may not be present.[69,70]

ENDOCRINE ABNORMALITIES

Ultrasound has become an integral part of evaluation of children with endocrine abnormalities. In the newborn with ambiguous genitalia, pelvic sonography can quickly determine the presence or absence of the uterus and vagina. Identification of the ovaries or testes is more difficult because normal neonatal ovaries are not seen on ultrasound. Using a high-resolution (12-17 MHz) linear transducer, the gonads may be found in the inguinal canal or in the ambiguous labioscrotal folds. **Differentiation of the gonads** between ovaries and testes may be possible because ovaries often have small, hypoechoic follicles and testes have a solid, homogeneous echotexture.[71]

Causes of Primary Amenorrhea

Sonographic assessment of the uterine size, shape, maturity, and ovarian development can provide a clue to the many causes of primary amenorrhea. A small or absent uterus may be an indication of **gonadal dysgenesis, chromosomal abnormalities, decreased hormonal states, testicular feminization,** or **isolated uterine hypoplasia or agenesis.** In **Turner's syndrome,** the most common form of **gonadal dysgenesis,** there is delayed or absent puberty associated with short stature, webbed neck, renal anomalies, and coarctation of the aorta. In those girls with pure 45,XO karyotypes, the ovaries may not be visualized sonographically although a prepubertal uterus may be demonstrated. In genetic mosaicism with 45,XO/46,XX karyotype, the ovaries can vary from nonvisualized streak ovaries to normal adult ovaries. The uterine configuration also varies from prepubertal to an intermediate length that is less than that of the normal adult female. Haber and Ranke[72] demonstrated in a group of 93 patients with Turner's syndrome that one or both ovaries were detected in 44%. Within the prepubertal group, the mean uterine volume and mean ovarian volume measurements were significantly lower than those of the normal controls ($p < 0.001$) (0.5 ± 0.2 mL versus 1.0 ± 0.3 mL and 0.3 ± 0.3 mL versus 0.6 ± 0.4 mL, respectively). In prepubertal girls, no significant relationship was found between age and uterine size or ovarian volume. Both uterine volume and ovarian volume of 19 women with spontaneous puberty increased during breast development, although mean uterine volume and mean ovarian volume were significantly ($p < 0.01$) lower than those of pubertal control patients.

Other forms of gonadal dysgenesis are also associated with nonvisualization of the ovaries as a result of absent or streak gonads. In **pure gonadal dysgenesis** (Swyer's syndrome), the patients have 46,XX or 46,XY karyotypes and normal height. **Mixed gonadal dysgenesis** is a genetic mosaic of karyotypes 45,XO/46,XY with a streak ovary and a contralateral intra-abdominal testicle. Both these forms of gonadal dysgenesis have an increased risk of gonadal tumors as a result of the presence of the Y chromosome. **Noonan's syndrome** (pseudo–Turner's syndrome) is characterized by phenotypic changes of Turner's syndrome, normal ovarian function, and normal ovaries on ultrasound.

Testicular feminization is another cause of primary amenorrhea. It is a sex-linked recessive abnormality, resulting in end-organ insensitivity to androgens. These patients are phenotypic females with a 46,XY karyotype. The uterus and ovaries are absent, the vagina ends blindly, and the testes are ectopic (usually pelvic or within inguinal canals or in labia majora).

Precocious Puberty

Sonography is an important imaging modality in the evaluation of children with precocious puberty. Precocious puberty is the development of secondary sexual characteristics, gonadal enlargement, and ovulation before age 8 years. In true precocious puberty, the endocrine profile is similar to that of normal puberty, with elevated levels of estrogen and gonadotropins. The uterus has an enlarged, postpubertal configuration (fundus/cervix ratio, 2:1 to 3:1) with a more prominent echogenic endometrial canal than seen in prepubertal females. The ovarian volume is greater than 1 mL, and functional cysts are often present. Precocious puberty is classified into two types: central and peripheral. **Central precocious puberty** (true precocious puberty) is gonadotropin dependent.[73] More than 80% of these cases are idiopathic. Intracranial tumors, usually a **hypothalamic glioma or hamartoma,** account for 5% to 10% of cases. There are occasional cases following development of increased intracranial pressure, such as **postmeningitis hydrocephalus.** The augmented uterine and ovarian volumes shown at ultrasound occur before the typical changes in secretion patterns of LH and FSH revealed with the LH-releasing hormone (LHRH) test. Follow-up pelvic sonography during treatment with long-acting gonadotropin-releasing hormone analogs will show decreased uterine and ovarian volume, and the hormonal status will become appropriate for age.[74,75]

In **pseudoprecocious puberty**, the peripheral type, the endocrine profile is variable because this type is gonadotropin independent. Usually, the estrogen levels are elevated and the gonadotropin levels are low. The cause is outside the hypothalamic-pituitary axis and is usually caused by an **ovarian tumor.** Granulosa theca cell tumor is the most common lesion. Other, less frequent causes are functioning ovarian cysts, dysgerminoma, teratoma, and choriocarcinoma. Ultrasound will identify the ovarian mass and a mature uterus. Although **feminizing adrenal tumors** are a rare cause of pseudoprecocious puberty, **sonographic examination of the adrenal areas should be performed in all patients with precocious puberty** who are referred for pelvic ultrasound. The liver should be examined as well because precocious puberty has been associated with **hepatoblastoma.** In isolated premature thelarche (breast development) or premature adrenarche (pubic or axillary hair development), sonography shows normal prepubertal uterus and ovaries.

NORMAL MALE ANATOMY

The Prostate

The configuration of the prostate is ellipsoid in boys compared with the more conical shape seen in adult males. The prostatic echogenicity is hypoechoic and more homogeneous than in the adult prostate, which is frequently heterogeneous secondary to central gland nodules, calcifications, and corpora amylacea.[76,77] Prostate volume may be calculated by using the following formula for a prolate ellipsoid:

$$\text{Length} \times \text{Width} \times \text{Depth (in cm)} \times 0.523$$
$$= \text{Volume (in mL)}$$

Ingram et al.[78] showed that in a group of 36 boys, age 7 months to 13.5 years (mean 7.7 years), the prostatic volume ranged between 0.4 and 5.2 mL (mean 1.2 mL). The seminal vesicles may be identified in young boys and adolescents and are best seen in the transverse plane as small, hypoechoic structures giving an appearance similar to the wings of a seagull (Fig. 56-28).

The Scrotum

Before sonographic examination of the scrotum, the clinician should carefully palpate the entire scrotum. The pediatric scrotum is examined with a high-frequency linear array broadband scanhead, generally a 12-5 MHz for children and teenagers and a 17-5io, small-footprint, "hockey stick" probe for very small testes in infants, young children, and atrophic testes. The probe should be equipped with gray-scale and duplex/color flow Doppler as well as power Doppler imaging. It is helpful to elevate and immobilize the testes by gently placing a rolled-up towel posterior to the scrotum in a vertical position between the legs. For accurate measurements of larger adolescent testes, a curvilinear, broad-bandwidth probe, either a 9-4 or 5-2 MHz, and a stepoff pad may be necessary. In infants or any patient with a painful scrotum, a stepoff pad is essential to obtain this valuable study. Both hemiscrota should be routinely examined so that differences in size and echogenicity of the intrascrotal contents can be recognized. Color flow Doppler

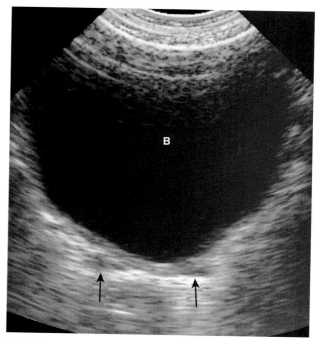

FIGURE 56-28. Seminal vesicles. Through a well-distended bladder *(B)*, the seminal vesicles *(arrows)* are seen as hypoechoic, bilaterally symmetrical structures.

imaging parameters should be optimized for the best detection of low-velocity and low-volume blood flow typically seen in the scrotum (color gain settings are maximized until background noise becomes visible, and wall filter and pulse repetition frequencies are adjusted to the lowest settings). Power mode Doppler imaging, with its increased sensitivity for the detection of blood flow, is useful for examination of slow flow states in the cooperative patient and particularly in very young children who normally have low testicular flow. In very small testes, power output may need to be increased to detect flow. Color flow in the two hemiscrota should be compared for symmetry. The addition of pulsed Doppler imaging allows for quantitative evaluation of arterial waveforms and measurements of velocity.

The Testes

The normal **newborn testes** have a homogeneous low- to medium-level echogenicity and are spherical or oval in shape with a length of 7 to 10 mm (Fig. 56-29). The epididymis and **mediastinum testis** are usually not seen in the neonate. By puberty, the testis contains homogeneous medium-level echoes and an echogenic linear structure along its superoinferior axis, which represents the mediastinum testis (Fig. 56-30). The testis measures 3 to 5 cm in length and 2 to 3 cm in depth and width after puberty. Studies of testicular sizes during infancy and adolescence performed using orchidometers report the range of mean testicular volumes as 1.10 mL (SD ± 0.14) and 30.25 mL (SD ± 9.64).[79] The author's personal experience, as well as references to testicular sizes in more recent radiologic articles, supports the existence of normal testes smaller than 1 mL in young infants and children.[80,81] The **tunica albuginea** may be seen as a thin echogenic line around the testis. Occasionally, a hypoechoic linear band is noted in the normal testis, usually in the middle third, corresponding to sites of **intratesticular vessels.**[82]

Both pulsed and color flow Doppler ultrasound can be used to assess the blood supply to the testis. The normal color flow Doppler appearance of the testes also changes with age. Despite optimized slow-flow settings, it may not be possible to detect color flow in normal, small, prepubertal testes.[80,81,83] Atkinson et al.[80] reported that centripetal arterial flow could be identified with color flow Doppler imaging in only 6 (46%) of 13 testes measuring less than 1 mL and in all testes measuring greater than 1 mL. When color flow is seen in prepubertal testes, it generally appears as pulsatile foci of color without the linear or branching pattern seen in adolescents or adults[80] (Fig. 56-30). The recurrent rami arteries are usually too small to be identified in children, although they may be seen in adolescents. Color Doppler imaging can demonstrate flow in 60% to 83% of prepubertal testes, and power Doppler imaging can demonstrate flow in up to 73% to 92% of prepubertal testes. Luker and Siegel[83] showed that power mode Doppler ultrasound improved depiction of intratesticular vessels in normal prepubertal and postpubertal testes, but that there was still a lack of flow in several normal prepubertal testes.

Normal pulsed wave Doppler testicular flow reflects its supply from the testicular artery, which has a low-resistance pattern (low peak systolic velocities and relatively high diastolic velocities). Flow in extratesticular vessels reflects supply from the cremaster and deferential arteries and has a higher resistance pattern (low diastolic flow). Because the periphery of the testis contains capsular branches of the testicular artery and branches of the cremasteric and deferential arteries, **the patency of the testicular artery can be established reliably only by placing the Doppler sample volume in the center of the testis.** The RI of the testicular artery in young men ranges from 0.48 to 0.75 (mean 0.62), and the RI of the capsular arteries ranges from 0.46 to 0.78 (mean 0.66). The RI of the supratesticular arteries varies from 0.63 to 1.00 (mean 0.84). The RI in intratesticular arteries is lower in postpubertal than in prepubertal boys.[84]

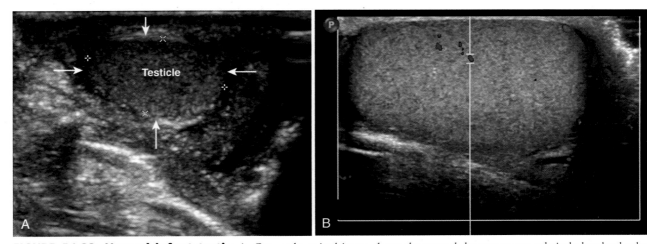

FIGURE 56-29. Normal infant testis. A, Gray-scale sagittal image shows the normal, homogeneous, relatively low-level echogenicity of this normal infant testis. **B,** Some color Doppler flow is demonstrated within the testis.

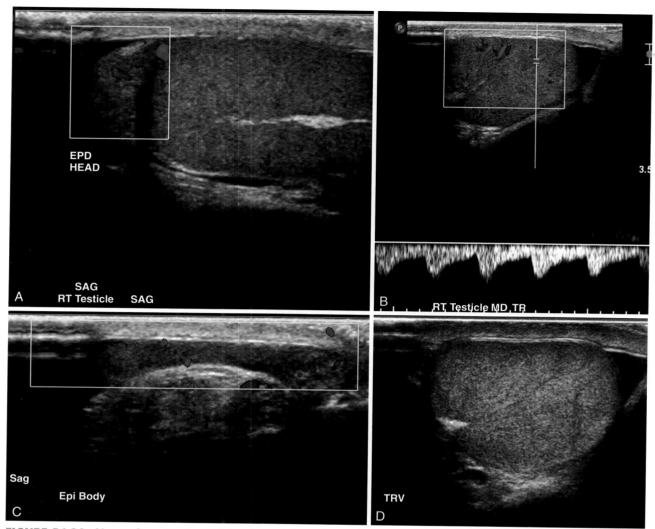

FIGURE 56-30. Normal postpubertal testis. A, Color flow Doppler image demonstrates flow within the head of the epididymis. The testis demonstrates normal homogenous echogenicity, with the mediastinal testis appearing as a white stripe. **B,** Normal duplex color Doppler flow in the centripetal arteries of this normal-appearing testis. **C,** There is also normal flow in the body and tail of the epididymis. **D,** Transverse image of testis. A small hydrocele is seen on all four images.

The examiner must compare the symmetry of color Doppler flow in both testes to detect disease more accurately and to ensure the system is optimally set to detect flow in the clinically normal testis. Absent flow may not be valid if the ultrasound equipment being used is insufficiently sensitive to detect low flow or if faulty technical settings are used (e.g., high wall filter, low gain, high pulse repetition frequency, low transducer frequency). Power Doppler is often better than color Doppler sonography in assessing symmetry of blood flow.[85]

The **epididymis** lies along the posterolateral aspect of the testis. The triangular-shaped epididymal head is isoechoic with the testis or slightly hyperechoic, whereas the echogenicity of the epididymal body is isoechoic or slightly hypoechoic in relationship to the testis. Flow may not be detected in the normal prepubertal epididymis but is generally seen on both color flow and power mode Doppler imaging in postpubertal epididymides.[83]

CONGENITAL MALE ABNORMALITIES

In **cryptorchidism** the testis does not descend through the inguinal canal into the scrotum as expected between the 25th and 32nd week of gestation. In most cases the testes are located within the scrotum at birth or within 4 to 6 weeks after birth. Undescended testes are seen in 4% of full-term newborns and in approximately 33% of premature male infants weighing less than 2500 grams. Testicular descent continues during the first year of life, so that by the end of the first year, only 0.7% to 0.8% of these infants have true cryptorchidism, and in 10% to 25%, it is bilateral cryptorchidism.[86] Although the malpositioned testis may lie anywhere along its course from the retroperitoneum to the scrotum, most testes (80%-90%) are located at or below the inguinal canal

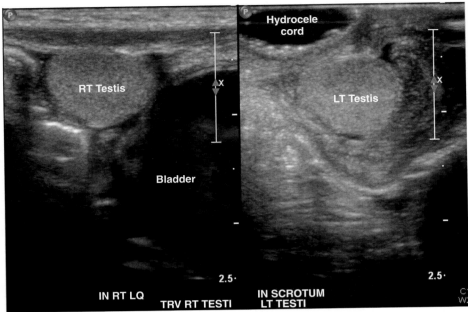

FIGURE 56-31. Undescended right testis. Normal-appearing right testis is located in the baby's pelvis anteriorly adjacent to the bladder. Normal-appearing left testis is located in the left hemiscrotum. A small hydrocele of the cord is located superficially.

and thus are amenable to sonographic localization[87] (Fig. 56-31). MRI may be employed for localizing intra-abdominal cryptorchid testes.[88] **Localization of the undescended testis** is important in disease prevention because cryptorchidism is associated with increased risks of malignancy, infertility, and torsion.[87] Rarely, the testis is found in the perineum or at the base of the penis. **Anorchidism,** bilateral testicular absence, occurs in 1 in 20,000 newborn males. **Monorchidism,** unilateral testicular absence, occurs in 1 in 5000 boys and is usually left sided. This is thought to result from an in utero torsion or vascular accident because of the associated blind-ending spermatic vessels and spermatic cords.[89]

The number of testes may vary and range from **anorchidism** to **polyorchidism** (testicular duplication), which normally presents in the older child as an asymptomatic scrotal mass. The testes share a common epididymis, vas deferens, and tunica albuginea. Usually, a single, small, **accessory testis is demonstrated within the scrotum in addition to two normal testes** (triorchidism).[90] Polyorchidism is usually an incidental finding, presenting as an asymptomatic scrotal "mass", but occasionally, it will present with pain due to torsion. A **bilobed testis** may mimic a duplicated testis. Polyorchid and bilobed testes have medium-level homogeneous echogenicity and are smaller than the contralateral testis.

Aberrations in testicular descent may result in **transverse testicular ectopia,** an anomaly in which both testes are located in the same hemiscrotum. Patients present clinically with a nonpalpable testis on one side and a scrotal "mass" on the other.[91] About 20% have associated anomalies, such as seminal vesicle cysts, renal dysplasia, hypospadias, ureteropelvic junction obstruction, and ipsilateral inguinal hernia.

Testes smaller than normal in size may result from cryptorchidism, torsion, inflammation, varicocele, prior inguinal hernia repair, radiation treatment, and trauma. Congenital causes include Klinefelter's syndrome and primary hypopituitarism. These small gonads may have normal, increased, or decreased echogenicity.[91]

True hermaphroditism is an intersex condition in which the patient has both ovarian and testicular tissue, either in the form of separate structures or an **ovotestis.** Ultrasound can demonstrate the textural difference within an ovotestis in that the testicular portion is more homogeneous with medium-level echoes, whereas the ovarian tissue is more heterogeneous with small, anechoic, cystic follicles interspersed with the low- to medium-level parenchymal echogenicity[92] (Fig. 56-32). These patients present either prepubertally with ambiguous genitalia or postpubertally with the development of gynecomastia, cyclic hematuria, or cryptorchidism in a patient reared as a boy, or amenorrhea in a patient reared as a girl (Fig. 56-33).

Cystic dysplasia of the testis is a rare congenital condition consisting of dilated rete testis and efferent ducts, as well as adjacent parenchymal atrophy. Patients typically present with painless scrotal enlargement at a mean age of 5.8 years.[93] The ultrasound appearance consists of multiple, small, anechoic, cystic structures seen predominantly in the region of the mediastinum testis (Fig. 56-34). The defect may result from an embryologic defect preventing fusion between the rete testis tubule (arising from the gonadal blastema) and efferent ductules (arising from the mesonephros). Several reported cases in children were associated with ipsilateral renal agenesis, multicystic dysplastic kidney, or renal dysplasia.[93,94] The appearance in the scrotum is similar to the incidentally noted condition of tubular ectasia of the rete testis described in adults, which probably represents an acquired condition secondary to prior inflammation or trauma[94,95] (Fig. 56-35). The lack of color flow within these cystic structures distinguishes tubular ectasia from **intratesticular varicocele,** which can have a similar gray-scale appearance but demonstrates venous flow on color flow Doppler imaging.[96] This condition may mimic a cystic neoplasm such as teratoma. If filled with mucoid material or debris instead of anechoic fluid, the cysts may mimic a solid mass.

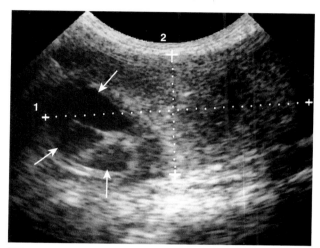

FIGURE 56-32. Ovotestis. Ovotestis in a 15-year-old phenotypic boy with bilateral gynecomastia, intermittent scrotal pain and swelling, and recent scrotal trauma. Sagittal sonography of the right hemiscrotum reveals a heterogeneous right gonad *(calipers)* with focal cystic areas representing follicles in the upper pole *(arrows).* This gonad contains pathologically proven ovarian and testicular tissue.

ACUTE SCROTAL PAIN OR SWELLING

The most common causes of acute pain and swelling in the pediatric scrotum include testicular torsion, epididymitis with or without orchitis, torsion of the testicular appendages, testicular trauma, acute hydrocele, and incarcerated hernia. Less common causes are idiopathic scrotal edema, Henoch-Schönlein purpura, scrotal fat necrosis, familial Mediterranean fever, or secondary scrotal involvement from abdominal pathology.[94-98] It is often impossible clinically to differentiate between the conditions that require conservative medical treatment and those that demand immediate surgery.[99] However, the combination of gray-scale and color flow Doppler sonography provides information about morphology and testicular perfusion.[100-103]

Testicular torsion and **epididymitis** (with or without orchitis) are the two most frequently encountered causes

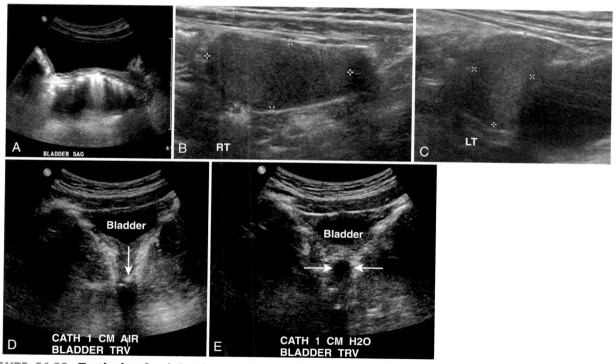

FIGURE 56-33. Testicular feminization syndrome. This 5-year-old girl underwent bilateral inguinal herniorrhaphies. At surgery, the tissue within each of the inguinal canals felt more firm than expected in the presence of normal herniated ovaries, and thus both were biopsied. **A,** Sagittal scan of the normal-appearing urinary bladder reveals no evidence of a uterus or ovaries. **B** and **C,** Male-type gonads are seen bilaterally, as evidenced by the homogeneity and lack of follicles in either gonad. Biopsy of both gonads revealed normal, male-type gonads. **D** and **E,** Using the bladder as a sonic window, the length of the vaginal canal was assessed by injecting air and then sterile water into the vaginal opening during sonographic observation. The vaginal canal was extremely short, approximately 1 cm in length. The catheter could be advanced only 1 cm into the vagina, implying an extremely short vaginal canal.

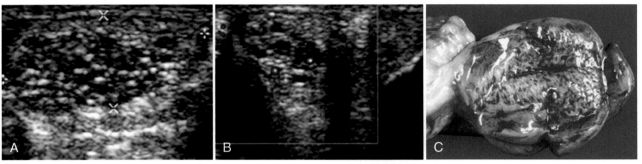

FIGURE 56-34. Cystic dysplasia of testis. A, Sagittal sonogram, and **B,** color Doppler sonography, show multiple tiny cysts in the testicle. **C,** Pathologic specimen shows tiny cysts. *(Case courtesy Janet Strife, MD, Cincinnati Children's Hospital.)*

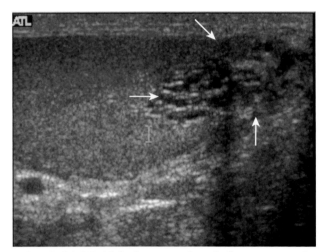

FIGURE 56-35. Tubular ectasia of the rete testis. This 9-year-old boy presented with left scrotal pain. Sagittal sonogram demonstrates a focal cluster of tiny, oval-shaped cysts in the symptomatic area.

ACUTE SCROTAL PAIN OR SWELLING

COMMON
Testicular torsion
Epididymitis with and without orchitis
Torsion of testicular appendages
Testicular trauma
Acute hydrocele
Incarcerated hernia

UNCOMMON
Idiopathic scrotal edema
Henoch-Schönlein purpura
Scrotal fat necrosis
Familial Mediterranean fever
Abdominal pathology

of the acute scrotum in the pediatric population. High-resolution ultrasound with color flow Doppler imaging has become the method preferred for distinguishing between these two entities.[100-109] This is crucial because testicular torsion is treated surgically and epididymitis with or without orchitis is treated medically. To confirm the diagnosis of testicular torsion unequivocally, the clinician must demonstrate absence of flow in the painful testis and normal flow in the asymptomatic normal testis,[81] keeping in mind that the presence of flow in the painful testis does not exclude torsion. In the patient with incomplete or partial spermatic cord torsion (twist of ≤360 degrees), normal arterial flow may be demonstrated, although it is usually quantitatively diminished compared with the asymptomatic contralateral testis.[107,109]

Torsion of the spermatic cord is found in 14% to 31% of children and adolescents presenting with an acute scrotum. Testicular torsion results when the testis and spermatic cord twist one or more times, obstructing blood flow. Torsion of the testis has the highest prevalence during two age peaks, infancy and adolescence.[81] Two types of torsion have been described: extravaginal and intravaginal, with the latter being more common. **Extravaginal torsion** is generally found in neonates at the level of the spermatic cord, which is poorly fixed in the inguinal canal. All the scrotal contents are strangulated in this type of torsion.[81,92,110] Extravaginal torsion is thought to occur in utero.[111] The loose attachment of the spermatic cord and testes to surrounding structures may account for increased mobility and may predispose to the extravaginal type of torsion seen in neonates (Fig. 56-36). The scrotum is swollen and red with a firm, painless enlarged testicle, which is generally unilateral. Surgical salvage at birth is unlikely because the testis is already necrotic, but occurrence of extravaginal torsion after birth demands emergency surgery.[112] The ultrasound findings vary according to the duration of the torsion. In more recent torsion, the testis is heterogeneously enlarged with hypoechoic and hyperechoic areas. When the torsion is more chronic, the testis may be normal or slightly enlarged, with peripheral echogenicity corresponding to calcifications in the tunica albuginea. There is often associated scrotal skin thickening and hydroceles.[110,111] There is no Doppler signal in the spermatic cord or the testis. Power Doppler sonography, with its greater sensitivity to minimal flow. may be useful in evaluating the presence or absence of flow in these very small testes.[112] Contralateral compensatory

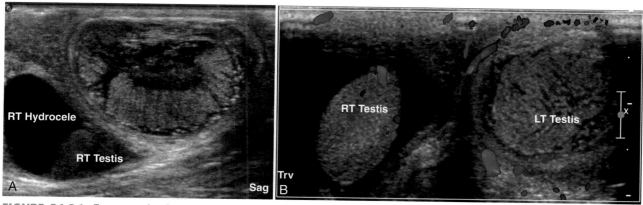

FIGURE 56-36. Extravaginal testicular torsion. Newborn with hard, nontender, left testicular mass. **A,** Sagittal sonogram of the scrotum reveals an enlarged, heterogenous left testis with dilated rete testes. There are multiple foci of bright echogenicity surrounding the left testis, suggesting an intrauterine torsion "missed" torsion. Note the normal right testis with surrounding anechoic hydrocele. **B,** Normal flow is shown in the normal-appearing right testis. However, a surrounding rim of color Doppler flow is seen around the avascular, swollen left testis.

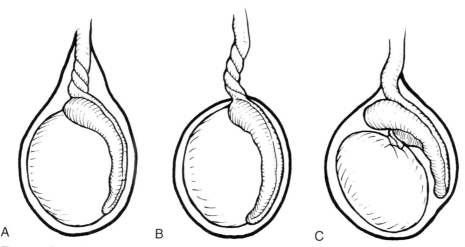

FIGURE 56-37. Types of testicular torsion. A, Intravaginal torsion above the epididymis. **B,** Extravaginal torsion. **C,** Torsion of the testis below the epididymis. *(From Leape LL. Torsion of the testis. In Welch KJ, Randolph JG, Ravitch MM, editors.* Pediatric surgery. *St Louis, 1986, Mosby.)*

hypertrophy may be seen.[113] Other conditions that mimic extravaginal torsion in patients who present with a swollen scrotum in the neonatal period include meconium peritonitis, intraperitoneal bleeding tracking through the patent processus vaginalis, and tumor.

With **intravaginal torsion** the tunica vaginalis completely surrounds the testis and inserts high on the spermatic cord, preventing fixation of the testis to the scrotum and allowing the testis to rotate freely on its vascular pedicle, known as the **bell-and-clapper deformity.**[114] Another, less frequently encountered type of intravaginal torsion is **torsion of the mesorchium,** the tissue attachment between the testis and epididymis[81,91,115] (Fig. 56-37). In this situation, the testis twists within the tunica vaginalis without torsion of the epididymis. **Torsion within the scrotal sac,** or intravaginal torsion, may occur in any age group but is seen more often in adolescents and young adults.[81] The boys present with sudden onset of scrotal or lower abdominal pain.

There is often a history of similar previous self-limited episodes, suggesting prior torsion and detorsion. Nausea and vomiting are more frequently seen in testicular torsion than in other causes of acute scrotum, with a positive predictive value of more than 96%. The boys may also have anorexia and low-grade fever. Physical examination is difficult because of severe tenderness. The affected hemiscrotum is swollen and erythematous with the affected testis often oriented transversely. The cremasteric reflex may be absent.[106] Most importantly, patients with suspected intravaginal torsion require emergency surgery to optimize testicular salvage. If it is clinically obvious that a patient has an acute torsion, emergency surgery should be done, even without imaging, because any delay in surgical treatment reduces the likelihood of testicular salvage. Some believe that closed manual detorsion may improve salvage rates and convert an emergent situation to an elective surgical procedure for future orchiopexy (Fig. 56-38); however, this is

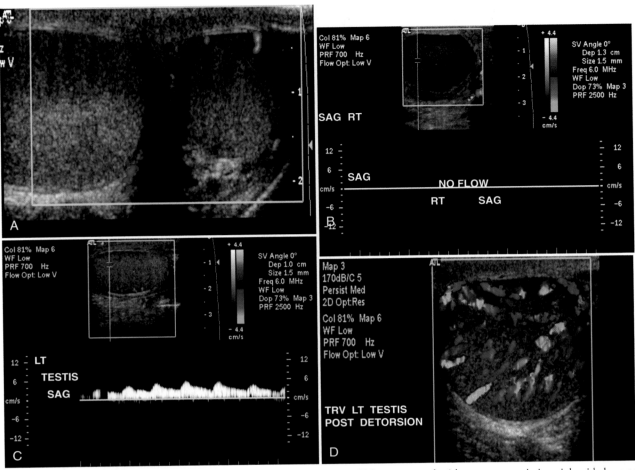

FIGURE 56-38. Acute testicular torsion. *A to C,* This 13-year-old boy presented with acute, excruciating right-sided scrotal pain. **A,** Transverse gray-scale image of both testes demonstrates enlargement of the avascular right testis. **B,** Absence of both color and pulsed Doppler flow is noted on this sagittal image of the right testis. **C,** Normal pulsed and color Doppler flow confirmed in asymptomatic, normal-appearing left testis. **D,** Teenage boy with acute left-sided testicular torsion. Closed manual detorsion of the left testis was done at diagnosis in the ultrasound suite. Color Doppler sonogram of the left testis obtained immediately after detorsion shows dramatic hyperemia throughout the left testis.

SONOGRAPHIC SIGNS OF TESTICULAR TORSION

TESTES
Normal early
Hypoechoic after 4 to 6 hours from edema
Heterogeneous after 24 hours from hemorrhage
  and infarction ("missed" torsion)

PERITESTICULAR
Hypoechoic epididymis
Reactive hydrocele
Skin thickening
Enlarged, twisted spermatic cord

---

controversial.[116,117] The best results are obtained in those who have immediate detorsion and fixation to the scrotal wall and orchiopexy of the contralateral testis.[91] There is virtually a 100% salvage rate when surgery is performed within 6 hours of the onset of symptoms; approximately 70% within 6 to 12 hours of symptoms; and only 20% if surgery is delayed for 12 to 24 hours after the onset of pain.[81,107] After 24 hours, the testis is virtually never salvageable. The sonographic features in testicular torsion depend on the duration and severity of the vascular compromise.

The gray-scale appearance of the torsed testis ranges from normal (early on) to enlarged and hypoechoic secondary to edema (usually after 4 to 6 hours) and then to a heterogeneous appearance with areas of increased echogenicity secondary to vascular congestion, hemorrhage, and ischemia (usually after 24 hours)[81,107] (Fig. 56-39). The latter appearance is also known as **"missed" torsion.** Surgical removal is recommended if the testis is clearly necrotic because if left in situ, the contralateral testis may be adversely affected because of a presumed antibody-induced immunologic process.[91] Other gray-scale findings in the presence of torsion include abnormal orientation of the testis within the scrotum (e.g., transverse lie) as well as abnormally thickened

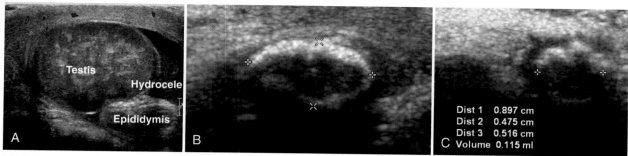

FIGURE 56-39. "Missed" testicular torsion. A, This 18-year-old male patient presented with a 2-day history of left scrotal pain and swelling. Sagittal sonogram demonstrates greatly enlarged (volume, 22.6 mL), hypoechoic, heterogenous left testis and epididymis with increased echogenicity and thickening of the tunica albuginea. There is no arterial or venous flow within the left testis or epididymis, although there is hyperemia around the testis. This constellation of findings is consistent with a "missed" testicular torsion of a subacute nature. A reactive hydrocele is seen around the left testis, which contains complicated fluid. **B** and **C,** Sagittal and transverse sonograms in 5-month-old male infant who presented with missed torsion of the left testis, with history since birth of a normal size right testis (not shown) and a small hard left testis. The tiny left testis (volume, 0.1 mL) is shown in the left hemiscrotum, with the tunica albuginea appearing brightly echoic and demonstrating partial shadowing of the ultrasound beam, consistent with delayed (missed) torsion, the insult presumably having occurred during intrauterine life.

paratesticular structures. The epididymis is usually enlarged because of vascular congestion and may be iso-, hypo-, or hyperechoic to the testis. There may be scrotal wall thickening and reactive hydrocele formation. Associated findings include an enlarged, hypoechoic epididymis, reactive hydrocele, skin thickening, and sometimes an enlarged, twisted spermatic cord.[108]

Color Flow Doppler Sonography in Testicular Torsion

To make the diagnosis of acute testicular torsion, the clinician must unequivocally demonstrate absent blood flow in the painful testis and normal blood flow in the contralateral asymptomatic testis. The color flow examination includes careful comparison of the symmetry of flow in both testes. The sensitivity of color flow Doppler for detecting acute testicular torsion in pediatric patients is 90% to 100%, whereas the sensitivity of scintigraphy approaches 100%.[116-118] In technically adequate studies performed on state-of-the-art equipment, the specificity of color flow imaging is almost 100%.[107] Again, importantly, presence of flow in the painful testis does not exclude the diagnosis of torsion.[119-121] In patients with incomplete or partial spermatic cord torsion (≤360 degrees), arterial flow may be demonstrated, although diminished in quantity compared with the asymptomatic testis.[121]

In cases of **detorsion,** color flow Doppler may demonstrate increased flow within the painful testis and paratesticular soft tissues caused by **reactive hyperemia.** This phenomenon may mimic the reactive hyperemia that occurs in inflammatory conditions such as epididymoorchitis.[121] The clinical findings should help to differentiate between torsion and inflammation. In the patient with acute scrotal pain that spontaneously resolves and in whom color Doppler imaging shows hyperemia,

detorsion is likely. Spontaneously or manually reduced torsion does not require emergency surgery, but these patients are at risk for subsequent torsion and can benefit from orchiopexy.[121,122] In cases of **late torsion** (>24 hours), color flow Doppler typically shows marked hyperemia of the scrotal wall and paratesticular soft tissues with absent testicular flow, analogous to the scintigraphic doughnut sign. Pulsed Doppler waveform analysis is unnecessary for the diagnosis of torsion. The sensitivity of pulsed Doppler for detecting torsion ranges from 67% to 100%. In small children, identification of flow can be difficult in normal testes because of the small size of the testicular arteries. In addition, it may be difficult to distinguish between paratesticular and intratesticular arterial pulsations, and thus scrotal wall hyperemia associated with torsion may be mistaken for normal flow.

With **chronic torsion** the testis will begin to atrophy after 14 days. During this phase, the testis may remain hypoechoic, or it may become hyperechoic if fibrosis or calcification develops.[121] The ipsilateral epididymis is often enlarged and echogenic, often with an accompanying hydrocele. Other causes of **testicular infarction** include trauma, polyarteritis nodosa, and subacute bacterial endocarditis. Extrinsic compression of the cord or testis leading to testicular infarction can occur with hernias,[107] hydroceles,[123,124] and epididymitis.

Acute epididymitis accounts for 28% to 47% of cases of acute scrotal pain in children and is more common in pubertal than prepubertal boys. It is thought that many cases of prepubertal epididymitis are actually cases of appendiceal torsion, especially in patients with a negative urine culture.[106] Patients with epididymitis typically have a more gradual onset of pain with fewer constitutional symptoms compared with patients with testicular or appendiceal torsion.[107,125]

On sonography, the inflamed epididymis may be focally or diffusely enlarged with coarse echoes. The

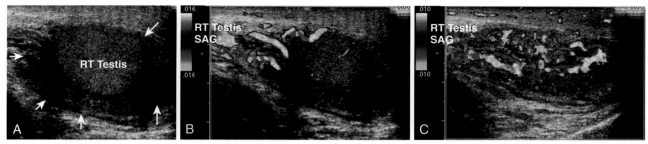

FIGURE 56-40. Acute epididymitis in 8-year-old boy with right scrotal pain. A, Gray-scale sagittal sonogram of the right testis shows a normal-appearing testis surrounded posterolaterally by a prominent, hypoechoic heterogeneous epididymis. **B,** Longitudinal color flow Doppler image of the scrotum reveals increased flow in the head of the epididymis with normal flow in the testis. **C,** Marked hypervascularity is noted throughout the body and tail of the epididymis. Skin thickening is noted on all three images.

overall echo pattern is usually decreased, but normal or increased echogenicity may be observed.[126] Associated orchitis is more often diffuse; when focal, however, it is usually close to the inflamed epididymis. The involved portion of the testis is usually hypoechoic and enlarged. On color flow Doppler imaging, the inflamed epididymis and testis are typically hyperemic (Fig. 56-40), although occasionally, normal flow may be seen in the involved organs.[14,125,126] Pulsed Doppler evaluation is not necessary to establish the diagnosis of acute epididymitis, but when performed, there is elevated diastolic flow in the epididymal arteries, a low-resistance waveform (RI <0.7 for epididymal arteries), and detectable venous flow.[126,127]

With **orchitis** there may also be abnormally decreased vascular resistance (RI <0.5) for testicular arteries. In testicular tumors, there may be hyperemia, but the RI is usually greater than 0.5. Therefore, **pulsed Doppler** may be useful to differentiate hyperemic tumor from testicular hyperemia.[125,127] Associated sonographic findings include reactive simple or complex hydrocele and skin thickening. Complications of severe epididymo-orchitis include abscess formation and ischemia leading to infarction. Testicular infarction secondary to severe epididymo-orchitis is indistinguishable from infarction secondary to torsion.

TORSION ON COLOR FLOW DOPPLER ULTRASOUND

Decreased or absent flow
Spontaneous detorsion causes normal or increased flow.
Incomplete torsion causes normal or decreased flow.

Because there is overlap in the gray-scale appearance of both testicular torsion and epididymo-orchitis, their differentiation depends on color flow Doppler imaging.[118,128] **Torsion** typically is characterized on Doppler imaging by decreased or absent flow within the involved testis. The classic appearance of **epididymitis and orchitis** is increased flow within the epididymis and the involved testis if orchitis is present.

EPIDIDYMITIS ON COLOR FLOW DOPPLER ULTRASOUND

Increased flow in epididymis
Increased flow in testes if also infected
Ischemia may cause decreased flow.

However, the overlap between the two may lead to false-positive or false-negative diagnoses. The hyperemia or normal color flow seen in testes with **spontaneous detorsion** may be confused for epididymitis.[125] **Incomplete torsion** of the testis may reveal normal or decreased color flow[108] (Fig. 56-41). **Ischemia** and **infarction** may also be seen with severe epididymitis, although this is usually less of a diagnostic dilemma because these patients also require surgery. Because Doppler imaging is limited in young patients with testes less than 1 mL, power and contrast agents may be helpful in distinguishing between torsed and normal testes.[116,118]

With **chronic epididymitis** the epididymis becomes enlarged and heterogeneous, and the testicular tunica becomes thickened, appearing as an echogenic hyperemic rim around the testis. Small calcifications may develop in the epididymis and the tunica albuginea. Ultimately, the testis may atrophy and become diffusely or focally hypoechoic.[91] **Isolated orchitis** is unusual and generally has a viral etiology. **Mumps orchitis** is generally seen in 30% of prepubertal boys infected with mumps. The testes are usually enlarged and hyperechoic bilaterally during the initial phase, resulting in testicular atrophy and reduced fertility.

Clinical findings should aid in the differentiation of detorsion and scrotal inflammation. Detorsion is more likely in the presence of spontaneously resolved acute scrotal pain and hyperemia on color Doppler imaging.

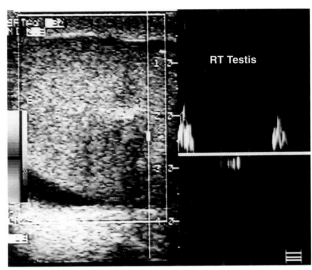

FIGURE 56-41. Incomplete testicular torsion in 14-year-old boy with 3 hours of right scrotal pain. Sagittal image of the right testis with color flow and pulsed wave Doppler sonograms demonstrates decreased intraparenchymal testicular flow on color flow Doppler imaging and an abnormally high-resistance pattern on pulsed Doppler imaging. (*Note:* The color seen on and above the mediastinum testis is artifactual.)

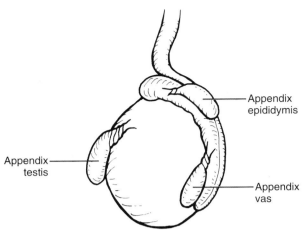

FIGURE 56-42. Testicular appendages. Appendix testis, appendix epididymis, and appendix vas (vas aberrans of Haller). (*From Leape LL. Torsion of the testis. In Welch KJ, Randolph JG, Ravitch MM, editors.* Pediatric surgery. *St Louis, 1986, Mosby.*)

Pulsed Doppler waveform analysis is not necessary to establish the diagnosis of epididymitis, but if used, it shows elevated diastolic flow in the epididymal arteries, a low-resistance waveform (RI <0.7 for epididymal arteries), and detectable venous flow. Abnormally decreased vascular resistance (RI <0.5 for testicular arteries) is also seen in orchitis.[127] When surgery is not done to remove an infarcted testis, the infarcted testis will begin to atrophy after 14 days. During this chronic phase, the testis may be hypoechoic, but when fibrosis and calcification develop, the gonad may become hyperechoic.

In younger boys, epididymitis is more often secondary to genitourinary abnormalities, such as ectopic ureter draining into the vas deferens or seminal vesicles. **Bladder outlet obstruction** (e.g., posterior urethral valve and dysfunctional voiding) can cause reflux of urine into the ejaculatory ducts and lead to epididymitis even if the urine is sterile.[119,129] Epididymitis may also follow **trauma.** With epididymitis, patients generally have a more gradual onset of symptoms and fewer constitutional symptoms than with torsion. There may be mild scrotal tenderness to severe scrotal pain and tenderness with fever and pyuria. In adolescent boys, most are secondary to **sexually transmitted organisms** (e.g., *C. trachomatis, N. gonorrhoeae*). In young boys, *Escherichia coli* is found in 10% to 25% of patients.[106,128]

Torsion of a testicular appendage, or appendix epididymis, is the most common cause of acute scrotal pain in prepubertal boys, with an incidence of 26% to 67% peaking between 6 and 12 years of age[80,130,131] (Fig. 56-42). Torsion of a testicular appendage may produce the same clinical signs and symptoms of testicular torsion

or epididymitis, but there is generally no nausea and vomiting. If the classic clinical finding of a small, firm, round, mobile, tender paratesticular mass, which often exhibits bluish discoloration visible through the skin **(blue-dot sign),** in the superior aspect of the scrotum is not found, then ultrasound is recommended to avoid unnecessary surgery.[91] The diagnostic sonographic appearance of a **torsed appendage** is that of a solid, ovoid mass with a variably sized hypoechoic center and hyperechoic rim adjacent to the superior aspects of a testis or epididymis with normal vascularity[131,132] (Fig. 56-43). Reactive hydroceles, scrotal skin thickening, testicular and epididymal enlargement, and hypoechogenicity may be seen as well.[132,133] In acute torsion of an appendix, the torsed appendix appears avascular and the epididymis hyperemic. In late torsion (>1 day), a zone of reactive hyperemia may surround the torsed appendage. Depending on the extent of the associated inflammatory process, the testis may have normal or increased vascularity.[82,132-135] The testicular appendages are embryologic remnants of blind-ending mesonephric tubules.[129] The **appendix testis** is attached to the tunica albuginea on the superior pole of the testis, and the **appendix epididymis** is located on the epididymal head. Both appendages are pedunculated and thus predisposed to torsion; 92% of males have an appendix testis, and 25% have an appendix epididymis.[91] Most torsed appendices atrophy, with resolution of symptoms with supportive care. Surgery is reserved for persistently symptomatic appendages. Eventually, infarcted appendages shrink in size, may calcify, and may break free to become **scrotoliths**.[82,130]

Trauma to the scrotum most often results from sporting injuries but may be seen in straddle or handlebar injuries, motor vehicle crashes, child abuse, or birth trauma. Trauma can cause a testicular hematoma, fracture, or rupture.[136,137] Testicular rupture is a surgical

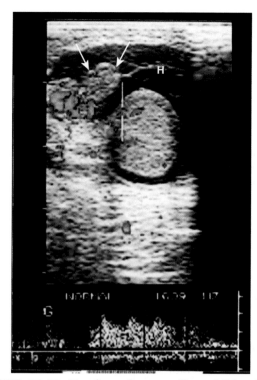

FIGURE 56-43. Torsion of appendix epididymis in 12-year-old boy with 10 hours of scrotal pain. Sagittal color flow and pulsed wave Doppler image of the scrotum reveals an enlarged avascular paratesticular mass *(arrows)* with increased flow in the adjacent epididymis. Normal testicular flow detected, excluding testicular torsion. A reactive, complex hydrocele *(H)* is seen. *(Case courtesy Heidi Patriquin, MD.)*

emergency. Improved salvage rates have been shown if surgery to repair a ruptured testis is performed within 72 hours of the traumatic event.[129] Sonographic findings of rupture (Fig. 56-44) include diffuse parenchymal heterogeneity with loss of a normal, smooth contour and disruption of the tunica albuginea, extrusion of seminiferous tubules, and nonvisualization of the testis. The presence of flow on color flow Doppler imaging in the traumatized testis is helpful in excluding testicular ischemia. **Testicular hematomas** appear as avascular masses, the echogenicity of which varies depending on the age of the hematoma.[82] Associated findings include scrotal hematomas, hematoceles, and wall thickening. Complications of testicular rupture include infarction, chronic pain, abscess, and infertility. Although ultrasound may aid in evaluating the traumatized scrotum, controversy surrounds its usefulness because some clinicians question its accuracy and recommend early surgical exploration even in the absence of testicular rupture.[136]

Acute **idiopathic scrotal edema** is a less common cause of scrotal edema that may involve one or both testes. This uncommon condition typically affects boys between 5 and 11 years of age, and patients present with scrotal swelling, erythema, and minimal pain (Fig. 56-45). Swelling may extend to the anterior abdominal wall and perineum. Sonographic findings include marked thickening of the scrotal wall, with normal testes and epididymides.[83,91,138] Color flow Doppler imaging may show normal or slightly increased flow to the scrotal wall

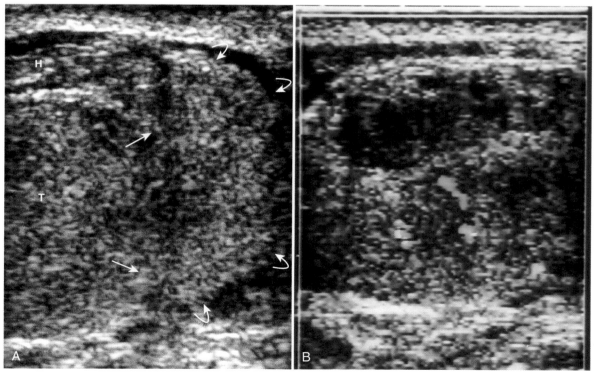

FIGURE 56-44. Testicular rupture in patient with scrotal pain after groin kick. A, Longitudinal view of the inferior aspect of the left testis shows disruption of the tunica albuginea *(straight arrows)* with extrusion of seminiferous tubules *(curved arrows)*. Associated hematocele *(H)* is present. *T,* Testis. **B,** Color flow Doppler image of the left testis reveals heterogeneity, representing contusion and hemorrhage within the testicular parenchyma. Intratesticular flow excludes infarction.

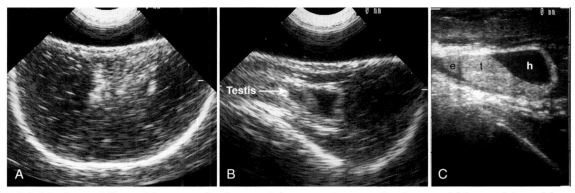

FIGURE 56-45. Acute idiopathic scrotal edema with normal testes in 4-year-old boy with sudden, painless, scrotal swelling. Transverse (**A**) sonogram of the scrotum and sagittal (**B** and **C**) images of the left hemiscrotum using a stepoff pad reveal marked scrotal swelling, normal right testis *(t)*, and epididymis *(e)* with an adjacent hydrocele *(h)*. The left testis and epididymis (not shown) were also normal.

with normal flow to the testes and epididymides.[114,138-140] Acute scrotal edema resolves spontaneously within several days without sequelae.

Scrotal or testicular involvement is estimated in 15% to 38% of patients with **Henoch-Schönlein purpura,** a vasculitis involving small vessels and affecting the skin, gastrointestinal tract, joints, and kidneys. Sonographic findings include diffuse swelling of the scrotum and contents with intact testicular flow, obviating the need for surgery in this entity, which usually resolves spontaneously and completely.[141] The echotexture of the testes is normal, but there is generally bilateral epididymal enlargement with a heterogeneous echo pattern, reactive hydrocele, and scrotal wall thickening.[139,140] Color flow Doppler imaging reveals hypervascularity, especially in the thickened scrotal wall and epididymis with normal intratesticular flow.[142] Careful examination for the classic purpuric rash over the buttocks, lower extremities, and perineum aids in diagnosis.[84]

Fournier's gangrene, also called "spontaneous gangrene," is a necrotizing infection of the scrotum that presents with erythema and edema of the scrotum and inferior penile surface.[143] There is obliterative endarteritis of the branches of the pudendal artery and scrotal wall edema. The testicular artery is not involved, and thus the testis and spermatic cord are unaffected and appear normal sonographically. The infection is caused by aerobes and anaerobes, including gas-forming organisms. Sonographically, the scrotal skin and soft tissues are thickened and heterogeneous, containing hypoechoic and hyperechoic areas that reflect the presence of edema and gas bubbles.

Scrotal swelling and pain may also be secondary to an intra-abdominal process, especially in neonates with a patent processus vaginalis. Various fluids, such as blood, chyle, pus, dialysis fluid, cerebrospinal fluid (CSF) from ventriculoperitoneal shunt, or other intraperitoneal fluids can drain into the scrotum. Blood from the abdomen can enter the scrotum through diapedesis into the tissue planes or through a patent processus vaginalis and can be the presenting signs in patients with

adrenal hemorrhage,[101] hepatic laceration, or delayed splenic rupture in a battered child. Scrotal swelling has been reported in association with inflammatory or infectious conditions, such as acute appendicitis, perforated appendicitis,[100] or Crohn's disease.[103] Another unusual cause for scrotal swelling is testicular vein thrombosis from a femoral venous line during cardiac catheterization. In the neonate with scrotal swelling and in older children with scrotal swelling of uncertain cause, abdominal sonography may help diagnose a primary abdominal event as the cause for secondary scrotal pathology.[101]

SCROTAL MASSES

Intratesticular Causes

Sonography plays an important role in the evaluation of scrotal masses by confirming the presence of a lesion, determining its site of origin, and characterizing its contents. Ultrasound has almost 100% sensitivity in detecting testicular tumors.[143,144] Ultrasound is able to distinguish intratesticular and extratesticular tumors in only 90% to 100% of cases.[95] This distinction is important because most intratesticular masses are malignant and most extratesticular masses are benign. Benign and malignant testicular tumors are the seventh most common neoplasm in children. **About 80% of testicular tumors are malignant.** In the pediatric age group, there are two peak incidences of testicular neoplasms: in children younger than 2½ years (60%) and in late adolescence (40%). The incidence of malignancy in a cryptorchid (abdominal) testis is increased by a factor of 30 to 50. Both **seminomas** (malignant) and **gonadoblastomas** (benign) often develop in dysplastic gonads associated with undescended testes, testicular feminization syndrome, male pseudohermaphroditism, and true hermaphroditism.[140]

Testicular tumors account for about 1% of all childhood neoplasms and for 2% of solid malignant tumors in boys.[145,146] **Primary testicular neoplasms** are divided

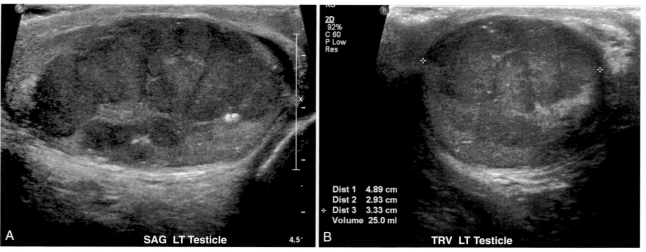

FIGURE 56-46. Seminoma in 18-year-old patient with painless left scrotal mass. A and **B,** Sagittal and transverse sonograms of the left testis demonstrate a testicular volume of 25 mL, with a lobulated, heterogeneous, relatively hypoechoic mass occupying most of the testis with a thin rim of normal testis and a few tiny clusters of calcification, as well as multiple, tiny, brightly echoic speckles both inside and outside the mass. The tiny speckles represent microlithiasis.

into those of germ cell and non–germ cell origin. In prepubertal children, 70% to 90% of primary testicular neoplasms are of germ cell origin, and most of these (66%-82%) are **endodermal sinus tumors** (yolk sac carcinomas). Yolk sac tumor is localized to the scrotum at presentation in most patients (≥80%).[145,146] The remaining 20% of patients present with lymphatic spread to regional and retroperitoneal lymph nodes or hematogenous spread to distant sites. Survival is about 70% or greater with disease restricted to testis.[145] Embryonal cell carcinomas, teratocarcinomas, and choriocarcinomas are more aggressive tumors and metastasize early through lymphatic and hematogenous routes. Endodermal sinus tumors occur primarily as a painless scrotal mass in infants 12 to 24 months of age. There may be an associated ipsilateral hydrocele (25%) or inguinal hernia (21%). The tumor may metastasize to the lungs, especially in older children, but retroperitoneal lymph node metastasis is rare. **Embryonal carcinoma** usually occurs in adolescence or young adulthood. It is highly malignant and usually spreads to retroperitoneal and mediastinal lymph nodes, with hematogenous metastases to the lung, liver, and brain.[140] Elevated serum alpha-fetoprotein levels are common in yolk sac and embryonal cell tumors, whereas elevated serum levels of β-hCG are seen most often with embryonal cell tumors and teratocarcinomas.[145,146]

The remaining germ cell tumors seen in adolescents and adults are benign teratomas, embryonal carcinomas, teratocarcinomas, and choriocarcinomas.[145] **Testicular teratoma** is the most common benign germ cell tumor of the testis in infants and young children. Teratomas are most often seen in children younger than 4 years. Patients with testicular neoplasms usually present with painless scrotal or testicular enlargement. Pain secondary to torsion or hemorrhage into the tumor is rare.[90] About 85% of benign teratomas contain well-differentiated elements from all three germ cell layers. There are poorly differentiated elements in approximately 15% of these tumors, but even so, the tumor usually has a benign course.[145] In pubertal patients, however, teratomas are often malignant and tend to behave more aggressively, necessitating orchiectomy.

Seminoma, the most common testicular tumor in adults, is rare in children, is most often associated with cryptorchidism, and when present, is usually in adolescents. Seminomas generally are uniformly hypoechoic masses, rarely containing areas of necrosis and hemorrhage[95,147] (Fig. 56-46). On the other hand, **teratomas** and **teratocarcinomas** are complex masses with hypoechoic areas from serous fluid and hyperechoic areas representing fat and calcifications.[95,146-148] The remaining germ cell tumors have nonspecific, variable appearances.[147] When the tunica is invaded by aggressive tumors, the testicular contour appears irregular. Testicular tumors are accompanied by reactive hydroceles in 20% to 25% of cases.[145,149] The scrotal skin is rarely thickened in the presence of tumors, and when observed in the presence of a mass, is generally indicative of an inflammatory process.

Doppler is useful in the evaluation of testicular tumors, with degree of vascularity dependent on tumor size. Larger tumors are usually hypervascular, but tumors less than 1.5 cm in diameter tend to be avascular or hypovascular.[150] One may demonstrate tumor vascular displacement or compression or a normal vascular course. In some cases a tumor may not be obvious on gray-scale imaging but is obvious with color flow Doppler imaging. RI determinations do not aid in diagnosis.[151]

The most common primary non–germ cell tumors of the testes are **Leydig cell and Sertoli cell tumors.**[152] These stromal tumors account for about 10% of

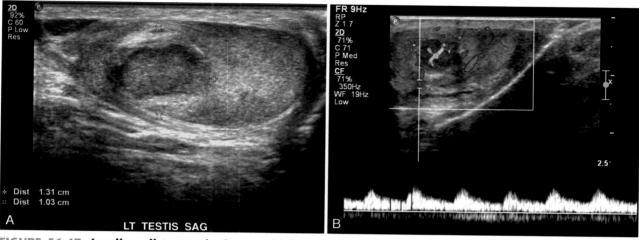

FIGURE 56-47. Leydig cell tumor in 8-year-old boy with 6-month history of precocious puberty. A, Gray-scale sagittal sonogram of left testis demonstrates a 1.3 × 1.0 × 1.0–cm hypoechoic, well-defined mass with peripheral areas of brighter echogenicity. **B,** Sonogram demonstrates arterial flow within the mass.

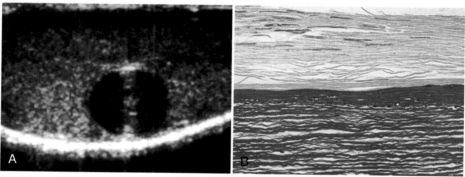

FIGURE 56-48. Epidermoid cyst. A, Sagittal, magnified sonogram shows a sharply defined lesion composed of multiple circular layers caused by epidermal tissue. **B,** Histologic specimen. *(Courtesy Janet Strife, MD, Cincinnati Children's Hospital.)*

testicular neoplasms and are usually hormone-secreting masses.[146] The Leydig cell tumors account for about 60% of the non–germ cell tumors and Sertoli cell tumors, about 40%. Leydig cell tumors are typically seen in patients age 3 to 6 years and produce testosterone, which results in precocious virilization. Patients with Sertoli cell tumors usually present with painless masses within the first year of life. Most are hormonally inactive, but some secrete estrogen that results in gynecomastia. Both these non–germ cell tumors are slow growing and virtually always benign in prepubertal patients.[140] These tumors are usually small, well-circumscribed hypoechoic lesions[95,147] (Fig. 56-47). In larger lesions, cystic spaces may develop secondary to hemorrhage and necrosis. Orchiectomy is curative, although tissue-sparing surgery is possible for Leydig cell tumors.

Another rare tumor is the **gonadoblastoma,** which is found in phenotypic females with streak gonads or in patients with a male karyotype and testes.[91,145,146] These tumors are usually small, well-circumscribed hypoechoic lesions.[95,147] In larger lesions, cystic spaces may develop secondary to hemorrhage and necrosis. These are

generally benign, solid, hypoechoic masses usually found at surgery to remove intra-abdominal dysplastic gonads.[145,153] Other benign testicular masses include hemangiomas, neurofibromas, lipomas, fibromas, epidermoids, and cysts.[145,154] There are also nonneoplastic lesions that resemble benign solid neoplasms, including cystic dysplasia, adrenal rests, hematomas, and Leydig cell hyperplasia.[155] The sonographic appearance is quite variable, but characteristically the **epidermoid cyst** is hypoechoic, well circumscribed, and contains internal echoes or an onion-skin lamellated appearance[156] (Fig. 56-48). **Adrenal rests** appear in the testes when fetal adrenal cortical cells migrate coincidentally with the gonadal tissue during embryologic development. Adrenal rests form tumorlike masses in response to increased levels of adrenocortical hormones, usually caused by **congenital adrenal hyperplasia** and **Cushing's syndrome.** At sonography, adrenal rests appear as round, variably sized, hypoechoic, solid intratesticular nodules, usually located near the mediastinum testis.[155,157,158] They are usually bilateral intratesticular nodules that may enlarge or regress over time.[158] The rests resemble

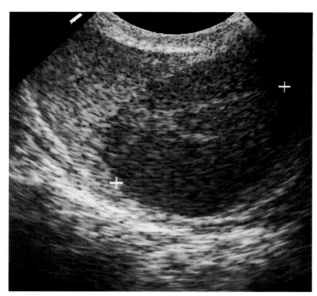

FIGURE 56-49. Leukemic infiltration of testis in 20-year-old man with acute lymphocytic leukemia relapse. Sagittal image reveals an enlarged right testis with an oval, hypoechoic mass *(calipers)* representing focal leukemic infiltration.

Leydig cell tumors histologically and sonographically, but the clinical setting of abnormal hormonal levels associated with hyperfunctioning adrenals usually clarifies the diagnosis.[159]

The testes are a well-known sanctuary site for **leukemia** and **lymphoma** (Fig. 56-49). Clinically silent testicular involvement may be seen in 25% of boys with newly diagnosed acute lymphoblastic leukemia. The testes may be enlarged, homogeneously hypoechoic, or contain focal hypoechoic masses.[160,161] Bilateral involvement is most common, and color Doppler flow is almost always increased, with a disorganized vascularity.[162] **Neuroblastoma, Wilms' tumor, Langerhans cell histiocytosis, retinoblastoma, rhabdomyosarcoma**, and **sinus histiocytosis** may metastasize to the testes.[163] The spread may be lymphatic or hematogenous, or by direct extension from contiguous tumor. The masses are painless and firm, or there may be diffuse testicular enlargement. The sonographic findings in all these testicular tumors are not specific. The involved testicle is usually enlarged with a globular or lobulated contour. Both primary and metastatic tumors may result in focal masses or diffuse involvement. The echogenicity ranges from hypoechoic to hyperechoic, and the parenchyma may be homogeneous or heterogeneous with areas of decreased echogenicity, reflecting hemorrhage or necrosis or areas of increased echogenicity reflecting calcification.[151,160,162,164,165] At times, the echogenicity will be normal.[162] Gray-scale abnormalities may be seen more frequently in the testes of older postpubertal patients with testicular tumors. This may reflect the histologically different tumors affecting different age groups.

Color flow Doppler imaging is helpful in the evaluation of pediatric testicular tumors. Disorganized hypervascular blood flow was seen in six (86%) of seven patients in a study of pediatric patients with testicular tumors by Luker and Siegel.[162] Although all the patients had testicular enlargement, the testicular echotexture in four (57%) of seven patients was normal; thus color flow Doppler was helpful in depicting the tumor in these patients. Hypervascularity with normal echogenicity may be seen in orchitis; however, orchitis without epididymitis is uncommon, especially in prepubertal children, and history helps in distinguishing the two entities because tumor frequently presents as an enlarged, nontender mass.[162] The management of testicular tumors in childhood has evolved during the last 20 years as a result of a multicenter retrospective survey that identified the preoperative and intraoperative criteria of nonmalignancy and analyzed the results of conservative management of a testicular mass. Valla[166] reported the findings of the Study Group in Pediatric Urology. A testicular tumor in children had a 50% chance of being benign, and ultrasound results were more conclusive than clinical criteria in limiting the preoperative diagnosis to teratoma, epidermoid cyst, and particularly, simple cyst. The group concluded that treatment selection according to clinical, biologic, radiologic, and frozen-section findings should allow appropriate decision making regarding testis-sparing surgery without additional oncologic risk, and with an esthetic, psychological, and functional benefit.[166] Patients with **solitary simple cysts**, which are uncommon testicular masses, present with painless scrotal enlargement.[167] These lesions are benign and thus may be followed with sonography. In infants, growth of the cyst may cause compression and replacement of testicular parenchyma. Thus, early conservative surgery with removal of the cyst and preservation of the adjacent parenchyma may be performed.[168] Simple enucleation suffices when sonography demonstrates that the cyst is undoubtedly simple. The cysts are anechoic masses with smooth walls, no nodular or solid elements, and increased sound transmission. They differ from epidermoid cysts and other cystic neoplasms that contain internal echoes.

Extratesticular Causes

Hydroceles are an abnormal collection of serous fluid in the scrotal sac and represent the most common cause of painless scrotal enlargement in children. Hydroceles may be congenital or acquired. In neonates and infants, virtually all hydroceles are congenital. As the testis descends into the scrotum, it becomes invested with a portion of peritoneum, the processus vaginalis. At birth, the processus vaginalis normally closes off proximally and forms the tunica vaginalis. A variable amount of peritoneal fluid may be trapped within the tunica vaginalis, forming a stable hydrocele in the neonate. This fluid is resorbed slowly during the first 18 months of life. If the processus vaginalis fails to close, an open communication exists between the peritoneal cavity and the scrotum. This can result in a scrotal hernia or a **communicating hydrocele** with a varying amount of fluid. Extension of the hydrocele into the pelvis can be seen in a communicating hydrocele. Surgical ligation is required to close the patent processus vaginalis.[169]

The usual sonographic appearance of a hydrocele is an anechoic, well-demarcated area with increased through-transmission (Fig. 56-50). In older children, hydroceles are generally acquired. The presence of echoes or septations in the fluid suggests a **reactive hydrocele** caused by infection, torsion, trauma, or tumor. Other collections, such as chronic hemorrhage or lymphoceles (associated with ipsilateral renal transplantation), may be seen and mistaken for a reactive hydrocele. These result from lymphatic disruption with leakage of lymph fluid into the tunica vaginalis or from direct extension of a periallograft lymphocele through the inguinal canal.[170] They appear on ultrasound as septated fluid collections surrounding the testes.

Hematoceles are collections of blood in the tunica vaginalis. Most are the result of surgery or trauma[169] but may also be secondary to bleeding disorders or malignant tumors.[171,172] They appear on sonography as fluid collections with low-level internal debris, septations, or fluid-debris levels. Scrotal wall thickening may be present with chronic hematoceles.

Scrotal hernia is a common mass in boys that is usually evident clinically. **Inguinal hernias** are almost always the result of a patent processus vaginalis (indirect hernia) into the scrotal sac. Hernias are more frequently right sided because the right processus vaginalis closes after the left. Sonography may demonstrate fluid- or air-containing bowel loops in the scrotum, normal testis, and epididymis, and an echogenic area representing herniated omentum[173] (Fig. 56-51). Lack of peristalsis within herniated bowel loops suggests ischemia. Ischemia and incarceration (nonreducibility of bowel loops) convert an elective procedure to emergent surgery. Extratesticular pathology, such as hematoceles, loculated hydroceles, scrotal abscesses, and urinomas, can mimic fluid-filled bowel loops, and herniated omentum can be confused for a primary scrotal mass. Thus, examination of the inguinal canal and the region of Hesselbach's triangle is recommended to evaluate for a hernia sac and exclude a primary scrotal pathology.

Other scrotal masses often identified in adolescent and postpubertal males are varicoceles, spermatoceles, and epididymal cysts.[173] **Varicoceles** represent dilated veins in the pampiniform plexus positioned posterior to the testis. The majority (85%-98%) are on the left side.[174] The presence of varicoceles in young boys is uncommon and may result from compression of the spermatic cord by tumor. Gray-scale sonographic evaluation reveals small, serpentine, anechoic structures that display flow on color Doppler imaging and venous waveforms on pulsed Doppler imaging. Augmentation of Doppler flow occurs with a Valsalva maneuver and upright positioning (Fig. 56-52). **Spermatoceles** occur in the epididymal head and consist of fluid, spermatozoa, and sediment. **Epididymal cysts** contain no spermatozoa and can occur in the epididymal head, body, or tail. Sonographic examination shows round structures with good through-transmission and well-defined back walls, which may contain debris (Fig. 56-53). They range in size from a few millimeters to several centimeters.[171] Other cystic lesions include **spermatic cord cysts** and **cysts of the tunica vaginalis**.

Paratesticular Tumors

Both benign and malignant paratesticular tumors are rare and generally involve the epididymis or spermatic

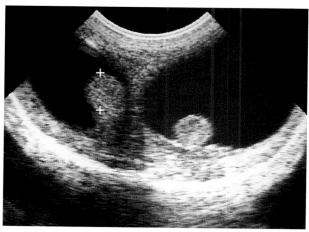

FIGURE 56-50. Bilateral hydroceles in newborn. Transverse view of the scrotum shows both testes outlined by large, anechoic fluid collections.

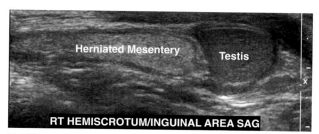

FIGURE 56-51. Inguinal hernia in baby with right inguinal mass. Sagittal sonogram of the right hemiscrotum/inguinal area demonstrates brightly echoic fatty mesentery extending from the peritoneal cavity into the right inguinal canal, abutting the right testis.

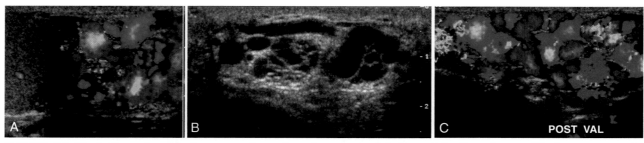

FIGURE 56-52. Left varicocele in postpubertal patient complaining of feeling "wormlike" structures in left side of scrotum. A, Transverse color Doppler sonogram of the left testis shows multiple areas filled with color in the paratesticular tissues lateral to the normal-appearing left testis. **B,** Sagittal scan of the paratesticular tissues demonstrates prominent, anechoic, tortuous, tubular structures. **C,** Exuberant color Doppler flow and enlargement of these paratesticular veins is seen after Valsalva maneuver.

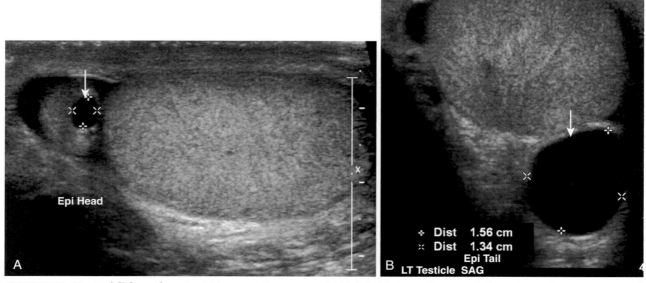

FIGURE 56-53. Epididymal cysts. This teenage boy presented with left-sided scrotal masses. **A,** Sagittal scan demonstrates a small cyst *(arrow)* in the head of the epididymis and a normal left testis. **B,** Transverse scan of the inferior aspect of the left testis demonstrates a larger cyst *(arrow)* in the adjacent tail of the epididymis. A small hydrocele is present.

cord. They may also arise in the appendix testis or testicular tunics. About 30% of spermatic cord tumors are malignant and generally are caused by **embryonal rhabdomyosarcoma**[145,175] (Fig. 56-54). This tumor usually appears as a rapidly growing, painless, intrascrotal mass in boys younger than 5 years. Up to 40% have retroperitoneal lymph node involvement at diagnosis.[175] Other malignant lesions include metastatic neuroblastoma, lymphoma, leiomyosarcoma, and fibrosarcoma.[164,176,177] They are usually well-defined, homogeneous or heterogeneous, hypoechoic solid masses. Benign paratesticular tumors include fibromas, hemangiomas, lipomas, leiomyomas, lymphangiomas, and neurofibromas. Both benign and malignant paratesticular tumors may appear hypoechoic or hyperechoic, and heterogeneity may be evident. Ultrasound cannot clearly distinguish benign from malignant lesions.[178] Increased vascularity on Doppler imaging in a paratesticular rhabdomyosarcoma may mimic that seen with epididymitis.[175] Thus, **clinical and sonographic follow-up should be performed in**

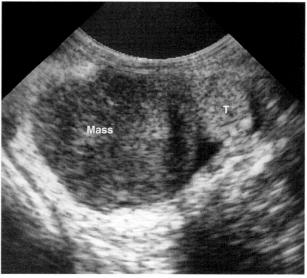

FIGURE 56-54. Paratesticular rhabdomyosarcoma. Large, solid mass was identified medial to left testis *(T)* with a small amount of free intrascrotal fluid in this 18-month-old boy.

cases of suspected epididymitis to ensure resolution of any mass because patients with rhabdomyosarcoma can present this way.[178]

The adenomatoid or fluid-filled masses, such as spermatoceles and cysts of the epididymis or tunica albuginea, are the most common benign paratesticular masses. **Adenomatoid tumors** are usually seen in the body of the epididymis and less often in the spermatic cord or testicular tunics. They are solid, well-circumscribed, variably echoic masses. **Epididymal cystadenomas** (associated with von Hippel–Lindau disease)[179] and **lymphangiomas** are septated cystic masses.[171,180] With **splenogonadal fusion**, a rare congenital anomaly, a mass of ectopic splenic tissue may be noted adjacent to the left testis.[181]

Focal calcifications from meconium periorchitis may appear as palpable scrotal masses (Fig. 56-55). These dystrophic calcifications result from in utero bowel perforation during the second or third trimester of gestation. Sterile intestinal contents (meconium) leak into the peritoneal cavity and enter the scrotum through a patent processus vaginalis and elicit a foreign body inflammatory response that results in focal calcifications. As with calcification elsewhere, these areas are echogenic with strong posterior shadows and may mimic a solid neoplasm, particularly a teratoma. Differentiation is based on the finding of additional intraperitoneal calcifications on sonography or plain film radiography of the abdomen.[178] Eventually, spontaneous regression of these calcifications occurs, and thus conservative management is recommended.[182] Differential diagnosis of scrotal or testicular calcifications in the pediatric patient includes teratoma, gonadoblastoma, Leydig cell tumor, testicular microlithiasis, calcified loose bodies, phleboliths, meconium peritonitis, calcified hematomas, and postinflammatory or infectious scrotal calculi.

Testicular microlithiasis is an asymptomatic condition that has a characteristic sonographic appearance and usually is discovered incidentally. It has been reported in normal patients, Down syndrome, cryptorchidism, and Klinefelter's syndrome. Testicular microlithiasis represents calcified debris within the seminiferous tubules. The cellular debris has a calcific core and surrounding lamellated collagen, resulting from a failure of Sertoli cell phagocytosis. On ultrasound there are tiny (1-3 mm), hyperechoic, most often nonshadowing foci[178] (Fig. 56-56). The number of echogenic foci within the testis can range from a few to many. Although a benign disease, testicular microlithiasis is associated with conditions that have an increased risk of malignancy, such as cryptorchidism, infertility, and testicular atrophy. In adults, Backus et al.[183] reported in a retrospective study the presence of germ cell neoplasms in 17 (40%) of 42 patients with microlithiasis. Until the association of testicular microlithiasis is better understood, clinical and sonographic monitoring of these patients is advised.

LOWER URINARY TRACT

Congenital Anomalies

Duplication anomalies of the collecting systems and ureters are the most common congenital anomalies of the urinary tract. In **complete ureteral duplication** the lower ureter inserts orthotopically into the trigone, often resulting in vesicoureteral reflux. The upper-pole ureter usually inserts ectopically in the bladder (at the bladder neck) or in the trigone (inferomedial to the normal location). It can also insert into the urethra, vagina, or uterus in girls, resulting in urinary dribbling. In boys the **ectopic ureter** can insert in the proximal urethra, seminal vesicle, vas deferens, or ejaculatory duct. Urinary incontinence is not a presenting symptom in boys because the ectopic insertion is always proximal to the external

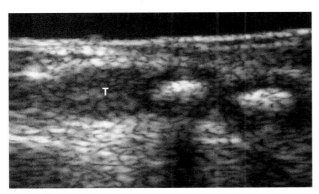

FIGURE 56-55. Meconium periorchitis in 5-year-old boy with painless scrotal masses. Sagittal view of the left hemiscrotum using a stepoff pad shows two well-defined, oval, brightly echogenic masses with hypoechoic halos and acoustic shadows, which lie inferior to the normal left testis *(T)*. *(From Mene M, Rosenberg HK, Ginsberg PC. Meconium periorchitis presenting as scrotal nodules in a 5-year-old boy. J Ultrasound Med 1994;13:491-494.)*

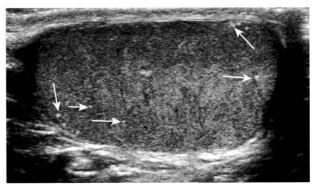

FIGURE 56-56. Testicular microlithiasis. Right testis in 18-year-old patient with seminoma shown in Figure 56-46. Multiple, tiny, hyperechoic foci are seen scattered throughout the right testis, some of which are indicated by very small arrows.

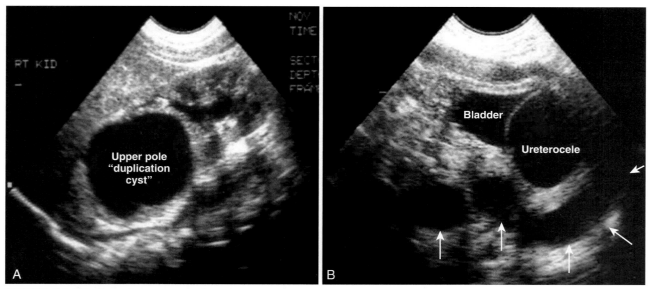

FIGURE 56-57. Ectopic ureterocele. Obstructed upper-pole moiety of a duplex kidney in a young baby with urinary tract infection. **A,** Sagittal sonogram of right kidney showing upper-pole "duplication cyst" and mild dilation of the intrarenal collecting system in the lower pole surrounded by normal parenchyma. **B,** Sagittal view of the pelvis demonstrates a large, ectopic ureterocele within the urinary bladder, which is in continuity with the greatly dilated, tortuous, upper-pole ureter *(arrows).*

sphincter. Duplication anomalies are often asymptomatic; **urinary tract infection** (UTI) is the most common initial presentation. The upper-pole moiety often becomes obstructed as a result of an **ectopic ureterocele.** Sonography demonstrates a dilated upper-pole collecting system and ureter that ends distally as a well-defined, thin-walled cystic protuberance into the bladder base (Fig. 56-57). The lower-pole system is often dilated secondary to reflux.[184] Less frequently, the lower-pole moiety may be dilated from obstruction of the ureteral orifice by the adjacent ectopic ureterocele or because of vesicoureteral reflux. About 10% to 20% of ectopic ureters are associated with a single collecting system (Fig. 56-58). The renal parenchyma associated with an ectopic ureter may be dysplastic (containing echogenic parenchyma, loss of corticomedullary junction, and variably sized cysts).

Sonography is well suited for screening siblings of patients with **vesicoureteral reflux** who are at greater risk of having reflux than the general population. Giel et al.[185] showed that given the seemingly innocuous nature of vesicoureteral reflux in older asymptomatic siblings of known patients with reflux, observation alone in this group is an acceptable form of management. Ultrasound can be used as a reliable alternative to voiding cystourethrography (VCUG) to screen these patients when the parent or physician is concerned about a particular child.

Posterior urethral valves are a common cause of urinary tract obstruction. Signs and symptoms at presentation include palpable flank masses caused by hydronephrosis or urinoma, poor urine stream, UTI, and failure to thrive. On sonography, the bladder has a thick, trabeculated wall, and the posterior urethra is dilated (Fig. 56-59). There may be marked hydronephrosis

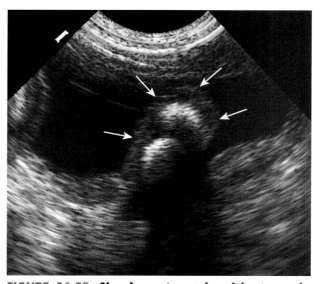

FIGURE 56-58. Simple ureterocele with stones in 7-year-old child with recent mild trauma. Sagittal view of the left side of the bladder demonstrates a simple ureterocele *(arrows)* protruding into the bladder lumen, containing two brightly echogenic, shadowing calculi.

CAUSES OF BLADDER OUTLET OBSTRUCTION

Posterior urethral valves
Prune-belly syndrome
Anterior urethral valves
Urethral duplication
Congenital urethral stricture
Anterior urethral diverticulum
Posterior urethral polyp

with dilated, tortuous ureters secondary to vesicoureteral reflux. Occasionally, the reflux is unilateral, resulting in ipsilateral hydroureteronephrosis. The renal parenchymal echogenicity may be abnormally increased as a result of long-standing reflux or obstructive nephropathy. Many infants with posterior urethral valves have secondary renal dysplasia, manifested on sonography as brightly

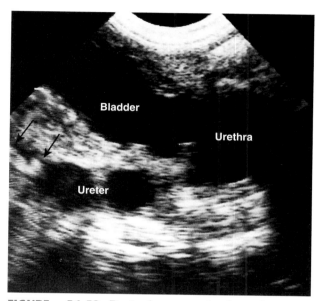

FIGURE 56-59. Posterior urethral valves in newborn boy. Midline sagittal scan shows irregularly thickened bladder wall (caused by obstruction), massively dilated posterior urethra, and moderately dilated tortuous distal ureter. Arrows show the serosal surface of the bladder wall. *(From Rosenberg HK. Sonography of pediatric urinary tract abnormalities. Part I. Am Urol Assoc Weekly Update Series 1986;35:1-8.)*

echogenic kidneys usually devoid of corticomedullary differentiation and often containing tiny cysts.[186] The appearance of the renal parenchyma has predictive value in infants with posterior urethral valves in regard to potential renal function.[187]

The **prune-belly syndrome** (abdominal muscle deficiency or Eagle-Barrett syndrome) is another common cause of urinary tract obstruction in infant boys. The syndrome is composed of a triad of absent abdominal musculature, bilateral hydroureteronephrosis, and cryptorchidism. There are three forms of urinary tract abnormality. In the most severe form, urethral atresia and renal dysplasia are present; these children have a very poor prognosis and generally die in infancy. Associated congenital anomalies are frequent and include intestinal malrotation or atresia, imperforate anus, Hirschsprung's disease, congenital heart defects, skeletal anomalies, and cystic adenomatoid malformation of the lung. In the less severe form of urinary tract abnormality, the bladder is large and atonic, and there is bilateral hydroureteronephrosis, impaired renal function, and no urethral obstruction. The changes are thought to be caused by a neurogenic dysfunction rather than a mechanical obstruction. There are usually no associated congenital anomalies, and these infants have a better prognosis.[188] In the mildest type of prune-belly syndrome, the urinary tract is only mildly affected.

Other uncommon forms of bladder outlet obstruction include **anterior urethral valves, urethral duplication, congenital urethral stricture, anterior urethral diverticulum, posterior urethral polyp**[189] (Fig. 56-60) and **stones**[190] (Fig. 56-61). Rarely, a giant bladder diverticulum many descend below the bladder neck and lead to

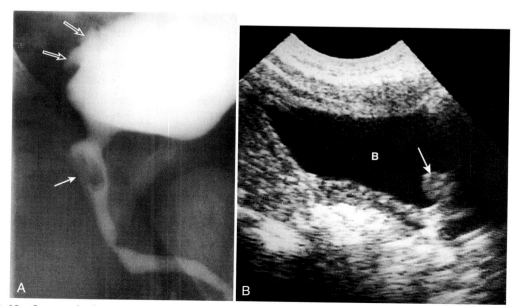

FIGURE 56-60. Congenital urethral polyp that caused prenatal hydroureteronephrosis in newborn boy.
A, Voiding cystourethrography (VCUG) demonstrates an oval, polypoid mass in the posterior urethra *(solid arrow)* and posterior bladder wall thickening *(open arrows).* **B,** Sagittal sonogram of the bladder *(B)* 4 months later shows a solid polypoid mass *(arrow)* protruding from the bladder neck into the bladder lumen. *(From Caro PA, Rosenberg HK, Snyder HM. Congenital urethral polyp. AJR Am J Roentgenol 1986;147:1041-1042.)*

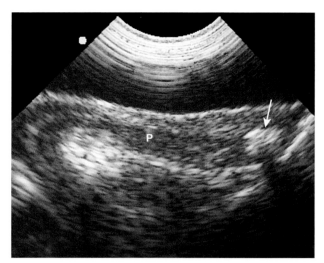

FIGURE 56-61. Urethral stone in fossa navicularis. Sagittal image of penis *(P)* using stepoff pad reveals a 7-mm calculus *(arrow)* in the distal urethra of this 6-year-old boy with gross hematuria, dysuria, and suprapubic pain.

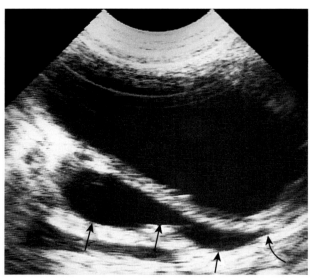

FIGURE 56-62. Congenital ureterovesical junction (UVJ) obstruction in infant with urinary tract infection. Sagittal sonogram of the bladder shows the dilated ureter *(straight arrows)*, which tapers inferiorly at the UVJ *(curved arrow)*.

bladder outlet obstruction.[191] VCUG, in addition to sonography, is usually necessary to identify these urethral obstructions.

The Ureter

The ureters cannot be visualized on ultrasound unless they are dilated. Real-time sonography can sometimes differentiate between mechanical obstruction and vesicoureteral reflux. In **ureterovesical junction obstruction** the distal ureter is dilated but may taper, making it difficult to visualize at the level of the bladder trigone, and at times, ureteral peristalsis is absent (Fig. 56-62). Sonography is useful for identification of a stone as the cause of distal ureteral obstruction (Fig. 56-63). With **vesicoureteral reflux** the ureterovesical junction is often gaping or patulous, and active peristalsis is demonstrated[86,192] (Fig. 56-64). In patients with a dilated tubular structure posterior to the bladder, duplex and color flow Doppler ultrasound can be used to differentiate a ureter, artery, or vein. In addition, color flow Doppler sonography allows reliable visualization of the **ureteric jet phenomenon.** Marshall et al.[193] found that the distance of the ureteric orifice from the midline of the bladder correlated with vesicoureteric reflux when the mean distance was 10.25 mm ± 2.40 SD. Jequier et al.[194] used color flow Doppler imaging to show that (1) the duration of the ureteric jet varied from 0.4 to 7.5 seconds and depended largely on fluid intake, (2) the direction of the normal jet was anteromedial and upward, (3) jets from refluxing ureters could appear normal, and (4) Doppler analyses of the ureteric jet do not allow either the diagnosis or the exclusion of vesicoureteral reflux.[194] Berrocal et al.[195] demonstrated that cystosonography with SH U-508A appears comparable to VCUG in the depiction of vesicoureteral reflux. Darge et al.[196]

showed that the number of VCUGs was significantly reduced as a result of implementation of voiding urosonography using the intravesical application of the ultrasound contrast agent Levovist.

Neurogenic or Dysfunctional Bladder

Urinary tract sonography has become a routine screening procedure in children with neurogenic or dysfunctional bladders. The most common cause of neurogenic bladder in children is **myelomeningocele.** Other acquired forms of dysfunctional bladder include **traumatic paraplegia, cerebral palsy, spinal cord tumor,** and **encephalitis** or **transverse myelitis.** These children have a higher incidence of UTI, bladder stones, and reflux. Sonography of a neurogenic bladder demonstrates an irregularly thickened, trabeculated bladder wall, often with multiple diverticula (Fig. 56-65). Echogenic material within the bladder lumen may represent complications of infection, hemorrhage, stone formation, or foreign body insertion via the urethra.[197] Ultrasound can also be used to assess the patient's ability to empty the bladder spontaneously or after Credé maneuver or catheterization. Residual urine volumes can be estimated as described earlier.[198]

Urachal anomalies can be identified on ultrasound when there is persistence of the embryonic tract between the dome of the bladder and umbilicus. Cacciarelli et al.[199] identified a normal urachal remnant in 62% of bladder sonograms in children.[10,200] A normal urachal remnant appears as a small (6.2 mm depth × 13 mm length × 11.8 mm width), elliptical, hypoechoic structure located posterior to the rectus abdominis muscle

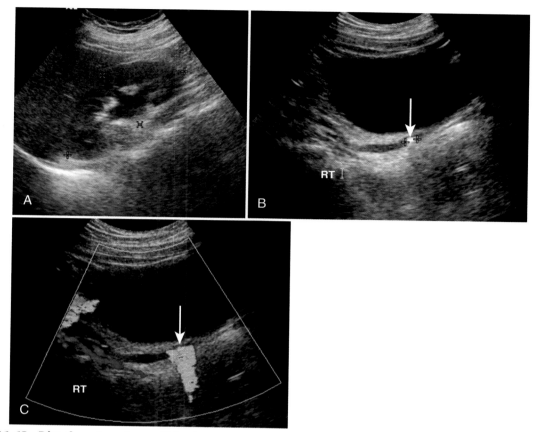

FIGURE 56-63. Distal ureter stone. This 14-year-old patient presented with hematuria and right flank pain that radiated to the right groin. **A,** Mild right-sided hydronephrosis. **B,** Small stone *(arrow)* is lodged in the mildly dilated distal ureter, with acoustic shadowing of the ultrasound beam. **C,** Color Doppler sonogram shows "twinkle" artifact, confirming the presence of a stone.

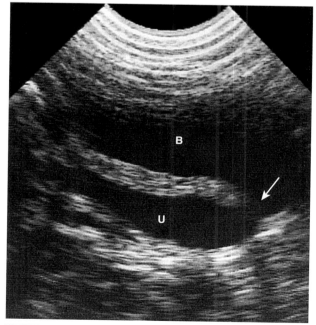

FIGURE 56-64. Vesicoureteral reflux. Moderately distended ureter *(U)* can be traced to patulous ureterovesical junction *(arrow); B,* bladder. *(From Sherman NH, Boyle GK, Rosenberg HK. Sonography in the neonate. Ultrasound Q 1988;6:91-150.)*

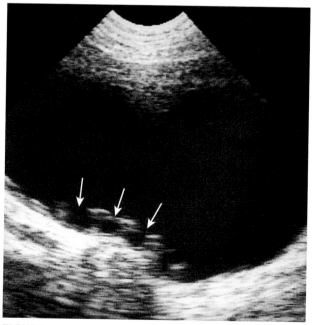

FIGURE 56-65. Neurogenic bladder in 14-year-old boy with spina bifida. Sagittal view of an overdistended bladder demonstrates multiple small diverticula *(arrows). (From Sherman NH, Rosenberg HK. Pediatric pelvic sonography. In Fisher MR, Kricun ME, editors. Imaging of the pelvis. Rockville, Md, 1989, Aspen.)*

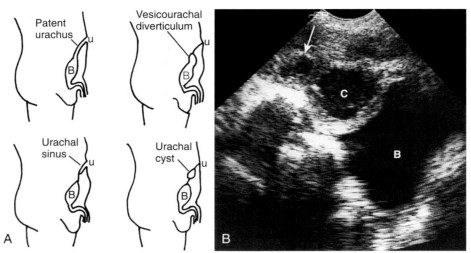

FIGURE 56-66. Urachal abnormalities. A, Patent urachus (urachal lumen communicates with both umbilicus and bladder); **vesicourachal diverticulum** (urachal lumen communicates only with bladder); **urachal sinus** (urachal lumen communicates only with umbilicus); and **urachal cyst** (does not communicate with bladder or umbilicus). **B, Infected urachal cyst.** This 6-year-old boy presented with lower abdominal pain, fever, intermittent diarrhea, polyuria, and dysuria. Sagittal midline scan of pelvis shows thick-walled cystic lesion *(C)* above the bladder dome *(B)* containing internal echoes caused by infectious debris. Smaller, hypoechoic area more superior *(arrow)* was caused by necrotic adenopathy. (*A from Boyle G, Rosenberg HK, O'Neill J: An unusual presentation of an infected urachal cyst: review of urachal anomalies. Clin Pediatr 1988;27:130-134.*)

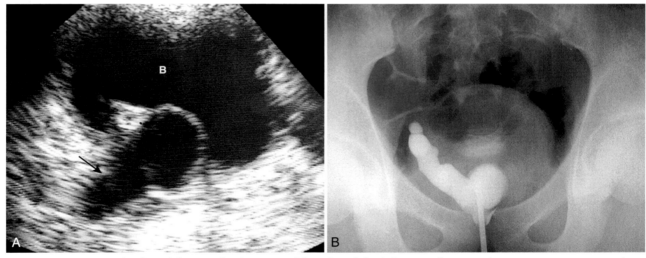

FIGURE 56-67. Seminal vesicle cyst in 17-year-old male with right renal agenesis. A, Transverse sonogram shows tubular structure *(arrow)* with a rounded portion projected over bladder *(B)*. **B,** Intraoperative cystoscopic retrograde injection of aqueous contrast material confirms the presence of a seminal vesicle cyst.

and on the midanterosuperior surface of the distended bladder. Involution of the urachus is not complete at birth and can be followed up on sonography during the first months of life. Thus, young infants with a discharging umbilicus or an infected urachus may benefit from a conservative approach using serial sonography as a guide because sonography can document spontaneous involution as well as abnormal development.[10] There are four types of urachal anomalies: **patent urachus** (completely open urachal lumen associated with urinary drainage from umbilicus), **urachal sinus** (opening to umbilicus), **urachal diverticulum** (opening to bladder),

and **urachal cyst** (urachus obliterated at both ends with extraperitoneal position of isolated cyst)[201] (Fig. 56-66, *A*). Two sonographic patterns have been described in urachal anomalies: (1) a cystic mass, often with internal echoes or septations caused by infection, and (2) an echogenic, thickened, tubular sinus tract (8-15 mm in diameter)[201] (Fig. 56-66, *B*).

Other anomalies of the lower urinary tract that can be identified on ultrasound include **ectopic pelvic kidney, seminal vesicle cysts** (Fig. 56-67), **müllerian duct** (prostatic utricle) **cysts** (Fig. 56-68), and congenital or acquired **bladder diverticula**[202] (Fig. 56-69).

Infection

Urinary tract infections are common in children, especially girls, and are usually the result of cystitis. Clinically, these children may present with urinary frequency, incontinence, dysuria, and/or hematuria.[203,204] The UTI is usually bacterial. **Hemorrhagic cystitis** can develop secondary to a viral infection (Fig. 56-70), chemotherapy with cyclophosphamide, or indwelling catheters. **Granulomatous cystitis** in a patient with chronic granulomatous disease of childhood can be detected on ultrasound. On sonography, the bladder may appear normal in mild cases of cystitis. More specific signs of cystitis are diffuse or focal bladder wall thickening and irregularity (Fig. 56-71). Echogenic material in the bladder lumen may represent purulent or hemorrhagic urine. **Bladder calculi** are more common with *Proteus* or *Pseudomonas*

infections. With **cystitis cystica** or **cystitis glandularis**, rounded, isoechoic or hypoechoic, polypoid lesions may protrude into the lumen, mimicking a bladder tumor (Fig. 56-72, *A* and *B*). Rosenberg et al.[205] reported children with hematuria, dysuria, and frequency plus cystographic or sonographic demonstration of a bladder with reduced capacity and circumferential wall thickening, or sonographic findings of isoechoic bladder wall thickening (focal, multifocal, or circumferential distribution), intact mucosa, and bullous lesions. These findings should strongly suggest inflammation and not malignancy. In addition, changing mass contour and thickness with increasing bladder filling are particularly suggestive of inflammatory thickening (Fig. 56-72, *C-E*). When an

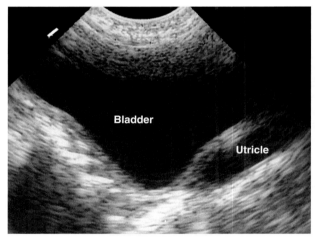

FIGURE 56-68. Utricle in 4-year-old true hermaphrodite. This child was reared as a boy after external genitalia reconstruction. Sagittal view of the bladder reveals a fluid-filled, tubular utricle posterior to the bladder base.

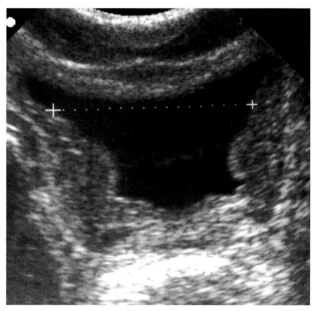

FIGURE 56-70. Viral cystitis in 11-year-old boy with frequency, hematuria, and dysuria. Transverse sonogram shows lobulated thickening *(cursors)* of the bladder wall.

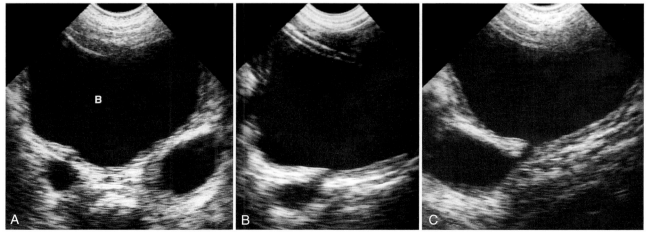

FIGURE 56-69. Bladder diverticula in 12-year-old boy. A, Transverse sonogram of the bladder *(B)* shows two oval structures inferolateral to the bladder base, which could be distal ureters. Sagittal views of right side **(B)** and left side **(C)** of the bladder demonstrate a neck from each connecting the diverticula to the bladder.

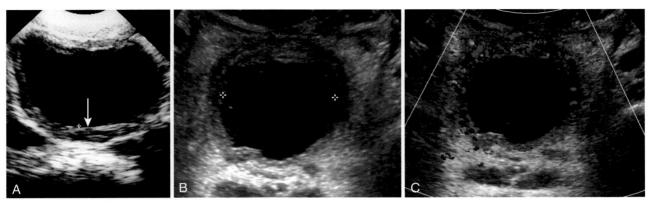

FIGURE 56-71. Cystitis. A, Chronic bacterial cystitis. Transverse sonogram demonstrates bladder wall thickening *(arrow)*. **B** and **C,** Cyclophosphamide (Cytoxan) cystitis in child after bone marrow transplant. The bladder wall is thickened and hyperemic. Some debris and septations are noted within the bladder lumen.

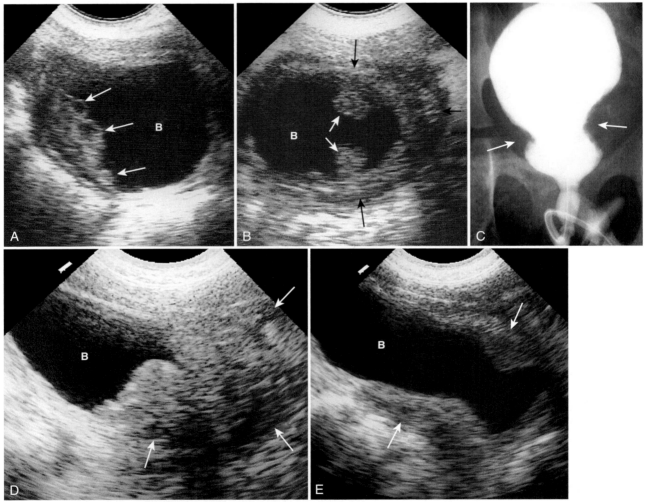

FIGURE 56-72. Bullous, benign cystitis from cytomegalovirus after 24 hours of dysuria and hematuria. A, Sagittal sonogram of the bladder *(B)*. Complex mass containing multiple, well-circumscribed, hypoechoic and anechoic, polypoid lesions *(arrows)* arising from the dome and projecting into the lumen. **B, Hemorrhagic cystitis.** Transverse view of the bladder *(B)* shows asymmetrical bladder wall thickening involving left half of bladder *(black arrows)* with polypoid-like protrusions of thickened wall *(small white arrows)* into bladder lumen. **C,** Frontal image from a voiding cystourethrography (VCUG) shows concentric irregular narrowing of the distal third of the bladder above the bladder base *(arrows)*. **D,** Sagittal sonogram with partial bladder *(B)* filling shows tremendous masslike thickening of the posteroinferior bladder walls *(arrows)*. **E,** Sagittal sonogram obtained after further bladder *(B)* filling shows a decrease in the size of the mass *(arrows)* with increased bladder distention. **(B** and **E** *from Rosenberg HK, Zerin JM, Eggli KD, et al. Benign cystitis in children mimicking rhabdomyosarcoma. J Ultrasound Med 1994;13:921-932.)*

inflammatory lesion is suspected, follow-up imaging should be performed in 2 weeks, which will preclude biopsy if normal.[205]

Neoplasm

Rhabdomyosarcoma is the most common tumor of the lower urinary tract in children, with 21% arising from the genitourinary tract. The most frequent primary site is the bladder trigone or prostate. Less frequent sites of origin are the seminal vesicles, spermatic cord, vagina, uterus, vulva, pelvic musculature, urachus, and paratesticular area.[39,206] There is a slight male predominance of 1.6:1. The peak incidence occurs at 3 to 4 years of age; a second, smaller peak is seen in adolescence. The most common rhabdomyosarcoma cell type is the embryonal form, of which **sarcoma botryoides** is a subtype. The alveolar form is next in frequency; **undifferentiated** and **pleomorphic types** are uncommon. Tumors arising from the bladder, prostate, or both usually present early with symptoms from urinary tract obstruction and hematuria. Rhabdomyosarcoma has been reported to be associated with neurofibromatosis, fetal alcohol syndrome, and basal cell nevus syndrome.

On sonographic examination, rhabdomyosarcoma appears as a homogeneous, solid mass with an echotexture similar to muscle. Anechoic spaces caused by necrosis and hemorrhage are occasionally seen (Fig. 56-73). Calcification is uncommon. Bladder lesions originate in the submucosa, infiltrate the bladder wall, and produce polypoid projections into the lumen (sarcoma botryoides). Tumors arising in the prostate cause concentric or asymmetrical enlargement of the prostate and often infiltrate the bladder neck, posterior urethra, and perirectal tissues (Fig. 56-74). Regional and retroperitoneal lymph node metastases are common. Rarely, leiomyosarcoma may arise from the bladder wall and is more likely to have calcifications (Fig. 56-75).

Benign tumors of the lower urinary tract are extremely rare and include **transitional cell papilloma** (Fig. 56-76), **neurofibroma, fibroma, hemangioma,** and **leiomyoma.**[207,208] Neurofibromatosis can be invasive, with diffuse involvement of the pelvic organs.[209] **Pheochromocytoma** of the bladder is a rare tumor that

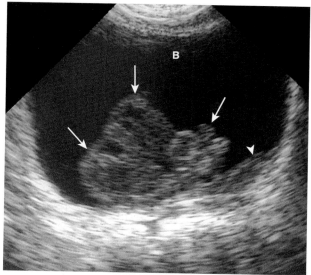

FIGURE 56-73. Rhabdomyosarcoma of bladder wall. Large, complex, polypoid-like mass *(arrows)* arises from base of the bladder *(B)* in this 9-year-old boy with painless hematuria. Asymmetrical bladder wall thickening was noted posterolaterally on patient's left *(arrowhead).*

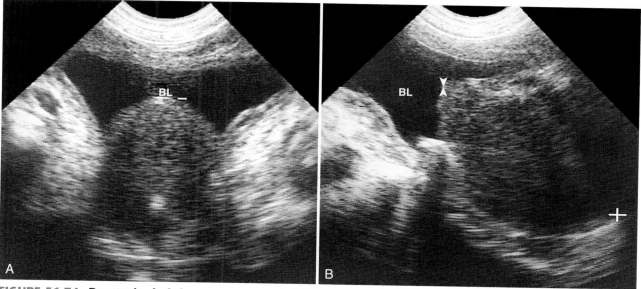

FIGURE 56-74. Prostatic rhabdomyosarcoma with bladder invasion in 11-month-old boy with pelvic pain. **A** and **B,** Transverse and sagittal sonograms of the pelvis demonstrate a large, solid mass arising inferior to the bladder neck *(BL)* invading the bladder base.

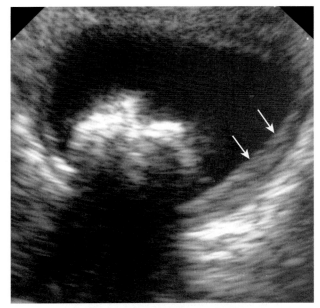

FIGURE 56-75. Leiomyosarcoma of bladder. Transverse scan of the bladder in a 14-year-old girl with bilateral retinoblastoma and severe dysuria shows a central, brightly echogenic, lobulated shadowing mass posteriorly and thickening of the left lateral wall of the bladder (arrows).

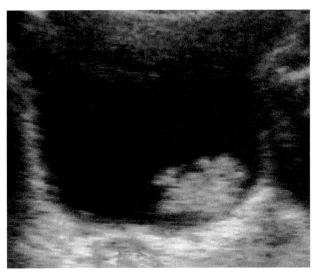

FIGURE 56-76. Transitional cell papilloma of bladder. Transverse sonogram of the bladder in a 7-year-old boy with hematuria reveals a polypoid, solid mass arising from the left posterior bladder wall.

probably arises in the paraganglia of the visceral (autonomic) nervous system and is located submucosally either in the dome or in the posterior wall close to the trigone. In children, 2% of bladder pheochromocytomas are malignant. Pheochromocytomas can be seen in the context of familial syndromes or diseases, which include neurofibromatosis, von Hippel–Lindau disease, Sturge-Weber syndrome, tuberous sclerosis, multiple endocrine neoplasia type A (medullary thyroid carcinoma and hyperparathyroidism), and multiple endocrine neoplasia

type IIB (medullary thyroid carcinoma, mucosal neuromas, and pheochromocytoma). Pheochromocytomas of the bladder may cause headache, blurred vision, diaphoresis, palpitations, intermittent hypertension (70%), and hematuria (6%). Any of these symptoms may be seen with micturition.[210] Benign polyps in the male urethra can arise from a stalk near the verumontanum and cause urinary tract obstruction.

Trauma

Trauma to the lower urinary tract in children is most often caused by blunt trauma. Foreign bodies and complications of surgery are less frequent causes. The bladder in children is in a more intra-abdominal position than in adults, and therefore bladder rupture is usually intraperitoneal. **Spontaneous bladder rupture** is rare in children and is seen primarily in neonates with urinary ascites secondary to urethral obstruction or neurogenic bladder. Preexisting abnormalities of the vesical wall, such as tumors, stones, tuberculosis, diverticula, and surgical scars, can predispose a child to spontaneous rupture of the bladder.[211] Sonography can demonstrate urinary ascites in cases of intraperitoneal rupture or a loculated fluid collection (**urinoma**) in the retropubic or perivesical space in extraperitoneal rupture.

Postoperative Bladder

Sonography has assumed an important role in the evaluation of the postoperative bladder. **Ureteral reimplantation** is a common surgical procedure for the correction of persistent vesicoureteral reflux. The reimplanted ureteral segment is submucosal and contiguous to the bladder mucosa. Sonograms reveal an echogenic, fixed, tubular, submucosal structure without acoustic shadowing at or just above the trigone. Occasionally, the reimplanted ureter appears only as an area of focal thickening of the posterior bladder wall.[212] Sonography is also useful for the demonstration of the echogenic mound present after treatment with Deflux (dextranomer–hyaluronic acid copolymer) as a first-line treatment for high-grade vesicoureteral reflux[213] (Fig. 56-77).

Bladder augmentation is now a widely accepted surgical procedure for the reconstruction of small-capacity bladders caused by exstrophy, neurogenic bladder, or tumor. Segments of bowel, usually the sigmoid, cecum, ileum, or the ileocecal segment, are anastomosed to the bladder to increase the size of the urinary reservoir. Sonography of the augmented bladder reveals a thick or irregularly shaped bladder wall (Fig. 56-78). Pseudomasses within the bladder lumen, representing bowel folds, mucous collections, or bowel that was surgically intussuscepted into the reconstructed bladder to prevent reflux, are a common finding. Fine debris and linear strands often float within the urine and probably represent mucus. Active peristalsis within the bowel segment

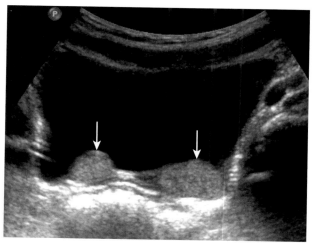

FIGURE 56-77. Bilateral injections of Deflux into ureterovesical junctions. This 2-year-old girl had a history of recurrent urinary tract infection and bilateral vesicoureteral reflux. Note the round, brightly hyperechoic mounds of Deflux *(arrows)* at the trigones bilaterally.

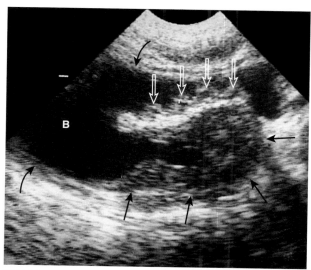

FIGURE 56-78. Augmented bladder. Transverse view of the bladder *(B)* shows the thick wall of the anatomic bladder *(straight black arrows)* and the large augmentation *(curved arrows); open arrows,* haustral markings.

can be identified on real-time imaging. Complications of bladder reconstructive surgery can be detected on ultrasound and include enterocystic **anastomotic strictures, ureteral reflux or obstruction, calculi, extravasation, abscess, urinoma, hematoma,** and large amounts of residual urine after voiding.[214,215]

GASTROINTESTINAL TRACT

Obstruction

Sonography has become an important imaging modality in the evaluation of the pediatric gastrointestinal

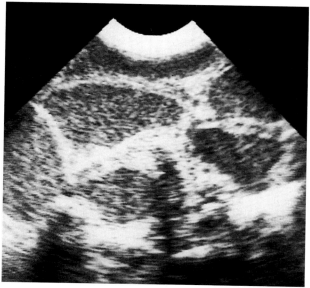

FIGURE 56-79. Meconium ileus. Transverse sonography of the right lower quadrant shows distended, meconium-filled, small bowel loops. *(From Sherman NH, Boyle GK, Rosenberg HK. Sonography in the neonate. Ultrasound Q 1988;6:91-150.)*

tract.[216-218] In the child with a distended abdomen, ultrasound is a useful diagnostic tool for the detection of ascites, dilated fluid-filled bowel loops, masses, abscess collections, and closed-loop obstructions that may not be evident on the plain abdominal radiographs.[217] In a distal bowel obstruction, real-time ultrasound shows active peristalsis in dilated, fluid-filled, tubular-shaped proximal bowel loops. The small bowel mucosal pattern and colonic haustrations become obliterated as the bowel lumen distends. The normal gut wall is uniform and compliant, with an average thickness of 3 mm when distended. Acutely, the thickness of the bowel wall is normal, but as the obstruction persists, the bowel wall thickens as a result of edema. In a paralytic ileus, peristaltic activity is greatly diminished, but the valvulae conniventes can be appreciated within discrete tubular loops.[216]

Distal bowel obstruction in the neonate results in the retention of meconium proximal to the obstruction. The meconium appears as echogenic material within the bowel lumen[86] (Fig. 56-79). The most common causes of neonatal distal bowel obstruction include **ileal atresia, meconium ileus, meconium plug syndrome,** and **Hirschsprung's disease** (Fig. 56-80). Although contrast enemas usually provide the diagnosis, ultrasound has been helpful in difficult cases. In meconium ileus the thick, tenacious meconium appears as brightly echogenic masses with little fluid within the small bowel lumen.[219] In contrast, the meconium in ileal atresia has a normal consistency, and the echogenic meconium is admixed with fluid-filled loops. In addition, sonography is useful for demonstration of a smaller than normal size caliber rectum.

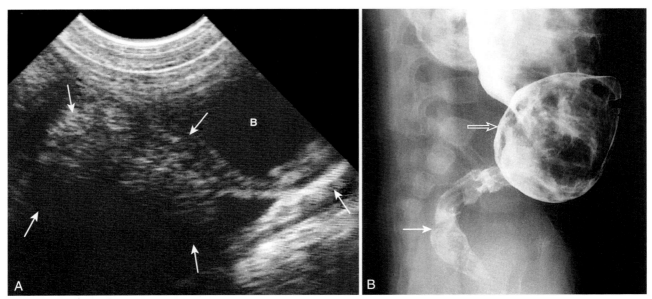

FIGURE 56-80. Hirschsprung's disease. This 9-month-old boy presented with hypotonia, weakness, normocytic anemia, and large abdomen. **A,** Sagittal sonogram of pelvis shows narrow, unfilled rectum *(thick arrow)*. Above this area is massively distended sigmoid *(thin arrows)* filled with tremendous fecal boluses that shadow the ultrasound beam. *B,* Bladder. **B,** Barium enema demonstrates collapsed aganglionic segment *(solid arrow)* and distended, feces-filled sigmoid colon *(open arrow)*. *(From Rosenberg HK, Goldberg BB. Pediatric radiology: sonography. In Margulis AR, Burhenne HJ, editors. Alimentary tract radiology. 4th ed. St Louis, 1989, Mosby, pp 1831-1857.)*

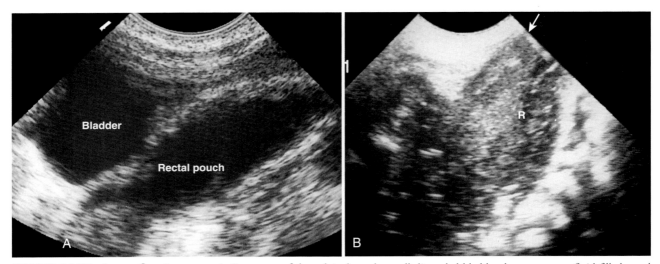

FIGURE 56-81. Imperforate anus. A, Sonogram of the pelvis through a well-distended bladder demonstrates a fluid-filled rectal pouch extending inferiorly, implying a low, imperforate anus. **B,** In same newborn as **A,** perineal scan shows that the rectal pouch is in fact a covered anus *(arrow)*; R, rectum. *(From Rosenberg HK, Goldberg BB. Pediatric radiology: sonography. In Margulis AR, Burhenne HJ, editors. Alimentary tract radiology. 4th ed. St Louis, 1989, Mosby, pp 1831-1857.)*

Imperforate Anus

Sonography has been used in the evaluation of imperforate anus to determine the level of the rectal pouch.[220,221] The position of the rectal pouch, in relation to the levator sling, determines the surgical approach. A direct perineal approach and pull-through technique is performed if the rectal pouch is low and passes through the levator sling.[221] In high lesions above the puborectalis muscle, a decompressive colostomy is performed initially. There is also a high association of renal and ver-

tebral anomalies and rectal fistulas with the genitourinary tract in high imperforate anus. Ultrasound has now been added to the radiologist's imaging armamentarium for the evaluation of this difficult problem. High-resolution, real-time sonography of the lower abdomen and the pelvis using a suprapubic approach, as well as a longitudinal midline transperineal scan, is useful for determining the level of the imperforate anus (Fig. 56-81). The distance between the fluid-filled rectal pouch and the perineum is measured, and if 1.5 cm or less, a low

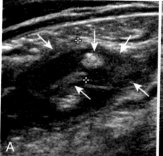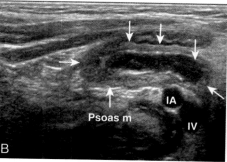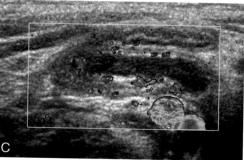

FIGURE 56-82. Acute appendicitis. Both patients presented with right lower quadrant pain, vomiting, loss of appetite and fever. **A,** Sagittal sonogram of the right lower quadrant/upper pelvis shows a thick-walled, dilated (8-mm cross-sectional diameter), noncompressible, fluid-filled, blind-ending tubular structure consistent with an appendix *(arrows)* that contains a bright, shadowing, echogenic focus within its lumen representing an appendicolith. **B** and **C,** Gray-scale and color Doppler images in the second patient also demonstrate a thick-walled, dilated, noncompressible, blind-ending tubular structure filled with hypoechoic fluid. The wall of this dilated appendix is hyperemic. *IA,* Iliac artery; *IV,* iliac vein.

imperforate anus is presumably present. We advise gentle scanning pressure to avoid compression reduction of the area of interest. On transabdominal images, the rectal pouch does not pass below the base of the bladder in high imperforate anus.

Cloacal malformation is an uncommon anomaly in which the rectum, vagina, and urethra end in a common terminal channel as the only outlet for the three systems. There is no anus; at times the external genitalia may be ambiguous; the sacrum is frequently deformed; and there may be associated uterine, vaginal, genitourinary tract (particularly vesicoureteral reflux), musculoskeletal, cardiovascular, genitointestinal, and central nervous system anomalies.[222]

APPENDICITIS: SONOGRAPHIC FINDINGS

Tubular, blind-ending mass
Noncompressible
Appendix >6 mm
Periappendiceal edema

Inflammation

Acute appendicitis is the most common cause of emergency surgery in children. Perforation with acute appendicitis is more common in children than adults. In infants, appendiceal perforation may occur in 80% of cases. In addition, the progression of disease from the onset of symptoms to perforation is more rapid in infants than in older children and adults.[223] Using the graded-compression technique,[224] the inflamed appendix can be directly visualized with high-resolution ultrasound. Ultrasound has been evaluated as a more cost-effective imaging modality to diagnose acute appendicitis in young children, without the risk of iodinated contrast material or radiation exposure.[225] At our institution,

focused sonography is routinely performed for the diagnosis of acute appendicitis in young children, adolescents, and young adults, with CT reserved for those individuals who are extremely obese or in whom the sonogram is inconclusive in the presence of strong clinical suspicion.

The inflamed appendix appears as a tubular, blind-ending structure with a hypoechoic center that is surrounded by an inner echogenic and outer hypoechoic layer.[226] The appendix is rigid, lacks peristalsis, has a maximum outer diameter greater than 6 mm, and does not compress when the examiner gently presses the abdominal wall with the transducer. Appendiceal wall thickening of greater than 2 mm is often asymmetrical.[227] Graded-compression sonography can also identify appendiceal calculi **(appendioliths)** and periappendiceal edema and abscess (Fig. 56-82). Evaluation of the pelvis is done in addition to sonography of the right lower quadrant to examine for focal and free fluid collections, as well as to exclude pelvic pathology that can mimic the sonographic findings of acute appendicitis (Fig. 56-83).

Three sonographic findings associated with appendiceal perforation are (1) a loculated pericecal fluid collection, indicating abscess; (2) prominent pericecal fat more than 10 mm in thickness; and (3) circumferential loss of the echogenic submucosal layer of the appendix.[228] Sonography is also helpful in the detection and follow-up evaluation of postappendectomy fluid collections.[229,230]

Quillin and Siegel[231] showed that the addition of color flow Doppler imaging to routine gray-scale imaging can

APPENDICEAL PERFORATION: SONOGRAPHIC FINDINGS

Loculated pericecal fluid or abscess
Prominent pericecal fat >10 mm thick
Loss of echogenic submucosa of appendix

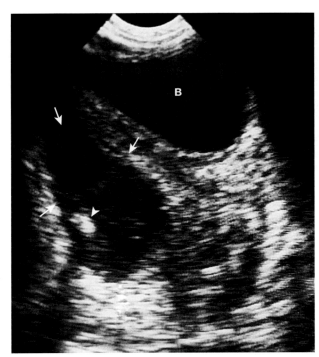

FIGURE 56-83. Appendiceal abscess. Loculated fluid collection *(arrows)* was noted in right lower quadrant, containing scattered internal debris and calcified appendicolith *(arrowhead);* B, bladder. *(From Fisher MR, Kricun ME, editors. Imaging of the pelvis. Gaithersburg, Md, 1989, Aspen.)*

APPENDICITIS ON COLOR FLOW DOPPLER ULTRASOUND

Hypervascularity of appendix
Hypervascularity of periappendix area
Hypervascularity around a fluid collection with perforation

increase the sensitivity of the ultrasound examination for detecting appendicitis to 95%. The normal appendix and periappendiceal tissues have minimal to no flow on color Doppler ultrasound. The presence of hypervascularity in the appendix or periappendiceal tissues reflects an infectious or inflammatory process. This proved useful in identifying inflamed appendices in 9% of patients in Quillin and Siegel's study, despite normal appendix size on gray-scale imaging.[231] Peripheral **appendiceal hyperemia** suggests the presence of nonperforated appendicitis.[232] The absence of appendiceal hyperemia, however, does not exclude appendicitis. Color flow Doppler predictors of appendiceal perforation include hyperemia in the periappendiceal soft tissues or around a periappendiceal or pelvic fluid collection. Bowel hyperemia may be seen in nonperforated appendicitis and in primary bowel disease and thus is not specific for perforation.[232]

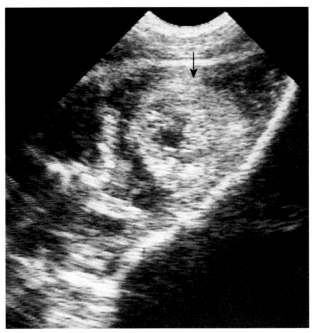

FIGURE 56-84. Psoas hematoma. Transverse view of left psoas muscle shows rounded, complex, echogenic mass *(arrow)* within muscle, which is consistent with psoas hematoma in this teenager with hemophilia.

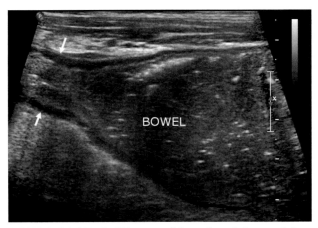

FIGURE 56-85. A 17-year-old male with vomiting and abdominal pain. Sagittal ultrasound image of right lower quadrant demonstrates marked thickening of the walls of the terminal ileum *(arrows)* with severe dilatation of the proximal bowel loop, consistent with stricture formation.

Other causes of acute right lower quadrant and pelvic pain can also be diagnosed with pelvic sonography, such as PID and ovarian torsion.[21] A **psoas abscess or hematoma** is usually confined to the psoas muscle, and the patient often presents with lower abdominal pain, pelvic pain, or both, which radiates to the groin and hip (Fig. 56-84). In **inflammatory bowel disease** the involved bowel loops have a thickened, hypoechoic wall with dense central echoes (Fig. 56-85). There is decreased mobility, compressibility, and peristalsis of the involved loop. The adjacent mesentery is thickened. Additional sonographic findings in **Crohn's disease** include adynamic ileus with distended, fluid-filled bowel loops; a complex heterogeneous mass caused by a conglomerate of matted, inflamed bowel loops; abscess; and secondary ureteral obstruction with hydronephrosis.[233]

Mesenteric adenitis and **acute terminal ileitis**, caused by *Yersinia enterocolitica* infection, often cause clinical symptoms identical to acute appendicitis. However, these entities are treated conservatively without surgical intervention. The graded compression technique can be used to differentiate these two diseases from appendicitis. The sonographic criteria of mesenteric adenitis includes multiple, round or oval, enlarged, tender mesenteric lymph nodes that demonstrate flow in the fatty hila with hyperemia of the nodes in some cases, and no evidence of an inflamed appendix.[234] With acute terminal ileitis, mural thickening (4-6 mm) of the terminal ileum and cecum may be seen along with diminished peristalsis (Fig. 56-86).

PRESACRAL MASSES

The presacral space is a potential space between the perirectal fascia and the fibrous coverings of the anterior sacrum. A lesion in the presacral space can usually be identified on routine transabdominal sonograms through a distended bladder. To confirm the origin of the mass, a water enema can be performed to identify the rectosigmoid colon in relation to the lesion. Additional scans through the buttocks are often helpful to determine the true extent of the tumor.

Sacrococcygeal teratoma is the most common presacral neoplasm in the pediatric age group. About 50% are noted at birth, with a 4:1 female/male incidence.

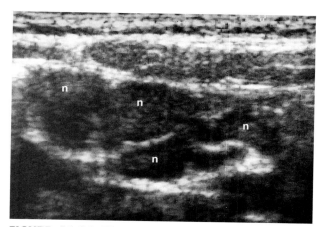

FIGURE 56-86. Mesenteric adenitis in 3-year-old boy with right lower quadrant pain and fever. Transverse ultrasound of the right lower quadrant and upper pelvis reveals multiple, ovoid, soft tissue masses representing lymph nodes *(n)*. The appendix was not visualized. The patient's symptoms resolved spontaneously.

PRESACRAL MASSES IN CHILDREN

SOLID
Sacrococcygeal teratoma
Neuroblastoma
Rhabdomyosarcoma
Fibroma
Lipoma
Leiomyoma
Lymphoma
Hemangioendothelioma
Sacral bone tumors

CYSTIC
Abscess
Rectal duplication
Hematoma
Lymphocele
Neurenteric cyst
Sacral osteomyelitis
Ulcerative colitis
Anterior meningocele

Sacrococcygeal teratoma arises from multipotential cells in Hensen's nodes that migrate caudally and come to lie within the coccyx. Radiographic evidence of bony abnormalities of the sacrum or coccyx may be present. There is a 75% incidence of associated congenital anomalies, most often involving the musculoskeletal system. These teratomas are most common in families with a high frequency of twins.[235]

Sacrococcygeal teratomas can be benign or malignant. Tumors detected before age 2 months are most likely benign. Those detected after 2 months have a 50% to 90% incidence of malignancy. Malignancy is more common in boys and in lesions that are predominantly solid on ultrasound and CT examinations. Cystic lesions are more likely benign. All teratomas have a malignant potential, regardless of their texture, location, or size. Recurrence of a benign teratoma after incomplete surgical removal leads to increased risk of malignant transformation; therefore the coccyx must be removed completely at surgery to prevent recurrence. Sacrococcygeal teratomas can be divided into the following four types, based on their location:

Type I: Predominantly external
Type II: External with a significant intrapelvic component
Type III: Small external mass with predominant intrapelvic portion
Type IV: Entirely presacral with no external component

Type I lesions are usually benign and appear at birth. Types II, III, and IV have a higher incidence of malignancy, probably because the large intrapelvic component goes unrecognized and undetected for longer periods than the large, exophytic masses.[235] Malignant teratomas are usually endodermal sinus tumors.

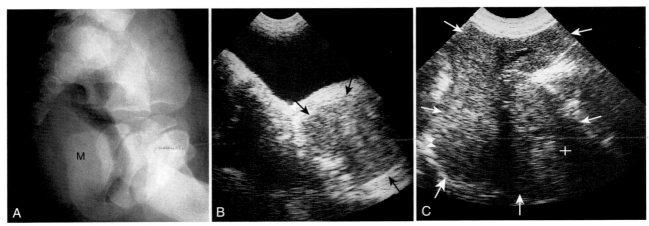

FIGURE 56-87. Sacrococcygeal teratoma in 2-year-old boy with palpable mass at base of spine. A, Lateral conventional radiograph of the pelvis shows lack of coccygeal ossification and large, retrorectal, soft tissue mass *(M)* with anterior displacement of the rectum. **B,** Sagittal ultrasound of the pelvis shows a solid mass *(arrows)* deep in the pelvis posteroinferior to the bladder. **C,** Transverse ultrasound over the base of the spine posteriorly shows a primarily solid mass *(arrows)* with one small, cystic area extending deep into the pelvis.

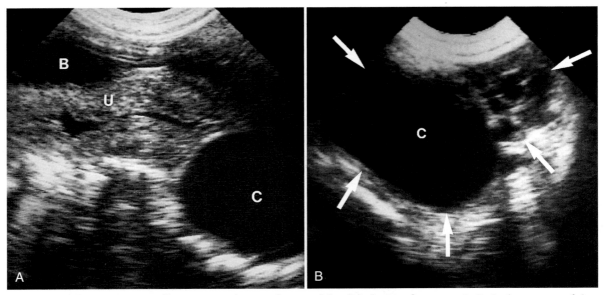

FIGURE 56-88. Sacrococcygeal teratoma in newborn girl with buttock mass. A, Sagittal sonogram of the pelvis demonstrates a large, cystic mass *(C),* deep in the pelvis, posteroinferior to the uterus *(U).* The small amount of fluid noted in the endometrial canal is secondary to residual material hormonal stimulation. *B,* Bladder. **B,** Transverse image over the base of the spine posteriorly demonstrates a complex mass *(arrows)* with a predominantly large cystic *(C)* component.

There is a wide spectrum of ultrasound appearances of sacrococcygeal teratomas, ranging from purely cystic to mixed or purely solid (Figs. 56-87 and 56-88). Calcifications, seen in one third of cases, can be amorphous, punctate, or spiculated and suggest the lesion is benign. Fat within the tumor appears as bright areas of heterogeneous echogenicity. Large tumors may displace and compress the bladder anteriorly and superiorly, causing urinary retention and hydronephrosis.

Neuroblastoma and other neurogenic tumors can arise in the presacral space in children. Five percent of neuroblastomas arise in the pelvis. Because of their midline location, they are considered stage III tumors. Pelvic neuroblastoma has a better prognosis than intra-abdominal neuroblastoma. The pelvic lesions have a similar sonographic appearance to the adrenal lesions. They are solid, echogenic, heterogeneous masses with a 70% incidence of calcification. Areas of cystic necrosis and hemorrhage are uncommon[236-238] (Fig. 56-89).

Rhabdomyosarcoma arising from the pelvic musculature can present as a solid presacral mass. It is usually an infiltrating tumor with poorly defined margins. Anechoic spaces within a predominantly solid mass suggest areas of necrosis and hemorrhage. Calcification

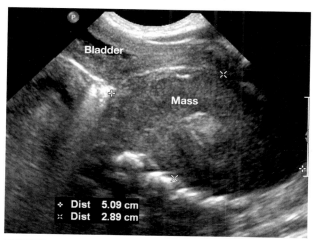

FIGURE 56-89. Neuroblastoma. Full-term male baby with a prenatal diagnosis of a large (5 × 3 × 4 cm), solid, deep, pelvic mass that contains a central, nonshadowing calcification. The mass flattens the urinary bladder while displacing it anteriorly.

is rare.[239] Ultrasound is an excellent method for identifying and staging rhabdomyosarcoma arising from the genitourinary tract. However, CT and MRI provide more complete information for those tumors arising from the pelvic side walls. Other predominantly **solid presacral masses** to be considered in the differential diagnosis include fibroma, lipoma, leiomyoma (and their malignant counterparts), lymphoma, hemangioendothelioma, and metastatic disease. **Sacral bone tumors**, such as Ewing's sarcoma, osteosarcoma, chondrosarcoma, giant cell tumor, and aneurysmal bone cyst, may also present as presacral masses. Chordomas of the sacrococcygeal region are rare in children.

Cystic presacral lesions, in addition to sacrococcygeal teratomas, can be detected on sonography. These include abscess, rectal duplication, hematoma, lymphocele, neurenteric cyst, sacral osteomyelitis, and ulcerative colitis. An anterior sacral meningocele also presents as a cystic presacral mass. It represents herniation of the meninges through an anterior defect in the sacrum. The sacrum usually has a scimitar- or sickle-shaped configuration. A solid mural nodule within the cystic meningocele represents glial or lipomatous tissue.

References

Sonographic Technique

1. Stranzinger E, Strouse PJ. Ultrasound of the pediatric female pelvis. Semin US CT MR 2008;29:98-113.
2. Garel L, Dubois J, Grignon A, et al. Ultrasound of the pediatric female pelvis: a clinical perspective. Radiographics 2001;21:1393-1407.
3. Female pelvis. In: Siegel MJ, editor. Pediatric sonography. 3rd ed. Philadelphia: Lippincott–Williams & Wilkins; 2002. p. 530-577.
4. Male genital tract. In: Siegel MJ, editor. Pediatric sonography. 3rd ed. Philadelphia: Lippincott–Williams & Wilkins; 2002. p. 579-624.
5. Cohen HL, Bober SE, Bow SN. Imaging the pediatric pelvis: the normal and abnormal genital tract and simulators of its diseases. Urol Radiol 1992;14:273-283.
6. Arbel-DeRowe Y, Tepper R, Rosen DJ, Beyth Y. The contribution of pelvic ultrasonography to the diagnostic process in pediatric and adolescent gynecology. J Pediatr Adolesc Gynecol 1997;10:3-12.
7. Teele RL, Share JC. Ultrasonography of the female pelvis in childhood and adolescence. Radiol Clin North Am 1992;30:743-758.
8. Rubin C, Kurtz AB, Goldberg BB. Water enema: a new ultrasound technique in defining pelvic anatomy. J Clin Ultrasound 1978;6:28-33.
9. Bellah RD, Rosenberg HK. Transvaginal ultrasound in a children's hospital: is it worthwhile? Pediatr Radiol 1991;21:570-574.
10. Jequier S, Rousseau O. Sonographic measurements of the normal bladder wall in children. AJR Am J Roentgenol 1987;149:563-566.
11. Zieger B, Sokol B, Rohrschneider WK, et al. Sonomorphology and involution of the normal urachus in asymptomatic newborns. Pediatr Radiol 1998;28:156-161.
12. Marchal GJ, Baert AL, Eeckels R, Proesmans W. Sonographic evaluation of the normal ureteral submucosal tunnel in infancy and childhood. Pediatr Radiol 1983;13:125-129.
13. Comstock CH, Boal DK. Pelvic sonography of the pediatric patient. Semin Ultrasound 1984;5:54-67.
14. Cohen HL, Susman M, Haller JO, et al. Posterior urethral valve: transperineal US for imaging and diagnosis in male infants. Radiology 1994;192:261-264.
15. Schiller VL, Grant EG. Doppler ultrasonography of the pelvis. Radiol Clin North Am 1992;30:735-742.

Normal Female Anatomy

16. Rosenberg HK. Sonography of the pediatric urinary tract. In: Bush WH, editor. Urologic imaging and interventional techniques. Baltimore: Urban & Schwarzenberg; 1989. p. 164-179.
17. Siegel MJ. Pediatric gynecologic sonography. Radiology 1991;179:593-600.
18. Cohen HL, Shapiro MA, Mandel FS, Shapiro ML. Normal ovaries in neonates and infants: a sonographic study of 77 patients 1 day to 24 months old. AJR Am J Roentgenol 1993;160:583-586.
19. Cohen HL, Tice HM, Mandel FS. Ovarian volumes measured by US: bigger than we think. Radiology 1990;177:189-192.
20. Orbak Z, Kantarci M, Yildirim ZK, et al. Ovarian volume and uterine length in neonatal girls. J Pediatr Endocrinol Metab 2007;20:397-403.
21. Quillin SP, Siegel MJ. Transabdominal color Doppler ultrasonography of the painful adolescent ovary. J Ultrasound Med 1994;13:549-555.

Ovarian Abnormalities

22. De Silva KS, Kanumakala S, Grover SR, et al. Ovarian lesions in children and adolescents: an 11-year review. J Pediatr Endocrinol Metab 2004;17:951-957.
23. Nussbaum AR, Sanders RC, Benator RM, et al. Spontaneous resolution of neonatal ovarian cysts. AJR Am J Roentgenol 1987;148:175-176.
24. Kuo HC, Lee HC, Shin CH, et al. Clinical spectrum of alimentary tract duplication in children. Acta Paediatr Taiwan 2004;45:85-88.
25. Riddlesberger MM Jr, Kuhn JP, Munschauer RW. The association of juvenile hypothyroidism and cystic ovaries. Radiology 1981;139:77-80.
26. Rosado Jr WM, Trambert MA, Gosink BB, Pretorius DH. Adnexal torsion: diagnosis by using Doppler sonography. AJR Am J Roentgenol 1992;159:1251-1253.
27. Lee EJ, Kwon HC, Joo HJ, et al. Diagnosis of ovarian torsion with color Doppler sonography: depiction of twisted vascular pedicle. J Ultrasound Med 1998;17:83-89.
28. Hurh PJ, Meyer JS, Shaaban A. Ultrasound of a torsed ovary: characteristic gray-scale appearance despite normal arterial and venous flow on Doppler. Pediatr Radiol 2002;32:586-588.
29. Graif M, Itzchak Y. Sonographic evaluation of ovarian torsion in childhood and adolescence. AJR Am J Roentgenol 1988;150:647-649.
30. Cass DL. Ovarian torsion. Semin Pediatr Surg 2005;14:86-92.
31. Servaes S, Zurakowski D, Laufer MR, et al. Sonographic findings of ovarian torsion in children. Pediatr Radiol 2007;37:446-451.

32. Harmon JC, Binkovitz LA, Binkovitz LE. Isolated fallopian tube torsion: sonographic and CT features. Pediatr Radiol 2008;38:175-179.
33. Baltarowich OH, Kurtz AB, Pasto ME, et al. The spectrum of sonographic findings in hemorrhagic ovarian cysts. AJR Am J Roentgenol 1987;148:901-905.
34. Hann LE, Hall DA, McArdle CR, Seibel M. Polycystic ovarian disease: sonographic spectrum. Radiology 1984;150:531-534.
35. Jeffrey Chang R, Coffler MS. Polycystic ovary syndrome: early detection in the adolescent. Clin Obstet Gynecol 2007;50:178-187.
36. Dolz M, Osborne NG, Blanes J, et al. Polycystic ovarian syndrome: assessment with color Doppler angiography and three-dimensional ultrasonography. J Ultrasound Med 1999;18:303-313.
37. Lee AR, Kim KH, Lee BH, Chin SY. Massive edema of the ovary: imaging findings. AJR Am J Roentgenol 1993;161:343-344.
38. Roth LM, Deaton RL, Sternberg WH. Massive ovarian edema: a clinicopathologic study of five cases including ultrastructural observations and review of the literature. Am J Surg Pathol 1979;3:11-21.
39. Sty JR, Wells RG. Other abdominal and pelvic masses in children. Semin Roentgenol 1988;23:216-231.
40. Sisler CL, Siegel MJ. Ovarian teratomas: a comparison of the sonographic appearance in prepubertal and postpubertal girls. AJR Am J Roentgenol 1990;154:139-141.
41. Patel MD, Feldstein VA, Lipson SD, et al. Cystic teratomas of the ovary: diagnostic value of sonography. AJR Am J Roentgenol 1998;171:1061-1065.
42. Stankovic ZB, Djukic MK, Sedlecki K, et al. Rapidly growing bilateral ovarian cystadenoma in a 6-year-old girl: case report and literature review. J Pediatr Adolesc Gynecol 2006;19:35-38.
43. Sherman NH, Rosenberg HK. Pediatric pelvic sonography. In: Fisher MR, Kricun ME, editors. Imaging of the pelvis. Rockville, Md: Aspen; 1989.
44. Bickers GH, Siebert JJ, Anderson JC, et al. Sonography of ovarian involvement in childhood acute lymphocytic leukemia. AJR Am J Roentgenol 1981;137:399-401.
45. Fleischer AC, Rodgers WH, Kepple DM, et al. Color Doppler sonography of benign and malignant ovarian masses. Radiographics 1992;12:879-885.
46. Carter J, Saltzman A, Hartenbach E, et al. Flow characteristics in benign and malignant gynecologic tumors using transvaginal color flow Doppler. Obstet Gynecol 1994;83:125-130.

Uterine and Vaginal Abnormalities
47. Rosenberg HK, Sherman NH, Tarry WF, et al. Mayer-Rokitansky-Kuster-Hauser syndrome: US aid to diagnosis. Radiology 1986;161:815-819.
48. Blask AR, Sanders RC, Gearhart JP. Obstructed uterovaginal anomalies: demonstration with sonography. Part I. Neonates and infants. Radiology 1991;179:79-83.
49. Blask AR, Sanders RC, Rock JA. Obstructed uterovaginal anomalies: demonstration with sonography. Part II. Teenagers. Radiology 1991;179:84-88.
50. Wilson SR, Beecham CT, Carrington ER, editors. Obstetrics and gynecology. 8th ed. St Louis: Mosby; 1987.
51. Brody JM, Koelliker SL, Frishman GN. Unicornuate uterus: imaging appearance, associated anomalies, and clinical implications. AJR Am J Roentgenol 1998;171:1341-1347.
52. Scanlan KA, Pozniak MA, Fagerholm M, Shapiro S. Value of transperineal sonography in the assessment of vaginal atresia. AJR Am J Roentgenol 1990;154:545-548.
53. Messina M, Severi FM, Bocchi C, et al. Voluminous perinatal pelvic mass: a case of congenital hydrometrocolpos. J Matern Fetal Neonatal Med 2004;15:135-137.
54. Fisher MR, Kricun ME, editors. Imaging of the pelvis. Gaithersburg, Md: Aspen; 1989.
55. Meglin AJ, Balotin RJ, Jelinek JS, et al. Cloacal exstrophy: radiologic findings in 13 patients. AJR Am J Roentgenol 1990;155:1267-1272.
56. Capito C, Echaieb A, Lortat-Jacob S, et al. Pitfalls in the diagnosis and management of obstructive uterovaginal duplication: a series of 32 cases. Pediatrics 2008;122:e891-e897.
57. Mirkovic L, Mirkovic D, Boskovic V, Markovic Z. Uterus didelphys with obstructed hemivagina and ipsilateral renal agenesis. Acta Chir Yugosl 2007;54:137-139.
58. Hu MX, Methratta S. An unusual case of neonatal peritoneal calcifications associated with hydrometrocolpos. Pediatr Radiol 2001;31:742-744.
59. Andrassy RJ, Wiener ES, Raney RB, et al. Progress in the surgical management of vaginal rhabdomyosarcoma: a 25-year review from the Intergroup Rhabdomyosarcoma Study Group. J Pediatr Surg 1999;34:731-734; discussion 734-735.
60. Lin EP, Bhatt S, Dogra VS. Diagnostic clues to ectopic pregnancy. Radiographics 2008;28:1661-1671.
61. Pellerito JS, Taylor KJ, Quedens-Case C, et al. Ectopic pregnancy: evaluation with endovaginal color flow imaging. Radiology 1992;183:407-411.
62. Yeh HC, Rabinowitz JG. Amniotic sac development: ultrasound features of early pregnancy–the double bleb sign. Radiology 1988;166:97-103.
63. Zinn HL, Cohen HL, Zinn DL. Ultrasonographic diagnosis of ectopic pregnancy: importance of transabdominal imaging. J Ultrasound Med 1997;16:603-607.
64. Lipscomb GH, Stovall TG, Ling FW. Nonsurgical treatment of ectopic pregnancy. N Engl J Med 2000;343:1325-1329.
65. Wherry KL, Dubinsky TJ, Waitches GM, et al. Low-resistance endometrial arterial flow in the exclusion of ectopic pregnancy revisited. J Ultrasound Med 2001;20:335-342.
66. Bulas DI, Ahlstrom PA, Sivit CJ, et al. Pelvic inflammatory disease in the adolescent: comparison of transabdominal and transvaginal sonographic evaluation. Radiology 1992;183:435-439.
67. Schoenfeld A, Fisch B, Cohen M, et al. Ultrasound findings in perihepatitis associated with pelvic inflammatory disease. J Clin Ultrasound 1992;20:339-342.
68. Dinerman LM, Elfenbein DS, Cumming WA. Clinical Fitz-Hugh-Curtis syndrome in an adolescent: ultrasonographic findings. Clin Pediatr (Phila) 1990;29:532-535.
69. Caspi B, Zalel Y, Katz Z, et al. The role of sonography in the detection of vaginal foreign bodies in young girls: the bladder indentation sign. Pediatr Radiol 1995;25(Suppl 1):60-61.
70. Deligeoroglou E, Deliveliotou A, Laggari V, et al. Vaginal foreign body in childhood: a multidisciplinary approach. J Paediatr Child Health 2006;42:649-651.

Endocrine Abnormalities
71. Goske MJ, Emmens RW, Rabinowitz R. Inguinal ovaries in children demonstrated by high resolution real-time ultrasound. Radiology 1984;151:635-636.
72. Haber HP, Ranke MB. Pelvic ultrasonography in Turner syndrome: standards for uterine and ovarian volume. J Ultrasound Med 1999;18:271-276.
73. Haber HP, Wollmann HA, Ranke MB. Pelvic ultrasonography: early differentiation between isolated premature thelarche and central precocious puberty. Eur J Pediatr 1995;154:182-186.
74. Ambrosino MM, Hernanz-Schulman M, Genieser NB, et al. Monitoring of girls undergoing medical therapy for isosexual precocious puberty. J Ultrasound Med 1994;13:501-508.
75. Jensen AM, Brocks V, Holm K, et al. Central precocious puberty in girls: internal genitalia before, during, and after treatment with long-acting gonadotropin-releasing hormone analogues. J Pediatr 1998;132:105-108.

Normal Male Anatomy
76. Mong A, Bellah R. Imaging the pediatric prostate. Radiol Clin North Am 2006;44:749-756, ix.
77. Shapiro E, Hartanto V, Perlman EJ, et al. Morphometric analysis of pediatric and nonhyperplastic prostate glands: evidence that BPH is not a unique stromal process. Prostate 1997;33:177-182.
78. Ingram S, Hollman AS, Azmy AF. Ultrasound evaluation of the paediatric prostate. Br J Urol 1994;74:601-603.
79. Daniel Jr WA, Feinstein RA, Howard-Peebles P, Baxley WD. Testicular volumes of adolescents. J Pediatr 1982;101:1010-1012.
80. Atkinson Jr GO, Patrick LE, Ball Jr TI, et al. The normal and abnormal scrotum in children: evaluation with color Doppler sonography. AJR Am J Roentgenol 1992;158:613-617.
81. Patriquin HB, Yazbeck S, Trinh B, et al. Testicular torsion in infants and children: diagnosis with Doppler sonography. Radiology 1993;188:781-785.
82. Fakhry J, Khoury A, Barakat K. The hypoechoic band: a normal finding on testicular sonography. AJR Am J Roentgenol 1989;153:321-323.
83. Luker GD, Siegel MJ. Scrotal ultrasound in pediatric patients: comparison of power and standard color Doppler ultrasound. Radiology 1996;198:381-385.

84. Paltiel HJ, Rupich RC, Babcock DS. Maturational changes in arterial impedance of the normal testis in boys: Doppler sonographic study. AJR Am J Roentgenol 1994;163:1189-1193.

85. Barth RA, Shortliffe LD. Normal pediatric testis: comparison of power Doppler and color Doppler ultrasound in the detection of blood flow. Radiology 1997;204:389-393.

Congenital Male Abnormalities

86. Sherman NH, Boyle GK, Rosenberg HK. Sonography in the neonate. Ultrasound Q 1988;6:91-150.

87. Christensen JD, Dogra VS. The undescended testis. Semin Ultrasound CT MR 2007;28:307-316.

88. Maghnie M, Vanzulli A, Paesano P, et al. The accuracy of magnetic resonance imaging and ultrasonography compared with surgical findings in the localization of the undescended testis. Arch Pediatr Adolesc Med 1994;148:699-703.

89. Gong M, Geary ES, Shortliffe LM. Testicular torsion with contralateral vanishing testis. Urology 1996;48:306-307.

90. Finkelstein MS, Rosenberg HK, Snyder 3rd HM, Duckett JW. Ultrasound evaluation of scrotum in pediatrics. Urology 1986;27:1-9.

91. Kogan S, Kadziselimovic F, Howards SS, et al. Pediatric andrology. In: Gillenwater JY, Grayback JT, Howards SS, et al, editors. Adult and pediatric urology. 3rd ed. St Louis: Mosby; 1996. p. 2623-2674.

92. Eberenz W, Rosenberg HK, Moshang T, et al. True hermaphroditism: sonographic demonstration of ovotestes. Radiology 1991;179:429-431.

93. Eberli D, Gretener H, Dommann-Scherrer C, et al. Cystic dysplasia of the testis: a very rare paediatric tumor of the testis. Urol Int 2002;69:1-6.

94. Piotto L, LeQuesne GW, Gent R, et al. Congenital cystic dysplasia of the rete testis. Pediatr Radiol 2001;31:724-726.

95. Hamm B, Fobbe F, Loy V. Testicular cysts: differentiation with ultrasound and clinical findings. Radiology 1988;168:19-23.

96. Weiss AJ, Kellman GM, Middleton WD, Kirkemo A. Intratesticular varicocele: sonographic findings in two patients. AJR Am J Roentgenol 1992;158:1061-1063.

Acute Scrotal Pain or Swelling

97. Pimpalwar A, Chowdhary S, Huskisson J, Corkery JJ. Cysts of the ejaculatory system: a treatable cause of recurrent epididymo-orchitis in children. Eur J Pediatr Surg 2002;12:281-285.

98. Galejs LE, Kass EJ. Color Doppler ultrasound evaluation of the acute scrotum. Tech Urol 1998;4:182-184.

99. Makela E, Lahdes-Vasama T, Rajakorpi H, Wikstrom S. A 19-year review of paediatric patients with acute scrotum. Scand J Surg 2007;96:62-66.

100. Friedman SC, Sheynkin YR. Acute scrotal symptoms due to perforated appendix in children: case report and review of literature. Pediatr Emerg Care 1995;11:181-182.

101. Yang WT, Ku KW, Metreweli C. Case report: neonatal adrenal haemorrhage presenting as an acute right scrotal swelling (haematoma)—value of ultrasound. Clin Radiol 1995;50:127-129.

102. Schroder CH, Rieu P, de Jong MC. Peritoneal laceration: a rare cause of scrotal edema in a 2-year-old boy. Adv Perit Dial 1993;9:329-330.

103. Simoneaux SF, Ball TI, Atkinson Jr GO. Scrotal swelling: unusual first presentation of Crohn's disease. Pediatr Radiol 1995;25:375-376.

104. Older RA, Watson LR. Ultrasound diagnosis of testicular torsion: beware the swollen epididymis. J Urol 1997;157:1369-1370.

105. Kilkenny TE. Acute scrotum in an infant: post-herniorrhaphy complication. Sonographic evaluation. Pediatr Radiol 1993;23:481-482.

106. Kadish HA, Bolte RG. A retrospective review of pediatric patients with epididymitis, testicular torsion, and torsion of testicular appendages. Pediatrics 1998;102:73-76.

107. Gronski M, Hollman AS. The acute paediatric scrotum: the role of colour Doppler ultrasound. Eur J Radiol 1998;26:183-193.

108. Hollman AS, Ingram S, Carachi R, Davis C. Colour Doppler imaging of the acute paediatric scrotum. Pediatr Radiol 1993;23:83-87.

109. Bhatt S, Dogra VS. Role of ultrasound in testicular and scrotal trauma. Radiographics 2008;28:1617-1629.

110. Brown SM, Casillas VJ, Montalvo BM, Albores-Saavedra J. Intra-uterine spermatic cord torsion in the newborn: sonographic and pathologic correlation. Radiology 1990;177:755-757.

111. Groisman GM, Nassrallah M, Bar-Maor JA. Bilateral intra-uterine testicular torsion in a newborn. Br J Urol 1996;78:800-801.

112. Zinn HL, Cohen HL, Horowitz M. Testicular torsion in neonates: importance of power Doppler imaging. J Ultrasound Med 1998;17:385-388.

113. Koff SA. Does compensatory testicular enlargement predict monorchism? J Urol 1991;146:632-633.

114. Klin B, Lotan G, Efrati Y, et al. Acute idiopathic scrotal edema in children—revisited. J Pediatr Surg 2002;37:1200-1202.

115. Leape LL. Torsion of the testis. In: Welch KJ, Randolph JG, Ravitch MM, editors. Pediatric surgery. St Louis: Mosby; 1986.

116. Paltiel HJ, Connolly LP, Atala A, et al. Acute scrotal symptoms in boys with an indeterminate clinical presentation: comparison of color Doppler sonography and scintigraphy. Radiology 1998;207:223-231.

117. Chen DC, Holder LE, Kaplan GN. Correlation of radionuclide imaging and diagnostic ultrasound in scrotal diseases. J Nucl Med 1986;27:1774-1781.

118. Coley BD, Frush DP, Babcock DS, et al. Acute testicular torsion: comparison of unenhanced and contrast-enhanced power Doppler US, color Doppler US, and radionuclide imaging. Radiology 1996;199:441-446.

119. Siegel MJ. The acute scrotum. Radiol Clin North Am 1997;35:959-976.

120. Deurdulian C, Mittelstaedt CA, Chong WK, Fielding JR. Ultrasound of acute scrotal trauma: optimal technique, imaging findings, and management. Radiographics 2007;27:3573.

121. Prando D. Torsion of the spermatic cord: the main gray-scale and Doppler sonographic signs. Abdom Imaging 2009;34:648-661.

122. Haynes BE, Haynes VE. Manipulative detorsion: beware the twist that does not turn. J Urol 1987;137:118-119.

123. Erbay N, Brown SL, Spencer RP. Hydrocele mimicking testicular torsion on radionuclide and ultrasound studies. Clin Nucl Med 1997;22:570-571.

124. Nye PJ, Prati Jr RC. Idiopathic hydrocele and absent testicular diastolic flow. J Clin Ultrasound 1997;25:43-46.

125. Nussbaum Blask AR, Rushton HG. Sonographic appearance of the epididymis in pediatric testicular torsion. AJR Am J Roentgenol 2006;187:1627-1635.

126. Horstman WG, Middleton WD, Melson GL. Scrotal inflammatory disease: color Doppler US findings. Radiology 1991;179:55-59.

127. Jee WH, Choe BY, Byun JY, et al. Resistive index of the intrascrotal artery in scrotal inflammatory disease. Acta Radiol 1997;38:1026-1030.

128. Lee JC, Bhatt S, Dogra VS. Imaging of the epididymis. Ultrasound Q 2008;24:3-16.

129. Bukowski TP, Lewis AG, Reeves D, et al. Epididymitis in older boys: dysfunctional voiding as an etiology. J Urol 1995;154:762-765.

130. Cohen HL, Shapiro MA, Haller JO, Glassberg K. Torsion of the testicular appendage: sonographic diagnosis. J Ultrasound Med 1992;11:81-83.

131. Lewis AG, Bukowski TP, Jarvis PD, et al. Evaluation of acute scrotum in the emergency department. J Pediatr Surg 1995;30:277-281; discussion 281-282.

132. Strauss S, Faingold R, Manor H. Torsion of the testicular appendages: sonographic appearance. J Ultrasound Med 1997;16:189-192; quiz 193-194.

133. Hesser U, Rosenborg M, Gierup J, et al. Gray-scale sonography in torsion of the testicular appendages. Pediatr Radiol 1993;23:529-532.

134. Monga M, Scarpero HM, Ortenberg J. Metachronous bilateral torsion of the testicular appendices. Int J Urol 1999;6:589-591.

135. Black JA, Patel A. Sonography of the normal extratesticular space. AJR Am J Roentgenol 1996;167:503-506.

136. Jeffrey RB, Laing FC, Hricak H, McAninch JW. Sonography of testicular trauma. AJR Am J Roentgenol 1983;141:993-995.

137. Corrales JG, Corbel L, Cipolla B, et al. Accuracy of ultrasound diagnosis after blunt testicular trauma. J Urol 1993;150:1834-1836.

138. Herman TE, Shackelford GD, McAlister WH. Acute idiopathic scrotal edema: role of scrotal sonography. J Ultrasound Med 1994;13:53-55.

139. Ben-Sira L, Laor T. Severe scrotal pain in boys with Henoch-Schönlein purpura: incidence and sonography. Pediatr Radiol 2000;30:125-128.

140. Sudakoff GS, Burke M, Rifkin MD. Ultrasonographic and color Doppler imaging of hemorrhagic epididymitis in Henoch-Schönlein purpura. J Ultrasound Med 1992;11:619-621.

141. Grainger AJ, Hide IG, Elliott ST. The ultrasound appearances of scrotal oedema. Eur J Ultrasound 1998;8:33-37.
142. Munden MM, Trautwein LM. Scrotal pathology in pediatrics with sonographic imaging. Curr Probl Diagn Radiol 2000;29:185-205.
143. Begley MG, Shawker TH, Robertson CN, et al. Fournier gangrene: diagnosis with scrotal US. Radiology 1988;169:387-389.

Scrotal Masses

144. Kocakoc E, Bhatt S, Dogra V. Ultrasound evaluation of testicular neoplasms. Ultrasound Clin 2007;2:27-44.
145. Castleberry RP, Cushing B, Perlman E, et al. Germ cell tumors. In: Pizzo PA, Poplack DG, editors. Principles and practice of pediatric oncology. 3rd ed. Philadelphia: Lippincott-Raven; 1997. p. 921-945.
146. Skoog SJ. Benign and malignant pediatric scrotal masses. Pediatr Clin North Am 1997;44:1229-1250.
147. Geraghty MJ, Lee Jr FT, Bernsten SA, et al. Sonography of testicular tumors and tumor-like conditions: a radiologic-pathologic correlation. Crit Rev Diagn Imaging 1998;39:1-63.
148. Liu P, Phillips MJ, Edwards VD, et al. Sonographic findings of testicular teratoma with pathologic correlation. Pediatr Radiol 1992;22:99-101.
149. Worthy L, Miller EI, Chinn DH. Evaluation of extratesticular findings in scrotal neoplasms. J Ultrasound Med 1986;5:261-263.
150. Horowitz MB, Abiri MM. Ultrasound case of the day. Benign cystic teratoma and testicular microlithiasis. Radiographics 1997;17:793-796.
151. Horstman WG, Melson GL, Middleton WD, Andriole GL. Testicular tumors: findings with color Doppler ultrasound. Radiology 1992;185:733-737.
152. Castleberry RP, Kelly DR, Joseph DB, et al. Gonadal and extragonadal germ cell tumors. In: Fernback VT, editor. Clinical pediatric oncology. 4th ed. Chicago: Mosby–Year Book; 1991. p. 577-594.
153. Luisiri A, Vogler C, Steinhardt G, Silberstein M. Neonatal cystic testicular gonadoblastoma: sonographic and pathologic findings. J Ultrasound Med 1991;10:59-61.
154. Hertzberg BS, Mahony BS, Bowie JD, Anderson EE. Sonography of an intratesticular lipoma. J Ultrasound Med 1985;4:619-621.
155. Seidenwurm D, Smathers RL, Kan P, Hoffman A. Intratesticular adrenal rests diagnosed by ultrasound. Radiology 1985;155:479-481.
156. Moghe PK, Brady AP. Ultrasound of testicular epidermoid cysts. Br J Radiol 1999;72:942-945.
157. Avila NA, Premkumar A, Merke DP. Testicular adrenal rest tissue in congenital adrenal hyperplasia: comparison of MR imaging and sonographic findings. AJR Am J Roentgenol 1999;172:1003-1006.
158. Avila NA, Shawker TS, Jones JV, et al. Testicular adrenal rest tissue in congenital adrenal hyperplasia: serial sonographic and clinical findings. AJR Am J Roentgenol 1999;172:1235-1238.
159. Walker BR, Skoog SJ, Winslow BH, et al. Testis sparing surgery for steroid unresponsive testicular tumors of the adrenogenital syndrome. J Urol 1997;157:1460-1463.
160. Mazzu D, Jeffrey Jr RB, Ralls PW. Lymphoma and leukemia involving the testicles: findings on gray-scale and color Doppler sonography. AJR Am J Roentgenol 1995;164:645-647.
161. Patriquin HB. Leukemic infiltration of the testis. In: Siegel BA, Proto AV, editors. Pediatric disease (fourth series) test and syllabus. Reston, Va: American College of Radiology; 1993. p. 667-688.
162. Luker GD, Siegel MJ. Pediatric testicular tumors: evaluation with gray-scale and color Doppler ultrasound. Radiology 1994;191:561-564.
163. Casola G, Scheible W, Leopold GR. Neuroblastoma metastatic to the testis: ultrasonographic screening as an aid to clinical staging. Radiology 1984;151:475-476.
164. Koseoglu V, Akata D, Kutluk T, et al. Neuroblastoma with spermatic cord metastasis in a child: sonographic findings. J Clin Ultrasound 1999;27:287-289.
165. McEniff N, Doherty F, Katz J, et al. Yolk sac tumor of the testis discovered on a routine annual sonogram in a boy with testicular microlithiasis. AJR Am J Roentgenol 1995;164:971-972.
166. Valla JS: Testis-sparing surgery for benign testicular tumors in children. J Urol 2001;165(Suppl 6):2280-2283.
167. Garcia CJ, Zuniga S, Rosenberg H, et al. Simple intratesticular cysts in children: preoperative sonographic diagnosis and histological correlation. Pediatr Radiol 1999;29:851-855.

168. Altadonna V, Snyder 3rd HM, Rosenberg HK, Duckett JW. Simple cysts of the testis in children: preoperative diagnosis by ultrasound and excision with testicular preservation. J Urol 1988;140:1505-1507.
169. Holloway BJ, Belcher HE, Letourneau JG, Kunberger LE. Scrotal sonography: a valuable tool in the evaluation of complications following inguinal hernia repair. J Clin Ultrasound 1998;26:341-344.
170. Dierks PR, Moore PT. Scrotal lymphocele: a complication of renal transplant surgery. J Ultrasound Med 1985;4:91-92.
171. Chung SE, Frush DP, Fordham LA. Sonographic appearances of extratesticular fluid and fluid-containing scrotal masses in infants and children: clues to diagnosis. AJR Am J Roentgenol 1999;173:741-745.
172. Miele V, Galluzzo M, Patti G, et al. Scrotal hematoma due to neonatal adrenal hemorrhage: the value of ultrasonography in avoiding unnecessary surgery. Pediatr Radiol 1997;27:672-674.
173. Aso C, Enriquez G, Fite M, et al. Gray-scale and color Doppler sonography of scrotal disorders in children: an update. Radiographics 2005;25:1197-1214.
174. Niedzielski J, Paduch D, Raczynski P. Assessment of adolescent varicocele. Pediatr Surg Int 1997;12:410-413.
175. Wood A, Dewbury KC. Case report: paratesticular rhabdomyosarcoma—colour Doppler appearances. Clin Radiol 1995;50:130-131.
176. Frates MC, Benson CB, DiSalvo DN, et al. Solid extratesticular masses evaluated with sonography: pathologic correlation. Radiology 1997;204:43-46.
177. Zwanger-Mendelsohn S, Shreck EH, Doshi V. Burkitt lymphoma involving the epididymis and spermatic cord: sonographic and CT findings. AJR Am J Roentgenol 1989;153:85-86.
178. Akbar SA, Sayyed TA, Jafri SZ, et al. Multimodality imaging of paratesticular neoplasms and their rare mimics. Radiographics 2003;23:1461-1476.
179. Choyke PL, Glenn GM, Wagner JP, et al. Epididymal cystadenomas in von Hippel–Lindau disease. Urology 1997;49:926-931.
180. Alaminos-Mingorance M, Sanchez-Lopez-Tello C, Castejon-Casado J, et al. Scrotal lymphangioma in children. Urol Int 1998;61:181-182.
181. Cirillo Jr RL, Coley BD, Binkovitz LA, Jayanthi RV. Sonographic findings in splenogonadal fusion. Pediatr Radiol 1999;29:73-75.
182. Mene M, Rosenberg HK, Ginsberg PC. Meconium periorchitis presenting as scrotal nodules in a five-year-old boy. J Ultrasound Med 1994;13:491-494.
183. Backus ML, Mack LA, Middleton WD, et al. Testicular microlithiasis: imaging appearances and pathologic correlation. Radiology 1994;192:781-785.

Lower Urinary Tract

184. Nussbaum AR, Dorst JP, Jeffs RD, et al. Ectopic ureter and ureterocele: their varied sonographic manifestations. Radiology 1986;159:227-235.
185. Giel DW, Noe HN, Williams MA. Ultrasound screening of asymptomatic siblings of children with vesicoureteral reflux: a long-term followup study. J Urol 2005;174:1602-1604; discussion 1604-1605.
186. Macpherson RI, Leithiser RE, Gordon L, Turner WR. Posterior urethral valves: an update and review. Radiographics 1986;6:753-791.
187. Hulbert WC, Rosenberg HK, Cartwright PC, et al. The predictive value of ultrasonography in evaluation of infants with posterior urethral valves. J Urol 1992;148:122-124.
188. Garris J, Kangarloo H, Sarti D, et al. The ultrasound spectrum of prune-belly syndrome. J Clin Ultrasound 1980;8:117-120.
189. Caro PA, Rosenberg HK, Snyder 3rd HM. Congenital urethral polyp. AJR Am J Roentgenol 1986;147:1041-1042.
190. Kessler A, Rosenberg HK, Smoyer WE, Blyth B. Urethral stones: ultrasound for identification in boys with hematuria and dysuria. Radiology 1992;185:767-768.
191. Shukla AR, Bellah RA, Canning DA, et al. Giant bladder diverticula causing bladder outlet obstruction in children. J Urol 2004;172:1977-1979.
192. Keller MS, Weiss RM, Rosenfield NS. Sonographic evaluation of ureterectasis in children: the significance of peristalsis. J Urol 1993;149:553-555.

193. Marshall JL, Johnson ND, De Campo MP. Vesicoureteric reflux in children: prediction with color Doppler imaging. Work in progress. Radiology 1990;175:355-358.

194. Jequier S, Paltiel H, Lafortune M. Ureterovesical jets in infants and children: duplex and color Doppler US studies. Radiology 1990; 175:349-353.

195. Berrocal T, Gaya F, Arjonilla A, Lonergan GJ. Vesicoureteral reflux: diagnosis and grading with echo-enhanced cystosonography versus voiding cystourethrography. Radiology 2001;221:359-365.

196. Darge K, Ghods S, Zieger B, et al. Reduction in voiding cystoure-throghraphies after the introduction of contrast enhanced sonographic reflux diagnosis. Pediatr Radiol 2001;31:790-795.

197. Benz MR, Stehr M, Kammer B, et al. Foreign body in the bladder mimicking nephritis. Pediatr Nephrol 2007;22:467-470.

198. Erasmie U, Lidefelt KJ. Accuracy of ultrasonic assessment of residual urine in children. Pediatr Radiol 1989;19:388-390.

199. Cacciarelli AA, Kass EJ, Yang SS. Urachal remnants: sonographic demonstration in children. Radiology 1990;174:473-475.

200. Choi YJ, Kim JM, Ahn SY, et al. Urachal anomalies in children: a single center experience. Yonsei Med J 2006;47:782-786.

201. Boyle G, Rosenberg HK, O'Neill J. An unusual presentation of an infected urachal cyst: review of urachal anomalies. Clin Pediatr (Phila) 1988;27:130-134.

202. Heaney JA, Pfister RC, Meares Jr EM. Giant cyst of the seminal vesicle with renal agenesis. AJR Am J Roentgenol 1987;149:139-140.

203. Hayden Jr CK, Swischuk LE, Fawcett HD, et al. Urinary tract infections in childhood: a current imaging approach. Radiographics 1986;6:1023-1038.

204. Rifkin MD, Kurtz AB, Pasto ME, Goldberg BB. Unusual presentations of cystitis. J Ultrasound Med 1983;2:25-28.

205. Rosenberg HK, Eggli KD, Zerin JM, et al. Benign cystitis in children mimicking rhabdomyosarcoma. J Ultrasound Med 1994;13: 921-932.

206. Wexler LH, Helman LJ. Rhabdomyosarcoma and the undifferentiated sarcomas. In: Pizzo PA, Poplack DG, editors. Principles and practice of pediatric oncology. Philadelphia: Lippincott-Raven; 1997. p. 799-829.

207. Williams JL, Cumming WA, Walker 3rd RD, Hackett RL. Transitional cell papilloma of the bladder. Pediatr Radiol 1986;16:322-323.

208. Bornstein I, Charboneau JW, Hartman GW. Leiomyoma of the bladder: sonographic and urographic findings. J Ultrasound Med 1986;5:407-408.

209. Shapeero LG, Vordermark JS. Bladder neurofibromatosis in childhood: noninvasive imaging. J Ultrasound Med 1990;9:177-180.

210. Crecelius SA, Bellah R. Pheochromocytoma of the bladder in an adolescent: sonographic and MR imaging findings. AJR Am J Roentgenol 1995;165:101-103.

211. Zerin JM, Lebowitz RL. Spontaneous extraperitoneal rupture of the urinary bladder in children. Radiology 1989;170:487-488.

212. Mezzacappa PM, Price AP, Kassner EG, et al. Cohen ureteral reimplantation: sonographic appearance. Radiology 1987;165:851-852.

213. Puri P, Pirker M, Mohanan N, et al. Subureteral dextranomer/hyaluronic acid injection as first line treatment in the management of high grade vesicoureteral reflux. J Urol 2006;176:1856-1859; discussion 1859-1860.

214. Hertzberg BS, Bowie JD, King LR, Webster GD. Augmentation and replacement cystoplasty: sonographic findings. Radiology 1987; 165:853-856.

215. Gundeti MS, Eng MK, Reynolds WS, Zagaja GP. Pediatric robotic-assisted laparoscopic augmentation ileocystoplasty and Mitrofanoff appendicovesicostomy: complete intracorporeal—initial case report. Urology 2008;72:1144-1147; discussion 1147.

Gastrointestinal Tract

216. Miller JH, Kemberling CR. Ultrasound of the pediatric gastrointestinal tract. Semin US CT MR 1987;8:349-365.

217. Carroll BA. Ultrasound of the gastrointestinal tract. Radiology 1989;172:605-608.

218. Gupta AK, Guglani B. Imaging of congenital anomalies of the gastrointestinal tract. Indian J Pediatr 2005;72:403-414.

219. Barki Y, Bar-Ziv J. Meconium ileus: ultrasonic diagnosis of intraluminal inspissated meconium. J Clin Ultrasound 1985;13:509-512.

220. Schuster SR, Teele RL. An analysis of ultrasound scanning as a guide in determination of "high" or "low" imperforate anus. J Pediatr Surg 1979;14:798-800.

221. Haber HP, Seitz G, Warmann SW, Fuchs J. Transperineal sonography for determination of the type of imperforate anus. AJR Am J Roentgenol 2007;189:1525-1529.

222. Jaramillo D, Lebowitz RL, Hendren WH. The cloacal malformation: radiologic findings and imaging recommendations. Radiology 1990;177:441-448.

223. Puylaert JB, van der Zant FM, Rijke AM. Sonography and the acute abdomen: practical considerations. AJR Am J Roentgenol 1997; 168:179-186.

224. Puylaert JB. Acute appendicitis: ultrasound evaluation using graded compression. Radiology 1986;158:355-360.

225. Wan MJ, Krahn M, Ungar WJ, et al. Acute appendicitis in young children: cost-effectiveness of US versus CT in diagnosis—a Markov decision analytic model. Radiology 2009;250:378-386.

226. Rosenberg HK, Goldberg BB. Pediatric radiology: sonography. In Margulis AR, Burhenne HJ, editors. Alimentary tract radiology. 4th ed. St Louis: Mosby; 1989. p. 1831-1857.

227. Kaneko K, Tsuda M. Ultrasound-based decision making in the treatment of acute appendicitis in children. J Pediatr Surg 2004; 39:1316-1320.

228. Borushok KF, Jeffrey Jr RB, Laing FC, Townsend RR. Sonographic diagnosis of perforation in patients with acute appendicitis. AJR Am J Roentgenol 1990;154:275-278.

229. Baker DE, Silver TM, Coran AG, McMillin KI. Postappendectomy fluid collections in children: incidence, nature, and evolution evaluated using ultrasound. Radiology 1986;161:341-344.

230. Gervais DA, Brown SD, Connolly SA, et al. Percutaneous imaging-guided abdominal and pelvic abscess drainage in children. Radiographics 2004;24:737-754.

231. Quillin SP, Siegel MJ. Appendicitis: efficacy of color Doppler sonography. Radiology 1994;191:557-560.

232. Quillin SP, Siegel MJ. Diagnosis of appendiceal abscess in children with acute appendicitis: value of color Doppler sonography. AJR Am J Roentgenol 1995;164:1251-1254.

233. Dinkel E, Dittrich M, Peters H, Baumann W. Real-time ultrasound in Crohn's disease: characteristic features and clinical implications. Pediatr Radiol 1986;16:8-12.

234. Puylaert JB. Mesenteric adenitis and acute terminal ileitis: ultrasound evaluation using graded compression. Radiology 1986;161: 691-695.

Presacral Masses

235. Rescorla FJ, Sawin RS, Coran AG, et al. Long-term outcome for infants and children with sacrococcygeal teratoma: a report from the Childrens Cancer Group. J Pediatr Surg 1998;33:171-176.

236. Miller JH, Sato JK. Adrenal origin tumors. In Miller JH, editor. Imaging in pediatric oncology. Baltimore: Williams & Wilkins; 1985. p. 305-340.

237. Kangarloo H, Fine RN. Sonographic evaluation of children with urinary retention caused by an extragonadal pelvic mass. Int J Pediatr Nephrol 1985;6:137-142.

238. Watanabe M, Komuro H, Kaneko M, et al. A rare case of presacral cystic neuroblastoma in an infant. J Pediatr Surg 2008;43:1376-1379.

239. Neifeld JP, Godwin D, Berg JW, Salzberg AM. Prognostic features of pediatric soft tissue sarcomas. Surgery 1985;98:93-97.

CHAPTER 57

The Pediatric Hip and Musculoskeletal Ultrasound

Leslie E. Grissom and H. Theodore Harcke

Chapter Outline

Ultrasound has been widely used in the diagnosis and management of developmental dysplasia of the hip (DDH), although many other applications for sonography of the pediatric musculoskeletal system have been developed. Ultrasound is ideally suited to the evaluation of the immature skeleton and associated soft tissues because of visualization of the cartilage found in large amounts in developing bones and because of the lack of ionizing radiation. Other advantages include the ability to perform dynamic evaluations and to examine children without sedation. With some applications, including DDH, sonography may replace other imaging studies; in other cases, sonography complements radiography to aid in the diagnosis. In this chapter we review the use of ultrasound in DDH and also describe briefly its use in other pediatric musculoskeletal conditions, including congenital, inflammatory, and traumatic abnormalities. Ultrasound of the pediatric spine is discussed in Chapter 51; fetal spine sonography is discussed in Chapter 35.

HIP ULTRASOUND

The use of ultrasound to assess the hip has gained wide acceptance and is the primary focus of this chapter. Hip sonography offers clear advantages over other imaging techniques in two specific areas in pediatrics: DDH and hip pain. **Developmental dislocation and/or dysplasia of the hip** (DDH), formerly called "congenital dislocation of the hip," usually manifests in the first year of life. At that age, the femoral head and acetabulum consist of cartilage components that are clearly identified by ultrasound. Real-time sonography allows assessment of the hip in multiple planes, both at rest and with movement. Ultrasound can replace radiographic studies and reduce radiation exposure to the young infant. **Hip pain** is a common presenting symptom throughout the pediatric age range and results from a number of inflammatory and traumatic conditions. Early in the course of these conditions, radiographic findings are absent or limited to subtle soft tissue changes. The sonographic detection of fluid in the hip joint is an important finding that may lead to diagnostic aspiration.

DEVELOPMENTAL DISLOCATION AND DYSPLASIA OF THE HIP

Clinical Overview

Early detection of an abnormality in the infant hip is the key to successful management. If treatment is begun at a young age, most of the sequelae that occur when DDH goes unrecognized until walking age can be prevented. Clinical screening programs have been instituted, and primary care physicians are taught to evaluate the hips as part of the newborn physical examination. Historically, infants with abnormal clinical examinations were referred for plain radiographic film examinations.

Ultrasound has now become the preferred technique for diagnosis and management of DDH in the first 6 to 8 months of life.[1]

The incidence of DDH varies throughout the world. In whites, overt dislocation is reported to be 1.5 to 1.7 per 1000 live births.[2,3] When lesser degrees of abnormality such as subluxation are included, as many as 10 infants per 1000 live births may show some features of the disorder.[4]

The cause of DDH is multifactorial, with both physiologic and mechanical factors playing a role. Maternal-fetal interaction influences the development of hip problems in both categories. Maternal estrogens and hormones that affect pelvic relaxation just before delivery are believed to lead to temporary laxity of the hip capsule in the perinatal period. Most fetuses are exposed to extrinsic forces in the later weeks of pregnancy because of their increasing size and the diminishing volume of amniotic fluid. It is theorized that these forces, although gentle, can lead to deformation if persistently applied.[5] There is an increased incidence of DDH in infants born in the breech position, infants with a positive family history of DDH, in firstborns, and in pregnancy with oligohydramnios. Infants with skull-molding deformities, congenital torticollis, and foot deformities are also at increased risk for DDH.[6]

RISK FACTORS FOR DDH

Family history of DDH
Firstborn child
Oligohydramnios
Breech delivery
Skull-molding deformities
Congenital torticollis
Foot deformities

DDH, Developmental dislocation and/or dysplasia of the hip.

The mechanism of a typical dislocation is thought to be a gradual migration of the femoral head from the acetabulum because of the loose, elastic joint capsule. In the newborn period, the head usually dislocates in a lateral and posterosuperior position relative to the acetabulum. The displaced femoral head can usually be reduced, and the joint components typically do not have any major deformity. When dislocation is not recognized in early infancy, the muscles tighten and limit movement. The acetabulum becomes dysplastic because it lacks the stimulus of the femoral head. Ligamentous structures stretch, and fibrofatty tissue occupies the acetabulum. Thus, it becomes impossible to return the femoral head to the acetabulum with simple manipulation; a **pseudoacetabulum** may form where the femoral head rests superolaterally.

There is some evidence of familial **acetabular dysplasia,**[7] although this is not considered a cause in most cases. Another form of hip dislocation and dysplasia is the **teratologic dislocation** that occurs early in fetal life. In these cases, the infant exhibits advanced adaptive changes in the pelvis and femoral head. The clinical and radiographic findings are more obvious, and this uncommon form of hip dislocation has a poor prognosis.[8]

Development of Hip Sonography

The first in-depth use of sonography was performed by Graf,[9] an Austrian orthopedic surgeon. He used an articulated-arm B-scan unit and developed an evaluation technique based on a coronal image of the hip. Scanning was performed from the lateral approach with the femur in its anatomic position. Graf's method established ultrasound's ability to distinguish the cartilage, bone, and soft tissue structures that compose the immature hip joint.

With real-time sonographic equipment, sonographers have experimented with different views. This has led to an alternative approach to hip sonography that emphasizes dynamic assessment of the hip in multiple positions.[10,11] Although two basic philosophies evolved, **morphologic** and **dynamic,** it is recognized that the two methods have common features. Both approaches recognize the need for critical landmarks of the femur and acetabulum. The dynamic technique, as proposed by Harcke et al.,[11,12] in addition to stressing positional relationships and stability, included assessment of critical acetabular landmarks. This formed the basis for an examination drawing on elements from both techniques,[12,13] which has become the technique recommended by the American College of Radiology (ACR)[14] and the American Institute of Ultrasound in Medicine (AIUM).[15]

Dynamic Sonographic Technique: Normal and Pathologic Anatomy

Technical Factors

Hip sonography should be performed with real-time linear array transducers. Although sector scanners were initially used with success,[16] current preference is for the linear configuration because of the greater accuracy of representation. Also, acetabular measurements reported in the literature are made with a linear transducer. One should use the highest-frequency transducer that provides adequate penetration of the soft tissues to the depth required. For infants up to 6 months of age, the 15-8 MHz broadband digital transducer is successful. A lower-frequency transducer may be required for infants older than 6 months.

All scanning is performed from the lateral or posterolateral aspect of the hip, moving the hip from the neutral position at rest to a position in which the hip is flexed. With the hip flexed, the femur is moved through a range of abduction and adduction, with stress views performed

MINIMUM ACR STANDARD EXAMINATION FOR DDH*

- The diagnostic examination for DDH incorporates two orthogonal planes: a coronal view in the standard plane at rest and a transverse view of the flexed hip with and without stress. This enables an assessment of hip position, stability,[1] and morphology when the study is correctly performed and interpreted. It should be noted that additional views and maneuvers can be obtained and that these may enhance the confidence of the examiner.
- Morphology is assessed at rest. The stress maneuvers follow those prescribed in the clinical examination of the hip and assess femoral stability.
- The attempts to dislocate the femoral head or reduce a displaced head are analogous to the Barlow and Ortolani tests used in the clinical examination. It is important that the infant is relaxed when hips are assessed for instability. It is acceptable to perform the standard examination with the infant in a supine or lateral position.[14]

*Modified from American College of Radiology standard for developmental dislocation and/or dysplasia of the hip.

in the flexed position. One aspect of hip sonography relevant to dynamic examinations is the shift of the transducer between the examiner's hands when examining the right and left hip. The infant is lying supine with the feet toward the sonographer. When examining the left hip, the sonographer grasps the infant's left leg with the left hand, and the transducer is held in the right hand. When the right hip is examined, we recommend that the sonographer hold the transducer in the left hand and use the right hand to manipulate the infant's right leg. Although sonographers find this awkward at first, ambidexterity is easily mastered. We found that this technique makes it possible to perform the stress maneuver more reliably and better maintain the planes of interest.

To obtain a satisfactory examination, the infant should be relaxed. Infants can be fed before or during the examination. Toys and other devices to attract the infant's attention are helpful and can be used as sonography is being performed. A parent can hold the infant's arms or head and can talk to the infant. There is no need for sedation. The upper body may remain clothed. Our standard practice is to leave the infant diapered and expose only the side of the hip being examined (strongly recommended for boys).

The anatomy is considered in four different views. It is our routine practice to record images in each of these views for permanent records. This standardizes the examination and, in our institution, provides a guideline for the technologist who performs the initial

examination. In describing the four views, we use a two-word combination that indicates the plane of the transducer with respect to the body (**transverse** or **coronal**) and the position of the hips (**neutral** or **flexed**).

It is the objective of the dynamic hip assessment to determine the position and stability of the **femoral head,** as well as the development of the **acetabulum.** With a normally positioned hip, the femoral head is congruently positioned within the acetabulum. Mild displacement, such as when the head is in contact with part of the acetabulum or is displaced but partly covered, is referred to as **subluxation.** The **dislocated hip** has no contact with or coverage by the acetabulum. A change in position of the femur may change the relationship of the femoral head and acetabulum. A hip that is subluxated in the neutral or rest position may not seat itself with flexion and abduction. A dislocated hip may improve its position and partially reduce to a subluxated position. This is, in fact, a principle of treatment.

The stability of the hip is determined through motion and the application of stress. The **stress maneuvers** are the imaging counterparts of the clinical Barlow and Ortolani maneuvers, which are the basis for the clinical detection of a hip abnormality. The **Barlow test** determines whether the hip can be dislocated. The hip is flexed and the thigh brought into the adducted position. The gentle push posteriorly can demonstrate instability by causing the femoral head to move out of the acetabulum.[2] The **Ortolani test** determines whether the dislocated hip can be reduced. As the flexed, dislocated hip is abducted into a frog-leg position, the examiner feels a vibration or "clunk" that results when the femoral head returns to the acetabulum.[8] During dynamic hip sonography, stress maneuvers are performed in a manner analogous to the Barlow and Ortolani clinical maneuvers. The **normal hip** is always seated at rest, with motion, and during the application of stress. The lax hip is normally positioned at rest and shows mild subluxation with stress. It must, however, invariably remain within the confines of the acetabulum. The **subluxable hip** is displaced laterally at rest and is loose, but is not dislocatable. When a hip is able to be pushed out of the joint, it is considered to be "dislocatable." A **dislocated hip** may be able to be returned to the acetabulum with traction and abduction. This hip is distinguished from the most severe form of DDH, in which the femoral head is dislocated and cannot be reduced.

At birth, the proximal femur and much of the acetabulum are composed of cartilage. On sonographic examination, **cartilage** is hypoechoic compared with soft tissue, so it is easy to distinguish. A few scattered specular echoes can be visualized within the cartilage when high-frequency transducers are used and technique adjustments are optimally set. The acetabulum is composed of both bone and cartilage. At birth, the bony ossification centers in the ilium, ischium, and pubis are separated by the **triradiate cartilage,** which has a Y configuration. A cartilaginous acetabular rim (the **labrum**) extends outward from the acetabulum to form the cup that normally contains the femoral head. Most of the acetabular cartilage has an echogenicity similar to the femoral head. It is still possible to determine the **joint line,** which distinguishes the cartilaginous acetabulum from the femoral head, by simply rotating the femur. More pronounced movement of the hip often creates echoes within the joint space, probably as a result of the formation of microbubbles. At the lateral margin of the labrum, the hyaline cartilage changes to fibrocartilage, and this shows increased echogenicity. The **echogenic hip capsule,** composed of fibrous tissue, borders the femoral head laterally. The bony components of the hip reflect all of the sound beam from their surface. This creates a bright linear or curvilinear appearance on the sonogram, indicating the contour of the osseous surfaces in that plane.

Radiographically, the **ossification center** of the femoral head is recognized between the second and eighth months of life. It is typically seen earlier in females than in males, and there is a wide normal variation for the time of appearance. Although some asymmetry between the left and right hips can be normal, both in time of appearance and in size, delayed appearance and development are associated with DDH. Hip sonograms reflect the development of the ossification center and can be used to document the development of the center.[17] The ossification center can be found by ultrasound several weeks before it is visible radiographically. Initially, a confluence of blood vessels produces increased echoes within the cartilage. This precedes actual ossification. As ossification begins, the calcium content is insufficient to produce a visible radiographic density; however, the sound waves are reflected. With maturation, the size of the ossification center increases. In early development, the echoes from the center have a punctate appearance, whereas later in the first year of life, the growth in size gives it a curvilinear margin. As the normal infant approaches 1 year of age, the size of the ossification center precludes accurate determination of medial acetabular landmarks. We believe that sonography of the hip is practical only up to 8 months of age, unless there is delayed ossification of the femoral head. Between 6 months and 1 year of age, radiography becomes more reliable. Usually by 1 year of age, the femoral ossification center is large enough to prevent good visualization of the acetabulum.[15] The presence and size of the ossific nucleus can be evaluated in all four views: coronal/neutral, coronal/flexion, transverse/flexion, and transverse/neutral.

Coronal/Neutral View

The coronal/neutral view, which forms the basis for the morphologic technique, is performed from the lateral aspect of the joint with the plane of the ultrasound beam oriented coronally with respect to the hip joint.

The femur is maintained with a physiologic amount of flexion. Graf[18] recommends the use of a special device that allows the infant to be maintained in a lateral decubitus position while the hip is being examined, but the coronal/neutral view can also be performed with the patient supine (Fig. 57-1, *A*). The transducer is placed on the lateral aspect of the hip, and the hip is scanned until a standard plane of section is obtained (Fig. 57-1, *A-C*). The plane must precisely demonstrate the midportion of the acetabulum, with the straight iliac line superiorly and the inferior tip of the os ilium seen medially within the acetabulum. The echogenic tip of the labrum should also be visualized. The alpha and beta angles, if measured, relate to fixed points on the bony and cartilaginous components of the acetabulum[18] (Fig. 57-1, *D*), and the exact plane must be obtained for the measurements to be reliable. The similarity can be noticed between the appearance of the acetabulum in this view and in the **coronal/flexion view** (Fig. 57-2, *C*). The difference is that the bony shaft (metaphysis) of the femoral neck is visualized below the femoral head in the coronal/neutral projection. In the coronal/flexion view, the femoral shaft is not in the plane of examination because the femur is flexed. A stability test can be performed in this view by gently pushing and pulling the infant's leg. This helps to verify deformity of the acetabulum and to identify craniodorsal movement of the femoral head under pressure. Zieger et al.[19] proposed a further adaptation of this view, advocating flexion and adduction of the hip to identify lateral displacement when instability is present. This is similar to the coronal/flexion stress view.

In the **normal coronal/neutral view** the femoral head is resting against the bony acetabulum. The acetabular roof should have a concave configuration and cover at least half the femoral head. The cartilage of the acetabular roof is hypoechoic and extends lateral to the acetabular lip, terminating in the labrum, which is composed of fibrocartilage and is echogenic (Fig. 57-1, *C*). When a hip becomes subluxed or dislocated, the femoral head gradually migrates laterally and superiorly, with progressively decreased coverage of the femoral head (Fig. 57-1, *E*). In hip dysplasia the acetabular roof is irregular and angled, and the labrum is deflected superiorly and becomes echogenic and thickened. When the hip is frankly dislocated, the labrum may be deformed. Echogenic soft tissue is interposed between the femoral head and the bony acetabulum. A combination of **deformed labrum** and **fibrofatty tissue (pulvinar)** prevents the hip from being reduced.

The acetabulum can be assessed visually or with measurements, noting the depth and angulation of the acetabular roof, as well as the appearance of the labrum (Fig. 57-1, *F*). This can be seen in both coronal/neutral and coronal/flexion views and is described in the report. Morin et al.[20,21] correlated coverage of the femoral head by the bony acetabulum with measurements of the

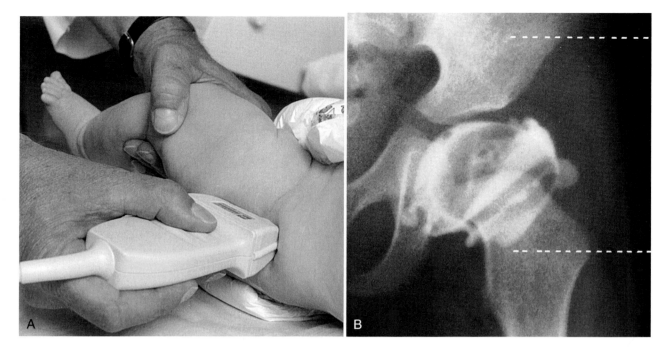

FIGURE 57-1. Coronal/neutral view. A, Linear array transducer is placed coronal and lateral with respect to the hip. The femur is in "physiologic neutral" for the infant (slight hip flexion). **B,** Scan area *(dotted lines)* on arthrogram.

acetabular angle. This assessment relates acetabular depth (d) to the diameter of the femoral head (D) and is expressed as percent (d/D × 100) coverage of the femoral head. These data showed that normal radiographic measurements always had a femoral head coverage that exceeded 58%, and that clearly abnormal radiographic measurements had coverage of less than 33%. This information should be used with caution because there is a significant group of intermediate values for which sonographic and radiographic measurements do not correlate. We have also noted cases in which sonography showed the acetabulum to be better developed than it appeared radiographically, and on occasion, we have seen an acetabulum that looked more well developed radiographically than on ultrasound.[22] This discrepancy occurs because the radiograph is a two-dimensional projection of the three-dimensional pelvis, and the sonogram is one selected coronal slice that may not match the projection.

Classification of hip joints may also be based on the measurement of the alpha and beta angles (Fig. 57-1, *D* and *F*). The **alpha angle** measures the inclination of the posterior and superior osseous acetabular rim with respect to the lateral margin of the iliac bone (baseline). The **beta angle** is formed by the baseline iliac bone and the inclination of the anterior cartilaginous acetabular roof, for which the tip of the labrum is its key landmark. Ultrasound units may contain software that facilitates measurement of these angles. Four basic hip types have been proposed on the basis of alpha and beta measurements.[18] Most of these subtypes have been subdivided,

and small changes in angular measurements can result in a change in category. The reproducibility of angular measurements and subtypes has been a point of considerable discussion. In Europe, classification by measurement has been based on large numbers of infants examined. Some examiners have experienced problems with the use of measurements,[19,20,23-25] but those who adhere strictly to the technique find acceptable reproducibility.[26-28]

Coronal/Flexion View

In the coronal/flexion view the transducer is maintained in a coronal plane with respect to the acetabulum (Fig. 57-2, *A*) while the hip is moved to a 90-degree angle of flexion. During the assessment in this view, the transducer is moved in an anteroposterior direction with respect to the body to visualize the entire hip. Anterior to the femoral head, the curvilinear margin of the bony femoral shaft is identified. In the midportion of the acetabulum, the normally positioned femoral head is surrounded by echoes from the bony acetabular components (Fig. 57-2, *B* and *C*). Superiorly, the lateral margin of the iliac bone is seen, and the transducer position must be adjusted so the iliac bone becomes a straight horizontal line on the monitor. This landmark (iliac bone line: flat and straight) is a key to accurately visualizing the midacetabulum and to obtaining the maximum depth of the acetabulum. When the transducer is positioned too anteriorly, the iliac line is inclined laterally, and if positioned too posteriorly, the iliac line exhibits some

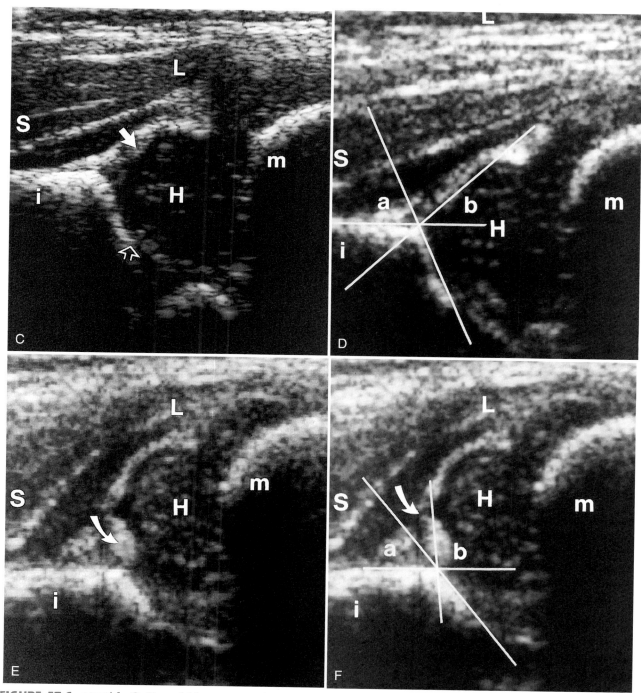

FIGURE 57-1, cont'd. C, Normal hip sonogram shows sonolucent femoral head *(H)* resting against the bony acetabulum. Note fibrocartilaginous tip of labrum *(solid arrow)* and junction of bony ilium and triradiate cartilage *(open arrow)*. **D, Normal hip** sonogram with alpha *(a)* and beta *(b)* angles used in measurement. **E, Dislocated hip** sonogram shows displacement of femoral head *(H)* laterally with deformity of labrum *(curved arrow)*. **F, Dislocated hip** sonogram with abnormal alpha and beta angles. *H,* Femoral head; *i,* iliac line; *L,* lateral; *m,* femoral metaphysis; *S,* superior.

concavity. When the plane is not correctly selected, it could be falsely concluded that the acetabulum is maldeveloped. A **normal hip** gives the appearance of a **"ball on a spoon"** in the midacetabulum. The femoral head represents the ball; the acetabulum forms the bowl of the spoon; and the iliac line is the handle. When the trans-

ducer is moved posteriorly and the scan plane is over the posterior margin of the acetabulum, the posterior lip of the triradiate cartilage becomes an easily recognized landmark. The bone above and below the cartilage notch is flat, and the normally positioned femoral head is not visualized (**Videos 57-1** and **57-2**).

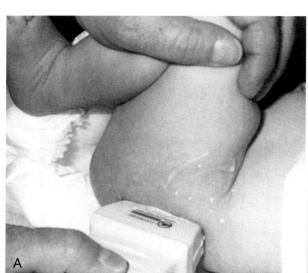
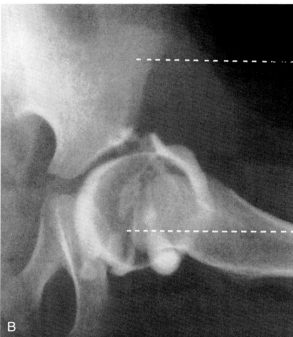

FIGURE 57-2. **Coronal/flexion view. A,** Linear array transducer is coronal to flexed femur. **B,** Scan area *(dotted lines)* on arthrogram. Coronal/flexion view.

In **subluxation** the femoral head is displaced laterally, posteriorly, or both, with respect to the acetabulum. Soft tissue echoes are seen between the femoral head and the bony reflections from the medial acetabulum. In **dislocation** the femoral head is completely out of the acetabulum (Fig. 57-2, *D*). With superior dislocations, the femoral head may rest against the iliac bone. In posterior dislocations, the femoral head is seen lateral to the posterior lip of the triradiate cartilage. The acetabulum is usually not visualized in a dislocation because the bony shaft of the femur blocks the view.

Dynamic examination in the coronal/flexion view has two components. The first is performed over the posterior lip using a **push-and-pull maneuver** (Fig. 57-2, *E* and *F*). In the normal hip the femoral head is never seen over the posterior lip of the acetabulum. When there is instability, a portion of the femoral head appears over the posterior lip of the triradiate cartilage as the femur is pushed. With a pull, the head disappears from the plane. In a dislocated hip the femoral head may be located over the posterior lip and may or may not move out of the plane with traction. The second component of the dynamic examination is performed over the midacetabulum. The Barlow-type maneuver is performed with **adduction** and gentle pushing against the knee. In the normal hip the femoral head will remain in place against the acetabulum. With subluxation or dislocation, the head will migrate laterally and posteriorly, and there will be echogenic soft tissue between the femoral head and the acetabulum (**Videos 57-3, 57-4, and 57-5**).

Transverse/Flexion View

Transition from the coronal/flexion view to the transverse/flexion view is accomplished by rotating the transducer 90 degrees and moving the transducer posteriorly so it is in a posterolateral position over the hip joint. The horizontal orientation of the scan plane with respect to the body is maintained (Fig. 57-3, *A*). The plane of the transducer and the landmarks are demonstrated on a computed tomography (CT) scan of a patient in a spica cast with a normal left and dislocated right hip (Fig. 57-3, *B*). Sonographically, the bony shaft and metaphysis of the femur give bright reflected echoes anteriorly, adjacent to the sonolucent femoral head. The echoes from the bony acetabulum appear posterior to the femoral head, and in the normal hip, a **U-shaped configuration** is produced by the metaphysis and the ischium (Fig. 57-3, *C*). The relationship of the femoral head and acetabulum is observed while the flexed hip is moved from maximum adduction to wide abduction. The sonogram changes its appearance in abduction and adduction. The deep, U-shaped configuration is produced with maximum abduction, whereas in adduction, a shallower, V-shaped appearance is observed. It is important to have the transducer positioned posterolaterally over the hip to see the medial acetabulum. When the transducer is not posterior enough, the view of the acetabulum is blocked by the femoral metaphysis, and the hip can appear falsely displaced. In **adduction** the hip is stressed with a **gentle posterior push** (a Barlow test). In the normal hip the femoral head will remain

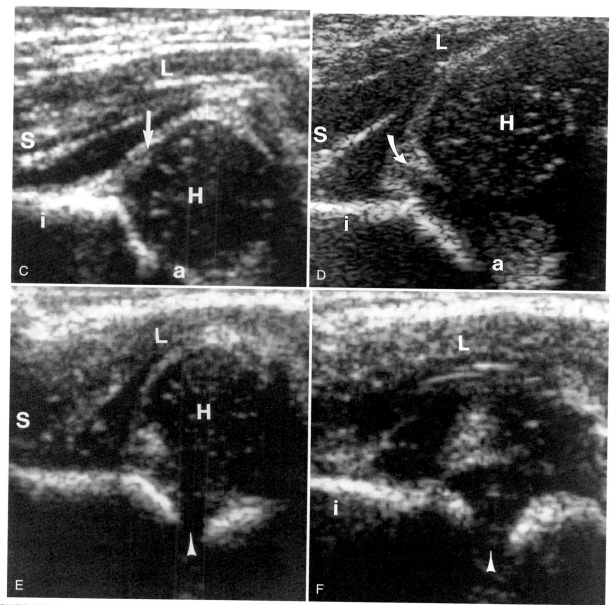

FIGURE 57-2, cont'd. C, Normal hip sonogram shows sonolucent femoral head *(H)* resting against bony acetabulum *(a)*. Note fibrocartilaginous tip of labrum *(arrow)*. *L,* Lateral; *S,* superior line; *i,* iliac line. **D to F, Dislocated hip** sonograms. **D,** Displacement of sonolucent femoral head *(H)* laterally and superiorly with deformity and increased echogenicity to labrum *(curved arrow)*. **E, Push maneuver** shows displacement of femoral head over posterior limb of triradiate cartilage *(arrowhead)*. **F, Pull maneuver** reveals head no longer positioned over triradiate cartilage *(arrowhead)* of posterior lip of acetabulum. (See also Videos 57-1 and 57-2: normal; Videos 57-3, 57-4, and 57-5: subluxation and dislocation.)

deeply in the acetabulum in contact with the ischium with stress. In **subluxation** the hip will be normally positioned or mildly displaced at rest, and there will be further lateral displacement from the medial acetabulum with stress, but the femoral head will remain in contact with a portion of the ischium. With **frank dislocation** the hip will be laterally and posteriorly displaced to the extent that the femoral head has no contact with the acetabulum, and the normal U-shaped configuration cannot be obtained (Fig. 57-3, *D*). The process of dislocation and reduction is able to be visualized in unstable hips in the transverse/flexion view. With abduction, the dislocated hip may be reduced, and this represents the sonographic counterpart of the Ortolani maneuver (**Videos 57-6, 57-7,** and **57-8**).

Transverse/Neutral View

The transition from the transverse/flexion view to the transverse/neutral view is accomplished by bringing the leg down into a physiologic neutral position. The transducer is directed horizontally into the acetabulum from

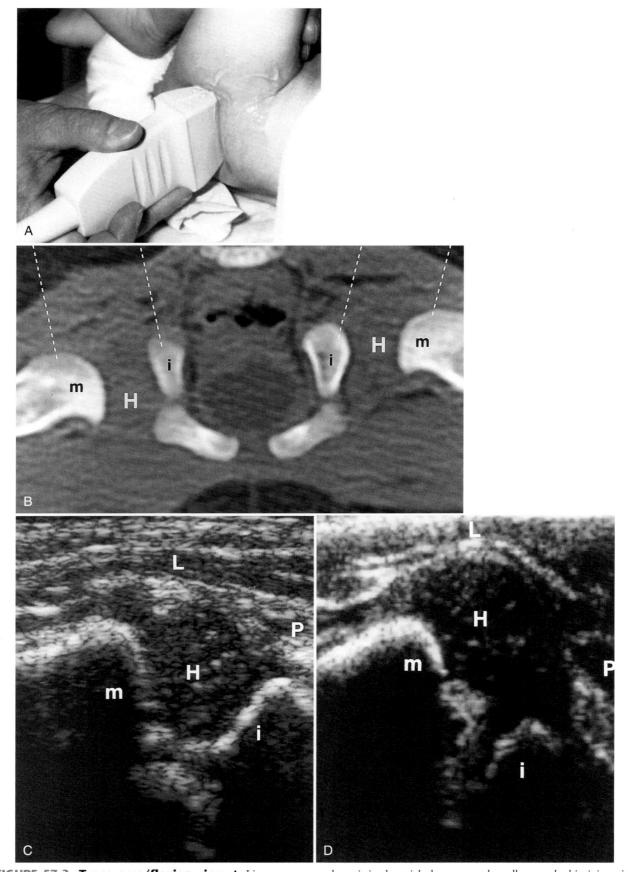

FIGURE 57-3. Transverse/flexion view. A, Linear array transducer is in the axial plane posterolaterally over the hip joint with the hip flexed. **B,** Scan area *(dotted lines)* on a prone CT scan. Scan demonstrates relationship of femoral head *(H)*, metaphysis *(m)*, and ischium *(i)* in a normal *(left)* hip, in the acetabulum, and dislocated *(right)* hip, femoral head displaced out of the acetabulum. **C, Normal hip s**onogram shows echolucent femoral head *(H)* surrounded by metaphysis *(m)* (anterior) and ischium *(i)* (posterior), forming a U around femoral head. *L,* Lateral; *P,* posterior. **D, Dislocated hip** sonogram shows sonolucent femoral head *(H)* displaced posterolaterally. The U configuration of normal metaphysis *(m)* and ischium *(i)* is not seen. (See also Video 57-6: normal; Video 57-7: subluxation; Video 57-8: dislocation.)

the lateral aspect of the hip (Fig. 57-4, *A*). The plane of interest is one that passes through the femoral head into the acetabulum at the center of the triradiate cartilage (Fig. 57-4, *B*). This can be located by beginning the examination caudally over the bony shaft of the femur. Moving cephalad, the transition from bone to cartilage in the proximal femur becomes apparent, and the circular cross section of the spherical femoral head is identified. In the normal hip the sonolucent femoral head is positioned against the bony acetabulum over the triradiate cartilage (Fig. 57-4, *C*). The elements of the sonogram resemble a flower. The **femoral head** represents the "bloom," and the echoes (from the **ischium** posteriorly and **pubis** anteriorly) form the "leaves" at its base. The "stem" is formed by echoes that pass through the **triradiate cartilage** into the area of acoustic shadowing created by the osseous structures. The cartilage over the pubis is thicker than over the ischium, so the head appears slightly displaced from the bone echoes anteriorly. When an ossific nucleus is present, echoes appear within the femoral head. The examiner must angle the plane of the transducer above or below the nucleus to identify the triradiate cartilage. Acoustic shadowing by the ossification center should not be mistaken for the triradiate cartilage because there are no echoes in the gap. The presence and size of an ossific nucleus can be evaluated in the transverse/neutral view. We do not use this view to assess acetabular development.

In the transverse/neutral view, malpositioned hips show soft tissue echoes between the femoral head and acetabulum (Fig. 57-4, *D*). The width and configuration of the gap depend on the nature of the displacement. With subluxation, the femoral head usually moves posteriorly and, in mild cases, remains in contact with the posterior aspect of the acetabulum. With more severe **subluxation**, lateral displacement accompanies the posterior migration. Most dislocations are lateral, posterior, and superior. Often, the **dislocated head** rests against some portion of the bony ilium. In this case, reflected echoes from the bone are apparent medially. **Inability to find the hypoechoic gap of the triradiate cartilage** distinguishes this hip from the normal hip. With some lateral dislocations, the femoral head does not rest against bone, and soft tissue echoes completely surround the sonolucent head.

ALTERNATIVE TECHNIQUES: ANTERIOR VIEWS

A number of anterior views have been described, and sonographers experienced in their use have indicated success with these views. In an early paper on real-time sonography, Novick et al.[10] reported an anterior view performed with the hip flexed and abducted. Gomes et al.[29] modified this approach with an anterior view that is also done with flexion and abduction but that

evaluates the hip in a slightly different plane. A dynamic stress test was incorporated to demonstrate the presence of instability. The anterior approach of Dahlstrom et al.[30] is performed with the patient supine and the hips flexed and abducted. The transducer is placed anterior to the hip joint and is centered over the femoral head with the plane of the sound beam parallel to the femoral neck. The image produced in a normal hip is an axial section through the acetabulum and a longitudinal section through the femoral head and neck[28] (Fig. 57-5, *A* and *B*). A Barlow or push maneuver can be performed to detect instability. *Complete dislocation* is considered to be present when femoral head displacement exceeds 50% of its diameter (Fig. 57-5, *C*). The anterior view is particularly useful in rigid abduction splints and casts in which the posterior aspect of the hip is covered.

Evaluation of the Infant at Risk

Sonography is most often used for evaluation of an infant with an abnormal physical examination or a DDH risk factor, such as positive family history, breech delivery, foot deformity, or torticollis. In these situations, ultrasound replaces the radiograph of the pelvis, which was routinely obtained in the past when hip abnormality was suspected. If a frankly dislocated hip is present, referral to orthopedics is appropriate. When the abnormal physical examination suggests less severe hip instability shortly after birth, sonography should not be done until at least 3 to 4 weeks of age because hip instability may resolve on its own. **Newborns with a risk factor for DDH should be checked at 4 to 6 weeks.** This avoids multiple examinations in cases of transient neonatal instability and immaturity related to maternal hormones. We examine each hip using the four dynamic sonographic views (Figs. 57-1 to 57-4) and report our findings with an emphasis on position and stability. **Femoral head position** is described as **normal, subluxed,** or **dislocated.** Dislocations are easy to determine, and we have had no difficulty with their identification. Sometimes it can be problematic to decide whether an abnormal hip, which is widely displaced, should be called subluxed or dislocated. Stability testing is reported as **normal, lax, subluxable, dislocatable** (for subluxed hips), and **reducible or irreducible** (for dislocated hips). When stress maneuvers are performed, it is important that the infant is relaxed; otherwise, inconsistency may be found between the sonographic and clinical examination findings and between serial ultrasound studies.

The **acetabulum** is assessed visually and is described as **normal, immature,** or **dysplastic.** More important are the development of the cartilaginous labrum and its coverage of the femoral head. Situations in which the bony component is steeply angled but the cartilage is well developed and covers the femoral head should be noted. Deformity and increased echogenicity of

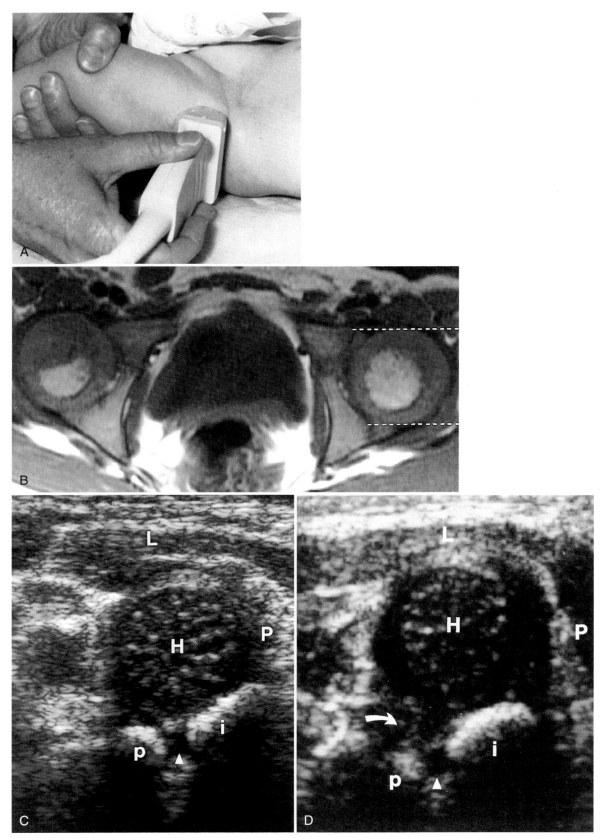

FIGURE 57-4. Transverse/neutral view. A, Linear array transducer is perpendicular to neutral femoral head in the plane of acetabulum. **B,** Scan area *(dotted lines)* on supine normal MRI. **C, Normal hip** sonogram shows sonolucent femoral head *(H)* centered over triradiate cartilage with pubis *(p)* (anterior) and ischium *(i)* (posterior). **D, Subluxed hip** sonogram shows sonolucent femoral head *(H)* displaced posterolaterally with gap between pubis *(p)* and femoral head *(arrow). Arrowhead,* Triradiate cartilage; *L,* lateral; *P,* posterior.

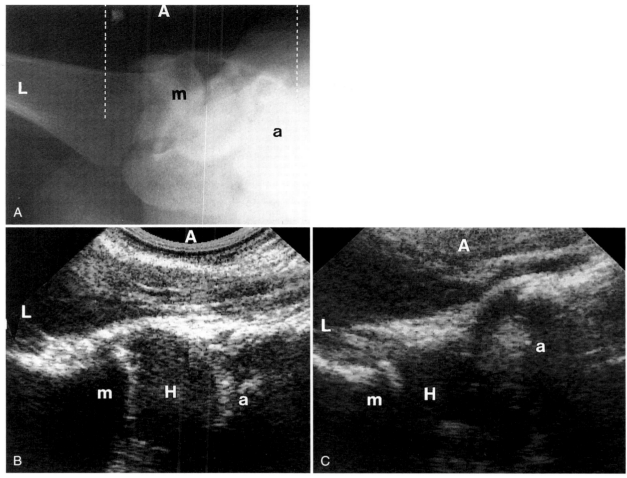

FIGURE 57-5. Anterior views (Dahlstrom). A, Scan area *(dotted lines)* on true lateral view of hip arthrogram; *A,* anterior; *L,* lateral; *m,* metaphysis; *a,* acetabulum. **B, Normal hip** sonogram shows sonolucent femoral head *(H)* bordered by metaphysis *(m)* laterally and acetabulum *(a)* medially. **C, Dislocated hip** sonogram shows posterior displacement of femoral head *(H)* and metaphysis *(m)*.

the cartilage are indications of more severe acetabular dysplasia.

Many reports attest to greater efficacy of sonography compared with the clinical and radiographic examination.[28-32] In young infants, ultrasound is able to detect hip laxity and malposition that is not apparent on the clinical and radiographic evaluations. Experience has indicated that most infants younger than 30 days have hip laxity that becomes normal after a few weeks without treatment. This is not a new observation; the phenomenon was recognized clinically by Barlow.[1] It identifies, however, a group of infants who need follow-up. Not all infants become normal, and these patients require continued observation.[28]

Evaluation during Treatment

The usefulness of sonography in the follow-up of infants with DDH, whether for observation of resolving abnormality or in conjunction with a defined treatment regimen, is widely accepted. Currently, sonography is routinely used to follow borderline cases, particularly in very young infants, before a commitment is made to a treatment regimen. When treatment is indicated, ultrasound is typically used to monitor hip position during treatment. Dynamic splints, such as the Pavlik harness, hold the hip in a flexed/abducted position. These restraints and similar devices are popular, and ultrasound has been tested as a way of monitoring hip position for infants in splint devices.[22,33,34] The sonographic examination in these patients is limited to the transverse/flexion and coronal/flexion views. The stress portion of the examination should not be performed unless requested. Typically, stress is not used until the conclusion of treatment, when weaning from the harness is instituted.

One of the problems with follow-up sonography has been its reliability in **morphologic assessment of the bony acetabulum.** Reports of discrepancies between the sonographic appearance of the bony acetabulum and the radiographic appearance indicate inexact correlation.[22] This may result from observer variation and the nature of the ultrasound measurements. We have chosen to include the pelvic radiograph as a baseline toward the end of the treatment protocol. The older the infant, the more we tend to consider radiography, particularly when the ossification centers are large. After successful treatment, continued monitoring of acetabular development by periodic radiographs is prudent. Residual acetabular dysplasia is reported in a small number of cases.[35]

At one time, in severe cases of DDH that required rigid casting, we removed a **plug** from the cast over the posterolateral aspect of the hip; this enabled us to evaluate the hip position using our standard views. Although this was successful for us and others,[15,36] there is a question of whether the reduction can be compromised by removal of the plaster plug. The use of anterior or groin views is possible; however, we have not been comfortable with those approaches. In our institution, infants in rigid casts are evaluated using CT. The localizer CT film enables the examiner to select one or two slices that are adequate to assess hip position. Attention to keeping the radiation dose low is key. Magnetic resonance imaging (MRI) is increasingly used and gives no ionizing radiation, although its high cost and unavailability are disadvantages.[37] Vascularity of the femoral head following reduction can be evaluated by adding contrast to the examination.[38]

Avascular necrosis of the femoral head is a recognized complication of DDH treatment devices. Both color and power Doppler ultrasound have been used to assess the vascularity of the femoral head during treatment. Because of the microvascular architecture in the cartilage canals, power Doppler sonography is thought to have the best potential. Normal hips show a radial pattern of flow from the center of the unossified head. The central collection of vessels is the precursor of the ossification center and is seen before the center is apparent on radiographs. Bearcroft et al.[39] reported that diminished flow can be demonstrated when the hip is placed in wide abduction, compressing the medial circumflex artery. This may correlate with development of avascular necrosis and has been proposed as an aid in determining a safe abduction position for treatment. The examination is technically difficult and currently performed primarily in the research arena.

Screening Program

The routine screening of all newborn infant hips with ultrasound has been a controversial issue. Based on a comparison between clinical and sonographic screening with sonography, Tonnis et al.[28] concluded that all newborns should be screened for DDH with ultrasound because it detects more pathologic joints than the clinical examination. In some European countries, routine screening has been tried on a regional basis. Critics of newborn screening programs note the high number of infants undergoing treatment or requiring follow-up studies (whether for minor instability or immaturity in acetabular development), but it is also recognized that studying only infants at risk will not eliminate late cases of DDH.[40,41] The current consensus in the United States is the net benefits of screening are not clearly established.

This opinion is based upon the fact that there is a high rate of spontaneous resolution of neonatal hip instability and dysplasia and lack of evidence that intervention affects outcomes for the population.[42] The American Academy of Pediatrics has published guidelines for pediatric examinations for the diagnosis of DDH.[43] Screening by clinical examination is recommended, and ultrasound is reserved for infants having an abnormal examination or risk factor.[44,45] According to the ACR 2008 practice guideline for the Performance of the Ultrasound Examination for Detection and Assessment of Developmental Dysplasia of the Hip,[14] indications for ultrasound of the infant hip include, but are not limited to, abnormal findings on physical or imaging examination of the hip, monitoring of patients with DDH treated with a Pavlik harness or other splint device, any family history of DDH, breech presentation regardless of gender, oligohydramnios and other uterine causes of postural molding and neuromuscular conditions.

INDICATIONS FOR HIP ULTRASOUND

1. Abnormal findings on physical or imaging examination of the hip.
2. Monitoring of patients with DDH treated with a Pavlik harness or other splint device.
3. Any family history of DDH.
4. Breech presentation regardless of gender.
5. Oligohydramnios and other uterine causes of postural molding.
6. Neuromuscular conditions.

DDH, Developmental dislocation/dysplasia of hip.

HIP JOINT EFFUSION

Clinical Overview

After 1 year of age, when sonography becomes unreliable for evaluation of DDH, it can be used to assess the painful hip. A variety of conditions cause hip pain in pediatric patients, including transient synovitis, osteomyelitis, Perthes' disease, slipped capital femoral epiphysis, fracture, and arthritis. Although radiography is performed initially and is often diagnostic, the plain radiographic film often is normal in the presence of small joint effusions. Sonography can be used to determine if an effusion is present and to guide arthrocentesis.

Sonographic Technique and Anatomy

The patient is examined in the supine position with the hips in the neutral position with as little flexion as possible. A high-frequency linear transducer is recommended. The hip is scanned in a sagittal, oblique plane along the long axis of the femoral neck (Fig. 57-6, *A* and *B*). The brightly echogenic anterior cortex of the femoral

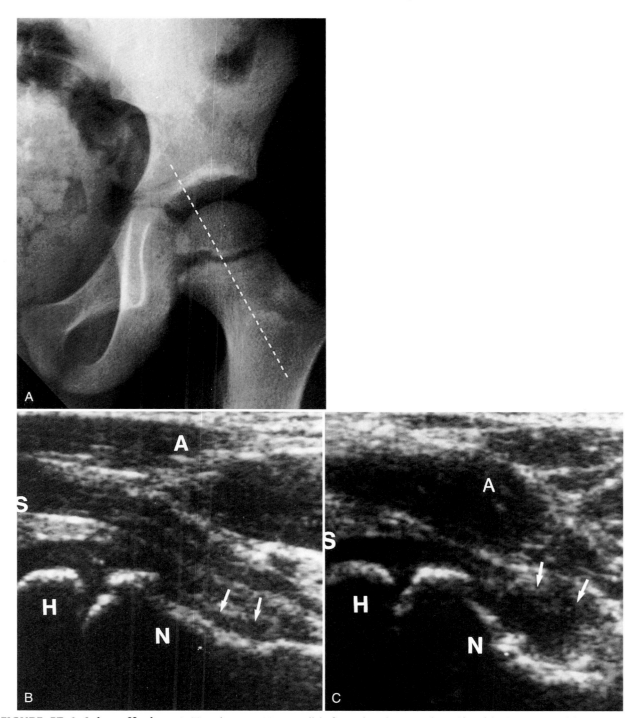

FIGURE 57-6. Joint effusion. A, Transducer position parallels femoral neck. Scan plane *(dotted line).* **B, Normal hip** sonogram shows joint capsule *(arrows)* following contours of femoral head *(H)* and neck *(N); A,* anterior; *S,* superior. **C, Hip effusion** sonogram shows bulging joint capsule *(arrows)* with mixed echogenicity within capsule caused by hemorrhage or inflammatory debris.

head and neck with the intervening echolucent physis is seen; the anterior margin of the bony acetabulum is visualized superiorly. The anterior recess of the joint capsule parallels the femoral neck in this area, with the outer margin forming an echogenic line anterior to the cortex of the femoral neck and extending over the femoral head (Fig. 57-6, *C*). The iliopsoas muscle is superficial to the capsule.

In the normal hip the joint capsule has a concave contour and the thickness of the capsule from the outer margin to the cortex of the femoral neck measures 2 to 5 mm. When there is a joint effusion, the anterior recess of the capsule becomes distended with a convex outer margin, and fluid is seen between the anterior and posterior layers of the joint capsule.[46] There is at least 2 mm of increased thickness of the abnormal joint capsule (Fig. 57-6, *C*) compared with the normal contralateral capsule[47-49] (Fig. 57-6, *B*). The use of measurements alone is problematic when both hips are abnormal, although this occurs infrequently.

Fluid of varying echogenicity is seen within the capsule. The echoes are created by inflammatory debris or hemorrhage.[48] Some studies have indicated specificity with regard to the appearance of the fluid. Zieger et al.[50] reported the fluid to be anechoic or hypoechoic in transient synovitis and more echogenic in septic arthritis, concluding that if the fluid is anechoic, the diagnosis of septic arthritis could be excluded. Other investigators have found the character of the fluid to be nonspecific,[47,51] describing echoes (probably representing hemorrhage) in the fluid in transient synovitis and anechoic fluid in cases of septic arthritis. Color Doppler sonography has also been used in an attempt to distinguish between infectious and noninfectious effusions, but the technique proved to be unreliable.[52]

When fluid is detected, **arthrocentesis** can be performed using sonographic guidance; a saline lavage can be used if fluid cannot be withdrawn. Although the procedure requires patient cooperation, it is relatively easy to perform and avoids the ionizing radiation required in fluoroscopic arthrocentesis. Some clinicians use arthrocentesis therapeutically in Perthes' disease because it reduces pain and allows a more normal range of motion.[48]

Other sonographic observations include fragmentation of the femoral head in Perthes' disease with thickened cartilage,[53] slippage of the head in slipped capital femoral epiphysis, and cortical disruption in fracture or osteomyelitis, but these findings are better evaluated radiographically. Soft tissue swelling and other soft tissue abnormalities outside the joint capsule have also been diagnosed.

Clinical Applications and Experience

Several large studies of sonographic hip joint **effusion** detection have been reported. They show the technique to be easy to master and rapidly performed. The results have been highly sensitive in the detection of effusion, with as little as 1 mm of fluid recognized experimentally. False-negative results have been reported in infants younger than 1 year,[50] probably because the femoral neck has not developed and the capsule is small. Fluid tends to surround the femoral head instead.

Although hip sonography is sensitive in the detection of effusion, its place in the workup of the painful hip varies from center to center. In one large series, although ultrasound facilitated early diagnosis or prompted further investigation in some patients, it altered the therapy or outcome in only 1% of the patients.[51] Another group recommends the use of a protocol to evaluate the painful hip using radiography, hip ultrasound, and scintigraphy as follows: when the radiographic findings are negative,

sonography is performed, to be followed by aspiration if there is an effusion or by bone scan if there is no effusion.[54]

At our institution, the workup of the **painful hip** is individualized, and we find hip sonography to be helpful in certain circumstances. When the clinical picture is unclear, the presence or absence of an effusion can guide the clinician in the diagnosis and the need for further evaluation. For example, in the patient with clinical and laboratory signs of transient **synovitis,** hip sonography may be used to demonstrate an effusion; however, the patient does not usually undergo joint aspiration. In a patient with hip pain and signs of **sepsis,** a bone scan or MRI is performed, regardless of the results of hip ultrasound, to exclude **osteomyelitis.** MRI provides a more detailed evaluation of localized disease, but bone scan has the advantage of global imaging of the skeleton.

OTHER PEDIATRIC MUSCULOSKELETAL ULTRASOUND APPLICATIONS

The sonographic technique used for pediatric musculoskeletal indications other than DDH is similar to hip ultrasound. Use of a high-frequency linear transducer is advised, with comparison to the contralateral unaffected side. Focal zones should be over the area of interest with the appropriate depth, and gain should be optimized for the tissues scanned.[55]

It is important for the sonographer to know the anatomy and obtain the proper landmarks to interpret the study correctly. In pediatric musculoskeletal sonography, knowledge of the normal appearance of cartilage and the ossification centers is essential (Fig. 57-7).

INFLAMMATION

Infection

Ultrasound can be used to evaluate pediatric patients for infection of the soft tissues. In infection of the osseous structures, it is used to supplement standard modalities.

Cellulitis (infection of subcutaneous soft tissues) and **pyomyositis** (infection of skeletal muscle) may be hematogenous or may originate from a puncture wound. Sonographically, there is heterogeneous soft tissue thickening and increased echogenicity in the affected area, and there may be regional adenopathy. If there is a puncture wound, foreign material may be present. Comparison to the contralateral unaffected side is helpful to make the diagnosis (Fig. 57-8). The inflammatory process can progress to abscess formation or necrosis. Although inflammatory debris within the abscess may be hypoechoic, it can also be isoechoic or even hyperechoic and difficult to appreciate.[56] In this situation, close

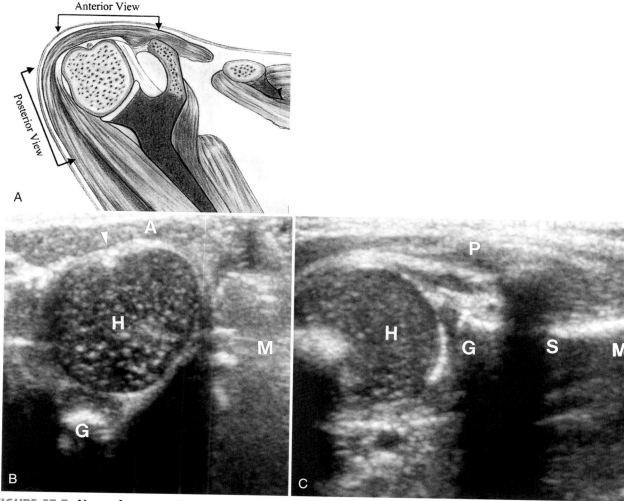

FIGURE 57-7. Normal neonatal shoulder. A, Illustration of anterior and posterior axial planes of interrogation of the shoulder. **B** and **C,** Sonograms of normal neonatal shoulder. **B,** Anterior axial image. Cartilaginous humeral head *(H)* anteriorly rests on glenoid *(G)* posteriorly. Biceps tendon *(arrowhead)* seen in the bicipital groove. **C,** Posterior axial image. Humeral head laterally and posterior margin of scapula medially. *A,* Anterior; *M,* medial; *P,* posterior; *S,* scapula. *(A from Grissom LE, Harcke HT. Infant shoulder sonography: technique, anatomy, and pathology. Pediatr Radiol 2001;31:863-868.)*

observation may reveal **movement of the echoes within the abscess.** Color and power Doppler may also assist in the diagnosis in that the rim of the abscess will demonstrate increased flow, and the debris within the cavity should be avascular.[57] If the fluid is mobile, motion may cause color or power signal on Doppler sonography, but spectral analysis will not reveal any true vascularity. Sonographic guidance can be used to biopsy or drain an abscess. A **recent hematoma, early myositis ossificans,** or a **necrotic mass** can have a similar appearance to an abscess, and the best way to distinguish infection from these entities is by clinical history and laboratory tests. In myositis ossificans and hematoma, after calcification develops, the echo pattern changes, and being mistaken for abscesses becomes unlikely.

Septic arthritis can be an isolated abnormality or can be secondary to infection in the adjacent soft tissues or bone. Fluid is seen in the joint, and debris may or may not be seen within it. When joint fluid is anechoic or hypoechoic, it is difficult to distinguish from the cartilage that caps the ends of the bones forming the joint. In addition, if there is debris in the fluid, it may be difficult to detect the septic effusion, similar to the soft-tissue abscess (Fig. 57-9). Movement of the joint will show the cartilage-fluid interface clearly. Application of pressure to the tissue around a joint will cause joint fluid to shift, making the fluid easier to recognize. Pressure from the sides and back of the knee, for example, can force fluid into the suprapatellar bursa, thereby confirming an effusion. Color or power Doppler sonography may help because there is hyperemia with infection, and the capsule may show increased flow,[58] but the absence of hyperemia does not exclude septic arthritis.[52] As with hip effusions, sonography can be used to aspirate fluid from the joints.[59]

Lyme disease, caused by the spirochete *Borrelia burgdorferi* and spread by deer ticks, can result in arthritis. This usually occurs in the subacute or chronic phase of

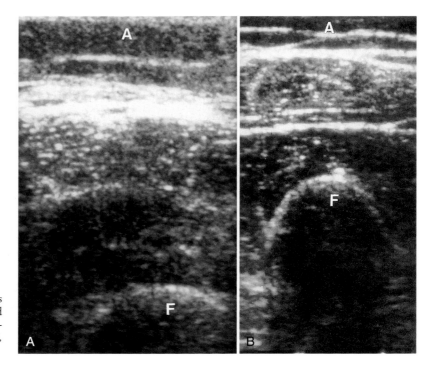

FIGURE 57-8. Cellulitis. Transverse images of the soft tissues of the thigh. **A,** Thickening and increased echogenicity of the soft tissues superficial to the femur *(F)* on the affected side; *A,* anterior. **B,** Normal side for comparison.

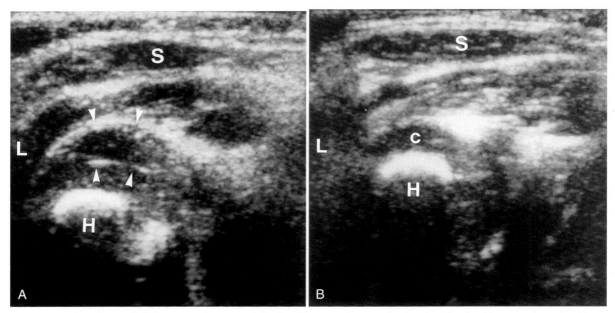

FIGURE 57-9. Septic arthritis. Coronal images of the shoulder. **A,** Echogenic fluid within the shoulder joint *(arrowheads)* superior to the humeral head *(H); c,* cartilage of humeral head; *L,* lateral; *S,* superior. **B,** Normal side for comparison.

the infection and is characterized by relapsing effusions, particularly in the knee joint. There may be synovial thickening, and cartilage loss is seen late in the course. This can be confused with juvenile rheumatoid arthritis, and the diagnosis should be considered in patients with oligoarticular joint effusions.[60]

Osteomyelitis typically occurs in the metaphyses of the long bones. The earliest sonographic sign is deep soft tissue swelling. Later signs are fluid along the cortex of the bone or, subperiosteally, fluid in the adjacent joint (either sterile or septic), and cortical disruption[61,62] (Fig. 57-10). Color and power Doppler sonography will show

increased flow at the margin of the elevated periosteum in advanced infection.[63] Osteomyelitis often spreads hematogenously in pediatric patients, so when it is detected in one location, examination of any other symptomatic areas is recommended. Some investigators examine all the extremities in this situation, particularly in infants who are difficult to assess clinically. A negative ultrasound does not exclude osteomyelitis.[64]

Cat-scratch fever is caused by a gram-negative bacillus and is characterized by fever and regional, sometimes suppurative, adenopathy occurring proximal to the affected area, for example, in the groin related to scratches

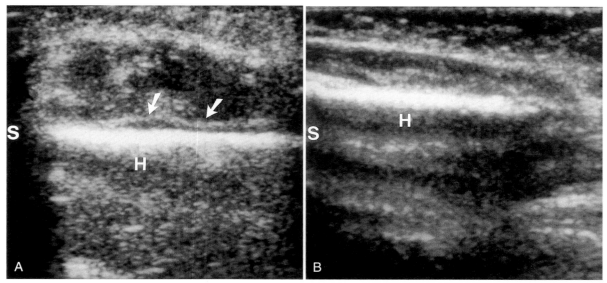

FIGURE 57-10. Osteomyelitis. Longitudinal sonogram of the humerus *(H)*; *S*, superior. **A,** Thickening and abnormal echogenicity of the soft tissues with fluid along the bone *(arrows)*. **B,** Normal side for comparison.

on the leg. These infected nodes are highly vascular[65] (Fig. 57-11). Patients with cat-scratch disease may also develop hypoechoic hepatic and splenic lesions.[66]

Noninfectious Inflammation

Sonography has been used to evaluate and to monitor the effects of treatment in pediatric patients with arthritis. **Synovitis** and **effusion** are often seen, and there is increased Doppler signal in the inflamed, thickened synovium. The cartilage can also be examined for decreased thickness, increased echogenicity, and erosive changes.[67-69] **Baker's cysts** occur in these patients, most often in the knee, and must be differentiated from a mass or deep venous thrombosis.

TRAUMA

Radiographs are the initial diagnostic modality used in evaluation of trauma, but sonography is a useful problem-solving tool when symptoms are present and radiographs are unrevealing. This applies to abnormalities such as growth plate fracture, soft tissue injury, retained non-opaque foreign body, and other soft tissue abnormalities, including Erb's palsy.

Sonography is an excellent means to detect a fracture through the growth plate, particularly in the infant when the epiphyses are not ossified. When searching for a fracture, it is important to study the bone from all possible angles. In the extremities, this may mean 360-degree visualization. By careful examination of the affected area and comparison to the contralateral normal side, one can confirm fracture findings and assess alignment. An **avulsion** or **metaphyseal fracture** may be detected that is not seen radiographically. This can be

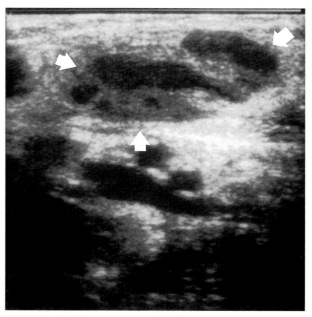

FIGURE 57-11. Cat-scratch disease. Enlarged inguinal lymph nodes *(arrows)* with increased vascularity *(gray areas)*.

especially useful in **nonaccidental trauma** (Fig. 57-12). The joint can be examined to differentiate fracture from dislocation and to diagnose secondary effusion. Care must be taken to distinguish fluid from cartilage because both are hypoechoic. Passive motion and compression help to eliminate confusion. With fracture, there is virtually always associated soft tissue abnormality, although this may be subtle and localized. The soft tissue planes become thickened by edema, and a small fluid collection may be present. **Hematoma** is initially hyperechoic with disruption of normal soft tissue planes, and later more

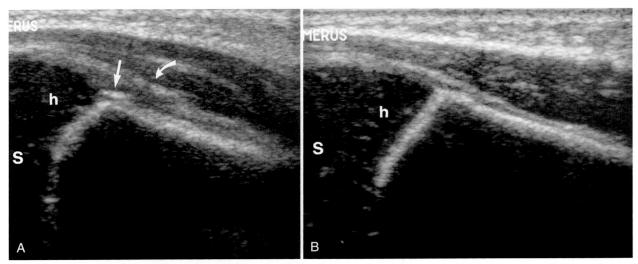

FIGURE 57-12. Infant with nonaccidental trauma. Longitudinal sonogram of shoulder. **A,** Metaphyseal fracture fragment *(straight arrow)* and soft tissue swelling *(curved arrow)* not detected on radiograph. **B,** Normal side for comparison. *h,* Humeral head; *S,* superior.

complex as it organizes and resorbs. If **myositis ossificans** develops, it will gradually ossify, starting peripherally, but the early appearance will be identical.[70,71]

Ultrasound is also useful in evaluation of soft tissue structures such as tendons, ligaments, and muscles. The musculoskeletal soft tissue components well visualized in adults can be seen in older children and adolescents, so techniques described in adult musculoskeletal sonography are generally applicable to pediatrics.[72,73] Although the larger tendons (e.g., Achilles, infrapatellar) can be seen at younger ages, the indications for ultrasound differ. For example, sonography can be used to diagnose and grade Osgood-Schlatter disease.[74,75]

Examination for retained nonradiopaque **foreign bodies** or localization of opaque foreign bodies is another indication for sonography. When foreign material is seen, the soft tissues can be examined for secondary inflammatory change, and sonography can provide guidance for removal and/or drainage[76] (Fig. 57-13).

Popliteal cysts often present in pediatric patients as a painless "swelling" or "soft tissue mass" behind the knee joint. Ultrasound is used to confirm the cystic nature of the mass. The cysts arise from the gastrocnemius-semimembranosus bursa and are lined with synovial fluid. They are deemed "idiopathic," and although many think these are posttraumatic, a trauma history is rarely elicited, and associated intra-articular pathology is rare.[77] Popliteal cysts are considered to be different from those found in childhood arthritis.[78] These cysts are usually oval with a few septations but no solid tissue, located posteromedially in the popliteal fossa. Popliteal cysts can persist for years but do not rupture or become symptomatic. The natural history is spontaneous regression, so typically no treatment is recommended.[79] Whenever a cyst is seen in the area of a joint, **ganglion cyst** should also be considered.[80]

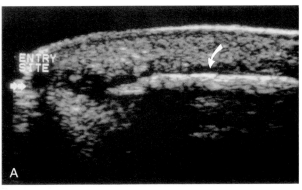

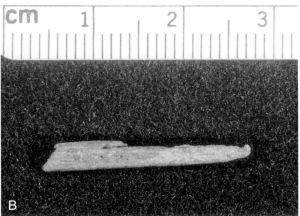

FIGURE 57-13. Foreign body. A, Sonographic image over a puncture wound in the foot. *Arrow,* Foreign body, entry site indicated. **B,** Linear foreign body proved to be a fragment of pencil.

Patients with Erb's palsy or **brachial plexus injury** from birth trauma present with a flaccid upper extremity, but patients with fractures of the metaphysis or clavicle can present similarly.[81] Scanning of the brachial plexus has been reported in infants. **Avulsed nerve**

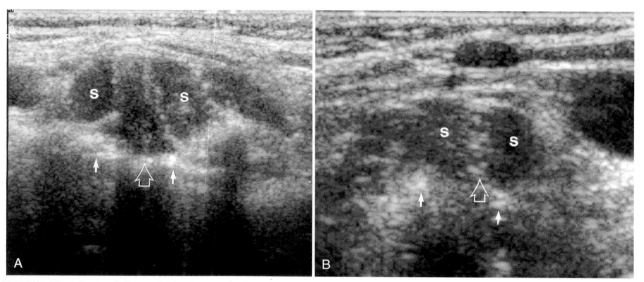

FIGURE 57-14. Avulsion of sixth cervical (C6) nerve root in an infant. Transverse image of interscalene region. *S,* Scalene muscle bony walls of the neural foramina *(solid arrows).* **A,** Thickened and hypoechoic injured nerve root *(open arrow).* **B,** Normal side for comparison. *(Courtesy Maura Valle, Genova, Italy.)*

roots, **meningoceles,** and **neurogenic tumors** can be demonstrated[82] (Fig. 57-14). Secondary subluxation or dislocation of the humeral head can be detected by scanning in multiple projections and using internal/external rotation of the humerus, again comparing the symptomatic and the contralateral normal sides. Normally the humeral head rests on the glenoid in all views. With subluxation the shoulder joint is widened with rotation, and in dislocation the humeral head will not be normally related to the glenoid.[83] Fractures of the clavicle or proximal humeral metaphysis can also be detected.

CONGENITAL ABNORMALITIES

Sonography can assist in characterizing congenital musculoskeletal abnormalities, including deficiency anomalies, such as **proximal femoral focal deficiency** (PFFD) and tibial hemimelia, congenital joint dislocations, teratologic hip dislocation, skeletal dysplasias with "atypical" hips, and fibromatosis colli. Ultrasound defines the cartilage and soft tissue elements that are not visible radiographically.

In PFFD and **tibial hemimelia,** there is a spectrum of abnormalities, and sonography can be used to define presence or absence of cartilaginous anlage and soft tissue structures that determine the subtype. When the subtype is established, the orthopedic surgeon can more accurately assess prognosis and treatment. Sonography is not intended to replace more definitive imaging, such as MRI, but to delay the need for this until the infant is older and treatment is being planned. In the case of PFFD, the presence and location of the femoral head and nonunion between the femoral head and the shaft are critical. The sonographic examination can be technically challenging because there is usually coxa vara and frequently also flexion contracture. There is the potential to misinterpret the elevated greater trochanter of the femur as a dislocated femoral head.[84] In tibial hemimelia the presence of patellar and tibial cartilage as well as the quadriceps tendon can be confirmed. Scanning from an anterior approach in the longitudinal plane, the cartilaginous patella is located, and, if present, the infrapatellar tendon can be traced to its distal insertion.[85] The cartilaginous tibial anlage can be measured. Voluntary and passive motion of the knee joint with real-time sonography is helpful in demonstrating function.

Congenital dislocations of the knee or elbow can be problematic radiographically because of the amount of cartilage making up the joints in the young infant. Often the question is not about the dislocation, but about the ability to reduce the dislocation and maintain stability with immobilization. Dynamic sonography provides a complete picture of the anatomic relationships and allows the joint components to be optimally positioned for splinting. Radial head dislocation can be anterior or posterior and is easily diagnosed sonographically, using a linear transducer and scanning the contralateral side for comparison. Knee dislocations result from in utero malposition (hyperextension). Dislocations can be evaluated sonographically for position and stability, as well as to establish the optimal degree of flexion before casting[86] (Fig. 57-15).

Foot anomalies, including **clubfoot** and **vertical talus,** have also been examined sonographically. Visualization of the unossified tarsal bones is possible, with studies focusing on these relationships and how readily they change with casting and surgery. Particular attention is given to the unossified tarsal navicular and its relationship to the medial malleolus.[87,88] In clubfoot (talipes) the navicular is medially displaced and smaller than normal; treatment by serial casting is intended to correct the alignment. Reports emphasize measurements of distance and angulation with the hope of differentiating feet that will respond to conservative treatment from those needing surgical correction.[89,90]

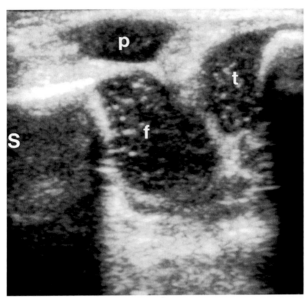

FIGURE 57-15. Knee dislocation. Anterior longitudinal view in extension; anterior displacement of the tibia corrected with partial flexion of the knee; *f,* distal femoral epiphysis; *p,* patella; *S,* superior; *t,* proximal tibial epiphysis.

Teratologic dislocation is considered a different entity than DDH. Teratologic hips are dislocated in utero and are seen in patients with various syndromes and neuromuscular disease. The sonographic findings at rest resemble those seen in the frank dislocations of DDH, but teratologic dislocation is more severe in that there is fixed positioning with minimal mobility. The dysplastic acetabula often cannot be accurately evaluated because they are obscured by the femoral shafts that project over the acetabula from dislocation of the femoral heads. The dynamic examination may be difficult because of soft tissue contractures.

While performing infant hip ultrasound examinations, the clinician occasionally encounters cases with morphologic features that vary from those typically seen in DDH. We use the phrase "atypical hip" to describe the findings in these hips, including echogenic cartilage and soft tissues, delayed ossification, and often coxa vara.[91,92] Patients with atypical hips include those with **spondyloepiphyseal dysplasia, meta-atropic dysplasia, cleidocranial dysplasia,** and **congenital myopathy.** In these conditions the hips are often dislocated with abnormal acetabula, mimicking DDH. As with PFFD, inexperienced sonographers can confuse the **elevated trochanter** with a laterally dislocated femoral head[84] (Fig. 57-16). The clue to the correct diagnosis is the increased echogenicity of the cartilage and of the muscles surrounding the hip joints.[91,93,94]

Fibromatosis colli is congenital thickening of the sternocleidomastoid muscle, usually secondary to

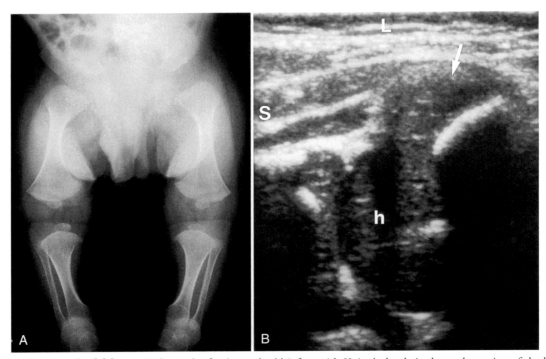

FIGURE 57-16. Atypical hip. A, Radiograph of a 4-month-old infant with Kniest's dysplasia shows shortening of the long bones and bulbous ends of the bones. **B,** Coronal neutral sonogram shows increased echogenicity of the cartilage and coxa vara with **elevation of the greater trochanter** *(arrow)* and narrowing of the acoustic window of the hip joint; *h,* femoral head; *L,* lateral; *S,* superior.

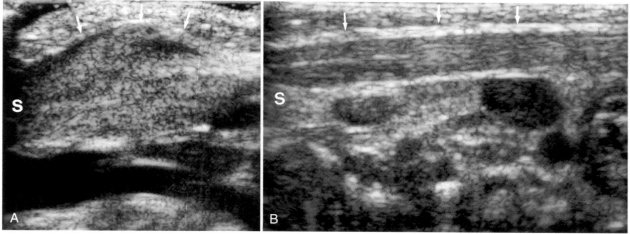

FIGURE 57-17. Fibromatosis colli. A, Longitudinal image of the sternocleidomastoid muscle *(arrows)* shows thickening and heterogeneous echogenicity. *S,* Superior. **B,** Normal side for comparison.

abnormal in utero positioning. These patients have an increased risk of DDH for the same reason. Patients usually present in the neonatal period with torticollis and are found on physical examination to have a unilateral anterior neck mass. Sonographic examination confirms the location of the mass in the muscle and demonstrates nodular and echogenic thickening of the muscle[95,96] (Fig. 57-17). The use of ultrasound can prevent more invasive testing and unnecessary biopsy when this benign condition is recognized.

CONCLUSION

Although DDH was the first and continues to be the most common single indication for musculoskeletal ultrasound in pediatric patients, many other uses have been explored and developed. The ability to discriminate between soft tissue structures and cartilage makes ultrasound especially helpful in pediatric patients. In this age of increasing concern regarding radiation, sonography has become an attractive alternative in the evaluation of the musculoskeletal system.

References

Developmental Dislocation and Dysplasia of the Hip

1. Harcke HT. Screening newborns for developmental dysplasia of the hip: the role of sonography. AJR Am J Roentgenol 1994;162:395-397.
2. Barlow TG. Early diagnosis and treatment of congenital dislocation of the hip. J Bone Joint Surg 1962;44B:292-301.
3. VonRosen S. Prevention of congenital dislocation of the hip joint in Sweden. Acta Orthop Scand 1970;130(Suppl):1-64.
4. Tredwell SJ, Bell HM. Efficacy of neonatal hip examination. J Pediatr Orthop 1981;1:61-65.
5. Dunn PM. Perinatal observations on the etiology of congenital dislocation of the hip. Clin Orthop Relat Res 1976:11-22.
6. MacEwen GD, Bassett GS. Current trends in the management of congenital dislocation of the hip. Int Orthop 1984;8:103-111.
7. Wynne-Davies R. Acetabular dysplasia and familial joint laxity: two etiological factors in congenital dislocation of the hip: a review of 589 patients and their families. J Bone Joint Surg 1970;52B:704-716.
8. Hensinger RN. Congenital dislocation of the hip: treatment in infancy to walking age. Orthop Clin North Am 1987;18:597-616.
9. Graf R. The diagnosis of congenital hip-joint dislocation by the ultrasonic Combound treatment. Arch Orthop Trauma Surg 1980;97:117-133.
10. Novick G, Ghelman B, Schneider M. Sonography of the neonatal and infant hip. AJR Am J Roentgenol 1983;141:639-645.
11. Harcke HT, Clarke NM, Lee MS, et al. Examination of the infant hip with real-time ultrasonography. J Ultrasound Med 1984;3:131-137.
12. Harcke HT, Grissom LE. Performing dynamic sonography of the infant hip. AJR Am J Roentgenol 1990;155:837-844.
13. Graf R. Ultrasonography of the infantile hip. In Sanders RC, Hill MC, editors. Ultrasound annual. New York: Raven Press; 1985. p. 177-186.
14. ACR practice guideline for the performance of ultrasound examination for detection and assessment of developmental dysplasia of the hip. American College of Radiology, 2008. www.acr.org.
15. American Institute of Ultrasound in Medicine (AIUM) practice guideline for the performance of an ultrasound examination for detection and assessment of developmental dysplasia of the hip. J Ultrasound Med 2009;28:114-119.
16. Harcke HT, Grissom LE. Sonographic evaluation of the infant hip. Semin Ultrasound 1986;7:331-338.
17. Harcke HT, Lee MS, Sinning L, et al. Ossification center of the infant hip: sonographic and radiographic correlation. AJR Am J Roentgenol 1986;147:317-321.
18. Graf R. Classification of hip joint dysplasia by means of sonography. Arch Orthop Trauma Surg 1984;102:248-255.
19. Zieger M, Hilpert S, Schulz RD. Ultrasound of the infant hip. Part 1. Basic principles. Pediatr Radiol 1986;16:483-487.
20. Morin C, Harcke HT, MacEwen GD. The infant hip: real-time US assessment of acetabular development. Radiology 1985;157:673-677.
21. Morin C, Zouaoui S, Delvalle-Fayada A, et al. Ultrasound assessment of the acetabulum in the infant hip. Acta Orthop Belg 1999;65:261-265.
22. Polanuer PA, Harcke HT, Bowen JR. Effective use of ultrasound in the management of congenital dislocation and/or dysplasia of the hip. Clin Orthop Relat Res 1990:176-181.
23. Zieger M. Ultrasound of the infant hip. Part 2. Validity of the method. Pediatr Radiol 1986;16:488-492.
24. Bialik V, Pery M, Kaftori JK, Fishman J. The use of ultrasound scanning in the management of developmental disorders of the hip. Int Orthop 1988;12:75-78.
25. Engesaeter LB, Wilson DJ, Nag D, Benson MK. Ultrasound and congenital dislocation of the hip: the importance of dynamic assessment. J Bone Joint Surg 1990;72B:197-201.

26. Langer R. Ultrasonic investigation of the hip in newborns in the diagnosis of congenital hip dislocation: classification and results of a screening program. Skeletal Radiol 1987;16:275-279.
27. Szoke N, Kuhl L, Heinrichs J. Ultrasound examination in the diagnosis of congenital hip dysplasia of newborns. J Pediatr Orthop 1988;8:12-16.
28. Tonnis D, Storch K, Ulbrich H. Results of newborn screening for CDH with and without sonography and correlation of risk factors. J Pediatr Orthop 1990;10:145-152.

Alternative Techniques: Anterior Views
29. Gomes H, Menanteau B, Motte J, Robiliard P. Sonography of the neonatal hip: a dynamic approach. Ann Radiol (Paris) 1987;30:503-510.
30. Dahlstrom H, Oberg L, Friberg S. Sonography in congenital dislocation of the hip. Acta Orthop Scand 1986;57:402-406.
31. Clarke NM, Harcke HT, McHugh P, et al. Real-time ultrasound in the diagnosis of congenital dislocation and dysplasia of the hip. J Bone Joint Surg 1985;67B:406-412.
32. Berman L, Klenerman L. Ultrasound screening for hip abnormalities: preliminary findings in 1001 neonates. Br Med J (Clin Res Ed) 1986;293:719-722.
33. Grissom LE, Harcke HT, Kumar SJ, et al. Ultrasound evaluation of hip position in the Pavlik harness. J Ultrasound Med 1988;7:1-6.
34. Dahlstrom H. Stabilization and development of the hip after closed reduction of late DDH. J Bone Joint Surg 1990;72B:9-12.
35. Alexiev VA, Harcke HT, Kumar SJ. Residual dysplasia after successful Pavlik harness treatment: early ultrasound predictors. J Pediatr Orthop 2006;26:16-23.
36. Boal DK, Schwenkter EP. The infant hip: assessment with real-time ultrasound. Radiology 1985;157:667-672.
37. McNally EG, Tasker A, Benson MK. MRI after operative reduction for developmental dysplasia of the hip. J Bone Joint Surg 1997;79B:724-726.
38. Tiderius C, Jaramillo D, Connolly S, et al. Post–closed reduction perfusion magnetic resonance imaging as a predictor of avascular necrosis in developmental hip dysplasia: a preliminary report. J Pediatr Orthop 2009;29:14-20.
39. Bearcroft PW, Berman LH, Robinson AH, Butler GJ. Vascularity of the neonatal femoral head: in vivo demonstration with power Doppler US. Radiology 1996;200:209-211.
40. Clarke NM, Clegg J, Al-Chalabi AN. Ultrasound screening of hips at risk for CDH. Failure to reduce the incidence of late cases. J Bone Joint Surg 1989;71B:9-12.
41. Rosendahl K, Markestad T, Lie RT. Ultrasound screening for developmental dysplasia of the hip in the neonate: the effect on treatment rate and prevalence of late cases. Pediatrics 1994;94:47-52.
42. Shipman SA, Helfand M, Moyer VA, Yawn BP. Screening for developmental dysplasia of the hip: a systematic literature review for the US Preventive Services Task Force. Pediatrics 2006;117:e557-e576.
43. Clinical practice guideline: early detection of developmental dysplasia of the hip. Committee on Quality Improvement, Subcommittee on Developmental Dysplasia of the Hip. American Academy of Pediatrics. Pediatrics 2000;105:896-905.
44. Boeree NR, Clarke NM. Ultrasound imaging and secondary screening for congenital dislocation of the hip. J Bone Joint Surg 1994;76B:525-533.
45. Harcke HT. The role of ultrasound in diagnosis and management of developmental dysplasia of the hip. Pediatr Radiol 1995;25:225-227.

Hip Joint Effusion
46. Robben SG, Lequin MH, Diepstraten AF, et al. Anterior joint capsule of the normal hip and in children with transient synovitis: ultrasound study with anatomic and histologic correlation. Radiology 1999;210:499-507.
47. Marchal GJ, Van Holsbeeck MT, Raes M, et al. Transient synovitis of the hip in children: role of ultrasound. Radiology 1987;162:825-828.
48. Alexander JE, Seibert JJ, Glasier CM, et al. High-resolution hip ultrasound in the limping child. J Clin Ultrasound 1989;17:19-24.
49. Kallio P, Ryoppy S, Jappinen S, et al. Ultrasonography in hip disease in children. Acta Orthop Scand 1985;56:367-371.
50. Zieger MM, Dorr U, Schulz RD. Ultrasonography of hip joint effusions. Skeletal Radiol 1987;16:607-611.
51. Miralles M, Gonzalez G, Pulpeiro JR, et al. Sonography of the painful hip in children: 500 consecutive cases. AJR Am J Roentgenol 1989;152:579-582.
52. Strouse PJ, DiPietro MA, Adler RS. Pediatric hip effusions: evaluation with power Doppler sonography. Radiology 1998;206:731-735.
53. Robben SG, Lequin MH, Diepstraten AF, et al. Doppler sonography of the anterior ascending cervical arteries of the hip: evaluation of healthy and painful hips in children. AJR Am J Roentgenol 2000;174:1629-1634.
54. Alexander JE, Seibert JJ, Aronson J, et al. A protocol of plain radiographs, hip ultrasound, and triple phase bone scans in the evaluation of the painful pediatric hip. Clin Pediatr (Phila) 1988;27:175-181.

Other Pediatric Musculoskeletal Ultrasound Applications
55. Harcke HT. Musculoskeletal ultrasound in pediatrics. Semin Musculoskelet Radiol 1998;2:321-330.

Inflammation
56. Loyer EM, DuBrow RA, David CL, et al. Imaging of superficial soft tissue infections: sonographic findings in cases of cellulitis and abscess. AJR Am J Roentgenol 1996;166:149-152.
57. Gottlieb RH, Meyers SP, Hall C, et al. Pyomyositis: diagnostic value of color Doppler sonography. Pediatr Radiol 1995;25(Suppl 1):109-111.
58. Breidahl WH, Newman JS, Taljanovic MS, Adler RS. Power Doppler sonography in the assessment of musculoskeletal fluid collections. AJR Am J Roentgenol 1996;166:1443-1446.
59. Fessell DP, Jacobson JA, Craig J, et al. Using sonography to reveal and aspirate joint effusions. AJR Am J Roentgenol 2000;174:1353-1362.
60. Lawson JP, Steere AC. Lyme arthritis: radiologic findings. Radiology 1985;154:37-43.
61. Mah ET, LeQuesne GW, Gent RJ, Paterson DC. Ultrasonic features of acute osteomyelitis in children. J Bone Joint Surg 1994;76B:969-974.
62. Nath AK, Sethu AU. Use of ultrasound in osteomyelitis. Br J Radiol 1992;65:649-652.
63. Newman JS, Adler RS. Power Doppler sonography: applications in musculoskeletal imaging. Semin Musculoskelet Radiol 1998;2:331-340.
64. Bureau NJ, Ali SS, Chhem RK, Cardinal E. Ultrasound of Musculoskeletal Infections. Semin Musculoskelet Radiol 1998;2:299-306.
65. Garcia CJ, Varela C, Abarca K, et al. Regional lymphadenopathy in cat-scratch disease: ultrasonographic findings. Pediatr Radiol 2000;30:640-643.
66. Danon O, Duval-Arnould M, Osman Z, et al. Hepatic and splenic involvement in cat-scratch disease: imaging features. Abdom Imaging 2000;25:182-183.
67. Aisen AM, McCune WJ, MacGuire A, et al. Sonographic evaluation of the cartilage of the knee. Radiology 1984;153:781-784.
68. Cooperberg PL, Tsang I, Truelove L, Knickerbocker WJ. Gray scale ultrasound in the evaluation of rheumatoid arthritis of the knee. Radiology 1978;126:759-763.
69. Van Holsbeeck M, van Holsbeeck K, Gevers G, et al. Staging and follow-up of rheumatoid arthritis of the knee: comparison of sonography, thermography, and clinical assessment. J Ultrasound Med 1988;7:561-566.

Trauma
70. Fornage BD, Eftekhari F. Sonographic diagnosis of myositis ossificans. J Ultrasound Med 1989;8:463-466.
71. Fornage BD. Muscular trauma. Clin Diagn Ultrasound 1995;30:1-10.
72. Read JW. Musculoskeletal ultrasound: basic principles. Semin Musculoskelet Radiol 1998;2:203-210.
73. Martinoli C, Bianchi S, Dahmane M, et al. Ultrasound of tendons and nerves. Eur Radiol 2002;12:44-55.
74. Lanning P, Heikkinen E. Ultrasonic features of the Osgood-Schlatter lesion. J Pediatr Orthop 1991;11:538-540.
75. Blankstein A, Cohen I, Heim M, et al. Ultrasonography as a diagnostic modality in Osgood-Schlatter disease: a clinical study and review of the literature. Arch Orthop Trauma Surg 2001;121:536-539.
76. Shiels 2nd WE, Babcock DS, Wilson JL, Burch RA. Localization and guided removal of soft tissue foreign bodies with sonography. AJR Am J Roentgenol 1990;155:1277-1281.

77. Seil R, Rupp S, Jochum P, et al. Prevalence of popliteal cysts in children: a sonographic study and review of the literature. Arch Orthop Trauma Surg 1999;119:73-75.
78. Szer IS, Klein-Gitelman M, DeNardo BA, McCauley RG. Ultrasonography in the study of prevalence and clinical evolution of popliteal cysts in children with knee effusions. J Rheumatol 1992;19:458-462.
79. Dinham JM. Popliteal cysts in children: the case against surgery. J Bone Joint Surg 1975;57B:69-71.
80. Helbich TH, Breitenseher M, Trattnig S, et al. Sonomorphologic variants of popliteal cysts. J Clin Ultrasound 1998;26:171-176.
81. Zieger M, Dorr U, Schulz RD. Sonography of slipped humeral epiphysis due to birth injury. Pediatr Radiol 1987;17:425-426.
82. Martinoli C, Bianchi S, Santacroce E, et al. Brachial plexus sonography: a technique for assessing the root level. AJR Am J Roentgenol 2002;179:699-702.
83. Grissom LE, Harcke HT. Infant shoulder sonography: technique, anatomy, and pathology. Pediatr Radiol 2001;31:863-868.

Congenital Abnormalities

84. Grissom LE, Harcke HT. Sonography in congenital deficiency of the femur. J Pediatr Orthop 1994;14:29-33.
85. Grissom LE, Harcke HT, Kumar SJ. Sonography in the management of tibial hemimelia. Clin Orthop Relat Res 1990:266-270.
86. Parsch K. [Ultrasound diagnosis of congenital knee dislocation]. Orthopade 2002;31:306-307.
87. Tolat V, Boothroyd A, Carty H, Klenerman L. Ultrasound: a helpful guide in the treatment of congenital talipes equinovarus. J Pediatr Orthop B 1995;4:65-70.
88. Chami M, Daoud A, Maestro M, et al. Ultrasound contribution in the analysis of the newborn and infant normal and clubfoot: a preliminary study. Pediatr Radiol 1996;26:298-302.
89. Hamel J, Becker W. Sonographic assessment of clubfoot deformity in young children. J Pediatr Orthop B 1996;5:279-286.
90. Coley BD, Shiels 2nd WE, Kean J, Adler BH. Age-dependent dynamic sonographic measurement of pediatric clubfoot. Pediatr Radiol 2007;37:1125-1129.
91. Grissom LE, Harcke HT. Ultrasonography of nondevelopmental dysplasia of the hips. Pediatr Radiol 1997;27:70-74.
92. De Pellegrin MP, Mackenzie WG, Harcke HT. Ultrasonographic evaluation of hip morphology in osteochondrodysplasias. J Pediatr Orthop 2000;20:588-593.
93. Lamminen A, Jaaskelainen J, Rapola J, Suramo I. High-frequency ultrasonography of skeletal muscle in children with neuromuscular disease. J Ultrasound Med 1988;7:505-509.
94. Heckmatt JZ, Pier N, Dubowitz V. Real-time ultrasound imaging of muscles. Muscle Nerve 1988;11:56-65.
95. Kraus R, Han BK, Babcock DS, Oestreich AE. Sonography of neck masses in children. AJR Am J Roentgenol 1986;146:609-613.
96. Crawford SC, Harnsberger HR, Johnson L, et al. Fibromatosis colli of infancy: CT and sonographic findings. AJR Am J Roentgenol 1988;151:1183-1184.

CHAPTER 58

Pediatric Interventional Sonography

Neil D. Johnson and William Shiels

Chapter Outline

GENERAL PRINCIPLES

The Patient

Unlike many adult patients, most pediatric patients are medically robust, without superimposed coronary, peripheral vascular, or cerebral disease. The smaller the patient, the more appropriate is the use of ultrasound guidance for interventional procedures, especially during the initial access phase. Physicians whose practice mostly involves adults often regard a baby or child as a fragile, dangerous patient. On the contrary, children tolerate levels of pH, creatinine, Po_2, and sedation that might cause major complications in adults. The pediatric patient typically is unconcerned about the details of the disease and treatment, and all but the sickest patients simply want to leave the imaging department with the most amount of play and least amount of anxiety and discomfort. The parents are often more difficult to manage than the child. Understanding of the different needs of the parents and the child is essential from the beginning of the interaction.

Personnel and Equipment

Adequate equipment and experienced assistants are essential for successful and safe pediatric intervention. Although most radiologists should be able to perform basic ultrasound-guided procedures on children, some cases are not appropriate for the inexperienced or occasional operator. A commitment to careful, graded learning, including the use of training phantoms, is needed, as is a good knowledge of regional anatomy or the willingness to learn and review the anatomy before attempting challenging procedures.

By its nature, the timing of interventional practice is not always predictable or convenient, and the general ultrasound department may resent calls for borrowing ultrasound equipment on short notice. Despite the inconvenience, the interventionist should aggressively insist on the best technical ultrasound equipment available. The ideal situation is to have dedicated interventional ultrasound equipment housed in the interventional suite. Some major pediatric radiology departments have moved the interventional suite to the operating room

(OR) environment. This integration of **interventional radiology services** within the OR environment has resulted in increased cooperation between interventional radiologists and surgeons, especially involving intraoperative ultrasound assistance during traditional surgical procedures.

GUIDANCE METHODS

Computed tomography (CT) is necessary for some procedures, especially those involving bone. In most other cases, however, ultrasound-guided access followed by ultrasound or fluoroscopic monitoring of wire and catheter placement is ideal (Table 58-1). Ultrasound can be used in the CT suite to complement a predominantly CT-guided procedure. Radiation dose to children undergoing CT procedures has recently aroused significant controversy, and use of ultrasound can reduce the need for CT.[1]

Multimodality Interventional Suites

The recent availability of cone-beam CT software on advanced angiography equipment, with virtual three-dimensional (3-D) guidance, enables combined complex interventional procedures involving ultrasound-guided access, CT-like 3-D imaging, live guidance **graticules** (superimposed over 3-D images), and conventional fluoroscopy, all in the same interventional radiology suite.[2]

Magnetic resonance imaging (MRI) guidance in pediatrics is used infrequently. Figure 58-1 provides an example of multimodality guidance; this 15-year-old boy presented with 3 months of left thigh pain initially treated as a knee sports injury. Later, radiographs and MRI demonstrated a multicystic lesion with fluid-fluid levels arising from the posterior femur. Ultrasound identified the soft tissue component of the lesion and the surrounding medium-caliber arteries, allowing avoidance of these vessels during initial ultrasound-guided placement of the biopsy device. Cone-beam CT with virtual guidance was then used to obtain initial soft tissue samples for frozen-section biopsy to minimize the risk of more aggressive biopsy of a malignant lesion. Frozen-section analysis revealed a benign lesion. Conventional fluoroscopy then allowed further sampling from all quadrants of the lesion.

ULTRASOUND TECHNIQUES

Transducers

A selection of transducers is essential. Small patient size and lack of subcutaneous fat in most children allow use of high-frequency transducers. Procedures performed around ribs, such as thoracentesis, are best done with small-footprint sector transducers. Vascular access procedures are best performed with a linear high-frequency transducer. Color Doppler ultrasound is useful for localization of major blood vessels. Transducers with good near-field resolution are used for superficial lesions and for initial accurate placement of local anesthetic on the peritoneum, deep fascia, or organ capsule.

One vs. Two Operators

Typically, inexperienced operators require the technologist or another radiologist to perform the ultrasound scanning. This should be vigorously discouraged. Although large, simple fluid collections can be drained this way, the necessary skills for accurate needle placement in small organs or near critical structures will never be learned. A single practitioner using an ultrasound transducer in one hand and the access needle or other device in the other hand is far superior to the "where's my needle now?" type of verbal communication required with two operators.

Freehand vs. Mechanical Guides

Most ultrasound equipment manufacturers supply well-designed mechanical guides that attach to a transducer and allow a predictable needle path to be visualized. These guides are useful for keeping the needle in the plane of the ultrasound beam and can be used for lesions with a simple approach path or a wide access window. Most devices require a disposable sterile kit when the device is used, adding to the cost of the procedure.

TABLE 58-1. COMPUTED TOMOGRAPHY VS. ULTRASOUND IN PEDIATRIC INTERVENTIONAL TECHNIQUES

	COMPUTED TOMOGRAPHY	ULTRASOUND
Radiation	Used; radiation dose to pediatric patients is an important issue in pediatric imaging.	None
Scan plane	Limited to axial (especially difficult near diaphragm)	Unlimited, except by bone or gas
Resolution	Excellent, although lack of fat in children can limit visualization	Excellent
Convenience	More difficult to schedule	High
Cost	High	Intermediate
Monitoring	By repeat scan; no real-time ability; recovery from kinked wires difficult	Real time
Gas and bowel	Excellent, especially with contrast	Poor

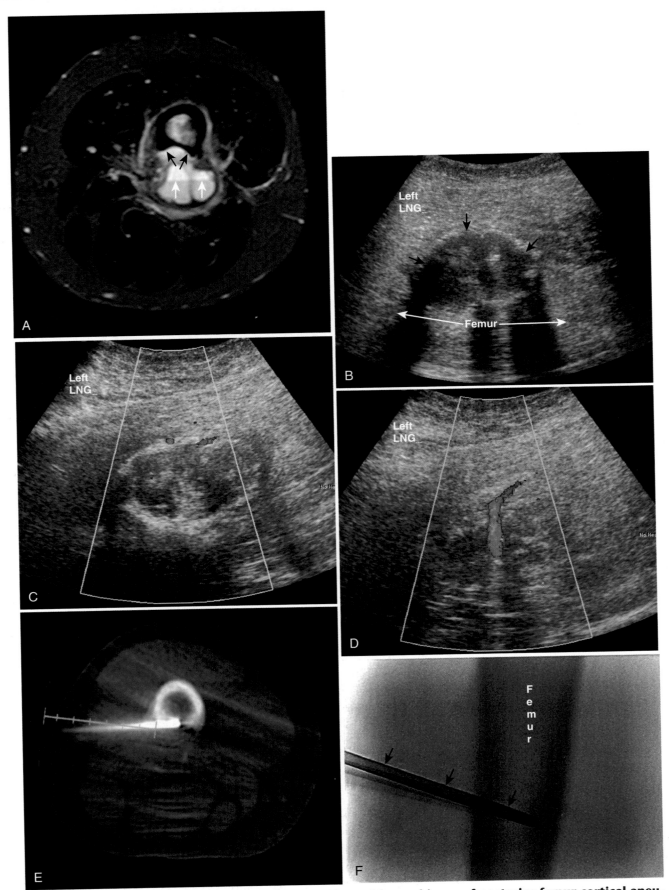

FIGURE 58-1. Multimodality interventional procedure guidance: biopsy of posterior femur cortical aneurysmal bone cyst. A, Transverse STIR magnetic resonance image of mid–left femur. *Black arrows,* Eroded posterior bone cortex; *white arrows,* fluid-fluid levels. **B,** Longitudinal sonogram shows the soft tissue component of the lesion *(black arrows).* **C,** Color Doppler ultrasound showed little internal blood flow, but **D,** moderate-sized peripheral arterial vessels were identified and avoided during the biopsy. **E,** Axial cone-beam CT shows initial guidance graticule and bone biopsy device entering the posterior bone cortex. **F,** Available fluoroscopy allowed sampling from multiple areas within the lesion.

Special needle guides are useful for the initial puncture for transrectal abscess drainage.[3]

Freehand guidance is more difficult to learn, but allows much more flexibility of approach. When the needle can be positioned 45 to 90 degrees to the beam, even fine, 30-gauge needles are easily visible. Freehand guidance allows the operator to choose the most advantageous transducer geometry and to steer the needle or biopsy device around other structures on the way to the lesion. Accurate placement of local anesthetic on the peritoneum, pleura, and other sensitive structures is made easier by freehand technique.

Color Doppler Ultrasound

Color Doppler sonography has been advocated for visualization of the moving needle during interventional procedures. In our experience, however, the potential for better visualization of the needle tip is outweighed by the degradation of the gray-scale image and flash artifacts when color Doppler is active. Various needle-tracking devices are available to enhance the visualization of the needle, but with the exception of the Yueh (Cook, Bloomington, Ind) and Skater (InterV, Stenlose, Denmark) type of sheathed access devices, which have tiny holes in the catheter tip, these devices all add complexity and expense and are generally unnecessary if accurate ultrasound technique is learned.

FREEHAND TECHNIQUE

Freehand technique requires that the transducer be held in one hand and the needle or biopsy device in the other. The interventional physician needs to be able to use either hand as the needle, or operating, hand. For example, a biopsy of the liver might be obtained by placing the transducer on the anterior abdominal wall using the right hand and making the needle approach from the patient's right lateral position, parallel to the table, using the left hand. A left-sided biopsy would best be done by using the left hand for the transducer and the right hand for the needle approach from the left flank. With some practice and some simple rules, it is not difficult to use the nondominant hand as the needle hand.

Initial Needle Placement and Localization

The most important technique to learn in freehand sonography is **needle localization.** These rules work equally well for a needle entry site near the transducer or at a distance (Fig. 58-2). The entry point is chosen after careful consideration of the anatomy and important structures such as ribs, large vessels, diaphragm, and bowel. Indentation of the entry site using a finger to compress the skin allows the exact entry site to be assessed (Fig. 58-3). Once the entry site is chosen, a last check can be made by placing the transducer exactly over the marked entry point for a "needle's-eye view" to ensure that there will be no surprises, such as the internal mammary artery, during mediastinal biopsy, which may be overlooked unless specifically localized. Once the entry path has been chosen, and after proper application of local anesthetic, the needle or biopsy device is placed through the skin toward the target. The needle and transducer need to be precisely in the same plane. This can be checked by looking directly down onto the top of the transducer and needle just before the initial placement is made (Fig. 58-4). The depth of the target should be measured and remembered before needle placement.

The needle should be initially advanced about one-half the distance to the target under direct ultrasound monitoring. If necessary, the preplanned distance of

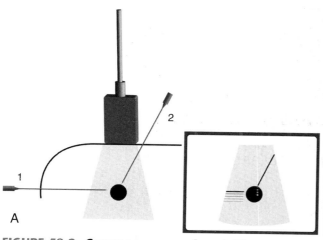
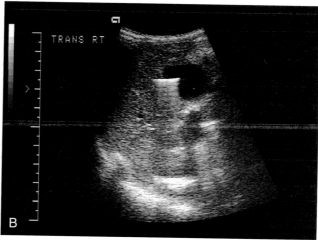

FIGURE 58-2. Common approaches. A, The most common entry sites are either *1,* lateral (parallel to the transducer face), or *2,* adjacent to the transducer. **B,** When the needle is parallel to the transducer face, a prominent reverberation artifact is seen or a "comet-tail" artifact is seen when the needle is not parallel. The needle can be more difficult to locate in position *2.*

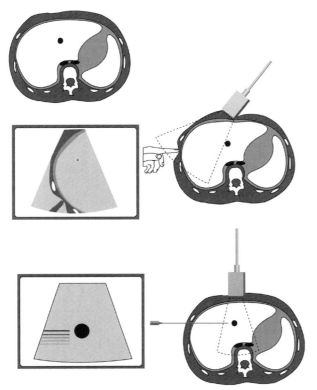

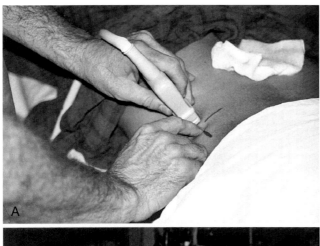

FIGURE 58-3. Locating the entry site laterally. The exact point of entry can be tested by rotating the transducer toward the body wall and palpating potential entry sites with a finger that is readily visible on the ultrasound real-time images.

insertion can be marked on the needle with a Steri-Strip. Inexperienced operators often obsessively keep pushing the needle, hoping somehow that it will magically make the needle visible. Radiologists who usually work with adults may not appreciate the short insertion distances required in small children and babies.

Locating Needle after Insertion

With experience, it is possible to keep the needle visible starting from the moment of insertion, but if not, the needle must be localized before further advancement. Check that the transducer and needle are parallel to each other by looking down the cable of the transducer with one eye closed. If the two are not parallel, adjust the position of the *transducer,* not the needle. Once the transducer and needle are parallel, keep the transducer in that plane, and move the transducer a few millimeters back and forth strictly in the plane of the needle (Fig. 58-5). It is often useful to anchor the transducer hand on the patient by placing the fourth and fifth digits or the hypothenar border of the transducer hand firmly on the patient's skin, using the thumb and the second and third digits to hold and move the transducer. It is important not to jab the needle in and out aggressively or move the needle and transducer in complex directions or angles all at once in a hopeful, and usually ineffective, attempt to localize the needle.

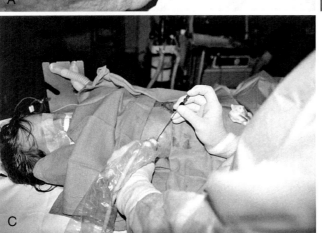

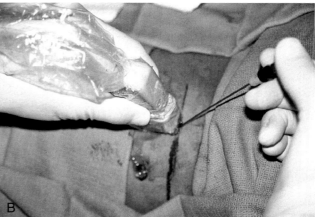

FIGURE 58-4. Needle alignment. A, After locating the entry site, the needle is inserted in a plane strictly parallel with the transducer, **B** and **C.**

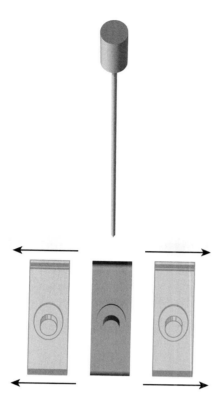

FIGURE 58-5. Transducer motion. After inserting the needle, if the needle is no longer visible on the ultrasound image, the transducer is translated backward and forward in the plane of the needle, without rotating the transducer, until the needle is localized. The actual amount of movement required is much less than shown in this diagram; typically, it is only a few millimeters.

If the whole length of the needle is not visible, it may be at an angle oblique to the plane of the transducer, resulting in an erroneous impression of the position of the needle tip (Fig. 58-6). Usually, only a few degrees of transducer rotation are required to obtain an image of the whole needle shaft.

The localization of the needle after initial placement must be a thoughtful and purposeful process that involves moving the transducer back and forth ("translation"), then adjusting and rotating its position in small increments until the whole length of the needle is visible.

If the needle and the target are visible, and the needle is pointing at the target, the needle is simply advanced toward the target. The needle may need a short, sharp jab to enter the target, particularly if the target is a normal structure such as the gallbladder, a calyx, or bile duct. The organs and tissue planes of children are soft and compliant and sometimes "float" away from the needle tip as it is advanced, but the short jab required to puncture such organs or structures must always be made purposefully and under control and. Some collagen disorders and prune-belly syndrome cause even greater difficulties in initial organ or structure puncture.

The most common problem is that the needle is not pointing at the target, or the target is no longer visible in the scan plane.

Correcting Needle Angle

If the needle and target are visible in the one image, but the needle angle is incorrect, do not attempt to change the angle radically while the needle is deep in an organ. Doing so, especially with a rigid biopsy needle, may result in significant bleeding and other complications. Instead, partly withdraw the needle until it is subcutaneous, adjust the angle, and reinsert the device under direct ultrasound monitoring as done previously (Fig. 58-7, *A-C*).

If the transducer is not vertical, it is sometimes difficult to decide which way to adjust the needle angle. This simple rule will always work: consider the position of the transducer cable, and move the needle in relation to it (Fig. 58-7, *D* and *E*). It is important, however, to know which side of the transducer belongs to which side of the ultrasound monitor screen. One should always test the orientation of the image before beginning a procedure by running a finger over the transducer face and noting where the finger appears on the screen. Otherwise, the image of the needle is expected on one side of the screen but is actually on the other side, where it is not noticed and is well on its way toward the aorta or other significant structure.

Correcting Off-Target Needle

If the needle is visible, but the target is not visible, move the transducer parallel to the plane of the needle, first one way and then the other, until the target is reestablished. Remember which way the transducer needed to be moved to reimage the target, then withdraw the needle to the skin, move the skin entry site in the same direction by moving the needle tip in the subcutaneous tissues, and advance the needle once again into the patient.

Training Aids for Freehand Sonographic Intervention

These techniques can be practiced on various **phantoms.** The most readily available and practical practice phantom consists of a turkey breast and various materials, such as beef kidney, olives, cocktail onions, or artificial cysts made by tying off the finger of a surgical glove that has been filled with water. These materials are placed in the plane between the pectoralis major and minor muscles while the turkey breast is under water.[4-6]

EQUIPMENT

Many types of needles and devices are available, and each practitioner should select and become familiar with a limited selection of these devices.

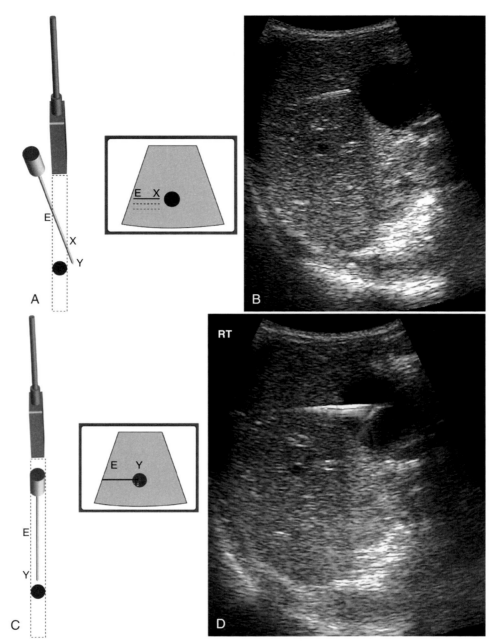

FIGURE 58-6. Off-plane needle position. A, This off-plane position results in a shortened view *(E-X)* of the needle and a false sense of needle tip position at point *X,* whereas the real position of the tip is at point *Y.* **B,** Off-plane view of part of the shaft of the needle during gallbladder puncture. **C,** With needle in the exact plane of the transducer, the whole of the needle *(E-Y)* is visible. **D,** It is now clear that the needle tip is actually in the gallbladder. Normally, the tip is accurately localized before puncture of the gallbladder. These images were obtained for illustration purposes, after successful gallbladder puncture.

Chiba Needles

The Chiba class of relatively safe, very useful, flexible, small-diameter (usually 22-gauge) needles is used for diagnostic contrast studies or for initial puncture of a target, especially if the target is near a vital structure. If the procedure involves subsequent placement of a guidewire or catheter, only a thin guide (typically 0.018 inch) can be placed through the needle. This is a relative disadvantage because a dilator will have to be placed over the 0.018-inch wire, and the thin wires are subject to kinking, especially when the dilator meets the deep fascia or capsule of an organ. We have found the Neff Set (Cook) to be especially useful and easy to use.

Drainage Catheters

Modern commercial catheters are of high quality, and usually a general-purpose or locking-loop catheter will suffice. For thick pus or old blood, a large-caliber catheter or even a chest tube may need to be placed.

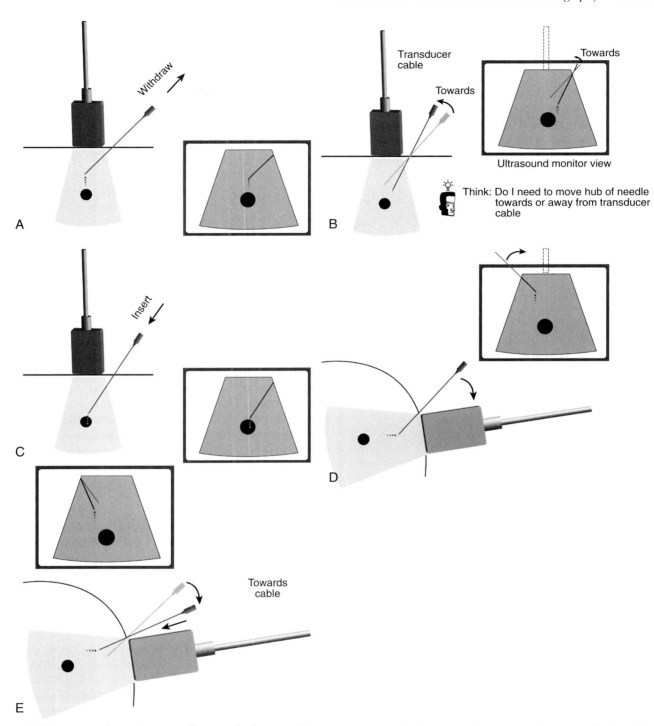

FIGURE 58-7. Changing needle angulation. A, If the needle, once localized, is not at the correct angle, the needle should be partly withdrawn. **B,** The hub is moved in relation to the position of the transducer cable. **C,** The needle is reinserted at the correct angle. **D** and **E,** The principle of moving the hub in relation to the transducer cable applies in any position of the transducer-needle combination.

Initial Puncture Device

Most drainage catheters need to be placed over at least a 0.035-inch-diameter guidewire. An initial puncture with a small-caliber needle and placement of a 0.018-inch wire requires an exchange maneuver, and each passage of a wire or dilator adds to the time and complexity of the procedure, increasing the risk of losing position or kinking the wire, especially with most 0.018 wires, which are not robust.

Various prepackaged exchange sets are available commercially. Some sets have a dilator/sheath that is placed over the 0.018 wire, and then the dilator is removed, leaving the larger sheath in place, which allows

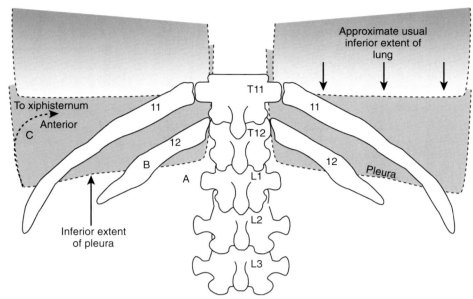

FIGURE 58-8. Surface anatomy of diaphragm, posterior view. The pleural space normally extends inferior to the 12th rib medially (position **A**), and superior to the lateral third of the 12th rib (position **B**). A line drawn from position **B** to the xyphoid process of the sternum (xiphisternum) (position **C**) will map out the surface markings of the peripheral attachment of both the normal and the pathologically elevated diaphragm. Even if the dome of the diaphragm is grossly elevated by a pathologic process, the peripheral attachment remains unchanged!

placement of the 0.035 wire. These systems are used for some biliary procedures or where vital structures are close to the target. The Yueh access device (Cook, Blooming-ton, Ind.) is a needle/sheath device with small holes drilled in the end of the catheter, making it more con-spicuous during ultrasound guidance.

Biopsy Devices

Aspiration cytology is not widely used in children because there is a much more diverse group of potential lesions in children than in adults. Many of the pediatric tumors depend partly on cellular arrangement for diagnosis, and pediatric pathologists are generally uncomfortable with making important diagnoses based on cytology specimens alone. Disposable, automated suction-core or slotted needle instruments are most often used. Although it may seem logical that small-diameter devices should be used in children, in general, 16 to 18–gauge needles are most often used in order to obtain sufficient material for pathology examination. The larger needles may seem more dangerous, but placement and monitoring under ultrasound guidance minimizes the risk.

ANATOMY

Diaphragm

A thorough knowledge of regional anatomy is essential. If a procedure will occur in an unfamiliar area, there is always time to look up the anatomy in a text before proceeding. The surface anatomy of the diaphragm must

be thoroughly understood (Fig. 58-8). It is important to remember that even if the apex of the diaphragm is grossly elevated by a mass or a subphrenic fluid collec-tion, the diaphragm is still attached to the chest wall in the same relative position as it was at birth. If the pleural space is to be avoided, one must still enter a subphrenic collection below the peripheral attachment of the dia-phragm. The diaphragm generally passes across the junction of the middle and outer thirds of the 12th rib posteriorly. From this point, a line drawn around the chest to the xiphoid process of the sternum (xiphi-sternum) will trace out the peripheral attachment of the diaphragm. It is important to be aware that the pleural space extends inferior to the inner third of the 12th rib.

Colon and Bowel

The colon lies just anterior to the kidneys and may be inadvertently punctured when entering from the pos-terolateral position during percutaneous nephrostomy. A nondistended colon may not be easily detectable by ultrasound, and one must be careful to avoid placing a nephrostomy too lateral or too anterior. If there is any doubt, a contrast enema can be performed, and the posi-tion of the colon can be localized by fluoroscopy before or during the procedure.

SEDATION

Few children under 12 years of age will cooperate during an invasive procedure, and a thorough familiarity with pediatric sedation is necessary, together with personnel and adequate resuscitation facilities. It is better to do a procedure under general anesthetic than to attempt the procedure without adequate sedation. If the child is uncomfortable or moving excessively, the sedation should be increased, help should be obtained, or the procedure should be terminated.

Our sedation protocol has been described.[7] Care must be used with all sedation medications, and fentanyl is generally not used in children younger than 12 months. Details of sedation are beyond the scope of this chapter. Specific publications should be consulted and training acquired before performing deep sedation in children. A well-organized and experienced team who perform sedation regularly, with appropriate guidelines and limits, is more important than which drugs are used. High-volume interventional groups are moving adjacent to or into the OR environment and are increasingly using the anesthesia service for sedation.

LOCAL ANESTHETIC TECHNIQUE

The most frequently used anesthetic agent is lidocaine (Abbott, Chicago) 1% solution. The usual maximum adult dose for local anesthesia is 4.5 mg/kg body weight (0.45 mL/kg of 1% solution). A maximum dose of 3 to 4 mg/kg (0.3-0.4 mL/kg of 1% solution) for children over 3 years of age is noted in the product-insert dosage recommendations, but there is no recommendation for younger children. We routinely use the 3 to 4 mg/kg (0.3-0.4 mL/kg of 1% solution) for all but extremely premature babies. Lidocaine is only chemically stable in a slight acid solution, so it is often used with sodium bicarbonate 8.4% solution in a 10:1 ratio immediately before injection, which effectively reduces the sensation of stinging as the local anesthetic is injected. Liberal use of topical local anesthetic creams is also useful, but must be applied 20 minutes before the procedure, and the entry site for a procedure is not always known in advance.

It is a common error to inject the local anesthetic and then immediately commence the procedure. All clinically useful local anesthetics work by diffusing across the lipid myelin and nerve cell membrane and paralyzing the sodium channel from the intracellular side of the sodium channel. It is therefore not surprising that lidocaine needs 5 to 8 minutes to achieve full effect. We usually place the local anesthetic, at least in the deep subcutaneous tissues, before gowning and gloving and preparing equipment. This allows time for the anesthetic to achieve maximal effect. Dentists are well aware of the time needed for maximal local anesthetic effect, but many physicians seem unaware of the need for waiting to achieve good local anesthesia. The description of an experimental, highly selective nociceptor (pain) agent without effect on motor or general sensation nerves is intriguing.[8]

The pain and stretch receptors are mostly in the epidermal layer. Discomfort associated with local anesthetic administration mainly results from the rapid stretching of the epidermal sensors, before the local anesthetic agent has had time to block the axons. Thus, the common practice of "raising a wheal" in the epidermis is contraindicated. Use of 30-gauge or smaller needles for initial slow, deep subcutaneous injection minimizes the discomfort and often allows initial injection without the patient being aware of the skin puncture. Initial local anesthetic application to the deep subcutaneous layers allows the agent first to block the axons of the pain and other epidermal sensory nerve endings. Once this has been achieved, later local anesthetic application to the epidermis is usually painless. Care must be taken to exclude air from the syringe and needle before injecting the local anesthetic; even the amount of residual air in a 30-gauge needle, injected subcutaneously, may seriously degrade the ultrasound image.

Ultrasound-Guided Deep Local Anesthetic Administration

One of the keys to successful percutaneous procedures in children is adequate local anesthetic control of deep sensation. Many practitioners anesthetize only the skin and subcutaneous tissues and are then surprised when the patient moves or complains vigorously as a dilator is passing through the peritoneum, deep fascia, or the capsule of the organ. The solution is to place the majority of the local anesthetic on the peritoneum, fascia, or capsule. In general, it is the external covering of an organ or muscle, the pleura, peritoneum, perimysium, or deep fascia that registers pain sensation. Subcutaneous fat, organs, and the muscle belly have few nerve endings. Deep local anesthetic application is best achieved by using sonographic guidance. Surprisingly, even 30-gauge needles can be easily identified close to the skin with high-quality 7- or 10-MHz transducers. The focal zone must be adjusted appropriately; with optimal conditions, however, the local anesthetic can be deposited where it will have the most effect. This reduces the depth of sedation required and the time required to complete some procedures, without the general anesthesia otherwise required (Fig. 58-9).

ANTIBIOTICS

Antibiotics are routinely needed only when draining an infected collection or when the patient is immunosuppressed. We usually use periprocedural antibiotics for liver and renal transplant patients. The choice of antibiotics is individualized after consultation with the referring service. Antibiotics are usually given intravenously at sedation or anesthesia induction. If a procedure involves obtaining material for microbiologic diagnostic

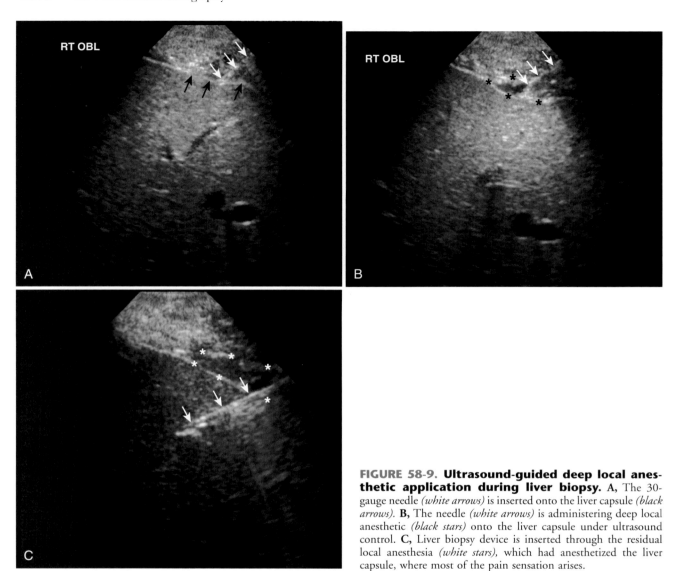

FIGURE 58-9. Ultrasound-guided deep local anesthetic application during liver biopsy. A, The 30-gauge needle *(white arrows)* is inserted onto the liver capsule *(black arrows).* **B,** The needle *(white arrows)* is administering deep local anesthetic *(black stars)* onto the liver capsule under ultrasound control. **C,** Liver biopsy device is inserted through the residual local anesthesia *(white stars),* which had anesthetized the liver capsule, where most of the pain sensation arises.

purposes, antibiotics are commenced only after the initial samples are obtained.

THE TYPICAL PROCEDURE

Prior Consultation and Studies

It is remarkable how many times interventional procedures are performed without complete knowledge of prior studies or procedures. The clinician should know the difficulties previously encountered or whether a contrast reaction occurred at a previous CT scan. Picture archiving and communication systems (PACS) with integrated radiology reports and other clinical data facilitate this effort. The interventionist is responsible for having a clear understanding of the clinical reasons for the procedure and the expected benefits. In large

institutions, the interventionist can become "sandwiched" between feuding clinical services, and if one simply accepts orders from a service without becoming knowledgeable about the case, some of the other services may not be supportive if a complication occurs. At times, it is the duty of the radiologist to insist on, or convene, a combined-care conference before undertaking a major procedure. This can be the greatest contribution a radiologist can make to the medical care of the child.

Clotting Studies

Clotting studies are indicated for most liver and deep-organ biopsies, but these are generally not necessary for simple diagnostic procedures or drainage procedures, unless there is a clear indication, as in liver transplant patients. A platelet count is usually obtained in oncology patients. Caution should be exercised when the platelet count is below 80,000, and it is important to remember that platelet function may be affected by some nonsteroidal anti-inflammatory agents, by uremia, and by other medical conditions. Patients with Wilms' tumor may rarely have an undiagnosed, transient, acquired von Willebrand's syndrome. Be cautious if the skin incision continues to bleed vigorously for more than 1 minute. It is better to cancel a procedure and do a full clotting workup than to continue and cause a major hemorrhage.

The kidney should always be regarded as a "sponge of blood." It is wise to approach each patient with confidence, modified by cautious optimism and common sense.

Aims and Expectations

Anticipation of problems is good practice, not a sign of weakness. No procedure should be undertaken without a clear understanding of the aims, the expected benefit, and a reasonably detailed plan for completing the task. If an abscess is difficult to localize by ultrasound (e.g., in the psoas muscle in a large adolescent), transfer to the CT suite should be considered. Fluoroscopy after initial ultrasound-guided access allows a kinked wire to be withdrawn into the dilator and replaced or advanced into the abscess. The kinked wire is much more difficult to recognize on CT because the procedure is not monitored in real time and there is little room for recovery. CT is essential in some areas, notably pelvic abscesses requiring transgluteal drainage.[9]

An alternate plan is important, especially in complex procedures, such as renal stone removal or ureteric stent placement. What happens if the patient moves, or the wire is dislodged? A second safety wire tucked up in an upper-pole calyx is always good insurance in complex renal procedures. Expect the unexpected, and the procedure will usually go as planned.

Initial Ultrasound Scan Should Occur before Sedation

Understand the individual patient's anatomy before sedation or general anesthesia. Spending enough time to consider the most effective approach and the adjacent anatomy is as important as proper needle placement. It is less-than-perfect technique to pass a needle through the colon when a little time and care would have avoided the problem. The radiologist should have a good three-dimensional understanding of the patient's regional anatomy before commencing a procedure.

Pus

Pus is the liquefied products of inflammation. **Liquefied** is the most important word for the interventionist.

Unlike CT, which generates a static image, real-time ultrasound allows exploration of the liquidity and therefore the drainability of a lesion. Urinomas are notoriously echogenic when first examined, but if the operator vigorously prods the collection with the ultrasound probe, the free-flowing nature of the collection becomes apparent. The urinoma can be drained by a simple 8-French catheter rather than the large-caliber sump catheter that might have been considered.

Difficult Catheter Fixation in Infants

Catheters are objects of wonder for small children and babies and are great chewing material if left in the grasp of tiny hands. Often, when a catheter "just falls out by itself," there has been some lapse in care on the part of professional staff. Either the catheter was not properly secured in the first place, or the nursing staff forgot to undo the safety pin when taking the child to the bathroom. Some methods of fixation include standard sutures, sutures secured to the catheter by waterproof tape, or various commercial skin fixation devices. If the catheter is stitched in place, the stitch must be placed deeply in the subcutaneous tissues. In infants the catheter is hidden out of reach, if possible, and secured with transparent plastic adhesive film. The joint between the catheter shaft and the hub of a drainage catheter is its weakest point, so we routinely affix the hub to the skin with adhesive tape or film, and train the patient's nurses always to retape this hub when performing routine catheter care.

Postprocedural Care and Follow-Up

Apart from bad communication skills, the quickest way to destroy an interventional referral pattern is to ignore the patient or the referring physician or surgeon once the patient has left the radiology department. The interventionist is responsible for accepting the patient, for confirming the procedure is justified and likely of significant benefit to the patient, and for both immediate postprocedural and long-term follow-up. Leaving a pager number in the medical notes may result in a few trivial calls, but overall it will benefit the patient and increase referrals and satisfaction. If a complication occurs, either deal with it or consult another service, but do the consultation personally, not through the junior intern messaging service.

Be cautious of blood loss in children after liver or other biopsy. A hematocrit before and 2 hours after biopsy is a prudent precaution. Blood loss is typically slow and self-limiting, but if bleeding persists, often the only objective signs are pain and a rising pulse rate. Children who are experiencing blood loss notoriously maintain blood pressure and brain perfusion until very late, then suddenly deteriorate.

SPECIFIC PROCEDURES

Abscess Drainage

When entering an abscess cavity, a pus sample is usually obtained for culture, but the cavity should not be aspirated completely before placement of the catheter. Once the catheter is in position, simple aspiration with ultrasound monitoring for completeness is all that is required. Flushing with large volumes of saline or performing a contrast study will only result in intravasation of infected material through the raw granulation tissue that always lines these abscesses. Contrast studies and flushing can be done later, once the cavity is healing, although we rarely do a postprocedural study for uncomplicated abscess drainage. During initial aspiration, blood return may be obtained near the end of aspiration. This is probably blood arising from the granulation tissue and, at times, can be alarming in amount. If active aspiration is halted, the bleeding usually stops. The catheter should be left in place until the aspirate is straw colored and less than a few milliliters per day.

Transrectal Drainage

Deep pelvic abscesses can be drained by surgery or by a catheter inserted under ultrasound control.[10] The ultrasound-guided method is particularly appropriate for high collections that are beyond the reach of surgeons, but at our institutions, ultrasound-guided transrectal abscess drainage has substantially replaced the surgical procedure (Fig. 58-10). The catheter can be withdrawn after complete aspiration of the cavity or left in place and secured to the leg with tape.[3]

PICC Catheters

Peripherally inserted central catheters (PICCs) are a useful way of obtaining safe central access for short- to medium-term use.[11] The catheters range from 2 French to 5 French in size, and various commercial units are available with insertion sets containing either a peel-away cannula similar to an IV catheter or a peel-away Seldinger-style sheath.

After insertion of the sheath into a peripheral vein (arm, leg, or scalp), the catheter is placed through the sheath and positioned in the central veins. Visual access to the arm veins is often easy in the older individual, but the veins of chubby babies can be notoriously difficult to identify and cannulate. Ultrasound guidance in these patients has become an essential skill for the PICC line service, and most PICC line nurses can successfully be taught the technique. In infants the technique of ultrasound guidance for venous access is different from previously described parallel techniques. Because of beam width issues, it is best to monitor the needle position by constantly adjusting the transverse position of the

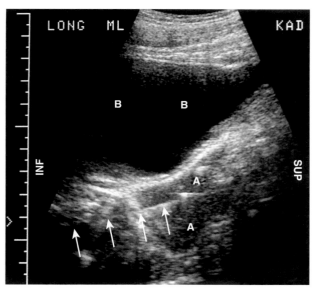

FIGURE   58-10. Ultrasound-guided   transrectal abscess drainage. The needle *(arrows)* has been inserted through the rectum and has punctured the high pelvic abscess *(A)* under ultrasound guidance. The bladder *(B)* is anterior to the abscess.

transducer in a sweeping manner (Figs. 58-11 and 58-12; **Video 58-1**). The veins are usually so small that monitoring the needle position with the transducer in the plane of the needle and vein usually results in malpositioning the needle because of the width of the ultrasound beam.

In older children with larger veins, scanning in the plane of the vein can be useful, and safe passage of the guidewire can be observed (Fig. 58-13).

Pleural and Peritoneal Drainage

Ultrasound-guided diagnostic aspiration of pleural fluid is a common and useful procedure. Simple catheter drainage of **parapneumonic complex fluid collection** or **empyema** has been described and can result in complete cure if performed early enough, although the pleura has a remarkable ability to thicken and produce fibrin. These infected collections often loculate and become difficult to drain using a simple catheter technique. CT scanning does not usually show the loculations, and therefore referring clinicians often believe that the parapneumonic fluid should be easy to drain. The administration of thrombolytics, typically tissue plasminogen activator (tPA) through the pleural tube to change the physical characteristics of the thick fluid,[12,13] is now a routine procedure. Any chest tube for empyema drainage must be monitored frequently by radiography, ultrasound, or occasionally postprocedure CT, to ensure that loculation has not recurred (Fig. 58-14).

Peritoneal fluid drainage for diagnostic or therapeutic reasons is usually not difficult and can often be

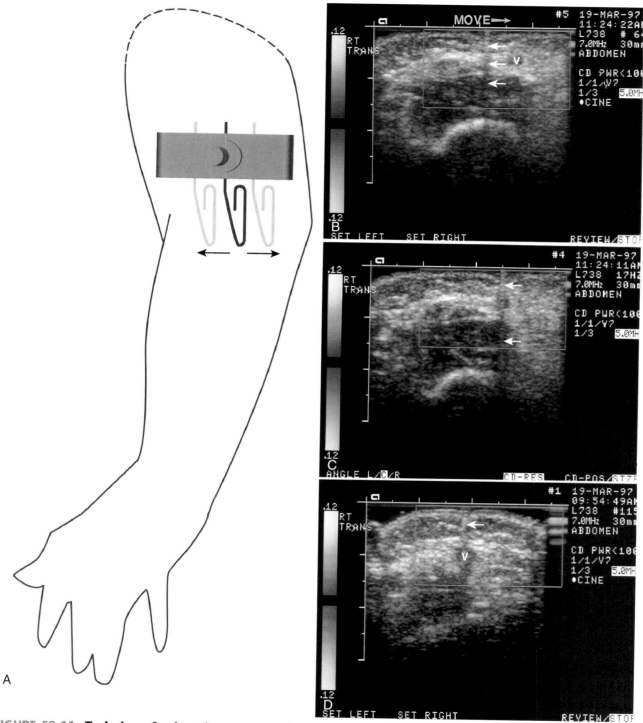

FIGURE 58-11. Technique for locating exact position of deep vein before PICC line placement. A, With the transducer held transverse to the direction of the target vein, a partly unfolded paper clip, placed between the skin and the transducer face, is moved backward and forward (**B** and **C**) to locate the vein for accurate application of subcutaneous local anesthetic. The transducer is held transverse to the needle path to avoid beam width errors. The thin, paper clip artifact *(arrows)* localizes the vein *(V)*. Note that with a tourniquet in place, especially in a small baby (**B-D**), color Doppler sonography may show no flow. A tight tourniquet in a baby can obstruct even arterial flow, resulting in erroneous placement of an intra-arterial PICC line, a dangerous event if unrecognized. *PICC,* Peripherally inserted central catheter.

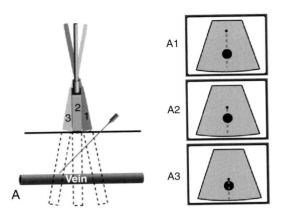

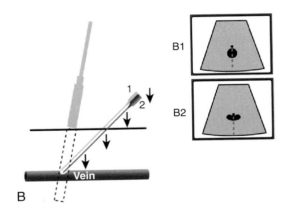

FIGURE 58-12. Localizing needle tip near vein.
A, As the needle is advanced toward the vein, the transducer is used in transverse orientation and rocked back and forth *(A1-A3)* to track the needle tip sequentially as it is advanced toward the vein. In the illustration the needle is only depicted as it is about to enter the vein (position *3*). **B,** Trapping and puncturing the vein. The needle can easily slip to the side of the vein if it is simply advanced, especially when attempting to puncture a deep brachial vein. The loose soft tissue surrounding deep veins allows the vein to slide out of the way of the needle. When the needle tip is positioned correctly, adjacent to the anterior wall of the vein *(B1)*, gentle downward movement of the needle, without trying to puncture the vein, will "trap" the vein with the needle tip *(B2)*. Once the vein is trapped, a quick thrust will puncture both walls. Careful withdrawal usually results in venous blood return through the needle, allowing successful PICC line placement.

achieved at the bedside with minimal or no sedation and good local anesthetic technique. When accessing the fluid through the lower quadrants, care must be taken to localize accurately and mark the position of the hypo-gastric vessels, which can cause substantial and difficult-to-control bleeding into the peritoneal fluid if injured during an otherwise "simple" aspiration procedure. Occasionally, debris obstructs the draining catheter and needs to be dislodged, either by vigorous movement of

the needle/catheter or by passage of a guidewire to dis-lodge the obstructing debris (**Videos 58-2** and **58-3**).

Percutaneous Cholangiography and Drainage

Percutaneous transhepatic cholangiography (PTC) can be successfully performed in children with or without duct dilation. Ultrasound is used to guide the Chiba needle toward the bile ducts, which lie in the portal tracts. The optimal diagnostic puncture site is at the junction of the middle and peripheral thirds of the duct, well away from the central portal veins and hepatic artery. If the ducts are dilated, the needle can be guided directly into the duct with the usual ultrasound tech-niques. Puncture should be made at a site and at an angle that will allow conversion of the track to a catheter drain should the diagnostic study reveal bile duct stenosis or complete obstruction, especially in liver transplant patients. Initial puncture of minimally dilated bile ducts in pediatric liver transplant patients is one of the most technically demanding ultrasound-guided procedures (Fig. 58-15).

Mediastinal Mass Biopsy

Lymphoma is a common childhood malignancy, often presenting with a mediastinal mass. In many cases, cervi-cal, abdominal, or axillary lymphadenopathy is seen at presentation enabling histologic diagnosis by surgical lymph node biopsy. In some cases, however, the patient presents with respiratory difficulty caused by tracheal compression, and no convenient enlarged lymph nodes are available for biopsy. Many of these patients are unable to lie flat without respiratory distress. The medi-astinal mass can enlarge rapidly, such that a child who could lie flat for initial CT scan cannot lie flat a few hours later. In these cases, ultrasound-guided mediasti-nal biopsy is often the safest option. Emergency radio-therapy and steroid administration can also be used to shrink the mass, but these maneuvers can result in inabil-ity to subtype the cells of the lymphoma, which is becoming more important for treatment decisions and prognosis.

Pediatric patients with lymphoma are managed in the OR in a semi-erect position and need to be supervised and sedated by experienced anesthesia staff. We typically use copious local anesthesia and only minimal IV seda-tion, avoiding intubation if possible.

Doppler ultrasound is used to locate and avoid the internal mammary artery and vein. The mass is usually approached through a paramanubrial intercostal space under direct ultrasound guidance using a small-footprint sector probe. The great vessels and lung must be clearly visualized before biopsy. Multiple samples can be obtained with remarkably low risk of complication (Fig. 58-16).

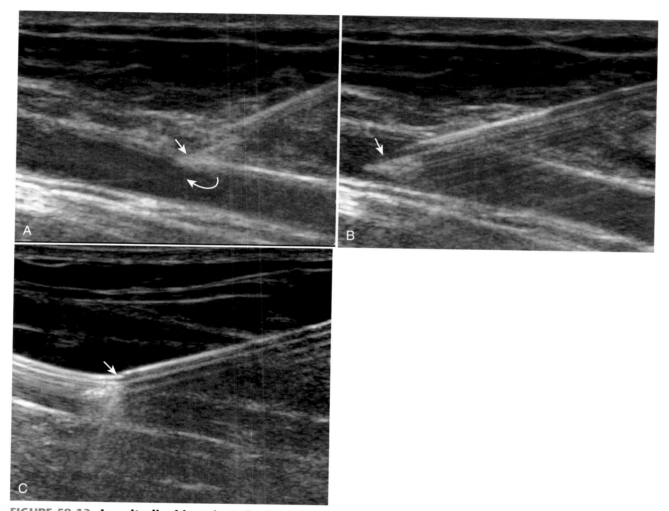

FIGURE 58-13. Longitudinal imaging of vein puncture for PICC line insertion. A, Access needle tip *(straight arrow)* about to enter the vein *(curved arrow).* **B,** Needle tip (with reverberation artifact) has entered vein. **C,** Guidewire leaving the needle tip *(arrow)* and clearly seen entering the vein.

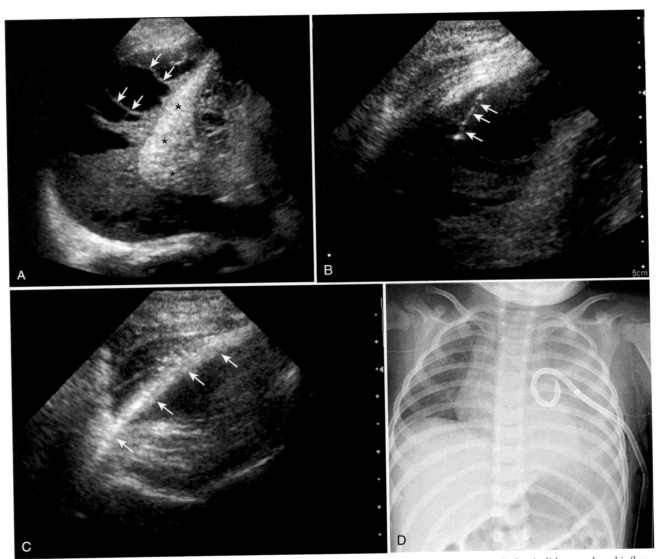

FIGURE 58-14. Ultrasound guidance for treatment of loculated chest empyema. A, Semisolid, extrapleural inflammatory material with septa *(white arrows)* is compressing the airless adjacent left lung *(black stars).* **B,** Access needle *(white arrows)* is seen entering the empyema. **C,** Left-sided chest tube is inserted for drainage and instillation of tissue plasminogen activator (tPA), a successful combined treatment for chest empyema, formerly treated by thoracotomy. **D,** Radiograph shows left-sided chest tube position.

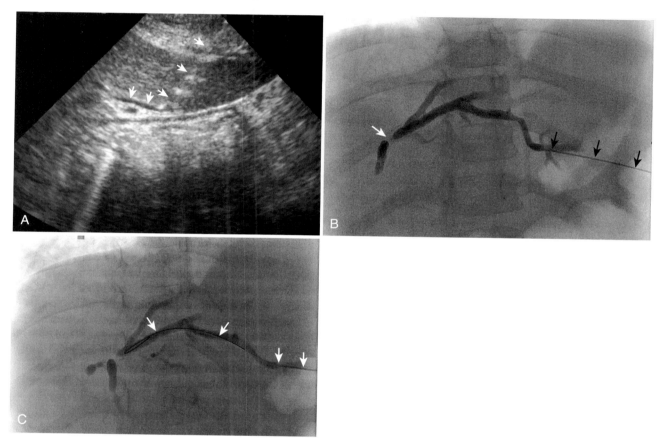

FIGURE 58-15. Access for drainage of obstructed bile ducts in liver transplant patient. A, Initial ultrasound-guided needle *(arrows)* placement shows the tip about to enter the slightly dilated left bile duct. **B,** Initial fluoroscopic image of the needle *(black arrows)* in the duct shows contrast outlining the severe duct stenosis *(white arrow).* **C,** The angle of puncture enabled by precise ultrasound guidance allowed easy passage of the initial Cope guidewire. The stenosis was later balloon-dilated and stented by the same route.

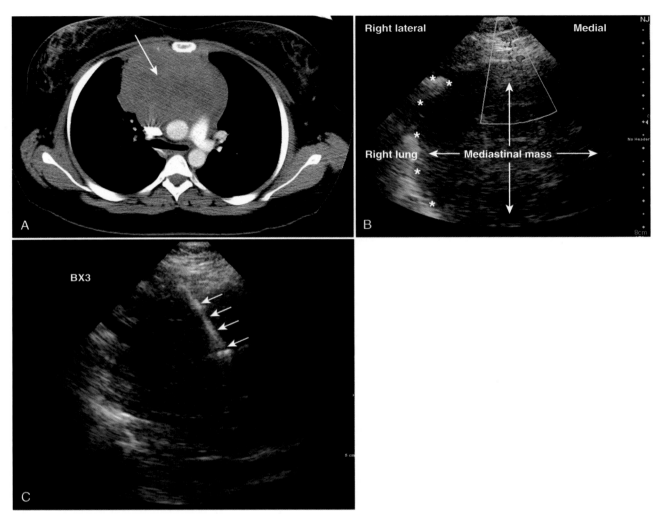

FIGURE 58-16. Biopsy of large mediastinal mass. A, CT image obtained 1 day previously shows the large mass compressing the carina; *arrow,* route of subsequent ultrasound-guided biopsy. **B,** Initial color Doppler ultrasound defines the mass and localizes the great vessels and the internal mammary vessels. **C,** Automated biopsy device *(arrows)* within the mass. Multiple biopsies were obtained to provide adequate tissue for advanced cell-typing studies of this B-cell lymphoma.

Appendiceal Abscess Drainage

Initial ultrasound-guided drainage of an appendix-associated abscess is a well-documented procedure. Occasionally, a secondary abscess occurs after interval endoscopic surgery for removal of the appendix, usually caused by a retained or unrecognized fecalith. Ultrasound guidance can also be used to drain these recurrent abscesses. In one case, we were able to target the retained fecalith precisely, drain the abscess, then remove the fecalith by a second interventional procedure using an Amplatz biliary sheath (Cook) and Fogarty balloon retrieval of the fecalith through the sheath (Fig. 58-17; **Video 58-4**).

Targeted Organ Lesion Biopsy

Ultrasound-guided specific organ biopsy, such as for routine liver or kidney interventions, is a well-established procedure. Targeted intraorgan lesion biopsy is more demanding. Each case must be assessed on its merits, but extra caution should be exercised for lesions close to the diaphragm or major intraorgan or extraorgan vasculature (Figs. 58-18 and 58-19).

Musculoskeletal Procedures

Although CT or cone-beam CT is the usual guidance modality for deep bone procedures, ultrasound can be useful for certain periosteal or cartilage-related lesions (Fig. 58-20; see also Fig. 58-1; **Videos 58-5, 58-6,** and **58-7**).

Steroid injection for local treatment of specific joints in diseases such as juvenile rheumatoid arthritis can be achieved by blind access in large joints, such as the knee. Increasingly, however, rheumatologists are referring patients for image-guided steroid injection for smaller or technically difficult joints, such as the subtalar or interphalangeal joints. Ultrasound guidance can be used for accurate access to these small joints. Ultrasound-guided steroid injection of tendon sheaths is a valuable procedure (Fig. 58-21; **Video 58-8**).

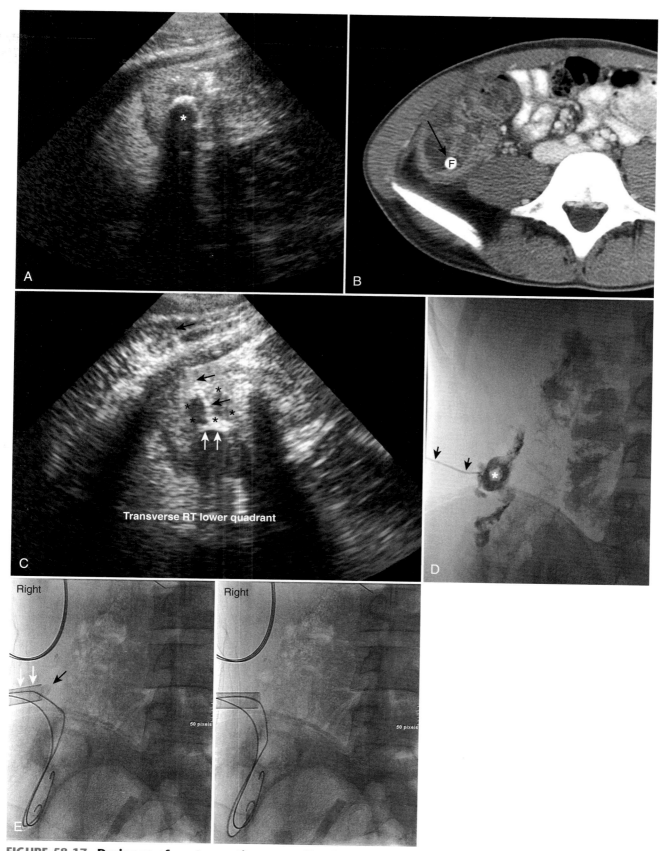

FIGURE 58-17. Drainage of postoperative appendiceal abscess. A, Retained echogenic fecalith *(asterisk)* in right lower quadrant was causing the abscess. **B,** CT scan shows identical area in **A;** *black arrow,* path of subsequent ultrasound-guided access. **C,** Initial ultrasound-guided needle *(black arrows)* access to the perifecalith abscess *(asterisks);* *white arrows,* anterior surface of fecalith. **D,** Fluoroscopy with contrast shows the sheath *(arrows)* adjacent to the fecalith *(asterisk).* **E,** Fluoroscopy images of an interval image-guided procedure show capture of the fecalith *(black arrow)* within the access sheath *(white arrows)* and subsequent fecalith removal through the sheath.

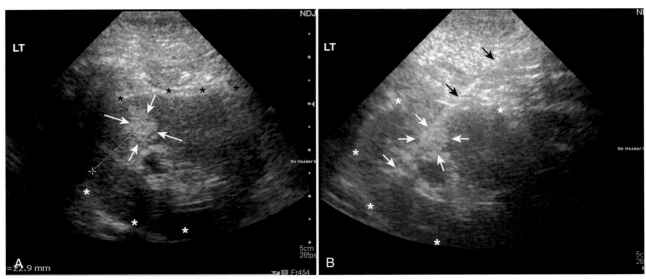

FIGURE 58-18. Targeted left upper-pole renal lesion biopsy. Patient had secondary renal cell carcinoma after prior treatment for cerebral tumor (PNET). **A,** Lesion high in the upper pole of the left kidney *(white arrows)*. Measurement calipers are estimating the depth of the biopsy to avoid puncturing the adjacent diaphragm *(white stars)* and spleen. **B,** Biopsy device *(black arrows)* is seen passing through the lesion *(white arrows)* and stopping short of the diaphragm.

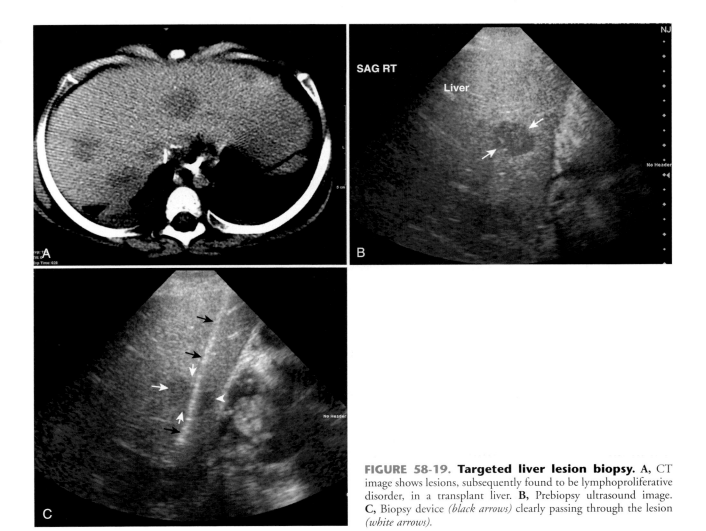

FIGURE 58-19. Targeted liver lesion biopsy. A, CT image shows lesions, subsequently found to be lymphoproliferative disorder, in a transplant liver. **B,** Prebiopsy ultrasound image. **C,** Biopsy device *(black arrows)* clearly passing through the lesion *(white arrows)*.

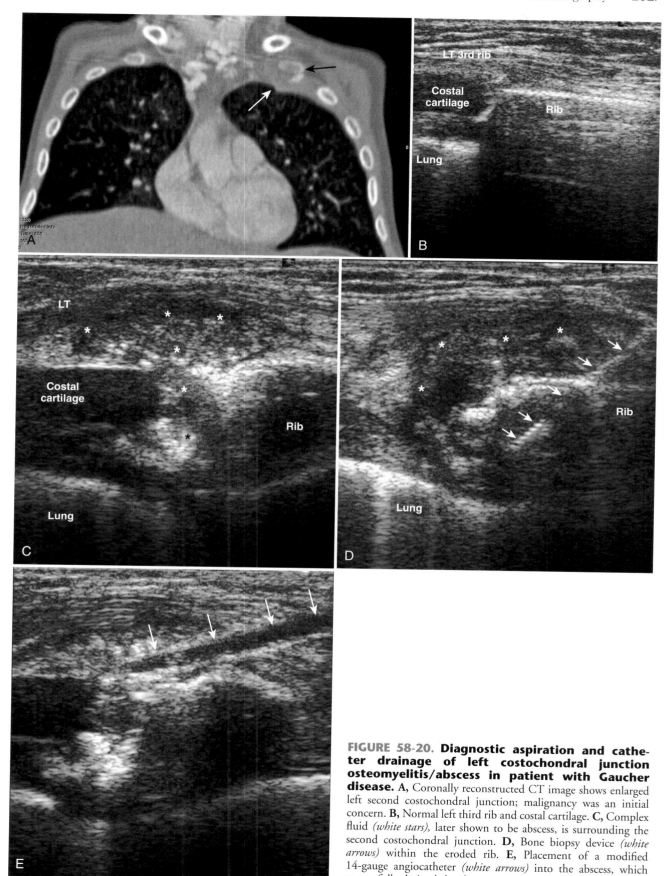

FIGURE 58-20. Diagnostic aspiration and catheter drainage of left costochondral junction osteomyelitis/abscess in patient with Gaucher disease. A, Coronally reconstructed CT image shows enlarged left second costochondral junction; malignancy was an initial concern. **B,** Normal left third rib and costal cartilage. **C,** Complex fluid *(white stars),* later shown to be abscess, is surrounding the second costochondral junction. **D,** Bone biopsy device *(white arrows)* within the eroded rib. **E,** Placement of a modified 14-gauge angiocatheter *(white arrows)* into the abscess, which successfully drained the abscess.

Some deep **foreign bodies** can be removed under ultrasound guidance (Fig. 58-22). It is important that the ultrasound-guided procedure be done before the wound is opened and probed in the emergency room or OR. Otherwise, air destroys the ability of ultrasound to visualize the foreign body, and the case must be canceled and rescheduled.

Head and Neck Lesions

Certain vascular and lymphatic malformations are amenable to ultrasound-guided access and treatment, usually by **sclerosing agents.**[14] Orbital lymphatic malformations are difficult to treat surgically, but respond well to percutaneous ultrasound-guided sclerotherapy (Fig. 58-23).

Ranulas are rare lesions consisting of saliva-containing cysts, most often caused by trauma or obstruction of the sublingual duct. The sublingual duct secretes saliva continuously, whereas the submandibular and parotid duct only secrete with oral stimuli such as eating, and therefore the sublingual gland is more prone to formation of ranula. **Plunging ranula** can be treated successfully by ultrasound and fluoroscopically guided sclerotherapy (Fig. 58-24).

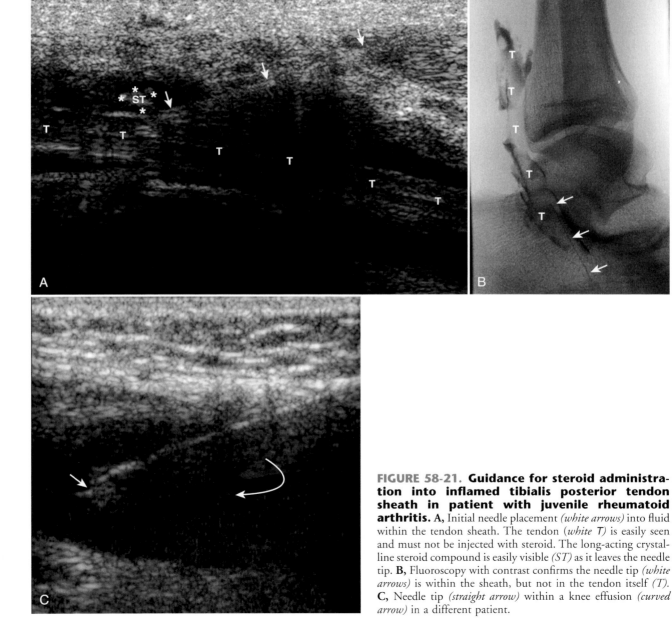

FIGURE 58-21. Guidance for steroid administration into inflamed tibialis posterior tendon sheath in patient with juvenile rheumatoid arthritis. A, Initial needle placement *(white arrows)* into fluid within the tendon sheath. The tendon *(white T)* is easily seen and must not be injected with steroid. The long-acting crystalline steroid compound is easily visible *(ST)* as it leaves the needle tip. **B,** Fluoroscopy with contrast confirms the needle tip *(white arrows)* is within the sheath, but not in the tendon itself *(T)*. **C,** Needle tip *(straight arrow)* within a knee effusion *(curved arrow)* in a different patient.

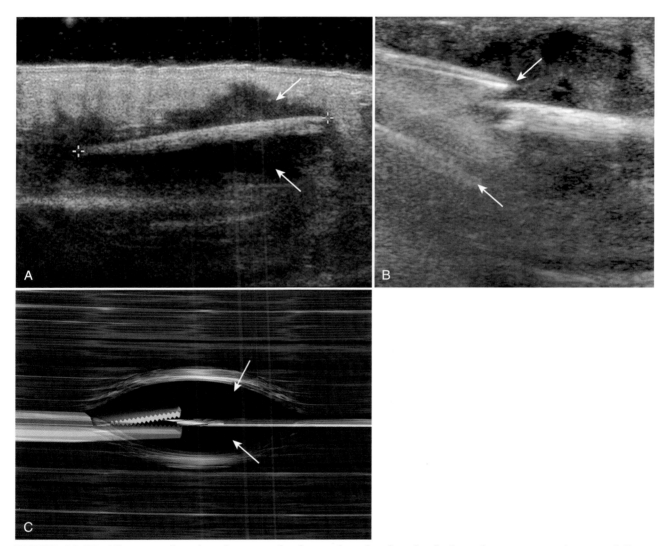

FIGURE 58-22. Ultrasound-assisted removal of wooden foreign body in subcutaneous tissues of foot. **A,** Wood *(cursors)* is demonstrated in the subcutaneous tissues, surrounded by pus *(arrows).* **B,** Hemostat with jaws open *(arrows)* approaching the foreign body under direct ultrasound monitoring. **C,** Diagram illustrates procedure and shows jaws closed on the wooden foreign body.

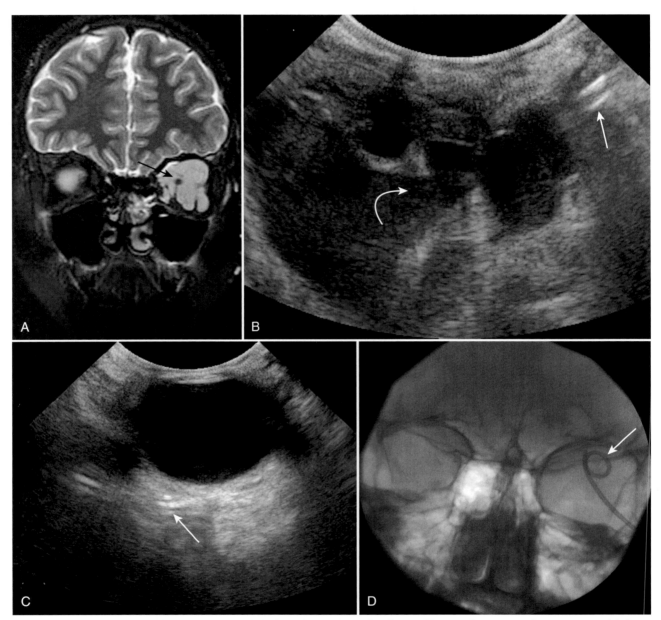

FIGURE 58-23. Successful treatment of left orbital lymphatic malformation (LM) in 13-year-old boy.
A, Coronal T2-weighted MR image demonstrates the lymphatic malformation with medium-intensity-signal fluid surrounding the left optic nerve *(arrow)*. **B,** Longitudinal sonogram of the left orbit with a 14-gauge angiocatheter needle *(straight arrow)* about to enter the macrocystic LM *(curved arrow)*. **C,** Transverse sonogram demonstrates the 5-French catheter *(arrow)* in the left orbital LM after aspiration of LM fluid. The anechoic fluid-filled structure is the globe. **D,** Fluoroscopic spot film demonstrates the 5-French pigtail catheter in place for sclerotherapy of the macrocystic element of the orbital LM.

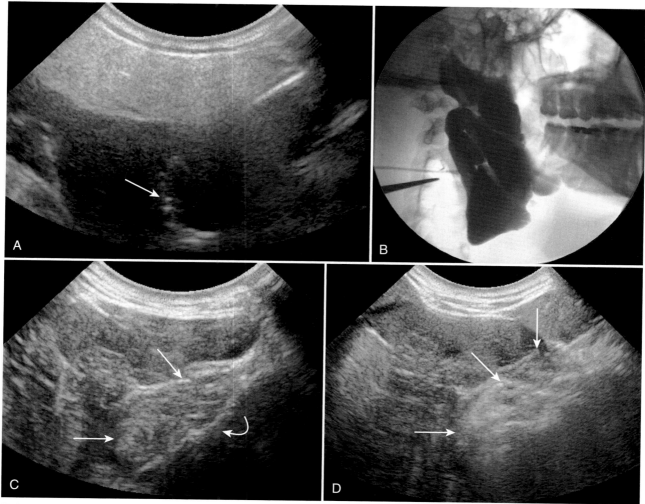

FIGURE 58-24. Percutaneous treatment of plunging ranula in left side of neck. A, Longitudinal sonography demonstrates a 5-French pigtail catheter *(arrow)* within the hypoechoic ranula fluid. **B,** Contrast material is filling the ranula sac. **C,** Transverse sonography demonstrates the left sublingual gland *(straight arrows)* adjacent to the left mandible *(curved arrow)* before ablation. **D,** Increased echogenicity in the left sublingual gland *(arrows)* during ethanol injection for ablation.

References

Guidance Methods

1. Slovis TL. The ALARA concept in pediatric CT: myth or reality? Radiology 2002;223:5-6.
2. Racadio JM, Babic D, Homan R, et al. Live 3D guidance in the interventional radiology suite. AJR Am J Roentgenol 2007;189: W357-W364.

Ultrasound Techniques

3. McGahan JP, Wu C. Sonographically guided transvaginal or transrectal pelvic abscess drainage using the trocar method with a new drainage guide attachment. AJR Am J Roentgenol 2008;191:1540-1544.

Freehand Technique

4. Gibson RN, Gibson KI. A home-made phantom for learning ultrasound-guided invasive techniques. Australas Radiol 1995;39: 356-357.
5. Georgian-Smith D, Shiels 2nd WE. Freehand interventional sonography in the breast: basic principles and clinical applications. From RSNA refresher courses. Radiographics 1996;16:149-161.
6. Harvey JA, Moran RE, Hamer MM, et al. Evaluation of a turkey-breast phantom for teaching freehand, ultrasound-guided core-needle breast biopsy. Acad Radiol 1997;4:565-569.

Sedation

7. Egelhoff JC, Ball Jr WS, Koch BL, Parks TD. Safety and efficacy of sedation in children using a structured sedation program. AJR Am J Roentgenol 1997;168:1259-1262.

Local Anesthetic Technique

8. Binshtok AM, Bean BP, Woolf CJ. Inhibition of nociceptors by TRPV1-mediated entry of impermeant sodium channel blockers. Nature 2007;449:607-610.

The Typical Procedure

9. Harisinghani MG, Gervais DA, Maher MM, et al. Transgluteal approach for percutaneous drainage of deep pelvic abscesses: 154 cases. Radiology 2003;228:701-705.

Specific Procedures

10. Pereira JK, Chait PG, Miller SF. Deep pelvic abscesses in children: transrectal drainage under radiologic guidance. Radiology 1996;198: 393-396.
11. Racadio JM, Doellman DA, Johnson ND, et al. Pediatric peripherally inserted central catheters: complication rates related to catheter tip location. Pediatrics 2001;107:E28.
12. Moulton JS, Moore PT, Mencini RA. Treatment of loculated pleural effusions with transcatheter intracavitary urokinase. AJR Am J Roentgenol 1989;153:941-945.
13. Ray TL, Berkenbosch JW, Russo P, Tobias JD. Tissue plasminogen activator as an adjuvant therapy for pleural empyema in pediatric patients. J Intensive Care Med 2004;19:44-50.
14. Shiels 2nd WE, Kenney BD, Caniano DA, Besner GE. Definitive percutaneous treatment of lymphatic malformations of the trunk and extremities. J Pediatr Surg 2008;43:136-139; discussion 140.

Index

Page numbers followed by *f* indicate figures; *t*, tables; *b*,
boxes.